Psychiatric Nursing

SEVENTH EDITION

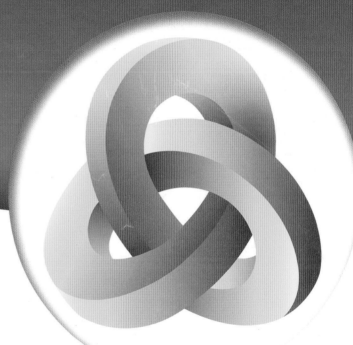

Norman L. Keltner, EdD, RN, CRNP
Professor, School of Nursing
University of Alabama at Birmingham
Birmingham, Alabama

Debbie Steele, PhD, RN, LMFT
Associate Professor
Christian Counseling
Golden Gate Baptist Theological Seminary
Mill Valley, California

ELSEVIER

ELSEVIER
MOSBY

3251 Riverport Lane
St. Louis, Missouri 63043

PSYCHIATRIC NURSING, SEVENTH EDITION   ISBN: 978-0-323-18579-0

Notice

Knowledge and best practice in this field are constantly changing. As new research and experience broaden our understanding, changes in research methods, professional practices, or medical treatment may become necessary.

Practitioners and researchers must always rely on their own experience and knowledge in evaluating and using any information, methods, compounds, or experiments described herein. In using such information or methods they should be mindful of their own safety and the safety of others, including parties for whom they have a professional responsibility.

With respect to any drug or pharmaceutical products identified, readers are advised to check the most current information provided (i) on procedures featured or (ii) by the manufacturer of each product to be administered, to verify the recommended dose or formula, the method and duration of administration, and contraindications. It is the responsibility of practitioners, relying on their own experience and knowledge of their patients, to make diagnoses, to determine dosages and the best treatment for each individual patient, and to take all appropriate safety precautions.

To the fullest extent of the law, neither the Publisher nor the authors, contributors, or editors, assume any liability for any injury and/or damage to persons or property as a matter of products liability, negligence or otherwise, or from any use or operation of any methods, products, instructions, or ideas contained in the material herein.

Library of Congress Cataloging-in-Publication Data
Keltner, Norman L., author.
   Psychiatric nursing/Norman L. Keltner, Debbie Steele. – Seventh edition.
      p. ; cm.
   Includes bibliographical references and index.
   ISBN 978-0-323-18579-0 (paperback : alk. paper)
   I. Steele, Debbie, author. II. Title.
   [DNLM: 1. Psychiatric Nursing. 2. Mental Disorders–drug therapy. 3. Nurse-Patient Relations.
4. Psychotherapy–methods. 5. Psychotropic Drugs–administration & dosage. 6. Vulnerable Populations–psychology. WY 160]
   RC440
   616.89'0231–dc23
                                                                        2014016516

Senior Content Strategist: Yvonne Alexopoulos
Senior Content Development Specialist: Lisa P. Newton
Publishing Services Manager: Jeff Patterson
Senior Project Manager: Anne Konopka
Designer: Margaret Reid

Printed in China

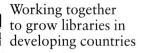

Working together
to grow libraries in
developing countries

www.elsevier.com • www.bookaid.org

Last digit is the print number: 9 8 7 6 5 4 3 2

Melanie Daniel, MSN, RN
Instructor
University of Alabama at Birmingham
Birmingham, Alabama

Jonathan S. Dowben, MD
Department of Behavioral Medicine
Brooke Army Medical Center
Fort Sam Houston, Texas

Susanne Astrab Fogger, DNP, CRNP, PMHNP-BC
Associate Professor
MSN Psychiatric Mental Health Specialty
Track Coordinator
School of Nursing
University of Alabama at Birmingham
Birmingham, Alabama

Joan S. Grant, PhD, RN, CS
Professor
School of Nursing
University of Alabama at Birmingham
Birmingham, Alabama

Karmie M. Johnson, MSN, PMHNP-BC
Instructor
School of Nursing
University of Alabama at Birmingham
Birmingham, Alabama

Teena M. McGuinness, PhD, CRNP, FAAN
Professor
School of Nursing
University of Alabama at Birmingham
Birmingham, Alabama

Gary Milligan, DNP, MSHA, APHN-BC
Assistant Professor
School of Nursing
University of Alabama at Birmingham
Birmingham, Alabama

Randy L. Moore, DNP, RN
Assistant Professor
Veterans Affairs Nursing Academic
Partnership with the School of Nursing
University of Alabama at Birmingham
Birmingham, Alabama

Donna C. Newell, MSN, PMHCNS-BC
Psychiatric Mental Health Clinical Nurse Specialist
Nurse Psychotherapist
Birmingham, Alabama

Gordon I.G. Pugh, MDiv, MPhil
Board Certified Chaplain
Children's Hospital of Alabama
Birmingham, Alabama

Aida J. Sapp, PhD, RN, PMHCNS-BC, LMFT
Professor of Nursing
University of Mary Hardin-Baylor
Belton, Texas

Lee Hilyard Schwecke, BSN, MSN, EdD
Associate Professor Emeritus
School of Nursing
Indiana University
Indianapolis, Indiana

Willie O. Smith, MSN, RN
Adjunct Associate Professor
Health Sciences Division
San Joaquin Delta College
Stockton, California

Richard A. Sugerman, PhD
Professor of Anatomy, Emeritus
Director, Service Learning Projects
College of Osteopathic Medicine of the Pacific
Western University of Health Sciences
Pomona, California

Nanci A. Swan, MSN
Instructor
University of Alabama at Birmingham
Birmingham, Alabama

David E. Vance, PhD
Associate Professor
School of Nursing
University of Alabama at Birmingham
Birmingham, Alabama

Barbara Jones Warren, PhD, RN, FAAN, CNS-BC, PMH
Professor of Clinical Nursing
Director of College of Nursing Psychiatric and
Mental Health Nurse Practitioner Specialty
Interim Director Doctor of Nursing Practice
Program Ohio State University
Columbus, Ohio

ANCILLARY WRITERS

Katherine M. Fortinash, MSN, APRN, PMHCNS
Advanced Clinical Specialist
Psychiatric Mental Health Nursing
Formerly: Clinical Specialist Sharp Hospital
Behavioral Health Services
Professor of Nursing Education
Grossmont College
San Diego, California
Powerpoint Presentations

Pamela E. Marcus, RN, APRN/PMH-BC
Associate Professor of Nursing
Prince George's Community College
Largo, Maryland
Advanced Practice Nurse Psychotherapist
Private Practice
Upper Marlboro, Maryland
Powerpoint Presentations

Linda Turchin, RN, MSN, CNE
Associate Professor of Nursing
Fairmont State University
Fairmont, West Virginia
Test Bank and NCLEX Review Questions

Linda Wendling, MS, MFA
Learning Theory Consultant
University of Missouri – St. Louis
TEACH for Nurses

Patty Bollinger, MSN, APRN-CNS
Bryan College of Health Sciences
Lincoln, Nebraska

Claudia Chiesa, PhD, RPh
Staff Pharmacist
Catalina Pharmacy Management Services
Tucson, Arizona

Phyllis Fentress, RNC, MSN
Professor of Nursing
Elizabethtown Community & Technical College
Elizabethtown, Kentucky

Debbie Fitzgerald, PhD, RN, CNE
Professor
Nursing & Allied Health
Joliet Junior College
Joliet, Illinois

Kimberly Ann Simpson, MSN, RN, CADC
University of Illinois at Chicago-Urbana Campus
College of Nursing
Urbana, Illinois

PREFACE

"Of making many books there is no end, and much study is a weariness to the flesh." Solomon said that way back in ~950 B.C. How did he know? I mean, he got it right on both ends. There are millions of books out there, and studying is hard, tiring work. But another way to look at it is this—what you are going through has been experienced by billions of people at least since Solomon's time.

With King Solomon in mind, we have attempted to write a book that you will enjoy reading—at least for a textbook. We have tried to write in a clear, concise style. Of course, you will be the judge of whether that objective has been met. We deliver what we believe is a straightforward approach to psychiatric nursing. It is the *psychotherapeutic management* approach consisting of three interlinking parts we describe as *Me, Meds, and Milieu*. We emphasize how you will interact with psychiatric patients, the medications you will give to your patients, and how you will assist in making their environment more therapeutic. We hope you actually enjoy reading this text, and, even more, we hope you learn from it. With those hopeful thoughts in mind, we practice clarity and conciseness right from the beginning—with this short preface. Good luck!

FOR INSTRUCTORS

Instructor Resources on Evolve, available at http://evolve.elsevier.com/Keltner/, provides a wealth of material to help you make your psychiatric nursing instruction a success. In addition to all of the Student Resources, the following are provided for instructors:

- *TEACH for Nurses* **Lesson Plans**, based on textbook chapter Learning Objectives, serve as ready-made, modifiable lesson plans and a complete roadmap to link all parts of the educational package. These concise and straightforward lesson plans can be modified or combined to meet your particular scheduling and teaching needs.
- **PowerPoint Presentations** are organized by chapter with approximately 400 slides for in-class lectures. These are detailed and include customizable text and image lecture slides to enhance learning in the classroom or in Web-based course modules. If you share them with students, they can use the note feature to help them with your lectures.
- **Audience Response Questions for i>clicker and other systems** are provided with one to three multiple-answer questions per chapter to stimulate class discussion and assess student understanding of key concepts.
- The **Test Bank** has more than 900 test items, complete with the correct answer, rationale, cognitive level of each question, corresponding step of the nursing process, appropriate NCLEX format, Client Needs label, and text page reference(s).

FOR STUDENTS

Student Resources on Evolve, available at http://evolve.elsevier.com/Keltner/, provides a wealth of valuable learning resources for students. The Evolve Resources page in the front of the book gives login instructions and a description of each resource.

- Updated **Evolve website for students** includes Appendixes, NCLEX-RN review questions, answers to Chapter Critical Thinking Questions, Psychotropic Drug Monographs, and Video Lectures.

As is true of all nursing text authors, our goal is to present accurate and meaningful information to the student without the distraction of sexist language. Where possible, we have made every attempt to avoid the use of sexist pronouns by using plural nouns and pronouns or "his or her" rather than risk stigmatizing by gender. To avoid awkwardness of style, we have sometimes referred to the nurse as "she" and the patient as "he."

Norman L. Keltner
Debbie Steele

ACKNOWLEDGMENTS

The fact that *Psychiatric Nursing* warrants a seventh edition humbles me. In these many years in the field of psychiatric nursing, numerous people have guided my thinking, encouraged me at the right time, or even pushed me to develop my philosophy of and approach to psychiatric nursing care. I remember these individuals and their contributions to my life. I attempted to list all of them in past editions. However, in this edition, I will mention the great institutions I have worked in. In these places, I have learned, formed lifelong friendships, and earned a living so that I could raise and support a family. A list of these important institutions follows:

Stockton State Hospital in Stockton, California (15 years)
United States Army
University of Wyoming (my first teaching position)
Baylor University
California State University, Bakersfield
University of Alabama at Birmingham (since 1990)

I am not sure how one thanks an institution, but I will try anyway.

Dear SSH, US Army, UW, BU, CSUB, and UAB: Thank you for giving me an interesting and rewarding career and for allowing me to provide a comfortable living for my family. Most sincerely, Norm

I also want to acknowledge my family of origin–my mom, Gladys (1914-1984), my dad, Lawrence (1910-1989), my brother Hode (Stockton, CA), and my sister Jennifer (Coeur d'Alene, ID). They all believed in me more than I did myself.

Finally, I dedicate this book to my four grandsons, Sam, Asher, Izzy, and Axel, and my three granddaughters, Addie, Millie Kate, and Audrey.

N.L.K.

I would like to thank Dr. Norman Keltner for the rich experience of collaborating on the 7th edition of his nursing textbook. I also want to acknowledge the extraordinary work of researchers, educators, and practitioners who have contributed to the development of this *Psychiatric Nursing* textbook.

D.S.

CONTENTS

CHAPTER

1

Me, Meds, Milieu

Norman L. Keltner

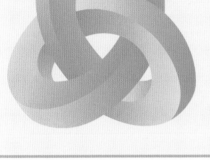

evolve WEBSITE

http://evolve.elsevier.com/Keltner

LEARNING OBJECTIVES

- Describe the components of psychotherapeutic management.
- Explain the way in which the balancing of psychotherapeutic management components forms a powerful therapeutic model of care.

- Recognize the relationship between the continuum of care and the psychotherapeutic management model.
- Identify the various levels of care within the continuum of care.

We dare not lengthen this book much, lest it be out of moderation and should stir men's antipathy because of its size.
Aelfric, Abbot of Eynsham (955-1020)

Where to start? You start with basics—the basic tools you need to work with people who have mental health problems. Whether as a student or as a seasoned psychiatric nurse, when you look in the mirror and ask yourself, "What are my tools?", the answer will be: "I have Me, Meds, and the Milieu." (Milieu is a fancy French word for environment, but because it is commonly used in psychiatry, we will use it too.) This text consistently advances this simplistic model and calls the model *psychotherapeutic management*. Most often, instead of "Me," we use the term *nurse-patient relationship*, but because you are the nurse in the nurse-patient relationship, the use of "Me" just helps make the point. The psychiatric nurse has three ways to work with her patients (we will probably use the pronoun "her" most often but will work in "him" sometimes as well for all of the politically correct reasons): her interpersonal skills, her medication skills, and her ability to enhance (or create or construct) a safe and therapeutic environment.

Thus, we delightedly use the attention-grabbing chapter title, "Me, Meds, Milieu."

Although we admit the model is simplistic, we do not believe it is simple to master. Learning to communicate therapeutically is a continuous process. Understanding psychiatric medicines is far from simple. It not only takes a lot of work, but it also hinges on how well you learned anatomy, physiology, and pharmacology. Anybody can give a pill, but a competent nurse understands the many dimensions of the drugs he gives. Finally, modifying an environment to make it both safe and therapeutic takes tremendous skill and consistency. The rest of this chapter explores the concept of psychotherapeutic management—a simple model of organizing your thinking and your care. Following that discussion, the chapter provides an overview of various sources of mental health care and support—the so-called *continuum of care*.

PSYCHOTHERAPEUTIC MANAGEMENT

Psychiatric nursing is in need of care delivery models that are not only effective for patient care but that also can capitalize on the uniqueness of the discipline. Psychotherapeutic management proposes a real-world approach to psychiatric nursing care that recognizes the interdependence of the mental health profession and exploits the strengths of psychiatric nursing. It seeks to answer the question, *"What do psychiatric nurses do that is different from other mental health professionals, particularly social workers, psychiatrists, and psychologists?"* Psychiatric treatment can be divided into five basic categories: (1) use of words, (2) use of drugs, (3) use of environment, (4) somatic therapies, and (5) behavioral conditioning. Psychotherapeutic management emphasizes the first three of these categories: (1) *words* from which nurses develop the nurse-patient relationship, (2) *drugs*, specifically psychotropic drugs, and (3) *environment* (as noted, the French word for environment, *milieu*, is often used). However, the nurse cannot effectively use these interventions unless she has a sound understanding of psychopathology (Figure 1-1).

Stated another way, the student has three intervention tools to rely on:
1. Me (nurse)
2. Meds
3. Milieu (or environment)

One Size Does Not Fit All!

The authors also plead with you not to overlook the power of this paradigm just because it looks simple. You can approach every patient with this model in mind. Simply (there's that word again), you can approach every patient by asking the following questions: "How should I talk with this patient?" "What kind of medicine should he be taking?" and "What are the environmental issues that will promote health and safety?"

One intervention might take priority over another depending on the situation. The particular approach depends on the patient's diagnosis (i.e., psychopathology) and level of functioning. For example, the nurse learns to use *different words* when he speaks with a patient with a diagnosis of schizophrenia as opposed to a patient with a diagnosis of depression. More than

likely, the patient with schizophrenia requires antipsychotic medications, whereas the depressed patient receives antidepressant drugs—hence, drug management is different. Finally, the patient with schizophrenia might need an environment that reduces stressors, whereas a key environmental concern for the patient with depression or bipolar disorder might be safety (e.g., suicide prevention). In other words, the psychotherapeutic management model recognizes that one size does not fit all.

NORM'S NOTES
STOP!! Take a good look at this chapter. It will make a lot of sense because it gives you a simple approach for conceptualizing what you are doing with patients. When you work with patients, you need to focus on three things: (1) ME: how *you* will interact with them, (2) MEDS: the *medications* they need, and (3) MILIEU: how you can affect their *environment*. This approach arms you with a strategy. Now, although the framework is simple, the basics of the psychotherapeutic management approach are not simple—far from it. You will spend the entire term understanding what goes into fleshing out this model.

Application of Psychotherapeutic Management Interventions

The application of psychopathology and the knowledgeable use of psychotherapeutic management skills extend beyond inpatient settings into various care settings, such as outpatient programs, residential services, and home care. The needs of the individual and the setting in which care is delivered influence the degree to which each component of psychotherapeutic management is provided within the continuum of care (Figure 1-2).

For example, individuals with depression in an inpatient setting benefit most when a therapeutic nurse-patient relationship, an antidepressant, and a well-managed milieu are available. When one component is missing from the equation, treatment is compromised. Just think about the possibilities when one part is missing. For example, what if the psychiatrist orders the right antidepressant (say, Lexapro), but the nursing staff does not carefully observe a potentially suicidal patient? The results could be disastrous! This simplistic example demonstrates that all components of the psychotherapeutic management equation should be present for patients to realize maximum benefit from nursing care.

PSYCHOTHERAPEUTIC MANAGEMENT: THREE INTERVENTIONS

Therapeutic Nurse-Patient Relationship

Distinguishing therapy from being therapeutic is crucial for the student of psychiatric nursing. Therapy is the focus of graduate-level psychiatric nursing training as well as the graduate programs in other disciplines. It is not taught at the basic nursing program level. What you will be taught is how to be therapeutic. Think about the difference and savor it. You can learn to be a therapeutic nurse in the short time you are

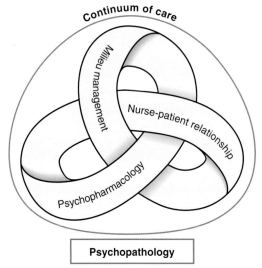

FIG 1-1 Psychotherapeutic management in the continuum of care.

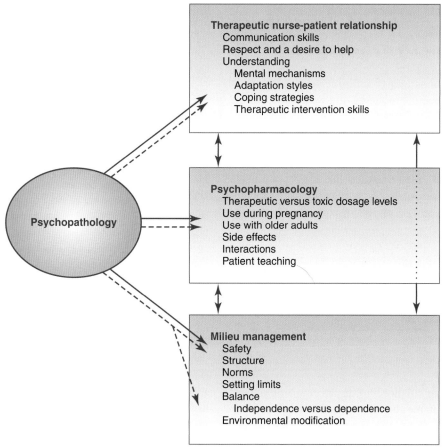

FIG 1-2 Psychotherapeutic management model.

taking this course. When this course is completed, the student is *not a therapist* but should possess *therapeutic skills*.

Unit II is devoted to the "Me" dimension of psychotherapeutic management. A new vocabulary of words and concepts are discussed within a relationship context. Specifically, general communication skills, the nature of the nurse-patient relationship, working with groups of patients, working with the families of patients, and other related concepts are discussed.

Psychopharmacology

Unit III is devoted to the contribution of psychotropic drugs to psychiatric care, the responsibilities of the nurse, and essential information about these drugs. Psychopharmacology is an important dimension in psychotherapeutic management because psychotropic drugs have enabled millions of people to live increasingly independent lives. *Drug intervention is neither always desirable nor appropriate.* However, when drug therapy is indicated, patients usually respond more rapidly than they would without drugs.

The nurse who uses the nursing process model can assess patients' responses to medication, plan to respond to side effects should they occur, implement those plans, and evaluate for desired results. The nurse's pivotal role, particularly in an inpatient setting, allows intervention before serious drug-related problems occur. Additionally, the nurse administers medications and makes decisions regarding as needed (prn)

medications. Finally, the nurse needs a sound foundation in psychopharmacology in order to teach patients about drugs. For these and other reasons, the nurse must have immediate access to information about psychotropic drugs.

Milieu Management

Milieu (or environmental) management is a proactive approach to care that forges therapeutic benefits from patients' surroundings, whether in the hospital, outpatient setting, or home. The six environmental elements that nurses must consider in creating a therapeutic milieu are the following:

1. Safety: keeping the patient free from danger or harm
2. Structure: the physical environment, regulations, and schedules
3. Norms: specific expectations of behavior (e.g., acceptance, nonviolence, privacy)
4. Limit setting: clear and enforceable limitations on behaviors
5. Balance: negotiating the line between dependence and independence
6. Environmental modification: changing the environment to promote mental health.

These elements might overlap; for example, safety is a component of all the dimensions of milieu. Various aspects of milieu management are discussed in Unit IV.

NCLEX Tip: Safety trumps all other patient concerns!

Other Important Components of Understanding Psychiatric Nursing
Psychopathology—the Key to Psychotherapeutic Management

Unit V discusses psychopathology and provides the foundation on which the three components of psychotherapeutic management rest. It lays the groundwork for an understanding of psychopharmacology, the nurse-patient relationship, and milieu management. Unit V includes information about the major mental disorders. Schizophrenia, depressive disorders, bipolar disorders, anxiety-related disorders, cognitive disorders, personality disorders, sexual disorders, substance-related disorders, and eating disorders are considered in separate chapters of Unit V.

 CRITICAL THINKING QUESTION

1. If you develop a mental health problem, which aspect of psychotherapeutic management would be most important to you?

Special Populations

In Unit VI, the problems and needs of special populations are discussed. Unit VI contains chapters on survivors of violent behavior, children and adolescents, older adults, and soldiers and veterans.

 CRITICAL THINKING QUESTION

2. Based on your clinical setting, what is your evaluation of the components of the psychotherapeutic management model that you have observed?

CONTINUUM OF CARE: ALL THE PLACES TO IMPLEMENT ME, MEDS, AND MILIEU

The continuum of care provides individuals with a wide range of treatment options. Not everyone needs admission to a hospital, and our economy cannot afford this level of care for the large number of people with mental health problems. The hope is to have an integrated approach that provides the most appropriate care within a seamless continuum. Figure 1-3 illustrates a decision tree for the continuum of care. The first step after a mental health problem is suspected is to confirm its existence. You would do the same thing if you heard a knocking sound in your car. Is there really anything wrong here? The next step is to ask this question: *Does this person require hospitalization?*

If the answer is *yes*, then it should happen even though it can be expensive. Also, to establish credibility, we have to admit that the bar is pretty high for admitting someone to a hospital—particularly against the will of the person. Our news media is full of stories depicting horrible crimes in which the perpetrator is said to have a mental disorder. Often the

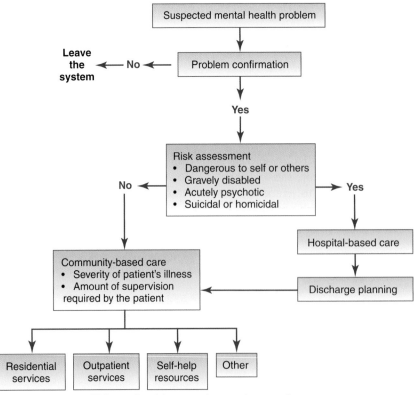

FIG 1-3 Decision tree for continuum of care.

family has tried to have the perpetrator hospitalized against his wishes (yes, these individuals are mostly "he's"), only to be rebuffed by a legal system that is reluctant to confine a person. The bar is high, and we cannot help but wonder if it might be lowered in the future.

If the answer is *no*, then several treatment alternatives are available. Figure 1-3 identifies residential services, traditional outpatient services, day treatment programs, and self-help resources. There are many other options as well. When hospitalization is necessary, discharge planning is started soon after admission, and on discharge the same continuum of treatment options is considered for the released individual.

The role of nurses and other professionals is to assess the individual's current level of functioning and direct (or escort) the individual to appropriate resources. Coordination of services for the individual necessitates multidisciplinary collaboration. Without this coordination, the continuum of care will not be seamless and may hinder the very thing it purports to help. Multidisciplinary care has been expanded to include not only professional staff but also nonprofessionals, patients (many treatment environments prefer the term *consumer*), family, peers, and various nonpsychiatric resources (e.g., representatives from Medicare, Medicaid, nursing homes, group homes, and medical clinics).

The decision tree in Figure 1-3 may seem boring to review, but is very helpful once grasped. It is used to match the needs of the individual with appropriate services based on safety requirements, intensity of supervision needed, severity of symptoms, level of functioning, and type of treatment needed. Following are some great examples:

1. An individual with auditory hallucinations telling her to kill her newborn infant needs inpatient hospitalization with 24-hour nursing care and supervision in a safe environment.
2. An individual with thoughts of suicide but without a plan might be managed effectively by attending a day treatment program 5 days a week for 2 weeks.
3. An individual with a diagnosis of schizophrenia with a history of not regularly taking his antipsychotic medication and who needs a place to live might be appropriately placed in a group home with 24-hour supervision.
4. An individual with alcoholism who has completed acute detoxification might need referral to outpatient counseling or a self-help group such as Alcoholics Anonymous.

For any individual, additional referrals along the continuum of care can be made if needs change. An individual might be referred to mental health services at the suggestion of a family physician, minister, police officer, family member, friend, or staff from any of the programs within the continuum. Self-referral is also a means whereby individuals can gain entry into the mental health system.

NORM'S NOTES
The idea of a "continuum of care" might not grab you like a chapter titled "Schizophrenia." However, this concept is very important. There must be different options and different levels of care for everyone. As said earlier in the chapter, one size does not fit all. Furthermore, people cannot just be dropped out of one program with nowhere else to turn. People with mental disorders should not have to fend for themselves. There needs to be a system in place, and, in most places in the United States, there is. The continuum of care provides resources for the neediest among us all the way to those who are almost ready to control all aspects of their lives.

Hospital-Based Care

Historically, hospitals were the point of entry into the health care system, whereas the point of entry now can be anywhere along the continuum of care. Patients admitted for psychiatric hospitalization 20 to 30 years ago stayed about 4 to 6 weeks. If you go back even further, patients admitted to large state hospitals could be hospitalized for years. Today, length of stay is typically 3 to 5 days; this is largely driven by economic decisions. As reimbursement has decreased, the goals, staffing patterns, acuity of patients, and discharge planning of hospitalization have changed as well.

- The goals are crisis intervention and safety.
- Staffing must be cost-effective while maintaining quality of service.
- Acuity of patients has increased.
- Discharge planning begins immediately after admission.

The highest priority for admission to hospital-based care is safety for self and others. When a patient is deemed a danger to himself (suicidal) or to others (homicidal), 24-hour supervision in a secure environment is required. Often these individuals are first seen in an emergency department. Other individuals who require hospitalization include those who are at risk for accidental harm—that is, individuals who are gravely disabled. For example, individuals who are acutely psychotic or who are confused and disoriented might not function well enough to meet their basic needs for food, clothing, shelter, medical care, or physical safety. In addition to safety and protection, hospitalization provides thorough medical and psychiatric evaluation to identify the underlying cause of presenting symptoms.

Another group that might be admitted includes individuals who are experiencing toxic reactions to medications or other substances and individuals who need medical intervention when withdrawal from substances might produce life-threatening conditions. Some individuals might be admitted for a medical evaluation or because a medical illness produces or complicates a psychiatric disorder. Types of hospital-based care include:

- Locked units (individuals cannot enter or leave without a key (or key card)
- Open or unlocked units
- Psychiatric intensive care units for high-acuity patients
- Specialty units (e.g., adult, geriatric, child and adolescent, substance abuse)

🔑 CRITICAL THINKING QUESTION

3. You are admitting a 15-year-old boy to an inpatient unit because of alcohol and marijuana abuse, risky sexual behaviors, and failing grades. These behaviors developed over the last 3 months after his father was diagnosed with terminal cancer. What issues need to be addressed during his hospitalization?

Residential Services

Residential services are available to help individuals who need temporary or long-term housing. Most states have long-term care facilities for individuals needing prolonged 24-hour supervision. The length of stay might be 3 to 6 months or longer.

Extended care facilities (e.g., nursing homes) are available for people who require 24-hour supervision and medical nursing care. This level of care is often required for individuals with severe developmental disabilities, dementia, or acute and chronic medical illnesses.

Group homes might provide temporary or permanent housing for individuals with chronic mental disorders. Depending on the needs of the residents, staff might be present for 24 hours a day or less. Some group homes provide group therapy and structured activities, whereas others might provide only meals, a bed, and laundry facilities.

Traditionally, *halfway houses* were available for individuals recovering from chemical dependency. Residents were expected to seek employment and participate in cooking and cleaning chores. Residents also attended self-help groups that met on site, such as Alcoholics Anonymous. Some halfway houses are now open to individuals with other mental health problems.

Apartment living programs provide varying degrees of supervision and programming. Staff might be on site on a daily basis, offering group sessions and activities, or they might visit periodically to provide medication assistance and facilitate attendance at various appointments.

Foster care and *boarding homes* are generally staffed by nonprofessionals but have professional supervision available on an intermittent basis. *Shelters* provide room and board to homeless people. Some homes might provide services for specific populations, such as victims of violence (e.g., abused women and their families) or individuals with addictions.

Traditional Outpatient Services

Outpatient treatment traditionally has occurred in mental health clinics and private offices. The person providing counseling might be a psychiatrist, psychologist, social worker, psychiatric nurse practitioner, nurse, or other professional. The number of visits per week or month varies according to the individual's needs. The typical pattern for an individual with a chronic mental illness might be a visit once a month with a counselor or case manager and periodic appointments with a psychiatrist for medication review. During these counseling visits, an assessment of needs for additional services is made to determine whether the individual requires more intensive treatment or a different type of treatment.

Clinical Example: Loss of self care abilities

Larry, a 31-year-old man with a diagnosis of chronic undifferentiated schizophrenia, attends a community support program. He meets with his case manager every other week after he receives his haloperidol decanoate injection (a long-acting form of the drug that is given once every 2 to 4 weeks) from the nurse. The nurse assesses for effectiveness of the medication and for side effects. Larry also participates in a social club, which offers lunch and social activities twice weekly. The psychiatrist meets with him every 3 months for medication evaluation.

Day Treatment Programs

Individuals who need minimal supervision, structured activities, and ongoing treatment might benefit from a day treatment program. These programs vary in length from 4 to 8 hours per day and 1 to 5 days per week. Programming can occur during the day, evening, and night. Depending on the community, these programs might provide treatment for specific populations based on age (child, adolescent, adult, or older adult) or type of problem (addiction or chronic mental illness).

Clinical Example: Loss of a life partner

John, a 52-year-old man with severe depression resulting from the unexpected death of his wife, is discharged from the hospital but is unable to return to work. He attends a partial program for 2 weeks that meets from 10 A.M. to 3 P.M., Monday through Friday. He attends groups that focus on exercise, spirituality, coping with losses, and self-esteem issues. Lunchtime provides an opportunity for socialization with program members.

Self-Help Groups

Self-help groups are another source of support on the continuum of care (Table 1-1). Self-help group meetings are conducted by members, not professionals, and may take place on a weekly basis.

TABLE 1-1	SELF-HELP GROUPS
TYPE OF GROUP	**EXAMPLES**
Addiction-based	Alcoholics Anonymous
	Narcotics Anonymous
	Overeaters Anonymous
Survivor-based	Survivors of Suicide
	Incest Survivors Anonymous
	Adult Children of Alcoholics
Disorder-based	Eating disorders
	Bipolar disorder
	Family and caregiver support groups
	National Alliance for the Mentally Ill
Loss-based	Grief, divorce, bereavement support groups
Medically based	Lupus, cancer, chronic fatigue syndrome, AIDS support groups
Prevention-based	Parenting, Boundaries in Relationships

Other Outpatient Programs

As noted in Figure 1-3, the previously described outpatient programs do not constitute an exhaustive list of treatment options available. Other programs available in most areas include *psychiatric home care*, which provides mental health services to people who are homebound because of their illness or disability. Many areas also provide *community outreach programs*, which were developed to reach individuals in places where there is a lack of traditional medical and social services. Sometimes these programs comprise *mobile crisis teams*, which seek to reach individuals who are homeless or transient. An even more aggressive approach to seeking those in need of mental health services is the *Assertive Community Treatment (ACT)* model, which mobilizes interprofessional teams (e.g., nurses, physicians, social workers) that are responsible for providing services 24 hours a day, 7 days a week. The team can go anywhere and provide mental health care or provide services as mundane (yet monumental for some patients) as helping with shopping, laundry, or transportation.

Clinical Example: Loss of intellect

Joe, an 80-year-old man with Alzheimer's disease, lives at home with his wife. The nurse assesses Joe's mental status and level of functioning. Assistance is given to Joe's wife in implementing safety measures in the home because of Joe's wandering behavior. The nurse assists with arranging respite care so that Joe's wife can go shopping and attend a weekly caregivers' support group.

PRIMARY CARE

We would be remiss if we did not acknowledge the role that primary care physicians and nurse practitioners play in treating individuals with mental health problems. General practitioners prescribe 65% of antianxiety medications, 60% of antidepressants, 50% of stimulants, and 35% of antipsychotic drugs (Mark, 2010; Mark et al., 2009). Individuals with mental health problems such as anxiety, depression, and other mental health issues seek help for these problems in primary care offices and clinics. Three reasons for this are:

1. Stigma of mental health care (no one will know)
2. Lack of knowledge about who to see and where to get help
3. Reduced access to care

Psychiatric medications are sometimes prescribed by primary care providers without a comprehensive history and assessment of the patient. The patient's immediate need might be addressed, but other modes of treatment that could benefit the patient might not be provided. The nurse working in primary care areas should provide the interventions (i.e., self, drugs, milieu) that benefit individuals with mental health needs. Thus, psychotherapeutic management is relevant in the primary care setting too.

? CRITICAL THINKING QUESTION

4. During one of your visits to a homeless shelter, you meet Ann, who is 19 years old. Ann has been homeless for 2 months and until recently had been living with friends. Ann has bipolar disorder, which was diagnosed 5 months ago. She lost her job as a waitress shortly after becoming ill and quickly emptied her small savings account to pay rent and buy food. She has not been taking her medication because of lack of money. Ann is motivated to work, but does not know how to go about finding a job and housing. She is feeling overwhelmed and is afraid that she will get sick again. What community resources in your area would be helpful to Ann?

Use of the Nursing Process in the Community

The nursing process is the foundation of case management. Effective use of the nursing process in the areas of psychiatric rehabilitation, crisis intervention, home care, therapy, consultation and liaison, resource linkage, and advocacy enhances these services to psychiatric patients (Figure 1-4). The nurse should be skilled in synthesizing these components in an understandable and useful manner for patients. The nursing process and the psychotherapeutic management model are readily adapted to outpatient psychiatric care.

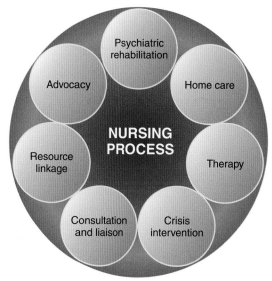

FIG 1-4 Case management components.

STUDY NOTES

1. Your tools as a psychiatric nurse are Me, Meds, and Milieu.
2. Psychotherapeutic management is a model of care that clarifies the nature of psychiatric nursing and distinguishes psychiatric nursing practice from the practice of other disciplines.
3. The components of psychotherapeutic management include a therapeutic nurse-patient relationship (Me), psychopharmacology (Meds), and milieu or "environment" management, all of which are supported by a basic understanding of psychopathology.
4. Psychopharmacologic understanding is important because nurses administer medication, make decisions about as needed (prn) medication, and evaluate for therapeutic and adverse responses to medication.
5. Because humans are incapable of not interacting with their environment, milieu management is an important nursing consideration. Nurses are uniquely responsible for developing the patients' treatment environment.
6. An understanding of psychopathology facilitates the nurse-patient relationship, lays the groundwork for understanding psychopharmacology, and provides a theoretical structure for milieu management.
7. In the continuum of care, the individual is guided to services based on specific needs at a given point in time.
8. Assessment of the individual's needs and level of functioning and the level of supervision that the individual requires determine referral to hospital-based or community-based care.
9. Most hospital-based care is now provided on a short-term basis, focusing on crisis intervention and safety.
10. Discharge planning begins at the time of admission and varies in complexity.
11. The psychotherapeutic management model is the most relevant approach to short-term hospitalization.
12. Continuum of care includes inpatient hospitalization, outpatient services, residential care, self-help activities, and other resources.
13. The nursing process and the psychotherapeutic management approach can be adapted in any setting along the continuum of care.

REFERENCES

Mark, T. L. (2010). For what diagnoses are psychotropic medications being prescribed? A nationally representative survey of physicians. *CNS Drugs, 24,* 319–326.

Mark, T. L., Levit, K. R., & Buck, J. A. (2009). Datapoints: Psychotropic drug prescriptions by medical specialty. *Psychiatric Services, 60,* 1167.

Historical Issues

Norman L. Keltner

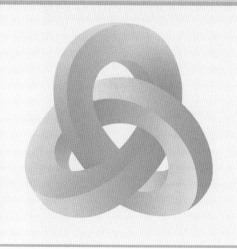

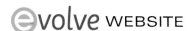 WEBSITE

http://evolve.elsevier.com/Keltner

LEARNING OBJECTIVES

- Describe the enormity of mental health concerns in both human and financial contexts.
- Explain the history of psychiatry as a foundation for current psychiatric nursing practice.
- Identify the significant changes that occurred during the period of the Enlightenment.
- Relate the contributions of early scientists to the current understanding of mental illness.

- Explain the impact of psychotropic drugs on psychiatric care.
- Analyze the immediate and long-term effects of the community mental health movement.
- Describe the impact of the Decade of the Brain on psychiatric care.
- Identify the specific strengths that enable psychiatric nurses to become effective in the new continuum of care.

Nescire autem quid ante quam natus sis acciderit, id est semper esse puerum.
Marcus Tullius Cicero (106-43 B.C.)

Epidemiologic evidence indicates 25% of American adults (>17 years old) meet the criteria for a mental disorder during any 12-month period with 50% experiencing these disorders when viewed over a lifetime (Kessler & Wang, 2008). Many of these disorders are considered mild in nature with most sufferers going untreated. However, many are not: four of the top medical disorders causing disability are psychiatric disorders (i.e., major depression, schizophrenia, bipolar disorder, and alcohol abuse) (Nasrallah, 2012a). About half of all mental disorders start by the midteens (Kessler et al., 2007). Table 2-1 provides a breakdown by diagnosis of the disorders prevalent over the course of 12 months in American society. The pervasiveness of these maladies and the tremendous costs that they incur indicate a great need for psychiatric health care professionals, including nurses, today and in the foreseeable future.

BENCHMARKS IN PSYCHIATRIC HISTORY

And a certain woman … had suffered many things of many physicians, and had spent all that she had, and was nothing bettered, but rather grew worse.
Mark 5:25-26, King James Version (1611)

NORM'S NOTES
Read Cicero's statement again. Oh, you didn't take Latin either. Well, let's put it in English— *"Not to know what happened before you were born, that is to be always a boy, to be forever a child."* Besides perhaps being a little sexist, Cicero makes a strong point. This chapter discusses history, and when you understand history, you understand context. Without an understanding of history, many things do not and cannot make sense. More than that, this chapter describes where we have been and how we got to where we are now. History can help you understand things better, such as the homeless man sitting on the sidewalk who is acting strangely or the incessant ads for antidepressants in the media. It provides a foundation for the rest of the book. Now if Cicero and I have not convinced you of the importance of history, read the summary of Rosenhan's study in Box 2-1. If it doesn't get you fired up, check your pulse!

The modern era of psychiatric care can be traced from events that occurred in England and France near the end of the eighteenth century, a time referred to as *the Enlightenment*. Before this time (or *Preenlightenment*), mentally ill people were often regarded as no better than wild animals. Confinement was the most restrictive method of coping with the mentally ill,

TABLE 2-1 12-MONTH PREVALENCE RATE OF MENTAL DISORDERS IN THE UNITED STATES*		
DISORDERS	**APPROXIMATE PERCENTAGE >17 YEARS OLD (%)*(UNLESS NOTED FOR CHILDREN)**	**GENDER OVERREPRESENTATION**
Anxiety Disorders	18.1 overall	
Agoraphobia	1.7	Female
Panic disorder	2.4	Female
Panic attacks	11.2	Female
Social anxiety	7	Female
Specific phobia	7-9	Female
Separation anxiety	1.2	Equal
Generalized anxiety disorder	2	Female
Posttraumatic stress disorder	3.4	Female
Obsessive compulsive disorder	1.2	Equal
Major depression	8.6	Female
Bipolar I and II	1.8	BD I: ~Equal BD II: Female
Autism Spectrum Disorders	1 in children	Male
Disruptive, Impulse Control, and Conduct Disorders	8.9 overall	
Conduct disorders *	4 in children	Male
Attention-deficit/hyperactivity disorder *	5 in children 2.5 in adults	Male
Substance Use Disorders	8.9 overall	
Alcohol use disorder	8.5 in adults 2.5 in 12-17 year olds	Male
Drug use disorders	1.4	Male
Schizophrenia	1.1	~Equal

*Not one source has all of this information. This information has been derived from the following sources: Kessler, R.C., et al. (2012). Twelve-month and lifetime prevalence and lifetime morbid risk of anxiety and mood disorders in the United States. *International Journal of Methods of Psychiatric Research*, 21, 169; Substance Abuse and Mental Health Services Administration. (2009). *Results from the 2008 national survey on drug use and health: national findings*; http://www.samhsa.gov/data/nsduh/2k8nsduh/2k8Results.htm Accessed November 13, 2013. American Psychiatric Association. (2013). *Diagnostic and statistical manual of mental disorders* (DSM 5). Arlington, VA: APA.

who were often chained. The mentally ill were thought to be immune to normal biologic stressors such as cold, heat, and hunger. Mentally ill individuals were often placed on display for the amusement of their caretakers and the paying public. For example, until 1770, a small fee was charged to visitors of St. Mary of Bethlem Hospital (aka "Bedlam") in England (McMillan, 1997). At Bicêtre in France, the attendants served as "ringmasters," using whips to "encourage" their patients to perform (Rosenblatt, 1984). These warehouses for the tormented discouraged outside intrusion and attracted employees who were at the bottom levels of society, both socially and morally.

As the late 1700s approached, a day of enlightenment dawned: the establishment of the asylum. Five periods stand out as benchmarks in the evolution of modern psychiatric care (Table 2-2):

Benchmark I: approximately 1790s

Benchmark II: mid to late 1800s

Benchmark III: 1950s

Benchmark IV: 1960s

Benchmark V: 1990s

During each of these periods, the way of thinking about the mentally ill underwent significant changes.

Benchmark I: Period of Enlightenment

To consider madness incurable … is constantly refuted by the most authentic facts.

Philippe Pinel, December 11, 1794 (cited in Weiner, 1992)

Pinel's comment captured a new way of thinking (people could get better) and launched a new era. The modern age of psychiatric care began with Philippe Pinel in France and another visionary, William Tuke, in England. In 1793, Pinel became the superintendent of the French institution Bicêtre (for men) and, later, the Salpêtrière (for women). Pinel was dismayed by the conditions he found and wrote of the patients, "They were abandoned to the incompetence of a callous director and to the cold brutality of servants …" (Weiner, 1992). Soon after assuming leadership, Pinel unchained the shackled, clothed the naked, fed the hungry, and abolished whips and other tools of abuse. Simultaneously, in England, Tuke was planning a private facility that would ensure moral treatment for the mentally ill after he witnessed the deplorable conditions in public facilities. In 1796, based on Quaker teachings, his York Retreat opened for patients, providing "a place in which the unhappy might obtain refuge—a quiet haven in which the shattered bark might find a means of reparation or safety" (Charland, 2007; Gollaher, 1995). Pinel and Tuke crafted this first benchmark of modern psychiatric care.

TABLE 2-2   BENCHMARK PERIODS IN PSYCHIATRIC HISTORY

PERIOD	KEY PEOPLE OR DEVELOPMENTS	SIGNIFICANT CHANGE IN THINKING	RESULT(S)
Enlightenment, ~1790s	Pinel (1745-1826)	Human dignity upheld	Asylum movement developed
	Tuke (1732-1822)		
Scientific Study, ~1870s	Freud (1856-1939): Emphasized the importance of early life experiences	Mental illness could be studied	Study of the mind and treatment approaches to psychiatric conditions flourished
	Kraepelin (1856-1926): Studied the brain		
Psychotropic Drugs, ~1950s	1949: Lithium	If some mental disorders are caused by chemical imbalances, then chemicals could restore the balance: people would no longer need to be confined	Destigmatization of mental illness occurred; parents and others not to blame
	1950: Thorazine		
	1952: MAOIs		
	1958: TCAs		
	1960: Benzodiazepines		
Community Mental Health, 1960s	Community Mental Health Centers Act (1963)	People have the right to be treated in their own community	*Advantage*: Intervention in familiar surroundings has helped many people and is less expensive *Disadvantage*: Homelessness linked to deinstitutionalization; many people "slip through the cracks" of the system
Decade of the Brain, 1990s	Congressional mandate	If we can understand the brain, we can help millions of people with mental disorders	Increase in funding for brain research, leading to new treatment strategies

MAOIs, Monoamine oxidase inhibitors (which are antidepressants); *TCAs*, tricyclic antidepressants.

Asylum

The concept of the asylum developed from the humane efforts of Pinel and Tuke. The term *asylum* can mean protection, social support, or sanctuary from the stresses of life. A touring Cuban gymnast pleading for asylum is a good example of this definition. More often, however, asylum most often provokes an image of mistreatment and neglect. It was the first definition that motivated Pinel, Tuke, and other similarly minded individuals. Understanding that mental illness worsened with deplorable conditions, these individuals sought to provide an environment relatively free from stressors. Their language is inappropriate today—"madness," "lunacy," "insanity," "idiocy," "feeblemindedness"—but these were the accepted terms of their day. These early reformers were driven by a desire to improve the lot of abandoned, mentally ill persons and to provide asylum or sanctuary.

Dorothea Dix (1802-1887), one of the first major reformers in the United States, was instrumental in developing the concept of asylum; she played a direct role in opening 32 state hospitals. Her efforts have been described as a crusade. Several years before launching her crusade, she visited Tuke's York Retreat. Undoubtedly, Tuke's moral treatment influenced her to confront the pain and suffering she had witnessed in the United States. Dix came to believe that the people of America had an obligation to their mentally ill brothers and sisters. She proposed to alleviate suffering with adequate shelter, nutritious food, and warm clothing. In Gollaher's biography of Dix (1995), he quotes from one of her Memorials, the documents she wrote to expose the terrible plight of the insane. From her Massachusetts Memorial, he notes:

> *Concord*: A woman from the [Worcester] hospital in a cage in the almshouse.
> *Lincoln*: A woman in a cage.
> *Medford*: One idiotic subject chained, and one in a close [or narrow] stall for 17 years ….
> *Granville*: One often closely confined … now losing the use of his limbs from want of exercise.

Although Dix is rightfully credited with being the first reformer to have a nationwide perspective, other, more regional sanctuaries had been established before she began her crusade. The first asylum in the United States was the Eastern Lunatic Asylum in Williamsburg, Virginia, founded in 1773.

Other institutions followed, such as the Frankford Asylum near Philadelphia (1813), the Bloomingdale Asylum in New York (1818), and the Hartford Retreat in Connecticut (1824). The Philadelphia and New York asylums were established under Quaker influence and thus can be traced to Tuke.

The period of Enlightenment was relatively short-lived. Within 100 years of the establishment of the first asylum, the reformers were being charged with misuse and abuse of their charges. State hospitals were beset with problems. The first definition of asylum (*sanctuary*) had materialized in the form of hospitals built in rural settings. Patients were isolated geographically and socially and, after release, from follow-up care. Patients were also isolated from public scrutiny, which enabled many large institutions to become closed systems. As might be guessed, the beneficence of the reformers was not shared by the many caretakers who followed. Within this relatively brief period, the meaning of asylum changed; it evolved from a *place of refuge* to a *place of torment.*

Today, a renewed interest in asylum as a place of rest and restoration exists. This concept can be considered in terms of the four *P*'s: parents, professionals, patients, and public, each of which has a stake in the discussion of asylum. Wasow (1993) has written persuasively of the need for asylum: "Some people's illnesses are so severe that they will always need asylum. A continuum of care is needed: from total freedom to total hospitalization, reflecting the diverse needs of mentally ill people."

? CRITICAL THINKING QUESTIONS

1. Which of the two definitions of *asylum* do you believe is more prevalent in psychiatric nursing today?
2. What are some negative outcomes of hospitalization that you have witnessed or with which you have been personally involved?

Benchmark II: Period of Scientific Study

Around 1850, however, a great transformation began as medicine moved from the clinic into the laboratory, and doctors increasingly shifted their interest from prognosis and care to diagnosis and cure.

George Makari, 2009.

The shift in focus from sanctuary to treatment is linked to the second benchmark in psychiatric care, personified by Sigmund Freud (1856-1939). Toward the last third of the nineteenth century, several scientists devoted themselves to understanding the mind and mental illness. The fruits of their labor held great promise, some of which is still unfulfilled. Nonetheless, the efforts forever changed the world's view: mental illness need not be suffered (however humanely patients were treated) but might be alleviated. In a sense, psychiatric care was popularized.

Early Scientists

Although Freud had the greatest impact on the world's view of mental illness, he neither thought nor worked in a vacuum. Other men and women had tremendous influence on this newly enthusiastic and optimistic approach to mental illness. Emil Kraepelin (1856-1926) made tremendous contributions to the classification of mental disorders. He was a true scientist whose classic descriptions of schizophrenia are valuable reading. Eugen Bleuler (1857-1939) coined the term *schizophrenia* and added a note of optimism to its treatment. Others, many of whom were colleagues or disciples of Freud, made significant contributions to the emerging field of psychiatry.

Freud's contributions still influence psychiatric care, although for a number of years belittling his thinking was popular. Paraphrasing a statement made by Sir Isaac Newton (1642-1727): "If we see far today, it is because we stand on the shoulders of giants." Freud was a giant.

Freud described human behavior in psychological terms. He developed a theory of motivation, established the usefulness of talking (catharsis), explained the importance of dreams, and proposed to unlock the hidden parts of the mind. He openly discussed sex and his ideas remain surprisingly relevant today. He introduced terms that have become part of our language—*psychoanalysis, id, ego, superego,* and *free association.* The work of others evolved from Freud's studies. Alfred Adler, Carl Jung, Ernest Jones, Otto Rank, Helene Deutsch, Karen Horney, and Anna Freud (Freud's youngest child) all made significant and, in most cases, lasting contributions to the field of dynamic psychiatry.

However, Freud's inspiration reached far beyond the people with whom he worked personally. Society in general is indebted to him, even though conflicting opinions about his ideas have emerged. Freud challenged society to look at human beings objectively and fostered a milieu of thinking about the mind and mental disorders. Unit II builds on these concepts and is devoted to the implementation of strategies for working with psychiatric patients.

Benchmark III: Period of Psychotropic Drugs

From this milieu of theory and scientific thought came the third benchmark, which began around 1950 with the discovery of psychotropic drugs. Chlorpromazine (Thorazine), an antipsychotic drug, and lithium, an antimanic agent, were introduced first, and imipramine (Tofranil), an antidepressant, was introduced a few years later. The impact of these drugs has been powerful. Patients who appeared beyond reach became less agitated and experienced a reduction in psychotic thinking. Depressed patients regained normal feelings. Hospital stays were shortened, and hospital environments improved. Psychotropic drugs have allowed many patients to be treated in less restrictive environments; however, ethical, moral, and legal questions have arisen with this treatment modality. Unit III is devoted to an understanding of the role of psychotropic drugs in the treatment of mental disorders.

Benchmark IV: Period of Community Mental Health

If the foregoing suggests the notion that one benchmark period ended entirely before the next one began, then we will clarify that misunderstanding. Trends tend to overlap as advocates of one view struggle to defend existing strategies while more dynamic forces emerge elsewhere. As the various treatment approaches were being developed in the milieu derived from Freud's theories, criticism grew, and the state hospital system continued its plunge into "psychiatric Siberia." The popular movie *The Snake Pit* (1948) portrayed a mindless, ineffective, and at times cruel system of care. In an even more devastating exposé, the book *The Shame of the States*, by Albert Deutsch (1948), vividly revealed with words and photographs the deplorable conditions in several large state hospitals in the United States.

Legislators were watching, reading, and listening; legislation was passed that would change the approach to psychiatric care. In 1946, President Truman signed the National Mental Health Act, enabling the establishment of the National Institute of Mental Health a few years later (in 1949). In 1947, the Hill-Burton Act legislated funds to build general hospitals that included psychiatric units (Table 2-3). This initiative began the effort for early intervention and helped shorten the length of hospitalization for psychiatric patients.

In 1961, the Joint Commission on Mental Illness and Health, appointed by President Kennedy, published a report entitled *Action for Mental Health*. It urged increased support for the state hospital system in recognition of the need for improved treatment of the mentally ill population. Opponents of the state hospital system overwhelmed supporters of this report. The more outspoken critics of state hospitals declared that these hospitals were actually the cause of mental illness. The era of the large state hospitals was over.

Rather than increasing monetary support for the state hospital system, a convergence of forces set the stage for this fourth benchmark period in psychiatric history:
1. The public's declining confidence in the state hospital system
2. The failure of various treatment approaches to eradicate mental illness
3. The legislative climate that had begun in the 1940s, emphasizing the civil rights of mentally ill people
4. The newfound faith in psychotropic drugs

These factors led to the enactment of the Community Mental Health Centers Act in 1963, which virtually destroyed the state hospital system. A deliberate shift was made from institutional to extrainstitutional care; the goal was

deinstitutionalization of the state hospital system population. The problem of geographic isolation was addressed with the establishment of community treatment centers and community living arrangements. Keeping the individual closer to the family addressed issues of isolation from family members. Isolation from follow-up care was remedied because various levels of care were available locally in the continuum of care (see Chapter 1). Eventually, community mental health programs were developed to meet the needs of all those living within the boundaries of a designated area.

Deinstitutionalization

The practice, over the past four decades, of releasing people with severe mental illnesses from institutions has been one of the largest social experiments in twentieth century America.

E. Fuller Torrey (1997)

Deinstitutionalization refers to the depopulating of state mental hospitals. State hospitals reached their peak population in 1955 and then slowly began the process of trimming their census rolls. This process began with growing concern about hospital "asylums" (i.e. a place of poor treatment or no treatment) and was nurtured by some of the negative events discussed earlier in the chapter. A more subtle influence was the growing disillusionment of psychiatry and psychiatric nursing with the chronically mentally ill and a turning to the worried well. Lest the importance of this statement escape the reader, the concept will be reworded. Nurses and physicians gravitated toward people with whom they could identify. *It is much easier to counsel and medicate a woman going through the crisis of divorce than to attempt to understand the babblings of a person with disorganized schizophrenia.*

These factors clearly laid the groundwork for deinstitutionalization; however, federal actions helped fully ignite the process. The first, as noted, was the Community Mental Health Center Act of 1963. The second federal action was legislation that provided mentally disabled persons with an income while living in the community. This legislation was named Aid to the Disabled and is now called Supplemental Security Income and Social Security Disability Insurance. The number of individuals with mental disorders receiving these benefits has increased dramatically in recent years.

Shifting the Cost of Mental Illness or "Follow the Money"

State governments soon found that Aid to the Disabled, even when supplemented by the state, was less expensive than public hospitalization because the federal government paid most of the costs. The federal share grew by 3100% between 1963 and 1994 (Torrey, 1997). Naturally, state financial incentives declined as the involvement of the federal government increased.

Perhaps the final event in the deinstitutionalization movement was the change in commitment laws. Out of concern for the civil rights of mental patients, involuntary commitment of individuals to a state hospital became

TABLE 2-3	**LEGISLATIVE EVENTS THAT CHANGED PSYCHIATRIC CARE IN THE UNITED STATES**
YEAR	**LEGISLATIVE ACT**
1946	President Truman signed the National Mental Health Act
1947	Hill-Burton Act allocated funds for general hospitals to develop psychiatric units
1949	National Institute of Mental Health established
1961	President Kennedy established Joint Commission on Mental Illness and Health
1963	Community Mental Health Centers Act

BOX 2-1   ON BEING SANE IN INSANE PLACES

Rosenhan wondered whether the "sane" could be distinguished from the "insane." He selected eight pseudopatients (people who pretended to be mentally ill) and instructed them to attempt to gain admission to public mental hospitals. The task was much easier than anyone had anticipated. Twelve hospitals in five states were used. The pseudopatient group consisted of a graduate student in psychology, three psychologists (including Rosenhan himself), a pediatrician, a psychiatrist, a painter, and a housewife; three were women, and five were men. No one in the hospital knew of the deception. The pseudopatients were trained to do the following:

1. Call the hospital and make an appointment.
2. On arriving at the hospital, tell the psychiatrist that they had been hearing voices.
3. On being asked to describe the voices, say that they were not sure but remembered the words *empty*, *hollow*, and *thud*.
4. Other than giving this false information and false information about their names, occupations, and employers, they were to be truthful and "normal" from that point forward.
5. Immediately on admission, they were to cease simulating abnormal behavior and behave "normally."
6. When asked how they were doing, they were told to respond "fine" and to inform the staff that they were no longer experiencing problems.

Despite behaving normally, none of the pseudopatients were discovered by the staff. However, approximately 25% of the other patients made comments about the pseudopatients' "sanity," and a few even guessed that the pseudopatients were doing some type of undercover work. Rosenhan noted reluctance by the staff to recognize mental health in their patients. He stated, "Having once been labeled schizophrenic, there is nothing the pseudopatients can do to overcome the tag." Pseudopatient histories were written to support their diagnoses. In other words, psychiatrists saw problems that had never existed.

The pseudopatients were also asked to write down their observations. At first, they followed elaborate precautions to avoid detection; however, they were soon jotting down observations in front of the staff. The pseudopatients discovered that no one was paying attention to them.

Another part of the experiment was to determine the amount of time spent with patients. This amount was difficult to measure; thus, a proxy behavior was substituted—time the nurses spent outside the nurses' station. Nursing attendants had the highest percentage of time spent outside the station (11.3%). Rosenhan found that measuring registered nurse time outside the nurses' station was impossible because it occurred so infrequently. Psychiatrists were even worse because they hid behind their closed office doors; at least the patients were able to see the nurses. Rosenhan concluded, "Those with the most power have least to do with patients, and those with the least power are most involved with them."

Rosenhan decried the powerlessness and the depersonalization experienced by the pseudopatients. He remembered how he was frequently awakened in the hospital to which he had been admitted: "Come on you m——f——s, out of bed."

The pseudopatients were hospitalized on average for 19 days before they were deemed well enough for discharge. The range of stay was from 7 to 52 days.

From Rosenhan, D.L. (1973). On being sane in insane places. *Science*, *179*, 250.

difficult. The state had to demonstrate that individuals brought for involuntary commitment were a clear danger to themselves or to others. These sweeping changes were reactions to years of injustice during which persons said to be mentally ill could be detained and involuntarily committed, with little recourse, for long periods. Rosenhan's (1973) classic study, summarized in Box 2-1, illustrates how difficult it was for a sane person to be discharged from a mental hospital. The stage was set for the rapid depopulation of state hospitals. Today, for many patients and families, getting into a state hospital is even harder. (Think of recent tragedies in which the families of perpetrators of horrendous crimes lament that they could not "get any help.")

Depopulation of State Hospitals

The state hospital population reached its peak in 1955, with 558,922 patients. Stated another way, in 1955, there was 1 psychiatric bed for every 300 Americans, but by 2010, there was only 1 bed for every 3000 Americans (Nasrallah, 2012b). Today, the state hospital population is about 70,000 patients, a decline of more than 85%. Perhaps 1 million people would be in state hospitals today if the proportions of 1955 were in effect. If this projection is correct, greater than 900,000 individuals who might have been hospitalized

TABLE 2-4   WHERE INDIVIDUALS WITH SEVERE MENTAL ILLNESS LIVE

Nursing homes
Prisons/jails
State hospitals
Homeless
Home with families, group or board-and-care homes, or on their own

From Torrey, E.F. (1997). The release of the mentally ill from institutions: a well-intentioned disaster. *The Chronicle of Higher Education*, *43*, B4.

years ago are currently living outside such institutions. This decline has resulted in the closing of many state hospitals. Patients hospitalized today require a high level of care, have few social relationships, are often psychotic, and are typically acutely ill young men. Table 2-4 provides insights into where mentally ill people outside of institutions might be living. Prisons and jails provide a significant amount of the mental health "care" in the United States. In fact, today there are 300% more patients with severe mental illness in jails and prisons than in hospitals in the United States (Torrey et al., 2010).

Community Effects—from Deinstitutionalization to Transinstitutionalization

The effects of deinstitutionalization are also evident in community agencies. For example, emergency department use by acutely disturbed individuals has increased dramatically in the absence of the previous system. Emergency psychiatric services are sagging from the load they now carry. Some general hospital psychiatric units are overwhelmed at times with a continuous flow of patients being admitted and discharged. Many professionals believe that the typical patient is also different. Compared with the patients of the 1960s and 1970s, today's patients are more aggressive, and many are armed when first seen in the emergency department. Puffenberger (2007) suggests that the term *deinstitutionalization* no longer captures what we are witnessing. The term *transinstitutionalization* more aptly depicts reality. The Los Angeles County Jail has been described as the largest mental health system in the world (Keltner and Vance, 2008).

? CRITICAL THINKING QUESTION

3. It has been stated that the fields of psychiatry and psychiatric nursing lost interest in the SMI and became more interested in working with the worried well. Do you believe that this is still true in psychiatric nursing? Support your answer.

Benchmark V: Decade of the Brain

The 1990s were declared the Decade of the Brain by the U.S. Congress. During this decade, a steep increase in brain research occurred that coincided with an increased interest in biologic explanations for mental disorders. That interest continues to the present moment. Just recently President Obama's *Brain Initiative* was launched with $110 million of federal funds earmarked for the year 2014 alone (Shen, 2013).

The impetus in 1990 for this benchmark was the significant changes in the *Diagnostic and Statistical Manual (DSM)-III* (see subsequent discussions in this chapter). However, in many ways, the emphasis on brain biology represented a completion of the circle started by Kraepelin 100 years before. Kraepelin believed brain pathology was at the root of serious mental disorders.

Significant changes in public awareness occurred because of the Decade of the Brain, which enabled clinicians to address complex topics with patients and families. Nursing responded to this challenge with a significant augmentation of psychobiologic content in academic nursing programs and a torrent of continuing education programs. In fact, psychiatric nursing textbooks published before 1990 provided very little, if any, information about psychobiology and psychopharmacology, leaving many nursing graduates of that period inadequately prepared. All textbooks now provide this information. Nurses educated in previous decades felt the pressure to upgrade their knowledge to remain viable in the workplace. Most have done so, and nurses who did not or could not for the most part have moved on.

The Decade of the Brain brought many challenges, but the benefits have been tremendous in terms of making psychiatric nursing a more viable specialty. It crystallized the fact that some behaviors are caused by biologic irregularities and not willful contrariness, or worse. It also enabled individuals to move beyond blaming toward a focus on what could be done. The Decade of the Brain brought nursing back into the mainstream of psychiatric care.

ISSUES THAT AFFECT THE DELIVERY OF PSYCHIATRIC CARE

Several important issues affecting the delivery of psychiatric care remain for discussion:

1. Although briefly discussed earlier in this chapter, the *paradigm shift* that has occurred in the way we think about and treat mental disorders is very important. The way we conceptualize a disorder informs all decisions about that disorder.
2. *Homelessness* is a problem that also influences psychiatric care. Vast numbers of individuals are standing on street corners with signs pleading for money, and studies have indicated that many of these people have a serious mental disorder.
3. The need for and the reality of *community-based care* is another issue. What mechanisms are in place to fortify the continuum of care?
4. Finally, we have developed a system of care that is driven by carefully described signs and symptoms. This *bible of diagnoses* is indispensable in our psychiatric care delivery system.

Paradigm Shift in Psychiatric Care

Psychiatry in general lost interest in the seriously mentally ill (SMI) as a result of the influx of psychoanalysts in the 1930s and 1940s (Miller, 1984). As Freud himself had discovered, his analytic approach was most helpful to persons with less severe problems and was not particularly helpful to psychotic patients. Thus, as Freudian thinking influenced more psychiatrists and psychiatric nurses, a natural withdrawal from the SMI and a refocusing on individuals more amenable to treatment occurred. "Asylum psychiatry, and the Kraepelinian model on which it was based, fell into relative decline" (Wilson, 1993).

Public mental hospitals lost prestige, as did the physicians and nurses working in them. Within the psychiatric nursing fraternity, staff nurses were not as highly valued as nurses who worked in the role of therapist. In many cases, as participants in a self-fulfilling prophecy, the devalued inpatient psychiatric nurses in public hospitals became what they were perceived to be. They were often derisively referred to as either '*crazy or lazy*'.

The mainstream of psychiatry and psychiatric nursing turned from chronically disturbed patients to individuals with lowered self-esteem, individuals who were striving to reach their potential, and individuals who were existentially unhappy (Detre, 1987). Psychiatry changed its focus from one extreme of the psychiatric care continuum (the SMI) to the other (the worried well) over a few decades. Social issues started to emerge as legitimate professional concerns. Psychiatry and psychiatric nursing became interested in issues such as poverty, racism, alternative lifestyles, and sexism at the professional level. Some clinicians believe that this process of enlightenment and social relevance further distanced the mainstream of psychiatric care from persons most in need of that care.

Psychiatry returned to its roots with the publication of the *DSM-III* in 1980. That edition has been described by Wilson (1993) as the "remedicalization of psychiatry." Psychiatric nursing was much slower to embrace research (i.e., evidence-based diagnosis) and the biologic underpinnings of the more severely mentally ill. However, as the Decade of the Brain (the 1990s) progressed, psychiatric nursing and psychiatric nursing textbooks reflected the "new" understanding.

Homelessness

Many psychiatric professionals believe that homelessness can be directly linked to benchmark IV. The most popular view 30 years ago was that homeless people (mostly white men) were skid row bums, alcoholics, and hobos who chose to be homeless. Current studies have altered that perception considerably. The current belief is that the homeless are people (including entire families) who have been displaced by social policies over which they have no control. One out of 50 children is homeless (Gerber, 2013).

Estimates concerning the prevalence of mental illness among this population also vary. However, the consensus of opinion is that 20% to 25% of the adult homeless population have a severe mental illness and that approximately 54% (women) to 84% (men) suffer from alcohol abuse (Gerber, 2013). Many suffer from drug abuse as well.

People who are homeless and mentally ill present a challenge to the mental health and political systems in the United States; these individuals are usually single or divorced and have a weak social support system. The homeless SMI are found in parks, airport terminals, soup kitchens, jails, and general hospitals and often present a troubling appearance. Furthermore, the economic turmoil experienced by most Americans in recent years has filtered down to the streets. Many homeless mentally ill persons have become bold in their efforts to survive, assaulting the sensitivities of passersby. From aggressive panhandling to embarrassing public elimination of bodily wastes, societal standards are being affronted. Although much of this alienating behavior is required for survival on the "mean" streets, it is behavior that offends mainstream America. The dilemma is real, and mental health professionals are searching for answers.

As mentioned, homeless people may live exclusively on the streets (so-called *street people*), or they may live in homeless communities, shelters, halfway houses, or board-and-care homes. A possible third group includes individuals who are able to stay for short periods in cheap hotels or with friends ("couch surfers"), alternating between this and nights in less accommodating surroundings. Another significant group moves among homeless shelters, rehabilitation programs, jails, and prisons.

Homelessness is an end product of chronic mental illness and probably exacerbates it as well. Stated another way, many chronically ill persons end up on the streets because of their inability to succeed in a competitive society, and once they are on the streets, the stresses of the homeless life compound their mental health problems; they are in a no-win situation. Proponents of deinstitutionalization argue that these particular problems are not inherently a part of depopulating state hospitals but have resulted instead because money has not followed patients into the community. They attempt to make the case that community mental health has never been allocated the resources necessary to realize its promise. Traditionalists point to the homeless and the disproportionate effect experienced by some minority groups as evidence of the need for change. These critics maintain that homelessness is more than a lack of shelter—it is a lack of support systems that are available in the public mental hospital system.

Community-Based Care

The future of psychiatric care and psychiatric nursing will be linked to continuing efforts to prevent mental health problems and to treat existing disorders more effectively. Because of economic realities, much of that will be a community-based effort as part of the continuum of care. Specific problems associated with community mental health were the liberalization of commitment laws, which allowed SMI patients to go untreated, and restrictive confidentiality rulings, which made discussing the difficult issues of treatment with family members a legal concern. As newspaper editorials, grassroots mental health organizations, and families have clamored about the obvious unmet needs of the SMI, the mental health and legal communities have rallied to respond. This insistence has culminated in thoughtful and deliberate dialog among mental health professionals, with the objective of making the mental health system work. The Recovery Model, which is discussed in Chapter 7, is an outcome of these discussions.

To make the system work, a seamless continuum of care that coordinates the activities of diverse treatment sources and facilitates movement between and among its entities is needed. Until this seamless continuum is developed, many patients will slip through the cracks of the system as both bureaucratic dysfunction and corporate self-interest drain energy away from programs. Box 2-2 suggests how the system is changing to develop this seamless continuum of care. Box 2-3 presents typical individual movement through the continuum of care, from the most restrictive to a less restrictive environment.

BOX 2-2 SYSTEMIC CHANGES

In the new health care reality, community mental health must move rapidly away from some practices and toward new ways of conceptualizing the system:

AWAY FROM	TOWARD
Symptom stabilization	Recovery and reintegration
Professionals having all the answers	Including consumers and families
Medication management	Holistic thinking (e.g., housing, finances)

BOX 2-3   EXAMPLE OF A CONTINUUM* OF CARE IN SMI PATIENTS

1. Commitment to a state hospital
2. Day treatment (five times per week) while living at a state or county licensed residential facility
3. Day treatment (1 to 3 days per week); seeking or beginning gainful employment
4. Scheduled follow-up with therapist and prescribing clinician; living in the community

* From *most* restrictive to *least* restrictive for a patient with a severe mental illness.

The Diagnostic Bible of Psychiatry

Labels provide a usually false yet comforting sense of being able to control the uncontrollable.

Allen J. Frances and Helen Link Egger (1999)

The *Diagnostic and Statistical Manual of Mental Disorders* (*DSM*) outlines the signs and symptoms required for clinicians to assign a specific diagnosis to a patient. Not only are diagnoses based on these criteria, but also all third-party payers insist on a *DSM* diagnosis before considering reimbursement payments. The *DSM* has been published in seven editions since its inception in 1952:

DSM-I	1952	106 diagnoses
DSM-II	1968	185 diagnoses
DSM-III	1980	265 diagnoses
DSM-III-R (Revised)	1987	292 diagnoses
DSM-IV	1994	361 diagnoses
DSM-IV-TR (Text Revision)	2000	361 diagnoses
DSM-5	2013	~376 diagnoses

The first edition was published in a spiral-bound notebook, cost only a few dollars, and described about 106 disorders. It was heavily influenced by Freudian or psychoanalytic thinking. As Grob (1987) has noted, the *DSM* relied on and reflected, "… an extraordinary broadening of psychiatric boundaries and a rejection of the traditional distinction between mental health and mental abnormality. To move from a concern with illness in institutional populations to the incidence in the general population represented an extraordinary intellectual leap."

The development of the third edition was turned over to Robert Spitzer, a psychiatrist in his mid-forties. Working for 6 years on the new manual, he finally pulled together a document that improved the reliability of psychiatric diagnosis (Spiegel, 2005). Historically this was a watershed moment. As one Freudian psychiatrist was heard to say, "The biologists have stolen psychiatry from us."

There are significant changes in thinking in the new *DSM-5*. The first noticeable change is the switch from Roman numerals (IV) to Arabic numerals (5). Also, it is the first major rewrite of the manual in over 20 years. Over 130 people worked on it with an advisory group of 400 available as backup resources. The *DSM-5* represents a paradigm shift toward an "etiopathophysiological" classification of psychiatric disorders that is, it is hoped, more clinically useful (Tandon, 2012). Nonetheless, many leaders in psychiatry cannot fully embrace the new thinking. A description of these changes and potential challenges is provided in Chapter 23.

Psychiatric Nursing Education: Three Firsts
First Psychiatric Nurse

The official history of psychiatric nursing in the United States began more than 120 years ago. Linda Richards, the first American psychiatric nurse, was a graduate of the New England Hospital for Women. Richards spent much of her professional career developing nursing care in psychiatric hospitals and directed a school of psychiatric nursing in 1880 at the McLean Psychiatric Asylum in Waverly, Massachusetts. Because of her efforts, more than 30 asylums had developed schools for psychiatric nurses by 1890.

First Psychiatric Nursing Textbook

In 1920, Harriet Bailey wrote the first psychiatric nursing textbook. The title of the book, *Nursing Mental Diseases*, reflects the appropriate terminology of the day. An important distinction for psychiatric nursing is that it was not brought into the greater nursing fold until the 1940s. Because psychiatric nurses were trained in state hospitals, they were allowed to work only in state hospitals. In 1937, the National League for Nursing (then called the National League for Nursing Education) recommended that psychiatric nursing be made part of the curriculum of general nursing programs.

First Psychiatric Nursing Theorist

In the 1950s, the views of Hildegard Peplau, an important figure in psychiatric nursing, shaped and gave direction to psychiatric nursing practice and contributed to the development of a professional climate. Peplau (1952, 1959) developed a model for psychiatric nursing practice. Her book, *Interpersonal Relations in Nursing* (1952), influences practice to this day; her approach, heavily influenced by Harry Stack Sullivan, emphasizes the interpersonal dimension of practice. Peplau also wrote a history of psychiatric nursing that carefully traced the unfolding of the profession. She might be the most important historical figure in psychiatric nursing.

SUMMARY

Even if we wanted to, we could not get away from psychiatric concerns. Our daily newspapers jog us from any indifference we might have with accounts of mentally disordered individuals committing crimes. Furthermore, the selective serotonin reuptake inhibitors (SSRIs; e.g., Prozac, Paxil, and Zoloft) are ubiquitous. Tens of millions of Americans are taking these drugs.

Humane psychiatric care started to develop in the late 1700s and has evolved through at least five distinct periods: Enlightenment, Scientific Study, Psychotropic Drugs, Community Mental Health, and Decade of the Brain. Initially, the biologic aspect of mental illness was embraced, but this understanding gave way to a Freudian or psychoanalytic view, which directed the clinician to search for what was behind the symptoms. Although this detective approach was intellectually stimulating and made for wonderful conversation, it conceptually missed the point. Many patients were not living out a dark drama from childhood but instead were suffering from present-day biologic disturbances (e.g., low norepinephrine levels). Finally, in the 1980s and 1990s, respectively, psychiatry and psychiatric nursing returned to their roots and acknowledged that many mental health problems are caused by biologic abnormalities.

The *DSM*, sometimes referred to as the bible of psychiatric diagnosis, is the *lingua franca* (i.e. unifying language) of psychiatry. To participate fully in clinical discussions, nurses need a basic understanding of its concepts.

❓ CRITICAL THINKING QUESTION

4. If it is the patient that truly counts, why get caught up in *DSM* terminology? Doesn't this serve to distance the nurse from the patient?

▌ STUDY NOTES

1. Understanding the principles of psychiatric nursing is important because mental health problems affect approximately 25% of the population.

2. Modern psychiatry can be traced through five benchmark periods: Enlightenment, Scientific Study, Psychotropic Drugs, Community Mental Health, and Decade of the Brain.

3. Historically, mentally ill people were often confined, but the period of Enlightenment ushered in an era in which the mentally ill were treated humanely.

4. The asylum movement (providing sanctuary from the hostile world) grew out of the humane emphasis of the period of Enlightenment and resulted in the development of state hospital systems.

5. During the period of scientific study, men such as Freud, Kraepelin, and Bleuler studied people objectively; this effort resulted in both psychodynamic and biologic understanding of mental disorders.

6. During the period of psychotropic drugs, antipsychotic drugs (early 1950s), antidepressant drugs (late 1950s), and other drugs were developed and greatly contributed to the treatment of specific mental disorders.

7. The period of community mental health began as a result of several converging factors, including:
   - Hostility toward state hospitals (sometimes warranted)
   - Psychotropic drugs
   - Civil rights
   - Financial incentives (which did not always materialize)

8. Deinstitutionalization, which changed the locus of treatment from large public hospitals to the community, is a product of the community mental health movement.

9. In 1955, more than a half million patients were in state hospitals; today, approximately 70,000 are in these hospitals.

10. A large percentage of the homeless in the United States has a diagnosable mental disorder. Critics of deinstitutionalization place some of the blame for homelessness on the community mental health movement.

11. Community mental health nurses have a major role in the continuum of care because of their specialized training in patient care, comprehensive services, patient education, and case management.

12. Psychiatric care and psychiatric nursing have evolved during the twentieth century. At one time, psychiatric nursing was closely associated with the care of the SMI, but, similar to psychiatrists, nurses in the field became professionally interested in the worried well. Beginning with the Decade of the Brain, many psychiatric nurses renewed their interest in understanding biologic variables affecting patients with mental disorders.

13. The *DSM* is the bible of psychiatric diagnosis. Nurses who seek to provide the best care and who want to advocate for patients most effectively learn these concepts.

REFERENCES

American Psychiatric Association, (2013). *Diagnostic and statistical manual of mental disorders* (5th ed.). Arlington, VA: APA.

Charland, L. C. (2007). Benevolent theory: Moral treatment at the York retreat. *History of Psychiatry, 18*, 61.

Detre, T. (1987). The future of psychiatry. *The American Journal of Psychiatry, 144*, 621.

Deutsch, A. (1948). *The shame of the states*. New York: Harcourt Brace.

Frances, A. J., & Egger, H. L. (1999). Whither psychiatric diagnosis. *The Australian and New Zealand Journal of Psychiatry, 33*, 161.

Gerber, L. (2013). Bringing home effective nursing care for the homeless. *Nursing, 43*, 32.

Gollaher, D. (1995). *Voice for the mad: The life of Dorothea Dix*. New York: Free Press.

Grob, G. (1987). The forging of mental health policy in America: World War II to the new frontier. *Journal of the History of Medicine and Allied Sciences, 42*, 410.

Keltner, N. L., & Vance, D. E. (2008). Incarcerated care and quetiapine abuse. *Perspectives in Psychiatric Care, 44*, 202.

Kessler, R. C., et al. (2012). Twelve-month and lifetime prevalence and lifetime morbid risk of anxiety and mood disorders in the United States. *International Journal of Methods of Psychiatric Research, 21*, 169, Substance Abuse and Mental Health Services Administration. (2009).

Kessler, R. C., et al. (2007). Age of onset of mental disorders: A review of recent literature. *Current Opinion in Psychiatry, 20*, 359.

Kessler, R. C., & Wang, P. S. (2008). The descriptive epidemiology of commonly occurring mental disorders in the United States. *Annual Review of Public Health, 29*, 115.

Makari, G. (2009). On the shifting boundaries of medicine. *The Lancet, 373,* 206.

McMillan, I. (1997). Insight into bedlam: One hospital's history. *Journal of Psychosocial Nursing and Mental Health Services, 35,* 28.

Miller, R. D. (1984). Public mental hospital work: Pros and cons for psychiatrists. *Hospital & Community Psychiatry, 35,* 928.

Nasrallah, H. (2012a). The hazards of serendipity. *Current Psychiatry, 11,* 14.

Nasrallah, H. (2012b). Psychiatry and the politics of incarceration. *Current Psychiatry, 11,* 4.

Peplau, H. (1952). *Interpersonal relations in nursing.* New York: Putnam.

Peplau, H. (1959). *American handbook of psychiatry, principles of psychiatric nursing* (Vol. 2). In S. Arieti (Ed.), (pp. 1840–1856). New York: Basic Books.

Puffenberger, G. (2007). *Pharmacy orientation (slide presentation for new pharmacists).* MHM Services, used with permission.

Rosenblatt, A. (1984). Concepts of the asylum in the care of the mentally ill. *Hospital & Community Psychiatry, 35,* 244.

Rosenhan, D. L. (1973). On being sane in insane places. *Science, 179,* 250.

Rosenheck, R. (1997). Disability payments and chemical dependence: Conflicting values and uncertain effects. *Psychiatric Services (Washington, D.C.), 48,* 789.

Shen, H. (2013). Brain storm. *Nature, 503,* 26.

Spiegel, A. (2005). The dictionary of disorder. *The New Yorker, 56,* 56.

Substance Abuse and Mental Health Services Administration (SAMSHA). (2009). http://www.samsha.gov Accessed 18.04.05.

Tandon, R. (2012). Getting ready for DSM-5: Part 1. *Current Psychiatry, 11,* 33.

Torrey, E. F., et al. (2010). *More mentally ill persons are in jails and prisons than hospitals: A survey of the states.* Arlington, VA: Treatment Advisory Center.

Torrey, E. F. (1997). The release of the mentally ill from institutions: A well-intentioned disaster. *The Chronicle of Higher Education, 43,* B4.

U.S. Department of Health and Human Services, (2000). *Healthy people 2010.* Washington, D.C.: USDHHS.

U.S. Surgeon General, (1999). *Mental health: A report from the surgeon general.* Washington, D.C.: USDHHS.

Wasow, M. (1993). The need for asylum revisited. *Hospital & Community Psychiatry, 44,* 207.

Weiner, D. B. (1992). Philippe Pinel's "memoir on madness" of December 11, 1794: A fundamental text of modern psychiatry. *American Journal of Psychiatry, 149,* 725.

Wilson, M. (1993). DSM-III and the transformation of American psychiatry: A history. *American Journal of Psychiatry, 150,* 399.

3

Legal Issues

Willie O. Smith, Norman L. Keltner

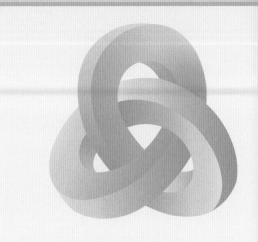

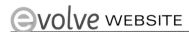 WEBSITE

http://evolve.elsevier.com/Keltner

LEARNING OBJECTIVES

- Define the terms that apply to legal issues in psychiatric care.
- Describe the liability of the nurse in issues such as wrongful commitment, duty to warn, and master-servant rule.
- Identify four landmark court rulings and their impact on psychiatric care.
- Define and discuss involuntary commitment issues and procedures.

- Define and apply the concept of least restrictive alternative.
- Define and apply the concept of confidentiality.
- Define and apply the concept of the right to treatment and the right to refuse treatment.
- Describe effects of mental illness on local, state, and federal justice systems

It is tempting to start off a chapter discussing psychiatric nursing legal issues with some reference to Newtown, Connecticut; Aurora, Colorado; or some other place where a person said to be mentally ill has killed many. We cannot or, more accurately, will not reduce those tragedies to an illustration in this textbook, so they are not discussed here. However, many of the principles covered in this chapter will apply to the legal proceedings of those accused.

The evolution of humane treatment of mentally ill persons roughly parallels that of advances made in the jurisprudence system. Historically, movement has been a slow, cautious process from viewing mentally ill people as demonic or weak-willed to viewing them as individuals with legitimate health care problems. Governmental systems and regulatory bodies thoughtfully attempt to achieve balance between the rights of individuals and the rights of society at large. Although most people are aware of the difficulty in reaching this goal in criminal cases, they are less aware of the struggle for such a balance in psychiatric care.

This chapter begins with a brief review of basic legal principles and sources of law that have influenced mental health delivery and serve as the basis for legally sound psychiatric nursing practice (Box 3-1). The following topics are reviewed:
1. Key legal terms
2. Common law, precedent-setting cases, statutory law, and administrative law

3. Tort law: negligence, assault and battery, false imprisonment, and related nursing liability

Additionally, the nurse's role in these and other legal issues is presented throughout the chapter to help the student understand the applicable legal, regulatory, and compliance issues.

SOURCES OF LAW

There are three basic sources of law: (1) common law, which is derived from judicial decisions; (2) statutory law, which is created by the federal and state legislatures; and (3) administrative law, developed by administrative agencies. When written laws are unclear or are contradictory to other laws, the

NORM'S NOTES
Legal stuff can put most of us to sleep, but there is something to be learned that will help you do something as simple as reading the paper. Almost daily, in any big city newspaper, you read about a mentally ill person who has committed a crime or about a legal defense strategy incorporating the laws mentioned in this chapter. What about the rights of the patient? People who have mental problems have important rights. One of the most important things you can do is understand the rights of people with mental health problems, whether it is your patient or a family member.

1. U.S. Constitution
2. Individual state and federal statutes
3. Precedent-setting legal cases
4. The Joint Commission (formerly The Joint Commission on Accreditation of Healthcare Organizations)
5. Centers for Medicare and Medicaid Services

judicial system is responsible for resolving these disputes. The resulting judicial decisions often influence legislative action to create an appropriate statute.

Common Law

The term *common law* is applied to the body of legal principles that has evolved and continues to evolve and expand from actual court cases. Many of these legal principles and rules have their origins in English common law.

The judicial system is necessary because having a law that covers every potential event that might occur is impossible. The judicial system serves as a mechanism for reviewing legal disputes that arise in the written law; it is an effective review mechanism for issues in which the written law is silent or confusing and for situations in which issues involving both written law and common law decisions occur.

Many of these rulings have influenced the current legal view of mental illness. Rules presented here, although they in no way form an exhaustive list of major court decisions, reflect decisions that have shaped the mental health treatment system and have served to improve patient care and protect the public.

1. The M'Naghten rule (1843) states that individuals who do not understand the nature and implications of murderous actions because of insanity cannot be held legally accountable for murder. This ruling was based on the case of Daniel M'Naghten, a Scotsman who felt persecuted by the ruling political party and attempted to kill the Prime Minister. Although he failed to kill the Prime Minister, he shot and killed the Prime Minister's secretary (Edward Drummond). He was ruled not guilty by reason of insanity and was committed to an asylum. This case has provided a basis for legal decisions in U.S. courts since 1851.
   Comment: When applied today, the M'Naghten criteria state generally that a person is not criminally responsible at the time of an act if, because of mental "disease or defect," the person did not know the nature and quality of the act, or if the person did know

CRITICAL THINKING QUESTION

1. "Not guilty by reason of insanity" is a phrase that evokes passion in many people. Jeffrey Dahmer, the cannabalist murderer, did not say that he didn't do it. He said he was not guilty because he did not know what he was doing. His lawyers said he was not guilty by reason of insanity. What do you think about this concept? Do you believe this legal defense is used too often? Is it reasonable to have such protection under the law?

it, he or she did not know that the act was wrong. Because this standard focuses on the knowledge of "right or wrong," it is occasionally referred to as the *cognitive standard*. It is estimated that this defense is successful in only 1% of cases (Moran, 2002).

Clinical Example: He didn't know what he was doing.

A: A 29-year-old man with a history of "mental health–related" contact with the police killed his mother, set her house on fire, and then shot randomly at passersby in a Southern California neighborhood before officers, who had confronted him as he attempted to flee by tractor, shot him dead. Police said the chaotic violence began to unfold shortly before 5 P.M. Saturday (August 24, 2013), when Ryan Carnan is believed to have shot his mother to death and set her home on fire in a Los Angeles suburb.

B: Charles McCoy, Jr., dropped building material off overpasses and then began shooting at automobiles on a major highway. He was responsible for 12 shootings and 200 acts of vandalism in the Columbus, Ohio, area in 2003 and 2004. He has pleaded innocence by reason of insanity to murder and 23 other counts. He said voices called him a "wimp."

---

2. *Wyatt v. Stickney*, 344 F Supp 373 (MD Ala 1972), confirmed a right to treatment. In this case, the entire mental health system of Alabama was sued for providing an inadequate treatment program. The court ruled that the Alabama mental health system must do the following at each institution:
   - Stop using patients for hospital labor needs.
   - Ensure a humane environment.
   - Develop and maintain minimal staffing standards.
   - Establish institutional human rights committees.
   - Provide the least restrictive environment for each patient.
   Comment: After nearly 30 years, this case was settled in 2000 under a consent decree that forced the state of Alabama to implement a wide range of mental health services at the local level.

3. *Rogers v. Okin*, 478 F Supp (D Mass 1979), determined the right to refuse treatment. In this case, the ruling prohibited Boston State Hospital from forcing nonviolent patients to take medications against their will. The court based its decision on the constitutional right to privacy. Furthermore, this decision required patients or their guardians to give informed consent before drug treatment could begin. This case has significant implications for nurses who are tempted to "force" patients to take medications for "their own good."

4. *Tarasoff v. The Regents of the University of California*, 17 Cal 3rd 425 (1976), ruled that mental health professionals have a duty to warn of threats of harm to others. In this case, a patient confided to the therapist that he intended to kill an unnamed but readily identifiable girl when she returned from spending the summer in Brazil. The therapist notified campus police and requested their assistance in confining the man. The officers took the patient into custody but released him because he appeared rational. Shortly after her return from Brazil, the man, Prosenjit Poddar,

(Box 3-2).

BOX 3-2 TIPS FOR MONITORING CONFIDENTIALITY

1. Keep all patient records secure.
2. Carefully consider the content of all written entries.
3. Release information only with written consent.
4. Disguise clinical material when it is used for educational purposes.
5. Share information only with people who need to know, not with friends or in public areas.
6. Guard written material taken outside the clinical area.
7. Do not access written or electronic information out of curiosity.
8. Note that fax transmissions to unsecured areas in which a receipt error is a possibility might be prohibited.
9. Know to whom you are talking when relating patient information on the phone; "family" might be a reporter, boss, or insurance attorney.

---

killed Tatiana Tarasoff on October 27, 1969. Her parents successfully sued the University of California, claiming that the therapist had a duty to warn their daughter of Poddar's threats.

Comment: The duty to protect endangered third parties is now a national standard of practice, although some jurisdictions still hold that any disclosure of confidential information is a violation of patient rights (Box 3-2).

Statutory Law

Statutory law is written law developed from a legislative body, such as a state legislature. A statute can abolish any rule of common law by specifically stating the rule. Statutory law follows a chain of command, with the Constitution of the United States being the highest in the hierarchy of enacted written law.

Article VI of the Constitution declares:

This Constitution, and the Laws of the United States which shall be made in Pursuance thereof; and all Treaties made, or which shall be made, under the Authority of the United States, shall be the supreme Law of the Land; and the Judges in every State shall be bound thereby, any Thing in the Constitution or Laws of any State to the Contrary notwithstanding.

This article means that the U.S. Constitution, federal law, and federal treaties take precedence over the constitutions and laws of states and local jurisdictions, such as state statutes.

Administrative Law

Administrative law is public law issued by administrative agencies authorized by statute to administer the enacted laws of federal and state governments. This branch of law controls the administrative operations of government. One example of these agencies is state boards of nursing. Monitoring and implementing these laws for federal and state legislative bodies is difficult. States boards of nursing have been created to issue guidelines for nursing practice, licensure, and compliance monitoring in the interest of public safety.

TORTS (CIVIL LAW)

Negligence

Negligence is a personal wrongdoing that is distinguished from a criminal law violation. Negligence is described as the failure to do or not to do what a reasonably careful person would do under the circumstances. Negligence is a form of conduct that is considered careless and is a departure from the standard of conduct generally imposed on reasonable persons.

The four elements that must be present for a plaintiff to recover damages caused by negligence are:
1. Duty to care
2. An obligation of reasonable care (i.e., standard of care)
3. Breach of duty
4. Injury proximately caused by a breach of duty

All four of these elements should be present for plaintiffs to prevail in suits involving a negligent act. If proof exists of all four elements of negligence, then the plaintiffs are said to have presented a *prima facie* case of negligence, which often enables them to win their case.

Duty to Care

Duty is defined as a legal obligation of care, performance, or observance imposed on a person who is in a position to safeguard the rights of others. This duty can arise from a special relationship, such as the relationship between a nurse and a patient. The duty to care can arise from a telephone conversation, or it can arise out of a voluntary act of assuming the care of a patient. Duty can also be established by statute or contract between the physician and patient.

Reasonable Care (Standard of Care)

A nurse who assumes the care of patients has the duty to exercise a standard of care, which is the degree of skill, care, and knowledge ordinarily possessed and exercised by other nurses in the care and treatment of patients. A nurse must be reasonable in the exercise of professional judgment regarding the care rendered; however, reasonable judgment must not present a departure from the requirements of accepted nursing practice. In court cases in which nurses are being sued for negligence, the question is always the following: "Did the nurse meet the standard of care?" Typically, expert nursing witnesses provide testimony to answer this question.

Breach of Duty

Breach of duty is the failure to conform to or the departure from a required duty of care owed to a person. The obligation to perform according to a standard of care might encompass either doing or refraining from doing a particular act.

Clinical Example: Nurses fail their duty.

A patient was admitted to a psychiatric facility late at night from a general hospital emergency department $1\frac{1}{2}$ hours away. The patient was known to have overdosed on a long-acting opioid drug. Although pronounced medically stable by the first hospital, the patient was noted to be semiconscious and incoherent, with an irregular respiration rate of 12 breaths/minute. The patient's respiratory irregularity did not improve, but neither the physician on call nor the paramedics were called. The patient died before morning of respiratory arrest. The nurses did not meet their obligation to meet the standard of care.

Proximate Cause or Causation

The fourth element necessary to establish negligence requires that a reasonable, close, and causal connection or relationship exists between the defendant's negligent conduct and the resulting damages suffered by the plaintiff. In other words, the defendant's negligence must be a substantial factor causing the injury. The mere departure from a proper and recognized procedure is insufficient to enable a patient to recover damages, unless the patient can show that the departure was unreasonable and the proximate cause of the patient's injuries. Foreseeability, as an element of negligence, is the reasonable anticipation that harm or injury is likely to result from an act or an omission to act. The test for foreseeability is whether anyone of ordinary prudence and intelligence should have anticipated the danger to another caused by his or her negligence.

Malpractice

A form of professional negligence is called *malpractice*. Malpractice claims can be brought against various professions, including nurses. These claims against nurses are often the result of the nurse's failure to take measures to prevent harm to patients or a failure to maintain the standard of care of nurses in the community.

The psychiatric nurse is responsible for many significant decisions in the care of psychiatric patients. Lapses in attention to specific legal issues related to nursing practice can result in liability and suits against the nurse and the nurse's employer. Areas of concern that can lead to suits include inappropriate dissemination of confidential information, illegal confinement, failure to obtain consent for medication and other treatments, inadequate treatment, medication errors, and the breach of duty to warn of threatened suicide or harm to others.

Understanding the concept of the *master-servant rule* is vital to both clinical nurses and supervisors. Simply stated, an employer is responsible for the acts of the employee as long as the employee is acting within the scope and authority of employment. A nurse who exceeds clinical boundaries or fails to act as a reasonable and prudent nurse would, in the same or similar circumstances, incurs liability to the employer. Similarly, it is critical to understand that unlicensed assistive personnel (UAPs) who exceed their clinical boundaries or authority and are under the direction or supervision of a nurse will cause liability to be incurred on the nurse.

Nursing Implications

With the push to reduce health care costs, the use of UAPs has increased significantly. More nurses are finding themselves with job responsibilities that include delegating tasks to UAPs. When a nurse delegates, the authority to carry out the act on behalf of the nurse is conveyed to the assistant; however, the nurse remains accountable for the consequences of the act and for the adequate supervision of the assistant. When delegating, the nurse at a minimum should:

1. Know and follow the local hospital procedures to stay within his scope and authority.
2. Ensure that UAPs assigned have been fully trained and are qualified to carry out the tasks they are expected to perform.
3. Know the limitations and responsibilities of nursing practice of his state.

Clinical Example: If you're in charge, it's on you!

Clara Meyers, a 40-year-old woman with a history of recent depression with sleep deprivation and suicidal ideation, is admitted to your unit, sedated, and placed on suicide precautions. The nurse assigns a new nursing assistant to check on the patient every 15 minutes for the entire shift. The nursing assistant, having checked the patient every 15 minutes for 2 hours and finding her asleep, decides that every 30 minutes is sufficient. The nurse who delegated this task was unaware that the new assistant had only general nursing assistant training and had never been oriented on a psychiatric unit. During the 30-minute period when the patient was left alone, she managed to get out of bed and go to the bathroom, where she fell and fractured her pelvis. In the subsequent lawsuit, the nurse was identified as being liable for the poor decision of the assistant that resulted in the fall.

Duty to Warn Others

Another area of importance to psychiatric nurses is the "duty to warn of threatened suicide or harm." As noted, this duty is derived in part from the landmark case of *Tarasoff v. The Regents of the University of California*. Before the Tarasoff ruling, mental health professionals had no legal duty to warn of threatened suicide or harm to others. In 1976, the California Supreme Court issued the Tarasoff ruling, which states that failure to warn, coupled with subsequent injury to the threatened person, exposes the mental health professional to civil damages for malpractice. Based on this case and other rulings, the mental health professional must balance a duty to protect confidentiality with a responsibility to warn society of possible danger.

Nursing Implications

A nurse who is aware of a patient's intention to cause harm to self or others must communicate this information to other professionals and take steps to protect the potential recipient of harm. Not all comments or vague threats should be reported. The Tarasoff ruling specifies that a specific threat to a readily identifiable person or persons must be made. Whenever possible, a decision to communicate confidential patient communications should be discussed with the clinical team before taking action to ensure that patients' rights are balanced with rights of third parties. Documentation in the patient's record is crucial for effective communication of this information. The nurse who fails to take prudent action can be held liable. See the following example.

Clinical Example: Better warn somebody!

Bud Hollman is a 36-year-old man with a history of mental illness that was successfully treated. He has maintained a steady job for the last 12 years. He has a history of abusing his wife over the last 7 years. His wife of 10 years has decided to divorce Mr. Hollman and end the abuse; she is currently in a safe house for abused women. Mr. Hollman is obsessed with his wife and with finding her. He goes to the homes of several friends and relatives searching for her. He is unsuccessful in finding her and becomes progressively more agitated. He is delusional, convinced that the only reason she left him is because she is possessed. When he fails to find her at her place of employment, he tells her fellow employees that she is possessed by a demon and that he intends to kill her. The police are called, and Mr. Hollman is arrested. He is involuntarily committed for a 72-hour evaluation and is found to have a psychosis manifested by delusions. Mr. Hollman specifically tells the therapist of his wife's demonic possession and his plans to remove the demon. On review, the police and Mrs. Hollman are warned of his threats.

Assault, Battery, and False Imprisonment

Assault

The distinguishing feature between assault and battery is that assault is the apprehension of physical contact or the person's mental security, and battery is the actual physical contact. An assault is the deliberate threat coupled with the apparent ability to do physical harm to another. No actual contact is necessary. Verbally threatening a patient that you are going to force him or her to take medication against the patient's will constitutes an assault.

Battery

A battery is an intentional touching of another's person, in a socially impermissible manner, without that person's consent. Battery is intentional conduct that violates the physical security of another. The receiver of the battery does not have to be aware that a battery has occurred. A clinical example of battery would be the force used in unlawful detention of a patient.

False Imprisonment

False imprisonment is the unlawful *restraint* of an individual's personal liberty or the unlawful restraint or confinement of an individual. The only necessity is that an individual who is physically confined to a given area

experiences a reasonable fear that force, which may be implied by words, threats, or gestures, will be used to detain or intimidate him or her without legal justification. Examples include the following:

1. Excessive force used to restrain a patient constitutes false imprisonment and battery.
2. Preventing a patient from leaving a health care facility constitutes false imprisonment.
3. Wrongfully committing a patient to a psychiatric facility constitutes false imprisonment.

A psychiatric facility should have a policy that defines the parameters of confinement, and the nurse must follow the policy guidelines. Please note that in example 2 in the list, a patient committed by a court proceeding can be prevented from leaving a facility, and doing so is legal—thus not false imprisonment.

COMMITMENT ISSUES

The decision to become a patient in a psychiatric facility is important. Patients must admit to themselves and to others that self-management is no longer a viable option for emotional stability. The paradox for individuals who require inpatient care is that the process of becoming a patient can itself cause anxiety and might be depressing. The psychiatric nurse should be aware of this aspect and of the legal status of the patients in her charge.

Voluntary Patients

Most people with mental health problems are voluntary patients—that is, they seek help voluntarily. Although specific procedures vary from hospital to hospital and from state to state, the basic procedure is that individuals or their therapists request admission, and patients sign the appropriate documents, including a consent to treatment. When individuals are ready to leave the treatment setting, they sign themselves out. Most states have a grace period of 48 to 72 hours to allow professional staff the time and opportunity to assess patients before they leave voluntarily. Voluntary patients who want to sign themselves out can be placed on an involuntary commitment status by the court when assessment of the staff indicates a need for further treatment.

Involuntary Patients (Commitment)

Mental illness is not equivalent to incompetence. Competence involves the patient's ability to comprehend. Involuntary treatment means that an individual who has the legal capacity to consent to mental health treatment refuses to do so. In every state, individuals who are considered dangerous to self or others because of a mental disorder can be involuntarily treated for that mental disorder (Table 3-1). However, the U.S. Supreme Court has repeatedly held that the civil commitment process is subject to the restraints of the Fourteenth Amendment of the U.S. Constitution. The state must produce clear and convincing evidence to prove that a person is both mentally ill and dangerous. Failure to comply with

TABLE 3-1	TYPES OF BEHAVIORS SUSCEPTIBLE TO INVOLUNTARY COMMITMENT	
ALL STATES	**SOME STATES**
Risk of harm through self-neglect, grave disability, or failure to meet basic needs	Risk of physical deterioration without commitment
Risk that a person might physically injure or kill himself	Potential danger to property
Risk that a person might physically harm other persons	Risk of relapse or mental deterioration

From Mossman, D.L. (2013). Psychiatric 'holds' for nonpsychiatric patients. *Current Psychiatry, 12,* 34.

these guidelines can render a commitment illegal. A third criterion—gravely disabled—is also cause (or required) for involuntary treatment. Involuntary treatment is divided into three common categories:

1. Emergency care
2. Short-term observation and treatment
3. Long-term commitment (3, 6, or 12 months)

Involuntary treatment is the area of psychiatric care from which most legal issues arise. Although involuntary commitment usually implies inpatient care, it can also be applied to outpatient treatment (e.g., group treatment as a consequence for driving under the influence of alcohol).

Emergency Care

Individuals who meet any one of three criteria (i.e., dangerous to self, dangerous to others, or gravely disabled) can be detained involuntarily for evaluation and emergency treatment in most states. An authorized person such as a police officer signs documents to place an individual under involuntary care. The length of the involuntary status varies from state to state; typically, 48 to 72 hours is the average. All states allow commitment of mentally ill individuals who pose a danger to themselves or others (Mossman, 2013).

Nursing Implications

Because the law determines the length of this involuntary treatment period, staff must scrupulously adhere to legal time constraints. The nursing staff must be absolutely aware of the point at which the emergency treatment period is over and prepare the patient for discharge at that time. Patients might be asked to remain voluntarily in the facility, and if they refuse, they might be asked to sign out against medical advice. The following clinical example provides a realistic scenario for involuntary detention.

Clinical Example: Acting "crazy."
Bill Wexler is a 52-year-old man who has been informed that his job of 30 years is being eliminated. Although the job loss is part of a larger downsizing effort, Mr. Wexler is deeply and personally affected. Within 1 week, he begins to decompensate. He stops bathing and wears the same suit every day. He shows up for work 2 weeks after being terminated, not having bathed or shaved for a week, and goes to his usual workstation. Another employee occupies the space, and Mr. Wexler demands that the worker move out of his space or he will throw him out. Efforts by other employees who know Mr. Wexler are unsuccessful in trying to calm him. He begins shouting that he is going to kill everyone in human resources and that he has a gun in the car and is going to get it. Security and the police are called, and after a brief struggle Mr. Wexler is successfully restrained. Mr. Wexler is taken to the county emergency department and involuntarily committed for 72 hours.

Short-Term Observation and Treatment

Each state has laws that provide for short-term observation and treatment for mental illness. These laws, which differ from state to state, authorize a qualified expert to determine whether a person has a treatable mental disorder. In most states, a qualified expert might be a physician, a psychiatrist, a psychiatric nurse practitioner, a social worker, or a psychologist. A treatable mental disorder indicates that the problem is amenable to and can improve with treatment. For example, a person who is hearing voices telling her to kill herself meets this criterion, whereas someone who is simply angry and threatening to kill someone might not.

During the emergency evaluation period, if it is suspected that further hospitalization is needed, a certification hearing takes place. A complaint or a probable cause statement is written, indicating that the person is a danger to self or others or is gravely disabled. The probable cause statement is required by the Fourth Amendment to the U.S. Constitution, which prohibits "search and seizure of a person without probable cause." In this context, probable cause means that known facts would lead an ordinary person to believe that the person detained is mentally disordered and is a danger to self or others or is gravely disabled. The probable cause hearing is not held to determine whether the person is mentally ill, but whether just cause exists to keep the person for treatment against his or her will.

If probable cause exists, individuals can be detained for observation and treatment. These individuals must be informed of their rights on being certified for this level of involuntary care. The lengths of the observation and treatment periods vary from state to state.

Nursing Implications

Patients must be released when no legal basis exists for continued confinement in the hospital. The hospital staff might suggest voluntary admission and might require patients to sign out against medical advice if voluntary admission is refused. The staff cannot hold someone simply because they believe that the individual needs to be protected from herself or himself.

Clinical Example: I want what I didn't have

Mr. Banks, a 65-year-old, well-nourished but dirty and smelly man, has been brought to the hospital by a social worker for psychiatric evaluation. Since his wife's death 3 years earlier, neighbors report that his house has been taken over by drug dealers and prostitutes. He is often seen outside at night, sleeping on the porch, despite cold weather. Furthermore, Mr. Banks has approached neighbors for food and has told them that the drug dealers have taken his social security check. Mr. Banks insists that he willingly allows others to live in his home, and he enjoys the sex and drugs that come with the arrangement. He is alert and oriented, and no evidence of psychiatric disorder is found during evaluation. He declines offers of assistance to find safe housing, stating that he wants to return to the lifestyle he missed during the years his wife kept him on the straight and narrow.

Long-Term Commitment

Long-term commitment is reserved for persons who need prolonged psychiatric care but refuse to seek such help voluntarily. These hospitalizations can last from about 90 days to much longer. Individuals are usually brought before a hearing officer, which is a major part of the system of checks and balances that decreases the possibility of someone being railroaded into a mental hospital.

Commitment of Incapacitated Persons

In most states, a procedure is required for establishing a conservator or guardian for a gravely disabled person (the conservatee) because adults are presumed competent before the law. The legal system in the United States maintains that although a person might be undergoing severe mental and emotional upheaval (as in the clinical example of Mr. Wexler), that person is nonetheless recognized as competent. A person who is identified as being gravely disabled is viewed by the legal system as incompetent. Once judged incompetent, the individual loses rights such as the right to marry, vote, drive a car, and enter into contracts.

Gravely disabled is defined as the inability to provide food, clothing, and shelter for oneself because of a mental illness. Not all people living on the streets are gravely disabled and thus should be hospitalized for their own good. However, people with money in their pockets who cannot negotiate arrangements for food or shelter are gravely disabled.

 CRITICAL THINKING QUESTION

2. What if a lucid patient, who will die without treatment, wants to leave the hospital? Does she have the right to refuse treatment and go home? Is wanting to go home to die in itself a sign of mental illness?

Conservators and Guardians

The appointment of a conservator or guardian is a serious legal matter, and full legal protection is provided for persons being evaluated for conservatee status. The proposed conservatee is entitled to representation by an attorney to challenge conservatorship. An appointed conservator or guardian can be given broad powers, including the right to order the conservatee to receive psychiatric treatment. Technically, although patients might receive treatment against their will, a legal distinction exists between this type of commitment and an involuntary commitment. That distinction is based on the premise that the conservator now speaks for the patient; hence, the treatment is not involuntary. Conservators are legally obligated to act in the best interests of conservatees.

Nursing Implications

Because conservators speak for conservatees, the nurse must obtain consent from conservators for decisions that are otherwise made by patients. A nurse who forgets to obtain conservator approval might face legal consequences.

Clinical Example: Somebody help her.

Ms. Park, a 73-year-old woman, is found by a social worker to be living in a filthy, roach-infested, older home. A neighbor who has not seen Ms. Park in several months calls the local department of human services. The neighbor explains that no one answers the door when she rings the doorbell. Ms. Park has lived there for years with her husband. Since he died 5 years ago, Ms. Park has lived alone. The stench of cats and cat feces is almost unbearable. Ms. Park is emaciated, incoherent, and paranoid. The social worker decides to initiate involuntary commitment for Ms. Park to evaluate her mental and physical condition and her need for a conservatorship hearing.

PATIENT RIGHTS

In addition to the information discussed in the following section, the *Federal Register*, published by the Centers for Medicare and Medicaid Services (CMS), is a good source of information about patient rights and regulations. Aside from the legal and patient care issues, these rights must be ensured for health care providers so that they can participate in the Medicare and Medicaid programs.

Right to Treatment with the Least Restrictive Environment

The concept of the least restrictive alternative or least restrictive environment is central to the ideology of the deinstitutionalization movement. People with mental health problems have the right to treatment of their problems in the least restrictive environment using the least restrictive means (e.g., without restraints and seclusion, unless necessary).

Nursing Implications

The nurse has treatment responsibilities and can be held liable if the patient does not receive adequate treatment. The following clinical example illustrates the issue of the right to treatment using the least restrictive alternative.

Clinical Example: He ain't heavy.

Joe Kelly is a 66-year-old Vietnam veteran who has post-traumatic stress syndrome characterized by periods of flashbacks and depression. After a flashback, Mr. Kelly is often confused and wanders about for days looking for friends he lost in the war. He poses no obvious danger to others or himself. His family is deceased, and he lives alone. When he is picked up by the police for loitering and evaluated by the social worker, Mr. Kelly insists on going home. His case is heard before the court, which rules that he does not need commitment to a psychiatric unit but does need a temporary structured environment. The social worker finds a halfway house with the Veterans Hospital, and Mr. Kelly agrees to temporary placement.

Right to Confidentiality of Records

And about whatever I may see or hear in treatment, or even without treatment, in the life of human beings—things that should not ever be blurted out outside—I will remain silent, holding such things to be unutterable.

From Hippocratic oath (from von Staden [1996]).

Patient information is privileged material and should be treated confidentially. Both voluntary and involuntary patients are granted this legal consideration. Maintaining confidentiality is not always as easy as it might appear; hence professional judgment is required. The guidelines in Box 3-2 provide a framework for mandatory confidentiality.

As straightforward as these guidelines are, they do not cover every situation or address exceptions. The rule of confidentiality is not absolute. For example, information about a patient at risk for self-harm must be made available to appropriate individuals. Keeping this type of information confidential constitutes professional malpractice.

Health Insurance Portability and Accountability Act

The Health Insurance Portability and Accountability Act (HIPAA) took effect in April 2003. Because modern technology is often a two-edged sword, concerns have arisen over its misuse. For example, even though computer technology speeds the transfer and storage of personal medical information, it has also proven to be a venue for invasion of privacy. HIPAA gives patients more control over their medical records. It also creates stiffer penalties for individuals who handle a patient's medical record in too cavalier a manner. Appelbaum (2002) outlined the four rights that patients have under HIPAA legislation:

1. Right to be educated about HIPAA privacy regulations
2. Right to access their own medical records
3. Right to correct or add to their medical records
4. Right to demand their authorization before their medical records are disclosed to others

Nursing Implications

The nurse should document all confidential information that is released in the nursing notes, including the date and circumstances under which disclosure was made, the names of the individuals or agencies receiving the disclosure and their relationships to the patient, and the specific information disclosed. To release information about patients, a consent form must be signed first. Most states provide legal redress for patients if a nurse willfully discloses confidential information without the proper signature. Confidentiality of the patient's records should not be confused with the doctrine of privileged communication. Under this doctrine, a psychiatrist is not obliged to reveal the contents of sessions with the patient, a privilege that is based on the understanding of the need for trust between physicians and patients. Most states do not include nurses under this provision.

The therapeutic modality of group therapy, which nurses often lead, is particularly vulnerable to violations of confidentiality. The group leader should always address this issue when starting a group or when a new member is introduced to the group. Nurses who lead group sessions must acknowledge the limitations to confidentiality that exist in the group format. After such a proclamation is made, forthrightness by group members concerning their thoughts, feelings, and behaviors might decline.

It is crucial that staff not discuss patients in settings in which individuals without a clinical need to know can overhear those conversations. *For example, several local students went to lunch and started discussing a patient. The patient's family was in the adjoining booth. The family heard the conversation and reported it back to the hospital. The students were reprimanded but were given a "second chance."*

❓ CRITICAL THINKING QUESTION

3. Confidentiality is stressed in nursing school, but it might be violated. What should you do when one of your classmates is discussing a patient inappropriately? Is it a violation of confidentiality to discuss a patient by name in a clinical conference?

Clinical Example: You are so special!

Students frequently find themselves in the following situation. After developing a relationship with a patient, the student might hear, "I want to tell you something, but I don't want anyone else to know." What is the proper response? Is it a breach of the patient's right to confidentiality to tell others or to record what is said in the patient's chart? The student must let the patient know that anything said within the context of the nurse-patient relationship will be shared with other team members when appropriate.

Right to Freedom from Restraints and Seclusion

Throughout history, mechanical restraints and segregation have been used to manage the out-of-control behavior that accompanies some psychiatric disorders. *Restraint* is a broad term used to characterize any form of limiting a person's movement or access to his or her own body. The limits can be the result of physical holds, bed rails, lap trays, restraint devices, or medications. *Seclusion* is defined as the process of isolating a person in a room in which he is physically prevented from leaving. The value of judiciously used restraint and seclusion to protect severely ill patients and individuals with whom they come into contact has been overshadowed in recent years by attention to injuries and deaths associated with their use. The U.S. Food and Drug Administration (FDA) has estimated that at least 100 restraint-related deaths occur each year. In some instances, restraints and seclusion have been substituted for more appropriate management interventions. When a patient's right to the least restrictive interventions to manage behavioral disturbances is violated, disability, injury, and death can result.

The 1987 Omnibus Reconciliation Act placed stringent limits on the use of physical and chemical restraints (e.g., antipsychotics, benzodiazepines) in nursing homes to ensure that their use is limited to medical necessity, not staff convenience. Many nursing homes have since implemented innovative strategies to preserve the safety of frail older adults, with a goal of becoming restraint-free. The Joint Commission (formerly known as the Joint Commission on Accreditation of Healthcare Organizations) has developed standards to guide efforts to reduce the use of restraints in both medical and psychiatric facilities. The CMS has also published within their Patients Rights document strict rules for restraint and seclusion use in hospitals that receive Medicare and Medicaid funds.

Clinical Example: Somebody needs to be fired!

Mr. Buck Tindal is a 75-year-old man who has been admitted to the geropsychiatric unit of a large teaching hospital for observation and treatment related to recent behaviors suggestive of dementia. Mr. Tindal, although confused at times, is able to feed himself, bathe without assistance, and self-manage toileting needs on admission. As do many men older than 60 years, Mr. Tindal experiences nocturia most nights. Because the staff is concerned about falling and consequent broken bones, Mr. Tindal has been "legally" restrained. Immediately, he begins wetting the bed, something he had not done since childhood. Within 2 weeks, Mr. Tindal is not able to feed and bathe himself and is described in his chart as incontinent.

Nursing Implications

Reduction in the use of restraints is difficult to achieve given the prevalent belief that a restrained patient is a safe one. Nurses who are aware of the potential negative physical, psychological, and legal consequences associated with restraint and seclusion are more apt to look for alternative strategies. The most valuable interventions are aimed at preventing a patient's escalation in behavior and loss of control. Attention to the nurse-patient relationship, therapeutic milieu, and principles of pharmacologic management can reduce the need for restrictive measures. Guidelines issued by the CMS for use of restraint and seclusion are substantially different in medically

necessary and behavioral control situations. Although laws differ from state to state, general guidelines for use in psychiatry include multiple elements important for the nurse to document, as follows:

1. Staff members involved in decisions to restrain or seclude and staff who apply or remove restraints must receive special training and demonstrate competency.
2. Alternatives must be considered before the use of restraint and seclusion.
3. Although nurses might be allowed to implement restraint or seclusion in emergent situations, a physician's order is required within 1 hour. Physician assistants and advanced practice nurses can also write restraint and seclusion orders.
4. The least restrictive method or device possible must be chosen.
5. Nurses should carefully document events leading to the intervention and justification for use.
6. Orders must contain the type of restraint, rationale for use, and time limitations.
7. As needed (prn) orders are not permitted. Each episode must be based on eminent risk.
8. Restraint and seclusion are used for the shortest possible time. The nurse must tell the patients what behaviors are expected before release and reevaluate the patients at least every 2 hours for continued need of restraint and seclusion.
9. Patients must be observed constantly during restraint and seclusion, with documentation of safety and comfort interventions at least every 15 minutes.
10. Patients must be debriefed after restrictive interventions.
11. Patients have the right to request notification of a family member or other person in the event that restraints or seclusion are implemented.
12. Death of any patient while in restraints, even when restraints did not contribute to death in the judgment of the health care provider, is required to be reported to the FDA.

? CRITICAL THINKING QUESTION

4. Some psychiatric professionals believe that the courts have gone too far in protecting the rights of patients and have actually set up barriers to effective mental health care. What do you think?

Clinical Example: Give me that old time religion.

Kim Young is a 28-year-old Korean national married to an American serviceman who is currently assigned overseas. Ms. Young is extremely well versed in the American culture and language, and she is exceptionally bright and talented. Ms. Young has performed endless hours of volunteer work in her community and church. She is viewed as a person with boundless energy who never appears to stop. Her volunteer hours continue to increase, and she begins to preach in local bars and taverns. Her language becomes incoherent at times, and English and

Clinical Example: Give me that old time religion.—cont'd

Korean are often mixed in the same sentence. When the owner of a local tavern calls the police after she refuses to leave, she begins to curse him and tries to hit him with a beer bottle. The police are able to restrain her, and she is involuntarily committed to a psychiatric unit. When approached by the staff, she spits, curses, and tries to strike them. Four-point physical restraint is ordered. Ms. Young requires seclusion and restraint thereafter for her aggressive behavior on several occasions. The nursing progress record (Box 3-3) and the restraint and seclusion nursing notes provide a record of her behavior and the nursing responses to that behavior.

Right to Give or Refuse Consent to Treatment

The right of voluntary patients to refuse treatment has been recognized for a long time. When voluntary patients believe that the treatment they are receiving is helpful, they can accept it; when they believe that the treatment is not helpful, they can refuse it. In contrast, involuntary patients have not always been understood to have the same right to refuse treatment (Box 3-4). Through the years, many involuntary patients have been forced to take medications against their will. Legally, involuntarily admitted patients do not lose their right to give informed consent to the administration of psychotropic drugs. The key issue is whether patients have the capacity to give informed consent to the administration of these drugs. After the court decides that a person is not competent to understand the need for treatment, medications can be imposed on that person. The way in which this decision is implemented varies from state to state. In cases of a psychiatric emergency, medications can be given without consent to prevent harm to the patient or to others.

BOX 3-3 NURSING PROGRESS RECORD FOR KIM YOUNG (CASE EXAMPLE)

TIME	FORMAT
0210	Patient continues to pace hallway, dayroom, and room; at 0235, asks for sleep medications; patient states that walking is the best way to get well.
0315	Patient refuses to go to room and tries to resist; paces dayroom and at times kneels as if in prayer.
0430	Patient is asleep on top of bed, naked; door is open.
0830	Patient refuses medication; appears very agitated.
0930	Patient is very agitated; tears up another patient's magazine and throws it into the trash; patient is placed in seclusion.
0945	Patient paces in room while praying loudly.
1000	Patient increases pacing and intermittently hits walls.
1015	Patient's agitation is escalated; when staff goes into room to check on patient, she swings at staff and attempts to bite the nurse; patient is placed in four-point restraint by four female and two male staff members; patient states that she is being "raped" and that "Christ lives in me"; Haldol 5 mg IM and Cogentin 2 mg IM are given.

BOX 3-4 A PRECEDENT SETTING CASE

Eleanor Riese, a 44-year-old woman, was first hospitalized at age 25 (in 1968) when she was given a diagnosis of schizophrenia. She was prescribed thioridazine (Mellaril), which brought her psychosis under control. After treatment, she was able to live alone for many years. Riese stopped taking her medication, and speculation asserted it was because of Mellaril-related bladder infections. Her psychosis returned, and she was in and out of psychiatric hospitals as a voluntary patient.

In 1985, Riese was admitted to Saint Mary's Hospital and Medical Center, San Francisco, California. Her status was eventually changed from voluntary to involuntary because she refused to take her medications. The American Civil Liberties Union (ACLU) sued on behalf of the rights of Riese and other involuntary patients to refuse medications.

The ACLU prevailed in the case, and it was determined that patients have the right to refuse treatment. If a mentally ill patient refuses to take medications, a court hearing must be scheduled to determine whether medications would benefit the patient in getting better. The hearing is called a Riese Hearing, and the judge determines if the patient would benefit from medications. This decision is based on input from the psychiatrist regarding treatment of the patient with psychotropic medications. Once the determination has been made, if the patient refuses oral medications, a substitute suitable injectable is given.

Adapted from *Riese v. St. Mary's Hospital and Medical Center, 259 Cal. Rptr. 669, 774 P2d 698.* (1989). <http://www.stanford.edu/group/psylawseminar/Riese.htm> Accessed September 13, 2013.

Nursing Implications

Nurses administer medications to patients. Because it is common for patients to refuse medications and for nurses to coax patients into taking medications, nurses must ensure that coaxing does not escalate to the point of forcing medication on a patient. Although it might be tempting to hide medications in food or liquid when patients refuse them, these actions are considered forcing. The deception is also counterproductive when trying to establish a therapeutic nurse-patient relationship. Also, factors that constitute a psychiatric emergency are not always clear. Nurses might be held liable if their interpretation of a psychiatric emergency differs from that of another professional or a judge.

Suspension of Patient Rights

Occasionally, suspension of rights for the protection of patients or others and for therapeutic purposes is necessary. For example, no units have unlimited telephone privileges, primarily because this policy might be nontherapeutic.

Nursing Implications

Suspension of a patient's rights requires the nurse to document clearly that allowing the patient to continue to exercise the specific right might result in harm to the patient or others. For example, a suicidal patient's right to access personal belongings might be suspended because it is believed that the patient might attempt to harm herself with those objects. The nurse must document the concern and suspension of this right in the nurse's notes.

PSYCHIATRIC ADVANCE DIRECTIVES

Most states have recognized the rights of individuals to choose the type of medical treatment they receive in case of a life-threatening medical condition, which is accomplished through the use of living wills and health care directives; 25 states have advance directives for psychiatric treatment (Luddington & Mossman, 2012). In spring 2005, the Terri Schiavo case brought this matter to the forefront. Ms. Schiavo had not executed a directive, and the world witnessed the drama that became her final days as her husband and the court decided to remove her feeding tube. Many people, inspired by this case, acted swiftly and legally to set forth their wishes in case of their incapacitation.

Luddington and Mossman (2012) report the case of Nancy Hargrove, a woman who lived in Vermont (where there is no separate psychiatric advance directive) and who was diagnosed with schizophrenia. In her durable power of attorney, she did clearly refuse "any and all anti-psychotic, neuroleptic, psychotropic, or psychoactive medications … and ECT [electroconvulsive therapy]." When she needed hospitalization and psychotropic medications, the big question was whether it was legal to administer involuntary medications to this patient. The authors report that although psychiatrists wanted to override her power of attorney, the courts ruled that Ms. Hargrove's decision to be medication-free must be honored. It should be noted that this decision would not be rendered in all states.

The U.S. Congress passed the Patient Self-Determination Act in 1990. This law requires all health care facilities that serve Medicare or Medicaid patients to provide each of their adult patients with written information regarding their right to make decisions about their medical care. These instructions must be consistent with the laws of each state. Patients are also made aware of the right to execute a living will or a durable power of attorney. Both the living will and the health care directive list specific actions that the patient can choose to implement or not under a life-threatening medical condition, such as mechanical ventilator support or artificial nutrition. A durable power of attorney is a written document in which one person (the principal) authorizes another person (the attorney in fact) to act on the principal's behalf in the event the principal becomes unable to act on his own behalf secondary to a physical or mental disability. The disability causes this type of power of attorney to take effect.

Advance directives for mental health treatment are similar to medical care advance directives in many ways, but they have additional challenges. The issue of ensuring competency when directives are executed is problematic, particularly for patients with fluctuating mental disorders. Nonetheless, in advance of a mental health crisis, individuals can issue directives about treatment in many areas, including, but not limited to, (1) the use of specific medications, including dose and route; (2) the use of specific treatment options, such as ECT; (3) the use of behavior management including restraint, seclusion, and sedation; (4) a list of the individuals who are to be notified and allowed to visit; (5) a consent to contact health care providers and obtain treatment records; and (6) a willingness to participate in research studies (Srebnik & LaFond, 1999).

? CRITICAL THINKING QUESTION

5. What if you learned from a patient during an individual session that his company was getting ready to launch a product that would cause the value of the company's stock to soar. Could you ethically use this information to enhance your investment savings?

Nursing Implications

Nurses should be aware of the patient's right to establish advance directives for both physical and mental health care in the form of written statement of preference or by legal documentation of a durable power of attorney. Nurses should also be familiar with and follow employer procedures and laws that govern how the patient is made aware of this right. The following actions are also important to ensure that the patient's right to self-determination is exercised:

1. Documentation in the medical record of either properly executed forms or a statement or signed waiver must be made indicating that the patient chooses not to exercise his or her right to provide advance directives.
2. The attorney in fact chosen by the patient is consulted before making decisions regarding the patient in areas specified by the document.
3. All members of the health care team are made aware of advance directives and that they are considered in treatment planning.

Effects of Mental Illness on Local, State, and Federal Justice System

Approximately 64% of local (jail) prisoners, 56% of state prisoners, and 45% of federal prisoners are reported to have mental health problems (James & Glaze, 2006). Most mentally ill prisoners do not receive adequate treatment. Some practitioners attribute this increase to deinstitutionalization and the subsequent decreased availability of care that leads to placement into the justice system.

The justice system is unable to meet the needs of prisoners with mental illness adequately. There are four overarching reasons for this.

First, the justice system was not designed to treat mental health problems. Psychiatric services are typically inadequate because of the relative paucity of psychiatric professionals and the anemic budgets that are squeezed from the facility's general budget.

Second, these staff and budget issues are compounded by the large number of inmates who pretend to have mental disorders to receive medications or to be "housed" in more comfortable (or safer) environments. Malingering has at least two downstream effects: (1) it diverts resources away from individuals who are truly mentally ill, and (2) it creates an antipathy toward mental illness by persons running these institutions.

Third, mentally ill individuals who need treatment frequently are fearful of taking medications because some medications have the potential to render them less able to defend themselves from fellow inmates. The irony of this development is that successful prison life demands adherence to rules (written and unwritten), and without the normalizing effects of psychotropic medications, many individuals are less able to respond appropriately. In other words, this reluctance to take medication may make individuals less capable of meeting the demands of prison.

Fourth, when a mentally ill inmate does receive treatment, there is a risk that these agents will be abused. Prisoners have been known to abuse the medication themselves, sell the drug to others, or have the drug taken from them by stronger inmates (Box 3-5). In a case report of one such incident, Hussain and colleagues (2005) describe a 34-year-old woman with polysubstance abuse and bipolar disorder who was found on morning rounds, sound asleep with a syringe still in her arm from a self-injection 12 hours earlier. She had crushed two 300-mg tablets of quetiapine (Seroquel) and injected them intravenously. She stated it was the best sleep she had ever had. Quetiapine is only one of many psychotropic drugs that can be abused.

BOX 3-5   THE FEAR FACTOR OF INCARCERATED LIFE

For the incarcerated individual
  Fear as a way of life
  Fear of being harassed
  Fear of being raped
  Fear of being hurt
  Fear of having dignity taken away (e.g., "You can't make me a zombie.")
For the psychiatric staff
  "Don't get caught down the hall by yourself."
  "I have contacts outside."
  Threats are often used to coerce psychiatric staff into making a mental health diagnosis or prescribing certain psychotropic medications.

From Audry Gorman, CRNP, Veterans Administration, Birmingham, Alabama (personal communication).

Nursing Implications

Nurses working within the justice system at local jails or state and federal prisons must have knowledge regarding care for the mentally ill prisoner, understanding of the disease process, psychopharmacologic treatment, and other treatment modalities. The nurse must recognize symptoms of mental illness and monitor for correct treatment and compliance to that treatment.

STUDY NOTES

1. The understanding of the rights of mentally ill persons has evolved over the centuries. Today, based on several precedent-setting legal decisions and laws, protection of the mentally ill person's rights has been established.

2. These landmark cases triggered several states to legislate the end of inappropriate, indefinite, and involuntary commitment to mental hospitals.

3. Three categories of commitment include:
   a. Voluntary patient: the person requests hospitalization and voluntarily agrees to be admitted.
   b. Involuntary commitment: a person with the legal capacity to consent refuses to do so and is treated against his will.
   c. Commitment of an incapacitated person: treatment of a person who does not have the legal capacity to consent to treatment.

4. Patients under psychiatric care have many rights guaranteed by the U.S. Constitution and the constitutions of individual states.

5. Seclusion and restraint are special procedures for coping with assaultive and dangerous patients; these patients can be isolated or mechanically restrained to prevent injury to the patient, other patients, or staff.

6. Patients, including involuntarily admitted patients, must give informed consent before they are given psychotropic drugs and retain the right to refuse medication. Except for emergency situations, involuntarily admitted patients cannot be given medication against their will without judicial approval.

7. Psychiatric patients have the right to be treated in the least restrictive alternative or least restrictive environment. In other words, if patients can receive appropriate care close to home in a community agency, they cannot be forced to go to a public mental hospital, far away from family and friends.

8. Mentally ill prisoners have a right to appropriate medical and nonmedical treatment while incarcerated.

REFERENCES

Appelbaum, P. S. (2002). Privacy in psychiatric treatment: Threats and responses. *American Journal of Psychiatry, 159*, 1809.

Highway assailant heard voices. *Birmingham News*, 3A. (2005, May 3).

Hussain, M. Z., Waheed, W., & Hussain, W. (2005). Intravenous quetiapine abuse. *American Journal of Psychiatry, 162*, 1755.

James, D. J., & Glaze, L. E. (September 2006). *Mental health problems of prison and jail inmates.* Bureau of Justice Statistics Special Report.

Luddington, N. S., & Mossman, D. (2012). Psychiatric advance directives: May you disregard them? *Current Psychiatry, 11*, 31.

Medicare and Medicaid Programs, (1999). Hospital conditions of participation: Patients' Rights; interim final rule. *Federal Register, 64*, 36069.

Moran, M. (2002). Insanity standards may vary, but plea rarely succeeds. *Psychiatric News, 37*, 24.

Mossman, D. L. (2013). Psychiatric 'holds' for nonpsychiatric patients. *Current Psychiatry, 12*, 34.

Srebnik, D., & LaFond, J. (1999). Advance directives for mental health treatment. *Psychiatric Services, 50*, 919.

von Staden, H. (1996). "In a pure and holy way": Personal and professional conduct in the Hippocratic oath. *Journal of the History of Medicine and Allied Sciences, 51*, a404.

4

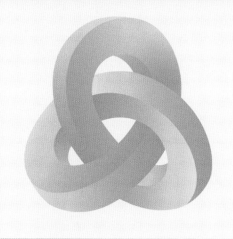

Psychobiologic Bases of Behavior

Richard A. Sugerman and
Jonathan S. Dowben

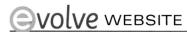
WEBSITE
http://evolve.elsevier.com/Keltner

LEARNING OBJECTIVES

- Describe the importance of the psychiatric nurse's understanding of brain biology.
- Identify and describe gross brain structures.
- Identify the role of specific neurotransmitters in schizophrenia, depression, anxiety, and dementia.

- Differentiate the functions of the sympathetic and parasympathetic nervous systems.
- Describe the function of the basal ganglia system and its significance for movement disorders.
- Discuss key psychobiologic assessment issues for the psychiatric nurse.

The central nervous system (CNS) comprises the brain and the spinal cord. The brain can be further divided into the cerebrum, the brainstem, and the cerebellum. The brain weighs approximately 3 pounds but contains 100 billion neurons, roughly the same as the number of stars in the Milky Way galaxy. The brain is incredibly complex, and a great deal concerning the functions of the brain remains to be discovered. What is known, however, is that many mental disorders that were formerly thought to be caused by psychosocial stressors, traumatic early life experiences, or both are the result of altered or disordered brain biology.

The U.S. Congress declared the 1990s as the Decade of the Brain. Before that time, psychiatric nursing had been influenced primarily by the dominant ideas of the nineteenth century—the ideas of Freud, Bleuler, and Jung—asserting that mental disorders originate from primarily psychodynamic causes. However, psychiatric nursing accepted the congressional mandate, and the 1990s witnessed significant changes in the education and practice of psychiatric nurses. Psychiatric nursing is now fully integrating biologic concepts and consequently is now being practiced holistically. The foundation of today's practice includes understanding basic neuroanatomy and neurophysiology.

The objective of this chapter is to present an overview of neurologic information so the student can become more engaged in the rest of this book, participate in interdisciplinary

discussions, and understand the psychiatric literature better. Understanding psychobiologic concepts enables the nurse to assess patients' behaviors better and plan appropriate nursing interventions. Specifically, the nurse should develop an appreciation for the neuroanatomy of the brain, neurons and neurotransmitters, the autonomic nervous system, and the ventricular system and should be able to apply this information to major psychiatric disorders in a clinical setting.

NORM'S NOTES
In Chapter 3, I mentioned that discussing legal parameters of mental illness might cause some of you to fall asleep. Well, maybe I jumped the gun. There is nothing like a good healthy dose of central nervous system pathways superimposed on a scintillating discussion of presynaptic and postsynaptic receptors to turn the most dedicated student into someone longing for the good old days of fundamentals. Well, it's funny that I should say that because learning some of the basics of brain biology is crucial to understanding the basics of mental illness. This is fundamental information.

NEUROANATOMY OF THE BRAIN

The nervous system is divided into the CNS and the peripheral nervous system (PNS). The CNS (Figure 4-1) can be divided

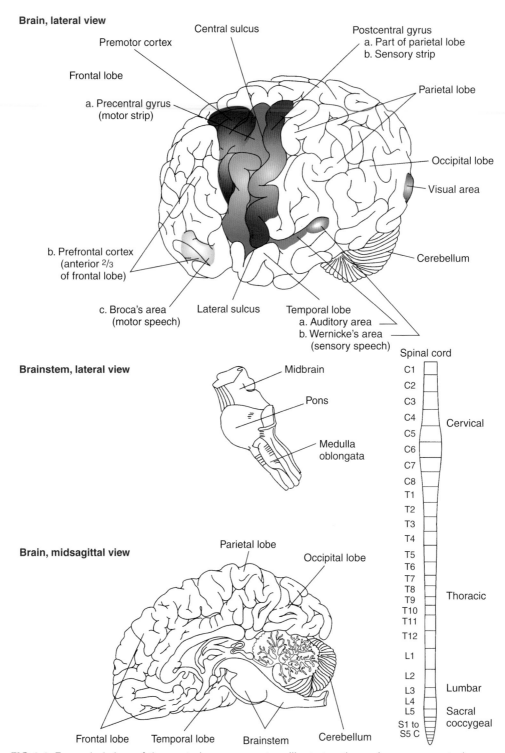

FIG 4-1 Expanded view of the central nervous system illustrates the major components (components are not to scale). (From Sugerman, R.A., Edmundson, M.J., & Robinson, S. [1979]. *Human anatomy*. Edina, Minnesota: Burgess.)

further into the brain and spinal cord. The brain comprises three areas: the cerebrum, the brainstem, and the cerebellum.

Cerebrum

The cerebrum is divided into two cerebral hemispheres and constitutes the bulk of the nervous system. The cerebral hemispheres are composed of a multitude of nervous system pathways, the cerebral cortex, certain limbic structures, the

basal ganglia, and the diencephalons. These structures are described in greater detail in the following section.

Nervous System Pathways

Some specialized neurons in the cerebral cortex transmit information via pathways throughout the CNS. A pathway is a bundle of these communicating neurons. In the CNS, a neuronal pathway (a bundle of neurons) may be called a *tract*, *fasciculus*, *peduncle*, or *lemniscus*. (In neuroanatomy, a single anatomic entity can have several names.) In the PNS, a neuronal pathway is called a *nerve*; cranial nerve (CN) III is part of the PNS.

Numerous large CNS pathways are readily apparent structures within white areas of the brain (white matter). Major pathways include the corpus callosum (Figures 4-2 and 4-3), the internal capsule in each hemisphere (Figures 4-3 and 4-4), and the corona radiata. Although a great deal of interest exists in differences between the right brain (visual-spatial, experiential tasks) and the left brain (language, mathematics, reasoning), many scientists now have a greater appreciation for the interrelatedness of the two hemispheres. The corpus callosum connects the two hemispheres and is the major communication pathway between them. When the corpus callosum is severed, split-brain syndrome develops. The internal capsule and the corona radiata are pathways through which motor and sensory information passes; for example, motor impulses from the motor cortex (precentral gyrus) to the foot pass through these pathways. In addition to these large pathways, many smaller tracts interconnect the four lobes of the cerebral cortex.

Cerebral Cortex

The cerebral cortex is the outermost part of the brain and is composed of gray matter. The gray matter, actually taupe (gray-brown) in color, does the work of the brain. Gray matter consists of neuronal cell bodies, dendrites, and synapses and is not myelinated. White matter consists of myelinated axons and transports information. The cerebral cortex is divided into four lobes: frontal, temporal, parietal, and occipital lobes (see Figures 4-1 and 4-2). Visual examination of the brain reveals the raised areas, or *convolutions*, and the grooves between these areas. Convoluted gray matter is referred to as a *gyrus* (plural, *gyri*), and the groove between two gyri is called a *sulcus* (plural, *sulci*). A deep sulcus is referred to as a *fissure*.

The net effect of this convoluted configuration is that a substantially greater surface area of gray matter can be provided to perform the work of the brain. This principle can be visualized by considering the coastline of Norway. If Norway did not have fjords, its coastline would be small (approximately 1600 miles). However, because of its fjords, the actual coastline of Norway is extraordinarily long for a country of its size (approximately 12,500 miles). The gyri and sulci of the cerebral cortex can be considered as the *fjords* of the brain. The indentations (sulci) provide for a much larger "coastline" of working gray matter (gyri) than would be the case if the surface of the brain were smooth. The four lobes of the cerebral cortex are divided by three sulci.

Frontal Lobes

The frontal lobes are divided into the *motor* (also called the *motor strip*), *premotor*, and *prefrontal areas*. The motor cortex lies immediately rostral to (in front of) the central

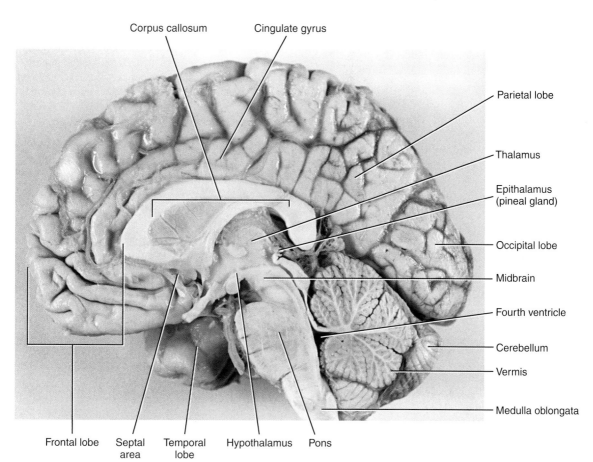

FIG 4-2 Midline view of right hemisphere with anatomic sites labeled. (Photograph by Berto Tarin, Multimedia Department, Western University of Health Sciences, Pomona, California.)

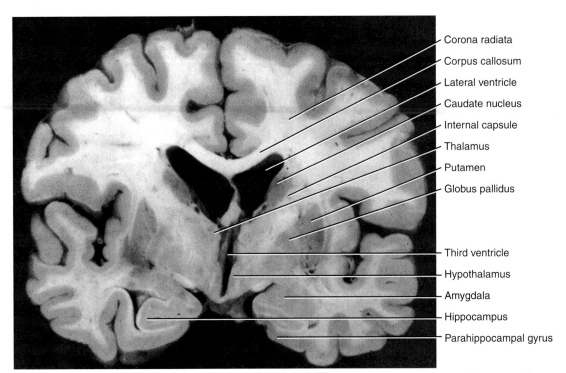

FIG 4-3 Coronal section of the cerebrum. The level of the hypothalamus is shown. (Courtesy of Richard E. Powers, MD, Brain Resource Program, University of Alabama, Birmingham, Alabama.)

sulcus (see Figure 4-1), which separates the frontal and parietal lobes. Because it lies in front of the central sulcus, the motor strip is also called the *precentral gyrus*. The motor cortex controls voluntary motor activity; from this area, the *corticospinal tract* (made up of axons) descends through the corona radiata and the internal capsule, crosses over toward the tail of the brainstem, and synapses in the spinal cord (see Figure 4-4). Approximately 80% of the corticospinal tract crosses over at the level of the lower brainstem (medulla oblongata), whereas the remaining 20% of the neuron axons descends down the spinal cord ipsilaterally (same side) before crossing over to the opposite side of the spinal cord. This remaining 20% of the corticospinal tract theoretically might be responsible for some limited motor recovery in patients with hemisected spinal cords; however, any significant long-term recovery is rare at best. From the spinal cord, spinal nerves branch out into the periphery and connect to muscles. The corticospinal tract is also referred to as the *pyramidal system* and controls voluntary motor movements. The term *pyramidal* is used because most neurons in this tract pass through the pyramids of the lower (or caudal) brainstem (medulla oblongata). The extrapyramidal motor system lies outside the pyramids.

Clinical Example

Think about wiggling your right big toe and then wiggle it. It is not known how a thought is translated into muscle movement, but what is known is that this voluntary movement is a two-neuron system; that is, neurons from the motor cortex descend as described and synapse with spinal neurons. The spinal neurons project as a spinal nerve

from the spinal cord and descend to the toe. The neurons from the motor cortex to the spinal cord are called *upper motor neurons* (see Figure 4-4). The neurons that project from the spinal cord down to the toe are called *lower motor neurons*. Whether a disease is an upper motor neuron disease (e.g., stroke) or a lower motor neuron disease (e.g., polio) is clinically significant. An upper motor lesion normally results in a contralateral (body side opposite of the lesion) Babinski's sign. A lower motor neuron lesion normally results in flaccid paralysis.

The premotor area is associated with programmed movement patterns for voluntary motor activity and with inhibiting lower motor neurons from overreacting to stimuli (Kandel et al., 2013). This area is not under conscious control. Many movement disorders, including disorders associated with long-term psychotropic drug use, such as tardive dyskinesia, arise from damage to the premotor cortex and extrapyramidal system. Both the motor cortex and the premotor cortex are organized systematically (Kandel et al., 2013). This arrangement is referred to as *somatotropic organization*, meaning that the area of the motor strip that controls a certain part of the body is relatively specific. This biologic reality has been visually depicted as a little person or, more commonly, as a homunculus (Figure 4-5; see Figure 4-4). Perhaps a word picture can best describe this specific pattern of voluntary motor localization. Think of a child hanging on the monkey bars with head down and feet hanging over the bar. Think of the top of the hemisphere as the bar, with the head hanging down laterally and one foot hanging down between the hemispheres. The area of the motor strip where the head is located controls head movements, the area where the foot hangs controls foot movements, and so on.

Cerebral hemispheres: frontal section

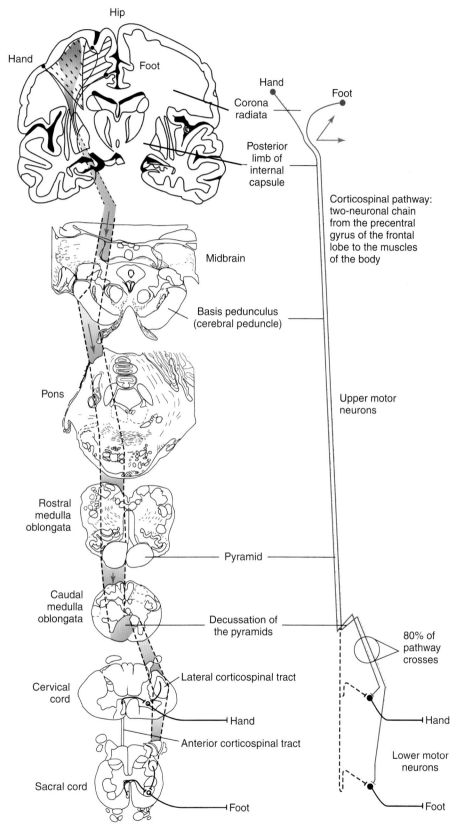

FIG 4-4 Distribution of the corticospinal tract. *Left*, Actual representation. *Right*, Schematic representation.

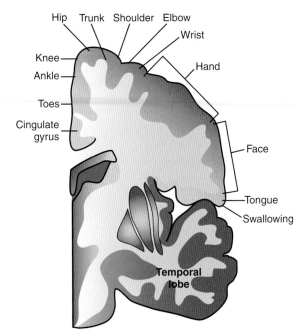

FIG 4-5 Homunculus of the precentral gyrus. Frontal section depicts the relative amount of cortex subserved in controlling the motor functions of various body areas.

The prefrontal area of the cerebral cortex is responsible for thought, goal-oriented behavior, and inhibition. The frontal poles represent the seat of the personality; injuries in this area result in personality changes. Injury to Broca's area, normally located in the left prefrontal lobe (see Figure 4-1), results in impaired motor speech production (Kandel et al., 2013).

Temporal Lobes

The temporal lobes lie inferior to the *lateral sulci* (or the *lateral fissures of Sylvius*). Each temporal lobe is divided into an olfactory area, a primary auditory receptive area, a secondary auditory association area, and a visual association area (Bear et al., 2007). Visual and auditory aphasias are the result of damage to the temporal lobe. Individuals with visual aphasia cannot recognize words in print that they previously understood; the words are as unrecognizable as printed Russian might be to most people. People with auditory aphasia hear sounds but cannot associate the sounds with meaning. Wernicke's area is normally located in the left temporal lobe (see Figure 4-1); a lesion in this area results in fluent speech but impaired comprehension (Kandel et al., 2013).

Parietal Lobes

The parietal lobes are posterior to the central sulcus. The postcentral gyrus (see Figure 4-1), which resides parallel to the precentral gyrus, is a sensory reception strip. The postcentral gyrus receives sensations. It has a homunculus similar to the motor strip. Caudal to this area are association areas, integrative cortical areas of the parietal lobes.

Occipital Lobes

The primary function of the occipital lobes is vision (see Figures 4-1 and 4-2). The occipital lobes are divided into primary visual cortex and association cortex. In contrast to temporal lobe lesions, which can produce various types of visual aphasias, lesions in the primary visual cortex of the occipital lobe result in loss of vision (blindness) from the contralateral visual field; that is, damage to the left side of the primary visual cortex results in loss of vision from the right visual field.

Limbic System

The limbic lobe forms the central core of the limbic system and is composed of the septal area, cingulate gyrus, and parahippocampal gyrus (see Figures 4-2 and 4-3). The limbic lobe is built on the olfactory (smell) system. *Limbic system* is a broad term, referring to the limbic lobe and the structures that function with it: frontal cortex, hypothalamus, amygdala, hippocampus, numerous tracts, brainstem nuclei, and autonomic system. The way in which emotions and motivation are generated in the limbic system remains unclear. No specific anatomic areas exist that can be correlated to emotions such as love, hate, aversion, or fear. Each emotion is likely diffusely linked to different limbic and nonlimbic areas. The limbic system is involved in feeding, memory consolidation, sense of pleasure, emotions, and motivational behaviors.

Limbic Olfactory Function

The first pathway discussed is the olfactory pathway, which is involved with odor detection and differentiation. This chapter does not discuss odor detection beyond its relationship to limbic functions. Understanding how significant smell relates to emotion is important. Smells have different effects on our motivational behaviors (e.g., perfumes and dirty socks).

Olfactory information is picked up by receptor neurons in the nasal cavity and transmitted to the olfactory bulbs, which are located directly under the surface of the frontal lobes. The olfactory bulbs project axons that synapse in the parahippocampal gyrus and in a subdivision of the amygdala (see Figure 4-3).

Feeding Functions

The hypothalamus is involved in several aspects of feeding (e.g., hypothalamic feeding and satiety centers). Experimentally, researchers can electrically stimulate or destroy these hypothalamic areas and affect whether an animal overeats or stops eating.

Memory Consolidation

The limbic system is crucial to memory. The amygdala and hippocampus, located deep in the temporal lobe, are key structures in the transfer of information from short-term to long-term memory (Bear et al., 2007), which are part of the *Papez circuit*. The *Papez circuit* consists of brain structures involved in the complex process whereby memories are created and stored. Discussion of the *Papez circuit* is beyond the scope of this book; however, the reader should recognize that lesions along this circuit cause memory problems. For example, a bilateral lesion of the hippocampal nuclei can result from anoxia, such as in near-drowning. Lesions of the mamillary bodies resulting in memory problems can occur in alcoholics because of a thiamine deficiency. In both situations, individuals frequently maintain long-term memory but cannot make new memories. Amnestic states, amnestic dementias, punch-drunk syndrome, herpes encephalitis, and Alzheimer's disease (AD) involve dysfunction of the hippocampus and possibly other limbic structures (Boss & Stowe, 1986).

Sense of Pleasure

Electric stimulation of the reward pathway can cause animals and people to feel pleasure. Rats press a bar repeatedly to receive electric stimulation to this pathway. The dopaminergic neurons projecting from the ventral tegmental area (Figure 4-6) are of particular importance. These brainstem neurons project rostrally to the cortical and limbic areas, particularly the nucleus accumbens. Investigators have hypothesized that cocaine and many other drugs of abuse produce their effects by increasing the action of dopamine in the nucleus accumbens (Figure 4-7), which is said to be one of the key pleasure centers of the brain. The nucleus accumbens is located in the septal area (see Figure 4-2). Additionally, electric stimulation of the septal area elicits sexual arousal in both animals and people. The nucleus accumbens is probably responsible for sexual arousal (Heath, 1972).

Emotions and Motivation Behaviors

The emotions and motivation behaviors include feelings about people, institutions, and life that affect behavior. Feelings help determine whether an act is right or wrong and good or bad and whether a particular act will be performed. These feelings can be referred to as *visceral aspects of behavior*. Electric stimulation of the amygdala, hypothalamus, or midbrain can elicit either rage or flight behavior. Bilateral destruction of the amygdala and selected areas in the hypothalamus can dull the visceral aspects of behavior and result in a calming effect.

Basal Ganglia

The basal ganglia (see Figure 4-3) comprise three major nuclei: the caudate nucleus, the putamen, and the globus pallidus. These structures are also involved in motor functions. The putamen and globus pallidus together are referred to as the *lentiform (lens-shaped) nucleus*. The basal ganglia and substantia nigra (see Figure 4-6) communicate back and forth about ongoing motor activity from the body. The substantia nigra produces and sends dopamine to the basal ganglia. The basal ganglia system, which includes the substantia nigra, the basal ganglia, and descending motor

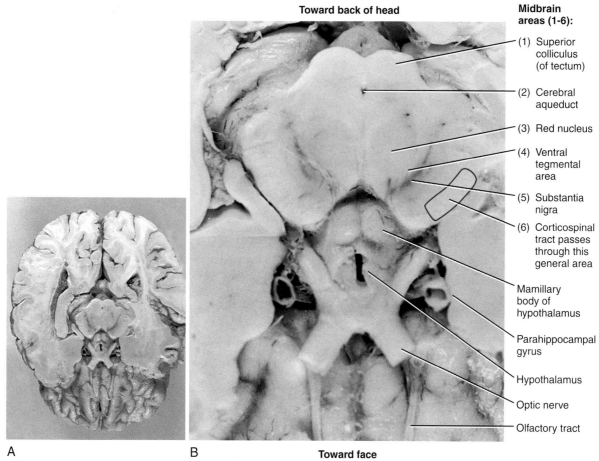

Toward back of head

Midbrain areas (1-6):

(1) Superior colliculus (of tectum)

(2) Cerebral aqueduct

(3) Red nucleus

(4) Ventral tegmental area

(5) Substantia nigra

(6) Corticospinal tract passes through this general area

Mamillary body of hypothalamus

Parahippocampal gyrus

Hypothalamus

Optic nerve

Olfactory tract

A   B   Toward face

FIG 4-6 A, Brain is sectioned transversely through the midbrain and parahippocampal gyri. **B**, Enlargement of the area through the midbrain is shown. (Photographs by Berto Tarin, Multimedia Department, Western University of Health Sciences, Pomona, California.)

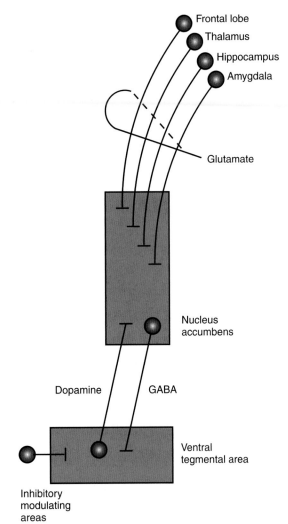

Frontal lobe
Thalamus
Hippocampus
Amygdala

Glutamate

Nucleus accumbens

Dopamine   GABA

Ventral tegmental area

Inhibitory modulating areas

FIG 4-7 The mesolimbic pathway (system) is identified as the primary pathway involved in substance abuse and in feeling pleasure. The ventral tegmental area projects dopamine neurons to the nucleus accumbens. Opioids inhibit the modulating areas that affect the ventral tegmental area and allow increased amounts of dopamine to be released into the nucleus accumbens, enhancing the reward aspects of the opioids. Glutamate neurons from the prefrontal cortex, thalamus, amygdala, and hippocampus project to the nucleus accumbens and are excitatory. A γ-aminobutyric acid (*GABA*) pathway also exists from the nucleus accumbens to the ventral tegmental area. The mesolimbic pathway includes many limbic structures. (From Alex, K.D., & Pehek, E.A. [2007]. Pharmacologic mechanisms of serotonergic regulation of dopamine neurotransmission. *Pharmacology & Therapeutics, 113*, 296-320.)

pathways, complements the pyramidal system. The pyramidal (or corticospinal) tract transmits commands for voluntary movement, and the basal ganglia system modulates these movements, maintains appropriate muscle tone, and adjusts posture. For example, when the hand is extended and the fingers are held still, slight oscillations of the fingers occur. The basal ganglia system, which includes some motor pathways, works with the pyramidal system to keep these movements small.

The basal ganglia system balances excitatory and inhibitory neurons that have different neurotransmitters. Acetylcholine is the primary excitatory neurotransmitter. γ-Aminobutyric acid (GABA) is an important inhibitory neurotransmitter in this system. Dopamine can be either excitatory or inhibitory. It modulates neuronal membranes, and its action depends on the receptors of the neuron it contacts. Any significant decrease or increase in the level of these neurotransmitters can result in basal ganglia (extrapyramidal) motor signs.

The basal ganglia system affects the contralateral side of the body. Because this system maintains muscle tone and posture, movements are most noticeable during rest. Parkinson's disease, an extrapyramidal disorder, manifests with a resting tremor. These unwanted movements diminish with concentration and intentional movement and are absent during sleep.

The pyramidal tract or corticospinal tract *controls* precise, voluntary movements; the basal ganglia, in conjunction with the cerebellum, *stabilize* motor movements. Lesions of the basal ganglia result in abnormal motor movements, such as those present in Parkinson's disease resulting from decreased dopamine bioavailability from the substantia nigra and in Huntington's disease (chorea) resulting from alterations in the GABA level and in the cholinergic system. All basal ganglia areas receive, integrate, and transmit motor information.

---

⑦ CRITICAL THINKING QUESTIONS

1. What disease is produced when dopamine from the substantia nigra is blocked from crossing the synapse at the next brain site (basal ganglia)?
2. What might happen to a person with an overproduction of cerebral dopamine?
3. How might a pituitary gland tumor affect a person's hormone production, body development, and behavior?
4. What signs or symptoms are used to differentiate a left-sided from a right-sided cerebral hemisphere stroke?

Diencephalon

The diencephalon (see Figures 4-2, 4-3, and 4-6) comprises the thalamus, hypothalamus, epithalamus (including the pineal gland), and subthalamus. Although all the nuclei of the diencephalon are important, only a brief review of the thalamus and the hypothalamus is provided in this text. All sensory pathways except the olfactory pathways synapse in the thalamus (Kiernan, 2007). The thalamus relays sensory information to the cerebral cortex via the internal capsule and corona radiata (see Figure 4-3). The hypothalamus maintains homeostasis and is the controller of the autonomic nervous system. The hypothalamus (Kiernan, 2007) is a tiny 4-g structure positioned below the thalamus that modulates visceral functions such as body temperature regulation, gastrointestinal activity, and cardiovascular functions. The hypothalamus also serves as a chemoreceptor by sampling cerebrospinal fluid and blood. It controls and influences functions such as food and water intake and endocrine secretion. The hypothalamus has two modes for affecting the pituitary gland (the following numbers refer to Figure 4-8). The first mode is through the

Two hypothalamic neurons

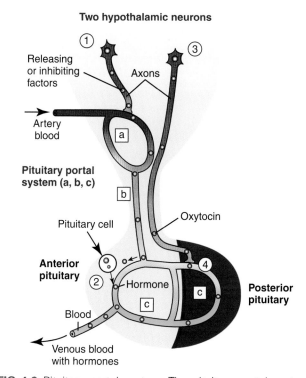

FIG 4-8 Pituitary portal system. The pituitary portal system has a capillary bed (a) at the base of the hypothalamus, a capillary bed (c) in the pituitary gland, and a portal vein (b) in between. Hypothalamic neurons (1, 3) make hormones (i.e., neurotransmitters). The neuron (1) releases its hormone into the capillary bed (a), and the hormone descends through the portal vessel (b) into the pituitary gland capillary bed (c). The hormone leaves the capillary bed and causes anterior pituitary gland cells to release specific hormones back into the capillary (2) for transport to glands or cells elsewhere in the body. A few hormones from the hypothalamus inhibit the production of pituitary gland cell hormones. The neuron (3) directly releases its hormone (e.g., oxytocin) into the posterior pituitary portion of the capillary bed (c). The hormone again leaves in the blood (4) and travels to glands or cells elsewhere in the body.

production of releasing and inhibiting hormones or factors that pass into the pituitary portal system, such as thyrotropin-releasing hormone or prolactin-releasing factor (1). These factors are transmitted to the anterior pituitary gland (2), where they cause the release or inhibition of anterior pituitary hormones into the blood of the pituitary portal system. The second mode is by the direct projection of hypothalamic neurons (3) into the posterior pituitary gland, where the neurons release their hormones (e.g., oxytocin) directly into the pituitary blood supply (4). Table 4-1 summarizes the hormonal cascade from the hypothalamus and some of the resulting clinical effects. Normally, all hormones are in careful balance.

Brainstem

The brainstem, cerebellum, and spinal cord are located beneath the cerebrum (see Figure 4-1). *Brainstem* is a collective term for the midbrain, pons, and medulla oblongata. The cerebellum is an expansive area attached to the posterior surface of the pons and resembles its Latin name, which means "little brain." The most caudal portion of the CNS is the spinal cord (not discussed in this chapter). The reticular formation is an important functional area that spans the brainstem.

Midbrain

The midbrain (see Figure 4-6), which represents the continuation of the CNS below the cerebrum, is approximately 1.5 cm in length and is relatively narrow. The red nuclei and substantia nigra are large structures in the midbrain that can be easily distinguished on gross examination. The red nuclei in freshly cut brains are large, reddish, round balls; the substantia nigra, as its name implies, is black. This black coloration is the result of melanin pigment found in substantia nigra neurons. Most of the brain dopamine is synthesized from these dark cells. In Parkinson's disease, these cells have become depigmented, and less dopamine is produced. Dopamine deficiency causes the extrapyramidal motor disorders associated

TABLE 4-1 HORMONAL CASCADE FROM THE HYPOTHALAMUS TO BEHAVIORAL EFFECTS			
HYPOTHALAMUS-MADE HORMONES	**PITUITARY GLAND**	**TARGET GLAND OR HORMONE**	**POSSIBLE BEHAVIORAL EFFECT**
Corticotropin-releasing hormone (CRH)	Stimulates production of two hormones: 1. ACTH 2. β-Endorphin	Adrenal gland—produces cortisol and cortisol-related hormones ACTH drives cortisol production	1. Stress causes release of cortisol 2. Depressed children have decreased diurnal cortisol secretory pattern 3. Depressed adolescents have increased cortisol around sleep onset 4. CRH increases in patients with PTSD 5. Patients with PTSD have a blunted ACTH response to CRH 6. β-Endorphin is involved in endorphin pleasure pathway and feeling good

(Continued)

TABLE 4-1	HORMONAL CASCADE FROM THE HYPOTHALAMUS TO BEHAVIORAL EFFECTS—CONT'D		
HYPOTHALAMUS-MADE HORMONES	**PITUITARY GLAND**	**TARGET GLAND OR HORMONE**	**POSSIBLE BEHAVIORAL EFFECT**
Thyroid-releasing hormone (TRH)	Stimulates production of TSH	Thyroid gland produces T_4 and T_3	1. Adding T_3 or T_4 to an antidepressant regimen may potentiate medication's response 2. In PTSD, T_3 level may be increased
Prolactin-releasing factor (PRF)	Stimulates production of prolactin	Mammary glands—produce milk	No significant effects; feminizing effect

Note. This table lists the following: (1) hypothalamic hormones—states whether they are releasing or inhibiting; (2) the specific hormones that they affect in the anterior pituitary gland (Griffin & Ojeda, 2004); (3) the way in which they affect hormone production; (4) the target glands or body cells affected; and (5) the proposed effects of the hormones on behavior (Charney et al., 2008).
ACTH, Adrenocorticotropic hormone; *PTSD,* posttraumatic stress disorder; *TSH,* thyroid-stimulating hormone; T_3, triiodothyronine; T_4, thyroxine.

with Parkinson's disease. The ventral tegmental area, which projects dopaminergic tracts to the limbic and cortical areas, is a midline structure medial and rostral to the red nucleus (see Figure 4-6, *B*).

Pons

The *pons* (literally means "bridge") forms a link between the midbrain and the medulla oblongata. The pons is a bulbous area approximately 2.5 cm in length that lies between the midbrain and the medulla oblongata and is anterior to the cerebellum. Some pathway fibers descending from the cerebrum pass through the midbrain and terminate in the pons. The pontine nuclei project motor and posture information to the cerebellum.

Medulla Oblongata

The medulla oblongata is approximately 3 cm in length and narrows until it becomes continuous with the cervical spinal cord. Corticospinal tracts (pyramidal tracts) travel on the anterior surface of the medulla oblongata in pyramid-shaped bulges known as *pyramids.* The decussation of the pyramids—that is, the crossing over of the now specified lateral corticospinal motor pathway contralaterally—takes place at the lower end of the medulla oblongata (see Figure 4-4). This crossing over is why a right brain stroke results in left-sided impairment. The medulla oblongata is responsible for many important functions, including respiration, regulation of blood pressure, partial regulation of heart rate, vomiting, and swallowing.

Reticular Formation

A multineural functional area called the *reticular formation* resides within the brainstem. This area is composed of a series of large nuclei, beginning within the midbrain and extending through the pons and the medulla oblongata. The reticular formation can be thought of as a primitive brain buried deep within the brainstem. Input from most sensory pathways passes into the reticular formation, where it is integrated and then projected to areas such as the thalamus and hypothalamus. The reticular formation affects motor, sensory, and visceral functions.

The reticular activating system (RAS), part of the reticular formation, serves as a screening device that allows individuals to tune out some stimuli and respond to other stimuli. The ability to tune out is important; otherwise, studying or even sleeping in some environments might be impossible. The RAS allows humans to fall asleep. It is activated by sensory stimuli, pain, movement, feedback from the cortex, muscle tone, and sympathomimetic drugs (stimulants). Any of these factors can help a person remain awake. Because of its many synapses, the RAS can be depressed easily. When a disruption occurs in the RAS and a person cannot sleep, psychosis can occur. However, when the RAS is turned off, coma results. Some people have had the RAS deactivated, but how to reactivate it is as yet unknown.

Cerebellum

The cerebellum (see Figures 4-1 and 4-2) consists of two hemispheres separated by a central portion called the *vermis.* The cerebellar hemispheres and most of the vermis simultaneously receive sensory input from muscles and joints and motor signals from the cerebral cortex, indicating how muscles are to be directed. Most of the cerebellum communicates with the cerebral cortex through the thalamus to coordinate the final motor activity. Walking without difficulty, writing with a pen, and shooting a basketball are possible because of a functioning cerebellum. Most of the cerebellum coordinates muscle synergy and activity but does *not* initiate movement. The second function of the cerebellum is maintenance of equilibrium. Differences between movement disorders associated with cerebellar dysfunction and movement disorders associated with basal ganglia dysfunction are presented in Box 4-1.

Cerebellar dysfunction can produce intention tremors on the same side of the body as the lesion. In contrast to basal ganglia resting tremors, which occur at rest, intention tremors occur when a person is asked to touch something, such as his own nose or a physician's moving finger. Such individuals have tremors when they attempt to concentrate on moving a limb.

BOX 4-1   DIFFERENCES BETWEEN BASAL GANGLIA AND CEREBELLAR MOVEMENT DISORDERS

General Difference
- Cerebellar dysfunction: Awkwardness of intentional movement
- Basal ganglia dysfunction: Meaningless, unintentional movement that occurs unexpectedly

Cerebellar Disorders
- Ataxia: Awkwardness of posture and gait; lack of coordination; overshooting the goal when reaching for an object; inability to perform rapid, alternating movements, such as finger tapping; awkward use of speech muscles, resulting in irregularly spaced sounds
- Decreased tendon reflexes on affected side
- Asthenia: Muscles tire easily
- Intention tremor: Noticed when intending to do something, such as reaching for a pencil
- Adiadochokinesia: Inability to perform fine, rapidly repeated coordinated movements

Basal Ganglia Disorders
- Parkinsonism: Rigidity, bradykinesia, resting tremor, masklike face, shuffling gait
- Chorea: Sudden, jerky, and purposeless movements (e.g., Huntington's disease, Sydenham's chorea)
- Athetosis: Slow, writhing, snakelike movements, especially of fingers and wrists
- Hemiballismus: A sudden, wild flailing of one arm
- Nystagmus: Involuntary rapid eye movements

Modified from Goldberg, S. (2003). *Clinical neuroanatomy*. Miami, Florida: MedMaster.

NEURONS AND NEUROTRANSMITTERS

Neurons are the basic subunit of the nervous system. A neuron is composed of a cell body with a large nucleus, an axon, and dendrites. The cell body and dendrites of the neuron make up the gray matter of the cortex and brain nuclei. Neurons transmit information by sending action potentials, or waves of electric depolarization, down their axon processes to other neurons. Two processes project from the cell body: *dendrites* and *axons*. The dendrites receive impulses from other neurons and transmit these impulses to the cell body. Axons carry impulses away from the cell body to another neuron, muscle, or gland. Each neuron usually projects only one axon. Some axons are 3 feet in length but are microscopically thin. Some axons can synapse with thousands of dendrites, and the dendrites of one neuron can receive impulses from the axons of thousands of other neurons (Bear et al., 2007). The brain is extremely complex, and research regarding this intricate wiring schematic continues.

Neurons can be divided into three basic types: (1) sensory neurons (or afferent neurons) send messages to the CNS, (2) motor neurons (or efferent neurons) send messages from the CNS to the periphery, and (3) association neurons (or interneurons) lie between sensory and motor neurons. Most CNS neurons are association neurons. Most impulses (action potentials) travel from one neuron to another by sending a chemical called a *neurotransmitter* across a 20-nm space (the synaptic cleft, which separates these cells) to affect postsynaptic receptors and evoke the next action potential (see Figure 4-2). The junction between two neurons, including two cell membranes and a synaptic cleft, is called a *synapse*. Many drugs have their site of action in the nervous system in or around the synapse.

Neurotransmitters are divided into four major groups or systems: cholinergics, monoamines, neuropeptides, and amino acids (Table 4-2). Specific examples for each group, where these specific transmitters are concentrated in the brain, and major brain pathways that use these neurotransmitters are indicated in Table 4-2. Neurotransmitters are thought to play major roles in some mental disorders (Table 4-3).

AUTONOMIC NERVOUS SYSTEM

The autonomic nervous system (Figure 4-9) is divided into the parasympathetic (craniosacral) and sympathetic (thoracolumbar) nervous systems. The parasympathetic nervous system, which is a cholinergic system, conserves energy and is divided into cranial and sacral portions. The cranial part has neuronal components in the oculomotor (CN III), facial (CN VII), glossopharyngeal (CN IX), and vagus (CN X) nerves; the sacral part is composed of neuronal elements located in the sacral spinal cord areas S2 to S4. Parasympathetic neurons are of particular interest to psychiatric nurses because of the many psychotropic drugs that have anticholinergic properties. Anticholinergic drugs block the function of these nerves. CN III affects pupil and ciliary body constriction; CN VII affects tearing (lacrimation) and salivation; CN IX affects salivation; and CN X affects the heart, gastrointestinal tract, and urinary system. Anticholinergic effects on these nerves cause dilated pupils, decreased lacrimation, dry mouth, tachycardia, and slowing of the bowels and bladder.

The sympathetic nervous system expends energy and forms a continuous column that runs from the first thoracic (T1) to the third lumbar (L3) spinal cord areas. Although sympathetic neuron cell bodies are confined within portions of the thoracic and lumbar spinal cord, sympathetic neurons innervate effector organs throughout the body.

Both the sympathetic and the parasympathetic systems contain two neurons between the spinal cord and the effector organs. The first neuronal cell body is in the spinal cord, and its myelinated axon extends from the spinal cord to synapse with a peripheral neuron. The first neuron in the system is referred to as the *preganglionic neuron*; the second is referred to as the *postganglionic neuron*. Preganglionic neurons secrete acetylcholine as their neurotransmitter (see Figure 4-9). Postganglionic neurons send their unmyelinated axons to effector organs—smooth muscle, cardiac muscle,

TABLE 4-2 CLASSIFICATION OF SELECTED NEUROTRANSMITTERS AND PATHWAYS

CATEGORY	NEUROTRANSMITTER	LOCATION IN CENTRAL NERVOUS SYSTEM	MAJOR PATHWAYS
Cholinergic	Acetylcholine	Basal nucleus of Meynert and in the pons	Basal nucleus of Meynert to cerebral cortex; septal area to hippocampus
Monoamines	Dopamine	Substantia nigra	Nigrostriatal
		VTA	Mesolimbic
		VTA	Mesocortical
		Hypothalamus	Tuberoinfundibular
	Norepinephrine	Locus ceruleus	Locus ceruleus (in pons) to thalamus, cerebral cortex, cerebellum, and spinal cord
	Serotonin	Raphe nuclei	Rostral (i.e going upward) raphe nuclei to thalamus, striatum, hypothalamus, hippocampus, nucleus accumbens, and prefrontal cortex
			Caudal (i.e. going downward) raphe nuclei to cerebellum and spinal cord
Amino acids	GABA	Most common inhibitory transmitter in brain	Purkinje cells to deep cerebellar nuclei; striatonigral
	Glutamate	Most common excitatory transmitter in brain	Widely distributed in central nervous system

Note. This table presents a simplified summary of many of the better known neurotransmitters and the general location where they are produced and released in the nervous system.

ACTH, Adrenocorticotropic hormone; *CCK,* cholecystokinin; *GABA,* γ-aminobutyric acid; *VIP,* vasoactive intestinal polypeptide; *VTA,* ventral tegmental area.

From Keltner, N.L., & Folks, D. (2005). *Psychotropic drugs* (4th ed.). St. Louis: Mosby.

TABLE 4-3 NEUROTRANSMITTERS AND RELATED MENTAL DISORDERS*

NEUROTRANSMITTER	MENTAL DISORDER
Increase (↑) in dopamine	Schizophrenia
Decrease (↓) in norepinephrine	Depression
Decrease (↓) in serotonin	Depression
Decrease (↓) in acetylcholine	Alzheimer's disease
Decrease (↓) in GABA	Anxiety

Note. This table is a simplified explanation. A more detailed explanation is offered in appropriate chapters.

GABA, γ-Aminobutyric acid.

or glands. Generally, parasympathetic postganglionic neurons secrete acetylcholine and sympathetic postganglionic neurons secrete norepinephrine as their neurotransmitters.

The hypothalamus has both sympathetic and parasympathetic functions and is considered to be the highest autonomic center in the CNS. The hypothalamus can drive both systems selectively (see Figure 4-9).

VENTRICULAR SYSTEM

The brain floats in approximately 140 mL (about the volume of a small cup of coffee) of cerebrospinal fluid (CSF); however, the CNS produces approximately 800 mL of fluid per day. CSF circulates around the brain in the subarachnoid space and inside ventricles in the brain. Three connective tissue layers, known as *meninges,* cover the brain. The subarachnoid space is a narrow space that is located between the middle meningeal layer (arachnoid) and innermost layer (pia mater) and adheres to the brain. The thick outer layer, the dura mater, attaches to the inner surface of many bones of the skull. The ventricles form four spaces within the brain (see Figure 4-3). One large ventricle resides in each cerebral hemisphere, and small third and fourth ventricles are located in the diencephalon and between the pons and the cerebellum, respectively. The fourth ventricle communicates with the subarachnoid space. Eventually, the CSF in the subarachnoid space enters the vascular system through arachnoid villi that protrude into the superior sagittal sinus on the superior surface of the brain. If the arachnoid villi are compromised for some reason, such as from a head trauma or meningitis, the CSF builds up quickly.

Enlargement of the ventricles occurs because of (1) blockage of the CSF outflow within or from the brain, (2) overproduction of CSF, (3) brain atrophy resulting from the death of large numbers of cortical neurons, and (4) neurodevelopmental problems. The first two problems are causes of hydrocephalus, whereas brain atrophy (neurodegeneration) is commonly found in chronic alcoholics and patients with AD. In the case of neurodegeneration, creation of new space results in the ventricles enlarging to fill the void. Neurodevelopmental problems resulting in ventricular variance are thought to be associated with schizophrenia (Charney et al., 2008).

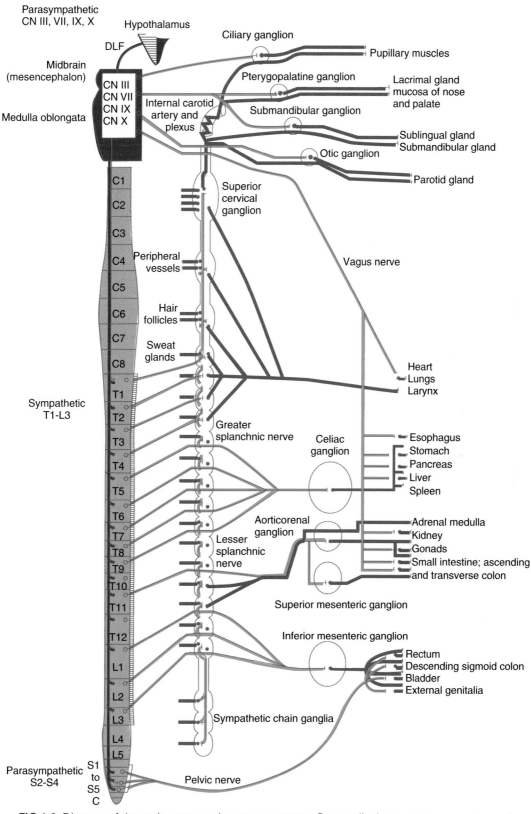

FIG 4-9 Diagram of the entire autonomic nervous system. Preganglionic neurons are represented as *green lines*; postganglionic neurons are represented as *blue lines*. The dorsal longitudinal fasciculus (*DLF*; represented as a *red line*) interconnects the hypothalamus with parasympathetic and sympathetic autonomic neurons down to the sacral spinal cord level. *CN*, Cranial nerve.

CLINICAL APPLICATION

As explained throughout this text, many mental disorders have biologic bases. A brief overview of these biologic influences is presented here, but more through discussions of these issues are presented in the chapters dealing with each respective disorder. This approach is consistent with our belief that the biologic context of mental disorders is inextricably linked to symptoms and behaviors and is part of a holistic approach to understanding patients with psychiatric disorders. Placing most of the specific discussion of the psychobiologic parameters of mental disorders in a separate chapter titled "Psychobiology" reinforces the perception that this etiologic view is only one of many from which the student can select. We believe differently. The student is urged to use this chapter as a foundation to the understanding of brain anatomy and physiology and to build on this foundation by applying this information to other chapters.

Schizophrenia

Several psychobiologic influences on schizophrenia have been proposed. First, some researchers have noted that an increase in ventricular size is apparent in many people with schizophrenia (Charney et al., 2008; Konrad & Winterer, 2008). As mentioned, ventricles enlarge for one of four reasons. In schizophrenia, increased ventricle size would be most likely related to neurodevelopmental factors; that is, the brain around the ventricles has failed to develop, and the ventricles have enlarged to fill the empty space. This phenomenon is referred to as an increase in *ventricular brain ratios*. In addition, in many individuals with schizophrenia, a decrease in the gray matter and white matter of the cortex and in the major subcortical nuclei is evident.

Other biologic differences found in people with schizophrenia include a decrease in cerebral blood flow, particularly in the prefrontal areas of the cortex. The term used to describe this condition is *hypofrontality* (Charney et al., 2008). Imaging technology that tracks blood flow and glucose metabolism has substantiated this physiologic change. These brain changes result in a decline in frontal cognitive functions, such as organizing, planning, learning, problem solving, and critical thinking.

The most celebrated and widely known biologic theory for schizophrenia is the dopamine hypothesis. According to this theory, schizophrenia is caused by alterations of dopamine levels in the brain. Chapter 24 elaborates on this theory and the biologically related genetic theory of schizophrenia. Antipsychotic medications are discussed in Chapter 14.

? CRITICAL THINKING QUESTION

5. In some patients with schizophrenia, a decrease in blood flow has been detected in the dorsolateral prefrontal area. Because this site is in the frontal lobe, what type of symptoms might you expect to see in general?

CASE STUDY

Schizophrenia

Specialist Gomez, a 20-year-old active duty soldier, presented to the Combat Stress Clinic in Afghanistan with two senior members of his command. His command was concerned because Specialist Gomez had requested to turn in his weapon earlier that day because he said he was worried that he might shoot one of his fellow soldiers. They also mentioned that Gomez had been "isolating himself more" the past several weeks and was beginning to smell a "bit rank" because he had stopped showering on a regular basis. On interview, the young specialist, who had immigrated to the United States from Venezuela as a teenager with his family for political reasons and to improve their standard of living, admitted that he had recently begun to hear the voice of Hugo Chavez. He was concerned because the voice of Chavez, a politician whom his family despised, was "starting to make sense." Gomez elaborated, "If Hugo is correct, then the Taliban terrorists may be correct." He added, "Hugo has been telling me to shoot my sergeant and some other soldiers. But I like the sergeant and my buddies. Hugo is telling me to be a man and not a wimp. So I thought the best thing I could do was to turn in my weapon." The young specialist was relieved of his weapon and was medically evacuated to Germany the following day.

Depression

Mood disorders are also thought to have a biologic basis. Decreased amounts of norepinephrine and serotonin, two important brain neurotransmitters, are thought to play a role in depression (see Table 4-3). Apparently, an overall deficiency exists in the concentration of these neurotransmitters, and psychopharmacologic treatment is based on restoring them to optimal levels. More recent findings suggest that other neurotransmitters might also be factors in depression. Some researchers have found evidence for the involvement of acetylcholine, dopamine, and GABA. Chapter 25 discusses these neurotransmitters and the roles of cell receptor, thyroid, hypothalamic, and pituitary function in depression.

CASE STUDY

Depression and Hypothyroidism

Mrs. Smith, a 65-year-old recently widowed grandmother, was admitted to the hospital because of increased difficulties with depression following the death of her husband of 40 years. She was noted to wring her hands constantly and spoke about how her family would be better off if she was placed on an ice floe and allowed to die. Her mood improved slightly after her medication for treatment of long-standing hypothyroidism was adjusted in response to an elevated thyroid-stimulating hormone level on admission. Her mood and general level of functioning markedly improved after she was started on fluoxetine, a medication that one of her two daughters was taking with benefit for her own depression.

Anxiety Disorders

Anxiety disorders appear to have a biologic basis as well. Research has indicated that drugs that activate GABA receptors, causing an inhibitory effect, can calm anxious patients. Other neurotransmitters, such as norepinephrine, dopamine, and serotonin, might also have roles in anxiety. When the sympathetic system is stimulated by epinephrine, norepinephrine, and dopamine (see Table 4-2), an anxietylike reaction occurs. Anxiety disorders are discussed in Chapter 27.

Dementias

Dementias are directly related to brain pathology. AD, the leading cause of dementia in the United States, is caused by brain atrophy, which has been demonstrated microscopically by the presence of neurofibrillary tangles and amyloid plaques. Patients with AD tend to have enlarged ventricles, narrowing of the cortical ribbon (gray matter), widening of the sulci, and decreases in the width of the gyri. A loss of cholinergic pathways also is found in patients with AD, contributing to memory problems. Patients with AD forget recent events, facts, how to use words, and how to use common objects. AD and other dementias are discussed in Chapter 28.

CASE STUDY

Dementia—Ventricular Size Change (Normal-Pressure Hydrocephalus)

George, a 70-year-old Korean War veteran and retired postal service employee, was brought to the geriatric evaluation unit of a Veterans Affairs hospital by his wife. She stated that she was concerned that her husband was having increasing trouble remembering; he had been brought home by the police 2 weeks ago after he had gotten lost when driving to their local grocery that was 5 blocks away. She said that for the past 1 to 2 years she was becoming "worn out" with having to do much more laundry because George often needed to change his clothes several times a day because he was "urinating on himself." George was admitted to the hospital. A computed tomography scan revealed some ventricular enlargement. A spinal tap was performed with only mild elevation in pressure noted. George was noted to have a wide-based gait and to walk in a shuffling manner. In the afternoon, he seemed to become more disoriented and was sometimes found by nursing staff to be "looking for bags of mail to pick up." He seemed to become less frustrated when he could help nursing staff deliver dinner trays to his fellow patients.

Degenerative Diseases

Parkinson's disease is a degenerative disease that affects motor function and emotional stability. In patients with parkinsonism, microscopic examination of the basal ganglia, specifically the caudate nucleus and globus pallidus, reveals degenerative changes. The most significant change is the deterioration of the substantia nigra, the primary site of synthesis of dopamine in the brain. The decreased availability of dopamine in the extrapyramidal system leads to resting tremors, bradykinesia, and rigidity. Parkinsonism is discussed in greater detail in Chapters 13 and 28.

Demyelinating Diseases

Multiple sclerosis is a demyelinating disease. In this disorder, the myelin and eventually the axons are attacked and eventually broken down by the body's own immune system (Brodal, 2010). This degeneration of myelin typically causes various problems, including loss of sensation, muscle weakness, fatigue, double vision, and tingling in the extremities. People with multiple sclerosis also experience psychological symptoms, undoubtedly related to demyelinization that occurs in the brain.

Anorexia Nervosa

Anorexia, a disorder characterized by the refusal to eat and various emotional problems, appears to be associated with hypothalamic dysfunction. Anorexia is discussed in more detail in Chapter 32.

Trauma

Individuals who have experienced CNS trauma can have brain insults similar to lesions found in dementia or parkinsonism. Victims of head trauma from automobile accidents and sport injuries (e.g., football) can exhibit symptoms based on the site, severity, and frequency of the traumas. Individuals with an injury to the temporal lobe might experience memory loss or aphasia; individuals with a prefrontal lobe injury might experience personality changes or psychosis. Dementia pugilistica (punch drunk syndrome, boxer's disease), a dementia syndrome with the same molecular pathology as AD, can result from repeated blows to the head such as occur in the sport of boxing (Kiernan, 2007).

Chemical Dependency

The biologic pathways that might be responsible for the control that addictive substances have on people are just beginning to be understood. Research studies have suggested that the nucleus accumbens might be an important piece of the addiction puzzle. Charney and colleagues (2008) discussed studies of the mechanisms involved in motivation and addiction.

Mitochondrial DNA Problems

Many people are aware of genetic diseases that affect the psychological health of individuals, such as Huntington's disease. Many other diseases are known to have a genetic predisposition, such as AD. These problems arise in the DNA of the chromosomes in each cell of the body. In 1988, scientists found that the DNA of mitochondria, the powerhouses of the human body, can mutate and give rise to physical and psychological problems (Schapira, 2012). These mutant mitochondria have been implicated in AD, MELAS syndrome (mitochondrial encephalopathy, lactic acidosis, and stroke-like episodes), and diabetes mellitus, among other entities.

In contrast to chromosomes, which are contributed by both parents, mitochondria are passed to the ovum only by the mother. Various mutant mitochondria can result in numerous diseases. The mutant mitochondria, which fail to produce the energy that cells need to function properly, increase in number over time and damage particular cells and body organs.

💡 CRITICAL THINKING QUESTION

6. From what you have read in this chapter, can you defend Kraepelin's view of schizophrenia as a dementia? Explain your answer.

Early Life Stress and Trauma

Another psychobiologic issue worth contemplating is the developmental impact of early life trauma or significant stress. As noted, the brain continues to develop after birth and becomes larger, more sophisticated, and more efficient. One aspect of this continued development is ongoing myelination. As individuals age, myelin thickens around axons, improving the precision and efficacy of connections among neurons. Myelination continues throughout the teenage years (Herrman, 2005), while pruning eliminates about 40% of synapses (Miller, 2005a). Even during late adolescence, parents and others should be aware of the good and bad possibilities of dynamic brain processes. Some of the very last connections to develop are connections that help individuals use good judgment, solve problems, and self-regulate (Miller, 2005a). Prolonged stress or significant trauma can compromise these processes.

At an even earlier age, stress and trauma increase cortisol levels. Excessive cortisol levels can cause atrophy of the hippocampus, impairing hippocampal activities such as memory and learning. Animal models consistently demonstrate that maternal deprivation or rejection causes profound behavioral changes in the animal's later life. Animals nurtured in good environments have lifelong advantages over deprived animals. Sustained or overwhelming early life stressors can lead to an increase in hypothalamic-pituitary-adrenal activity. Increased hypothalamic release of corticotropin-releasing factor causes increased release of adrenocorticotropic hormone from the anterior pituitary gland and results in a subsequent elevation of systemic cortisol. An elevated cortisol level is associated with increased heart rate, muscle tension, anger, anxiety, fear, and depression (Miller, 2005b). When adulthood is reached, an individual who has experienced years of elevated cortisol is likely to be burdened with a hypersensitive hypothalamic-pituitary-adrenal system that overreacts to stress and often leads to a life of depression and anxiety. Significant stress, trauma, maternal behavior, and maltreatment during childhood and adolescence are mental health issues because they have the potential to alter the structure and chemistry of the brain permanently.

CASE STUDY

Lucy was a 21-year-old college student who was referred by her primary care physician because of increased mood and anxiety difficulties and problems sleeping. At the initial appointment, Lucy, who was cachectic (very thin) in appearance, stated that she was "paranoid" about men and sometimes saw images of "ghosts and shadowy men." Occasionally, when she was very tired, one of the images that she saw would berate her and call her "a slut." She revealed that she had been sexually victimized as a young child and again when she was in high school "by a different man." She stated that she had been hospitalized for anorexia as a teenager and still "sometimes cut" on herself when feeling very overwhelmed. She related that she had long-standing difficulties sleeping and as a result sometimes smoked marijuana. She also used "bath salts" (a synthetic cocainelike substance) to wake up to take care of her "foster care" dogs. She stated that these dogs were her only reason for remaining alive. She was failing in her college studies, but she had a part-time job modeling exotic lingerie. She was initiated on a very low dose of risperidone, a neuroleptic medication, with some benefit. She slept better and experienced a decrease in paranoid ideations and hallucinations. Her mood was improved, and she was less anxious. However, she gained a little over a pound in weight in the 10 days since she started taking risperidone. She quipped that her parents with whom she resided were pleased that she was "eating better." She was concerned that an increase in weight would damage her nascent modeling career and asked that she be changed to a different medication.

HIGHLIGHTING THE EVIDENCE

Are the Brains of Men and Women the Same?

Men and women possess differences in their brains in terms of the relative size of their anatomic structures, levels of neurotransmitters and hormones, and how various neural structures function. For example, a few structural differences are that men have some larger areas in the parietal lobes, which are involved in spatial perception, whereas women have some larger areas in the frontal lobes and limbic areas, which are concerned with higher cognitive functions. The hippocampus, a structure involved with memory, is larger in women than in men. The neurotransmitter serotonin, a major chemical involved in setting moods, is 52% higher in men than in women. Could this be why women have a higher incidence of depression? The last point is an example of differences in brain function. In a positron emission tomography study on recall of disturbing films, subjects demonstrated that the right amygdala in men and the left amygdala in women were selectively activated 1 week after testing. These findings indicate that a patient's gender can be a factor in treatment for such problems as addiction, schizophrenia, depression, and post-traumatic stress disorder (Cahill, 2005).

STUDY NOTES

1. The brain is a complex organ composed of 100 billion neurons, and changes in its anatomy or physiology affect behavior. Holistic nursing care requires an understanding of the impact of brain dysfunction on behavior.

2. Many mental disorders that were formerly thought to have psychological etiologic factors are now known to be influenced by brain dysfunction.

3. The nervous system is divided into the CNS and the PNS.

4. The CNS is divided into the brain and the spinal cord.

5. The nervous pathways in the brain are composed of myelinated axons (white matter) that connect and communicate among brain nuclei (gray matter).

6. The cerebral cortex is the outer layer of gray matter of the brain. The gray matter consists of neuronal cell bodies and is responsible for the work of the brain.

7. The two major neurotransmitters in the extrapyramidal system are dopamine (inhibitory and excitatory) and acetylcholine (excitatory).

8. The pyramidal motor system controls precise movement; the basal ganglia motor system stabilizes motor movement.

9. The RAS involves degrees of consciousness. Sensory stimuli received in this system are forwarded to the thalamus. As stimulation of the RAS increases, the level of alertness increases.

10. Neurons are the basic subunits of the nervous system. A neuron consists of a cell body; *dendrites* that transmit information to the cell body; and a process called an *axon*, which transmits impulses away from the cell body.

11. Impulses travel from one neuron to another by sending a chemical called a *neurotransmitter* across a microscopic gap, known as a *synaptic cleft*.

12. The dopamine hypothesis postulates that schizophrenia results from alterations of levels of dopamine in the brain.

13. The neurotransmitter theory of depression states that depression is related to decreased levels of norepinephrine, serotonin, or both.

14. Anxiety disorders might be related to alterations in GABA levels.

15. Dementias, specifically AD, are related to brain atrophy and are characterized by microscopic changes in the cortical neurons and a buildup of neurofibrillary tangles and amyloid plaques. A deficiency in the neurotransmitter acetylcholine also occurs.

REFERENCES

Bear, M. F., Connors, B. W., & Paradiso, M. A. (2007). *Neuroscience: Exploring the brain* (3rd ed.). Philadelphia: Lippincott Williams & Wilkins.

Boss, B. J., & Stowe, A. C. (1986). Neuroanatomy. *The Journal of Neuroscience Nursing, 18*, 214–230.

Brodal, P. (2010). *The central nervous system* (4th ed.). New York: Oxford University Press.

Cahill, L. (2005). His brain, her brain. *Scientific American, 292*, 40–47.

Charney, D. S., Nestler, E. J., & Bunney, B. S. (2008). *Neurobiology of mental illness* (3rd ed.). New York: Oxford University Press.

Griffin, J. E., & Ojeda, S. R. (2004). *Textbook of endocrine physiology* (5th ed.). New York: Oxford University Press.

Heath, R. G. (1972). Pleasure and brain activity in man: Deep and surface electroencephalograms during orgasm. *The Journal of Nervous and Mental Disease, 154*, 3–18.

Herrman, J. W. (2005). The teen brain as a work in progress: Implications for pediatric nurses. *Pediatric Nursing, 31*, 144–148.

Kandel, E. R., Schwartz, J. H., & Jessell, T. M. (2013). *Principles of neural science* (5th ed.). New York: McGraw-Hill.

Kiernan, J. A. (2007). *Barr's the human nervous system: An anatomical viewpoint* (9th ed.). Philadelphia: Lippincott Williams & Wilkins.

Konrad, A., & Winterer, G. (2008). Disturbed structural connectivity in schizophrenia primary factor in pathology or epiphenomenon? *Schizophrenia Bulletin, 34*, 72–92.

Miller, C. M. (2005a). The adolescent brain: beyond raging hormones. Neuroscience research is suggesting some reasons why teenagers are that way. *The Harvard Mental Health Letter, 22*, 1–3.

Miller, C. M. (2005b). The biology of child maltreatment. How abuse and neglect of children leave their mark on the brain. *The Harvard Mental Health Letter, 21*, 1–3.

Schapira, A. H. (2012). Mitochondrial diseases. *The Lancet, 379*, 1825–1834.

5

Cultural Issues

Barbara Jones Warren

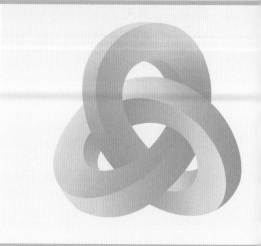

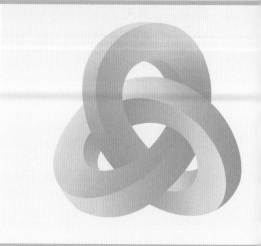

evolve WEBSITE

http://evolve.elsevier.com/Keltner

LEARNING OBJECTIVES

- Understand the importance of the effect of cultural variables on health and health care.
- Describe the components of cultural competence.
- Describe the factors involved in patients' and nurses' cultural perspectives.
- Articulate the differences in and the importance of worldview perspectives.

- Explain how incorporation of cultural competence can enhance psychiatric nursing clinical excellence.
- Analyze the symptoms suggestive of culture-bound syndromes.
- Apply understanding of ethnopharmacology as it might relate to a specific drug and a specific ethnic group.

Culture is a critical component of patients' lives that affects their health care attitudes and actions as well as their ability to understand and use the interventions that psychiatric nurses develop (Campinha-Bacote, 2007; Warren, 2007). *Culture* is the internal and external manifestation of learned and shared values, beliefs, and norms of a person, group, or community used to help individuals function in life and understand and interpret life occurrences (Leininger & McFarland, 2006). The cultural perspectives and patterns of both the nurse and the patient influence the nurse-patient interaction. These perspectives and patterns also affect a patient's level of mental health. For example, a patient's behaviors might be labeled as *pathologic* if a nurse misinterprets the patient's normal or culturally relevant beliefs and health care actions (Warren, 2007). A patient labeled as *noncompliant* might not be receiving culturally competent care (Purnell, 2009). The purpose of this chapter is to explain the role of the nurse and the connection between culture and cultural competence as they relate to psychiatric nursing.

BASIC CONCEPTS

Importance of Cultural Competence

Cultural competence is the process whereby the nurse shows proficiency in developing cultural awareness, knowledge, and skills to promote effective health care. A culturally competent

psychiatric nurse not only possesses knowledge about the process of cultural competence but also incorporates cultural competence into interactions with peers, students, patients, families, and communities. The use of cultural competence in conjunction with the psychotherapeutic management model serves as an evidenced-based health care approach that can enhance clinical excellence and promote recovery of psychiatric patients. Research on the use of culturally competent mental health strategies has indicated that cultural competence is key to patients' recovery process (Anthony, 1993; Warren, 2008a, 2008b, 2013b).

NORM'S NOTES
Nurses must be culturally relevant. In many parts of the United States, nurses might work with five or more distinct cultural groups on an ongoing basis. How can you do this and provide the type of nursing care that takes into account the various cultural backgrounds? Dr. Warren has spent many years helping nurses learn this. This chapter outlines some basic nursing behaviors to help you help all patients.

Culture and Psychiatric Nursing

The U.S. Surgeon General's report on mental health has emphasized the need for culturally competent mental health care (U.S. Surgeon General, 2001). Nurses provide services to a multitude of patients from diverse cultures. The term *cultural diversity* might encompass areas such as age, gender, socioeconomic status, religion, race, ethnicity, mental illness, and physically challenging conditions (Andrews & Boyle, 2007; Campinha-Bacote, 2007; De la Cruz, 2013; Giger & Davidhizar, 2008; Institute of Medicine, 2003; Leininger & McFarland, 2006; Munoz et al., 2007; Spector, 2004). The *Diagnostic and Statistical Manual of Mental Disorders, Fifth Edition (DSM-5)* has incorporated additional information regarding specific cultural features for each diagnostic category and a chapter on cultural formulation that includes specific assessment forms for the interviewer and the informant (American Psychiatric Association, 2013; Warren, 2013a).

Barriers to Culturally Competent Care

A growing knowledge and research base has indicated that patients' adherence to treatment increases when cultural needs are incorporated into health care planning (American Psychiatric Association, 2013; U.S. Surgeon General, 2001; Warren, 2012). Because nurses are often the gatekeepers for health care systems, knowledge of cultural factors related to psychiatric care is important.

The most common barrier to the delivery of culturally competent nursing care involves miscommunication between nurses and patients. A nurse might lack knowledge and sensitivity regarding a patient's cultural beliefs and practices; the nurse might not recognize the importance and value of these beliefs to the patient as they relate to health care practices. Similarly, patients might be unaware of the nurse's cultural perspectives and misinterpret health care recommendations from the nurse (Diala et al., 2001). Consequently, to facilitate successful relationships with their patients, nurses must understand their own cultural beliefs and values and how these beliefs and values influence patient care. This cultural awareness facilitates the psychotherapeutic relationship and the nursing process (Warren, 2008a).

❓ CRITICAL THINKING QUESTION

1. How would a nurse use the best evidence therapeutically and in a culturally competent manner in his care of a patient who is refusing to follow a nursing care plan because it does not align with the patient's cultural belief system?

Another barrier to culturally competent care results from failure to assess the patient's cultural perspective. A variety of clinical cultural assessment tools and models are available for assessing cultural perspective (Warren et al., 1994). Finally, barriers to culturally competent nursing care are primarily grounded in differences between nurses' and patients' cultural worldviews (Tables 5-1 to 5-4). These differences can increase miscommunication and negatively affect the nurse-patient relationship and interaction.

Cultural Etiology of Illness and Disease

Nurses' and patients' health care actions and beliefs are generally formulated by three factors: (1) their definition of health,

TABLE 5-1	**EUROPEAN-AMERICAN WORLDVIEW**
COMPONENT	**PERSPECTIVE**
Cultural value	Value is placed on the member or object or on the attainment of the object
Knowledge	Knowledge is acquired according to proof of the existence of anything— that is, the ability of an individual to see, hear, touch, taste, or smell it
Logic	Dichotomous mode of reasoning is used
Relationship	Relationships are developed based on the perceived need for them

TABLE 5-2	**AFRICAN, AFRICAN-AMERICAN, HISPANIC, AND ARABIC WORLDVIEW**
COMPONENT	**PERSPECTIVE**
Cultural value	Value is placed on the development and maintenance of interpersonal relationships
Knowledge	Knowledge bases are developed through the use of the affective or feeling senses
Logic	Reasoning ability is based on the union of opposites
Relationship	Development of interpersonal relationships is based on the fact that all relationships are interrelated across all continua

TABLE 5-3	**ASIAN, ASIAN-AMERICAN, AND POLYNESIAN WORLDVIEW**
COMPONENT	**PERSPECTIVE**
Cultural value	Value is placed on the balance between member and group interactions
Knowledge	Knowledge bases are developed in striving for transcendence of the mind and body
Logic	Reasoning ability is based on the belief that the mind and body can exist independently of the physical world
Relationship	Development of relationships is grounded in the belief that everyone and everything in the physical and spiritual worlds are related

(2) their perception of how illness occurs, and (3) their cultural worldview (Carter, 1995; Diala et al., 2001; Herrera et al., 1999). Nurses and patients might define *health* quite differently.

Closely connected to a nurse's or patient's definition of health is his or her belief of how illness and disease occur. The nurse or patient might believe that illness and disease are created by natural, unnatural, or scientific causes. A person who believes in the concept of *natural* cause of illness or disease believes that everyone and everything in the world is interrelated and that a disruption of this connectedness (e.g., a tornado) causes

TABLE 5-4	NATIVE-AMERICAN WORLDVIEW
COMPONENT	PERSPECTIVE
Cultural value	Value is placed in the context of a person's relationship to a Greater or Supreme Being
Knowledge	Knowledge bases are developed on the basis of a person's understanding of an individual's relationship with the Greater or Supreme Being
Logic	Reasoning ability is grounded in the belief that every person is innately good and has no evil within
Relationship	Development of relationships with another person, group, or community is grounded in the idea that the Greater or Supreme Being is in every person; hence, all persons should be valued

an illness or disease (Giger & Davidhizar, 2008; Spector, 2004). Conversely, nurses or patients might believe that *unnatural* or outside forces create illness and disease. An individual might believe that another person enlists the services of a magician, witch, ghost, or supernatural being to cast a spell or hex on him or her. Finally, nurses or patients might believe in the *scientific* cause of illness—specific, concrete explanations exist for every illness and disease (i.e., the entrance of pathogens such as viruses, bacteria, and germs into the body) (Campinha-Bacote, 2007; Warren, 2007). The scientific model is the typical model taught in most Western culture schools of nursing. However, many non-Western cultures acknowledge and teach health care providers the importance of natural and unnatural causes of illness.

Patients' health care beliefs and actions are related not only to the way in which health, illness, and the cause of illness are defined but also to individual worldviews. There are four primary worldviews: (1) analytic, (2) relational, (3) community, and (4) ecologic. The primary worldview is often the one that individuals express or are comfortable with when they are with family or significant others or during stressful times. Many individuals use a mixture of the four worldviews or adopt another worldview when they are in another environment, such as a work or business setting. The nurse's failure to understand the patient's primary worldview might negatively affect the nurse-patient relationship and impede successful interventions and mental health outcomes. Overarching worldviews that may be associated with ethnic populations are presented in Tables 5-1 to 5-4.

? CRITICAL THINKING QUESTION

2. A nurse enters a patient room and is ready to do the daily morning assessment. However, the patient is not responsive to the nurse's immediate need to conduct the assessment. The nurse complains that the patient is "noncompliant." The patient says "the nurse is always in a hurry and never listens to me." Are the worldviews of the patient and nurse in conflict? What are two suggestions you can make that would help the situation between the nurse and the patient?

Four Worldviews

A person who expresses the analytic worldview values detail to time (e.g., being on time, starting on time, ending on time), individuality, and possessions. A person with this view prefers to learn through written, hands-on, and visual resources. The relational worldview is grounded in a belief in spirituality and the significance of relationships and interactions between and among individuals. The preferred learning style is through verbal communication. An individual who expresses the community worldview believes that community needs and concerns are more important than individual ones. The valued learning style includes quiet, respectful communication as well as meditation and reading. The ecologic worldview is based on a belief that a form of interconnectedness exists between human beings and the earth and that individuals have a responsibility to take care of the earth. Learning is accomplished through quiet observation and contemplation, and verbal communication is minimized.

Worldviews form the basis for the expression of culturally bound mental health and wellness issues. For example, a patient or nurse using an analytic worldview perspective might espouse specific detail to time, calculations, individuality, and the importance of acquiring material objects. Being on time for appointments, immediately getting to the purpose of a health visit, and using printed pamphlets and books for health education are valued. Nurses and other health care professionals must be extremely accurate and precise when providing care for these patients. The components of the analytic worldview including individuality and valuing material goods are often embodied in traditional values, beliefs, and actions of American society.

An individual with a relational worldview values the development of interactions and relationships, usually prefers learning through verbal communication, and views spirituality as an important context for living life. These individuals might want to chat for a moment before getting to the heart of the health visit. They might desire the involvement of relatives, friends, or spiritual and religious advisors during the health visit or during the nurse's development of the nursing process. Individuals from African-American or Hispanic cultures often possess the relational worldview (Warren, 2007).

Individuals with a community worldview value the importance and needs of the community over the individual. People with this perspective often use meditation and contemplation techniques. A patient with this view is respectful and polite regarding health care advice and might not want to question a nurse or physician. This reticence might occur even if the patient does not understand the nurse's recommendation. People from some Asian cultural groups often embody these philosophies (Warren, 2007).

Finally, a patient or nurse with an ecologic worldview values interconnectedness with other people and the universe, takes responsibility for others and the world, and feels a need to maintain peace and tranquility. These individuals prefer a quiet, restful approach in interactions with others. Conversation is respectful, concise, and often kept to a minimum. Individuals from some of the indigenous or Native-American cultures might embrace this worldview.

💡 **CRITICAL THINKING QUESTION**

3. How can a nurse form a therapeutic relationship with a patient who is from Navajo culture and lives life using an ecologic worldview?

CULTURE-BOUND MENTAL HEALTH ISSUES

Culture-bound syndromes are recurring patterns of behavior that create disturbing experiences for individuals (American Psychiatric Association, 2013). These behaviors might or might not be congruent with symptoms presented in *DSM-5* for various diagnostic categories. However, because these behaviors can be culture-based, nurses must be aware of the symptoms to assess patients who are from racially and ethnically diverse cultures accurately. The Cultural Formulation Tool from *DSM-5* is a valuable assessment tool for nurses because it can assess both the nurse and the patient.

People from racially and ethnically diverse cultures often use culturally specific language to describe mental distress that they experience (Munoz & Luckmann, 2005; Ross, 2001; Taylor, 2003). One example involves the description of depressive symptoms and the actual symptomatology (Pouissaint & Alexander, 2000). Native Americans might state that they are "having heart pain" or are "heartbroken" when they experience depressive symptoms (Warren, 2007). A person of Hispanic descent might say that her "soul was lost" (*susto*) because of another person's ability to cause a frightening experience or to place an "evil eye" (*mal ojo*) on her (American Psychiatric Association, 2013; Campinha-Bacote, 2007). Someone who is experiencing a lost soul might be lethargic, have appetite and sleep changes, and have multiple physical complaints. Because good health is contingent on the restoration of a person's equilibrium, an ill person might initially consult a healer or "root doctor" to help break the spell of the evil eye and return the lost soul (Giger & Davidhizar, 2008). Traditional Western health care might be the last resource that the person contacts. Nurses must be knowledgeable about and sensitive to these beliefs.

People from diverse cultural groups often describe psychotic symptoms differently. Individuals from Malaya and Laos use the term *running amok*. People from certain Native-American nations might use the term *ghost sickness*. African-American and Appalachian-American individuals might say a *spell* has been cast on them. A more inclusive description of culture-bound syndromes can be found in *DSM-5* (American Psychiatric Association, 2013).

Clinical Example

A 33-year-old woman who is from Appalachian culture is worried because she is sure her illness is due to a hex placed on her by another woman in the community. How would you, as a nurse, provide care for her? Do you attempt to convince her that her ideas are wrong and there is no such thing as a hex?

The assessment of possible culture-bound syndromes and the cultural expression of psychiatric symptoms must be part of the psychotherapeutic and nursing processes. This additional assessment can provide important information that the nurse needs to provide culturally competent services for patients.

ALTERNATIVE THERAPIES

People from racially and ethnically diverse groups often use alternative therapies. These treatments might include the use of acupuncture, acupressure, nutritional therapies, skin scraping, moxibustion, and cupping. Acupressure and acupuncture restore balance by stimulating linear and circular lines throughout the body, known as meridians, with the use of needles (*acupuncture*) or pressure (*acupressure*) (Giger & Davidhizar, 2008). *Nutritional therapies* might include the use of certain foods or herbs. *Skin scraping* or *coining*, *moxibustion*, and *cupping* are used to restore balance by bringing heat to the skin surface, which allows the release of the toxin or evil spirit from the affected body area (Giger & Davidhizar, 2008). In the case of skin scraping or coining, a person (generally a healer in the community) uses a coin and briskly rubs or scrapes the skin surface. In moxibustion, a cotton ball containing a substance known as *moxa* is ignited with a match in a small glass or cup, which is then placed on the skin above a meridian. The belief is that the illness or evil is released from a person's body when heat is generated within the meridians. However, skin abrasions and contusions, often occurring on the skin as a result of skin scraping or coining, moxibustion, or cupping, might provide a climate for infection.

Certain cultural groups (e.g., Hispanic, South American) believe that certain liquids, foods, or medicines must be taken in balance to restore health (Fontaine, 2005). A medicine might be labeled as being *hot* and might need to be taken in conjunction with a *cold* liquid or food to be effective. The terms *hot* and *cold* do not refer to temperature but instead indicate how the substance reacts within the body to restore equilibrium.

ETHNOPHARMACOLOGY

Ethnopharmacology is the study of pharmacogenetic, pharmacodynamic, and pharmacokinetic influences based on different ethnic, racial, and cultural groups (Herrera et al., 1999; Munoz & Hilgenberg, 2006; Warren, 2007, 2008a, 2013c, 2013d). Culturally competent care is enhanced when this type of cultural knowledge is incorporated into patient care.

Individuals react to pharmacologic interventions based on their normal biologic makeup, environmental influences, and cultural influences (Herrera et al., 1999; Keltner & Folks, 2005). Specific ethnic, racial, and cultural differences affect a patient's medication options and dose requirements.

Variation in metabolism is most often cited as the cause of cross-ethnic differences in response to medications. Herrera and associates (1999) indicated that individuals from certain racial and ethnic groups have a genetically based pharmacokinetic variation that causes them to be fast or slow metabolizers. Drugs might accumulate in a patient's body when medications are metabolized too slowly. For example, people of Asian (about 50%) and Native-American descent are more sensitive to the effects of alcohol than people from other ethnic and racial backgrounds. This sensitivity is based on their relative deficiency of aldehyde dehydrogenase, resulting in slowed metabolism of the highly toxic intermediate product, acetylaldehyde (Herrera et al., 1999). Symptoms include a reddened flush to the neck and face, tachycardia, and a burning sensation in the stomach.

Most psychotropic drugs are metabolized by the cytochrome P-450 system (Munoz et al., 2007). Basically, only two cytochrome P-450 enzymes (see Chapter 12 for this discussion), 2D6 and 2C19, appear to have extensive cross-ethnic variability. Substrates of these enzymes are metabolized more slowly (poor metabolizers) in a certain percentage of each of these cultural groups (Keltner & Folks, 2005). This cross-ethnic variability is shown in Table 5-5.

TABLE 5-5	METABOLISM BY 2D6 AND 2C19 ENZYMES: CROSS-ETHNIC VARIABILITY	
ETHNIC GROUP	**2D6-POOR METABOLIZERS (%)**	**2C19-POOR METABOLIZERS (%)**
African-Americans	~2	~19
Whites	3-9	2.5-6.7
Hispanics	1-4.5	~5
Native Americans	0-5.2	0
East Asians	0-2.5	17-22

Modified from Keltner, N.L., & Folks, D.G. (2005). *Psychotropic drugs* (4th ed.). St. Louis: Mosby.

NURSE'S ROLE IN CULTURAL ASSESSMENT

Nurses not only should use the process of cultural competence in their practice settings, but they also should help others understand the need for culturally competent health care. One skill every nurse must develop is the ability to integrate cultural factors into the health assessment (Munoz & Luckmann, 2005; Warren, 2005).

Cultural Assessment Issues

Nurses must include some basic elements within their cultural assessments of patients, including communication, orientation, nutrition, family relationships, health beliefs, education, spiritual or religious views, and biologic or physiologic elements. Table 5-6 provides a handy assessment sheet to consider when evaluating culturally relevant information.

Questions and observations relative to cultural issues must be smoothly and sensitively incorporated into the nursing assessment process to ensure that the nurse does not appear rude or intrusive. Including someone from the patient's community or from the same cultural background during the assessment interview might be appropriate. Cultural preservation, cultural negotiation, and cultural repatterning are other culturally competent techniques that nurses might use during assessment and in care planning.

Cultural preservation is the nurse's ability to acknowledge, value, and accept a patient's cultural beliefs. *Cultural negotiation* is the nurse's ability to work within a patient's cultural belief system to develop culturally appropriate interventions.

TABLE 5-6	CULTURAL ASSESSMENT WORKSHEET
ASSESSMENT AREA	**QUESTIONS OR AREAS OF INQUIRY**
Communication	1. Do you speak any foreign languages? 2. Is English your first language? 3. Does the patient speak English fluently? 4. Does the patient prefer an interpreter? 5. Does the patient believe that appropriate touching is acceptable? 6. Does the patient use ethnic behaviors?
Orientation	1. How long have you lived where you now live? 2. Where were you born? 3. With which ethnic, racial, or cultural group do you identify yourself? 4. How closely do you follow the traditional values, beliefs, and practices of your self-identified group? 5. What are the patient's thoughts on the following: human nature, development of knowledge, work ethic, relationship with nature?
Nutrition	1. Do you have certain foods you prefer? 2. What kind of foods do you eat when you are ill? 3. Do you avoid certain foods because of your beliefs?
Significant others and family	1. Who do you consider as important to you? 2. Is there anyone that you would like me to contact or not contact while you are here for treatment? 3. How are decisions made in your home environment? 4. In your home, what are the roles for children, women, and men? 5. What are some of the social customs or practices that you do at home? 6. Share with me three of your most important values.

TABLE 5-6 CULTURAL ASSESSMENT WORKSHEET—CONT'D

ASSESSMENT AREA	QUESTIONS OR AREAS OF INQUIRY
Health	1. What brought you here for treatment today? 2. What do you think will help you feel better or get well? 3. Have you used treatments in the past that were helpful for you? 4. What type of treatments do you not like or feel uncomfortable receiving? 5. Is there something you think I can assist you with to help you improve? 6. Who do you usually go to for help or treatment when you are ill? 7. What do you think causes physical and mental problems?
Education	1. How do you prefer to learn new things and tasks (e.g., reading, watching television or videos, talking with someone)? 2. How have you received your education (e.g., in school, by self-instruction)? 3. How would you prefer to pay for your treatment?
Spirituality and religion	1. Do you consider yourself spiritual or religious? If so, what does that mean to you? 2. Do you have a religious preference? 3. Are there certain individuals you like to talk with regarding your spiritual views, religious beliefs, or health care? Are there certain practices in which you like to participate?
Biology and physiology	1. Do you have any specific health problems or disease conditions in your family of origin? 2. Are there certain medications, herbs, or therapies that you avoid because they make you ill? 3. Are there specific skin, hair, grooming, or health care needs that you prefer? 4. Are you taking any medications now? (Include an examination of vitamin, nutritional, and herbal approaches.) 5. How many cigarettes do you smoke every day? 6. How many glasses of wine do you drink per week? 7. How many cans or bottles of Coke, root beer, or beer do you drink per week? 8. How many cups of tea or coffee, or both, do you drink every day? 9. Are there any other beverages that you drink every day? 10. How many bars or pieces of chocolate do you eat every day?

From Warren, B.J., Campinha-Bacote, J., & Munoz, C. (1994). *Cultural assessment worksheet*. Columbus, Ohio: Authors.

Cultural repatterning is the nurse's ability to incorporate cultural preservation and negotiation to identify patient needs, develop expected outcomes, and evaluate outcome plans (Leininger & McFarland, 2006). The Critical Thinking Questions and Clinical Example in this chapter provide examples of how these three techniques might be incorporated into the care of a patient.

SUMMARY

Cultural competence is an important part of effective psychiatric nursing. Important components for the development of culturally competent nursing care include the nurse's understanding of the concepts of a worldview, culture-bound syndromes, and ethnopharmacology and the nurse's role in assessing patients for cultural variables that might affect patient care.

■ STUDY NOTES

1. Culture is the manifestation beliefs, values, and norms of an individual, group, or community used for daily life functioning.
2. Cultural competence is the process whereby the nurse develops cultural awareness, knowledge, and skills to promote effective health care for patients.
3. Cultural diversity refers to unique differences in areas such as age, gender, socioeconomic status, religion, race, and ethnicity.
4. A person's worldview is a perspective reflecting what the person values in how she functions and interacts with others on a daily basis.
5. Barriers to culturally competent care include miscommunication, failure to assess for a cultural perspective, and differences in worldview.
6. Illness can be viewed as resulting from natural, unnatural, or scientific (i.e., explainable) causes.
7. Four worldviews are analytic, relational, community, and ecologic.
8. Culture-bound syndromes are recurring patterns of behavior that create disturbing experiences for people.
9. Patients from non-Western cultures might use acupuncture, acupressure, nutritional therapies (e.g., herbal remedies), skin scraping, moxibustion, and cupping to treat illness.
10. Ethnopharmacology involves the study of genetic and culture-related factors that can affect metabolism of medications.
11. An important nursing role is the incorporation of cultural knowledge into addressing health and health care.

REFERENCES

American Psychiatric Association, (2013). *Diagnostic and statistical manual of mental disorders* (5th ed.). Arlington, Virginia: APA.

Andrews, M. M., & Boyle, J. S. (2007). *Transcultural concepts in nursing care* (5th ed.). Philadelphia: Lippincott.

Anthony, W. A. (1993). Recovery from mental illness: The guiding vision of the mental health services in the 1990s. *Psychiatric Rehabilitation Journal, 2,* 17.

Campinha-Bacote, J. (2007). *The process of cultural competence in the delivery of healthcare services: The journey continues* (5th ed.). Cincinnati: Transcultural C.A.R.E. Associates.

Carter, R. T. (1995). *The influence of race and racial identity in psychotherapy: toward a racially inclusive model.* New York: Wiley & Sons.

De la Cruz, M. S. D. (2013). Gender differences in health-related quality of life in patients with bipolar disorder. *Archives of Womens Mental Health, 16,* 317–323.

Diala, C. C., et al. (2001). Racial/ethnic differences in attitudes toward seeking professional mental health services. *American Journal of Public Health, 91*(5), 805–807.

Fontaine, K. L. (2005). *Complementary and alternative therapies for nursing.* Upper Saddle River, New Jersey: Prentice-Hall.

Giger, J. N., & Davidhizar, R. E. (2008). *Transcultural nursing: Assessment and intervention* (5th ed.). St. Louis: Mosby.

Herrera, J. M., Lawson, W. B., & Sramek, J. J. (1999). *Cross cultural psychiatry.* New York: Wiley & Sons.

Institute of Medicine, (2003). *Unequal treatment: confronting racial and ethnic disparities in healthcare.* Washington, D.C.: National Academy Press.

Keltner, N. L., & Folks, D. G. (2005). *Psychotropic drugs* (4th ed.). St. Louis: Mosby.

Leininger, M., & McFarland, M. R. (2006). *Cultural care and diversity and universality: a world-wide nursing theory* (2nd ed.). Boston: Jones & Bartlett.

Munoz, C., & Hilgenberg, C. (2006). Ethnopharmacology: understanding how ethnicity can affect drug response is essential to providing culturally competent care. *Holistic Nursing Practice, 20,* 5.

Munoz, C., & Luckmann, J. (2005). *Transcultural communication in nursing.* New York: Thomson Delmar.

Munoz, R., et al. (2007). *Life in color: Culture in American psychiatry.* Chicago: Hilton Publishing.

Pouissaint, A. F., & Alexander, A. (2000). *Lay my burden down: unraveling suicide and the mental health crisis among African Americans.* Boston: Beacon Press.

Purnell, L. D. (2009). *Guide to culturally competent health care* (2nd ed.). Philadelphia: F.A. Davis.

Ross, H. (2001). *Office of Minority Health publishes final standards for cultural and linguistic competence. Closing the gap, cultural competency part II.* http://www.omhrc.gov/assets/pdf/checked/Final%20Standards%20for%20Cultural%20and%20Linguistic%20Competence.pdf, Accessed September 2, 2013.

Spector, R. (2004). *Cultural diversity in health and illness* (6th ed.). Upper Saddle River, New Jersey: Prentice-Hall Health.

Taylor, J. S. (2003). The story catches you and you fall down: tragedy, ethnography, and "cultural competence." *Medical Anthropology Quarterly, 17,* 159.

U.S. Surgeon General, (2001). *Mental health: Culture, race, and ethnicity, a supplement to mental health: A report of the Surgeon General.* Washington, D.C.: U.S. Department of Health and Human Services.

Warren, B. J. (2013a). How culture is assessed in the DSM-5. *Journal of Psychosocial Nursing, 51,* 40–45.

Warren, B. J. (2013b). Many shades of blue: Body and spirit: Into the light: Interview as told to Jeannine Amber. *Essence, 3,* 116–119.

Warren, B. J. (2013c). Culturally sensitive psychopharmacology. In L. G. Leahy & C. G. Kohler (Eds.), *Clinical manual of psychopharmacology for nurses* (pp. 379–402). Washington, D.C.: American Psychiatric Publishing, Inc.

Warren, B. J. (2013d). Ethnopharmacology. In B. Cockerman (Ed.), *Blackwell encyclopaedia health and society medical anthropology.* Somerset, New Jersey: Wiley.

Warren, B. J. (2012). Guest Editorial: Shared decision making: A recovery cultural process. *Journal of Psychosocial Nursing and Mental Health Services, 50,* 4–5.

Warren, B. J. (2008a). Ethnopharmacology: The effect on patients, healthcare professionals and systems. *Urologic Nursing, 28,* 4.

Warren, B. J. (2008b). Cultural and ethnic considerations. In D. Antai-Otong (Ed.), *Psychiatric nursing: biological and behavioral concepts.* New York: Delmar.

Warren, B. J. (2007). Cultural competence in psychiatric nursing: an interlocking paradigm approach. In N. L. Keltner, L. H. Schwecke, & C. E. Bostrom (Eds.), *Psychiatric nursing* (pp. 164–172) (5th ed.). St. Louis: Mosby.

Warren, B. J. (2005). The cultural expression of dying. *The Case Manager, 16,* 44.

Warren, B. J., Campinha-Bacote, J., & Munoz, C. (1994). *Cultural assessment worksheet.* Columbus, Ohio: Authors.

Spiritual Issues

Gordon I.G. Pugh

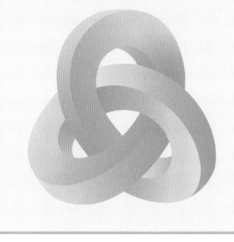

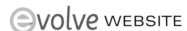 WEBSITE

http://evolve.elsevier.com/Keltner

LEARNING OBJECTIVES

- Describe two general uses of the term *spirituality*.
- Explain three helpful theoretical constructs regarding spirituality.
- Discuss and evaluate benefits and concerns of including spiritual care in patients' treatment.
- Be familiar with the *Diagnostic and Statistical Manual of Mental Disorders, Fifth Edition* (*DSM-5*) and the NANDA International diagnoses of spiritual care issues.

- Know two pieces of practical advice from psychiatric patients themselves regarding communication about spiritual concerns.
- Identify how the nurse can intervene, including using the HOPE or FICA questions.
- Know how and when to make a referral to a spiritual care professional.

One criticism of some psychological theories is that they are psychology without the psyche, and this suits people who think they have no spiritual needs or aspirations. But here both doctor and patient deceive themselves…. In a word, they do not give enough meaning to life, and it is only meaning that liberates (Jung, 1984 p. 198).

How does nursing address, or even approach, concepts such as forgiveness, peace, trust, fear, alienation, hope, love, grief, transcendence, discovery, meaning, purpose, relationship, or gratitude? These notions fall within the concept of spirituality and will be explored in this chapter.

There is no single common, agreed-on definition of spirituality, so research about "spirituality" is impossible. Instead, Koenig (2008b) contended that research can measure religious expressions, of which spirituality should be understood as a subset. In a nursing context especially, we want to be sure we understand what a patient means when talking of spiritual concerns or needs. For clinical practice, Koenig (2008b) advocated taking a spiritual history about beliefs that are used to cope (or that are a source of distress) by asking whether a patient is part of a supportive community, identifying spiritual needs, and supporting the patient's beliefs. "If patients indicate from the start that they are not religious or spiritual, then questions should be re-directed to asking

about what gives life meaning and purpose and how this can be addressed in their health care" (Koenig, 2008b).

People hold strong opinions about spirituality and religion (Pargament, 2013), but a significant number of Americans have changed their religious affiliation (Pew Research Center, 2008). A person's experiences with particular religions can be positive or negative or both. People born between 1945 and 1980 (Baby Boomers and Generation Xers) have likely heard people say that they are "spiritual but not religious." By contrast, Smith and Denton (2005) in their National Study for Religion and Youth found that most modern American teenagers they interviewed "had never heard this phrase before, and the vast majority, even if they had heard this phrase, said that they had no clue what it meant." Their research indicates that most teens in the United States are "rather positive about and conventional in living out religion" (Smith & Denton, 2005).

More than 80% of adults in the United States identify with a monotheistic religion (Pew Research Center, 2008). However, greater than 16% of American adults identify themselves as "unaffiliated with any particular religion" (see Table 6-1). A 2012 survey found that one third of adults younger than 30 years old were currently religiously unaffiliated (Pew Research Center, 2012). One could say that the second largest "religious group" in the United States comprises individuals with no religious

TABLE 6-1	MAJOR RELIGIOUS TRADITIONS IN THE UNITED STATES	
AMONG ALL ADULTS		**%**
Christian		78.4
Protestant		51.3
Evangelical churches		26.3
Mainline churches		18.1
Historic black churches		6.9
Catholic		23.9
Mormon		1.7
Jehovah's Witness		0.7
Orthodox		0.6
Greek Orthodox		<0.3
Russian Orthodox		<0.3
Other		<0.3
Other Christian		0.3
Other religions		4.7
Jewish		1.7
Reformed		0.7
Conservative		0.5
Orthodox		<0.3
Other		0.3
Buddhist		0.7
Zen Buddhist		<0.3
Theravada Buddhist		<0.3
Tibetan Buddhist		<0.3
Other		0.3
Muslim*		0.6
Sunni		0.3
Shia		<0.3
Other		<0.3
Hindu		0.4
Other world religions		<0.3
Other faiths		1.2
Unitarians and other liberal faiths		0.7
New Age		0.4
Native-American religions		<0.3
Unaffiliated		16.1
Atheist		1.6
Agnostic		2.4
Nothing in particular		12.1
Secular unaffiliated		6.3
Religious unaffiliated		5.8
Don't know/refused		0.8
Total		100.0†

*From *Muslim Americans: middle class and mostly mainstream.* (2007). Pew Research Center. http://www.pewresearch.org/2007/05/22/muslim-americans-middle-class-and-mostly-mainstream/ Accessed November 19, 2013.
†Because of rounding, figures may not add up to 100, and nested figures may not add up to the subtotal indicated.
From Pew Research Center. (2008). *U.S. religious landscape survey: Religious affiliation: Diversity and dynamic.* The Pew Forum on Religion & Public Life. <http://religions.pewforum.org/pdf/report-religious-landscape-study-full.pdf> Accessed November 19, 2013.

affiliation. However, even this group is widely diverse, ranging from atheists to people who say that religion is "somewhat important" or "very important" in their lives; 68% of "unaffiliated" individuals say that they believe in God. In times of crisis, people often turn to positive religious coping (Pargament, 2013).

It is hoped that this chapter will help you understand how to consider the spiritual concerns of patients and families. First, we discuss understandings and uses of spirituality. Next, we examine how spiritual concerns can look within different nursing contexts. Finally, we look at specific ways for you as a nurse to help with spiritual concerns.

NORM'S NOTES
Spiritual care—what is it? We all have a spirit, and we can feel it. Spiritual care attempts to go beyond the facts of psychiatry and brain biology and deal with that intangible part of our being that we call a spirit, but it can get tricky. You cannot impose your spiritual worldview on a patient, but how can you talk about spiritual issues without bringing your own values to the discussion? This chapter attempts to show how to deal with these competing forces—without reducing spiritual care to a meaningless behavior.

TOWARD AN UNDERSTANDING OF SPIRITUALITY

Psychiatry Based on Greek *Psyche* (The Soul)

The word *psychiatry* comes from two Greek words, *psyche* (soul) and *iatreia* (healing)—"healing of the soul." *Psyche* has a variety of meanings—the breath of life, the seat of feelings and emotions, and the part of human beings that transcends the earthly. The term *spirituality* is used to describe things beyond mere biologic existence.

Common Understandings of Spirituality

Spirit refers to something not strictly physical, which gives life, depth, and meaning to existence (Jung, 1980). Common understandings of spirituality have to do with making sense of life; with hopes, plans, and fears; with things that people value; with the way in which individuals relate to others; and with issues of meaning and belonging. Instead of a strict definition, a description of spirituality for clinical use is a better approach. In Great Britain, the Royal College of Psychiatrists (2013) describes spirituality as something to help us find meaning and purpose; hope; and the best relationship with "ourselves, others, and what lies beyond." Spirituality "emphasizes the healing of the person, not just the disease" and "views life as a journey."

The word *spirituality* is generally used in two ways. The first way sees the human spirit as inextricably connected to a transcendent source (God or a higher power or a universal spirit) and is often expressed within the individual's religious community. The second way seeks to distinguish spirituality from a religious perspective by emphasizing aspects of the human spirit and its relationship to other human spirits in ways that are not dependent on the notion of a higher power.

Spirituality in Relation to a Transcendent Spirit (Theistic View)

The first view is exemplified in the creation story of the world's three largest monotheistic religions (Christianity, Islam, and Judaism). God constructed the world, including human beings. God "breathes life" into a human being, who becomes a living soul. Therefore, the first understanding is that human lives are inspired (literally, breathed into) by a Supreme Being. This view is often marked by a sense of gratitude for basic existence.

Spirituality in Relation to Human Spirit (Humanistic View)

Jung (1980) described *spirituality* as "the sum total of intellectual and cultural possessions…." This understanding includes how people attempt to bring meaning to meaning in their lives apart from a religious community or an understanding of God. The emphasis is on the human spirit, both individually and collectively. This understanding emphasizes not a transcendent source but self-transcendence in particular, sometimes in relationship with others. The two understandings (theistic and humanistic) are not mutually exclusive; however, the latter understanding deemphasizes (and sometimes completely rejects) the theistic approach.

Other Helpful Perspectives for the Psychiatric Nurse
Clinical Understanding

Xavier (2008), a clinical psychiatrist, offered a useful distinction from his psychiatric experience between "healthy spirituality" and "sick religiosity." People sometimes have a negative opinion of institutional religion (e.g., church, synagogue, mosque) because of some painful or dehumanizing experience at the hands of someone who claimed religion. Xavier (2008) stated that sick religiosity is marked by "a sense of exclusiveness and absolutism." However, Xavier recognized that many religious expressions are healthy and beneficial. This reminder is especially important to his fellow psychiatrists, who seem to see a greater amount of psychopathology characterized by manifestations of sick religiosity than would presumably be found in the general population. There is also a positive correlation between mental health and spiritual well-being that is sometimes ignored (Freshwater, 2006).

Making Meaning in Suffering by Finding Hope

Viktor Frankl was a psychiatrist who experienced intense suffering as a prisoner in Nazi concentration camps during World War II. He recognized that although individuals cannot always choose their circumstances, they always have a choice about their attitudes toward their experiences. He witnessed overwhelming helplessness at the death camps. He noticed that prisoners who had no desire to live first gave up hope, then life. For example, prisoners who did not exchange their cigarettes for food "were those who had lost the will to live and wanted to 'enjoy' their last days" (Frankl, 1984). Many of the prisoners who found a reason to live maintained hope and were able to survive.

Trust and the Spirituality of Human Development

Loder (1989) postulated that early developmental experiences set the stage for later spiritual dynamics within the individual. He pointed out that in the biblical languages the words for "face" also mean "presence." At the age of 3 months, infants begin to recognize faces. The most important face in the development of trust is the primary caregiver, typically the mother. The primal response to this presence is a smile. At this point in development, the infant does not yet have a concept of time. However, by age 9 months, the infant understands when the mother is not present and experiences anxiety at her absence. For the infant who is 3 to 6 months old (who has not yet developed a sense of time or absence), basic needs are met by one whose presence is always assumed, who loves unconditionally, and who orders the infant's whole world. The infant's burgeoning capacity to trust is strengthened by the presence (face) of the nurturer. Loder (1989) contended that the spiritual search many people later experience is connected with the desire to experience in a new way the nature of being "given a place in the cosmos, confirmed as a self, and addressed by the presence of a loving other." Loder (1989) noted that the infant experiences no shame when gazing at this face, so this model can be useful in helping deal with issues of abandonment and shame.

PATIENT SPIRITUALITY AND THE PSYCHIATRIC NURSE

Importance of Spiritual Care

People often look for meaning when they are in a situation that requires nursing care. Nursing, medical, and accrediting groups have recognized this importance. The NANDA International nursing diagnoses (NANDA International, 2012) refer to several areas under the Life Principles domain, including recognizing hope and hopelessness, religiosity, spiritual well-being and distress, and being at risk for such distress. Under the Ego Integrity domain, NANDA International refers to several areas that are of spiritual concern—coping, denial, grieving, powerlessness, resilience, and anxiety about death, all of which can have a spiritual component.

Levine and Ion (2002) identified four factors of resilience essential for coping, which they called the "Four B's": Being, Belonging, Belief, and Benevolence. They discovered these factors through examining the experiences of resilient children who endured war, affliction, trauma, poverty, or prejudice. *Being* is related to self-respect and self-acceptance. *Belonging* has to do with being a part of a supportive, accepting group and often includes a family or religious community or both. *Belief* is about one's mission, vision, and purpose. Levine and Ion (2002) stated, "Belief embodies the questions about our fundamental existence, beyond material success. Highly personal, virtually indefinable, belief sustains when even being and belonging fail." *Benevolence* is more commonly exhibited by individuals who have experienced need. "We are kind because people have been kind to us" (Levine & Ion, 2002). These sources of strength can be important elements in a spiritual history and in helping people find and use their spiritual resources.

In its mission to relieve pain, palliative care medicine recognizes four domains of suffering: physical, psychological (emotional), social, and spiritual distress. Each of these is mentioned in various Joint Commission standards of care (National Consensus Project for Quality Palliative Care, 2009). In this context, "spiritual" can refer to cultural, religious, or existential concerns.

The *DSM-5* (American Psychiatric Association, 2013) has a diagnostic category dedicated to a "Religious or Spiritual Problem" (see *DSM-5* and NANDA International box). The Joint Commission (Ehman, 2013) has maintained that patients have a basic right to care that respects their cultural factors, religious beliefs, and spiritual values. For both of these accreditation groups, the spiritual aspect is viewed as unique and separate from the cultural, mental, emotional, psychosocial, and religious aspects.

DSM-5 AND NANDA INTERNATIONAL DEFINITIONS OF SPIRITUAL PROBLEMS

DSM-5

Religious or Spiritual Problem*

This category can be used when the focus of clinical attention is a religious or spiritual problem. Examples include distressing experiences that involve loss or questioning of faith, problems associated with conversion to a new faith, or questioning of spiritual values that might not necessarily be related to an organized church or religious institution.

NANDA

From NANDA Life Principles Domain†

Moral distress: Response to the inability to carry out one's chosen ethical or moral decision or action

Hope, readiness for enhanced: Pattern of expectations and desires that is sufficient for mobilizing energy on one's own behalf and can be strengthened

Hopelessness: Subjective state in which one sees limited or unavailable alternatives or personal choices and is unable to mobilize energy for problem solving on one's own behalf

Religiosity, impaired: Impaired ability to rely on beliefs or participate in rituals of a particular faith tradition

Religiosity, readiness for enhanced: Ability to increase reliance on religious beliefs or participate in rituals of a particular faith tradition

Religiosity, risk for impaired: At risk for an impaired ability to rely on beliefs or participate in rituals of a particular faith tradition

Spiritual distress: Impaired ability to experience and integrate meaning and purpose in life through one's connectedness with self, others, art, music, literature, nature, or a power greater than oneself

Spiritual distress, risk of: At risk for an impaired ability to experience and integrate meaning and purpose in life through one's connectedness with self, others, art, music, literature, nature, or a power greater than oneself

Spiritual well-being, readiness for enhanced: Ability to experience and integrate meaning and purpose in life through connectedness with self, others, art, music, literature, nature, or a power greater than oneself that can be strengthened.

---

*American Psychiatric Association. (2013). *Diagnostic and statistical manual of mental disorders* (5th ed.). Arlington, Virginia: APA.
†NANDA International. (2012). *Nursing diagnoses: definitions and classifications 2012-2014*. <http://www.fchs.ac.ae/fchs/uploads/Files/Semester%201%20-%202011-2012/NANDA%20group%20list.pdf> Accessed November 19, 2013.

Clinical Attention to Spiritual Concerns

Despite the emphasis on the importance of spiritual care, spiritual concerns rarely seem to be the focus of clinical attention. Nazir (2010) stated that 50% of the British psychiatrists responding to her survey reported taking a spiritual history and that the histories were sporadic and usually in the context of assessing delusions. Another study in the United States found that 60% of adolescent psychiatric inpatients reported that they had never been asked about their religious or spiritual beliefs by any mental health professional (other than the chaplain) (Grossoehme, 2001). Grossoehme (2001) made the following observation concerning the disparity between the professed importance of spiritual care and the actual treatment that psychiatric patients generally receive:

> A study of the relationship between psychiatrists' religious beliefs and their practice documented that the majority of them believe spirituality to be an area with which psychiatrists may appropriately be concerned. However, over half of the psychiatrists in that study inquired about their patients' religious beliefs "occasionally" or even less frequently; those that did assess this area generally did not have any interventions based upon their findings (p. 139).

Psychiatrists tend to be less religious personally and are more likely to identify themselves as spiritual but not religious. However, one study suggests that they are also more likely than other physicians to ask about and to address spiritual concerns in a clinical setting, to be more comfortable talking about patients' spiritual concerns, and to note associated "negative emotions that lead to increased patient suffering" (Curlin et al., 2007). The primary investigator of this study said that "attention to patients' spiritual concerns … may help patients identify the resources in their own religious traditions that can help them cope with the suffering caused by mental illness" (University of Chicago Medical Center Psychiatrists, 2007). Bender reports Lu's caution that one "…error a psychiatrist can make is to incorrectly judge certain behaviors or symptoms as related to a patient's cultural background instead of to psychopathology" (Bender, 2004).

INTERSECTION OF SPIRITUALITY AND MENTAL OR EMOTIONAL DISTRESS

Mental illness is a distressing situation that can give rise to important spiritual questions. Oates (1978) identified how aspects of schizophrenia affect the patient's spiritual perspective. The incapacity to symbolize—that is, the patient's concrete thinking—can cause special problems because "religious language is symbolic by nature." Oates related the story of a schizophrenic patient who decompensated while at a Pentecostal religious gathering: "She was terrified at the thought of Jesus 'entering her heart.' To her this was a literal invasion of her body."

Möller's (1999) participants reported being especially frustrated by their own concrete thinking and with the clergy's lack of understanding of this phenomenon. Oates (1978) stated that although religion can be a common theme in hallucinations and delusions and that these vary among cultures, the diminished capacity for trust tends to be consistent cross-culturally. Peteet and colleagues (2011) noted that it is important to ask, "What about this disorder is important to understand in order to distinguish religious/spiritual experiences from psychopathology?" This trust is built on consistently demonstrated, genuinely compassionate behavior on the part of the caregiver. The most practical advice comes from patients themselves, who reported that they want most of all for their spiritual care provider to (1) be authentic, caring, and respectful and (2) speak slowly and in concrete terms.

> **? CRITICAL THINKING QUESTION**
>
> 1. Psychiatric patients describe concrete thinking during a psychotic episode. How can these patients be open to spiritual care when spiritual language is by nature symbolic?

Pargament (2013) and Koenig (2008a) noted that studies about spirituality have proliferated since 2000. These authors confirmed "positive associations" of religion and mental health and noted that most studies do not show the kinds of connections between religion and mental illness in the general population that psychiatry has traditionally assumed. Vaillant (2008) associated spirituality with "positive emotions," noting that psychiatric textbooks do not mention emotions such as joy and gratitude. He identified six other positive emotions: love, hope, forgiveness, compassion, trust, and awe. Vaillant (2008) emphasized, "Of enormous importance is the fact that none of the eight are 'all about me.'" Brown and colleagues (2013) examined the relationship between religious coping styles and spiritual well-being with the psychological variables of anxiety and depression. Their study showed that people who report "higher levels of religiosity and spiritual well-being may also experience a reduction in mental and emotional illness."

HEALTH CARE APPLICATIONS

Suffering and Illness Elicit Crises

We recognize that not everyone who reads this textbook will become a psychiatric nurse and that there are a variety of situations in which nurses will encounter patients who express spiritual needs. These issues are important in psychiatric settings, but patients with chronic medical conditions, patients with acute disease, and patients needing end-of-life care, whether in an outpatient or inpatient setting, are also likely to have spiritual concerns, as are their loved ones. Even during a patient's "routine" visits to a health care provider, the nurse can encounter some level of spiritual concern.

A major life crisis, such as facing one's own mortality, is among the most difficult points in a person's life. Suffering, distress, illness, death, and grief can induce an existential urgency that causes people to consider their own mortality and their sense of belonging. Although this type of crisis might

be common, it almost always comes unexpectedly. At these critical life junctures, people have the opportunity to become more acutely aware of and interested in issues of meaning and their place in the world. Walsh (2012) noted that when such concerns arise, individuals can examine the impact of their beliefs beyond a narrow view of the immediate problem for which they are seeking help.

How Can the Nurse Assess and Intervene in a Realistic Way?

The issues of trust and compassion are at the core of providing quality spiritual care. The discussion in this chapter can help you to identify spiritual strengths and concerns but cannot equip you to address complex long-term needs. "Referrals to professionals with specialized knowledge or skills in spiritual and existential issues are made available when appropriate" (National Consensus Project for Quality Palliative Care, 2009).

Koenig (2008b) reminded nurses that they should do five things regarding spiritual care: (1) take a spiritual history; (2) support and show respect for the patient's beliefs; (3) pray with the patient if the nurse is comfortable doing so *and* if the patient wants *and* requests it; (4) provide spiritual care by being kind, gentle, sensitive, and compassionate; and (5) refer to pastoral care. Koenig (2008b) stated that nurses and chaplains are "natural allies," not competitors in providing spiritual care.

Even apart from a psychiatric setting, taking note of the patient's spiritual concerns is important. A simple spiritual history should be taken. Many spiritual assessment tools of different lengths and complexity are available from various disciplines. Among the simplest and easiest to use is the HOPE questions. Two physicians at Brown University School of Medicine developed a tool that can provide the health care professional with four concepts to discuss with patients, given the easy to remember acronym *HOPE* (Anandarajah and Hight, 2001). The answers can be an opportunity for further exploration of the spiritual issues involved.

H: Sources of *hope*, strength, comfort, meaning, peace, love, and connection
O: The role of *organized* religion for the patient
P: *Personal* spirituality and *practices*
E: *Effects* on medical care and *end-of-life* issues

Puchalski's FICA questions are another convenient way for a health care professional to take a spiritual history (Koenig, 2007):

F: Faith—what is your *faith* tradition?
I: Importance—how *important* is your faith to you?
C: Church/Community—what is your *church* or *community* of faith?
A: Address—how might we *address* your spiritual needs?

If you have time for only one simple question that will demonstrate respect for the patient's spiritual concerns, give you valuable information, and allow for future conversations, Koenig (2007) suggested: "Do you have any spiritual needs or concerns related to your health?"

CRITICAL THINKING QUESTION

2. What do you see as the similarities and differences of the HOPE and FICA questions?

USING CLERGY RESOURCES

Community clergy are usually not trained to address the spiritual needs of psychiatric patients. Given staff concerns about psychiatric patients' religious delusions, and given patient reports that they desire competent spiritual care, having a clinically trained professional chaplain as an integral component of the health care team makes sense. Psychiatric health care settings do a disservice to patients when they leave untrained people to provide spiritual care. Even so, patients will likely return to their community of faith, where they can be involved in an ongoing way. Smolak and associates (2013) discussed how family members and caregivers of patients with schizophrenia often influence treatment by preferring to interact with religious-based professionals and have "caution toward mental health professionals."

Patients with spiritual concerns should be referred to a clinically trained spiritual care professional (usually a chaplain), and this person should be part of an interdisciplinary health care team. Health care facilities provide and use chaplains in many different ways, ranging from community clergy to highly trained board-certified chaplains who serve on multidisciplinary teams. Having a first-hand understanding of what a professional chaplain does can greatly expand your practice and the resources available to help. "Shadowing a chaplain can be a key component of the spiritual education program" for a variety of disciplines (Galanter, 2008). As a nursing student, you can ask to shadow a chaplain to see what chaplains do and how they fit into the health care team. Koenig (2008b) recommended that hospital staff become acquainted with their chaplains and that they refer all but the simplest of spiritual needs.

 CRITICAL THINKING QUESTIONS

3. How can the HOPE or FICA questions provide an opportunity for further exploration of spiritual issues for a patient who is not involved with organized religion?
4. Did any of the following words catch your attention as you read this chapter? How many of these would you identify as spiritual issues as you care for a patient? Why or why not?
   abandonment anxiety awe belonging compassion faith forgiveness gratitude grief helplessness hope joy love place presence relationship trust

 CRITICAL THINKING QUESTION

5. Why do you think so many people want to draw a distinction between religion and spirituality?

STUDY NOTES

1. Spirituality is generally understood to be a major component of mental health and psychiatric care.
2. Spirituality is more broadly defined today in our postmodern culture than it was in the past.
3. At its most basic, spirituality has to do with making sense of life, with hopes, plans, and fears; with things that people value; with the way in which individuals relate to others; and with issues of meaning and belonging.
4. There are two basic views of spirituality: (1) transcendent view, in which life is ordered and given meaning by a source greater than humankind, and (2) humanistic view, in which life is ordered and given meaning by humankind.
5. This chapter discusses three different models for clinical application: (1) a difference between "healthy spirituality" and "sick religiosity," (2) making meaning through freedom to choose, and (3) acknowledging a presence that orders the world.
6. NANDA International, *DSM-5*, and The Joint Commission recognize the importance of and encourage a spiritual component to nursing care.
7. Some nurses and other professionals believe that nurses are not prepared to provide in-depth spiritual interventions.
8. Nurses can use a spiritual assessment tool to help patients identify spiritual issues. Two brief tools are included in this chapter, and many facilities have their own approach to spiritual assessment.
9. Although often discussed by clinicians, spiritual care remains a neglected component of psychiatric care. Nurses should not be afraid of patients' desires to discuss these issues.
10. There is evidence of the clinical benefits of a healthy spirituality.
11. There is evidence of the harmful consequences of sick religiosity.
12. A clinically trained spiritual care professional should be part of the health care team.
13. Patients experiencing physical distress and facing death often find comfort in the transcendent view of spirituality, although these issues can arouse a sense of discomfort for health care providers.
14. Patients with psychiatric disorders frequently present with conditions with spiritual themes.
15. Nurses can provide comfort, companionship, conversation, and consolation.
16. Nurses can take a spiritual history, pray for the patient under certain conditions, provide spiritual care, and refer to pastoral care.
17. Nurses are encouraged by psychiatric patients to be authentic, caring, and respectful and to speak slowly and in concrete terms.

REFERENCES

American Psychiatric Association, *Diagnostic and statistical manual of mental disorders* (5th ed.). (2013). Arlington, Virginia: APA.

Anandarajah, G., & Hight, E. (2001). Spirituality and medical practice: Using the HOPE questions as a practical tool for spiritual assessment. *American Family Physician, 63,* 81.

Bender, E. (2004). Psychiatrists urge more direct focus on patients' spirituality. *Psychiatric News, 39,* 12.

Brown, D. R., et al. (2013). Assessing spirituality: The relationship between spirituality and mental health. *Journal of Spirituality in Mental Health, 15,* 107–122.

Curlin, F. A., et al. (2007). Religion, spirituality, and medicine: psychiatrists' and other physicians' differing observations, interpretations, and clinical approaches. *American Journal of Psychiatry, 164,* 1825.

Ehman, J. (2013). *References to spirituality, religion, beliefs, and cultural diversity in JCAHO's 2013 Comprehensive accreditation manual for hospitals.* http://www.uphs.upenn.edu/pastoral/resed/JCAHOrefs.pdf, Accessed 19.11.13.

Frankl, V. E. (1984). *Man's search for meaning.* New York: Touchstone.

Freshwater, D. (2006). *Mental health and illness: Questions and answers for counsellors and therapists.* Chichester, United Kingdom: John Wiley & Sons.

Galanter, M. (2008). Addressing patients' spirituality in medical treatment. *Primary Psychiatry, 15,* 82.

Grossoehme, D. H. (2001). Self-reported value of spiritual issues among adolescent psychiatric inpatients. *Journal of Pastoral Care, 55,* 139.

Jung, C. G. (1980). *The archetypes and the collective unconscious* (R.F.C. Hull, Trans.). New York: Princeton University Press and Bollingen Foundation.

Jung, C. G. (1984). *Psychology and Western religion* (R.F.C. Hull, Trans.). New York: Princeton University Press.

Koenig, H. G. (2007). *Spirituality in patient care: Why, how, when, and what* (2nd ed.). Philadelphia: Templeton Foundation Press.

Koenig, H. G. (2008a). Religion and mental health: What should psychiatrists do? *Psychiatric Bulletin, 32,* 201.

Koenig, H. G. (2008b). Religion, spirituality and health: Research and clinical applications, Presented at North American Association of Christians in Social Work, February 5, 2008. Orlando, Florida.

Levine, S. E., & Ion, H. W. (2002). *Against terrible odds: Lessons in resilience from our children.* Boulder, Colorado: Bull Publishing.

Loder, J. E. (1989). *The transforming moment.* Colorado Springs, Colorado: Helmers & Howard.

Möller, M. D. (1999). Meeting spiritual needs on an inpatient unit. *Journal of Psychosocial Nursing and Mental Health Services, 37,* 5.

NANDA International, (2012). *Nursing diagnoses: Definitions and classifications 2012–2014.* http://www.fchs.ac.ae/fchs/uploads/Files/Semester%201%20-%202011-2012/NANDA%20group%20list.pdf, Accessed 19.11.13.

National Consensus Project for Quality Palliative Care, *Clinical practice guidelines for quality palliative care* (2nd ed.). (2009). http://www.nationalconsensusproject.org/guideline.pdf.

Nazir, S. (2010). *What proportion of psychiatrists take a spiritual history?* Psychiatry Special Interest Group of the Royal College of Psychiatrists. http://mhspirituality.org.uk/assets/June2011/Saliha%20Nazir%20What%20proportion%20of%20Psychiatrists%20take%20a%20spiritual%20history%20Edited.z.pdf, Accessed 19.11.13.

Oates, W. E. (1978). *The religious care of the psychiatric patient.* Philadelphia: Westminster Press.

Pargament, K. I. (2013). *What role do religion and spirituality play in mental health?* American Psychological Association. http://www.apa.org/news/press/releases/2013/03/religion-spirituality.aspx, Accessed 19.11.13.

Peteet, J. R., Lu, F. G., & Narrow, W. E. (Eds.), (2011). *Religious and spiritual issues in psychiatric diagnosis: A research agenda for DSM-V.* Arlington, Virginia: APA.

Pew Research Center, *U.S. religious landscape survey: Religious affiliation: Diversity and dynamic.* (2008). The Pew Forum on Religion & Public Life. http://religions.pewforum.org/pdf/report-religious-landscape-study-full.pdf, Accessed 19.11.13.

Pew Research Center, (2012). *"Nones" on the rise: One-in-five adults have no religious affiliation.* The Pew Forum on Religion & Public Life. http://www.pewforum.org/2012/10/09/nones-on-the-rise/, Accessed 19.11.13.

Royal College of Psychiatrists, *Spirituality and mental health.* (2013). http://www.rcpsych.ac.uk/expertadvice/treatmentswellbeing/spirituality.aspx, Accessed 19.11.13.

Smith, C., & Denton, M. L. (2005). *Soul searching: The religious and spiritual lives of American teenagers.* New York: Oxford University Press.

Smolak, A., et al. (2013). Social support and religion: Mental health service use and treatment of schizophrenia. *Community Mental Health Journal, 49,* 444–450.

University of Chicago Medical Center Psychiatrists, (2007). Least religious but most interested in patients' religion. *Press release,* December 12, 2007.

Vaillant, G. E. (2008). Positive emotions, spirituality and the practice of psychiatry. *Mens Sana Monographs, 6,* 48.

Walsh, J. (2012). Spiritual interventions with consumers in recovery from mental illness. *Journal of Spirituality in Mental Health, 14,* 229–241.

Xavier, N. S. (2008). Conscience: The ultimate guide for good relationships, Presented at Alabama Chaplains Association Conference, Birmingham, October 14, 2008.

CHAPTER

7

Models for Working with Psychiatric Patients

Debbie Steele

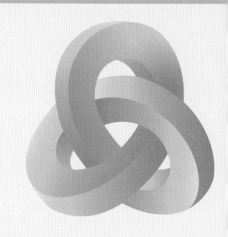

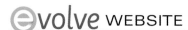 WEBSITE

http://evolve.elsevier.com/Keltner

LEARNING OBJECTIVES

- Compare and contrast major therapeutic models that contribute to the understanding of psychiatric patients and their needs.
- Identify key concepts of the major therapeutic models.
- Describe the relevance of each therapeutic model to psychiatric nursing practice.

This chapter provides an overview of some of the mental health models on which psychiatric nursing has been based. A basic knowledge of the following models is essential in guiding the therapeutic relationship and nursing care. The following models have been selected for discussion in this chapter because they provide essential concepts for working with psychiatric patients: recovery, psychoanalytical, developmental, interpersonal, and cognitive-behavioral. These models are summarized in Table 7-1 and discussed throughout the chapter.

RECOVERY MODEL

The recovery model is well known among most mental health care professionals. It is paramount that nurses delivering services within the mental health care system have a good working knowledge of this model. To understand the recovery model, nurses must recognize that a paradigm shift is required. In particular, the recovery model moves the mental health care system away from the medical model, which is widely used within the health care industry. The medical model of treatment focuses on a person's disease and dysfunction, whereas the focus of the recovery model is on improving a person's competencies, not simply alleviating symptoms. Generally, recovery from a mental disorder does not involve a cure but rather movement toward a meaningful way of life.

Key Concepts

Recovery is defined as "a process of change whereby individuals work to improve their own health and wellness and to live a meaningful life in a community of their choice while striving to achieve their full potential" (SAMHSA, 2011). The 10 guiding principles of the recovery model include the following: (1) person-driven, (2) occurs via many pathways, (3) holistic, (4) supported by peers, (5) supported through relationships, (6) culturally based and influenced, (7) supported by addressing trauma, (8) strength-based, (9) based on respect, and (10) emerges from hope.

Recovery-oriented care is person-driven and self-directed, exemplified by mental health professionals collaborating with consumers instead of telling them what to do. Empowerment includes encouraging consumers to try new things, while taking responsibility for their own care as they navigate their unique journey. Recovery is nonlinear, meaning that setbacks

TABLE 7-1 THERAPEUTIC MODELS

MODEL	ASSUMPTIONS	GOALS AND APPROACHES	DIALOGUE
Recovery	Consumers are the experts with identifiable strengths and abilities.	The consumer and family define and manage treatment options.	*Recovery-oriented responses:* "What are your treatment goals?" "How can I assist you in meeting the goals of your treatment plan?"
		Empower consumers by helping them explore personal options and action plans.	
Psychoanalytical (Freud)	Individuals are motivated by unconscious desires and conflicts. Personality is developed by early childhood.	*Insight* into unconscious conflicts and processes	*Patient:* "All women hate me." *Immediate response:* "Tell me about one woman with whom you are having trouble."
	Illness results from childhood conflicts, and ego defenses are inadequate to cope with anxiety.	Personality reconstruction	*Insight-oriented response:* "Tell me about your relationship with your mother."
	Change is a process of *insight.*	Using free association, dream analysis, and analyses of transference and resistance	
Developmental (Erikson)	Biologic, psychological, social, and environmental factors influence personality development throughout the life cycle.	Mastering developmental tasks through achievement of insight; continued development through death; analyzing developmental issues, fears, and barriers to *growth* to achieve insight	*Patient:* "I can't do anything right. Help me." *Immediate response:* "I hear your doubt in yourself; but I did see you make a positive decision this morning."
	Growth involves resolution of critical tasks at each of the eight developmental stages.		
	Lack of resolution of tasks causes incomplete development and difficulties in relationships.		
	Change involves reexperiencing and resolving developmental crises. Change is a process of *growth.*	Facilitating mastery of developmental tasks with support and problem solving	*Growth-oriented response:* "I can help you look at ways to develop your self-confidence."
Interpersonal (Sullivan, Peplau)	Interpersonal relationships and anxiety facilitate development of the self-system.	Developing satisfactory relationships and maturity; relative freedom from the interference of anxiety; learning effective interpersonal skills	*Patient:* "I can't sit still. I'm too nervous." *Immediate response:* "Let's take a walk for a few minutes."
	Development occurs in stages with changing types of relationships.		
	Faulty patterns of relating interfere with security and maturity.		
	Security operations protect against anxiety and interfere with learning.		
	Change is a process of *reeducation.*	Examining current interpersonal difficulties; using nurse-patient relationships as a vehicle for analyzing interpersonal processes and testing new skills; consensual validation, reality testing, and reflecting positive appraisals	*Reeducation response:* "Let's talk about what kind of things you get nervous about and what you can do about them."

(Continued)

TABLE 7-1 THERAPEUTIC MODELS—CONT'D

MODEL	ASSUMPTIONS	GOALS AND APPROACHES	DIALOGUE
Cognitive-behavioral (Beck, Ellis)	Individuals have value simply because they exist.	Substituting *rational* beliefs for irrational ones	*Patient:* "My wife makes me so angry." *Immediate response:* "What did your wife do that you didn't like?"
	Individuals have potential *rational* and irrational thinking. Irrational beliefs produce irrational emotions and behaviors. Change involves changing beliefs to change feelings and behaviors.	Eliminating self-defeating behaviors Increased responsibility for feelings, behaviors, and change Challenging irrational beliefs; cognitive homework	*Cognitive-behavioral response:* "What is self-defeating about the statement you just made?"
	Change is a process of *rational* thinking.	Role playing and testing out new behaviors	

are not considered failures. Rather, there is an understanding that symptoms may return, and mental health care services may be necessary for a period of time. During this period, it is important to create an atmosphere of hope, emphasizing consumer strengths and abilities. Respect is demonstrated with mental health care personnel taking care not to identify a person by his diagnosis. The individual is not "bipolar" but is the consumer who is experiencing depressive or manic symptoms.

Within the recovery model, the goal of treatment is to help consumers develop meaningful roles in their communities, not to develop long-term relationships with the mental health care system. Support systems, including family, peer, and community members, are central to attaining and maintaining recovery (Berger, 2004). Peer support is an essential element in the recovery process. Peer counselors are individuals who have experience with mental illness within their self-directed journey of recovery. They hold a unique perspective that informs and provides insight for mental health providers, consumers, and their families. After training and certification, peer counselors provide direct support to consumers and educate and provide feedback to mental health care professionals (Ahmed et al., 2012).

Recovery-oriented care is provided in a culturally competent manner that sensitively addresses consumers' race, ethnicity, language preference, age, gender, sexual orientation, religious or spiritual beliefs, and disability. In addition, structural inequities are considered, such as stigmatization, poverty, and homelessness. Recovery-oriented services include social supports, such as housing, income security, employment options, accessible transit systems, paid parental leave, language classes, and educational opportunities.

Relevance to Nursing Practice

Based on the recovery model, there are several key values that inform nursing care of individuals with emotional and behavioral problems. Ideally, individuals need to be regarded as partners in addressing their needs. Assessment of the consumer's general perception of his mental health and desire to make changes provides important insights as nurses

partner with the individual in the recovery process. Mental health consumers are active agents in their own recovery as the nurse aids them in exploring personal options and action plans (Camann, 2010).

The recovery movement has faced resistance from health care professionals who are accustomed to providing services to patients based on what they think is best for them. When patients do not comply with professional directives, they have been labeled noncompliant, unmotivated, treatment-resistant, and uncooperative. Health care professionals who practice recovery-oriented care understand that a patient's resistance can be a good sign—they have some ideas of their own. Collaboration becomes paramount as nurses learn to listen first and then help patients move ahead with their preferred plans. This approach is consistent with the recovery model, whose slogan is "Nothing about us without us!" This slogan translates into incorporation of consumers at every level of planning, training, delivery, policy, and evaluation of mental health care services.

PSYCHOANALYTICAL MODEL

The psychoanalytical model (Brill, 1938; Freud, 1936; Freud & Strachey, 1960) was a theory of the personality originated by Sigmund Freud that emphasized unconscious processes or psychodynamic factors as the basis for motivation and behavior. Freud believed that an individual's drives, instincts, and defenses are formed early in life and are crucial to an understanding of the personality.

In the 1980s, the field of psychoanalysis shifted from the individualism of Freudian theory to a more relationship-oriented self psychology and object relations theory. The essence of self psychology is that every human being longs to be appreciated. Children who are raised by parents who are responsive and accepting develop confidence, whereas children who are rejected move through life forever craving attention. Along the same vein, object relations theory proposes that individuals relate to others based on expectations formed by early experience. Early parent-child interactions determine an individual's mode of relating to other people throughout life. These theories emphasize the prominence of relationships and attachment as key issues in human development (Nichols, 2013).

KEY CONCEPTS

The parents' capacity to provide security for a child's development depends on whether they themselves feel secure. To very young children, parents are not separate individuals but *self objects*, experienced as part of themselves. As parents *mirror* understanding of the child and convey deep appreciation of how their children feel, they validate their child's inner experience. In addition, as the children *idealize* their powerful and strong parents, this identification adds to an already secure sense of self. In essence, if the early parental relationships are secure and loving, the child grows up feeling secure in relationships.

Disruptions in the early parent-child relationship lead to future relationship problems for the children. According to the psychoanalytical theories, relationship problems stem from how people distort their perceptions of others by attributing the qualities of parents to everyone else. This phenomenon is well known as *transference* and *projective identification*. An example of transference is when a patient displaces distrustful feelings for her father onto her male psychiatrist and refuses treatment. Projective identification is interactional by nature, exemplified by a mother who is terrified her teenage daughter will get pregnant, the same thing that happened to the mother at age 16. The anxious mother does not allow her 16-year-old to date boys. Consequently, the teenage daughter begins to sneak out of the house and gets pregnant by her boyfriend. In the end, the teenager is stigmatized, and the parent's overreaction is justified. Parents' inability to accept that their children are separate beings can have dire consequences. The outcome may be continued dependence or violent rebellion. Either way, the children are ill-equipped for mature relationships.

> **NORM'S NOTES**
> The recovery model is a new addition to this chapter that highlights the importance of understanding the meaning individuals have of their health and treatment choices. The Psychiatric-Mental Health Nursing: Scope and Standards of Practice adopted the recovery model, whose slogan is "Nothing about us without us!" I, for one, appreciate this approach and find the slogan refreshing.

Consciousness

Freud's concepts of the levels of consciousness are central to understanding problems of the personality and behavior. *Consciousness*, or material within an individual's awareness, is only one small part of the mind. The unconscious is a larger area and consists of memories, conflicts, experiences, and material that have been repressed and cannot be recalled at will. Preconscious material refers to memories that can be recalled to consciousness with some effort. Freud believed that uncovering unconscious material generates an understanding of behavior that enables individuals to make choices about behavior and improve their mental health. Insight into the meaning of symptoms facilitates change.

Defense Mechanisms

The ego usually copes with anxiety through rational means. However, when anxiety is too painful, the individual copes by using defense mechanisms to protect the ego and diminish anxiety. When these mechanisms are used excessively, individuals are unable to face reality and do not solve their problems. Defense mechanisms are primarily unconscious behaviors; however, some are within voluntary control. Common defense mechanisms are described in Table 7-2.

Painful feelings connected with childhood conflicts are often repressed. Later in life, as similar conflicts are experienced again, repression fails, and these feelings emerge, causing anxiety and discomfort. Freud defined three types of anxiety that form the

TABLE 7-2 DEFENSE MECHANISMS

DEFENSE MECHANISM	DEFINITION	PATIENT EXAMPLE
Denial	*Unconscious* refusal to admit an unacceptable idea or behavior	Mr. Davis, who is alcohol-dependent, believes that he can control his drinking if he so desires.
Repression	*Unconscious* and involuntary forgetting of painful ideas, events, and conflicts	Ms. Young, a victim of incest, no longer remembers the reason she always hated the uncle who molested her.
Suppression	*Conscious* exclusion from awareness anxiety-producing feelings, ideas, and situations	Ms. Ames states to the nurse that she is not ready to talk about her recent divorce.
Rationalization	*Conscious* or *unconscious* attempts to make or prove that one's feelings or behaviors are justifiable	Mr. Jones, diagnosed with schizophrenia, states that he cannot go to work because his coworkers are mean, instead of admitting that his illness interferes with working.
Intellectualization	*Consciously* or *unconsciously* using only logical explanations without feelings or an affective component	Ms. Mann talks about her son's death from cancer as being merciful and shows no signs of her sadness and anger.

(Continued)

TABLE 7-2 DEFENSE MECHANISMS—CONT'D

DEFENSE MECHANISM	DEFINITION	PATIENT EXAMPLE
Dissociation	The *unconscious* separation of painful feelings and emotions from an unacceptable idea, situation, or object	Ms. Adams recalls that when she was sexually molested as a child, she felt as if she were outside of her body watching what was happening without feeling anything.
Identification	*Conscious* or *unconscious* attempt to model oneself after a respected person	Ms. Kelly states to the nurse, "When I get out of the hospital, I want to be a nurse just like you."
Introjection	*Unconsciously* incorporating values and attitudes of others as if they were your own	Without realizing it, Mr. Chad talks and acts similarly to his therapist, analyzing other patients.
Compensation	*Consciously* covering up for a weakness by overemphasizing or making up a desirable trait	Mr. Hahn, who is depressed and unable to share his feelings with other patients, writes and becomes known for his expressive poetry.
Sublimation	*Consciously* or *unconsciously* channeling instinctual drives into acceptable activities	Mr. Smith, a former perpetrator of incest who fears relapse, forms a local chapter of Sex Addicts Anonymous.
Reaction formation	A *conscious* behavior that is the exact opposite of an *unconscious* feeling	Ms. Wren, who unconsciously wishes her mother were dead, continuously tells staff that her mother is wonderful.
Undoing	*Consciously* doing something to counteract or make up for a transgression or wrongdoing	After accidentally eating another patient's cookies, Ms. Donnelly apologizes to the patient, cleans the refrigerator, and labels everyone's snack with their names.
Displacement	*Unconsciously* discharging pent-up feelings to a less threatening object	A husband comes home after a bad day at work and yells at his wife.
Projection	*Unconsciously* or *consciously* blaming someone else for one's difficulties or placing one's unethical desires on someone else	An adolescent comes home late from a dance and states that her date would not bring her home on time.
Conversion	*Unconscious* expression of intrapsychic conflict symbolically through physical symptoms	A student awakens with a migraine headache the morning of a final examination and feels too ill to take the test. She does not realize that 2 hours of cramming left her unprepared.
Regression	*Unconscious* return to an earlier and more comfortable developmental level	A 6-year-old child has been wetting the bed at night since the birth of his baby sister.

basis of many mental illnesses: (1) reality anxiety, stemming from an external real threat; (2) neurotic anxiety, dealing with the fear that instincts will cause a person to do something to invite punishment, such as being promiscuous; and (3) moral anxiety, such as the guilt experienced when an individual acts contrary to his conscience, such as by stealing money from a friend.

Nurse's Role

The goals of Freudian psychoanalytical therapy and other psychodynamic therapies are to bring the unconscious into consciousness, enabling individuals to work through the past and understand their past and present behaviors. By overcoming repression and resistance to exploring feelings and thoughts, childhood experiences can be analyzed. Uncovering the causes of current behaviors leads to insight (Miller, 2004a). Only then can individuals decrease their self-defeating behaviors and improve their mental health.

In traditional long-term psychoanalysis, the nurse therapist uses free association (allowing the patient to say everything that comes to mind) so that repressed material can be identified and interpreted for patients. Dream analysis helps patients uncover the meaning of their dreams, which also increases awareness

about present behavior. Patients' inconsistencies and resistance to therapy are confronted. Transference (an unconscious emotional reaction based on previous experiences) that occurs in the current relationship with the therapist is used to encourage working through feelings that would otherwise remain unconscious. Transference is also discussed in Chapter 9.

Although its roots are in psychoanalytical and psychodynamic therapy, *supportive psychotherapy* was developed for ill patients who were unable to tolerate the intense probing of intrapsychic conflicts, defenses, and transference issues. It involves interaction with the patient (not silent listening) and emphasizes a focus on the present (not on the past). Questioning is less challenging and critical, and the approach conveys empathy and understanding (Miller, 2004b).

Relevance to Nursing Practice

In brief therapeutic encounters, the nurse must recognize and understand the maladaptive defense mechanisms that patients use. The nurse carefully shares observations regarding these mechanisms and works with patients to increase awareness about these behaviors to increase adaptive behaviors. For example, an individual who denies a problem with alcohol must recognize that an arrest for public intoxication, a pending divorce, and three job losses are related to drinking and that abstinence from alcohol is the major adaptive coping mechanism needed. In long-term relationships, patients can be assisted with learning to think, feel, and behave according to their own individual values, beliefs, and needs, not according to someone else's. As an example, a college student who is pursuing an engineering degree at the insistence of a domineering parent can be assisted in deciding her career goals, while developing the ego strength to withstand parental pressures. Patients might also need assistance with accepting their desires and drives as normal, for which they need not feel guilt or shame, and with choosing acceptable ways of expressing their desires and drives.

Clinical Example

A young divorced woman, who has repressed her memories of childhood sexual abuse, projects blame for her divorce onto her husband instead of looking at her painful feelings about sex. She is beginning a new intimate relationship but has not learned to accept her sexuality and desires as normal.

Nursing interventions focus on her feelings about being molested, examining the role of these feelings in fostering the divorce, and accepting her sexual desires as a normal part of being human. The patient might also need guidance in selecting healthy, adaptive outlets for her feelings and desires.

DEVELOPMENTAL MODEL

Erikson's psychosocial theory of development was built on Freud's psychoanalytical model; however, it included the impact of environmental factors, parents, and society on personality development from childhood to adulthood. According to Erikson's theory, every person must pass through a series of eight interrelated stages over the life cycle from birth to death. Each of the stages is associated with two possible outcomes. According to the theory, successful completion of each stage leads to a healthy personality, coupled with successful interactions with others. Failure to complete a stage successfully can result in a reduced ability to grow psychologically and relationally. Table 7-3 outlines adult manifestations of Erikson's eight developmental stages.

TABLE 7-3 ADULT MANIFESTATIONS OF ERIKSON'S STAGES OF DEVELOPMENT

LIFE STAGE	ADULT BEHAVIORS REFLECTING MASTERY	ADULT BEHAVIORS REFLECTING DEVELOPMENTAL PROBLEMS
I. Trust vs. mistrust (0-18 mo)	Realistic trust of self and others	Suspiciousness or testing of others
	Confidence in others	Fear of criticism and closeness
	Optimism and hope	Dissatisfaction and hostility
	Sharing openly with others	Denial of problems
		Withdrawal from others
		or
		Overly trusting of others
		Naive and gullible
		Sharing too quickly and easily
II. Autonomy vs. shame and doubt (18 mo-3 yr)	Self-control and willpower	Self-doubt or self-consciousness
	Realistic self-concept and self-esteem	Dependence on others for approval
	Pride and a sense of good will	Feeling of being exposed or attacked
	Simple cooperativeness	Sense of being out of control of self and one's life
	Knowing when to give and take	Ritualistic behaviors
	Delayed gratification when necessary	Projection of blame and one's feelings
		or
		Excessive independence or defiance, grandiosity
		Reckless disregard for safety of self and others
		Unwillingness to ask for help
		Impulsiveness or inability to wait
III. Initiative vs. guilt (3-5 yr)	An adequate conscience	Excessive guilt or embarrassment
	Initiative balanced with restraint	Passivity and apathy
	Appropriate social behaviors	Avoidance of activities or pleasures
	Curiosity and exploration	Rumination and self-pity
	Healthy competitiveness	Assuming a role as victim or self-punishment
	Original and purposeful activities	Reluctance to show emotions
		Underachievement of potential
		or
		Multiple incomplete projects
		Little sense of guilt for actions

(Continued)

TABLE 7-3   ADULT MANIFESTATIONS OF ERIKSON'S STAGES OF DEVELOPMENT—CONT'D

LIFE STAGE	ADULT BEHAVIORS REFLECTING MASTERY	ADULT BEHAVIORS REFLECTING DEVELOPMENTAL PROBLEMS
		Excessive expression of emotion
		Labile emotions
		Excessive competitiveness or showing off
IV. Industry vs. inferiority (6-12 yr)	Sense of competence	Feeling unworthy and inadequate
	Completion of projects	Poor work history (quitting, being fired, lack of promotions, absenteeism, lack of productivity)
	Pleasure in effort and effectiveness	Inadequate problem solving and follow-through on plans
	Ability to cooperate and compromise	Manipulation of others or violation of others' rights
	Identification with admired others	Lack of friends of the same sex
	Sense of direction	or
	Balance of work and play	Overly high achieving
		Perfectionistic/obsessive-compulsive
		Reluctance to try new things for fear of failing
		Feeling unable to gain love or affection unless totally successful
		Being a workaholic
V. Identity vs. role diffusion (12-20 yr)	Confident sense of self	Lack of or giving up of goals, beliefs, values, productive roles
	Commitment to peer group values	Feelings of confusion, indecision, and alienation
	Emotional stability	Vacillation between dependence and independence
	Development of personal values	Superficial short-term relationships with opposite sex
	Sense of having a place in society	or
	Establishing relationship with the opposite sex	Dramatic overconfidence
	Testing out adult roles	Acting-out behaviors (including alcohol and drug use)
		Seductive or "macho" behaviors
VI. Intimacy vs. isolation (18-30 yr)	Ability to give and receive love	Persistent aloneness or isolation
	Commitments and mutuality with others	Emotional distance in all relationships
	Collaboration in work and affiliations	Prejudices against others
	Sacrificing for others	Lack of established vocation; many career changes
	Responsible sexual behaviors	Seeking of intimacy through casual sexual encounters
	Commitment to career and long-term goals	or
		Possessiveness, jealousy, abusiveness to loved ones
		Dependency on parents or partner or both
VII. Generative lifestyle vs. stagnation or self-absorption (30-65 yr)	Productive, constructive, creative activity	Self-centeredness or self-indulgence
	Personal and professional growth	Exaggerated concern for appearance and possessions
	Parental and societal responsibilities	Lack of interest in the welfare of others
		Lack of civic and professional activities or responsibilities
		Loss of interest in marriage, extramarital affairs, or both
		or
		Too many professional or community activities to the detriment of the family or self
		Taking care of others, not oneself
VIII. Integrity vs. despair (65 yr to death)	Feelings of self-acceptance	Sense of helplessness, hopelessness, worthlessness, uselessness, meaninglessness, or all of these
	Sense of dignity, worth, and importance	Withdrawal and loneliness
	Adaptation to life according to limitations	Regression
	Valuing one's life	Focusing on past mistakes, failures, and dissatisfactions
	Sharing of wisdom	Feeling too old to start over
	Exploration of philosophy of life and death	Giving up on oneself and life
		or
		Inability to reduce amount of activities when needed
		Overtaxing strength and abilities
		Feeling indispensable
		Acting as if life lasts forever

Developed by Schwecke, L., & Wood, S. Indiana University. Revised 2005.

Key Concepts

Each stage in Erikson's model comprises developmental crises as a result of positive and negative experiences. Mastery of critical tasks in each of the stages affects an individual's ability to master future stages. Erikson believed that the drive of humans to live and grow is opposed by a drive to return to more comfortable earlier states and behaviors, known as regression. Regression is common during times of trauma, prolonged or severe stress, and physiologic or psychiatric illnesses.

Implied *but not clearly described* in Erikson's model is the concept of partial mastery of critical tasks in development. The degree of mastery of each stage is related to the degree of maturity that the adult attains. Deficits in development carried from one stage to the next progressively interfere with functioning until the individual is no longer capable of growing without returning emotionally to an earlier stage to resolve life's crises. For example, a person might develop enough trust in others to engage in superficial relationships but may be unable to maintain intimacy with a spouse. Another person might have enough initiative to secure a job but lack the industry to stay with it. An environmental or social tragedy can shake the early foundations of development, such as when divorce from a spouse threatens the children's sense of trust in others and results in self-doubt.

The regression and lack of mastery of developmental tasks seen throughout the life cycle are not necessarily permanent. Individuals can return to earlier stages to master the missing critical tasks. For example, a young teenage mother may not have developed a healthy sense of identity and intimacy as a result of the responsibilities of caring for a child. This young mother is likely to be drawn back to the issues of identity and intimacy as she relates to her child and others in her new adult world. This crisis creates an inherent conflict in roles, feelings, and behaviors. Mastery of the critical tasks of each stage occurs more easily when it is chronologically appropriate. Overcoming delayed or incomplete development is possible but difficult.

Relevance to Nursing Practice

Most patients with psychiatric disorders demonstrate only partial mastery of the developmental stages consistent with their chronologic age. The nurse conducts an assessment of the patient's level of functioning through the interpretation of verbal and nonverbal behaviors and identifies the degree of mastery of each stage up to the patient's chronologic age. The behavioral manifestations of problems reveal issues to be addressed in working with the patient. For example, an adolescent is overwhelmed with shame about being sexually abused as a child. Mature intimate relationships will not be achievable until the shame and doubt are resolved by processing the memories, thoughts, and emotions related to the abuse. Patients diagnosed with schizophrenia are often struggling with trust issues exhibited by suspiciousness and fear of closeness. The nurse must concentrate on trust-building strategies with these patients.

Although Erikson focused on the polarity of each developmental stage (e.g., trust vs. mistrust) as if the positive pole were the desirable task to be accomplished, it is now recognized that the extremes of either pole produce problems in functioning. For example, being overly trusting can result in being repeatedly taken advantage of by others. Having too much industry might result in working 14 to 16 hours a day without any time for recreation. Nursing interventions involving specific developmental issues are discussed in the chapters on specific disorders.

Clinical Example

A patient was admitted because of multiple cuts on the wrists. She says, "My boyfriend kicked me out. I just want to die. I knew I shouldn't trust anyone, ever!" She later reveals a history of abuse and neglect in her birth family and growing up in a series of foster homes. She admits to a fear of closeness, anger outbursts, and a sense of being out of control in regard to her emotions and her life in general. She acknowledges her inability to trust anyone and a sense of shame and guilt about being abused as a child. As she begins to trust the nurse, she agrees to work on (1) how to evaluate the trustworthiness of others, (2) sources of anger and ways to express it appropriately, (3) positive ways to get approval from others, (4) a realistic self-concept and self-esteem, (5) taking control of her life with healthy coping strategies, and (6) developing a healthy support system.

INTERPERSONAL MODEL

Sullivan (1953) developed a comprehensive explanation of interpersonal and intergroup relationships called the *interpersonal theory of psychiatry*, which he believed could be applied to international relations (Brody, 2004). Sullivan, whose background was psychoanalytical, believed that the *interactional* was more important than the *intrapsychic*. Sullivan considered the healthy person a social being with the ability to live effectively in relationships with others. Mental illness was viewed as any degree of lack of awareness or skill in interpersonal relationships. Relationships are viewed as sources of anxiety, maladaptive behaviors, and negative personality formation.

Today, interpersonal psychotherapy (IPT) is used in the treatment of depression and other mood disorders. Systematic studies on IPT, in conjunction with pharmacology, have been promising (Weissman, 2009). Additionally, these studies have emphasized the familial and genetic components of depression. IPT has been adapted for use with other disorders, including eating disorders and anxiety disorders.

Key Concepts

IPT addresses the stressful social and interpersonal dynamics associated with the onset of depressive symptoms. IPT does not propose that the only cause of depressive symptoms is interpersonal; rather, depressive symptoms occur within an interpersonal context that is mutually dependent within the illness. The goal of IPT is to improve social functioning by examining interpersonal disputes, role transitions, grief, and interpersonal deficits.

Interpersonal disputes and role transitions often occur in family, social, or work settings; there may be differing outlooks and expectations. For example, if a wife's attempt to return to work after giving birth led to conflict with her spouse, nurse therapist would explore the dispute, work with the wife to improve communication regarding the conflict, examine the expectations of both spouses, and offer negotiation and problem-solving skills that may improve the situation. When patients experience role transitions (e.g., divorce, caring for aging parents, caring for a chronically ill child), IPT teaches that these transitions are seen as losses, may involve a grieving process, and contribute to depressive symptoms. IPT promotes reappraisal of the inevitable stress related to transitions and changing roles. Additionally, IPT examines the number and quality of relationships, including the therapeutic relationship with the therapist. Interpersonal difficulties can be identified and addressed within the therapeutic relationship, serving as a model for change.

Nurse's Role

The nurse using IPT focuses on a patient's current interpersonal relationships and experiences. The goal of therapy is to develop mature and satisfactory relationships that are relatively free from anxiety. The nurse-patient relationship is a vehicle for analyzing the patient's interpersonal processes and testing new skills in relating. However, the focus of therapy is on the patient's interpersonal issues and distortions created by past experiences. The nurse helps correct these distortions with clear communication, consensual validation, and a warm and collaborative relationship. In challenging a negative self-image, the nurse presents an appraisal of the patient as a worthwhile, respectable individual with rights, dignity, and valuable abilities. The focus of sessions is often on loneliness, fear of rejection, clarifying emotions and their causes, using anxiety for learning about the self and others, managing interpersonal frustrations, and developing self-respect. Sessions are time-limited and rarely last more than 3 months.

Relevance to Nursing Practice

Peplau (1952, 1963) played a significant role in applying Sullivan's original concepts regarding interpersonal relationships to nursing practice. Peplau saw a major goal of nursing as helping patients reduce their anxiety and convert it to constructive action. Peplau (1963) elaborated on and applied Sullivan's concept of degrees of anxiety to nursing (pure euphoria, mild anxiety, moderate anxiety, severe anxiety, panic, terror states, and pure anxiety). Peplau described the effects of mild anxiety through panic levels on perception and learning (see Chapter 27 for a detailed explanation of these processes). She saw the nurse's role as helping patients decrease insecurity and improve functioning through interpersonal relationships that can be seen as microcosms of how patients function in other relationships. For example, a patient says, "My wife always knows when I'm upset and wants to help me, but I just say nothing." The nurse might say, "What are you anxious about when you think about telling her the truth?" Peplau's focus on the patients, their issues, and their interpersonal relationships is especially relevant for

patients with psychosis dealing with delusions, hallucinations, and distorted thinking. Understanding what patients are saying about themselves and their situations and helping them develop coping skills are always important aspects of patient care (Smoyak, 2004).

Clinical Example

The nurse recognizes that a patient experiences increased anxiety whenever he is beginning a relationship with a woman. The patient complains about not knowing what to say or do when he is alone with a woman (lack of interpersonal skills). "I'm so afraid of acting like an idiot that I get tongue-tied and sweaty (anxiety). It's no wonder that I never see her again." Nursing interventions focus on specific sources of anxiety, overcoming insecurities, rehearsing social conversations with the nurse, and practicing social skills in a small group of patients.

COGNITIVE-BEHAVIORAL MODELS

Beck's cognitive therapy (1967, 2005) and Ellis' rational-emotive therapy (1973) models focus on thinking and behaving rather than on expressing feelings. These models use a cognitive approach based on individuals' abilities to think, analyze, judge, decide, and do. Ellis and Beck view individuals' present perceptions, thoughts, assumptions, beliefs, values, attitudes, and philosophies as needing modification or change (Beck, 1976, 2005; Ellis, 1973). Individuals' interpretations of events and expectations of themselves and others (not the actual event or people) are seen as causing the maladaptive responses (Reilly & McDanel, 2005). Even distorted thinking learned from others in childhood can be unlearned.

Key Concepts

Beck and Ellis believe that individuals think both rationally and irrationally and that irrational or illogical beliefs are responsible for causing problems. In theory, irrational thoughts lead to self-defeating behaviors. Individuals are capable of understanding their limitations and can change their values and beliefs while challenging their self-defeating behaviors. The recurrence of irrational thoughts produces emotional disturbances that keep dysfunctional behaviors operant. Rational-emotive therapy teaches individuals to stop blaming themselves and to accept themselves as they are, with flaws and imperfections. Rational-emotive therapy attacks problems from a cognitive, emotive, and behavioral standpoint by using the *A-B-C* theory of personality. *A* is the activating event, *B* is the belief about *A*, and *C* is the emotional reaction. *A* (event) does not cause *C* (emotions); rather, *B* (irrational beliefs about *A*) causes *C*. Intervention is aimed at *B* (irrational beliefs) and is called *D* (disputing and changing irrational beliefs) (Ellis, 1973). The outcome is *E* ("the end result or *profound and effective new philosophies*" or beliefs) (Sacks, 2004). Similarly, cognitive therapy (Beck, 1976, 2005) examines the distorted perceptions, erroneous beliefs, self-deceptions, and blind spots that lead to "excessive, inappropriate emotional reactions" to events or stimuli. Reality testing and problem solving are aimed at correcting faulty cognitions and processes; the individual develops "more realistic appraisals of himself and his world" (Beck, 1976, 2005).

According to Ellis (1973, 2005) and Beck (1976, 2005), most individuals subscribe to at least some of the following irrational beliefs and ineffective rules for living:

- One should feel loved and approved by everyone.
- One must be totally competent to be considered worthwhile.
- Individuals have little ability to change or to control their feelings.
- Influences of the past should determine feelings in the present.
- Rejection or unfair treatment has catastrophic consequences.
- One is disliked when a disagreement exists with another.
- One "should" never make mistakes.
- Individuals who are obnoxious "ought" to be judged as rotten or bad.
- Being passive in life is easier than confronting difficulties and responsibilities.

Cognitive therapy has been adapted for individuals who have experienced traumatic events that often undermine basic assumptions about oneself and life, such as a view of the self as weak rather than strong and the world as threatening and fearful rather than benevolent. The focus of therapy is to challenge these latter assumptions and associated automatic thoughts to help individuals develop more logical assumptions, thoughts, feelings, and behaviors (Robertson et al., 2004).

Cognitive therapy has also been adapted for use on the Internet for patients with substance use disorders (Carroll et al., 2009) and for treatment of depression (Wright et al., 2005):

> *The computer program contains a variety of interactive self-help exercises designed to build skills for using the cognitive and behavioral therapy. Video, audio, graphics, and checklists are used extensively .... Specific content from the program [is] provided at each session: 1) orientation, basic cognitive model; 2) identifying automatic thoughts and cognitive errors using thought records; 3) revising automatic thoughts, finding rational alternatives; 4) behavioral methods, scheduling activities and pleasant events; 5) further behavioral exercises, graded task assignments; 6) identifying and modifying core beliefs; 7) review and further rehearsal (pp. 1158-1159).*

Cognitive-behavioral therapy (CBT) builds on cognitive therapy by incorporating techniques based on learning principles (Geffken et al., 2004) and behavior therapy techniques, including exposure (in vivo or imaginal), response prevention, skill training, and reinforcement. The goal is to work on directly changing behaviors as well as changing faulty thinking. CBT has been used to treat patients of all ages and their families (Suveg et al., 2009). Additionally, CBT with seriously ill patients might use a *multicomponent program*, which could include psychoeducation, medication education, problem solving about daily realities, social skills training, and cognitive skill practice.

Motivational enhancement therapy, a variation of CBT, is more widely used in the treatment of individuals with addictions. The goal is to enhance the patient's readiness and willingness to change habits related to the addictions, using *motivational interviewing*. This nonconfrontational approach includes expressing empathy, pointing out discrepancies between current behaviors and future goals, "rolling with resistance," and promoting self-efficacy. Motivational interviewing uses the concepts of "stages of change ... precontemplation, contemplation, preparation for action, and maintenance" (Miller, 2005).

Dialectical behavior therapy (DBT) (Linehan, 1993) was developed for the treatment of borderline personality disorder, which also has been viewed as complex posttraumatic stress disorder (Herman, 1992). DBT especially focuses on "parasuicidal" patients who have self-mutilation and suicide attempts in their histories (Oldham, 2004). It concentrates on ways to change these behaviors through concurrent individual therapy and group skills training. Contact with the therapist might be included between sessions for intervention with self-harm behaviors. DBT includes interventions related to dissociation, distress tolerance, affect regulation, and core mindfulness (using meditative practices to focus attention on bodily sensations, feelings, and conscious thoughts) (O'Haver Day & Horton-Deutsch, 2004; Robertson et al., 2004).

Nurse's Role

The nurse-patient relationship is viewed as a collaborative effort to achieve goals for improved self-esteem, coping, relationships, and lifestyles (Beck, 1976, 2005). Because patients have many irrational *shoulds*, *oughts*, and *musts*, the nurse therapist actively and directly challenges these beliefs. The nurse therapist demonstrates the degree to which the patient's thinking is irrational and illogical. Humor is often used to confront the patient's ineffective thinking. The nurse therapist explains ways to replace irrational thinking with rational thinking to reduce dysfunctional feelings and behaviors. The process of therapy focuses on the present. Patients learn to take responsibility for their irrational thoughts, feelings, and behaviors and eventually replace them with more productive ones. The nurse therapist accepts patients as they are and does not allow patients to rate or condemn themselves. Homework assignments are given to promote focusing on positive statements and behaviors and on skill development. New, positive self-statements are encouraged to enable patients to begin to think, feel, and behave differently. Role playing, modeling, and reinforcement are also used.

Relevance to Nursing Practice

Nurses help patients change irrational beliefs and reduce stress and anxiety through effective problem solving. Patients have many self-deprecating or negative feelings about themselves that the nurse can dispute by pointing out and reinforcing specific positive attributes. For example, after listening to a patient discuss all of her weaknesses, a nurse might say, "Let's work on a list of your positive qualities and strengths" to facilitate the patient's beliefs that she is worthwhile and has valuable qualities. One message is, "All of us make mistakes at times. Learning from these mistakes helps us grow and become more effective in relating to others." Patients who project blame for all of their problems onto others can be shown that they alone are responsible for their behaviors. Patients with alcoholism are skillful at blaming others for their problems when they alone are responsible for continuing to drink and for the problems that result from drinking. Other patients who continually function according to *shoulds*, *oughts*, and *musts* can be taught to act according to their personal wants and beliefs; they need not condemn themselves for being their own person, and their anxiety and hostile feelings toward themselves and others can be eliminated when they can achieve feelings of comfort about themselves.

Clinical Example

A depressed young man says to the nurse, "My friends have stopped coming around to see me. They say I'm always bragging about myself, but I feel like I have to prove myself to them and myself (irrational belief)." Nursing interventions focus on the acceptance of himself as a worthwhile person with a few weaknesses but many positive qualities. Interventions also challenge his beliefs that he "must" be totally competent in front of others and never make mistakes.

Clinical Example

A male patient is admitted several weeks after his mother has been diagnosed with terminal cancer. He is exhausted and showing symptoms of misperceptions of reality, delusions, and hallucinations. The patient says, "I can't live without her. I'll lose the house. I can't work if she isn't there to get me up and going in the morning. No one else will help me." The nurse develops a care plan that focuses on (1) protecting the patient from harm and reducing the anxiety level, (2) offering emotional and stress management strategies, (3) engaging the patient in anticipatory grief work, (4) developing a new support system, and (5) designing specific plans for getting up and being ready each morning to be on time for work.

INTEGRATIVE APPROACH

Most psychiatric nurses adopt an integrative approach in regard to the therapeutic models presented in this chapter. Concepts from various models that best explain a patient's behavior, problems, and needs are selected. For example, a recently divorced patient states, "I've screwed up my life. All I do is sit at home, cry, and sleep." The nurse might use the psychoanalytical model to identify that the patient is experiencing guilt and regression, the developmental model to understand the patient's dissatisfaction with self and withdrawal from others, or the cognitive-behavioral model to identify the irrational belief that one should never make mistakes. In the interpersonal model, the behavior of crying would be seen as a wish for contact with others and sleep as somnolent detachment. In addition, psychiatric nurses recognize that the key component in any therapeutic model is the *patient-nurse relationship*. This important component is discussed in depth in Chapter 9. The *therapeutic alliance* is often the best predictor of the outcome of any treatment approach (Bender, 2005).

 CRITICAL THINKING QUESTION

1. Which concepts and strategies derived from each of the therapeutic models have you observed being used with patients?

 CRITICAL THINKING QUESTION

2. Read the following case study. Using the models presented in this chapter, what goals would you help this patient achieve?

CASE STUDY

Ms. Levy has been admitted after a suicide attempt. During the admission assessment, she says that she recently began having nightmares about her sexual abuse as a child. She reports a lack of trust of men, yet always seeks their approval. Her interpersonal relationships with women are also stormy. Her anxiety interferes with her work performance. She admits to intense anger about the effect of the abuse on her life but believes that "women shouldn't show their anger." She says that she is afraid to "grow up and be responsible for herself" because she feels overwhelmed by life's stresses.

STUDY NOTES

1. Concepts from various models provide frameworks for understanding patients' behaviors and problems.
2. Recovery-oriented care provides a paradigm shift that emphasizes that the nurse must partner with clients to help them achieve their preferred future.
3. According to Freud, extensive use of defense mechanisms and maladaptive coping behaviors is assessed and understood by the nurse as inhibiting healthy or adaptive responses. The nurse helps patients develop adaptive coping responses or behaviors.
4. Unresolved developmental issues (Erikson) interfere with a patient's ability to solve problems and meet his own needs. These issues must be addressed in the nurse-patient relationship and interventions.
5. Sullivan created the interpersonal model to explain children's and adolescents' skills used in developing healthy adult interpersonal relationships. He also focused on sources of anxiety and coping skills.
6. Peplau used Sullivan's concepts of anxiety as a critical part of her framework in the nurse-patient relationship.

STUDY NOTES—CONT'D

Her goal was to help patients manage anxiety and use it for learning interpersonal skills through the nurse-patient relationship.

7. According to the cognitive-behavioral model, replacing irrational beliefs with rational beliefs can reduce stress and anxiety and self-defeating behaviors.

8. Multiple variations of cognitive and cognitive-behavioral therapies have been developed for specific populations.

9. An integrative approach allows the use of concepts from many models so that different aspects of patients' thoughts, feelings, behaviors, problems, and needs can be explained more thoroughly. No patient "fits" neatly into only one model.

REFERENCES

Ahmed, A., Mabe, A., & Buckley, P. (2012). *Peer specialists as educators for recovery-based systems transformation: The project GREAT experience.* http://www.psychiatrictimes.com/display/article/10168/2028364, Accessed 27.10.12.

Beck, A. T. (1967). *Depression: Chemical, experimental and theoretical aspects.* New York: Noeber Medical Division, Harper & Row.

Beck, A. T. (1976). *Cognitive therapies and the emotional disorders.* New York: International Universities Press.

Beck, A. T. (2005). The current state of cognitive therapy: A 40-year retrospective. *Archives of General Psychiatry, 62,* 953–959.

Bender, D. S. (2005). The therapeutic alliance in the treatment of personality disorders. *Journal of Psychiatric Practice, 11,* 73.

Berger, N. (2004). *How to accomplish practice change in behavioral healthcare in less than one year.* www.bbs.ca.gov/pdf/mhsa/resource/recovery/practice_change.pdf, Accessed October 27, 2012.

Brill, A. A. (Ed.). (1938). *The basic writings of Sigmund Freud.* New York: Random House.

Brody, E. B. (2004). Harry Stack Sullivan, Brock Chisholm, psychiatry, and the World Federation for Mental Health. *Psychiatry, 6,* 38.

Camann, M. A. (2010). The psychiatric nurse's role in application of recovery and decision-making models to integrate health behaviors in the recovery process. *Issues in Mental Health Nursing, 31,* 532–536.

Carroll, K. M., et al. (2009). Enduring effects of a computer-assisted training program for cognitive behavioral therapy: A 6-month follow-up of CBT4CBT. *Drug and Alcohol Dependence, 100,* 178–181.

Ellis, A. (1973). *Humanistic psychotherapy: The rational-emotive approach.* New York: Julian Press.

Ellis, A. (2005). Why I (really) became a therapist. *Journal of Clinical Psychology, 61,* 945–948.

Freud, S. (1936). *The problem of anxiety.* New York: Norton.

Freud, S. & Strachey, J. (Eds.). (1960). *The ego and the id.* New York: Norton.

Geffken, G. R., et al. (2004). Cognitive-behavioral therapy for obsessive-compulsive disorder: review of treatment techniques. *Journal of Psychosocial Nursing and Mental Health Services, 42,* 44–51.

Herman, J. (1992). Complex PTSD: a syndrome in survivors of prolonged and repeated abuse. *Journal of Traumatic Stress, 5,* 377.

Linehan, M. M. (1993). *Cognitive behavioral treatment of borderline personality disorder.* New York: Guilford.

Miller, M. C. (Ed.). (2004a). Interpersonal psychotherapy. In *The Harvard Mental Health Letter, 21,* 1.

Miller, M. C. (Ed.). (2004b). Supportive psychotherapy. In *The Harvard Mental Health Letter, 20,* 1.

Miller, M. C. (Ed.). (2005). Motivational interviewing. In *The Harvard Mental Health Letter, 21,* 5.

Nichols, M. (2013). *Family therapy: Concepts and methods.* Upper Saddle River, New Jersey: Pearson Education.

O'Haver Day, P., & Horton-Deutsch, S. (2004). Using mindfulness-based therapeutic interventions in psychiatric nursing practice—part I: Description and empirical support of mindfulness-based interventions. *Archives of Psychiatric Nursing, 18,* 164.

Oldham, J. M. (2004). Borderline personality disorder: The new treatment dilemma. *Journal of Psychiatric Practice, 10,* 204.

Peplau, H. E. (1952). *Interpersonal relations in nursing.* New York: Putnam.

Peplau, H. E. (1963). A working definition of anxiety. In S. F. Burd & M. A. Marshall (Eds.), *Some clinical approaches to psychiatric nursing* (pp. 323–327). Toronto: Macmillan.

Reilly, C. E., & McDanel, H. (2005). Cognitive therapy: A training model for advanced practice nurses. *Journal of Psychosocial Nursing, 43,* 27.

Robertson, M. F., Humphreys, L., & Ray, R. (2004). Psychological treatment for posttraumatic stress disorder: Recommendations for the clinician based on a review of the literature. *Journal of Psychiatric Practice, 10,* 106.

Sacks, S. B. (2004). Rational emotive behavior therapy. *Journal of Psychosocial Nursing, 42,* 23.

SAMHSA. (2011). *Recovery defined—a unified working definition and set of principles.* http://blog.samhsa.gov/2011/05/20/recovery-defined-a-unified-working-definition-and-set-of-principles/, Accessed 27.10.12.

Smoyak, S. A. (2004). The construction of reality or the deconstruction of the self. *Journal of Psychosocial Nursing, 42,* 6.

Suveg, C., et al. (2009). Cognitive-behavioral therapy for anxiety-disordered youth: Secondary outcomes from a randomized clinical trial evaluating child and family modalities. *Journal of Anxiety Disorders, 23,* 341–349.

Sullivan, H. S. (1953). *Interpersonal theory of psychiatry.* New York: Norton.

Weissman, M. (2009). Depression. *Annals of Epidemiology, 19,* 264–267.

Wright, J. H., et al. (2005). Computer-assisted cognitive therapy for depression: Maintaining efficacy while reducing therapist time. *American Journal of Psychiatry, 162,* 1158.

Learning to Communicate Professionally

Susanne Fogger

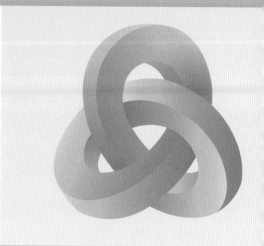

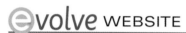 WEBSITE

http://evolve.elsevier.com/Keltner

LEARNING OBJECTIVES

- Understand major influences on communication.
- Distinguish between social and therapeutic communication.
- Identify goals of therapeutic communication.
- Discuss critical therapeutic communication issues.

- Describe various techniques that facilitate patient-centered communication.
- State common causes of interference with therapeutic communication.

Most communication is a two-way process between two or more individuals. In nursing, this process is focused on patients' needs and problems. Professional or therapeutic communication is one of the means whereby the nursing process is implemented to achieve quality patient care. In psychiatric nursing, therapeutic communication is one of the most important tools that nurses can use for building trust, developing therapeutic relationships, providing support and comfort, encouraging growth and change, and implementing patient education.

Nurses rely on verbal, written, telephone, and electronic (computer) communication for sharing information, analyzing data, collaborating with other disciplines, and delivering services. Consequently, nursing requires a solid foundation in effective communication concepts and skills. For nurses who work with patients with problems processing information because of alterations in thinking, feelings, and behavior, the challenge of communicating is even greater. The goal is not only to understand patients' meaning and ensure that they understand the nurse but also to teach patients more effective communication skills for improved outcomes.

CATEGORIES OF COMMUNICATION

Communication is an interaction between two or more people that involves the exchange of information between a sender and a receiver. The product of communication is the message, which is to be interpreted by the receiver. Words (verbal or written) and behaviors (nonverbal) are the primary channels for communication.

Written Communication

Because written material is a primary means of acquiring and sharing information, all professions require written reports, instructions, or sharing of findings and ideas. The skill of mastering vocabulary, grammar, and organization of ideas is critical.

NORM'S NOTES
How important is clear communication? Well, go visit a divorce court, or human relations department hearing, or a malpractice court ("Hey, doc, was that clonidine or Klonopin?"). In many of these cases, poor communication can be identified. Poor communication is a major enemy of human happiness and well-being. When you add a person with a mental disorder or an emotional problem to the equation of human interaction, even more "stuff" can be misconstrued or damaging. Take a good look. You can't go wrong if you thoroughly understand this material.

Telephone Communication

Telephones have provided patients access to crisis and suicide services (hotlines) for many years. Community mental health centers also might provide phone numbers so that patients can call in between visits for information or emergencies. Dealing with patients' perceived or real emergencies by telephone often prevents an inpatient admission. Case management for high-risk patients can use phone contact to facilitate discharge planning and increase adherence to follow-up appointments and treatment, reducing recidivism. The increase in smartphones or pay-as-you-go phones helps individuals who are isolated remain connected with others (Chen et al., 2009). Text messages can also remind patients of upcoming appointments or check-in reminders.

Electronic Communication

Electronic communication requires special attention. E-mail communication or texting is fast and direct. Often the sender and receiver can communicate instantly. However, the ease of communication needs to be balanced with appropriate use. Writing pointed or heated e-mails is a fast and easy way to vent annoyances, but the intelligent nurse will save the message rather than send it when emotions run high. Careers and friendships have been ended by pushing the send button (McGuinness, 2007). In contrast, a study by Leong and associates (2005) found that patient satisfaction with services increased significantly when patients were able to contact their physicians by e-mail. However, the physicians were not equally satisfied; security and privacy concerns, legal and ethical issues, guidelines and standards, and managing the volume of e-mail were some of the problems identified.

Technology also has made long-distance therapy available for patients who do not live near a therapist's office. Patients visit a satellite clinic and interact with the therapist via video contact (Martin et al., 2011; Miller, 2005). The therapist is able to assess the patient's verbal and nonverbal communication even though there may be hundreds of miles between the patient and therapist.

Inpatient and outpatient medical records are increasingly electronic only, but the nurse must ensure documentation accurately reflects the patient's condition, moods, and emotional needs. Extra precautions are required to preserve privacy and confidentiality, such as special screens that prevent people passing by from "accidentally viewing" confidential information.

In addition, wireless connections and smartphones have increased the number of people who use the Internet to access consumer health information. Medical reports, self-diagnostic tools, and other "self-help information" present new challenges for the nurse's role as patient educator. Nurses serve as patient advocates to help sift through the volume of information and offer help in interpreting health information and determining its accuracy.

Health Information Privacy

Whether nurses communicate patient information via written form, telephone, or electronically, all these forms of sharing patient information must comply with the Health Insurance Portability and Accountability Act. The *Standards for Privacy of Individually Identifiable Health Information* (U.S. Department of Health and Human Services, 2013) established a set of national standards for the protection of certain health information. These standards address the use and disclosure of individuals' health information. This information is called *protected health information* by organizations. It is paramount that nurses understand the standards and procedures adopted by their individual work setting for handling patient information.

Speech and Behavior

In addition to sound, oral communication includes the mannerisms and emotional tone that modify the message. The timbre and tone of voice have meaning. The rate and emphasis of speech affect the message. Body language can enhance or change the meaning of words. Verbal and nonverbal communication must match. Behaviors can negate a verbal message; for example, a patient is not likely to (and should not) believe a nurse who says, "Yes, I will help you," with a frown and an angry tone of voice. Often a confused or delirious patient cannot interpret what the nurse is saying but can be soothed by a gentle smile and pleasant affect.

Dynamics of Therapeutic Communication

Therapeutic communication requires attention to multiple, interacting factors. At the core of therapeutic communication are the words and nonverbal behaviors that relate to patients' health needs and are exchanged between patients and the nurse. Carl Rogers, one of the leaders in psychotherapy of the twentieth century, viewed patients with unconditional positive regard as well as with nonjudgmental acceptance. Figure 8-1 illustrates the key variables in communication for the patient and the nurse. Viewing the patient and the nurse as a whole that operates within an environmental context is important. Communication is influenced by the following factors: (1) an individual's personal experiences, gender, culture, values, and beliefs; (2) the purpose of the interaction; and (3) the physical and emotional context of the interaction. The nurse must communicate on patients' levels (according to their vocabulary, educational backgrounds, and the effects of their illnesses) without using a patronizing, condescending, or stigmatizing manner.

"Elderspeak" is a style of discrimination used with elderly patients based on stereotyping older adults as less competent. It usually involves changes in the rate, tone, and volume of speech and a simpler vocabulary and grammar, which are perceived as demeaning or like baby talk (Talerico, 2005). Good communication with someone thought to be hard of hearing requires assessing the individual's hearing before assuming the person is deaf. The nurse should speak clearly and position himself in front of the patient to assist with conversation.

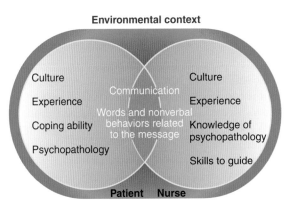

FIG 8-1 Essential and influencing variables of the therapeutic communication environment.

Interpretation of Communication

Interpretation of a message is filtered through an individual's knowledge, experience, and biases. Some aspects of communication are more commonly understood than others. Words are generally understood more precisely than behaviors. However, anyone who has studied a foreign language appreciates that nuances are often lost in translation because of the limitations of words. Both the nurse and the patient bring their own experiences to the relationship, which are different lenses through which each views an event. Having a broad knowledge of the effects of cultures is important if the nurse is to interpret accurately and respond appropriately to patient communications.

Themes in Patient Communications

Patient communications often convey indirect messages or underlying themes about content, mood, or interaction issues. Themes are reflected in patients' thoughts, which engender feelings and then produce behaviors. *Content themes* go beyond the words that a patient is saying and examine underlying messages about patients' perceptions of themselves and their problems over time. Their messages relate to beliefs and values, self-concept and self-esteem, a sense of helplessness and hopelessness, suspiciousness, risk for suicide, and disturbances in thinking or processing of information and beliefs. *Mood themes* relate to affect and the feelings conveyed while patients discuss their issues and concerns. Feelings often reflect shame, guilt, anger, sadness, and fear, which might or might not match the content theme. Affect can be flat, blunted, full range, euphoric, labile, congruent, or incongruent. Assessing for *interaction themes* involves examining the ways in which patients relate to family, friends, other patients, and staff. A patient might call the crisis center each time her roommate is out of town to complain about nervousness and loneliness. When her roommate returns, the patient is comfortable again. The interaction theme might be assessed as one of dependency. The patient who plays one staff member against another and seeks attention by complaining about all the other patients might be showing an interaction theme of manipulation.

In another example, a patient might spend 30 minutes describing his divorce of 3 years ago, two other broken relationships since then, having been laid off from his job, having to sell his house, and feeling as though he is a failure. The underlying *content theme* might be interpreted as a series of major losses. As he describes all these losses, he might convey anger, guilt, or both. These *mood themes* would be congruent with the content theme. Feelings do not always match the content theme. If the patient were laughing as he described his losses, his happiness would be considered as an *incongruent mood theme*. The *interaction theme* might be abandonment or social isolation. Themes are frequently the source of nursing diagnoses on which care plans are based, such as hopelessness, powerlessness, chronic low self-esteem, risk for suicide, denial, anxiety, fear, interrupted family processes, risk for loneliness, noncompliance, or impaired social interaction.

Environmental Considerations

The environment can facilitate or impede therapeutic communication. Factors such as noise level, privacy, type of furniture, space, and temperature can affect the quality of communication.

Ensuring privacy for the patient's conversation is important to the communication between the nurse and patient. Decreasing background noise can provide for clearer communication, especially for individuals hard of hearing. Proxemics refers to the way in which people perceive and use environmental, social, and personal space during interactions. Typically, boundaries of personal space for public and social communication are more distant compared with boundaries for intimate or therapeutic communication. Illness; emotional factors such as suspiciousness, anxiety, perceptual distortions, or aggressiveness; the genders of the two parties; and personal comfort also influence the amount of space needed between the patient and the nurse. Patients are generally more comfortable when the nurse is at their eye level rather than standing over them. Some patients might require sitting at an angle to the nurse or might need a table or empty chair between themselves and the nurse to feel safe enough to talk.

Physical Considerations

Patients with certain physical problems might experience communication difficulties. Patients with certain sensory limitations, such as hearing loss, might have compromised communication necessitating compensatory measures, such as slow, face-to-face speech for lip reading. Developmental disabilities might seriously limit the ability of patients to comprehend and remember. Simple sentences with a single main idea might have to be repeated several times. Speech impediments or other problems might interfere with the nurse's ability to understand the patient's needs. Asking for repetition, clarification, and validation is important, but this can increase a patient's frustration when the practice becomes excessive. Having patients write their answers is an alternative when they are able to read and write. Acute physical pain often interferes with patients' abilities to think clearly and concentrate. Pain may affect the sense of priority regarding problems to be addressed.

Kinesics Considerations

Kinesics is the study of body movements. Culturally based body language is another means by which individuals express their emotional state. Avoiding prolonged eye contact is often used to disengage or ignore communication. In some cultures, eye contact is avoided, and direct eye contact is considered rude. Crossing the arms over the chest often occurs when a person feels defensive (however, this also might occur when a person is cold). The nurse must be sensitive to these cues and interpret them in a global context of therapeutic communication. If the message appears inconsistent or confusing, then exploring the meaning of body language might be useful. For example, the nurse might say, "Many times, when people back away from someone, it is because they are afraid.

Are you afraid right now?" Body language might communicate feelings or emotions or merely reflect a habit. Behaviors in the nurse that communicate caring, confidence, and calmness as well as conveying hope should be cultivated. Reading body language to understand emotions can be a learned process and improves with experience (Minardi, 2013).

> ### ❓ CRITICAL THINKING QUESTION
>
> 1. Ann Williams has multiple facial injuries with both eyes patched, is breathing with a ventilator, and has been sedated. In what ways would you modify your techniques to facilitate communication with her?

THERAPEUTIC COMMUNICATION

Therapeutic versus Social Communication

The focus of therapeutic communication is on helping patients. Social communication involves equal disclosure of personal information and intimacy, and both parties have equal opportunities for spontaneity, with the expectation of mutual confidentiality. Therapeutic communication focuses on the patient but is planned and directed by the professional. During social exchanges, both participants seek to have personal needs met, whereas therapeutic communication focuses on the needs of the patient only. Therapeutic communication guides the patient to explore current personal issues and occasionally painful feelings. Remaining professional means maintaining a calculated emotional distance, near enough to be involved but objective enough to be helpful. Although confidentiality must be respected outside the treatment setting, a professional is obligated to share patient information with the treatment team, so the nurse needs to make it clear that she cannot keep secrets for the patient. The nurse is a patient's advocate, not a patient's friend.

Therapeutic Use of Self

In psychiatric nursing, the nurse, using verbal and nonverbal communication, is the primary therapeutic agent with psychiatric patients (compared with treatment procedures and physical interventions used by the medical-surgical nurse). The nurse's communication is a major vehicle that helps patients achieve productive thinking and good emotional and behavioral outcomes. Use of self, medications, and the environment are the major components of psychotherapeutic management.

Using silence and therapeutic listening are important components of the therapeutic use of self with patients; these are crucial for getting to know patients as individuals as well as their needs and concerns. Therapeutic listening has been described as being composed of the following attributes (Kemper, 1992):

- Being actively alert
- "Hearing" with all the senses
- Using eye contact
- Exhibiting an attending posture

- Ensuring concentration
- Being patient
- Displaying an openness to receive information
- Offering empathy and support
- Asking questions
- Assimilating verbal and nonverbal information
- Organizing, synthesizing, and interpreting information
- Validating and clarifying information
- Responding verbally and nonverbally to encourage patients to continue
- Summarizing important points
- Giving feedback appropriately

> ### ❓ CRITICAL THINKING QUESTION
>
> 2. Select three or four of the previous behaviors and communicate with a friend. What difference do you see in the way your friend responds?

Therapeutic use of the self requires the sensitivity to recognize important cues and make decisions about the priority of these cues. Objectivity is the process of remaining open to as many aspects of patients, their problems, and potential solutions as possible. Objectivity requires self-awareness by nurses to decrease their self-consciousness, blaming themselves (Horton-Deutsch & Horton, 2003), and their own feelings. Nurses must not allow their own issues and biases to influence their interactions with patients and should avoid being swept away by patients' emotions and perceptions.

Communicating empathy is an essential skill of the nurse. Empathy is the ability to recognize and understand the patient's feelings and point of view objectively. Empathy, expressed verbally and nonverbally, conveys caring, compassion, and concern for patients but never implies that the nurse can fully experience patients' feelings. Empathy helps patients to be more accepting of their feelings and express them more readily.

Being therapeutic includes being genuine and sincere, as conveyed by congruent verbal and nonverbal behaviors, authenticity, and honesty (without total self-disclosure by the nurse). Patients must feel respected, valued, and accepted by the nurse, even when all their behaviors are not tolerated. The nurse should not evaluate patients' thoughts, feelings, and behaviors as right or wrong; rather the nurse helps patients evaluate the effects or consequences of these factors. However, the nurse must also set limits on destructive behaviors to protect the integrity and dignity of patients as well as the safety and rights of other patients.

Touching is a complex issue. The meaning of touch varies widely among cultures, individuals, and patients with different diagnoses. Touching a patient's hand or shoulder or giving a light hug can convey caring, empathy, support, and acceptance. However, touching can be misinterpreted as a violation of personal space or privacy or as a sexual gesture or aggressive move. The use of touch with patients must be approached with caution. Patients' behaviors can provide clues to their ability to tolerate and benefit from touch. For example, a patient who is unable to sit close to the nurse is less likely to want to be touched. A patient who is trusting of the nurse is more likely to accept being touched. A patient who is sexually preoccupied might misinterpret any type of touch. With many patients (particularly patients who have been sexually or physically abused), asking permission before giving a gentle hug is appropriate: "What do you think about getting a hug from me?"

Techniques

Therapeutic techniques are a means of helping patients move toward productive goals but are not goals in themselves. The communication techniques presented in Table 8-1 are arranged in a way that facilitates patients' learning, problem solving, and change. Interactions with patients do not involve using all these techniques sequentially. Many nurse-patient interactions do not use a complete nursing process in a single session, but they always involve using therapeutic techniques. Occasionally, interactions have primarily a social or recreational focus rather than being a problem-solving process, but these still might be beneficial to the patient. Every encounter with a patient can be therapeutic with or without full use of the nursing process.

INTERFERENCE WITH THERAPEUTIC COMMUNICATION

In the same manner that therapeutic communication guides the patient toward goals, certain messages and behaviors interfere with reaching these goals. Some behaviors occur frequently because of nervous mannerisms or result from

TABLE 8-1 THERAPEUTIC TECHNIQUES IN PSYCHIATRIC NURSING

Techniques Fostering Description

Offering self: Making self available and showing interest and concern	"I'll sit with you for a while." "I'll stay with you."
Active listening: Paying close attention to verbal and nonverbal communications, patterns of thinking, feelings, and behaviors	Face the patient; maintain eye contact; be open, alert, and patient; respond appropriately.
Silence: Planned absence of verbal remarks to allow patients to think and say more	Maintain eye contact; convey interest and concern in facial expressions.
Empathy: Recognizing and acknowledging patients' feelings	"I can hear how painful it is for you to talk about this."
Questioning: Using open-ended questions to achieve relevance and depth in discussion (not closed/yes-no questions)	"Who?" "What?" "Where?" "What did you say?" "What happened?" "Tell me about it."
General leads: Using neutral expressions to encourage patients to continue talking	"Go on; I'm listening." "I hear what you are saying."
Restating: Repeating the exact words of patients to remind them of what they said, to let them know that they are heard	"You say you are going home soon." "Your mother wasn't happy to see you?"
Verbalizing the implied: Rephrasing patients' words to highlight an underlying message	*Patient:* "There is nothing to do at home." *Nurse:* "It sounds as if you might be bored at home."
Clarification: Asking patients to restate, elaborate, or give examples of ideas or feelings	"What do you mean by 'feeling sick inside'?" "Give me an example of feeling 'lost.'"

Techniques Fostering Analysis and Conclusions

Making observations: Commenting on what is seen or heard to encourage discussion	"You seem restless." "I noticed you had trouble making a decision about ...."
Presenting reality: Offering a view of what is real and what is not without arguing with the patient	"I know the voices are real to you, but I don't hear them." "I don't see it the same way."
Encouraging description of perceptions: Asking for patients' views of their situations	"What do you think is happening to you right now?" "What do you think is the issue with your wife?"
Voicing doubt: Expressing uncertainty about the reality of patients' perceptions and conclusions	"Is that the only way to interpret it?" "What other conclusion could there be?"
Placing an event in time or sequence: Asking for relationships among events	"When did you do this?" "Then what happened?" "What led up to ...?" "What is the connection between ...?"
Encouraging comparisons: Asking for similarities and differences among feelings, behaviors, and events	"How does this compare with the last time?" "What is different about your feelings today?"
Identifying themes: Asking patients to identify recurrent patterns in thoughts, feelings, and behaviors	"What do you do each time you argue with your wife?" "What feeling do you get when you see your father?"
Summarizing: Reviewing main points and conclusions	"Let's see, so far you have said ...."

TABLE 8-1 THERAPEUTIC TECHNIQUES IN PSYCHIATRIC NURSING—CONT'D

Techniques Fostering Interpretation of Meaning and Importance

Focusing: Pursuing a topic until its meaning or importance is clear

"Explain more about ...."
"What bothers you about ...?"
"What happens when you feel this way?"

Interpreting: Providing a view of the meaning or importance of something
Encouraging evaluation: Asking for patients' views of the meaning or importance of something

"It sounds as if this is very important to you."
"You seem to get in trouble when you ...."
"So what does all this mean to you?"
"How serious is this for you?"
"How important is it to change this behavior?"

Techniques Fostering Problem Solving and Decision Making

Suggesting collaboration: Offering to help patients solve problems
Encouraging goal setting: Asking patients to decide on the type of change needed
Giving information: Providing information that will help patients make better choices

"I can help you understand this better."
"Let's see if we can find an answer."
"What do you think needs to change?"
"What do you want to do differently?"
"I can tell you about your medicines."
"There are self-help groups available."
"What would be the advantage of trying ...?"
"What might happen if you tried ...?"

Encouraging consideration of options: Asking patients to consider the pros and cons of possible options
Encouraging decisions: Asking patients to make a choice among options
Encouraging the formulation of a plan: Probing for step-by-step actions that will be needed

"Which is the best alternative for you?"
"What would work best?"
"What exactly will it take to carry out your plan?"
"What else do you need to do?"

Techniques Fostering Completion of Plans
Testing New Behaviors and Evaluating Outcomes

Rehearsing: Requesting a verbal description of what will be said or done
Role playing: Practicing behaviors; the nurse plays a particular role
Supportive confrontation: Acknowledging the difficulty in changing but pushing for action
Limit setting: Discouraging nonproductive feelings and behaviors and encouraging productive ones

"Tell me exactly what you will say to your wife on Friday."
"I'll play your wife. What do you want to say to me?"
"I know this isn't easy to do, but I think you can do it."
"It's hard, but give it a try."
"You're slipping into your aggressive tone again. Try it again."
"That is a negative comment about yourself. Tell me something positive about yourself."

Feedback: Pointing out specific behaviors and giving impressions of reactions
Encouraging evaluation: Asking patients to evaluate their actions and the outcomes
Reinforcement: Giving feedback on positive behaviors
Repeating steps of the nursing process if needed: Using the steps of the nursing process to get a description of what happened, the degree of success, and ideas for change

"I thought you conveyed anger when you said ...."
"When you said ..., I felt ...."
"How well did it work when you tried ...?"
"What was your husband's reaction?"
"This new approach worked for you. Keep it up."
"What would help you do even better next time?"
"If things didn't go well, what do you want to do differently this time?"

social expectations in the therapeutic situation. The nurse must recognize and overcome any habitual communication problems that might interfere with effective therapeutic communication.

Nurse's Fears and Feelings

Because therapeutic communication involves the use of self, many personal feelings are naturally evoked and can be disturbing. A nurse might easily develop a feeling of fear when communicating with individuals who are experiencing psychotic symptoms or physical distress. Fear compromises therapeutic communication. The nurse might have

concerns such as, "Could this be me someday?" or "My brother does this sometimes; does that mean he's crazy?" or "What if this patient gets angry with me?" Therapeutic communication relies on coming to terms with these types of issues. Individuals become patients because of serious and ongoing difficulties in functioning, not because of an occasional dysfunctional behavior. The nurse should avoid personalizing what patients say and do. Patients who abruptly end a conversation with a nurse are probably responding to their own thoughts or anxieties rather than to something the nurse said. Nurses can benefit not only from analyzing the technique and content of interactions with patients but also from analyzing their own feelings and reactions. Using peers to discuss thoughts and feelings can help prevent internalizing interactions with patients.

Occasionally, a nurse is afraid of harming patients by saying the wrong thing. Patients do not fall apart or act out because of a nurse's single mistake, particularly when the nurse's overall attitude is positive and helpful; however, patients are sensitive to malicious intent and rejection. A mistake can become a therapeutic encounter because the nurse can represent a role model for the proper way to admit and apologize for an error. Many people, including patients with mental illness, have trouble recognizing and correcting mistakes with those who are significant to them. In many situations, a sincere apology, when warranted, can strengthen the relationship.

Another concern is invasion of privacy. Psychiatric nurses investigate personal areas of patients' lives intensely, such as values, beliefs, feelings, intimate relationships, and sexuality, or legally sensitive areas, such as incest, partner abuse, and drug use. Secrets the patient could not or would not discuss with friends or family are important to explore, especially if shame is an underlying emotion. Although patients must address these issues, they are not easy to discuss. The nurse can enhance patients' abilities to be open and honest by explaining the need to know about a sensitive area, by asking questions in a kind and matter-of-fact manner, by conveying empathy, and by reiterating a desire to help.

Ineffective Responses

Learning and consistently using effective communication techniques require practice. In particular, the nurse should work toward decreasing the number of yes-no questions (closed questions) asked of patients. Yes-no answers provide little new information and necessitate asking more questions. The nurse's response to messages should be based on assessment and knowledge of the situation as well as the dynamics of patients' illnesses and problems.

However, beginning nurses might not always interact as effectively as desired. A nurse might become defensive and withdraw from patients who are cursing angrily, rather than discussing the behavior. A patient might pick up on a nurse's anxiety and say, "Are you scared of crazies?" There is a tendency to deny this instead of being more truthful and saying, "I am afraid of saying something that might upset you."

Nurses might get caught up in the unfounded fears and accusations of paranoid patients and inadvertently reinforce the symptoms. Distinguishing between fact and distortion in what patients say is often difficult; the nurse must avoid premature conclusions. For example, staff members did not believe a patient who said he had written the theme song for a popular play. The patient finally brought in his original handwritten sheet music and the list of credits from the play's manuscript for the staff to see. Obtaining information from family members to validate information or waiting until medications help clear delusional thinking is beneficial.

Nurses might be preoccupied with what they want to say next rather than with listening to patients, or a nurse might be listening to a patient but not really hearing or understanding what the patient is saying. Nodding one's head as a patient talks might convey, "I hear you" or "I agree with you"—an important difference. Pretending to care is often easily interpreted by the patient as not being genuine and interferes with the process (Salmon & Young, 2011).

Overuse of one or two therapeutic skills, such as reflecting or restating, can stagnate communications when no movement toward analyzing and problem solving is evident. Giving advice to patients rather than helping them evaluate and choose their own solutions can also impede problem solving. False reassurances, such as, "Everything will be all right" or "Things are bound to get better," are basically promises that the nurse cannot keep. Box 8-1 lists other responses and behaviors that are generally ineffective or inappropriate. Mistakes by the nurse generally can be corrected, explanations given, and damage to the relationship reversed. Patients usually evaluate nurses by their overall attitude of caring and concern rather than by a single inappropriate response.

BOX 8-1   INEFFECTIVE OR INAPPROPRIATE RESPONSES AND BEHAVIORS

Not fully listening; not paying attention
Looking too busy; ignoring the patient
Seeming uncomfortable with silence; fidgeting
Being opinionated; arguing with the patient
Avoiding sensitive topics; changing the topic
Being superficial or using clichés
Having a closed posture; avoiding eye contact with the patient
Making false promises or reassurances
Giving advice or talking too much
Laughing or smiling inappropriately
Showing disapproval or being judgmental
Belittling feelings or minimizing problems
Being defensive or avoiding the patient
Making flippant or sarcastic remarks
Lying or being insincere
Texting with cell phone

■ STUDY NOTES

1. Therapeutic techniques are skills to help people but are not goals in themselves.
2. Therapeutic communication occurs with a plan and a purpose, whereas social communication involves equal levels of intimacy, sharing, and the opportunity for spontaneity.
3. Therapeutic communication differs from social communication because the focus is on the patient rather than on a give-and-take experience.
4. Goals of psychiatric nursing are to understand patients, ensure that patients understand the nurse, and teach more effective communication skills.

5. Listening is a therapeutic communication technique that requires careful concentration to guide the conversation toward a goal.

6. Nurses are responsible for therapeutic communication and must recognize communication barriers, including self-awareness of their own limitations.

7. Some common causes of interference with therapeutic communication are fear, lack of knowledge, insecurity, not being genuine, and inappropriate responses.

REFERENCES

Chen, G., et al. (2009). *MPCS: Mobile-based patient compliance system for chronic illness care.* In *Proceedings of the international workshop on ubiquitous mobile healthcare applications (MobiCare)* (pp. 1–7): IEEE Computer Society Press. http://www.cs.dartmouth.edu/~dfk/papers/chen-mpcs.pdf, Accessed 12/3/13.

Horton-Deutsch, S. L., & Horton, J. M. (2003). Mindfulness: Overcoming intractable conflict. *Archives of Psychiatric Nursing, 17,* 186.

Kemper, B. J. (1992). Therapeutic listening: Developing the concept. *Journal of Psychosocial Nursing and Mental Health Services, 30,* 21.

Leong, S. L., et al. (2005). Enhancing doctor-patient communication using email: A pilot study. *The Journal of the American Board of Family Practice, 18,* 180.

Martin, A., et al. (2011). Differences in readiness between rural hospitals and primary care providers for telemedicine adoption and implementation: Findings from a statewide telemedicine survey. *The Journal of Rural Health, 28,* 8–15.

Miller, M. C. (Ed.). (2005). Long-distance psychotherapy. In *The Harvard Mental Health Letter, 21,* 7.

Minardi, H. (2013). Emotion recognition by mental health professionals and students. *Nursing Standard, 27,* 41–48.

McGuinness, T. (2007). How to fail at e-mail. *Perspectives in Psychiatric Care, 43,* 161–162.

Salmon, P., & Young, B. (2011). Creativity in clinical communication: From communication skills to skilled communication. *Medical Education, 45,* 217–226.

Talerico, K. A. (2005). Enhancing communication with older adults: Overcoming elderspeak. *Journal of Psychosocial Nursing and Mental Health Services, 43,* 12.

U.S. Department of Health and Human Services. (2013). *Standards for privacy of individually identifiable health information* http://www.hhs.gov/ocr/privacy/index.html, Accessed 01/30/2014.

CHAPTER

9

Working with an Individual Patient

Melanie Daniel

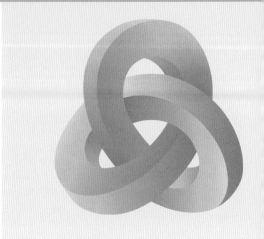

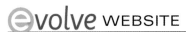

@volve WEBSITE

http://evolve.elsevier.com/Keltner

LEARNING OBJECTIVES

- Describe the meaning of being therapeutic.
- Describe the stages of a therapeutic nurse-patient relationship.
- Apply the nursing process to psychiatric nursing practice.
- Identify the components of the mental status examination.
- Describe the importance of a specific nursing diagnosis and care plan.
- Understand the importance of discharge planning.

Peplau (1952) defined nursing as "a significant, therapeutic, interpersonal process. Nursing is an educative instrument, a maturing force, that aims to promote forward movement of personality in the direction of creative, constructive, productive, personal, and community living." The nurse's relationship with patients consists of a series of goal-directed interactions through which the nurse assesses patients' problems, elicits patient input, selects interventions, and evaluates the effectiveness of care. In psychiatric nursing, the nursing process is grounded in the knowledge of the nature of therapeutic relationships, psychopharmacology, and milieu management, all of which are based on an understanding of concepts and processes of psychopathology. Developing the nurse-patient relationship is the first, and often the most pivotal, step in effective psychotherapeutic management (McCarthy & Aquino-Russell, 2009). Building this relationship (or therapeutic alliance) is vital, especially in the early phases of treatment (Bender, 2005).

THERAPEUTIC RELATIONSHIPS

Many factors influence the relationship between the nurse and the patient, and various therapeutic activities can be used within the relationship to facilitate successful patient outcomes. Each person is a unique, valuable individual who is struggling with internal needs and external realities; the nurse offers presence and engages in a relationship to support the individual's challenges and recognize unique strengths

(McCarthy & Aquino-Russell, 2009). Caring is an essential component of nursing that promotes patients' growth.

NORM'S NOTES
This chapter takes the material presented in Chapter 8 and amplifies it within the context of the nurse-patient relationship. Between your instructor and this textbook, you should learn to be therapeutic—not a therapist, mind you, but therapeutic. Learning to be therapeutic is an enormous gift, and you can use it in all types of situations. For example, how do you react to an angry person or someone who is actively hallucinating? How do you react when a friend learns that her husband is leaving her? This chapter provides some time-tested ideas for common situations that you might face as a nurse and as a friend.

Collaboration

Patients have a right to make decisions about their care. When patients recognize their problems, desire to change, and ask for assistance, the nurse is able to work with them on goals and plans. Collaboration generally produces more effective and enduring change than coercion or simple compliance. However, situations arise during which collaboration is not possible, such as when patients have an obvious disturbance in their thought processes (e.g., severe hallucinations or delusions). Occasionally, the only goal to which a patient will agree is "to get out of the hospital." However, even this goal provides an opening for discussion of behavioral changes that are necessary before discharge can occur. Patients with chronic illnesses might be able to agree to only small changes. Unless the nurse is tolerant, flexible, and realistic, the patient might feel overwhelmed.

Social versus Therapeutic Relationships

The establishment and maintenance of objectivity and goal-directedness is crucial in therapeutic relationships. Patients, particularly individuals with a history of unsatisfying relationships, might misinterpret the nurse's interest and concern. Patients often ask the nurse to be a friend or to go out on a date. In this situation, reminding the patient of the nurse's role and the patient's need for friendship, love, and support becomes necessary—for example, "I realize you would like to date. As a nurse I can help you find ways to form friendships that can offer you emotional support."

BEING THERAPEUTIC VERSUS PROVIDING THERAPY

The nurse's basic education provides the knowledge and skills for being therapeutic in encounters with patients. Psychiatric advanced practice nurses receive specialized training that might focus on a particular therapeutic model that attempts to explain the causes of mental illness or offers specialized techniques for achieving desired outcomes. Advanced practice nurses are also more interested in formalized, ongoing sessions that have a specified time, place, and length and are process-oriented.

In contrast, nurses who engage in therapeutic activities, in an inpatient setting or outpatient program, recognize that each encounter with patients is part of an overall therapeutic picture—a therapeutic milieu. Patients discuss problems and practical solutions and practice skills needed in real-life situations. Brief encounters offer an opportunity for patients to process feelings and thoughts as they occur. Validation and feedback from the nurse are available quickly. Many patients cannot tolerate intense, ongoing therapy but can benefit from consistent therapeutic encounters with nurses, even when their hospitalization lasts only a few days.

Informal or recreational encounters with patients (e.g., card games, craft classes, holiday parties) might be spontaneous but must be therapeutic. For example, the nurse might observe inappropriate social behaviors or a lack of social skills. Helping the patient develop appropriate social and verbal skills, test reality, and solicit feedback and support for new behaviors is appropriate for the nurse. Informal encounters are also opportunities for the nurse to demonstrate ways of handling situations: "Well, we didn't win this hand, but I'm enjoying the game anyway." "I've made that mistake before, too. I can show you how to correct it."

Brief therapeutic relationships are not as formalized as therapy but are planned, patient-centered, and goal-directed. The nurse purposefully and carefully guides conversations with patients toward the exploration of problems, issues, and needs. The nurse might share some personal data, such as age, marital status, or title, but should rarely disclose personal problems. Occasionally, a *brief self-disclosure* might

help patients clarify specific issues, feel less vulnerable, or feel more normal: "When I feel depressed, it's usually because I'm angry and not talking about it. What kinds of things do you get angry about?" or "Sometimes I'm afraid to tell my wife something because I don't know how she will react. What is hard for you to talk about with your wife?" Therapeutic self-disclosure facilitates comfort, honesty, openness, and risk taking but never burdens patients with the nurse's problems.

STAGES OF DEVELOPMENT OF A THERAPEUTIC RELATIONSHIP

When psychiatric care was provided primarily in long-term hospitals, Peplau believed that the nurse and the patient began as strangers and moved in stages to become collaborators in problem solving. In the *stage of orientation*, patients recognize needs and seek help. The nurse helps patients understand their problems and accept the help that is available. The nurse works actively to foster trust and to develop the relationship. In the *identification and exploration stage*, or *working stage*, clarification of perceptions and expectations about the relationship takes place. Problems and identification of tentative solutions are further defined. Patients become more motivated to take advantage of available resources to resolve problems. Patients might test the nurse and might fluctuate between dependence and independence. Peplau believed that the *resolution stage*, or *termination stage*, needs close attention to avoid destroying the benefits gained from the relationship. Focus in this stage is on the growth that occurred and on helping the patient develop self-responsibility for setting new goals. The entire relationship is viewed as promoting growth and as a learning experience for the nurse and for patients (Peplau, 1952).

Therapeutic relationships vary in depth, length, and focus. A brief therapeutic encounter might last only a few minutes, focusing on patients' *immediate needs*, *current feelings*, or *observed behaviors*. In a longer term hospitalization or program, the relationship might last 1 to 3 months with regular meetings that focus on underlying causes of behaviors, developmental issues, or long-term problems.

In this era of brief hospitalization and time-limited outpatient care, the phases of the nurse-patient relationship are not a sequence of processes; rather, they are a matter of different emphases or goals. The nurse concentrates on nursing approaches in a particular phase, depending on the status and needs of individual patients. For example, approaches used in the orientation phase have priority when a patient is highly suspicious because a need exists to develop trust with the patient. For a patient with good insight and motivation, approaches in the working phase are most important because they concentrate on problem solving and change. If the patient is to be admitted for only 3 days, approaches used in the termination phase are critical because of the need for formalizing plans for follow-up care and referrals to other services along the continuum of care.

Moving in and out of the three phases might depend on the patient's ability to cope with various issues (Gauthier, 2000). The patient might be ready to work on divorce issues but might be unable to process incest issues until more trust has been established. Regardless of the phase of the relationship that is most appropriate at any given time, events can alter the patient's situation, necessitating a major change in the nurse-patient relationship. For example, if the patient experiences a crisis event, then the nurse must employ crisis intervention strategies.

Stage I: Orientation Stage

The orientation stage involves nurses learning about patients and their initial concerns and needs (Gauthier, 2000). Patients also learn about the roles of the nurse during this first stage. The initial purpose might be stated as broadly as "identifying a problem on which you want to work," or "helping you figure out what has been happening to you lately." After the problems become more evident, the nurse collaborates with patients to define more specific areas to pursue—for example, learning to be assertive or processing feelings about a divorce. Nurses also help patients look at realistic options so that patients can make their own decisions.

In a longer term outpatient relationship between the patient and the nurse, arrangements are made about the time, length, and frequency of meetings. The session might be for 30 to 60 minutes once a week in a clinic or office or in the patient's home. It is helpful for patients to know the length of time the nurse can spend with them and that the relationship will end at the time of discharge or transfer to another level in the continuum of care.

Building Trust

Trustworthiness is built when the nurse is honest regarding intentions, is consistent, and follows through on actions. Mutual respect and trust are crucial goals. Warmth, interest, and concern are conveyed with words and congruent body language. Clear, specific communications decrease confusion and suspiciousness. Confidentiality is explained in terms of patient information being shared *only* with the immediate unit or program staff and not with anyone outside the treatment setting without the patient's consent and being consistent with Health Insurance Portability and Accountability Act regulations (Grace, 2004).

Because many patients are afraid or unable to approach the nurse, it is important for the nurse to reach out and initiate conversations. Quiet, withdrawn patients are often overlooked because they cannot ask for assistance. An offer to listen and help conveys to patients that they are worthwhile individuals who are respected. Initially, the nurse is nonconfrontational by not openly challenging statements that the patient makes. Such a challenge would interfere with trust.

Beginning Assessment

The initial sessions provide an opportunity to begin an assessment of patients' needs, coping strategies, defense mechanisms, and adaptation styles. Patients' recurring thoughts, feelings, and behaviors (*themes*) are clues to problem areas. Assessing the degree of a patient's awareness of problems and the ability and motivation to change is important.

Although assessment is ongoing and progresses over time, tentative goals are based on the most immediate needs or problems—for example, suicidal or homicidal thoughts, hallucinations, self-mutilation, or acting out.

Managing Emotions

At the time of admission to a unit or a program, patients typically experience painful thoughts and emotions, such as fear, grief, anger, ambivalence, confusion, shame, embarrassment, and guilt. Patients are often afraid of losing control of themselves or of being viewed as weak for expressing their feelings. A way to keep patients from feeling overwhelmed is to talk about their emotions directly. Because patients are likely to try to conceal or minimize feelings, the nurse must be alert to indirect references, nonverbal cues, and voice tones. The nurse can then identify the feeling and ask for validation: "Your voice is loud. You seem tense. What are you feeling right now?"

To cope effectively with feelings, particularly anger, the nurse should remember that the feeling is created not by the nurse but by some situation or significant person in the patient's life. A patient might displace anger onto the nurse at first. If questioned about the anger, however, the patient is more likely to recognize the real source of his or her emotions. Patients must understand that feelings are natural, but that the way they are expressed can cause a problem. Belittling or minimizing a patient's emotions is inappropriate, as is false reassurance, such as saying "Everything will be all right." Patients might feel worse for a while as they begin to face their problems and feelings, and such reassurance is dishonest as well as inappropriate.

Empathy is an objective understanding of the way in which patients see their situation. It can also convey hope for improvement: "I hear how painful this is for you and would like to try to help you deal with the situation in a productive way." Wheeler (2008) sees empathy as one of the most important components of a therapeutic relationship. However, sympathy is the nurse having the same feelings as the patient, and objectivity is lost. Sympathy often leads to comforting, reassuring, or pitying patients. After patients are able to talk directly about emotions, the focus can be on coping more effectively with them. In the orientation stage, resolving the problem that created the feelings is not possible, but temporarily reducing the feelings to a tolerable level by using palliative coping mechanisms is possible. Explaining the experiences and feelings to an empathic listener helps, but when ventilation intensifies the feelings, distracting patients from that topic for a while might be more therapeutic.

Providing Support

Support begins in the orientation stage and continues throughout the nurse-patient relationship. Support confirms patients' worth and rights as human beings and includes the nurse avoiding value judgments of patients (e.g., as bad, stupid, crazy, lazy), even when patients have made poor choices. Support acknowledges that no one is perfect, that making mistakes is human, and that learning from mistakes is beneficial. Support focuses realistically and concretely on patients' abilities and strengths—for example, the nurse would not say, "You're a good person," but rather, "I'm glad you were able to share your feelings in group today." Patients need recognition of their healthy actions and feelings.

Providing Structure

A major strategy in the orientation stage is to provide structure for patients. When patients lose control of their thoughts, feelings, or behaviors, it is the nurse's responsibility to take temporary control. The action might mean offering an as needed (prn) medication; directing patients to a quieter, less stimulating place; or staying with patients at a comfortable distance. If these measures are ineffective, then seclusion or restraints might be indicated. However, providing structure also includes decreasing the withdrawal and isolation of quiet, nonparticipating patients. Spending time with these patients, even in silence, is important. The nurse also can suggest activities, such as watching television or taking a walk with the patient. A major facet of providing structure is *limit setting*. Decreasing or stopping dysfunctional behaviors is in the best interest of patients. Limit setting involves pointing out behaviors and their negative effects and suggesting alternative behaviors. For example, when a patient is self-deprecating, the nurse points out the negative comments and how they affect the patient's self-esteem. The nurse also suggests that the patient identify something positive about himself or herself.

Behaviors that typically require immediate intervention are verbal and physical aggression, self-destructive behaviors, setting fires, noncompliance with rules and medications, alcohol or drug abuse, manipulation of others, inappropriate touching of others, indecent exposure, attempts to leave the hospital without permission, and failure to eat or sleep. Continuous rumination over painful feelings and disturbed thought processes are nonproductive and self-perpetuating. The nurse first listens to the content and the process of negative feelings or thoughts long enough to understand the messages or themes they convey and then distracts the patient with more productive suggestions. Limit setting is a kind but firm strategy: "I know you are angry right now, but I'm having trouble understanding the situation because of all the swearing; please stop" or "I realize that these thoughts are really important to you, but there are other areas I need to know about so I can help you."

The transition from the orientation stage to the working stage is not smooth or firmly defined. Patients' anxiety might increase when they are working on issues, and they might return to more superficial matters for a while. Some patients with chronic illnesses or multiple hospitalizations might need more of a focus on orientation stage interventions because of their difficulty in forming relationships.

Stage II: Working Stage

When patients are ready, the work toward changing their thoughts, feelings, and behaviors can begin. However, drastic changes might not be the goal for some patients, particularly chronically ill patients. Stabilization with medications, reduction of symptoms, and development of supportive relationships are valid goals (Miller, 2005). For patients with chronic schizophrenia in particular, the ability to relate to someone is an important goal. Some patients might be hospitalized several times before they can accept the painful fact that they have a chronic illness and need ongoing treatment (McGorry & McConville, 2000). Most patients have sufficient awareness, motivation, and trust in the nurse to begin to explore problems, identify possible solutions, and test new behaviors (Gauthier, 2000).

In-Depth Data Collection

The nurse facilitates awareness, analysis, and interpretation through in-depth (but selective) exploration of issues and identification of priority issues. Focusing on too many problems at once might overwhelm patients. The nurse directs the data collection and focuses on manageable and changeable issues. In-depth data collection increases the nurse's knowledge of patients' strengths, needs, and problems and of factors that can enhance or interfere with treatment.

Reality Testing and Cognitive Restructuring

Reality testing is an important strategy in the analysis, interpretation, and planning of steps. It helps patients see reality more clearly and objectively and allows patients to consider other options. Reality testing is constructive, not destructive, feedback: "I know the voices seem real to you, but I don't hear any" or "You sound as if you think all women are alike; that has not been my experience."

The goal of reality testing is *cognitive restructuring*—helping patients to cope with negative thoughts and beliefs and to recognize other viewpoints that help them come to more realistic conclusions (Wells-Federman et al., 2001). Patients might need to give up an irrational belief in favor of a more rational one—for example, changing from "I have to be perfect" to "It's okay to make mistakes; I can learn from them." This approach might also mean giving up an unrealistic goal for a more appropriate one.

Writing and Journaling

Having patients write down their thoughts and feelings each day is often useful. This exercise can be a release for emotions and can facilitate a more objective analysis of issues (Wells-Federman et al., 2001). The nurse asks patients to write a homework assignment between sessions—for example, making a list of their positive qualities and strengths. Patients might also write letters (that are *not* sent) to others with whom they are having problems.

Promoting Change

In addition to problem solving, facilitating change can be accomplished through the use of motivational interviewing. Motivational interviewing is a patient-centered, directive approach for enhancing intrinsic motivation to change by exploring and resolving ambivalence. Ambivalence is important to explore because lasting change is difficult to achieve until the patient endorses the necessity for change.

The therapeutic relationship between the nurse and the patient is the means through which feelings are processed using certain basic principles inherent to motivational interviewing. These principles include expressing empathy, developing discrepancy, rolling with resistance, and supporting self-efficacy (Levensky et al., 2007).

The principle of developing discrepancy establishes a cognitive dissonance between the patient's current behavior and his or her desired goals. This conflict is essential in building the foundation for the patient's level of intrinsic motivation. The patient reflects on current behaviors and behaviors he or she would like to adopt. The nurse facilitates the patient's exploration of reasons for change. The struggle to change is called *resistance*, and the nurse's strategy during this phase is supportive. The nurse invites the patient to problem solve possible solutions to the obstacles involved in change, while instilling hope and avoiding confrontation. Self-efficacy is the patient's own belief and confidence that he or she can make and sustain changes in behavior. The nurse's role is to boost the patient's confidence and provide ongoing encouragement.

Prochaska and Norcross (2002) describe five stages of the change process: *precontemplation, contemplation, preparation, action,* and *maintenance*. During precontemplation, the patient has yet to acknowledge that there is a problem and does not plan to change any of his or her own behaviors. During early hospitalization, patients are often in this stage. The most successful intervention is to engage the patient and begin to raise his or her awareness of possible issues. The nurse learns the extent to which patients understand their problems by asking for in-depth, detailed descriptions of situations, thoughts, feelings, and behaviors. Once aware of an issue, the patient enters the stage of contemplation. The patient begins to see that there is a problem and thinks about some action but is not committed to any course of action. Ambivalence is the predominant feeling. When the patient is imminently ready to work on change, he or she has entered the preparation stage.

The nurse does not give advice but helps patients solve their own problems. The nurse encourages short-term, realistic, and achievable daily goals. When the patient initiates a change, he or she moves to the action stage. For example, if a patient's goal is to lose weight, he or she may remain in the preparation stage for some time while thinking about and preparing to begin the process of weight loss. The action stage begins when modifications are made to the patient's daily schedule. The maintenance stage is when the patient has met his or her desired goals and can avoid slipping back into familiar patterns or relapsing into the original behavior. Effective behaviors are more likely to continue when the benefits of the behaviors are discussed and reinforcement is given.

Stage III: Termination Stage

In acute inpatient settings and short-term outpatient programs, the patient's work and changes are rarely completed. Patients are discharged or transferred to another level of care, and nurses change units or jobs. If all the nurses involved with the patient are not available to discuss termination, then the nurse who is assigned to discharge or transfer the patient can implement the strategies.

Evaluation and Summary of Progress

The nurse guides discussions to help patients identify *for themselves* the specific changes in thoughts, feelings, and behaviors that have occurred. Even small steps toward long-term goals are discussed. Reinforcing the changes in and strengths of patients is important. Areas or issues that need more work are outlined, while cautioning patients to avoid trying to change everything at once. Patients are encouraged to set priorities for these issues and to establish reasonable time frames for action.

Synthesizing the Outcomes

Synthesizing focuses on the more indirect outcomes of the nurse-patient relationship, such as more open communications or more appropriate expression of feelings. As a result of the relationship, patients often feel more comfortable with initiating interactions, making requests, and expressing opinions. As the nurse points out the benefits from the relationship, patients are encouraged to form other relationships with future nurses, counselors, and new friends.

Referrals

For problems that need continuing attention after discharge, referrals to appropriate resources are finalized. Providing written discharge instructions and ensuring patients understand them is a nursing responsibility to help facilitate seamless care. If the patient speaks a language other than English, then the instructions can be translated into the patient's native language.

Discussion of Termination

Regardless of the length, frequency of contact, or intensity of the nurse-patient relationship, discussing the participants' reactions to the relationship is important. Feelings might be positive, ambivalent, or negative and may vary in degree. Patients might experience anger or fear related to losing the support and acceptance that the nurse provides. Some patients might avoid any discussion of termination. Nonetheless, the nurse should attempt to make it official by saying "goodbye" and stating his or her feelings about the relationship—for example, "I'm glad I had a chance to work with you."

INTERACTIONS WITH SELECTED BEHAVIORS

The purpose of this section is to discuss interventions that are appropriate in brief encounters with patients to address specific troublesome behaviors. The behaviors included here are behaviors the nurse might encounter with any patient, regardless of the patient's diagnosis. Certain problem behaviors, such as anger and withdrawal, have already been discussed.

Violent Behavior

Fear of violent behavior and of being injured is a concern with the few patients who do not respond to staff efforts at verbal diffusion of anger. The following are a few precautions that can be taken for protection:

- Stay out of striking distance (this also reduces the threat to the patient).
- Avoid touching patients without approval.
- Change the topic temporarily if a patient's behavior is escalating.
- Suggest time out for the patient in a quiet area with fewer stimuli.
- Avoid entering a room alone with a patient who is not in control of his or her behavior.
- Leave temporarily if the patient is agitated and asking to be left alone.
- Call for staff assistance if the patient is losing control.

Hallucinations

Interventions with a patient with hallucinations generally occur in a sequence with newly admitted patients:

1. The initial approach with patients who appear to be listening to or talking with voices is to comment on their behavior: "You look as if you are listening to something. What do you hear?"
2. If the patient acknowledges hearing something that the nurse cannot hear, then the nurse can say, "I don't hear anything. Tell me what you hear."
3. The next step is assessment of hallucinations based on the content of the messages, which often reveals the dynamics of the patient's illness and typically revolves around *themes* of powerlessness, hatred, guilt, or loneliness.
4. After the content is known, focusing on the hallucinations is unnecessary; doing so might reinforce them: "I know the voices are important to you, but let's talk about your loneliness right now."
5. Eventually, the hallucinations are ignored, and the patient is distracted to become engaged in more productive activities or is taught how to distract himself or herself with activities, music, or interactions with others.

The exception is with hallucinations that command patients to harm themselves or others or to do other destructive acts. In such a case, the nurse should contract with patients to avoid acting on the commands they hear and to tell the staff. Another exception is with patients with dementia or severe cognitive impairments. These patients are not likely to be able to process the content or themes of the hallucinations. For them, the strategy of "ignore and distract" is more useful.

Delusions

The initial approach with respect to delusions is clarification of meanings for example, "Who do you think is trying to hurt you?" or "Tell me about this power you think you have." Similar to hallucinations, delusions are not discussed after the meanings are clarified. Arguing with a patient about delusions is ineffective and inappropriate, and it might strengthen the patients' belief in them. The underlying *themes* reflected in the delusions are more appropriately addressed in interventions that help the patient; for example, the nurse would use interventions to help a patient who says she is a queen feel important in realistic ways. Careful monitoring is needed if the delusions might lead patients to harm themselves or others; for example, a patient who does not want to eat because he believes all the food is poisoned needs to be monitored. With patients with dementia or severe cognitive impairments, ignoring and distracting might be more effective.

Conflicting Values

Occasionally, nurses and patients encounter conflicts with their beliefs or values. Nurses must understand the patient's point of view as the patient sees it. Nurses should encourage patients to examine the effects or outcomes of their beliefs on their lives, relationships, and happiness. For example, a patient might believe that she has the right to drink as much and as often as she wants because drinking is legal. Supportive confrontation can help her examine the effects of drinking on her marriage, job, health, and economic status.

Usually, patients need not change a belief or behavior that is not causing problems for them or for others around them. Beliefs and behaviors that have positive effects need reinforcement.

Severe Anxiety and Incoherent Speech Patterns

Disturbed thought processes are occasionally evident in speech, especially with patients who are upset, confused, or psychotic. When these processes occur, the typical approach is to clarify the meaning of the communications. However, severely ill or anxious patients might be unable to be clearer, and repeated questions only increase their anxiety. It is more effective to key into their feelings and underlying *themes*, rather than trying to make sense of the content of their speech. Spending frequent, brief time intervals with these patients (without pressuring or frustrating them) offers support and builds trust.

Manipulation

Common manipulations are a means to gain attention, sympathy, control, and dependence. Manipulation often is not recognized until it has already worked. The nurse might then experience anger or embarrassment. The initial approach is to address what is happening (or has happened):

- "I'm getting the impression that you would like me to tell you what to do. What scares you about this decision?"
- "You are experiencing a lot of emotional pain and would like me to relieve it for you. Let's talk about what *you* can do to relieve it."
- "I see you asking for a lot of attention. What is it that you really want?"

Limit setting is useful with manipulative patients. A power struggle with the patient is useless. Helping patients to express their needs directly to others is more productive.

Crying

Unless crying is a manipulative gesture or is prolonged and unproductive, it should be allowed and encouraged, verbally and nonverbally. By saying, "It's okay to cry" or quietly offering a tissue, the nurse gives patients permission to cry and relieve tension. Privacy should be provided. The nurse should be as quiet and unobtrusive as possible until the crying has ceased. The nurse should then offer the patient an opportunity to discuss the circumstance that precipitated the tears.

Sexual Innuendos or Inappropriate Touch

Patients generally stop inappropriate behaviors when asked and should be reminded that the actions are inappropriate. The nurse then discusses the underlying need. If the behaviors continue, setting limits can be stronger: "I want to talk to you but not if you continue to touch me." "If you don't stop, I will have to leave and come back later." The nurse should refrain from touching patients who have sexual or boundary issues. The nurse is responsible for maintaining professional boundaries in the relationship, especially when the patient is having difficulty with his or her own boundaries (Gutheil, 2005).

Denial and Lack of Cooperation

Patients can be uncooperative with the nurse in working toward treatment goals for many reasons. A common reason is severe disturbances in thought processes (e.g., hallucinations, delusions, disorientation, confusion). With some patients, the disturbances are less evident, but denial of any problems remains, and insight into their problems and recognition of the need for treatment are lacking (McGorry & McConville, 2000). Occasionally, a patient might admit to the need for help but disagrees with the type of treatment offered. Other patients might be afraid of changing, even though they realize that their behaviors are nonproductive or harmful. Listening, clarifying, and verbalizing thoughts that have been implied are appropriate for identifying the underlying causes of a lack of cooperation. The causes, fears, and outcomes of patients' behaviors are then discussed directly: "What are you afraid will happen if you have to give up alcohol as a way of avoiding your problem?" Trust is often an issue for these patients (Bender, 2005); measures to increase trust and a great deal of patience from the nurse are needed.

Depressed Affect, Apathy, and Psychomotor Retardation

When patients express sadness, helplessness, hopelessness, lack of energy, or a negative attitude about everything, the nurse uses patience, frequent contact, and empathy as effective ways for dealing with these feelings. Even when patients realize the change that must be made, they do not always have the energy to make the adjustment quickly. Improvement in personal hygiene, proper nutrition, and a gradual increase in activities are encouraged. Major decisions are postponed until emotions have subsided and thinking is more logical.

Suspiciousness

When patients are suspicious, they might be afraid of everyone. The nurse must communicate clearly, simply, and congruently. Misinterpretations by patients are clarified, but arguments over differences in opinion are avoided. Simple rationales or explanations for rules, activities, occurrences, noises, and requests are offered regularly. Participation of patients is encouraged but not forced, avoiding an increase in their fears.

Hyperactivity

Excessive physical and emotional activity of patients is upsetting to other patients, staff, and hyperactive patients themselves. Patients might unintentionally harm themselves or others. These patients should be in a quiet area, with minimal auditory and visual stimulation. The nurse must remain calm, speak slowly and softly, and respect patients' personal space. Occasionally, prn medications are required, including one to promote sleep.

Transference and Countertransference

Transference involves the unconscious emotional reaction that patients have in a current situation that is based on previous relationships and experiences (Evans, 2007). For example, a patient perceives the nurse as acting the way that his mother did, regardless of how the nurse is truly acting. Transference might be severe, in the form of delusions, or it might be subtle, as in stereotyping all males as aggressive and all females as submissive. Transference can be positive if patients view the nurse as helpful and caring. Negative transference is more difficult because of unpleasant emotions that interfere with treatment, such as anger and fear. Some authors have suggested that transference is an overgeneralization in thinking (Rabinovich & Kacen, 2009).

Countertransference might occur in response to a patient's transference (Jones, 2004). For example, when a patient criticizes the nurse, the nurse might relive feelings that were experienced when a teacher gave negative feedback to him or her in class. Another nurse might remember a favorite teacher who challenged him or her to improve. This range of both positive and negative feelings may interfere with the ability to be therapeutic (Satir et al., 2009).

The first intervention is to recognize the transference or countertransference, which is difficult because of the unconscious processes involved. Coworkers are more likely than others to recognize the phenomenon initially and give feedback to the nurse about it. Nurses must examine their strengths, weaknesses, prejudices, and values before they can interact more appropriately with patients. The transference reactions of patients must also be examined, gently but directly. Limit setting is useful when patients act inappropriately toward the nurse.

NURSING PROCESS

The use of the nursing process has the same goal in psychiatric nursing as it has in other areas of nursing: patient-centered, goal-directed action that facilitates health promotion, primary prevention, treatment, and rehabilitation. Nursing care must be adapted to the unique needs of each patient. Individualized care begins with a detailed assessment.

ASSESSMENT

Initial Patient Assessment

The assessment begins on admission to a unit or program. Each psychiatric hospital, unit, clinic, and program has its own version of an intake or nursing assessment form. Box 9-1 provides a sample of the type of information included in the initial assessment. Although a newly admitted patient might be "medically cleared," both physical and mental health assessment should be the focus of nursing care. Typically, the term *medical clearance* indicates that a cursory examination was performed.

A multidisciplinary team including at least a nurse, psychiatrist, psychologist, social worker, pharmacist, and dietitian is the foundation for quality care (Zwarenstein et al., 2009). A chaplain also might be included on the team to add the component of a spiritual assessment (O'Reilly, 2004). Because most facilities use intake forms or checklists, the results of

---

BOX 9-1 INITIAL PATIENT ASSESSMENT

- **Demographic data:** Full name, gender, age, date of birth, address, marital status, and names and ages of family members, partner, or significant other
- **Admission data:** Date and time of admission and type of admission (voluntary or committed)
- **Reason for admission:** Current problems as perceived by the patient; include stressors, difficulty with coping, developmental issues, "emergency behaviors" (suicidal or homicidal ideas and attempts, aggression, destructive behaviors, risk of escape), and family history
- **Previous psychiatric history:** Dates, inpatient or outpatient, reasons for and types of treatment and their effectiveness, current medications, and compliance
- **Current medical problems and medications:** Allergies, results of laboratory tests, x-rays, and examinations
- **Drug and alcohol use or abuse:** Amount, frequency, duration of past and present use of legal and illegal substances, date and time of last use, and potential for withdrawal symptoms
- **Disturbances in patterns of daily living:** Sleep, intake, elimination, sexual activity, work, leisure, self-care, and hygiene
- **Culture and spirituality:** Ethnicity, beliefs, practices, and religious preference
- **Support systems:** Amount of contact, nature and quality of relationships, and availability of support

---

the interviews do not have to be written in narrative form. Critical facts about the patient should be summarized in an admission note; the admission note is intended to aid other practitioners asked to see the patient.

Mental Status Examination

The mental status examination (MSE) is a very important component of patient assessment in psychiatric settings. The MSE focuses on the patient's current state in terms of thoughts, feelings, and behaviors. The information related to each of the categories includes the following:

- General appearance: Type, condition, and appropriateness of clothing (for age, season, setting), grooming, cleanliness, physical condition, and posture
- Behaviors during the interview: Degree of cooperation, resistance, and engagement
- Social skills: Friendliness, shyness, or withdrawal
- Amount and type of motor activity: Psychomotor agitation or retardation, restlessness, tics, tremors, hypervigilance, or lack of activity
- Speech patterns: Amount, rate, volume, tone, pressured speech, mutism, slurring, or stuttering
- Degree of concentration and attention span
- Orientation: To time, place, person, and situation and level of consciousness
- Memory: Immediate recall, recent, remote, amnesia, and confabulation
- Intellectual functioning: Educational level, use of language and knowledge, abstract versus concrete thinking (proverbs), and calculations (serial sevens)
- Affect: Labile, blunted, flat, incongruent, or inappropriate
- Mood: Specific moods expressed or observed—euphoria, depression, anxiety, anger, guilt, or fear
- Thought clarity: Coherence, confusion, or vagueness
- Thought content: Helplessness, hopelessness, worthlessness, suicidal thoughts or plans, homicidal thoughts or plans, suspiciousness, phobias, obsessions, compulsions, preoccupations, poverty of content, denial, hallucinations (auditory, visual, olfactory, gustatory, tactile), or delusions (of reference, influence, persecution, grandeur, religious, nihilistic, somatic)
- Thought processes reflected in speech: Ambivalence, circumstantiality, tangentiality, thought blocking, loose associations, flight of ideas, perseveration, neologisms, or word salad
- Insight: Degree of awareness of illness, behaviors, problems, and their causes
- Judgment: Soundness of problem solving and decisions
- Motivation: Degree of motivation for treatment

Some patients are too ill to participate in or complete the assessment interview. In these cases, objective data, such as patient behaviors and reports by family members, are used. During the initial assessment, behaviors can be described without knowing or identifying their causes—for example, anxiety level, degree of withdrawal, thought disturbances reflected in speech, voice tone, and general appearance.

Clinical Example

Anita Jarvis, a 46-year-old patient, is separated from her husband, who asked for a divorce and left her 1 week ago. Her son and daughter brought Anita to the hospital after they visited her and found that she had not been getting out of bed to shower or eat. They reported that their mother stated that she wished she were dead. Anita admits to feeling suicidal but denies having any suicide plans. She has no history of medical or psychiatric illnesses and takes no medications. Anita stated that she stopped seeing her friends 1 month ago and does not want to do anything anymore. She is not close to her parents, who live out of state. She called the school in which she teaches 4 days ago and said she was sick. She admits to staying in bed "all the time" but sleeping only 3 to 4 hours a night. Anita was admitted to the hospital with an initial diagnosis of depression.

Mrs. Jarvis and her situation are used in the chapter examples of a process recording (see Table 9-1), MSE (see Box 9-2), progress note (see Box 9-3), and care plan (at the end of the chapter). The process recording is an example of part of an initial assessment with Mrs. Jarvis.

Ongoing Assessments

Even when the initial assessment is complete, each encounter with a patient involves a continuing assessment that might or might not be congruent with the initial assessment. No one acts or feels the same way 24 hours a day, 7 days a week. The ongoing assessment often involves an investigation of patients' statements and actions at the moment: "You have been sitting alone for a while. What have you been thinking about?" When the nurse decides to investigate a patient's specific behavior, exploring the following might be valuable:

- Context or situation that precipitated the behavior
- Patient's thoughts at the time
- Patient's feelings then and now
- Whether the behavior makes sense in that context
- Whether the behavior was adaptive or dysfunctional
- How this episode fits with the total picture of the patient
- Whether a change is needed

A sample MSE with Mrs. Jarvis is presented in Box 9-2.

NURSING DIAGNOSIS

A nursing diagnosis is the identification of patients' problems based on conclusions about the dynamics evident in verbalizations and behaviors. It is directly related to the content, mood, and interaction themes. Emergency behaviors (e.g., suicidal or homicidal ideas or attempts, aggression, destructive behaviors, risk of arson or escape) are given priority in establishing nursing diagnoses and in negotiating no-harm agreements with patients. Suicidal intent should be regularly assessed, whether or not a patient agrees to a no-harm contract (Lynch et al., 2008). The diagnosis should be specific and indicate a desired outcome for the patient. In this text, NANDA International diagnoses are used because they are the most widely accepted and commonly used nursing diagnoses. NANDA International diagnoses suggest a statement format that has the following three components:

1. Risk for actual problems
2. Contributing, causative, or etiologic factors
3. Defining characteristic or behavioral outcome

The statement is typically written as follows: (Problem) related to (contributing factor) as evidenced by (behavioral outcome)—for example, "Anxiety, moderate, related to marital problems as evidenced by ineffective problem solving."

Actual or potential problems are identified from the list approved by NANDA International. Contributing or causative factors can include stressors, losses, past experiences, developmental issues, environmental circumstances, relationship issues, and self-perceptions. Defining

---

BOX 9-2   MENTAL STATUS EXAMINATION WITH MRS. JARVIS

- **General appearance:** Dressed appropriately for season; clothes are clean but not pressed; hair is unwashed and uncombed; slouched shoulders; pale, blank expression
- **Behaviors during interview:** Degree of cooperation, resistance, and engagement—slow to respond but cooperative
- **Social skills:** Withdrawn, no unusual habits, reduced socialization, poor eye contact
- **Amount and type of motor activity:** Slowed, crying at times, no tics or tremors noted
- **Speech patterns:** Amount is reduced with slowed rate and soft tone
- **Degree of concentration and attention span:** Decreased concentration, easily distracted by stimuli, slight shortening of attention span
- **Orientation:** Aware of person, place, and time; responsive
- **Memory:**
  - **Immediate recall:** Remembers nurse's name
  - **Recent:** Difficulty organizing sequence but mostly complete except for last week
  - **Remote:** Good detail on birth of children
- **Thought clarity:** Clear, coherent
- **Thought content:** Expressing helplessness, hopelessness, and suicidal thoughts without a plan; fears being alone; no evidence of hallucinations or delusions
- **Thought process:** No disturbances noted
- **Intellectual functioning:** College education evident in vocabulary, calculations and proverbs were not done, abstract thinking evident in discussion of love and fidelity
- **Affect:** Blunted
- **Mood:** Depressed, anxiety level moderate, guilt and covert anger expressed
- **Insight:** Aware of problems in facing divorce but not yet able to describe factors leading to separation
- **Judgment:** No impairment until last 2 weeks, when she became unable to make decisions, take action, or seek support
- **Motivation for treatment:** Wants help with depression, fatigue, and handling divorce; unable to state what type of help she needs

characteristics or behavioral outcomes are the verbal and nonverbal cues that reflect the patient's actual or potential problems. These maladaptive behaviors or cues are the focus of the nursing interventions—behaviors that it would be helpful to change. Nursing diagnoses do not include medical diagnoses in any of the three parts of the diagnostic statement.

OUTCOME IDENTIFICATION

A goal or outcome specifies an adaptive behavior to replace one that is dysfunctional. Expecting patients to change a negative self-image to a positive self-image during a short inpatient stay or outpatient program is unrealistic. A more realistic behavioral goal would be to ask patients to write a list of their strengths, abilities, and positive qualities. This goal is achievable and measurable. Short-term goals or outcomes are those achievable in perhaps 4 to 6 days for hospitalized patients and longer for patients in other settings. Long-term goals or outcomes relate to issues that require follow-up counseling after discharge to another type of service within the continuum of care. For example, a patient's short-term goal might be to identify difficulties in intimate relationships. The longer term goal is to practice how to respond to anxiety-provoking dating situations; by increasing awareness of fears, the patient might be better able to address these types of situations.

In establishing goals and outcomes *with* a patient (*collaboration*), the nurse must understand the problems the patient wants to address and the goals the patient wants to achieve. Patient desires and motivation play a major role in attaining outcomes (Atreja et al., 2005).

PLANNING AND INTERVENTION
Nursing Care Plans

Nursing staff, on units or in programs, often develop standardized care plans with expected outcomes for certain types of patient problems. These care plans might focus on psychiatric diagnoses (e.g., major depression) or more specific problems (e.g., self-mutilation). Standardized care plans are also called *clinical pathways, critical pathways*, or *multidisciplinary care plans*. The initial care plan might be updated at any time but begins with one or two behavior-oriented problems to be addressed immediately (e.g., suicide, aggression, arson, escape, withdrawal or isolation, delusions, hallucinations, impulsive or compulsive acts, suspiciousness, uncooperativeness, or altered thought processes). For example, a patient who has suicidal ideation (problem) would be expected to sign a no-harm agreement (outcome) within 24 hours (time constraint) and to verbalize a plan for dealing with suicidal ideation (outcome) by day 3 of admission (time constraint). Related nursing interventions would include (1) an agreement with the patient for safety, (2) removal of dangerous objects from the patient and the patient's room, and (3) assessment for suicidal ideation during every shift.

Given the current managed care climate, a goal of standardized care plans is to expedite treatment activities to achieve patient outcomes in a cost-effective manner (i.e., quickly). Nursing interventions focus particularly on "safety, structure, support, and symptom management." However, the nurse must remember that each patient is an individual, even when some of the patient's problems fit into a standardized plan. A patient's unique problems and needs must not be ignored when formulating the plan of care.

There is an increasing recognition of the chronic disease that many people who live with mental illness experience because these people tend to die from chronic diseases many years earlier than their counterparts without psychiatric illness. Medical conditions are undertreated in the psychiatric setting, and the life expectancy for individuals with serious psychiatric disorders is approximately 30% shorter than that of the general U.S. population (Fagiolini & Goracci, 2009). Psychiatric nurses must use both interpersonal skills and health assessment skills on behalf of their patients.

Nevertheless, the focus of psychiatric nursing is often on the verbal strategies that are used to guide patients in solving problems for themselves and achieving desired outcomes. Psychiatric nurses are primarily facilitators and educators. Patients might need help with developing specific and concrete plans for reaching their goals. For example, a patient might set a goal of finding a new apartment but needs assistance in locating rental options and evaluating the pros and cons of each option.

Progress Notes and Shift Reports

The style of charting progress notes (written or electronic) varies in each setting, but the components are basically the same: the patient's statements and the nurse's observations, analyses, and plans. Charting and shift reports are important ways of communicating with team members to ensure continuity of care. These reports are also ways of evaluating the effectiveness of treatment plans and progress toward short-term and long-term patient outcomes. The nurse must remember that the entire chart is a legal document subject to review by peer review agencies, quality improvement staff, and accreditation bodies (Oermann & Huber, 1999). Box 9-3 details the components of a progress note and provides a sample note for Mrs. Jarvis. Shift reports are a concise, focused, and abbreviated list of the items included in the progress notes.

EVALUATION
Patient Progress

The more realistic and measurable the goals are, the greater is the likelihood that patients and nurses will have a sense of progress. A major problem arises with evaluating care in psychiatric nursing when too much change is expected too soon. When the patient or nurse becomes aware of a lack of progress toward goals, evaluation should lead to reassessment.

BOX 9-3   PROGRESS NOTE COMPONENTS

- **Subjective content:** The patient's statements about his or her own thoughts, feelings, behaviors, and problems.
- **Objective data:** The nurse's observations or measurements, such as the patient's appearance, nonverbal behaviors, and vital signs.
- **Analysis or conclusions:** The nurse's impressions of what the patient is experiencing or demonstrating in behavioral or descriptive terms (not medical diagnoses); defenses, mood, and issues are identified; depressed mood and paranoid ideas can be discussed, but "depression" and "paranoia" are not listed as illnesses; conclusions about changes (regression or progression) in the patient and medication responses are described.
- **Plans:** Actions that nurses or other team members can take to intervene with the problems described in the progress note.

Sample Progress Note for Mrs. Jarvis

Date and time: 02/03/2014, 1600.

S: Patient states that she is a little less tired. States she is still unsure of what led to the separation and cannot face living alone. Still has thoughts of suicide but no plan: "I still wish I were dead." Verbalizes a "no-suicide contract." Verbalizes that she still does not know what to do about impending divorce and being alone in the future. Said she called her school to extend her sick leave and called her son and daughter, who will visit this evening.

O: Exhibits blunted, depressed affect; slowed motor activity; and slowed speech. Attended one therapeutic group and a craft activity but participated only briefly. Napped for only 2 hours this shift.

A: Patient cannot describe her thoughts and feelings, but guilt, helplessness, and hopelessness are evident. Anger is barely evident at this point. Suicidal but lacks energy to plan. Support is available from her adult children.

P:

1. Approach and sit with patient frequently.
2. Encourage verbalization of feelings, especially anger.
3. Monitor energy level and suicidal ideation.
4. Continue medications as ordered.
5. Encourage participation in group meetings and activities.

Evaluating patient progress is important in determining patient referrals to other levels of care and supervision within the continuum of care. The issue of prior nonadherence with medications and treatments needs to be addressed early in the admission. This issue might affect the type of referrals made for outpatient care (Julius et al., 2009).

In addition to evaluating the progress of patients, nurses evaluate the quality of their interventions and their professional behaviors.

Discharge Summaries

Many facilities and programs expect nurses to participate in writing transfer or discharge summaries and discharge instructions that are given to patients. Summaries usually identify outcomes that the patient has achieved and outcomes that must still be addressed. Medication (including dosages and times), follow-up appointments (with dates and times), and referrals to other services are often included in the discharge instructions. It is important to assess the patient's ability to read and understand the discharge instructions (Atreja et al., 2005).

Process Recordings

Peplau (1968) used process recordings in her writings to show applications of concepts and examples of interventions. Process recordings are tools for the nurse, particularly for the student nurse, to learn about working with patients effectively. The use of communication skills via process recordings is emphasized as a means of helping patients learn and solve problems.

This method provides a means of assessing and analyzing communication skills, identifying patient themes, and evaluating the effectiveness of interventions (Festa et al., 2000). Audiotape or videotape recordings are more accurate compared with written reports, but it is not always possible to obtain them in most settings or with many patients. A process recording is a record of an encounter with a patient that is as verbatim as possible. The recording generally includes the nonverbal behaviors of the nurse and the patient as well as the verbal interaction.

Analysis of content, mood, and interaction themes might be included next to each written statement or summarized at the end of the process recording. Videotaped nurse-patient clinical simulations also can be used (Festa et al., 2000). A sample written process recording with Mrs. Jarvis is presented in Table 9-1.

? CRITICAL THINKING QUESTION

1. For the patient, Mrs. Jarvis, can you identify two additional nursing diagnoses, two additional short-term goals, two additional long-term goals, and four additional nursing interventions?

CARE PLAN

Name: Anita Jarvis   ***Admission Date:*** _____
DSM-5 Diagnosis: Major Depression

Assessment	**Areas of strength:** Has family who cares, had good work record, has asked for help, is thinking abstractly.
	Problems: Is unable to get out of bed and care for self, has suicidal thoughts but no plan, exhibits decreased socialization and support, impending divorce.
Diagnoses	Risk for suicide related to impending divorce and wish to be dead.
	Anxiety related to anger and fear of living alone, as evidenced by expressed helplessness.
	Hopelessness related to lowered self-esteem, as evidenced by not caring for self.
Outcomes	**Short-term goals**
Date met: _____	Patient will agree to talk with staff when she thinks about wanting to be dead.
Date met: _____	Patient will verbally express anger at husband and situation.
Date met: _____	Patient will telephone friend, employer, and children for assistance.
	Long-term goals
Date met: _____	Patient will state where she will live after discharge.
Date met: _____	Patient will verbalize confidence in her ability to support self.
Date met: _____	Patient will describe resources available to her, especially if she becomes suicidal again.
Planning and Interventions	**Nurse-patient relationship:** Initiate suicide precautions as a nursing measure, monitor energy level and suicidal ideas, encourage activities of daily living, teach relaxation techniques, offer support as feelings are expressed, reinforce strengths, assist in compiling a list of resources.
	Psychopharmacology: Fluoxetine 20 mg PO every morning.
	Milieu management: Encourage patient to stay out of room; request patient attendance at grief and loss, self-esteem, assertiveness, problem-solving, and recreational groups.
Evaluation	Patient will stay with daughter after discharge; patient called employer and requested extended sick leave.
Referral	Patient made appointment for outpatient counseling; patient has information on divorce recovery group and a 24-hour crisis and suicide hotline.

TABLE 9-1 SAMPLE PROCESS RECORDING WITH MRS. JARVIS

Nurse introduces himself to Mrs. Jarvis and leads the way to the office, walking slowly but slightly ahead of the patient. The patient follows without looking at the nurse. In the office, the nurse sits in a chair at a desk and opens a folder of papers. The patient sits in a chair at the side of the desk, holding her purse with both hands on her lap.

NURSE		PATIENT		ANALYSIS	
VERBAL	**NONVERBAL**	**VERBAL**	**NONVERBAL**	**THEMES**	**THERAPEUTIC TECHNIQUES**
What do you prefer to be called, Mrs. Jarvis or Anita?	Has pen in hand, other hand is flat on desk; is looking at patient.	*(pause)* Anita.	Is looking at floor.	Content—oriented to person	Questioning, active listening
Anita, we will be better able to help you if we know more about you. What has happened in your life recently?	(Same as above.)	*(pause)* I couldn't get out of bed. *(pause)* I was so tired.	Is turning head slightly, still looking at the floor; is not smiling or frowning.	Content—describes fatigue and effects	Giving information, questioning
				Mood—sadness Interaction—opens up with nurse	
How long have you been feeling so tired?	Is writing, then looking at patient.	I don't know. *(pause)* A week, I guess.	(Same as above.)	Content—unsure of time frames, marital separation, possible divorce	Placing event in time or sequence, active listening

(Continued)

TABLE 9-1   SAMPLE PROCESS RECORDING WITH MRS. JARVIS—CONT'D

NURSE		PATIENT		ANALYSIS	
VERBAL	NONVERBAL	VERBAL	NONVERBAL	THEMES	THERAPEUTIC TECHNIQUES
What happened a week ago? I can see this is difficult for you to talk about.	Leans toward patient. Moves tissue box. Looks at patient; both arms are on lap.	(pause) My husband (pause) left.	Tears are in eyes; tries to open purse. Is nodding head; raises eyes slightly; is still not looking at the nurse. Starts to cry; gets tissue. Sobs occasionally.	Mood—sadness, guilt	Focusing, using empathy and silence, questioning
(pause) What did he say when he left?		That he was fed up. (pause) That he wanted a divorce.		Interaction—in conflict with husband, is more trusting of nurse	
What did you say to him?	Leans slightly toward patient. One arm is on lap, the other is on arm of chair.	I don't know. I don't remember. (pause) Maybe I asked him to stay.	Is crying quietly.	Content—difficulty describing situations, short-term memory disturbance	Focusing, active listening
Then what happened?	(Same as above.)	It's all a blur; I think I cried all day.	(Same as above.)	Mood—sadness, guilt Interactions— abandonment, loneliness	Focusing
Who did you talk to?	(Same as above.)	No one. (pause) My kids are married and gone. I just stayed in bed.	Is the same but crying less often.	Content—did not ask for help, avoidance of divorce issue Mood—sadness Interaction— perceived lack of support	Focusing
When you were feeling so tired, did you have thoughts of killing yourself?	(Same as above.)	(pause) I was so scared of being alone. I thought I'd rather be dead.	Looks at nurse for the first time; both hands are in lap.	Content—aware of fears, suicidal ideation but no plan, difficulty with problem solving	Questioning
How did you think about killing yourself?	(Same as above.)	I couldn't think of anything. I didn't know what to do.	Looks at floor again; fumbles in purse.	Mood—sadness, depression Interaction— abandonment, lack of support, open with nurse	Focusing
Are you still thinking about suicide?	Hands patient a tissue.	Not really. But (pause) I still wish I were dead. I don't know what to do.	Blows nose and then puts hands in lap; looks at nurse.	Content— minimizing suicidal ideation but ambivalent, helplessness Mood—sadness	Focusing
While you are here, we are going to help you consider some options about what to do so you won't feel so alone and scared. (pause)	Leans forward. Looks at patient. Both hands on lap.	(Silence)	Looks at floor; crying has stopped; looks at nurse.	Interaction— asking for help	Suggesting collaboration, verbalizing the implied, active listening
It will help us if I ask you some questions.	Turns back to papers. Is ready to write.	Okay.	Looks at nurse.		Giving information

STUDY NOTES

1. To be therapeutic, the nurse uses verbal and nonverbal communication to convey a willingness to listen, genuine respect, desire to help, and understanding of the patient as a person with unique problems and needs.

2. The nurse-patient relationship is a series of goal-directed interactions that focus on the patient's thoughts, feelings, behaviors, and potential solutions to problems.

3. The nurse-patient relationship is a tool that the nurse can use to assess the patient's problems, select and carry out specific interventions, and evaluate the effectiveness of care.

4. Each stage of the nurse-patient relationship (orientation, working, termination) involves specific tasks that are employed according to the needs and problems of each patient at a given time.

5. Issues and patient behaviors that interfere with the progress of the nurse-patient relationship must be addressed by the nurse.

6. The nursing process (a systematic approach to treatment) is relevant in psychiatric nursing practice.

7. The nursing process is a tool used by the nurse to assess each patient's problems systematically, select and carry out specific nursing interventions, and evaluate the effectiveness of the interventions on patient outcomes.

8. The initial patient assessment is holistic and includes data from all members of the multidisciplinary team, the patient, and the family.

9. Written patient assessments, care plans, and progress notes provide an important means of ensuring consistency and continuity of care.

10. Evaluation of patient progress is a foundation for discharge planning and for referrals to other services within the continuum of care.

11. Process recordings are learning tools used to clarify communication and facilitate professional growth.

REFERENCES

Atreja, A., Bellam, N., & Levy, S. R. (2005). Strategies to enhance patient adherence: Making it simple. *MedGenMed Medscape General Medicine, 7*, 4.

Bender, D. S. (2005). The therapeutic alliance in the treatment of personality disorders. *Journal of Psychiatric Practice, 11*, 73.

Evans, A. M. (2007). Transference in the nurse-patient relationship. *Journal of Psychiatric and Mental Health Nursing, 14*, 189.

Fagiolini, A., & Goracci, A. (2009). The effects of undertreated chronic medical illnesses in patients with severe mental disorders. *Journal of Clinical Psychiatry, 70*(Suppl. 3), 22.

Festa, L. M., et al. (2000). Maximizing learning outcomes by videotaping nursing students' interactions with a standardized patient. *Journal of Psychosocial Nursing and Mental Health Services, 38*, 37.

Gauthier, P. A. (2000). Use of Peplau's interpersonal relations model to counsel people with AIDS. *Journal of the American Psychiatric Nurses Association, 6*, 119.

Grace, P. J. (2004). Patient safety and the limits of confidentiality. *American Journal of Nursing, 104*, 33.

Gutheil, T. G. (2005). Boundary issues and personality disorders. *Journal of Psychiatric Practice, 11*, 88.

Jones, A. C. (2004). Transference and countertransference. *Perspectives in Psychiatric Care, 40*, 13.

Julius, R. J., Novitsky, M. A., Jr., & Dubin, W. R. (2009). Medication adherence: A review of the literature and implications for clinical practice. *Journal of Psychiatric Practice, 15*, 34.

Levensky, E. R., et al. (2007). Motivational interviewing: An evidence-based approach to counseling helps patients follow treatment recommendations. *American Journal of Nursing, 107*, 50.

Lynch, M. A., et al. (2008). Assessment and management of hospitalized suicidal patients. *Journal of Psychosocial Nursing and Mental Health Services, 46*, 45.

McCarthy, C. T., & Aquino-Russell, C. (2009). A comparison of two nursing theories in practice: Peplau and Parse. *Nursing Science Quarterly, 22*, 34.

McGorry, P. D., & McConville, S. B. (2000). Insight in psychosis. *The Harvard Mental Health Letter, 17*, 3.

Miller, M. C. (Ed.). (2005). Motivational interviewing. In *The Harvard Mental Health Letter, 21*, 5.

Oermann, M. H., & Huber, D. (1999). Patient outcomes: A measure of nursing's value. *American Journal of Nursing, 99*, 40.

O'Reilly, M. L. (2004). Spirituality and mental health clients. *Journal of Psychosocial Nursing, 42*, 44.

Peplau, H. E. (1952). *Interpersonal relations in nursing.* New York: Putnam.

Peplau, H. E. (1968). Psychotherapeutic strategies. *Perspectives in Psychiatric Care, 6*, 264.

Prochaska, J. A., & Norcross, J. C. (2002). Stages of change. In J. C. Norcross (Ed.), *Psychotherapy relationships that work* (pp. 303–313). New York: Oxford University Press.

Rabinovich, M., & Kacen, L. (2009). Let's look at the elephant: Metasynthesis of transference case studies for psychodynamic and cognitive psychotherapy integration. *Psychology and Psychotherapy, 82*, 427.

Satir, D. A., et al. (2009). Countertransference reactions to adolescents with eating disorders: Relationships to clinician and patient factors. *The International Journal of Eating Disorders, 42*, 511.

Wells-Federman, C. L., Stuart-Shor, E., & Webster, A. (2001). Cognitive therapy: Applications for health promotion, disease prevention, and disease management. *Nursing Clinics of North America, 36*, 93.

Wheeler, K. (2008). Psychotherapy for the advanced practice psychiatric nurse. In K. Wheeler (Ed.), *The initial contact and therapeutic communication* (pp. 57–80). St. Louis: Mosby.

Zwarenstein, M., Goldman, J., & Reeves, S. (2009). Interprofessional collaboration: Effects of practice-based interventions on professional practice and healthcare outcomes. *The Cochrane Database of Systematic Reviews*, (3), CD000072.

Working with Groups of Patients

Susanne A. Fogger

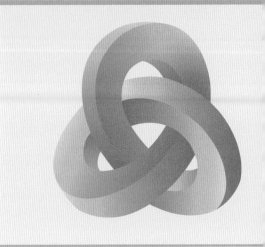

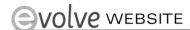 WEBSITE

http://evolve.elsevier.com/Keltner

LEARNING OBJECTIVES

- Describe specific therapeutic benefits of groups.
- Identify the major purpose of each type of group.
- Recognize qualities that the nurse leader of groups should have.

- Identify intervention strategies for common management issues in groups.

Working with groups of patients is an integral component of both inpatient and outpatient psychiatric care. Nurses have 24-hour accountability for patient care on the inpatient psychiatric unit and often are responsible for leading patient groups. This responsibility dictates economic use of nursing personnel; working with groups of patients addresses staff concerns while providing a proven therapeutic intervention. Similarly, working with groups in the community or outpatient arena has increased because of brief inpatient psychiatric hospital stays and the demand of managed care for the least expensive, most effective care. Therapies that help the patient to stabilize quickly and function optimally are currently used (Potter et al., 2004).

Patients with mental illnesses face problems in their daily living similar to problems of others but with the complication of symptoms of mental illness. Although mental illness interferes with the way patients can cope with their problems, conflicts, and interpersonal relationships, patients have the capacity to learn techniques to cope with and negotiate life's problems. Groups deal with current here-and-now issues and stressors. Patients gain awareness and knowledge about their maladaptive behaviors and thoughts. They learn how these behaviors impede communication and coping and become aware of alternatives that help them make better decisions and choices. On inpatient units and in community settings, nurses lead numerous educational and skill-development groups. Nurses also lead groups for patients' families to teach them about mental illness and help them cope with the mentally ill family member. This chapter addresses two questions:

1. Given a patient population that has serious interpersonal and cognitive disturbances, how does group work benefit the individual?
2. What can the nurse realistically expect to accomplish through formal and informal group work with patients?

Because groups typically have short-term, goal-oriented sessions and may be composed of acutely ill patients or patients with persistent and severe mental illness, nurses must have relevant information for developing group strategies. Issues regarding benefits of groups, types of groups, leadership of groups, and common group management are addressed to provide this information. Because working effectively with groups of patients is inextricably related to milieu management, the nurse is encouraged to read Chapters 20 through 22.

NORM'S NOTES
You will frequently work with groups of patients—it is economical, it is practical, and it has therapeutic advantages. Although a traditional group therapy session is rarely seen these days, psychoeducational and support groups are very common. Beyond such relatively formal atmospheres, you will have many opportunities for informal group activities as patients, clients, or consumers congregate in gathering places. A subtle message given in this chapter is that you are always on duty. Even in a day room environment, where patients are mingling casually, your interactions are important and should be therapeutic.

BENEFITS OF GROUPS

Benefits that patients receive from any group experience include the following:

- Patients gain knowledge about ways to relate to and communicate with others (Yalom & Leszcz, 2005).
- Patients gain acceptance, reassurance, and support from their peers and the group leader.
- Patients gain feelings of hopefulness and a sense of power regarding their ability to help themselves and others in the group.
- Patients are provided the opportunity to test out new behaviors with others during their treatment.
- Patients can share their feelings, problems, concerns, and ideas with others in a safe, structured environment.
- Patients' strengths that can enhance self-esteem are affirmed and developed further.
- Patients experience a sense of importance and an increased sense of worth.

These benefits might occur at different times for individual patients and in different group situations. Each group, depending on its goal or purpose, might focus on one particular outcome. For example, an activity group for art might focus on acceptance; no matter what the patients paint, they will be accepted and praised for their work.

THERAPEUTIC FACTORS

Yalom described 11 therapeutic factors that help patients, regardless of the therapeutic group (Box 10-1) (Yalom & Leszcz, 2005). Patients experience certain factors or benefits, depending on the type of group in which they participate; the patients as individuals deem these to be beneficial and important to them. Yalom originally related the therapeutic factors to psychotherapy groups but developed their application to brief, one-time–only groups along the continuum of care. It is important for the nurse to understand the meaning of these therapeutic factors and their significance to patients. The nurse who understands the ways groups help patients is more likely to initiate, lead, and participate in formal and informal groups. Nurses do not make therapeutic factors happen, but they facilitate the development and occurrence of these factors for patients.

TYPES OF GROUPS

Making the inpatient group a positive, beneficial experience for patients is of primary importance. Each session should be treated as a separate entity, with the patient feeling that something positive has been attained during the group session (Yalom & Leszcz, 2005). Patients must believe that they have gained something for themselves during their hospitalization. A positive inpatient group experience favorably predisposes patients to seek treatment on an outpatient basis. After discharge, follow-up care in the community is the setting in which most ongoing treatment occurs.

BOX 10-1   YALOM'S THERAPEUTIC FACTORS

- **Instillation of hope:** Patients receive hope from observing others who have benefited from the group experience.
- **Universality:** Patients experience relief in knowing that they are not alone and unique but that others experience similar problems, feelings, and concerns.
- **Imparting of information:** Patients learn or are provided information about areas related to their needs.
- **Altruism:** Patients experience themselves as helpful or useful to others.
- **Corrective recapitulation of primary family group:** Patients review previous dysfunctional family patterns and learn that these patterns can be changed to meet their present needs effectively.
- **Development of socializing techniques:** Patients are taught appropriate social skills.
- **Imitative behavior:** Patients selectively model healthy behaviors of the leader and other group members.
- **Catharsis:** Patients not only are allowed to express feelings but also are taught ways to express them appropriately.
- **Existential factors:** Patients share feelings about "ultimate concerns" of existence, such as death or isolation, and learn to accept that there is a limit to their control of these issues.
- **Cohesiveness:** Patients experience feelings of being accepted, valued, and part of a group experience.
- **Interpersonal learning:** Patients learn how their behaviors affect others and more appropriate ways of relating in the supportive atmosphere of the group.

From Yalom, I., & Leszcz, M. (2005). *The theory and practice of group psychotherapy* (5th ed.). New York: Basic Books.

Numerous types of groups can be offered in both inpatient and outpatient settings, including psychoeducational, maintenance, and activity. Cognitive behavior therapy, self-help or special problem groups, and multifamily or couple groups are also available in some treatment settings. Traditional therapy groups, such as insight-oriented groups and psychodrama, are no longer offered today because of brief inpatient stays and reimbursement issues. Frequent patient turnover on inpatient units necessitates focusing on topics that can stand independently and deal with patients' immediate needs (Potter et al., 2004).

Psychoeducational Groups

Nurses who work in inpatient or outpatient settings lead groups to offer patients and their families a variety of content and skills. Typically, groups deal with medication, the dynamics and management of illness, problem solving, stress management, anger management, social skills, basic living skills, and relapse prevention (Table 10-1). Groups run by a psychiatric nurse practitioner may include cognitive behavior therapy or other types of therapy. Patients have expressed increased satisfaction with inpatient care when psychoeducational groups focused on illness management, substance abuse, outpatient treatment, and living skills (Hackman et al., 2007). The reduction in inpatient hospitalization has increased the need for patients to learn skills that help them

TABLE 10-1	PSYCHOEDUCATIONAL GROUPS	
TYPE	**NURSE'S PURPOSE OR ROLE**	**EXAMPLES**
Illness	Teach patients and families the content related to dynamics of illness, symptoms of illness, signs of relapse, management of illness, and dealing with crises	Addiction processes, coping with symptoms, management of moods, causes and treatments of illnesses, trigger recognition, relapse prevention, community resources
Medication	Administer medications Assess symptoms and side effects Explain type and purpose of medication, dosage, therapeutic effects, and side effects Provide support measures to prevent relapse	Groups based on category of medications (e.g., antipsychotics vs. antidepressants, intramuscular vs. oral)
Problem solving	Help identify and describe current problems, discuss and develop solutions and their effects, decide on an alternative method and how to try it Evaluate and choose another method, if necessary	Milieu issues, conflict resolution, job concerns, relationship issues, discharge planning, housing issues
Stress management	Teach and facilitate adaptive coping behaviors	Lifestyle balance and management, relaxation training, tension reduction strategies, anger management, mindful meditation
Social skills	Teach, develop, and practice skills to enhance interactions with others; focus on realistic, day-to-day patient needs	Assertiveness training, handling social interactions (e.g., meeting new people, going on interviews, negotiating the return of a purchase)

manage their illnesses and their lives in the community. Increasing inpatient attendance in groups can result in improved patient outcomes and decreased readmission rates (Page & Hooke, 2009).

Group sessions vary in length but typically last 30 to 60 minutes for content presentation and discussion. How long the group meets varies, depending on the patients' level of cognitive and behavioral impairment. An inpatient group might be a 40-minute discussion of medication management, whereas an outpatient group on social skills or a supportive group might be 60 to 90 minutes in length. Nurses must collaborate with patients in treatment planning and developing educational programs based on the patients' needs and interests. The nurse's expertise, empathy, and support help patients learn that they can successfully take care of their illnesses and themselves.

Nurses also provide psychoeducational programs for families of mentally ill individuals. Families are interested in the content on illnesses, medication benefits and side effects, communication with the ill family member, ways to manage crisis situations with patients, and ways to negotiate with the mental health system and managed care to have needs met. Families benefit not only from the information they receive in groups but also from the high level of support that these groups provide. The benefits that families receive from group participation are similar to the patient benefits discussed earlier. Additionally, families experience less anger and have improved relationships with family members as they learn new family communication skills. Families also learn about available resources along the continuum of care and look to the nurse as an advocate and expert to help them arrange for needed services.

Maintenance Groups

The very nature of nursing implies support. The nurse supports patients in therapeutic interactions. Support means accepting, empathizing, and showing concern while listening and talking with patients. The nurse's presence, genuine interest, and encouragement facilitate the expression of patients' feelings and concerns. The nurse is instrumental in helping patients cope with their feelings and situations. Support is useful in many types of group situations.

The purpose of the support group is to reinforce or maintain existing strengths of patients, rather than to confront or change behaviors or defenses. Patients in a support group can be acutely or chronically ill. Group members might need a great deal of reassurance and emotional support during their hospitalization. These patients also need to reduce their anxiety to mild or moderate levels, and management techniques can be taught in group.

The reality orientation group is an example of a support group frequently found in inpatient settings. Patients who exhibit confusion and short attention spans resulting from some psychopathologic factor can benefit from participation in this type of group. The professional must provide an atmosphere of safety and security because these patients might be frightened, unsure, anxious, uncomfortable, and isolated. The reality orientation group can assist patients with decreasing isolation and increasing their self-esteem. Focusing on the here and now provides a framework with structure, social support, and reality testing. The nurse, as leader of this group, facilitates orientation to time, person, and place; rules and routines of the unit; and behavioral expectations, including some limit setting. Feeling valued, respected, and important as human beings is a feeling these patients might not have experienced for some time.

Activity Groups

The general goals of activity groups are to help patients increase self-esteem, expression of feelings, and social interaction. Withdrawn, depressed, and regressed patients benefit from these groups; because these individuals have experienced isolation and have difficulty with interpersonal relationships when interpersonal communication increases, focus on the activity per se decreases. The activity is a vehicle or means to facilitate (1) self-expression of both positive and negative feelings in a creative way, (2) patient interaction, and (3) enjoyment.

Recreation groups provide the opportunity for fun and relieve tension. Exercise groups or groups that foster physical activity benefit individuals mentally and physically by improving physical health and reducing psychiatric and social disability. These groups enable patients to experience a sense of participation, acceptance, and accomplishment. Individuals with serious mental illness often have sedentary lifestyles and possibly comorbid physical health problems. Psychiatric medications can induce weight gain, and diet modification with exercise can decrease the weight gain. Integration of a structured program, such as a walking group or exercise group, can be helpful. Individuals with serious mental illness value exercise as a component of their treatment (Richardson et al., 2005).

Self-Help and Special Problem Groups

Many groups focus on helping individuals with special problems; examples are weight loss, child abuse, anorexia and bulimia, and diabetes. These groups are homogeneous, meaning that all group members share the same problem. Members feel accepted and understood by the group and are more willing to share concerns and ask questions. Information is shared as well as personal feelings and difficulties. Members assist each other with helpful strategies; they do not feel alone or isolated but learn that others with the same problem or need are coping effectively. The nurse who leads special problem groups is interested, knowledgeable, and skilled in working with patients with specific problems.

Traditional self-help groups are also homogeneous but are not professionally organized and led. Self-help groups are organized and led by group members who share a similar problem. Self-help is based on the belief that an individual with a problem can be truly understood and helped only by others who have the same problem. Millions of people participate in hundreds of self-help groups. In some groups, such as Alcoholics Anonymous, individual 24-hour support is available. Members of self-help groups understand each other's lifestyles and needs, help each other solve problems and cope with stress, and confront each other about dysfunctional behaviors.

Professionals might be invited to a self-help group for a specific purpose, such as providing an educational program. Nurses commonly refer individuals to self-help groups and must be knowledgeable about the self-help groups in their area. For information about the availability of groups, individuals can call their local mental health organizations or Mental Health America and the National Alliance for the Mentally Ill (NAMI). NAMI can be very helpful as a support for families of patients affected by mental illness. Their website is a helpful reference for families (http://www.nami.org/).

GROUP MANAGEMENT ISSUES

Group Leadership

Group leadership functions range from formal to informal. The inpatient psychiatric nurse might engage in spontaneous, informal interactions with a group of patients in a card game or participate formally in a planned, structured group session in a special setting. An informal card game provides the nurse with an opportunity for therapeutic interpersonal interaction, socialization, and role-modeling behavior. Another example might be responding to medication questions that arise in small informal groups; the nurse reinforces compliance with medication and attempts to alleviate anxiety or concerns. These informal, spontaneous interventions with groups of patients occur repeatedly during the course of a day on an inpatient unit.

Although degrees of formality and types of patients vary, the nurse invariably uses group leadership skills to meet patients' interpersonal needs in the therapeutic milieu. As managers and providers of patient care (24 hours a day), nurses intervene with groups of patients. Consequently, nurses must use effective communication skills to interact with groups of patients (described later in this chapter).

Nurses on inpatient units should be aware of factors that influence the clinical setting. Short-stay inpatient hospitalization affects group work in many ways. For example, short hospitalizations result in a rapid turnover of patients in groups; expecting trust and cohesion to develop in such a group is unrealistic. Patients might also have acute symptoms of serious illnesses. The nurse must quickly assess the mental status of patients to determine whether they can tolerate a group session and involve patients in groups based on their level of functioning. Severely depressed or actively psychotic patients may not be appropriate group members. Charting patient progress in the group is an important nursing responsibility for both therapeutic and legal reasons.

Similarly, in outpatient care and in the community, nurses must consider realistic factors that impinge on treatment. Patients might be limited to a specific number of visits because of payment providers, or participation in day treatment or substance-related programs might be limited to a specific number of days during the course of a year. For patients in rural areas, transportation issues may affect the ability of patients to participate.

Confidentiality must be explained to group participants; that is, patients must understand that what is said or takes place in the group setting must remain private. However, statements within group sessions might be shared with staff members or the treatment team because of their responsibility for patient care. Personal information *is* shared in the group but should not leave the unit or care facility. In reality, group confidentiality can be difficult to ensure because trust and cohesion might not be fully developed. Content, or what is learned in group settings, such as information about medication, can be shared outside of the treatment setting.

Physical Setting

Physical arrangements are important considerations in creating an atmosphere that is conducive to group work. Finding adequate space or a private room is often difficult but is nevertheless important to ensure privacy and a quiet atmosphere. Adequate lighting, comfortable temperature, ample seating, and proper equipment also contribute to successful group functioning. Forming a circle of chairs allows patients to see each other and indicates an expectation that patients will relate to the leader and other group members. Chairs in rows might be appropriate for a didactic group but does not allow for effective interpersonal communication flow. A blackboard, dry marker board, or other media such as a DVD player can enhance learning. Handouts or printed materials might be useful for patients and families to take home for future reference.

Nurse leaders must be active, empathic, and able to provide structure. Because of time constraints, leaders cannot afford to be nondirective or to allow the group to be free-floating. The nurse must be goal directed and focus on the here and now in each inpatient or outpatient group session. The leader succinctly states the group's purpose at the beginning of the session, and most of the session is spent on the work to be accomplished. Patients generally prefer leaders who provide the group "with an active structure" (Yalom & Leszcz, 2005). The final 5 to 10 minutes are used to summarize and close the session. The summary should have a positive focus and include information that the patients have learned or gained from the group. The leader gives positive feedback to the group regarding progress during the session.

Expectations in the form of group rules must be explicit, such as patients are expected to arrive on time and remain for the entire group session, if possible. For an inpatient group, the group leader might permit patients to pace or leave the room and then return when they are able. The inability to sit still for an extended period might be the result of anxiety or medication side effects (usually akathisia). The decision to exclude patients from the group should be made carefully. The nurse might exclude patients who are acutely manic, disoriented, and too psychotic to benefit from group. Patients who are hostile and verbally threatening are also inappropriate for group sessions.

COMMON MANAGEMENT ISSUES

Basic interventions for groups are based on facilitative communication techniques (see Chapter 8). Nurses use these skills with patients individually and within groups. Nurses who facilitate group interactions on a therapeutic level help enable patients to share thoughts, feelings, and problems.

Basic communication skills that are useful for nurse leaders are detailed in Table 10-2. These skills are not unique to the group setting but are skills that can be used on a daily basis. These general interventions are therapeutic, regardless of the type of group. The use of positive feedback helps patients in their attempt to use new skills. For example, in an attempt to use a particular assertiveness skill, the patient goes off on a tangent. The nurse might say, "You have done well, Sam. When you gave us the example of saying to your boss, 'I need to talk with you about my work schedule,' you used an excellent example of 'I' statements." The nurse chooses to repeat the portion of Sam's statement that is realistic and is a correct example of an "I" statement for emphasis and clarity. As a result, the patient feels a sense of accomplishment and increased self-esteem.

For the group experience to be successful, the nurse leader must recognize and manage process and content areas (Puskar et al., 2012; Rindner, 2000). The combination of teaching didactic material (psychoeducation) with managing process issues requires knowledge and skill. For the group experience to be beneficial, the structure of the group session must include a balance between content to be taught and group process.

TYPES OF PATIENTS IN GROUPS

Dominant Patient

The dominant patient monopolizes the entire group session to the extent that other patients might believe that they do not have the opportunity to participate. The nurse uses gate-keeping techniques to offer all patients the opportunity to contribute to the group. For example, the nurse can say, "Cathy, you are doing well in contributing to our session today, but I would like to hear what others are thinking about at this time." This intervention can forestall monopolization of the group by a single patient without putting her down, while providing others with the opportunity to express themselves. The other patients in the group might be unable to handle this patient or might be too afraid. If the group leader is afraid or cannot control the patient, the integrity of the group is compromised.

Uninvolved Patient

The uninvolved patient presents another challenge to the nurse leader. The patient might be quiet because of anxiety or fear. Patients with chronic schizophrenia find relating in group sessions to be difficult and threatening. The nurse can say, "It's hard to talk about ourselves in the group, but I know that everyone here has something to share that can help someone else." The nurse recognizes that patients are mistrustful and anxious but can relate the message that each individual is important and capable of helping another.

Some patients who are uninvolved in the group might believe themselves to be at a higher level of functioning than the other members. These patients might believe that they are not as sick as the others, do not belong in the group, and would

TABLE 10-2 COMMUNICATION SKILLS: ELICITING, QUALIFYING, AND CLARIFYING COMMUNICATION

TECHNIQUES OF THE LEADER(S)	GROUP MEMBER RESPONSE	OUTCOME
1. **Giving information**: "My purpose in offering this group experience is ..."	Further validates his assumptions: "How is this going to happen?"	Leader(s) and member(s) enter into a dialogue in which member(s) get more information that helps them make decisions and build trust in group experience.
2. **Seeking clarification**: "Did you say you were upset with John because he said that?"	Might try to restate his thoughts or feelings: "Yes, I guess I was upset."	Member becomes aware that he was unclear and learns to identify thoughts and feelings more precisely, at the same time taking responsibility for them.
3. **Encouraging description and exploration** (delving further into communication or experiences): "How did you feel when Joann said that to you?"	Elaborates on his message: "I was angry."	Member deals in great depth with an experience in the group and again takes responsibility for his reactions. (This example also places events in time or in sequence, lending further perspective to group events.)
4. **Presenting reality**: "Would other members think Joann was unstable if they interviewed her for a job? You don't appear shaky to me."	Listens and considers other possibilities.	Member compares perception of self with others' perceptions of him.
5. **Seeking consensual validation** (seeking mutual understanding of what is being communicated): "Did I understand you to say that you feel better now than you did last week?"	Further clarification: "Well, yes, I'm better than last week but not as good as I'd like to be."	Group and leader(s) learn how member views his progress and how they should receive his evaluation of himself.
6. **Focusing** (identifying a single topic to concentrate on): "Could we identify one problem you have and talk more about that?"	Channels thinking: Members might think of the most puzzling problem they have.	Group leader(s) identify specific topics that they can resolve before the meeting ends. They increase their understanding of one problem before jumping to others.
7. **Encouraging comparison** (asking members to compare and contrast their experiences with others in the group): "How did the rest of the group handle this problem?"	Group members share their experiences as they relate to the topic.	Leader(s) and members gain greater insight into their commonalities and differences and learn from one another alternative ways of responding to problems.
8. **Making observations**: "You look more comfortable now, John, than you did at the beginning of the meeting." *or* "The group has been silent for the last 5 minutes."	Group members have something to respond to: "I feel more at ease now." *or* "I think we are quiet because we are bored."	Group members and leader(s) place attention on significant events and can elaborate on their meanings.
9. **Giving recognition or acknowledging**: "John, you are new to the group. Perhaps we can introduce ourselves."	Feels acknowledged and included: "Yes, I'm John, and I came here because ..."	Members view specific instances as important, and the leader(s) reinforce the behavior or event that they choose to notice—in this case, the desire to come to group.
10. **Accepting** (not necessarily agreeing with but receiving communication with openness): "Yes, I hear you say that you don't know if you want to be in the group or not."	Feels heard and understood without fear of attack.	Members learn that even "nonacceptable" attitudes can be talked about, and perhaps any thought is not so horrible that they cannot share it.
11. **Encouraging evaluation** (asking the group as a whole or individual members to judge their experiences): "When Marilyn gives you support, do you feel better?" *or* "How did we do in helping Joann with her problem?"	Member reflects on progress made: "Not exactly, because I don't know if I can trust her to be honest." *or* "It was hard. I'd like to know from her."	The criteria for success become clearer to members, and new directions might be formulated as a result of the discussion.
12. **Summarizing** (encapsulating in a few sentences what has occurred): "The group discussed several issues and problems today. They were ..."	Members recall significant points and events and block out onsideration of new or extraneous topics.	Members and leader(s) place in perspective and identify salient points of a group session. Such a summary can lead to a better understanding of group process.

From Van Servellen, G. (1983). *Group and family therapy.* St. Louis: Mosby.

not benefit from the session. The nurse leader might give attention to these members by giving them a job to perform for the group—for example, arranging chairs for the session or calling other group members to remind them of the group. Respect and recognition by the nurse is therapeutic for these patients because they will believe that they can contribute to the group.

? CRITICAL THINKING QUESTIONS

1. During a group session on medication management, a patient states, "I learn more by listening." How would you involve this patient in the group discussion?
2. During a group session, the nurse observes two patients whispering and snickering to each other. How would you handle this situation?

Hostile Patient

Hostility might mask a patient's fear, self-anger, or unresolved anger toward others. To help this patient verbalize feelings of anger appropriately, the nurse can say, "Melody, you sound angry today. What happened?" or "Tell us about it." The nurse directly confronts this patient in a supportive manner and attempts to help the patient deal with her feelings. Allowing verbal or nonverbal hostility to continue jeopardizes the progress of the group session. Unchecked hostility causes discomfort and uneasiness and impairs the ability of other patients to attend to the group's work. Patients might also mistakenly interpret anger as being directed toward them.

Distracting Patient

Some patients' behaviors and verbalizations sometimes can be very distracting to other members of the group. Others become distracted when inappropriate comments are made and when delusions are voiced or someone hallucinates in group. For the patient who has verbalized a delusion, the nurse could use empathy, focus on the underlying need, present reality, and refocus the group. For example, the patient might state, "Everyone here is against me." The nurse could reply, "It must upset you to feel that way. I don't think that anyone here is against you." The nurse ultimately brings the group members back to the topic being presented and discussed.

For the patient who is hallucinating, the nurse directs the patient to focus on reality and the topic of discussion. A simple statement to the group such as, "We are talking about side effect management of atypical antipsychotics. Let's review what we've talked about so far." The nurse does not confront the individual in group but may meet with the patient after group for one-to-one interaction.

The patient who verbalizes a sexually inappropriate comment can be handled by the nurse using limit setting. For example, the nurse could state, "Jim, that comment is inappropriate. We are discussing symptoms that could indicate relapse."

These group interventions help the nurse develop as a group leader. Patients quickly recognize the group leader's empathy, understanding, and respect for each patient as caring behaviors. Even though some patients make only minimal progress toward their individual treatment goals, interacting with the nurse who possesses and exhibits these traits can increase the patients' feelings of worth as human beings.

▌ STUDY NOTES

1. The psychiatric nurse interacts and intervenes with patients and families in informal groups as well as in formally structured sessions in inpatient and community settings.
2. Patients benefit from group experiences by gaining acceptance, hopefulness, and support from others. Through mutual sharing of feelings and problems, patients learn how their communication methods and behaviors interfere with relationships. Their strengths are reinforced and accumulated.
3. Families of mentally ill patients benefit from the information and support they receive in a group.
4. Nurse leaders must be active, empathic, goal directed, and comfortable keeping in the "here and now" for each group session.
5. Various types of groups exist in inpatient and outpatient settings that can benefit patients with acute and chronic illnesses. Typical groups include psychoeducational, maintenance, activity, and self-help or special problem groups. Psychoeducational and self-help groups are available for families of mentally ill patients.
6. As group leaders, nurses use facilitative communication techniques and role-modeling behaviors.
7. The nurse leader structures the group session by attending to content and process issues.
8. The nurse leader intervenes therapeutically with dominating, uninvolved, hostile, and distracting patients, while continuing to be respectful, guiding patients to improved communication skills.

REFERENCES

Crane-Okada, R. (2012). The concept of presence in group psychotherapy: An operational definition. *Perspectives in Psychiatric Care, 48*, 156–164.

Echternacht, M. (2001). Fluid group: Concept and clinical application in the therapeutic milieu. *Journal of the American Psychiatric Nurses Association, 7*, 39.

Hackman, A., et al. (2007). Consumer satisfaction with inpatient psychiatric treatment among persons with severe mental illness. *Community Mental Health Journal, 43*, 551.

Page, A. C., & Hooke, G. R. (2009). Best practices: Increased attendance in inpatient group psychotherapy improves patient outcomes. *Psychiatric Services (Washington, D.C.), 60*, 426.

Potter, M., Williams, R., & Costanzo, R. (2004). Using nursing theory and a structured psychoeducational curriculum with inpatient groups. *Journal of the American Psychiatric Nurses Association, 10,* 122.

Puskar, K., et al. (2012). Understanding content and process: Guidelines for group leaders. *Perspectives in Psychiatric Care, 48,* 225–229.

Richardson, C. R., et al. (2005). Integrating physical activity into mental health services for persons with serious mental illness. *Psychiatric Services (Washington, D.C.), 56,* 324.

Rindner, E. (2000). Combined group process-psychoeducation model for psychiatric clients and their families. *Journal of Psychosocial Nursing and Mental Health Services, 38,* 3.

Van Servellen, G. (1983). *Group and family therapy.* St. Louis: Mosby.

Yalom, I., & Leszcz, M. (2005). *The theory and practice of group psychotherapy* (5th ed.). New York: Basic Books.

11

Working with the Family

Debbie Steele[*]

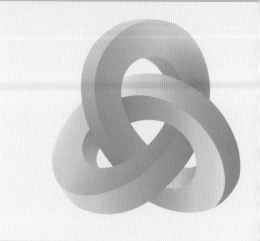

⊝volve WEBSITE

http://evolve.elsevier.com/Keltner

LEARNING OBJECTIVES

- Define the terms *family* and *family systems*.
- Discuss characteristics of healthy families.
- Evaluate the effects of mental disorders on the family system.
- List the factors to assess when working with families.
- Describe the skills necessary for working therapeutically and collaboratively with families.
- Explain the effects of mental illness on families.
- Discuss the issues associated with caring for psychiatric patients within a family context.

The family unit is the building block of society, functioning not only for procreation but also to transmit the values, protection, and nurturing needed for human survival. Most individuals maintain their ties to the family of origin into adulthood; the extended family continues to provide support in times of crisis. During times of illness or injury, families generally supply the required care and support to members both financially and emotionally (Kim & Salyers, 2008). When a family member experiences a mental illness, the family is likely to be the major source of assistance for the mentally ill member. Families are affected by the mental illness of a family member in numerous ways. Often, they are the first to observe the changes in behavior accompanying the illness, have been confused and concerned by their family member's actions, and often have tried desperately to obtain care for their family member. Nurses who care for individuals with mental disorders need to understand family functioning in order to work collaboratively with families to promote family adjustment to the effects of the mental disorder and improve chances for long-term effective management.

This chapter explores characteristics of families, the effects of mental disorders on the family system, and strategies for working therapeutically with families in various settings. The emphasis is on understanding and assessing families as a basis for therapeutic interactions, family conferences, education, support, and referrals, rather than family therapy.

DEFINITION OF FAMILY

The definition of family has changed over the years to reflect the rapidly occurring changes within society. There is more than one acceptable definition of *family*, which makes it essential to clarify what family means not only to the patient but also to the nurse. Today, the definition of family focuses more on the roles and functions of the family rather than the relationships between its members. McGoldrick and Carter (2003) stated that "Families comprise persons who have a shared history and a shared future." This statement speaks to the permanence of families, regardless of the family form or structure.

NORM'S NOTES
Where would you be without your family? I would not want to consider such a life, and you might not either. When a family member develops mental health problems, other family members are affected. A fundamental role of nurses and other psychiatric professionals is to help families to cope with and assist a family member with a mental health disorder and to understand how they contribute either to the problem or to the solution. Remember this, because I think it is humbling: When you have done what you know how to do, the family will almost always still be there dealing with the outcomes, whether good or bad.

---

*This chapter was previously written by Debra Wilson.

FAMILY SYSTEMS THEORY

The view of the family as a "system" is an important theoretical framework useful for health care professionals, particularly nurses and other professionals who work with mental disorders. The family is conceived as a collective unit made up of individual parts (Nichols, 2013). Every family member plays a critical, albeit unique, role in the system. It is impossible for change to affect one member of the system without causing a ripple effect of change among the other family members. The following clinical example helps illustrate the family system concept.

Clinical Example

Gordon is a 14-year-old high school freshman who reports being depressed for approximately 1 year. Recently he has been experiencing suicidal ideation without a realistic plan. During the assessment, Gordon mentions that he experiences a lot of anxiety at home, especially because his mother screams a lot at him and his siblings. He feels like his mother has high expectations of him and never seems to be satisfied with his efforts. He also explains that his mother and father don't seem to get along and seldom go anywhere together. He also hears his mother frequently yelling at his father. He tends to spend most of his time in his room, isolating himself.

In this clinical example, Gordon would be identified as the patient, and the focus would be on his suicidal ideation. From a family systems view, the family would be the "identified patient," and changing Gordon's mood would require a change in the family system. If his mother understands how her behavior (screams, yelling) causes Gordon to feel anxious and depressed, then she can make it a point of learning new ways of communicating with her husband and children. In addition, when Gordon's parents understand the effect their fighting has on the children, they can seek marital counseling. In time, as Gordon's parents change their behavior, Gordon's symptoms are likely to be ameliorated. The changes made by the parents would also have a positive effect on the other children in the home.

The family systems approach provides a solid framework for understanding how families function and how to support their change. Most importantly, the systems view deemphasizes blaming the family's problems on a given family member, particularly a child whose "acting-out" behavior may be a natural reaction to a distressing set of circumstances. With accurate identification of the process that sustains painful or stressful conditions in the family, positive outcomes can be both profound and permanent. For more information on the family systems framework, see the family systems definitions listed in Box 11-1.

CONTEMPORARY FAMILIES

The nuclear family is no longer the predominant family structure in contemporary life. Divorce, remarriage, and same-sex marriages have led to single-parent families, blended families,

---

BOX 11-1 FAMILY SYSTEMS DEFINITIONS

Parentification is the process of role reversal whereby a child takes on adult responsibilities within the family. Parentification takes many forms: (1) the child is obliged to act as parent to his or her *own* parent (i.e., helping a drunk mother get into bed); (2) the child or adolescent takes on the role of a confidant or mediator for (or between) parents (occurs frequently when parents are divorced); and (3) the child is coerced into taking the adult role (i.e., cases of incest).

Scapegoat refers to a member of the family, usually the identified patient, who is to blame for the conflict in the family. Family members focus on trying to fix the identified patient, rather than dealing with and resolving the real issues.

Enmeshed refers to a family structure that resists the demands for change. For example, attempts on the part of one member to change elicits immediate resistance from other family members. In addition, individual boundaries are not respected (e.g., newly married couple expected to go on family vacation with parents).

Disengaged refers to a family structure where members are distant and disconnected. Family relationships tend to be chaotic, and parental authority is relatively absent. Boundaries tend to be excessively rigid, meaning that the behavior of one family member does not affect other members (i.e., "don't call me if you end up in jail").

Triangulation occurs when there is a conflict between two family members and they attempt to involve a third person who is asked to take a side. For example, conflicted parents may each attempt to garner their child's favor, sympathy, or support.

---

and families with two parents of the same gender. Some people believe that these changes undermine the integrity of the family, whereas others believe that these new structures demonstrate the flexibility of the family system, allowing the family to remain viable and effective as a vehicle for raising children and maintaining family interpersonal support amid the stresses of modern life (Walsh, 2003a).

Alterations in family structure parallel other societal changes that have affected how families function. Economic pressures have made two-wage earner families the norm, necessitating out-of-home care for children and leaving a gap in the supervision of older children and adolescents after school. Statistically, 50% of marriages end in divorce in the United States, which encourages increasingly complex family interactions with parents, stepparents, grandparents, and step-grandparents, not to mention half-siblings and stepsiblings.

Adult children might continue living in their parents' home for an extended time because of divorce, job loss, or financial hardship. Relationships between parents and adult children living in the same household can become strained and, even if cordial, require significant effort to remain harmonious and stable over time as roles and functions shift from what they had been while the children were growing up. Young adults who choose to live independently of their parents often live with a roommate or partner for economic as well as personal reasons (Walsh, 2003a).

Society has become more culturally diverse as a result of immigration, intermarriage, and cross-cultural adoption. Issues of assimilation, integration, and maintaining one's cultural identity all affect the structure and function of families. With regard to immigration, cross-cultural marriage, and adoption, the involved parties must balance allegiance to their cultural heritage against the values, norms, and behaviors in the new culture in which they find themselves. Immigrant parents are faced with decisions regarding how much to focus on their own culture and how to free their Americanized children to fit into the U.S. culture. The children of immigrants easily adopt the customs of the culture in which they are living, often causing distress and feelings of loss in their immigrant parents. Assimilation of the younger generation into the new society is necessary for them to fit into the new culture and feel successful but might come at a price in terms of their cultural identity (Walsh, 2003a).

Discrimination and racism are faced by many immigrants, especially if their cultural norms and appearance are very different from the dominant culture in their new country. Lack of familiarity with the culture, difficulty speaking the language, and lack of job access can cause a ripple effect of low wages and economic hardship that can weaken the family structure.

Alterations in family structure and function, along with societal changes, can create stress in the family. In today's world, communications technology makes everyone constantly aware of world events, which can fuel fear about the future and one's own personal safety and make it more difficult for families to feel secure. In most major cities, random acts of violence, gang wars, and racism result in individuals and their families restricting their daily activities. Such constraints make it more difficult for families to function optimally, although most have shown great resiliency in dealing with such threats (Walsh, 2003a).

Nurses working with individuals with a diagnosis of a mental disorder must be aware of the needs of modern families. For example, families are more likely to be culturally diverse, requiring the nurse to learn about the values, beliefs, and customs of families from another culture. Information in this chapter and in Chapter 5 can assist nurses in understanding and responding to culturally diverse families.

FAMILY CHARACTERISTICS

The extreme variation in family structure prompts questions about the characteristics of a normal family. "What does a normal family look like, and how do they act?" Healthy families can be defined by their effectiveness in building caring and committed relationships. According to Walsh (2003a), healthy families can be contrasted to unhealthy families by their ability to adapt to societal changes as well as the changes that naturally occur within the family cycle.

To define a healthy or functional family, it is necessary to consider the defining characteristics of successful families of all types. Healthy, well-functioning families nurture and support their members and provide stability and cohesion in a rapidly changing world. It is often said in families that "Home is the place you can go and be accepted when the rest of the world rejects you." In today's fast-paced, high-stress society, such nurturing is invaluable. Everyone needs someone to care for them and help them when facing challenges. Knowing that the family will remain together and provide predictability in an unpredictable world can buffer the stresses that individuals face every day.

Successful families also protect their members from dangers by caring for vulnerable members whose age or condition renders them unable to care for themselves independently. For example, infants and children require many years of parental care and supervision. Family members who experience acute or chronic physical and emotional conditions benefit from family care and support. Elderly individuals experiencing physical and mental decline also receive care that is generally provided by family members.

The family of origin provides the platform of truth for children. It is where new members of the family learn what is needed to function in the world, from communication and socialization to values and roles required within the family and in the outside world. Children learn language, communication skills, and religious and secular beliefs as well as how to be a child, sibling, student, and parent from interactions within the family. In healthy, functional families, communication is open, lines of authority are clear, socialization is encouraged, and respect for self and others is taught as well as how to relate to each other and others outside the family. Family units serve as a vehicle where members are cared for, valued, and prepared to cope with the society in which they live. The nurturing of individuals as they grow and develop leads to a well-functioning, healthy adult.

These characteristics provide the basis for the family to cope effectively with internal pressures, such as the illness of a member, or external pressures, such as the loss of a job by a parent. During times of stress, a family might experience disruption in one or more of these desirable characteristics; however, the support of caregivers, the extended family, and friends can help the family weather the disruption and remain resilient. For example, job loss by the father causes an initial economic and personal crisis. However, if his wife can move to full-time employment and the family can problem solve the crisis together, the father can return to school to retrain for a better position to improve the family's long-term stability.

STAGES OF FAMILY DEVELOPMENT

Duvall and Miller (1985) defined the stages of family development based on the people and developmental tasks involved in a family at different periods of life. Initially, the single individual marries and becomes part of a "beginning family" (a couple). If a child enters the family, the stage changes to the "early childbearing family" when the oldest child is a toddler or preschooler and the family concentrates on incorporating the child into the family, introducing him or her to the outside world but controlling contact with others. As the oldest child enters elementary school—"families with schoolchildren"—parents must accept increased contact of their children with the outside world and focus on education, socialization, and monitoring contact with the outside world. "Families with teenagers" have their oldest child encountering increasing independence and planning for the future as the child negotiates high school and work or college. After the oldest child reaches the end of the teenage years, plans are made for the child to begin a life on his or her own—"launching center families." This stage is followed by "families in midlife," in which the couple readjusts to life without children (the empty nest). In the final stage, "families in retirement," the couple deals with issues of adjusting to retirement, becoming grandparents, and facing the eventual death of spouse and friends (McGoldrick & Carter, 2003). One critique of this model is its failure to consider the variation in structure of modern families.

Families are not static, but knowing the stage of family development with which a family is dealing can give the nurse an idea of potential issues and problems that the family might be facing. If a family has children of widely varying ages, the family might be dealing with developmental tasks at several levels at the same time. For example, in a blended family, one or both spouses might have adolescents and school-age children from a previous marriage, while also dealing with a newborn from their current union. Nurturing an infant and simultaneously guiding an adolescent to self-sufficiency requires different parenting techniques and might create stress in the family. Knowledge of appropriate child behavior at each developmental stage of childhood is also an important part of successful parenting that can contribute to the strength of family ties.

? CRITICAL THINKING QUESTION

1. Can healthy families have members with a mental disorder?

EFFECTS OF MENTAL DISORDERS ON THE FAMILY

Caring for an ill family member is stressful, but the diagnosis of a mental disorder is particularly disturbing for the family. The diagnosis of a mental disorder in a family member can elicit feelings of guilt over possible genetic transmission of the disease to the ill family member by parents, concern over the prognosis and course of the disease, and worry among other family members that they might become mentally ill. The stigma of mental illness leads to shame or embarrassment about how others might view the family (Fujino & Okamura, 2009; Rose et al., 2006). In cases of major depression, anxiety, and psychotic disorders, the family may face dangerous behavior, such as suicidal and homicidal threats or actions. In addition, the family member with a mental disorder diagnosis might exhibit feelings of sadness, anger, or resentment related to the disorder. Other feelings may include guilt about the difficulties caused to the family or resignation and hopelessness about the prognosis of the disorder (Oyebode, 2003).

The family must deal with the ill member's behavior as well as with agencies and institutions available to assist the family member. Law enforcement agencies, courts, social service agencies, schools, hospitals, clinics, and churches are among the many agencies having differing rules and procedures with which the family must negotiate. These agencies might be consulted in the process of obtaining needed care, or contacts might be made as a result of dangerous behavior related to the family member's mental disorder. For example, the family member who is paranoid might believe that a neighbor is planning to harm him or her and consequently might make a threat against the neighbor. This action would bring the family into contact with the local law enforcement agency and the courts. If the family member is committed for treatment, mental health agencies and hospitals might become involved in the person's care. Issues that might surface as a result of a family member's mental disorder include the following:

- Medication usage—presence and treatment of side effects of medication
- Lack of energy to complete activities of daily living
- Social isolation, avoidance of contact with others
- Acting-out behaviors, particularly threatening or paranoid behavior
- Mood swings
- Denial of disorder, lack of appropriate reasoning or judgment
- Inappropriate or incomprehensible communication
- Persistence of dangerous behavior (e.g., drug or alcohol abuse)
- Manipulation of others to achieve desired goals

When an individual is diagnosed with a mental disorder, the family must deal with various grief issues, which include a change in family functioning. Income might be lost if the family member has been a wage earner. Stress on the individual and others in the family can increase and affect everyone's school or work performance. The future of both the individual and the family might also be jeopardized (Conn & Marsh, 1999; Rose et al., 2006). The diagnosis of a mental illness can break apart a family—for example, when a spouse can no longer live with and subject children to an alcoholic or abusive partner—or it can bring family members together. Kay Redfield Jamison, a professor of psychiatry who also has manic-depressive illness, spoke of her mother in her autobiography (1995) in the following terms:

She could not have known how difficult it would be to deal with madness: had no preparation for what to do with madness—none of us did—but, consistent with her ability to love and her native will, she handled it with empathy and intelligence (p. 9).

? CRITICAL THINKING QUESTION

2. If the family of a child with a mental illness diagnosis is told that the disorder has a biologic-genetic component, what effect is that statement likely to have on the thoughts and feelings of the parents and siblings of the child?

FAMILY REACTIONS TO PSYCHIATRIC TREATMENT AND HOSPITALIZATION

The diagnosis of a mental disorder and possible admission to a psychiatric facility result in various reactions from family members. Relief might be felt among family members and sometimes by the patient. The immediate family might not want others to know about the hospitalization, fearing a negative reaction from distant family and friends. The family might be exhausted because of difficulty coping with the patient's bizarre behavior or concern about the safety of all family members.

When the individual must be involuntarily committed to a facility, conflicting emotions can arise on the part of the family. The family might want the person admitted, but all members may not concur with the degree of coercion used to force the patient into admission. The patient might desire help and agree to be admitted, or the patient might want help but refuse admission to an inpatient facility.

Frequent admissions might cause the family to experience burnout. When stress in the family is high, the family might wish the family member to be hospitalized to provide relief for the family system. Admission might be helpful to the entire family if the treatment provided meets the current safety and security needs of the patient and family. However, in the event family members are encouraging hospitalization because of their own stress and anxiety, the patient may be made to feel responsible for the mental health of the entire family. In any case, family therapy is encouraged for members of the family when conflict between the patient and family cannot be mediated by the nurse or other health care staff (Merrell, 2001). Family therapy should be carried out by a professional who has been prepared at the master's or doctoral level because of the complexity of the issues and the skills needed to carry out the treatment. Professionals who are qualified for family therapy are social workers, marriage and family therapists, psychologists, and advanced practice psychiatric nurses. Family therapy is beyond the scope of practice of the baccalaureate-prepared nurse.

When abuse or assault is discovered in the family by the health care team, it is important to refer for appropriate treatment. Abused members might experience relief that the *secret* has finally been revealed but might also experience anger, rejection, or humiliation from exposure of abuse. Fear about the future, fear of retribution, or fear of legal consequences of the abuse might be of concern to family members who have been victimized by another family member. Ensuring the safety of abused family members is necessary for them to confront the pain and suffering caused by the abuse. See Chapter 33 for further information.

NURSE RESPONSE TO PATIENTS AND FAMILIES SEEKING TREATMENT

When a family seeks treatment for any of the problems listed in Box 11-2 or for other problems, the nurse must listen to all parties involved and withhold judgment until all points

---

BOX 11-2	REASONS FOR A FAMILY TO SEEK TREATMENT FOR MENTAL HEALTH ISSUES

- Situational crises, such as loss of job or divorce
- Developmental crises, such as a child leaving home for the first time
- Relationship problems and conflicts, such as abuse of one or more family members
- Conflicts between families of origin and current family (family of marriage)
- Addition of family members through remarriage, adoption, and foster care
- Family conflicts over treatment when a family member has another type of illness
- Custody conflicts and issues
- Family exploitation of an ill family member
- Family confrontation or conflict with caregivers
- Acute or chronic mental disorder of a family member

---

of view have been examined. The nurse should refrain from perceiving one family member or an entire family as problematic. The nurse and other caregivers must refrain from placing blame either directly or implicitly on an individual family member. The family is not the cause of the mental disorder, and the family member with a mental disorder diagnosis is not the cause of the family's problems.

The family member diagnosed with a mental disorder may not be the sickest member of the family. The term "scapegoating" refers to the family process of identifying one member as the object of displaced conflict or criticism (Nichols, 2013). Often, the individual with the diagnosis is the one who is most sensitive to the disruptions in family life and most desirous of obtaining help to overcome the problem (Walsh, 2012). The nurse can ameliorate some of the scapegoating that might be occurring in a family by consulting directly with the patient and other family members during assessment and treatment. The nurse can offer positive reinforcement about the patient's willingness to engage in the treatment process. Even if the patient is only minimally cooperative with treatment, positive reinforcement can serve to improve the patient's cooperation and boost his or her self-esteem.

ABILITIES NEEDED WHEN WORKING WITH FAMILIES

The nurse must possess several important skills and characteristics to work effectively with patients and their families. Self-knowledge, spirituality, assessment skills, and communication skills allow the nurse to collaborate with patients, families, and caregivers and to provide appropriate care and possible referrals.

Self-Knowledge

The nurse must recognize and accept his or her own values, beliefs, and biases related to the importance of families and their involvement in the care of their member with a mental disorder diagnosis. The nurse must also avoid allowing personal concerns to become involved with the problems of patients and families. To do this, the nurse must be aware of and acknowledge his or her own family history and appreciate that all families have strengths and needs (Walsh, 2012). The nurse must model adaptive self-care and stress management techniques, such as regular exercise, healthy eating, and strong support and nurturance from friends and family. Such self-care activities prepare the nurse to assist patients and families in learning healthier coping skills to manage their lives.

Assessment

Interactions among all family members are the raw material for problem solving by the family and nurse. The nurse must become the family's partner in assessment and decision making so that the family can own and be invested in problem solving (Johnson et al., 2002). A family assessment guide (Box 11-3) can help the nurse obtain information about family strengths and the problem or problems for which they seek assistance so that the nurse can base problem solving on these and available resources while addressing family needs. Individual and family strengths are used to overcome deficits, helping family members to see themselves as capable of change rather than suffering at the mercy of their circumstances and problems. Additionally, by participating in assessment of their problems, the family learns valuable skills for managing future issues they might encounter.

Assessments include the following:
- Family characteristics in both the family of origin and the present family
- Developmental stage of the family at the present time
- Family's accomplishment of developmental and daily tasks
- Patient's and family's reasons for seeking treatment and reactions to care
- Effects of mental illness on family members and on the family as a whole
- Family strengths
- Family's understanding of the mental disorder
- Current coping skills for managing life
- Other health issues of the patient, family members, or significant others that might affect care

The nurse's observational skills are important when interacting with members of the family. The nurse should observe the behavior and words of all family members and consider how members relate to each other and to the nurse, rather than focusing on the actions of one individual (the patient) alone. The nurse must consider all available information, its relevance, and its impact before arriving at conclusions about a family. If conclusions are drawn too quickly and with too little information, the solution is not likely to be effective; this might discourage the family from seeking help with family problems in the future.

Therapeutic Communication

Therapeutic interactions should be based on the nurse's understanding of the following: families are generally functioning as well as possible, in light of their available resources and abilities; families are capable of solving their problems with the guidance and support of caregivers; all families have strengths that can be applied to solving their issues; placing blame does nothing to solve the family's problems and serves only to diminish the self-esteem of family members and the family as a whole; and family members act out frustration or pain when they are unable to face their issues directly (Conn & Marsh, 1999). Nurses should also remember that every interaction with a patient and family represents an opportunity to be therapeutic. Therapeutic interviewing skills include the ability to display respect for all family members and an ability to be nonjudgmental about the family members and the issues they face.

Specific therapeutic communication techniques used with families by the nurse vary depending on the stage of the relationship with the family but are likely to include active listening, eye contact, expressions of empathy and support, sensitivity to verbal and nonverbal cues, validating and clarifying information, summarizing, and reinforcing the family's efforts. Chapter 8 presents more information concerning therapeutic communication.

Family Education

Nurses, who have always educated patients and families, can serve as a support to families in both treating and

---

BOX 11-3   FAMILY ASSESSMENT GUIDELINES: POSSIBLE QUESTIONS TO ASK

Family Membership and Development
- "Tell me about the members of your immediate (nuclear) family, including ages and gender (male or female)."
- "What other relatives do you have? How are they involved with your immediate family?"

Family Strengths and Needs
- "What do you think is a strength in your family?"
- "What is something you would like to change about your family?"

Family Coping
- "Describe a problem that your family has dealt with successfully."
- "What helped you to deal with this problem successfully?"

Family Problem Identification
- "What is your perception of the current family problem?"
- "How do you think the current problem should be resolved?"

Family Use of Resources
- "What resources or agencies have you used successfully in the past in dealing with this type of problem?"
- "What does your family do to stay healthy? What does your family do to treat or control mental, emotional, and physical illness?"
- "What type of help would you like from me (the nurse) in resolving the current problem?"

preventing mental health problems. For at-risk families, preventive education can enhance functioning and prevent the occurrence of mental health problems. Nardi (1999) demonstrated that a parenting education program such as *Systematic Training for Effective Parenting* (*STEP*) can diminish the use of harsh discipline; promote parent-child attachment; and encourage parents in a low-income, high-violence geographic area to play with their children. Nurses can promote a therapeutic partnership by acting as a family educator about topics of interest and need for specific families. Wilson and Hobbs (1999) described this type of nursing role with patients with a new diagnosis of psychosis and their families. The nurse explains the disorder and symptoms that might be frightening to patients and their families, which eases the shock and distress that occurs when patients begin to act and talk in odd ways. This role involves partnership and advocacy of the family with the treatment team and community, reinforcement of family strengths, and facilitation of transition to postdischarge rehabilitation. Programs of family education, such as those presented by Wilson and Hobbs (1999), are similar to the rehabilitation programs that patients and family members go through in medical settings after a family member experiences a stroke or heart attack. Such programs not only speed recovery from acute episodes of the disorder but also enable the patient and family to manage the acute symptoms more effectively, with fewer relapses.

Effective education of patients and families requires knowledge of learning styles and the ability to present information in a variety of ways, such as through oral and written communication, pictures, and stories. The most successful educators adapt information to the preferred method of learning of the patient and the family. For example, if the nurse must educate a family whose members have a low level of formal schooling, pamphlets written at an elementary school reading level with pictures to illustrate important information can be helpful. Interpreters or pamphlets written in Spanish are helpful for a family who has just arrived from Mexico. The proliferation of information on the Internet provides rich educational resources for the nurse and family, although the nurse must evaluate the quality and accuracy of Internet information and determine whether it comes from reliable sources before offering it to the patient and family.

The National Alliance on Mental Illness (NAMI) and other groups such as the National Mental Health Association advocate effectively for the rights of patients and their families. These groups also provide information about the availability of new treatments; effectiveness of certain treatments; risks and benefits of specific treatments; cost-benefit ratio of specific services; availability of services such as mutual support groups; and assistance in negotiating insurance or with mental health systems and other bureaucracies. The NAMI Family to Family program is a good example of an effective educational and support program for families of mentally ill individuals (Dixon et al., 2001).

Spirituality

By demonstrating empathy, support, patience, and hope, the nurse facilitates care and provides a spiritual dimension to treatment, enriching interventions that have been implemented (Sperry, 2000). Because of their close and frequent contact with patients and families, nurses are adept at providing spiritual care by partnering with the patient and family, sharing their pain and joy, and respecting the values and beliefs of the patient and family. The nurse can encourage contact with spiritual resources, such as a minister, priest, or rabbi, when needed or desired by the patient or family. If a family's spiritual beliefs conflict with the prescribed treatment, the nurse should accommodate the beliefs whenever possible. For example, some patients and families are wary of using medication to alter mental function and prefer to rely on prayer as a treatment. However, when a patient is experiencing hallucinations, a reduction in symptoms is more likely to occur with the aid of antipsychotic medication. Nursing care that respects the values and beliefs of the family is more likely to be well received and appreciated, in light of the difficult decisions family members face. For example, as the nurse encourages the use of prayer because it is a valued and important component of a family's lifestyle, the family will be more likely to discuss the advantages and disadvantages of medication geared to reduce symptoms.

Collaboration

The nurse must work with patients, families, and colleagues in providing care for families and helping families reach their goals. Nurses must collaborate with multidisciplinary teams and agencies to advocate for patients and achieve positive family outcomes.

Competencies of mental health care workers have been identified by members of the Adult Panel of the Managed Care Initiative coordinated by the Center for Mental Health Policy and Service Research at the University of Pennsylvania (Coursey et al., 2000). Of the 12 competencies developed by the panel, 3 relate to collaboration. The first competency mentions engaging adults with serious mental disorders as full collaborators in planning, delivering, and evaluating their care. The second competency indicates that family members and others who care about the adult with a serious mental disorder should be involved in all aspects of care. The ninth competency directs caregivers to work collaboratively with all sectors of the service delivery system. The focus on collaboration demonstrates that interdisciplinary collaboration is essential for the delivery of quality mental health care.

To collaborate successfully with all stakeholders in providing comprehensive mental health care, nurses need to recognize their skills; acknowledge the contributions of other team members; involve the patient, family, and other health care workers in problem identification and problem solving; be knowledgeable about resources; and work cooperatively with all involved to attain quality mental health care for the patient and family.

Referrals and Family Support

Referrals are helpful when working with families who have unmet needs. The nurse must have the knowledge and skills to support families as they enter the health care system to ensure that they can receive the assistance they require for their specific issues. The nurse must be knowledgeable about the resources to which he or she refers families. The referral is most effective when the patient and family know where to go, whom to meet, the reason for the referral, and what to expect when they get there. If the nurse merely gives the patient and family the name and address of a facility or support person, the probability that the patient and family will follow up is low. The family might not know how to get to the location, might be afraid that the treatment will be harmful or costly, or might fear that the family member will be taken away from them and hospitalized against their wishes. The extra effort made by the nurse to personalize and individualize a referral pays dividends in better continuity of care and better mental health for the entire family.

APPLICATION OF THE NURSING PROCESS TO THE FAMILY

Assessment

The assessment process begins within the context of the nurse-patient-family relationship. Assessment provides the nurse, patient, and family an opportunity to discuss each family member's perspective of how well family members are functioning. Questions might be asked when the patient and the family are together, when only some family members are present without the patient, or when only the patient is available. Obtaining the viewpoint of as many family members as possible greatly enhances treatment.

Patients who seek treatment might live with their intact family of origin, a parent who has remarried, adoptive parents, foster parents, other relatives, a spouse, or significant other; by themselves; or in a residential facility. The nurse must consider living arrangements and the persons supporting the patient who are involved in his or her treatment. Current problems might be an extension of problems that began with the original family or might represent new issues not related to the family of origin.

An assessment should also consider other physical and mental health issues within the family that occur as members cope with a chronic mental disorder. Family members may find themselves losing sleep, not eating healthy meals, and becoming more susceptible to the effects of increased anxiety. Possible symptoms may include headaches, indigestion, ulcers, hypertension, and other stress-related physical problems. Puchelak (2003) indicated that among parents of mentally ill adults in the Family Association in Poland, the most distressing and burdensome feelings include feeling helpless and fearful, losing dreams for the future of their mentally ill child, and the necessity of changing plans they had made before the onset of serious symptoms (Lively et al., 2004; Smith et al., 2000).

A family assessment guideline can help the nurse think of the family as a system when conducting a family assessment. Examples of questions that the nurse might wish to ask are listed in Box 11-3. These questions are designed as triggers to help the family tell their story, rather than respond to standardized questions that might not reflect the family's issues and concerns. Through nurse-guided discussions, families can be actively engaged in decision making regarding health priorities.

Nursing Diagnosis

Based on the family assessment, the nurse develops priority nursing diagnoses from those approved by the NANDA International classification system. Examples of some typical diagnoses are ineffective family therapeutic regimen maintenance, impaired parenting, interrupted family processes, and risk for caregiver role strain. These nursing diagnoses help define the problems that the family is facing, providing a foundation for outcome identification. Although nursing diagnoses are generally stated in terms of deficits, the assessment should include a determination of patient and family strengths that can be used to help overcome deficits or prevent risks for deficits becoming actual patient problems (NANDA International, 2005).

Outcome Identification

The nurse works with patients and their families to establish goals to be accomplished during treatment that are based on the family assessment. These goals might be individual goals for a specific family member, goals for the family as a whole, or both. The outcomes or goals identified must be specific, measurable, and achievable within an explicit time frame and under the control of the individual family members. When establishing goals with highly distressed families, the nurse must consider how other agencies will be involved in the treatment process. Agency contact might focus on economic issues, protection for one or more family members, reporting of abuse to a state agency, contacts with police, or actions of a court order.

Planning and Implementation

The skills needed for therapeutic interactions have already been specified earlier in this chapter. Other interventions that the nurse might use when working with patients and their families individually and in groups are listed in the Key Nursing Interventions for Working with Families box. Through the process of understanding the patient's and family's perspective concerning the stresses of living with a mental disorder, the nurse can develop interventions that help all parties involved. Parents in the Mental Health Family Association in Poland determined that relief of caregiver burden involved providing information to help them understand the disease process; hope that the family member's life could improve; and supportive family, friends, and professionals to talk to about their concerns (Puchelak, 2003).

KEY NURSING INTERVENTIONS FOR WORKING WITH FAMILIES

- Provide respect, empathy, support, and acceptance to patients and families.
- Advocate for patients and families in their interactions with other providers, institutions, and organizations.
- Help the family build the patient's self-esteem, yet be realistic in their expectations of the patient, themselves, and others.
- Facilitate resolution of normal developmental crises of individuals and families.
- Help families use more adaptive coping skills, facilitating future problem solving.
- Provide referrals to support groups and resources for families who are experiencing normal developmental issues of family life as well as families dealing with more serious crises.
- Empower families by teaching problem-solving, limit-setting, and conflict resolution skills.
- Help families validate, clarify, negotiate, and communicate feelings appropriately.
- Assist families in recognizing and coping with abuse issues to maintain safety of all family members.
- Offer feedback to patients and families concerning their progress in dealing with their problems.
- Negotiate role flexibility between patients and their families in response to family needs.
- Provide support for families through referral to brief, problem-focused, and psychoeducational groups.
- Be honest with patients and families if abuse must be reported.
- Teach communication and parenting skills.
- Teach families about the causes, manifestations, and treatment of mental disorders.
- Teach families about the desired effects and side effects of medications and symptoms to report to professionals to prevent or minimize relapse.
- Teach and model the management of difficult behaviors of patients.
- Include the patient and family in goal setting and treatment planning.
- Teach and encourage family members to practice self-care as well as care for the patient.

Evaluation

Outcomes of working with patients and their families can be measured by determining whether treatment goals have been met and whether patients and families have developed effective solutions. Periodically throughout treatment, the nurse and family must evaluate progress toward the resolution of issues defined by the nurse, patient, and family. When appropriate, the nurse can assist patients and families in reformulating goals and creating posttreatment goals toward which the family can work after the patient's discharge from an inpatient unit or outpatient program. Ongoing nursing evaluation of patient progress and outcome achievement is essential for successful treatment and represents one of the most important phases of the nursing process.

Resources Available to Families

The nurse can assist families in finding helpful resources and arranging for appropriate services. These services might include medical services, social welfare agencies, churches, emergency food services, voluntary agencies, support groups, community health services, and psychiatric home care services. Resources for families include the following:

- Al-Anon/Alateen: Available at http://www.al-anon.org
- Alcoholics Anonymous: Available at http://www.aa.org
- Families Anonymous: Available at http://www.familiesanonymous.org
- Narcotics Anonymous: Available at http://www.na.org
- NAMI and NAMI-CAN (Child/Adolescent Network): Available at http://www.nami.org
- Parents Anonymous: Available at http://www.parentsanonymous.org
- Alzheimer's Association: Available at http://www.alz.org
- Mental Health America: Available at http://www.nmha.org

? CRITICAL THINKING QUESTIONS

3. What family-oriented approaches would you use with a family having difficulty coping with increasing suicidality of a severely depressed member?

STUDY NOTES

1. Nurses who work with families see many types of contemporary families and should respect their diversity and resilience.
2. Difficulties in accomplishing family tasks and developmental stages reflect the complexities and issues of modern life in a family.
3. The family of origin influences the communication skills, self-esteem, and coping skills that a person brings to the current family. However, healthy problem-solving and interaction skills can be developed with the assistance of health care professionals and community resources.
4. Having a family member with a mental disorder inevitably changes the dynamics within a family.
5. The nursing process with families requires that the nurse possess self-knowledge; assessment, therapeutic, communication, spiritual, and collaboration skills; and skills regarding referrals and family support to help family members cope with the diagnosis of a mental disorder.
6. The nurse must collaborate with the family to assess the function of the family and refer the family to the most appropriate resource for assistance.

REFERENCES

Conn, V. S., & Marsh, D. T. (1999). Working with families. In C. A. Shea, et al. (Eds.), *Advanced practice nursing in psychiatric and mental health care* (pp. 371–385). St. Louis: Mosby.

Coursey, R. D., et al. (2000). Competencies for direct service staff members who work with adults with severe mental illness: Specific knowledge, attitudes, skills, and bibliography. *Psychiatric Rehabilitation Journal, 23,* 370.

Dixon, L., et al. (2001). Evidence-based practices for services to families of people with psychiatric disabilities. *Psychiatric Services, 52,* 903.

Duvall, E., & Miller, B. (1985). *Marriage and family development* (6th ed.). New York: Harper & Row.

Fujino, N., & Okamura, H. (2009). Factors affecting the sense of burden felt by family members caring for patients with mental illness. *Archives of Psychiatric Nursing, 23,* 128–137.

Jamison, K. R. (1995). *An unquiet mind.* New York: Vintage.

Johnson, L. N., Wright, D. W., & Ketring, S. A. (2002). The therapeutic alliance in home-based family therapy. *Journal of Marital and Family Therapy, 28,* 93.

Kim, H. W., & Salyers, M. P. (2008). Attitudes and perceived barriers to working with families of persons with severe mental illness: Mental health professionals' perspectives. *Community Mental Health Journal, 44,* 337.

Lively, S., Friedrich, R. M., & Rubenstein, L. (2004). The effect of disturbing illness behaviors on siblings of persons with schizophrenia. *Journal of the American Psychiatric Nurses Association, 10,* 222.

McGoldrick, M., & Carter, B. (2003). The family life cycle. In F. Walsh (Ed.), *Normal family processes* (pp. 375–398) (3rd ed.). New York: Guilford.

Merrell, J. (2001). Social support for victims of domestic violence. *Journal of Psychosocial Nursing, 39,* 30.

NANDA International, (2005). *NANDA nursing diagnoses: Definitions and classifications, 2005.* Philadelphia: NANDA International.

Nardi, D. A. (1999). Parenting education as family support for low-income families of young children. *Journal of Psychosocial Nursing, 37,* 7.

Nichols, M. N. (2013). *Family therapy: Concepts and methods* (10th ed.). Boston: Allyn & Bacon.

Oyebode, J. (2003). Assessment of carer's psychological needs. *Advances in Psychiatric Treatment, 9,* 45.

Puchelak, R. (2003). *The face of family burden,* Newsletter of the World Fellowship for Schizophrenia and Allied Disorders, First Quarter, 10.

Rose, L. E., Mallinson, R. K., & Gerson, L. D. (2006). Mastery, burden, and areas of concern among family caregivers of mentally ill persons. *Archives of Psychiatric Nursing, 20,* 41.

Smith, G. C., Hatfield, A. B., & Miller, D. C. (2000). Planning by older mothers for the future care of offspring with serious mental illness. *Psychiatric Services, 51,* 1162.

Sperry, L. (2000). Spirituality and psychiatry: Incorporating the spiritual dimension into clinical practice. *Psychiatric Annals, 3,* 518.

Walsh, F. (2003a). Changing families in a changing world: Reconstructing family normality. In F. Walsh (Ed.), *Normal family processes* (pp. 3–26) (3rd ed.). New York: Guilford.

Walsh, F. (2012). Clinical views of family normality, health, and dysfunction: From deficit to strengths perspective. In F. Walsh (Ed.), *Normal family processes* (4th ed.). New York: Guilford.

Wilson, J. H., & Hobbs, H. (1999). The family educator: A professional resource for families. *Journal of Psychosocial Nursing and Mental Health Services, 37,* 22.

CHAPTER

12

Introduction to Psychotropic Drugs

Norman L. Keltner, David E. Vance

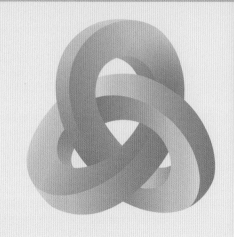

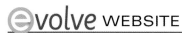 **WEBSITE**

http://evolve.elsevier.com/Keltner

LEARNING OBJECTIVES

- Define the role of psychopharmacology in psychotherapeutic management.
- Identify the nurse's responsibilities in administering psychotropic drugs.
- Describe pharmacokinetic and pharmacodynamic processes as they relate to clinical practice.
- Describe the function and inactivation of neurotransmitters.

- Discuss the function of the blood-brain barrier and the significance of lipid solubility.
- State the benefits of teaching patients about psychotropic drugs.
- Describe common reasons why psychiatric patients might not comply with prescribed drug regimens.

Above all, do no harm.

Hippocrates

The United States is a drug-taking society. People take all types of drugs: drugs to sleep, drugs to wake up, drugs to fight infections, drugs to lower blood pressure, drugs to lower cholesterol, and drugs to lose weight. People take drugs for all types of reasons. People take prescription drugs, over-the-counter drugs, legal drugs, and illegal drugs. Drugs, drugs, drugs! Drugs are taken to fix mental and emotional problems.

Among the drugs taken to "fix things" are drugs that treat delusions and hallucinations (antipsychotics), slow down runaway thinking (mood stabilizers or antimanic agents), improve mood (antidepressants), calm nerves (antianxiety drugs), and improve thinking (drugs for Alzheimer's disease). There are also drugs to correct problems caused by some of the drugs just listed (e.g., antiparkinsonian drugs).

The introductory quote from Hippocrates (460-370 BC) coupled with the pejorative tone of the opening paragraph would suggest a negative view of psychotropic drugs by the authors of this text. Nothing could be further from the truth. However, the following six points must be made:

1. Drugs are not always warranted.
2. Drugs are not always effective.
3. Effective optimal outcomes typically occur when other interventions are coadministered (e.g., counseling in addition to medication).
4. Psychotropic agents can be used (by both patients and clinicians) to avoid the hard work of getting better.
5. Many psychotropic drugs have significant or even life-threatening side effects, drug interactions, or both.
6. Finding the right drug regimen is often a trial-and-error exercise.

Ideally, psychotropic drugs should be prescribed based on an accurate diagnosis and taken until an acceptable mental

NORM'S NOTES
Take a good look at this chapter. If you read it thoroughly, it will help you really understand psychotropic drugs. If you don't understand such basics as pharmacokinetics and pharmacodynamics, you will have to memorize each drug. You shouldn't have to do that! You have often heard that nurses need to know the reason for some treatment, some side effect, or some adverse response. The basics found in this chapter form the foundation for understanding the actions of a drug. So, take your time—Norm's key to learning important information is REPETITION, REPETITION, REPETITION.

or emotional state can be maintained. At that point, it is hoped that the patient can be withdrawn from the medication and proceed with his or her life. However, this scenario does not always occur. Some individuals recover and never need medications again; others become dependent on psychotropic agents to function, finding it difficult to quit; and still others might need the chemistry-correcting properties of these drugs for the remainder of their lives. Some individuals, especially patients with severe mental illness, might improve enough to warrant drug continuation (the drug is helping) but never improve enough to be functionally independent.

Chapter 2 presented a brief historical review of the development of psychotropic drugs. Box 12-1 summarizes significant points during the evolution of psychopharmacology. Antipsychotics, antidepressants, and antimanic agents all were

BOX 12-1	**SIGNIFICANT POINTS IN THE HISTORY OF PSYCHOTROPIC DRUGS: 1949-1990s**
1949	Lithium is "discovered" in Australia.
1951	Chlorpromazine, the first antipsychotic, is "discovered" in France.
1952	Monoamine oxidase inhibitors are "discovered" when a tuberculosis drug is found to improve mood.
1958	Tricyclic antidepressants article is published in the *American Journal of Psychiatry*.
1960	Harris publishes the first article on the effectiveness of benzodiazepines in the *Journal of the American Medical Association*.
1980s	A new class of antidepressants, selective serotonin reuptake inhibitors (SSRIs), is developed. The first SSRI marketed is fluoxetine (Prozac).
1990s	Clozapine (Clozaril), the first truly new antipsychotic agent in 40 years, is released in the United States. Risperidone (Risperdal), olanzapine (Zyprexa), quetiapine (Seroquel), ziprasidone (Geodon), and aripiprazole (Abilify) follow over the next decade.
1990s	Drugs used to treat patients with Alzheimer's disease are made available.
Present-day	New agents and new concerns about psychotropic agents continue to emerge.

"discovered" serendipitously before 1960. Although many related drugs were eventually synthesized from the prototypes of each class, the clones were remarkably similar to the original. However, since the 1990s, several substantially different types of drugs have emerged. Clozapine (Clozaril) and other atypical antipsychotic medications differ from the traditional antipsychotics, and selective serotonin reuptake inhibitors (SSRIs) (e.g., fluoxetine [Prozac]) and other newer antidepressants (e.g., venlafaxine [Effexor]) are quite different from the earlier antidepressants. Finally, drugs in the treatment of Alzheimer's disease (e.g., donepezil [Aricept], rivastigmine tartrate [Exelon], memantine [Namenda]) are providing hope and encouragement to many patients and families affected by this illness. These examples point to the continuing efforts by clinicians and researchers to address mental, emotional, and addictive disorders, which affect approximately 25% of Americans, effectively. These exciting developments in psychopharmacology should challenge every nurse to understand psychopharmacologic concepts and apply them to practice.

NURSING RESPONSIBILITIES

Psychopharmacology is the second component of the psychotherapeutic management model (see Chapter 2 to review this model, if needed). The effectiveness of treatment with antipsychotic, antidepressant, antimanic, and antianxiety drugs has been well established. These drugs have enabled millions of individuals to live increasingly satisfying and productive lives. The least restrictive alternative or environment, a concept that reflects the community mental health effort to allow individuals to live their lives in an unrestrictive atmosphere, has largely evolved as a result of the impact of these drugs.

The nurse must understand key dimensions of psychotropic drug use. Because nursing provides 24-hour care, the nurse is responsible for assessing drug side effects, evaluating desired effects, and applying preventive care to reduce potential problems. Additionally, the nurse usually makes decisions concerning as needed (prn) medications.

Unit III provides a discussion of pharmacologic effects (desired effects), pharmacokinetics administration, side effects (undesired effects), and drug interactions. Chapter 34 discusses the use of psychotropic drugs in children and adolescents. Understanding psychopharmacology involves more than memorizing facts. It should be noted that *memorization* is not a dirty word. Some basics of pharmacology must be memorized, but the nurse who tries to get by on memorization alone *is a medication error waiting to happen*. Because of our strong belief in the importance of nurses understanding the basics of psychopharmacology, we review the following important concepts:

- Pharmacokinetics
- Pharmacodynamics
- Drug-drug interactions
- Blood-brain barrier
- Neurons and neurotransmitters
- Receptors

This chapter concludes with a few general strategies for helping patients and families understand important considerations in regard to psychotropic drug use. Drug-specific patient teaching content is presented in each chapter.

> ### ? CRITICAL THINKING QUESTION
>
> 1. Some nurses might have little knowledge about some drugs they administer. Do you consider this unethical, unprofessional, unsafe, or simply a reality of the nursing profession? Because no one can know every drug, what basic information should a nurse know before giving medication?

PHARMACOKINETICS: WHAT THE BODY DOES TO THE DRUG

Pharmacokinetics is defined as the effects that the body has on a drug. The four aspects of pharmacokinetics are the following:

- *Absorption*—getting the drug into the bloodstream
- *Distribution*—getting the drug from the bloodstream to the tissues and organs
- *Metabolism*—breaking the drug down into an inactive and typically water-soluble form
- *Excretion*—getting the drug out of the body

Absorption

Drugs taken orally must get out of the gastrointestinal (GI) tract and into the bloodstream to have an effect. For a drug to get out of the GI tract, the drug molecule must pass through the stomach or small intestinal wall into blood vessels. Molecules pass through cell membranes (composed of a phospholipid bilayer) in the following three ways:

1. Small molecules can fit through pores or channels in the membrane.
2. Some drug molecules have special transport systems to ferry them through the membrane.
3. Lipid-soluble drugs (most drugs are lipophilic) can pass through the phospholipid membranes.

Only a certain percentage of an oral drug reaches the systemic circulation, whereas 100% of a drug given intravenously reaches the systemic circulation. The percentage of an oral drug that reaches the systemic circulation is a drug's *bioavailability*. Bioavailability is only a fraction of the dose for many drugs given orally because of incomplete absorption and first-pass metabolism. (First-pass metabolism is the enzymatic breakdown of drugs before they reach systemic circulation.) First-pass metabolism occurs during passage through the gut wall and in a presystemic hepatic exposure. The latter exposure occurs because the capillaries in the GI tract do not behave as do most capillaries (i.e., dumping into venules) but instead connect with hepatic portal veins, shunting drugs directly from the GI tract to the liver before they reach the general circulation. Some drugs are substantially "used up" in this manner. For example, buspirone (BuSpar), an antianxiety drug, has a bioavailability of 1% to 4%, which means that most of this drug is metabolized before it gets into general circulation. If the first pass through the liver could be eliminated for buspirone by some mechanism, its dose would have to be dramatically reduced.

Clinical relevance: Only absorbed drugs can have an effect. Drugs with a high first-pass metabolism must be significantly reduced in dose level if given intramuscularly or intravenously.

Distribution

Distribution is the process of the body getting the drug out of the bloodstream and into tissues and organs. If a psychotropic drug cannot leave the bloodstream, it cannot have a therapeutic effect. Lipid-soluble molecules can penetrate capillary membranes as easily as they can penetrate other cell membranes. However, water-soluble (or polar) molecules also leave circulation because of significant gaps between the cells of the capillary wall. Essentially, because molecules are innately active, water-soluble molecules bounce around inside the capillary until they hit a gap and move into extracellular fluid. Another distribution issue involves protein binding. Most drugs bind to plasma proteins (mostly albumin) to some degree or another. For example:

Familiar Psychotropic Drugs	Drug Protein Binding (%)
Sertraline (Zoloft)	99
Diazepam (Valium)	98
Fluoxetine (Prozac)	95
Lorazepam (Ativan)	92
Escitalopram (Lexapro)	55
Venlafaxine (Effexor)	23

Protein binding is important because molecules that are bound to proteins cannot leave circulation—that is, the protein is simply too large to pass through the gaps in the capillary wall. Protein-bound drugs do not have a pharmacologic effect, cannot be metabolized, and cannot be excreted. Specifically, diazepam (Valium) (with 98% protein binding), which has a calming (or anxiolytic) effect, produces its results because of the 2% or so of active drug. Taking Valium with another drug that can reduce its protein binding to 96% would literally double its effect.

Clinical relevance: Both desired and undesired effects of highly protein-bound drugs result from the activity of the relatively few free drug molecules in circulation. Drug combinations that compete for protein binding sites have the potential of causing significant increases in levels of the free or active drug.

Metabolism

Metabolism is the process whereby the body breaks down a drug molecule. Most drugs are metabolized to inactive and water-soluble states in preparation for excretion from the body in the urine. It is important to note that not all drugs are broken down into inactive forms, not all drugs are converted into water-soluble particles, and not all drugs are eliminated via the renal system. More detailed descriptions of metabolism can be found in a general pharmacology text.

Most metabolism occurs in the liver, but it is not the only site; some metabolic activity occurs in the kidneys, lungs, GI tract, and plasma. Enzymes facilitate the metabolic processes and are said to be catalysts because they provoke reactions yet are unaffected by the biochemical reaction. An enzyme is much larger (perhaps 100 times larger) than the drug molecule and is configured in such a way that only molecules matching that specific configuration (i.e., the enzyme's substrates) can be metabolized. A single enzyme performs its metabolic task over and over very rapidly. For example, each molecule of cholinesterase, the enzyme that degrades acetylcholine, metabolizes 5000 molecules of acetylcholine per second (Purves et al., 1997).

Two enzyme systems are of particular importance to nurses who administer psychotropic drugs: (1) the monoamine oxidase (MAO) system and (2) the cytochrome P-450 (CYP-450) system. The MAO system metabolizes monoamines, which include dopamine, norepinephrine, and serotonin. The other system, CYP-450, breaks down most psychotropic drugs.

Monoamine Oxidase System

MAO is the enzyme that rapidly inactivates monoamines (e.g., serotonin, dopamine, norepinephrine) and slowly metabolizes noncatecholamines (e.g., ephedrine, phenylephrine). MAO is located in the liver, intestinal wall, and central nervous system (CNS) in the terminals and synapses of neurons containing serotonin, norepinephrine, or dopamine (Nestler et al., 2009). In the liver, MAO inactivates tyramine, which is found in many foods, and the biogenic amines found in some drugs. When liver MAO is prevented from metabolizing these amines, serious sympathetic effects can develop. MAO is present in two forms: (1) MAO-A, which inactivates norepinephrine and serotonin, and (2) MAO-B, which inactivates dopamine. Some psychotropic drugs inhibit both

MAO-A and MAO-B and are correctly described as *nonselective* MAO inhibitors (these are the agents warned about on so many over-the-counter drug containers). A few drugs are selective and inhibit either MAO-A or MAO-B. These agents are described as *selective* MAO inhibitors.

Cytochrome Enzyme System

Beyond being involved in the metabolism of psychotropic drugs, the CYP-450 enzyme system is the point at which most drug interactions occur. Box 12-2 lists psychotropic drugs that are substrates for these enzymes as well as inhibitors.

The CYP-450 enzyme system has been traditionally referred to as the *hepatic microsomal enzyme system*. This complex name can be broken down as follows: *cyto* stands for microsomal vesicles, *P* stands for pigmentation (because the enzymes contain red-pigmented heme), and *450* refers to the wavelength (in nanometers) at which light absorption occurs (Cozza et al., 2003). Although this much information is probably more than you want to know, it is included here for two reasons: (1) This is the same system that older texts refer to as the *hepatic microsomal system*, and (2) it outlines the reasoning behind an otherwise intimidating name.

CYP-450 enzymes contain 12 families, with more than 40 individual enzymes found in humans (Lehne, 2012). Six enzymes account for approximately 90% of CYP-450 enzymes in humans: 1A2, 3A4, 2C9, 2C19, 2D6, and 2E1 (Sandson et al., 2005). These enzymes are sometimes referred to as *isoenzymes* or *isozymes*. This text uses only the more generic but equally accurate term, *enzymes*.

Clinical relevance: Most drugs must be metabolized to an inactive and water-soluble form to be excreted from the system. Certain conditions (e.g., liver disease, kidney disease) or drug combinations that inhibit metabolism can lead to significant or even deadly results. Mago (2012) developed a mnemonic to remember antidepressants that are relatively "safe" from CYP-450 interactions: *Various Medicines Definitely Co-mingle Very Easily* for *V*enlafaxine (Effexor), *M*irtazapine (Remeron), *D*esvenlafaxine (Prestiq), *C*italopram (Celexa), *V*ilazodone (Viibryd), and *E*scitalopram (Lexapro). In other words, these antidepressants are less likely to have CYP-450-related drug interactions.

Smoking: Another significant issue when administering psychotropic drugs is the influence tobacco smoke has on drug pharmacokinetics. Cigarette smoking causes the induction of CYP-450 1A2 (i.e., causes more of this enzyme to be synthesized). Table 12-1 lists the names of psychotropic drugs that are substrates of CYP-450 1A2. Maximum enzyme induction occurs with 7 to 12 cigarettes per day for some agents (e.g. clozapine, olanzapine), which leads to a 40% to 50% reduction in their serum level (Fankhauser, 2013). The serum level of other drugs may not decline by this much unless the patient is a heavy smoker (≥30 cigarettes per day). Regardless, a patient who smokes a half a pack or more of cigarettes per day requires more medication than the patient would have required if he or she did not smoke. Depending on the drug, this could lead to toxic levels developing if the medication is not titrated downward as the patient stops smoking. These same effects can occur from secondhand smoke as well.

DOPAMINE

Activation (Agonists)
Schizophrenia-like symptoms
Psychosis
Dyskinesias
Hallucinations
Delusions
Nausea
Vomiting
Addictive behaviors
Sexual function enhancement

Antagonism
Antipsychotic effect
Negative symptoms of schizophrenia
Temperature dysregulation
Antiemetic effect
Parkinsonism and extrapyramidal side effects
Cognitive problems
Sexual dysfunction
Neuroendocrine dysregulation
Depression, anhedonia
Lack of energy, motivation

BOX 12-2   PSYCHOTROPIC SUBSTRATES AND GENERAL INHIBITORS AND INDUCERS OF SELECTED CYTOCHROME P-450 ENZYMES

1A2
1A2 Substrates
Antidepressants
Amitriptyline
Imipramine
Fluvoxamine
Mirtazapine
Clomipramine

Antipsychotics
Clozapine
Haloperidol
Olanzapine
Phenothiazines

Other Drugs
Caffeine
Tacrine

1A2 Inhibitors
Fluvoxamine
Fluoroquinolones
Beta-estradiol
Ciprofloxacin
Erythromycin
Grapefruit juice

1A2 Inducers
Carbamazepine
Cigarette smoke
Omeprazole
Phenobarbital
Primidone (anticonvulsant)
Rifampin (tuberculosis drug)

2D6
2D6 Substrates
Antidepressants
Some tricyclic antidepressants (e.g., desipramine, nortriptyline)
Venlafaxine
Fluoxetine
Paroxetine
Trazodone
Mirtazapine

Antipsychotics
Thioridazine
Risperidone
Haloperidol
Clozapine

2D6 Inhibitors
Paroxetine
Fluoxetine
Fluphenazine
Sertraline (>100 mg)
Quinidine
Haloperidol
Cimetidine
Thioridazine
Amitriptyline
Oral contraceptives
Clomipramine
Desipramine

3A4
3A4 Substrates
Antidepressants
Amitriptyline
Imipramine
Clomipramine
Sertraline
Mirtazapine
Bupropion

Antipsychotics
Clozapine
Haloperidol
Quetiapine

Benzodiazepines
Alprazolam
Diazepam

3A4 Inhibitors
Fluvoxamine
Sertraline (>100 mg)
Cimetidine
Diltiazem
Verapamil
Ketoconazole
Erythromycin
Fluoxetine
Progestagens
Grapefruit juice
Paroxetine

Adapted from Keltner, N.L., & Folks, D.G. (2005). *Psychotropic drugs* (4th ed.). St. Louis: Mosby.

Question: What might happen when a heavy smoker who is taking olanzapine is hospitalized on a nonsmoking unit?

Answer: After a few weeks of nonsmoking, his CYP-450 1A2 level would return to normal with a subsequent increase in serum levels unless the dose is reduced. With some drugs, this could be dangerous.

? CRITICAL THINKING QUESTION

2. As stated, most psychotropic drug interactions occur as a result of the effects on the CYP-450 system. If an inhibitor of the CYP-450 3A4 enzyme is given (e.g., grapefruit juice), which psychotropic drugs would be affected? What is the effect? (Refer to Box 12-2 to answer this question.)

TABLE 12-1	**PSYCHOTROPIC DRUGS THAT INTERACT WITH TOBACCO SMOKE**

Caffeine
Clozapine
Doxepin
Duloxetine
Fluvoxamine
Mirtazapine
Olanzapine
Riluzole (glutamate antagonist)
Thiothixene
Trifluoperazine

Adapted from Fankhauser, J.P. (2013). Drug interactions with tobacco smoke: implications for patient care. *Current Psychiatry, 12*, 12.

Half-Life of Drugs

The half-life of a drug is the amount of time required for 50% of the drug to disappear from the body. If drug X has a half-life of 4 hours, then 50% of the drug will be out of the system in 4 hours. In another 4 hours, only 25% of the original dose will remain. In most cases, it would not matter whether the patient took 100 mg or 300 mg: the amount of drug in the body would decrease by 50% every 4 hours. This action is referred to as *linear kinetics*, and most drugs follow this pattern. This rule has exceptions, most notably in the case of alcohol, in which only a set amount of the drug is metabolized in a given period, regardless of the amount ingested (i.e., nonlinear kinetics). If the nurse gives the same drug dose (e.g., 100 mg) at the same time (e.g., three times a day), a steady state is achieved in four half-lives. When discontinuing a drug, four half-lives are required to eliminate 96% of the drug. This period is referred to as the *washout period*.

> ### ❓ CRITICAL THINKING QUESTION
>
> 3. Prozac has a half-life of approximately 10 days or longer (when including its active metabolite, norfluoxetine). How long is the washout period? If a drug known to interact with Prozac is to be given, how long should the interval be between stopping Prozac and beginning the new drug?

Excretion

The kidney excretes most drugs in the urine, but other routes of excretion exist, such as breast milk, bile, feces, saliva, sweat, and the lungs. Factors that can affect excretion include kidney disease, age, and drug competition for active tubular transport.

Clinical relevance: Drugs that are not adequately excreted (e.g., because of kidney disease), particularly drugs excreted unchanged (a few drugs are not metabolized [lithium, amphetamine]), have a more pronounced effect compared with drugs that are excreted.

PHARMACODYNAMICS: WHAT THE DRUG DOES TO THE BODY

Pharmacodynamics is the effect that a drug has on the body. The two global responses to drugs are the desired effects and the side effects. Drugs that activate receptors are called *agonists*, and drugs that block receptors are called *antagonists*. Some psychotropic drugs are agonists, whereas many others are antagonists. Pharmacodynamic effects of particular interest to this discussion are down-regulation of receptors and pharmacodynamic tolerance.

Down-Regulation

Down-regulation of receptors is an important concept, primarily because chronic exposure to certain psychotropic drugs causes receptors to change. For example, consistent use of antidepressants causes postsynaptic receptors to decrease in number. Because this down-regulation occurs at about the same time that the antidepressant effect develops (approximately 2 to 4 weeks), it is thought by some that reduction in postsynaptic receptors might provide a better explanation for mood elevation than increases in neurotransmitters.

Pharmacodynamic Tolerance

Pharmacodynamic tolerance describes a reduction in receptor sensitivity (or desensitization). A good example is a chronic drinker of alcohol. When the newspaper reports a person driving a car with a blood alcohol level (BAL) of 0.35, the story is likely about a case of pharmacodynamic tolerance. This person's receptors are no longer responding to the ethanol in the way a normal person's receptors would respond. Although at first glance this idea might appear appealing, it really is not. Tolerance to a BAL that could cause deadly respiratory depression does not occur. A person who is functioning at an elevated BAL might drink only a little more alcohol and wind up dead.

Clinical relevance: Knowledge of down-regulatory functions helps the nurse explain the lag time between initiating drug therapy and clinical improvement. Knowledge of pharmacodynamic tolerance aids in teaching patients and families about drug tolerance to some drug effects but little, if any, tolerance to some lethal effects (e.g., respiratory depression) at just slightly higher doses.

Drug-Drug Interactions

There are two types of drug-drug interactions: pharmacokinetic interactions and pharmacodynamic interactions. Pharmacokinetic interactions occur when one of the four pharmacokinetic processes is inhibited or induced. An example of how each pharmacokinetic process might play into a drug interaction follows:

Absorption: Drug A is taken with another drug that changes stomach pH, affecting absorption of drug A.

Distribution: Two drugs are both highly protein bound. Drug A "hogs" most of the binding sites, leaving more of drug B available. Drug B would have a greater pharmacologic effect.

Metabolism: Two drugs are metabolized by the CYP-450 enzyme 2D6. One or both drugs could have a higher blood level.

Excretion: Drug A alters the urinary pH, speeding or hindering the excretion of another drug.

Enzyme induction usually takes several days to weeks to develop, whereas enzyme inhibition develops almost immediately (Sandson et al., 2005).

Pharmacodynamic interactions are straightforward. On the one hand, two drugs with anticholinergic properties have the potential to have a synergistic or additive effect. On the other hand, two drugs can oppose each other, basically reducing their effectiveness.

BLOOD-BRAIN BARRIER

The blood-brain barrier is also an important concept for understanding psychotropic drug activity. The brain, more than other organs of the body, requires a constant internal milieu. Although other parts of the body experience fluctuations in body chemistry, even small changes in the brain produce serious problems. The brain is protected from fluctuations by the blood-brain barrier. This barrier regulates the amount and speed of substances in the blood entering the brain. Water, carbon dioxide, and oxygen readily cross the barrier; other substances are excluded from the brain.

The blood-brain barrier has three dimensions: (1) an anatomic dimension, (2) a physiologic dimension, and (3) a metabolic dimension. The anatomic dimension is the structure of the capillaries that supply blood to the brain and prevent many molecules from slipping through. There are no gaps.

The physiologic dimension is a chemical and transport system that recognizes and allows certain molecules into the brain. Lipid solubility is the most important of the chemical properties that determine whether a molecule can pass through the blood-brain barrier. Highly lipid-soluble substances pass the blood-brain barrier with relative ease. Highly water-soluble substances penetrate this barrier slowly and in insignificant amounts. Nicotine, ethanol, heroin, caffeine, and diazepam (Valium) are examples of highly lipid-soluble substances. This characteristic is clinically important because only drugs that can pass through this barrier in significant amounts are effective in treating a psychiatric or medical disorder of the brain. Certain non–lipid-soluble substances such as glucose, which is the brain's primary energy source, and essential amino acids, which are needed for the synthesis of neurotransmitters, are required for normal brain function. Special transport systems carry these essential substances across the blood-brain barrier.

P-glycoproteins: Another dimension to the physiologic barrier is the *P-glycoprotein efflux transporter system.* This system has various substrates and ferries these molecules back out of the cell about as fast as they enter it. For instance, the P-glycoprotein efflux transporters cause second-generation antihistamines to be nonsedating. These antihistamine drug molecules are transported out of the CNS before they can have a sedating effect (Cozza, et al., 2003). Some drugs induce the P-glycoprotein system (e.g., venlafaxine) to produce even greater efflux of certain substrates, causing some drugs to be less effective (Levin, 2012). What is particularly perplexing is that a drug that inhibits P-glycoproteins can cause an increased central effect without causing a change in serum levels. How? By inhibiting P-glycoproteins, more of drug X gets into the brain even though more of the drug has not been taken by the patient. The serum level is unchanged, but the effect can be significantly greater. Table 12-2 lists P-glycoprotein substrates, inhibitors, and inducers.

TABLE 12-2	SELECTED PSYCHOTROPIC DRUGS THAT AFFECT P-GLYCOPROTEIN EFFLUX TRANSPORTERS	
SUBSTRATES	**INHIBITORS**	**INDUCERS**
Amitriptyline	Amitriptyline	Phenothiazines
Carbamazepine	Carbamazepine	Trazodone
Chlorpromazine	Chlorpromazine	Venlafaxine
Citalopram	Desipramine	
Nortriptyline	Disulfiram	
Olanzapine	Fluoxetine	
Paroxetine	Haloperidol	
Quetiapine	Imipramine	
Risperidone	Paroxetine	
Sertraline	Sertraline	
Venlafaxine		

Adapted from Levin, G.M. (2012). P-glycoproteins: why this drug transporter may be clinically important. *Current Psychiatry, 11,* 38.

The metabolic barrier prevents molecules from entering the brain by enzymatic action within the endothelial lining of the brain capillaries. For example, levodopa can pass the blood-brain barrier, but much of it is changed to dopamine before it can pass completely through the capillary wall into the brain. The metabolic product, dopamine, does not readily pass this barrier, thus illustrating the third way that the brain protects itself from substances in peripheral circulation.

Understanding the blood-brain barrier helps the nurse conceptualize, administer, and monitor drug therapy accurately as well as understand addiction to highly lipid-soluble substances such as alcohol and heroin. A comparison of systemic penicillin and dopamine serves as an example for understanding this important principle. If penicillin were the only antibiotic available (which was true at one time), then large doses would be needed to treat a CNS infection, because this water-soluble drug does not pass through the blood-brain barrier easily. When a large dose of penicillin is given, only a fraction of that dose enters the brain. Most of the penicillin stays in the peripheral system, which does not cause alarm because penicillin has relatively few adverse effects. However, dopamine has many adverse effects on the body. The dose needed to penetrate the blood-brain barrier and affect the brain adequately (a central effect) is so large that it would have serious adverse effects on the rest of the body (e.g., cardiac stimulation, a peripheral effect).

NEURONS AND NEUROTRANSMITTERS

Nerve cells, or neurons, compose the basic unit of the nervous system. Nerve cells are designed to receive and give information. Dendrites are the projections from the neuron that receive information and transmit it to the cell body. Axons send information from the nerve cell to the dendrites, axons, or cell bodies of other neurons. Axons of one cell are separated from the dendrites, axons, or cell body of another by a microscopic space known as a *synapse* (Figure 12-1). Figure 12-2 depicts the relationships among neurotransmitters, neurons, and psychotropic drugs.

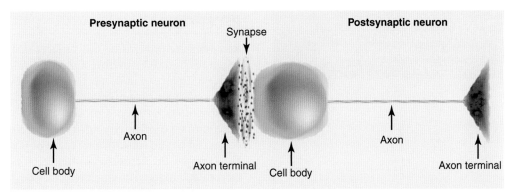

FIG 12-1 This two-neuron chain shows presynaptic and postsynaptic neurons interconnected by a synapse. The synapse is composed of a synaptic bouton (triangle) or presynaptic terminal, the synaptic cleft, and the postsynaptic membrane, which, in this example, is the dendrite or cell body (circle) of the postsynaptic neuron.

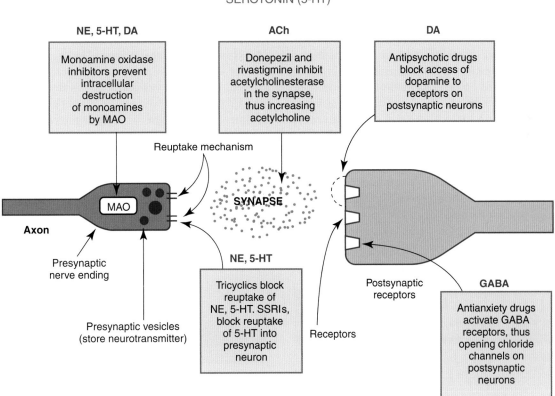

FIG 12-2 Explanation of the way psychotropic drugs affect five major neurotransmitters. (Modified from Stuart, G., & Sundeen, S. (1995). *Principles and practice of psychiatric nursing* (5th ed.). St. Louis: Mosby.

Information, in the form of an electrochemical excitation, is communicated between cells in a specific manner. An electrochemical impulse runs from the cell body through the axon to the synaptic terminal. Neurotransmitters are stimulated and released from the synaptic terminal into the synaptic cleft and combine with receptors on the postsynaptic neuron, evoking a neuronal response. Remember, however, that neurons are not strung throughout the brain end on end. The neuronal system is highly complex, with most neurons receiving input from thousands of other neurons. The arborization, or branching, of dendrites continues into late adolescence and early adulthood. It is when most of these connections are finally complete that who we are truly emerges.

BOX 12-3 CATEGORIES OF NEUROTRANSMITTERS* THAT ARE IMPORTANT IN PSYCHIATRY

Monoamines
Dopamine
Norepinephrine
Serotonin

Cholinergic
Acetylcholine

Amino Acids
Gamma-aminobutyric acid (GABA)
Glutamate

*Peptides not included.

Neurotransmitters are synthesized from natural precursors (e.g., amino acids) in the body (Box 12-3). These precursors are extracted from the bloodstream and synthesized in the cell into neurotransmitters. Neurotransmitters are stored in storage vesicles in the presynaptic terminals of the cell. Neurotransmitters come in many forms, and they combine with specific receptors. For example, the neurotransmitter norepinephrine combines with a norepinephrine receptor. After norepinephrine electrochemically stimulates the norepinephrine receptor, information is transmitted to the cell body, which communicates to the next neuron, and so on. After it is in the synaptic cleft, the neurotransmitter can, until it is inactivated, continue to stimulate the postsynaptic receptor. Neurotransmitters are inactivated by enzymes in the synaptic cleft or by enzymes in the presynaptic terminal or are taken up into surrounding glial cells. Knowledge of this inactivation process has facilitated the evolution of psychopharmacology. The most important neurotransmitters for psychiatric nursing students to understand along with related mental disorders are presented in Table 12-3.

RECEPTORS

Receptors are proteins on cell surfaces that respond to endogenous ligands or to drug molecules. A ligand is a transmitter substance or molecule that fits and evokes a response from a receptor. Examples of ligands include drugs, neurotransmitters, hormones, prostaglandins, and leukotrienes. Receptors are configured so that only precisely shaped molecules can fit and subsequently cause or prevent a response. For example, the neurotransmitter serotonin fits serotonin receptors, but acetylcholine molecules do not fit serotonin receptors.

Four primary receptor processes exist (Lehne, 2012). The two most commonly addressed processes in psychopharmacology literature are the ligand-gated ion channel (or first-messenger) process and the G-protein–coupled (or second-messenger) process. When the ligand-gated receptor is activated, an ion channel, such as a sodium, calcium, or chloride channel, opens, and the respective ion flows through into the cell. Depending on the ion, this action causes cell depolarization (the cell fires) or hyperpolarization (cell firing slows down, or the cell does not fire). The process is extremely rapid, usually occurring within milliseconds. Acetylcholine (at nicotinic receptors only), gamma-aminobutyric acid (GABA), glycine, and glutamate use the first-messenger system. The G-protein–coupled receptor is a more complex process—a biologic cascade of intracellular reactions develops and is slower compared with the first-messenger system. Norepinephrine, serotonin, dopamine, acetylcholine (at muscarinic receptors only), and peptides couple with G-protein or second-messenger receptors. Consequences of selected receptor activation or antagonism are listed in Boxes 12-4, 12-5, and 12-6.

Psychotropic drugs can affect neurotransmitters in several ways:
1. **Block** metabolism (e.g., some antidepressants and drugs for Alzheimer's disease)
2. **Block** reuptake (e.g., SSRIs and other antidepressants)
3. **Block** receptors (antagonists)

TABLE 12-3 NEUROTRANSMITTERS AND RELATED MENTAL DISORDERS*

NEUROTRANSMITTER-RELATED STATE	MENTAL DISORDER
Increase in dopamine	Schizophrenia
Decrease in norepinephrine	Depression
Decrease in serotonin	Depression
Decrease in acetylcholine	Alzheimer's disease
Decrease in GABA	Anxiety
Increase in glutamate	Excitotoxicity leading to neuronal death
Decrease in glutamate	Psychotic thinking

GABA, Gamma-aminobutyric acid.
*Although this explanation is overly simplistic, this information nevertheless serves to convey the basic neurotransmitter theories for each related mental disorder and continues to drive drug treatment for those disorders.

BOX 12-4 RESULTS OF ACTIVATING AND ANTAGONIZING SEROTONIN RECEPTORS

SEROTONIN ACTIVATION	SEROTONIN ANTAGONISM
Antidepressant effect	Depression
Anxiety	Dysthymia
Nausea	Suicidality
Vomiting	Aggressiveness
Other GI disturbances	Obsessive thinking
Sexual dysfunction	Sleep-wake cycle disruption
Reduced appetite and weight loss	Pain
Insomnia	Compulsive behavior
Movement disorders	Anxiety
Temperature dysregulation	Panic
Psychotic thinking	

BOX 12-5   RESULTS OF ACTIVATING AND ANTAGONIZING ACETYLCHOLINE RECEPTORS

ACETYLCHOLINE ACTIVATION	ACETYLCHOLINE ANTAGONISM
Pupil contraction	Pupil dilation
Decreased heart rate	Increased heart rate
Constriction of bronchi	Dilation of bronchi
Increased respiratory secretions	Decreased respiratory secretions
Increased voiding	Decreased voiding
Salivation	Dry mouth
Increased gastric secretions	Decreased gastric secretions
Increased defecation	Constipation
Sweating	Decreased sweating
Enhancement of cognitive processes	Cognitive slowing

BOX 12-6   RESULTS OF ACTIVATING AND ANTAGONIZING NOREPINEPHRINE RECEPTORS

NOREPINEPHRINE ACTIVATION	NOREPINEPHRINE ANTAGONISM
Antidepressant effect	Depressive effect
Vasoconstriction (alpha-1)	Vasodilation (alpha-1 antagonism)
Increased heart rate (beta-1)	Decreased heart rate (beta blocker)
Bronchial dilation	Sexual dysfunction
Other physical effects	Other physical effects

4. **Stimulate** or **block** autoreceptors (see following discussion on autoreceptors)
5. **Stimulate** receptors (agonists)
6. **Stimulate** receptor affinity (benzodiazepines cause GABA receptors to have a greater attraction for GABA)
7. **Stimulate** the release of a neurotransmitter (e.g., amphetamine stimulates the release of dopamine).

The following terms relating to receptors are defined to facilitate understanding of information presented in the drug chapters.

Receptor antagonism. Receptor antagonism is the process in which receptor function is compromised related to blocking of that receptor by a psychotropic drug. Antagonists prevent the endogenous ligand from activating the receptor.

Receptor agonist. A receptor agonist is a drug that fits and activates the receptor in the same manner as the naturally occurring ligand.

Autoreceptor. An autoreceptor is the negative feedback mechanism that neurons use to increase or decrease the release of a neurotransmitter; they are typically, but not always, found on the presynaptic neuron. Autoreceptor agonists tell the neuron that enough of the neurotransmitter is

present; a decrease in the release of the neurotransmitter occurs. Autoreceptor antagonists tell the receptor to release more of the neurotransmitter.

Receptor affinity. Receptor affinity is the attraction or strength of attraction between neurotransmitters and receptors.

Receptor life cycle. Receptors are continually being formed and continually breaking down. The life cycle of the average receptor is short.

Receptor modulation. Some neurotransmitters do not have a direct effect but modify (or modulate) the effect of another neurotransmitter (Figure 12-3). The following scenario might help in the understanding of receptor modulation. Picture, if possible, one neuron (#1) synapsing with the synaptic terminal of a presynaptic neuron (#2), which is synapsing in the traditional way with a third neuron (#3). Neuron #1 influences the release of neurotransmitter from #2, which then affects the amount of neurotransmitter released into the synapse between #2 and #3. Neuron #1 is modulating neuron #2 (see Figure 12-3).

PATIENT EDUCATION

The importance of patient and family education cannot be overemphasized. Historically, many psychiatric patients and their families have demonstrated little understanding of their medications. Although the emphasis on education has partially remedied this problem, teaching about these potent drugs will always be a nursing priority. In addition, many rehospitalizations are related to patients' nonadherence to medication schedules. As knowledge deficits are removed, better compliance can be anticipated.

Despite a certain risk associated with discussing medications and side effects with patients, nurses have a professional duty to do so with knowledge and sensitivity—that is, with balance. The nurse might frighten patients with too much or inappropriate information. Good professional judgment is important, including teaching patients about what effects are visible, what can be felt, and what the possibilities are of becoming drug-dependent. The nurse should also emphasize the need for regular checkups and tests. Specific areas of education include the following (Malone et al., 2004):

1. Discussion of side effects:
   - Side effects can directly affect the patient's willingness to adhere to the drug regimen; for example, SSRIs, such as sertraline (Zoloft), are known to reduce libido and sexual functioning. Thus, these drugs indirectly affect spouses as well.
   - Side effects can cause medical problems or even death.
   - Some drugs cause patients to experience emotional flattening, dulling responses to the environment, counseling, and family.
   - Some drugs cause cognitive slowing.
   - The nurse should always inquire about the patient's response to a drug—both therapeutic responses and adverse responses.

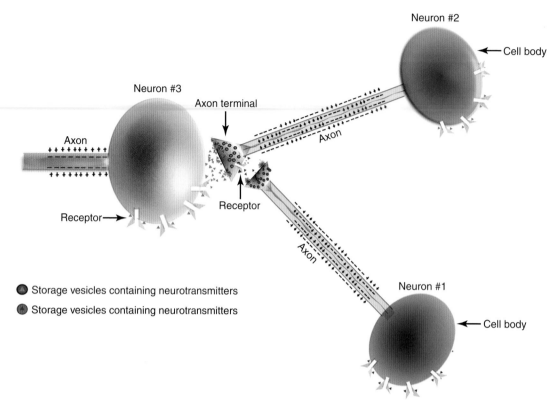

FIG 12-3 Neuronal modulation.

2. Discussion of safety issues:
   - Does the patient take the drug as prescribed?
   - Do the patient and family know which effects should be reported to the nurse or physician?
   - Because some drugs, such as tricyclic antidepressants and lithium, have a narrow therapeutic index, thoughts of self-harm must be discussed.
   - Does the drug have potential for abuse or dependence?
   - Can the drug be discontinued abruptly without effect? Patients should know that many drugs must be tapered gradually.
   - Because many psychotropic drugs cause sedation or drowsiness, discussions concerning use of hazardous machinery and driving must occur.

3. Attitudes of patient and nurse about medications:
   - Because many patients and families believe that the use of medications is a sign of weakness or lack of faith in God, the nurse must discuss these issues.
   - Some nurses do not really "believe" in psychotropic medications either. These nurses must examine their own views and perhaps work in areas of nursing that do not involve psychotropic drugs.
   - For patients and families who are resistant to the use of psychotropic agents, the nurse must discuss the potential ramifications of noncompliance.
   - Issues of dependence and long-term medication use must be discussed.
   - Because many patients and families do not want to become addicted, the nurse must point out the specific addiction potential of any specific drug. Most psychotropic drugs are not addicting.

4. Drug interactions:
   - Patients and families must be taught to discuss the effects of the addition of over-the-counter drugs, alcohol, and illegal drugs to currently prescribed drugs.
   - Patients who see more than one clinician must make potential prescribing professionals aware of all drugs that are currently being taken.

5. Instructions for older adult patients or children of older adult patients:
   - Because older individuals have a different pharmacokinetic profile than younger adults, special instructions concerning side effects and drug-drug interactions should be tailored for this population.

6. Instructions for pregnant or breast-feeding patients:
   - Because pregnant or breast-feeding patients have special risks associated with psychotropic drug therapy, special instructions should be tailored for these individuals.

7. Awareness of metabolic differences in diverse races and ethnicities:
   - Because of genetic differences as well as diet, cultural beliefs and expectations, and lifestyle, patients of different races may achieve the same therapeutic outcome from lower doses of medication than others.
   - Gene expression and mutation of certain enzymes (e.g., CYP-450 2D6) have been shown to alter the rate at which medications are metabolized, with some resulting in being poor metabolizers and others being ultrarapid metabolizers. Different doses must be considered to achieve the optimal therapeutic outcome.

Teaching patients about their medications enables them to be mature participants in their own care and decreases undesirable

BOX 12-7 COMMON REASONS FOR PATIENTS NOT TAKING MEDICATION AS PRESCRIBED

Sexual dysfunction
Specific side effects (e.g., dry mouth, insomnia, sleepiness)
Emotional dulling
Cognitive slowing
Denial of need
Fear of becoming addicted
Religious reasons
Interference with work
Inability to use alcohol or other recreational drugs
Pregnancy
Illness (suspiciousness, delusions of conspiracy)

side effects. Effective teaching can reduce noncompliance, or the failure to take medications as prescribed. Box 12-7 lists common reasons that patients give for not taking their medication as prescribed. Each chapter in this unit outlines patient education issues specific to each class of drugs discussed.

? CRITICAL THINKING QUESTION

4. In this chapter, we state that the nurse should use balance when giving information to a patient about a drug. What is the balance between arousing unneeded apprehension in a patient who is vulnerable to suggestion (i.e., giving complete information) and treating that adult patient as a child (i.e., withholding information to protect the patient)? In your role as student and later as nurse, you would not want to do either.

STUDY NOTES

1. Psychopharmacology is the second component of psychotherapeutic management. Psychotropic drugs have enabled millions of people to live more productive lives in the least restrictive environment.

2. Nurses assess for drug side effects, evaluate desired effects, and make decisions about prn medications.

3. Pharmacokinetic processes include absorption, distribution, metabolism, and excretion of drugs.

4. Absorption is the process whereby drugs leave the GI tract and get into the bloodstream.

5. Bioavailability is the percentage of a drug that reaches the systemic circulation.

6. Distribution refers to the process of drug molecules leaving the bloodstream to reach tissues and organs. Drugs that do not leave the bloodstream cannot have a psychiatric effect.

7. Lipid solubility is a property that affects absorption and distribution. Highly lipid-soluble drugs easily penetrate the blood-brain barrier.

8. Protein binding, the propensity of a drug to bind to serum proteins, also affects drug distribution. Drugs that are bound to serum proteins cannot leave the bloodstream.

9. Metabolism is the process whereby the body breaks down a drug to remove the drug from the body.

10. The liver is the site of most drug metabolism.

11. The two major enzyme systems associated with psychotropic drugs are the MAO system and the CYP-450 system.

12. An individual enzyme breaks down thousands of drug molecules per second.

13. The CYP-450 system is mentioned often in current psychotropic drug literature. Older texts referred to the CYP-450 system as the *hepatic microsomal enzyme system.*

14. Most drug-drug interactions are related to interference with the CYP-450 system.

15. The half-life of a drug is the length of time required for the body to remove 50% of the original dose. If a single dose of a drug is given and the drug has a half-life of 4 hours, 50% of the drug will remain in the body after 4 hours, 25% of the drug will remain after 8 hours, and 12.5% of the drug will remain after 12 hours.

16. Excretion is the removal of drug from the body through the kidneys via the urine.

17. Pharmacodynamics involves the effects of the drug on the body.

18. Drug effects are typically categorized as desired effects or side effects.

19. Down-regulation of a receptor refers to a decrease in the number of receptors or to decreased receptor sensitivity.

20. Pharmacodynamic tolerance is a state in which receptors become less sensitive to agonists.

21. Highly lipid-soluble drugs, such as ethanol, heroin, and diazepam (Valium), pass the blood-brain barrier with ease. This characteristic partially accounts for the widespread abuse of these drugs.

22. Only drugs that pass the blood-brain barrier can affect the CNS.

23. Neurotransmitters, which are neurochemical substances in the brain, evoke a neuronal response, are synthesized by cytoplasmic enzymes, and are usually stored in storage vesicles in the presynaptic terminals of the neuron.

24. Both neurotransmitter deficiency and neurotransmitter excess are related to mental disorders; psychotropic drugs are effective because they cause an increase or decrease in the brain's ability to use a specific neurotransmitter.

25. Receptors are proteins on the cell surface that respond to specific ligands.

26. The two receptor processes most important for psychiatric nurses to understand are the first-messenger system and the second-messenger system.

27. The first-messenger system causes a cellular response when a ligand couples with the receptor, which immediately opens an ion channel.

28. The second-messenger system is more complex compared with the first-messenger system. The initial ligand-receptor

coupling initiates a series of events that culminate in a neuronal response.

29. The blood-brain barrier protects the brain from the physiologic fluctuations that the body experiences and regulates the amount of substances entering the brain and the speed with which they enter.

30. The P-glycoprotein efflux transporter system ferries molecules out of the cell. Inhibitors of this system allow more of a substrate to stay in the cell, whereas inducers potentiate P-glycoproteins to remove an even greater amount of the substrate.

31. Teaching patients can decrease the incidence of side effects and increase adherence to the drug regimen. The nurse should use good clinical judgment when deciding what to share with patients and their families.

REFERENCES

Cozza, K. L., Armstrong, S. C., & Oesterheld, J. R. (2003). *Drug interaction principles for medical practice*. Washington, D.C: American Psychiatric Publishing.

Fankhauser, J. P. (2013). Drug interactions with tobacco smoke: Implications for patient care. *Current Psychiatry, 12*, 12.

Keltner, N. L., & Folks, D. G. (2005). *Psychotropic drugs* (4th ed.). St. Louis: Mosby.

Lehne, R. A. (2012). *Pharmacology for nursing care* (8th ed.). Philadelphia: Saunders.

Levin, G. M. (2012). P-glycoproteins: Why this drug transporter may be clinically important. *Current Psychiatry, 11*, 38.

Mago, R. (2012). Reducing CYP-450 drug interactions caused by antidepressants. *Current Psychiatry, 11*, 55.

Malone, K., et al. (2004). Antidepressants, antipsychotics, benzodiazepines, and the breastfeeding dyad. *Perspectives in Psychiatric Care, 40*, 133.

Nestler, E. J., Hyman, S. E., & Malenka, R. C. (2009). *Molecular neuropharmacology* (2nd ed.). New York: McGraw-Hill.

Purves, D., Augustine, G. J., & Fitzpatrick, D. (1997). *Neuroscience*. Sunderland, MA: Sinauer Associates.

Sandson, N. B., Armstrong, S. C., & Cozza, K. L. (2005). An overview of psychotropic drug-drug interactions. *Psychosomatics, 46*, 464.

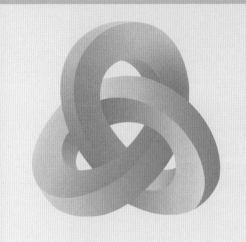

Antiparkinsonian Drugs

Norman L. Keltner

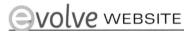 WEBSITE

http://evolve.elsevier.com/Keltner

LEARNING OBJECTIVES

- Differentiate between Parkinson's disease (PD) and parkinsonism.
- Discuss the causes and symptoms of parkinsonism.
- Identify the two neurotransmitters primarily associated with PD.

- Describe the biochemical relationship between PD and extrapyramidal side effects (EPSEs).
- Discuss the side effects of antiparkinsonian drugs.

PARKINSON'S DISEASE AND EXTRAPYRAMIDAL SIDE EFFECTS

Extrapyramidal side effects (EPSEs) are serious and sometimes dangerous complications of treatment with psychotropic drugs. Antipsychotic agents typically cause these adverse responses, but other drugs can also produce EPSEs. Historically, it has been assumed that the newer antipsychotic drugs (called atypical or second-generation antipsychotic agents) were less likely to cause EPSEs (Haddad et al., 2012). However, large meta-analyses suggest these differences are more imagined than actual (Peluso et al., 2012). EPSEs are the result of the biochemical changes similar to those found in Parkinson's disease (PD).

PD is a progressive, chronic, degenerative disease of un-known cause that involves the functional area of the brain called the *extrapyramidal system*. Approximately 1% of people older than age 60 are affected by this disorder, with an annual cost in the United States of about $2 billion (Fritsch et al., 2012). A well-regulated extrapyramidal system is needed for normal coordination of involuntary movement, which sup-ports voluntary movement. When a person walks down the street, numerous involuntary movements facilitate the volun-tary movements associated with walking. PD is characterized by four cardinal symptoms: (1) tremors, (2) bradykinesia, (3) rigidity, and (4) postural instability. A balance of two neurotransmitters—acetylcholine (ACh) and dopamine—is required for normal functioning of the extrapyramidal system. The four primary symptoms and other associated symptoms (e.g., difficulty swallowing, drooling, weight loss, choking, impaired breathing, urinary retention, constipation) occur when these two neurotransmitters are out of balance.

> ## ❓ CRITICAL THINKING QUESTION
>
> 1. How are the associated or secondary symptoms of PD linked to the primary symptoms? (For example, excessive saliva or drooling is related to difficulty swallowing, which is secondary to rigidity.)

Dopamine is synthesized in the midbrain by pigmented cells in an area called the *substantia nigra* (Latin for "black sub-stance"). Cell bodies are located in the substantia nigra, and their axons project to a specific area of the extrapyramidal sys-tem called the *basal ganglia* (also known as the *corpus striatum*). The axon terminals of these neurons release dopamine, which activates the dopamine receptors there. This pathway, from the midbrain to the basal ganglia, is known as the *nigrostriatal tract*. In PD, the pigmented neurons of the substantia nigra lose their pigmentation ("blackness"), signifying a decline in dopamine production. A deficiency in dopamine and a subsequent de-crease in dopamine transmission to the basal ganglia result in an imbalance with ACh in the basal ganglia. The basal ganglia are shown in Figure 13-1 in what is referred to as a *coronal* cut of the brain (this is a slice that runs from top to bottom with

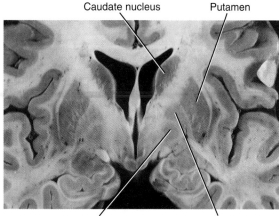

FIG 13-1 Basal ganglia. The basal ganglia are composed of several subcortical (below the surface of the outer brain gray matter or cortex) nuclei, including the caudate nucleus, putamen, and globus pallidus. The globus pallidus can be divided further into the globus pallidus externa and the globus pallidus interna. (Courtesy of Richard E. Powers, Director, Brain Resource Program, University of Alabama at Birmingham.)

the outer edges of this view being close to the ears). Figure 13-2 illustrates the depigmentation occurring in PD by comparing the substantia nigra and locus ceruleus (where norepinephrine is synthesized) of a young man (Figure 13-2, *A*) with those of an older man without PD (on the right) and an older man with PD (on the left). This figure clearly shows that normal aging results in a loss of pigmented neurons and that PD dramatically accelerates the process.

NORM'S NOTES

As you might have guessed, I love understanding how drugs work and how a certain category of drug helps treat a specific mental disorder. I always start teaching my students about psychotropic drugs by discussing the antiparkinsonian drugs. Studying these drugs and Parkinson's disease (PD) itself provides a perfect vehicle for explaining neurotransmitter imbalance (and balance) and neuronal tract degeneration. In some ways, PD could be considered the opposite of schizophrenia, and overtreating schizophrenia can cause PD-type side effects. This is a great place to start.

EPSEs are also caused by an imbalance between ACh and dopamine (Figure 13-3) but with an important difference. PD is related to neurodegeneration of the substantia nigra at the beginning of the dopamine tracts, whereas EPSEs are caused by the blockade of dopamine receptors in the basal ganglia at the end of the dopamine tracts.

PD is treated with antiparkinsonian agents that increase dopamine (or dopaminergic) levels, such as levodopa/carbidopa (Sinemet) and levodopa, with anticholinergic agents (e.g., benztropine [Cogentin]), or with both. EPSEs are treated only with anticholinergics because psychosis is thought to be related to an increase in dopamine levels. To give a dopamine-enhancing drug such as levodopa to a patient with schizophrenia would potentially cause psychotic

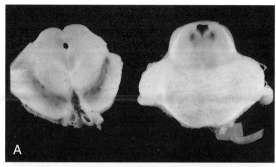

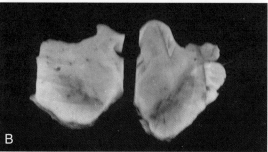

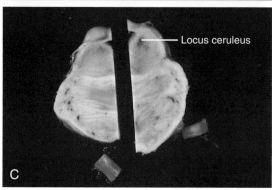

FIG 13-2 The effects of aging and disease on catecholamine centers in the brainstem. **A,** Normal pigment in the substantia nigra *(left)* and locus ceruleus *(right)* of a young man. **B,** Mild age-related loss of pigment in the brainstem of a normal individual *(right)* and loss of pigmented neurons in the brainstem of an individual with Parkinson's disease *(left)*. **C,** Mild depigmentation of the locus ceruleus (site of norepinephrine synthesis) in an aged individual *(right)* and severe depigmentation in an individual with Parkinson's disease *(left)*. (Courtesy of Richard E. Powers, Director, Brain Resource Program, University of Alabama at Birmingham.)

symptoms to increase. A careful review of Table 13-1 will facilitate your understanding of the central point of this chapter.

? CRITICAL THINKING QUESTION

2. What is the connection between PD and schizophrenia from a neurotransmitter perspective? (*Hint:* You might need to look at the next chapter.)

Specific Extrapyramidal Side Effects

Although EPSEs are biochemically related to PD, they are not the same as PD. EPSEs are divided into at least seven distinct types. Table 13-2 provides further information on these disorders.

- *Akathisia:* Akathisia is a subjective feeling of restlessness that elicits restless legs, jittery feelings, and nervous energy. Akathisia is the most common EPSE and responds poorly to treatment.

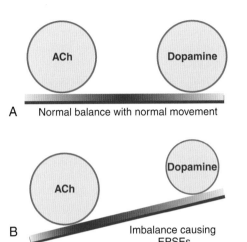

A Normal balance with normal movement

B Imbalance causing EPSEs

FIG 13-3 A, Balance between acetylcholine (ACh) and dopamine, resulting in normal movement. **B,** Imbalance (too little dopamine) results in extrapyramidal side effects (EPSEs).

- *Akinesia and bradykinesia:* Akinesia refers to an absence of movement, but a slowed movement (i.e., bradykinesia) is more likely. Symptoms include weakness, fatigue, painful muscles, and anergia. Akinesia often responds to anticholinergics.
- *Dystonias:* Dystonias are abnormal postures (i.e., muscle freezing) caused by involuntary muscle spasms. Symptoms manifest as sustained, twisted, and contracted positioning of the limbs, trunk, neck, or mouth. Dystonias tend to appear early in treatment (within about 3 days) and respond to anticholinergic drugs. These agents occasionally must be given parenterally because of the gravity of the situation. Types of dystonias include:
  - Torticollis—contracted positioning of the neck
  - Oculogyric crisis—contracted positioning of the eyes upward
  - Laryngeal—pharyngeal constriction (potentially life-threatening)
- *Drug-induced parkinsonism:* The cardinal symptoms of PD are experienced—tremor, rigidity, bradykinesia, and postural instability.
- *Tardive dyskinesia (TD): Tardive* means "late appearing." This EPSE tends to develop late, after about 6 months of

TABLE 13-1	MODEL FOR DRUG-INDUCED PARKINSONISM		
CLINICAL MANIFESTATION	**THEORETICAL UNDERSTANDING**	**POSSIBLE INTERVENTION**	**EFFECT OF INTERVENTION**
Positive symptoms of schizophrenia	Increased levels of dopamine given	Dopamine (D_2) receptor blockers	Improvement of psychotic symptoms and possible development of EPSEs
EPSEs	Drug-induced imbalance between ACh and dopamine has occurred	Anticholinergic	Continued improvement in psychotic symptoms and amelioration of EPSEs (restored balance between dopamine and ACh)

ACh, Acetylcholine; *EPSEs,* extrapyramidal side effects.

TABLE 13-2	EXTRAPYRAMIDAL SIDE EFFECTS CAUSED BY ANTIPSYCHOTIC DRUGS AND NURSING INTERVENTIONS
EPSE	**NURSING INTERVENTIONS**
Akathisia	Be patient and reassure patient who is "jittery" that you understand the need to move and that appropriate drug interventions can help differentiate akathisia and agitation. Because akathisia is a major cause of nonadherence with antipsychotic regimens, switching to a different class of antipsychotic drug might be necessary to achieve adherence.
Akinesia/bradykinesia	May or may not respond to anticholinergics. May want to reduce dose or change antipsychotics.
Dystonias	If a severe reaction (e.g., oculogyric crisis, torticollis) occurs, give antiparkinsonian drug (e.g., benztropine [Cogentin]) or antihistamine (e.g., diphenhydramine [Benadryl]) immediately, as needed. Offer reassurance. If an order for intramuscular administration has not been written, call the physician at once to obtain the order. When an order for an antiparkinsonian drug is warranted for less severe dystonias, notify the physician.
Drug-induced parkinsonism	Assess for major parkinsonism symptoms (tremors, rigidity, and bradykinesia); report to physician. Antiparkinsonian drugs are probably indicated.
TD	Assess for signs by using AIMS. Drug holidays might help prevent TD. Anticholinergic agents can worsen TD; question their indiscriminate prophylactic use.
Neuroleptic malignant syndrome	Be alert for this potentially fatal side effect. Routinely take temperatures, and encourage adequate water intake for all patients on a regimen of antipsychotic drugs; routinely assess for rigidity, tremor, and similar symptoms.
Pisa syndrome	Treat with antiparkinsonian drugs.

AIMS, Abnormal inventory movement scale; *EPSEs,* extrapyramidal side effects; *TD,* tardive dyskinesia.

antipsychotic therapy. The dopamine-ACh imbalance per se does not cause TD; consequently, anticholinergics are not administered for treatment. Anticholinergics generally worsen TD. Long-term use of antipsychotics is thought to cause dopamine receptors in the basal ganglia to become hypersensitive. Symptoms are bothersome and can be embarrassing. Typical symptoms include tongue writhing, tongue protrusion, teeth grinding, and lip smacking. TD stops with sleep. Although TD movements can be suppressed willfully for a short time, they soon reappear. TD is often irreversible but if caught in time can be averted. No satisfactory pharmacologic treatment has yet been developed. Prevention remains the most important approach to this disorder.

- *Neuroleptic malignant syndrome:* Neuroleptic malignant syndrome is a potentially lethal side effect of antipsychotic agents. Less than 1% of patients taking antipsychotics develop this problem, but 5% to 11% of patients who are untreated die (Benzer, 2005). The incidence was much higher in the past, but careful scrutiny of patients by nurses and physicians has reduced both incidence and mortality. Cardinal symptoms include hyperthermia (temperature typically 101° F to 103° F but can increase to 108° F), rigidity, and autonomic dysfunction. Neuroleptic malignant syndrome can be treated with muscle relaxants (e.g., dantrolene [Dantrium]) and with centrally acting dopaminergics (e.g., bromocriptine [Parlodel]).
- *Pisa syndrome:* Pisa syndrome is a condition marked by the patient leaning to one side. It can be acute or tardive, and older adults are more vulnerable.

Women and elderly adults are more vulnerable to developing EPSEs than others. Box 13-1 lists populations at a higher risk for developing EPSEs from antipsychotics.

ANTICHOLINERGICS TO TREAT EXTRAPYRAMIDAL SIDE EFFECTS

Anticholinergic drugs are used to treat EPSEs and work by restoring the imbalance caused by antipsychotic drugs. As noted in this chapter and in the next chapter, antipsychotic agents block (or antagonize) dopamine receptors. This dopamine receptor antagonism causes an artificial or iatrogenic parkinsonian-like syndrome, the aforementioned EPSEs. However, restoring the balance with a dopaminergic is inappropriate because, as the chapter on schizophrenia emphasizes, a compelling hypothesis for schizophrenia is the presence of excessive amounts of dopamine. Instead, anticholinergics (drugs that block cholinergic receptors) are used to restore the balance.

The following outline is repetitive but might be helpful:
1. Schizophrenia is linked to excessive dopamine.
2. Antipsychotic drugs block dopamine.
3. Blocked dopamine receptors can cause EPSEs.
4. Antiparkinsonian drugs can fix the problem that antipsychotics create.
5. If dopaminergic antiparkinsonian drugs are given, schizophrenia might worsen.
6. Anticholinergic drugs are given to restore ACh-dopamine balance.

Several anticholinergic drugs are available to treat EPSEs. The site of action of these drugs for relieving EPSEs is the central nervous system (CNS). They also have pronounced peripheral effects. The prototype drug for this class of drugs is atropine, but it is not used to treat EPSEs. Atropine is most commonly used to reduce aspiration during surgery. Benztropine (Cogentin) is the most commonly prescribed anticholinergic for EPSEs, but diphenhydramine (Benadryl) is also effective. The relative anticholinergic potency of selected psychotropic drugs is given in Table 13-3. (Table 13-4 lists the adult dosages of anticholinergics.)

Pharmacologic Effects

Anticholinergic drugs primarily block ACh receptors, preventing ACh stimulation of the cholinergic excitatory pathways. Anticholinergics are used alone in the treatment of EPSEs.

TABLE 13-3	**ANTICHOLINERGIC EFFECT OF FREQUENTLY PRESCRIBED PSYCHOTROPIC DRUGS COMPARED WITH BENZTROPINE**	
DRUG	**EQUIVALENT (mg)**	**TYPICAL USE**
Atropine	0.5	Given before surgery
Benztropine (Cogentin)	1	Antiparkinsonian
Trihexyphenidyl (Artane)	2	Antiparkinsonian
Biperiden (Akineton)	1	Antiparkinsonian
Amitriptyline (Elavil)	10	Antidepressant
Nortriptyline (Pamelor)	60	Antidepressant
Imipramine (Tofranil)	75	Antidepressant
Desipramine (Norpramin)	150	Antidepressant
Clozapine (Clozaril)	15	Antipsychotic
Chlorpromazine (Thorazine)	370	Antipsychotic
Diphenhydramine (Benadryl)	50	Antihistamine

Note: According to this table, 50 mg of Benadryl has the same anticholinergic effect as 1 mg of benztropine.
Modified from de Leon, J., et al. (1994). A pilot effort to determine benztropine equivalents of anticholinergic medications. *Hospital & Community Psychiatry, 45,* 606.

TABLE 13-4	ANTICHOLINERGIC ADULT DRUG DOSAGES FOR EXTRAPYRAMIDAL SIDE EFFECTS
ANTICHOLINERGIC	**DOSAGE**
Benztropine (Cogentin)	EPSEs: 1-4 mg PO or IM once or twice a day For acute dystonic reactions: 1-2 mg IM/IV, then 1-2 mg PO twice a day
Trihexyphenidyl (Artane)	Start with 1 mg daily, then increase Usual dosage range: 5-15 mg/day

EPSEs, Extrapyramidal side effects; *IM,* intramuscularly; *IV,* intravenously; *PO,* orally.

Antipsychotic drugs block dopamine receptors, frequently causing EPSEs. Many of the symptoms associated with naturally occurring PD—tremors, rigidity, and bradykinesia—are present in drug-induced parkinsonism, along with related symptoms such as akathisia, dystonia, and dyskinesia. Blockade of dopamine receptors in the basal ganglia (i.e., nigrostriatal tract) produces EPSEs. High-potency antipsychotic agents such as haloperidol (Haldol) cause EPSEs more often than low-potency or atypical agents. Additionally, several nonpsychiatric drugs cause EPSEs. These symptoms contribute to the discomfort, anxiety, and frustration of these already troubled patients and are major contributors to nonadherence. Patients taking antipsychotic drugs can experience a gradual or sudden onset of EPSEs.

? CRITICAL THINKING QUESTION

3. Although you have not read the chapter on antidepressants yet (Chapter 15), it is known that selective serotonin reuptake inhibitors (SSRIs, such as fluoxetine [Prozac] or paroxetine [Paxil]) can cause EPSEs. Can you figure out why this is so?

Side Effects

Although clinicians tend to consider anticholinergic side effects less significant than EPSEs, not all patients agree (Ozbilen & Adams, 2009). Anticholinergic drugs produce both CNS and peripheral nervous system (PNS) side effects (Table 13-5). CNS effects include confusion, cognitive impoverishment, agitation, dizziness, drowsiness, and disturbances in behavior. Because the cholinergic system contributes to memory and learning, anticholinergic drugs affect these cognitive functions as well. Ingesting drugs with anticholinergic properties can often explain recent changes in cognition in older adults (Campbell et al., 2009). Because cognitive decline is a major symptom domain in schizophrenia, giving anticholinergics to patients with schizophrenia has proven to worsen mental abilities (Desmarais et al., 2012).

TABLE 13-5	PERIPHERAL NERVOUS SYSTEM SIDE EFFECTS AND NURSING INTERVENTIONS FOR ANTICHOLINERGICS
SIDE EFFECTS	**NURSING INTERVENTIONS**
Dry mouth	Offer sugarless hard candy and chewing gum; encourage frequent rinses; take medication before meals.
Nasal congestion	Recommend over-the-counter nasal decongestant, if approved by physician.
Urinary hesitation	Introduce running water, privacy, warm water over perineum.
Urinary retention	Catheterize for residual fluids; encourage frequent voiding.
Blurred vision, photophobia	Provide reassurance (normal vision typically returns in a few weeks); encourage sunglasses; advise caution when driving (tolerance develops). Pilocarpine (a muscarinic agonist that causes pupil constriction) eye drops may be given.
Constipation	Give laxatives, as ordered; encourage diet with fiber; recommend 2500-3000 mL of water daily.
Mydriasis	If eye pain develops, undiagnosed narrow-angle glaucoma might be the cause; immediate attention is warranted.
Decreased sweating	Decreased sweating can lead to fever; take temperature; if fever occurs, reduce body temperature (e.g., sponge baths).
Fever	Advise limited strenuous activity; encourage patient to wear appropriate clothing.

From Desmarais, J.E., Beauclair, L., & Margolese, H. (2012). Anticholinergics in the era of atypical antipsychotics: short-term or long-term treatment? *Journal of Psychopharmacology (Oxford, England), 26,* 1167.

? CRITICAL THINKING QUESTION

4. Why do older individuals have a more intense response to anticholinergics? (See Box 13-3 for answer.)

PNS anticholinergic effects, such as dry mouth, blurred vision, nausea, and nervousness, occur in 30% to 50% of patients. Basically, peripheral anticholinergic side effects result from blocking the parasympathetic system (a cholinergic [ACh] system) (Table 13-6). Blurred vision results from pupils that dilate because of the blocking of ACh receptors of the third cranial nerve (CN III; oculomotor nerve). CN III constricts the pupil; when it is blocked, the pupil dilates. Dry mouth results when CN VII and CN IX (facial and glossopharyngeal nerves) are blocked from causing salivation. Decreased tearing is related to blockage of CN VII.

TABLE 13-6	ANTICHOLINERGIC EFFECTS ON CRANIAL NERVES WITH PARASYMPATHETIC FUNCTIONS	
CRANIAL NERVE	**PARASYMPATHETIC FUNCTION**	**ANTICHOLINERGIC EFFECT**
III	Constricts pupils	Mydriasis (dilates pupils), blurred vision
	Alters shape of lens	Impairs accommodation
VII	Salivation	Dry mouth
	Lacrimation	Decreased tearing
	Nasal mucous secretion	Dry nasal passage
IX	Salivation	Dry mouth
	Nasal mucous secretion	Dry nasal passage
X	Slows heart rate	Tachycardia
	Promotes peristalsis	Slows peristalsis; constipation
	Constricts bronchi	Dilates bronchi
	Promotes urination	Urinary hesitancy or retention

Although these problems are annoying, they are not usually major health hazards. However, when CN X (vagus nerve) is blocked, tachycardia can occur and cause serious problems. Why? See Norm's Notes for the answer.

NORM'S NOTES
The sinoatrial node has a rhythm of 100 to 120 impulses per minute. Hearts do not beat this fast because the parasympathetic system provides a braking action. When anticholinergic drugs are given, part of the brake is removed, which can result in major problems, particularly for older individuals.

Constipation, a problem with patients with parkinsonism secondary to rigidity, can be worsened by anticholinergics as well. Urinary hesitance and retention and decreased sweating are other PNS effects. Patients who drool or perspire excessively might welcome dry mouth and decreased sweating. However, because of the risk of hyperthermia, reduced sweating may be a significant issue. Box 13-2 lists the more serious risks associated with anticholinergic use.

Nursing Implications for Anticholinergic Drugs
Therapeutic versus Toxic Dose Levels
Therapeutic dose ranges are listed in Table 13-4. Doses above therapeutic ranges can cause toxic effects. Overdose might result in CNS hyperstimulation (confusion, excitement, hyperpyrexia, agitation, disorientation, delirium, or hallucinations) or CNS depression (drowsiness, sedation, or coma). The cardiovascular, urinary, and gastrointestinal systems are particularly involved. The eyes are also affected. High fevers are the result of the CNS effects of anticholinergics and their ability to decrease sweating.

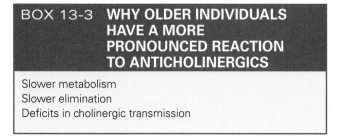

BOX 13-2	RISKS ASSOCIATED WITH ANTICHOLINERGIC USE

1. Might be lethal in overdose
2. Might induce dependence
3. Might exacerbate tardive dyskinesia
4. Might induce psychosis
5. Might cause erectile dysfunction
6. Might cause paralytic ileus

From Houltram, B., & Scalan, M. (2004). Extrapyramidal side effects. *Nursing Standard, 18,* 39.

BOX 13-3	WHY OLDER INDIVIDUALS HAVE A MORE PRONOUNCED REACTION TO ANTICHOLINERGICS

Slower metabolism
Slower elimination
Deficits in cholinergic transmission

From Ozbilen, M., & Adams, C.E. (2009). Systematic overview of Cochrane Reviews for anticholinergic effects of antipsychotic drugs. *Journal of Clinical Psychopharmacology, 29,* 141.

Use during Pregnancy
Anticholinergics should be used cautiously during pregnancy. Theoretically, these drugs would decrease milk flow during lactation.

Use in Older Adults
As this chapter and other chapters in this text have emphasized, older individuals are particularly sensitive to anticholinergic agents (Box 13-3). Cognitive, cardiovascular, and gastrointestinal side effects are more pronounced in older patients compared with younger patients. Difficulties in older men with prostatic enlargement can be exacerbated with the use of these agents. Cognitive impairment is also associated with anticholinergic drugs (Desmarais et al., 2012).

Side Effect Interventions
Numerous annoying side effects are associated with anticholinergic drugs (see Table 13-5). Several nondrug alternatives to help the patient are listed in Table 13-5.

Interactions with Anticholinergic Drugs
The nurse should alert the patient to the dangers of over-the-counter drugs and other prescription drugs that intensify the atropine-like effects of centrally acting anticholinergics. Other interactions include an intensification of sedative effects when combined with CNS depressants and a decrease in absorption when combined with antacids and antidiarrheal drugs.

Teaching Patients
In addition to teaching appropriate information about side effects, the nurse should emphasize certain points. The patient and family should be advised of the following:

- Avoid discontinuing these drugs abruptly. Tapering off over a 1-week period is advised.
- Avoid driving or other hazardous activities until tolerance develops and drowsiness and blurred vision diminish.
- Avoid over-the-counter medications (e.g., cough and cold preparations) that have anticholinergic or antihistamine properties; alcohol, which exacerbates CNS depression; and antacids, which interfere with the absorption of anticholinergics.

Selected Anticholinergic Drugs

Benztropine

Benztropine (Cogentin) is used to treat all parkinsonian-like disorders, including drug-induced EPSEs. Benztropine, which is the most frequently prescribed anticholinergic antiparkinsonian drug, is usually given orally but can be given intramuscularly for nonadherent psychotic patients and intramuscularly or intravenously for acute dystonic reactions.

Diphenhydramine

Diphenhydramine (Benadryl), the prototype antihistamine, is effective for most parkinsonian-like disorders. Diphenhydramine can cause considerable sedation in some individuals and little in others; it is considerably less potent than benztropine (see Table 13-3).

Trihexyphenidyl

Trihexyphenidyl (Artane) was the first anticholinergic used extensively for EPSEs. Because trihexyphenidyl is unavailable in parenteral form, its use for acute dystonias is limited.

OTHER TREATMENT OPTIONS FOR EXTRAPYRAMIDAL SIDE EFFECTS

Drugs

Although anticholinergic agents are the mainstay of treatment and prophylaxis of EPSEs, several other agents are available as well, including the following:

- Dopamine agonist—amantadine (Symmetrel)
- Beta blocker—propranolol (Inderal)
- Benzodiazepines—diazepam (Valium), lorazepam (Ativan), clonazepam (Klonopin)

Vitamins

Both vitamins E and B_6 have some empirical support for their abilities to diminish symptoms associated with TD. Anecdotal evidence also suggests that some patients benefit from vitamin E. Whether this vitamin actually reduces TD symptoms or prevents further deterioration has been debated by many nurses and physicians.

PREVENTION

The best approach to treating EPSEs is prevention. By following a few simple guidelines, both the prescriber and the nurse can reduce EPSE incidence (Houltram & Scalan, 2004). Enhanced patient care requires the following (in about this order):

1. Establish whether the patient is from a high-risk group (see Box 13-1).
2. Obtain baseline information about EPSEs using a validated tool.
3. Choose an antipsychotic with a lower probability of causing EPSEs (although this is disputed):
   a. High-risk agents—haloperidol (Haldol), fluphenazine (Prolixin), and maybe other traditional antipsychotics.
   b. Lower risk agents—clozapine (Clozaril), quetiapine (Seroquel), and perhaps other atypical antipsychotics.
4. Monitor the patient on a regular basis.
5. If EPSEs develop, consider switching to an atypical drug, or if the patient is already taking an atypical drug, lower the dose or change to another atypical drug with a better side effect profile. Add an antiparkinsonian agent.

CASE STUDY

A 25-year-old woman who is taking an antipsychotic drug (haloperidol) starts to experience psychomotor slowing as she walks down the hallway of the hospital. Before she reaches the end of the hall, she requires assistance. Within 2 minutes of sitting down, her neck becomes rigidly hyperextended, and her eyes roll upward in a fixed stare. Her breathing becomes labored because of the position of her neck, and she is frightened. Because she is also delusional, it is difficult to imagine what this frightening side effect of her medication represents to her. Benztropine, 2 mg, is given intramuscularly and repeated in 15 minutes because she did not respond as quickly as was hoped. Within another 5 minutes, she was back to her "normal" self.

▋ S T U D Y   N O T E S

1. PD is related to degeneration of the substantia nigra, the dopamine-generating portion of the brain; however, the cause is unknown.
2. EPSEs, a type of parkinsonism (cause known), develop when dopamine receptors in the basal ganglia are blocked by antipsychotic or other drugs.
3. Normal muscle activity requires a balance between dopamine and ACh; consequently, a dopamine deficiency is responsible for symptoms of PD.
4. The four primary symptoms associated with PD are tremors, bradykinesia, rigidity, and postural instability.

5. Drug treatment of PD is based on reestablishing a balance between dopamine and ACh.

6. Drug treatment for EPSEs is based on blocking ACh receptors. Administering a dopaminergic drug could exacerbate psychotic symptoms.

7. The three major anticholinergic antiparkinsonian drugs are benztropine (Cogentin), trihexyphenidyl (Artane), and the classic antihistamine diphenhydramine (Benadryl).

8. Anticholinergic drugs have many side effects. Older individuals are particularly sensitive to these side effects.

REFERENCES

Benzer, T. I. (2005). *Neuroleptic malignant syndrome in emergency medicine.* http://emedicine.medscape.com/article/816018-overview, Accessed 12.02.13.

Campbell, N., et al. (2009). The cognitive impact of anticholinergics: A clinical review. *Clinical Interventions in Aging, 4,* 225.

de Leon, J., et al. (1994). A pilot effort to determine benztropine equivalents of anticholinergic medications. *Hospital & Community Psychiatry, 45,* 606.

Desmarais, J. E., Beauclair, L., & Margolese, H. (2012). Anticholinergics in the era of atypical antipsychotics: Short-term or long-term treatment? *Journal of Psychopharmacology (Oxford, England), 26,* 1167.

Fritsch, T., et al. (2012). Parkinson disease: Research update and clinical management. *Southern Medical Journal, 105,* 651.

Haddad, P. M., et al. (2012). Antipsychotic drugs and extrapyramidal side effects in first episode psychosis: A systematic review of head-head comparisons. *Journal of Psychopharmacology (Oxford, England), 26,* 15.

Houltram, B., & Scalan, M. (2004). Extrapyramidal side effects. *Nursing Standard, 18,* 39.

Keltner, N. L., & Folks, D. G. (2005). *Psychotropic drugs* (4th ed.). St. Louis: Mosby.

Ozbilen, M., & Adams, C. E. (2009). Systematic overview of Cochrane reviews for anticholinergic effects of antipsychotic drugs. *Journal of Clinical Psychopharmacology, 29,* 141.

Peluso, M. J., et al. (2012). Extrapyramidal motor side-effects of first-and second-generation antipsychotic drugs. *British Journal of Psychiatry, 200,* 387.

Antipsychotic Drugs

Norman L. Keltner

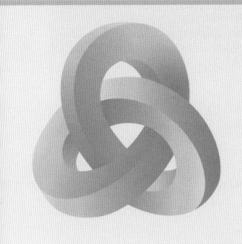

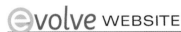 **WEBSITE**

http://evolve.elsevier.com/Keltner

LEARNING OBJECTIVES

- Explain the concept of neurotransmitters, specifically dopamine, in relation to psychosis.
- Identify the clinical uses of first-generation and second-generation antipsychotic drugs.
- Recognize differences between high-potency and low-potency traditional antipsychotic drugs.
- Identify representative high-potency, low-potency, and atypical antipsychotic drugs, including the specific side effects and interactions of each drug.

- Describe the two theories of atypicality for second-generation antipsychotics.
- Describe signs and symptoms associated with extrapyramidal side effects.
- Describe potential interactions of antipsychotic drugs.
- Discuss implications for teaching patients about antipsychotic drugs.

Antipsychotic drugs are used to treat schizophrenia, schizoaffective disorder, bipolar disorder, and psychotic depressions as well as various other psychiatric disorders (Box 14-1). Additionally, these drugs have numerous off-label uses, such as the treatment of insomnia, tics, delirium, and stuttering (Tripathi & Macaluso, 2013). Because of their widespread use, spending on antipsychotics in the United States has reached $16.1 billion annually making antipsychotics one of the top five categories of drugs sold in this country (Berkrot, 2010; Mark, 2010).

Antipsychotics were discovered accidentally around 1950. A French scientist was hoping to develop a new antihistamine and in the process formulated chlorpromazine, which was initially used to calm presurgery jitters but was soon found to possess antipsychotic properties. Chlorpromazine is considered the first antipsychotic drug.

Before the introduction and acceptance of chlorpromazine and of many related drugs, hundreds of thousands of patients with severe psychiatric disturbances were hospitalized, many never to be released. These patients were isolated, physically restrained, and occasionally subjected to psychosurgery (lobotomy). These treatments rarely restored patients to a state that enabled them to function productively or to interact in a reasonably normal way with others.

Although all the hopes for antipsychotic drugs have not been realized, these drugs have had a dramatic impact on psychiatric care. The use of antipsychotic drugs resulted in the abandonment of most of the ineffective treatments and dramatically reduced long-term hospitalizations. The drugs discussed in this chapter are generally called *antipsychotic agents*, but historically they have also been referred to as *major tranquilizers*, *ataractics* (drugs that produce calmness or serenity), and *neuroleptics* (Greek for "neuron clasping").

NORM'S NOTES
There are two categories of drugs that dominate psychiatric care—antipsychotics and antidepressants. I think that the antipsychotics are the more important category. Many years ago, when I worked in a large state hospital, the antipsychotics had only recently been discovered. Some of the staff had worked there since the 1930s, and I was fascinated with their stories of the pre-Thorazine days, when the hospital could only be described as a madhouse— so much pain, so much agony. Although not without some problems, what a difference antipsychotics have made in many people's lives.

BOX 14-1 HOW ANTIPSYCHOTICS ARE USED

98.9% for psychiatric conditions
39%—mood disorders
35%—psychoses
7%—delirium, dementia, and similar disorders
6%—ADHD, conduct disorders, and disruptive behavior disorders
5.5%—anxiety disorders
2.3%—in children (e.g., autism)

From Mark, T.L. (2010). For what diagnoses are psychotropic medications being prescribed? A nationally representative survey of physicians. *CNS Drugs, 24*, 319–326.

BOX 14-2 CLASSIFICATION OF TRADITIONAL ANTIPSYCHOTIC DRUGS BASED ON POTENCY

High-Potency Drugs
Fluphenazine (Prolixin)
Haloperidol (Haldol)
Thiothixene (Navane)
Trifluoperazine (Stelazine)

Moderate-Potency Drugs
Loxapine (Loxitane)
Perphenazine (Trilafon)

Low-Potency Drugs
Chlorpromazine (Thorazine)
Thioridazine

CLASSIFICATION SYSTEMS

Antipsychotic drugs are generally conceptualized in two ways. The two categories are (1) traditional antipsychotics, or first-generation antipsychotics, and (2) atypical antipsychotics, or second-generation antipsychotics. Antipsychotic drugs are listed under these headings in Table 14-1. Antipsychotics have diverse chemical properties, but all effectively reduce various psychiatric symptoms. The type, intensity, and frequency of side effects vary among these drugs because of intrinsic differences.

Traditional antipsychotic drugs, developed between 1950 and 1990, are further divided based on potency (Box 14-2). Subclassification based on potency has support because of its clinical utility. Essentially, the effects of traditional antipsychotics are related to the blockade of a specific type of dopamine receptor (D_2) (Box 14-3). Clinical effectiveness occurs when 60% to 70% of these receptors are blocked in a certain area of the brain (which we discuss later in the chapter).

TABLE 14-1 MAJOR TRADITIONAL AND ATYPICAL ANTIPSYCHOTIC DRUGS

DRUG	USUAL ADULT MAINTENANCE RANGE (mg/day)	RATE OF EPSEs	RATE OF ANTICHOLINERGIC EFFECTS	RATE OF ORTHOSTASIS	RATE OF SEDATION	RATE OF WEIGHT GAIN
Traditional (First Generation)						
High-Potency Drug						
Fluphenazine (Prolixin)	0.5-40.0	High	Low	Low	Low	Low
Haloperidol (Haldol)	1-15	High	Low	Low	Low	Low
Moderate-Potency Drug						
Perphenazine	12-64	High	Low	Low	Moderate	Low
Low-Potency Drug						
Chlorpromazine (Thorazine)	200-1000	Moderate	Moderate	High	Moderate	High
Thioridazine	200-800	Low	High	High	High	High
Atypical (Second Generation)						
Aripiprazole (Abilify)	10-30	Low	Low	Low	Low	Low
Asenapine (Saphris)	10-20	Low	Low	Low	Moderate	Moderate
Clozapine (Clozaril)	75-900	Low	High	High	High	High
Iloperidone (Fanapt)	12-24	Low	Moderate	Moderate	Moderate	Moderate
Lurasidone (Latuda)	40-80	Low	Low	Low	Low	Low
Olanzapine (Zyprexa)	5-20	Low	Moderate	Low	High	High
Paliperidone (Invega)	3-12	Low	Low	Moderate	Moderate	Moderate
Quetiapine (Seroquel)	200-800	Low	Low	Moderate	Moderate	Moderate
Risperidone (Risperdal)	0.5-6.0	Low*	Low	Moderate	Moderate	Moderate
Ziprasidone (Geodon)	40-160	Low	Low	Low	Low	Low

Note: Costs obtained from Consumer Reports Best Buy Drugs (2009) and Citrome (2011). Prices based on brand name for atypical agents.
*However, EPSEs develop at high doses.
EPSEs, Extrapyramidal side effects.

BOX 14-3 EFFECTS OF DOPAMINE D_2 ANTAGONISM

60% to 70%—optimal clinical effect
~70%—elevated prolactin
~80%—extrapyramidal side effects

Jindal, R.D., & Keshavan, M.S. (2008). Classifying antipsychotic agents: need for new terminology. *CNS Drugs, 22,* 1047.

Some of the drugs have *high milligrams but low potency*. For example, approximately 100 mg of chlorpromazine (a low-potency traditional drug) is required to achieve the same clinical effect, or block the same number of D_2 receptors, as 2 mg of haloperidol (a high-potency traditional drug). This classification system is not perfect. A few traditional drugs do not fall comfortably into either a high-potency or a low-potency group (hence a moderate-potency category). Nonetheless, this dichotomy is clinically significant because low-potency drugs tend to cause more intense anticholinergic effects (e.g., dry mouth, blurred vision) and antiadrenergic effects (e.g., orthostatic hypotension), whereas high-potency drugs cause more extrapyramidal side effects (EPSEs) and prolactin elevation. Knowing this difference prepares the nurse for the most likely set of side effects. As a general rule, drugs with increased anticholinergic effects, such as chlorpromazine, produce fewer EPSEs (see Table 14-1). Table 14-2 outlines the theoretical effects of specific receptor blockade.

TABLE 14-2 THEORETICAL EFFECTS OF RECEPTOR BLOCKADE

RECEPTOR	EFFECTS
D_2	Mesolimbic tract: Antipsychotic effect (all antipsychotic drugs antagonize D_2)
	Nigrostriatal tract: EPSEs
	Tuberoinfundibular tract: Prolactin level elevation
	Mesocortical tract: Secondary negative symptoms (symptoms caused by antipsychotic drugs themselves)
$5\text{-}HT_{2A}$	Improves negative symptoms; decreased EPSEs
M_1	Anticholinergic side effects; can restore ACh-dopamine balance, particularly for EPSEs caused by FGAs
H_1	Sedation, orthostasis, weight gain
Alpha-1	Orthostasis, dizziness, sedation
Alpha-2	Sexual dysfunction
GABA	Lowers seizure threshold; produces anxiety

ACh, Acetylcholine; *EPSEs,* extrapyramidal side effects; *FGAs,* first-generation antipsychotics; *GABA,* gamma-aminobutyric acid; $5\text{-}HT_{2A}$, 5-hydroxytryptamine 2A; M_1, cholinergic muscarinic receptors. From Bezchlibnyk-Butler, K.Z., & Jeffries, J.J. (2007). *Clinical handbook of psychotropic drugs* (14th ed.). Seattle: Hogrefe & Huber; Keltner, N.L. (2000). Neuroreceptor function and psychopharmacologic response. *Issues in Mental Health Nursing, 21,* 31.

The second category is different. The newer agents (from 1990 on) are referred to as *atypical* because of the following characteristics:
1. Reduced risk for EPSEs
2. Increased effectiveness in treating negative symptoms
3. Minimal risk of tardive dyskinesia (TD)
4. Reduced risk for elevated prolactin

NEUROCHEMICAL THEORY OF SCHIZOPHRENIA

The neurochemical theory affords the best explanation for the effectiveness of antipsychotic agents. This theory states that increased levels of dopamine in the limbic area of the brain cause schizophrenia and its positive symptoms (e.g., hallucinations, delusions). Because antipsychotic drugs are dopamine blockers, it follows that their effectiveness can be attributed to this dopamine-blocking activity. This theory of schizophrenia is supported by clinical observations and clinical research, both of which demonstrate that high doses of the dopaminergic drugs levodopa and amphetamine can produce schizophrenic symptoms.

However, this explanation does not answer all the questions surrounding the issue, most specifically questions regarding *negative* and cognitive symptoms. Figure 14-1 provides additional useful information. As shown in Figure 14-1, the brain has four major dopaminergic tracts. Dopamine is synthesized primarily in the substantia nigra and ventral tegmental area and is delivered to distant sites via dopaminergic tracts. To appreciate the complexity of psychopharmacologic treatment of schizophrenia fully, the student must recognize the existence of dopamine-dependent areas of the brain that communicate with dopamine-synthesizing areas (substantia nigra and ventral tegmental areas in the midbrain) via different neuronal tracts.

Tract 1: The nigrostriatal tract is involved in movement. Traditional antipsychotic blockade can *cause EPSEs*.

Tract 2: The tuberoinfundibular tract modulates pituitary function. Traditional antipsychotic blockade can lead to *elevation in prolactin levels*.

Tract 3: The mesolimbic tract is involved in emotional and sensory processes. Traditional antipsychotic blockade normalizes these processes in individuals with schizophrenia, *relieving or eliminating hallucinations and delusions*.

Tract 4: The mesocortical tract is involved in cognitive processes. Traditional antipsychotic blockade can *intensify negative and cognitive problems*.

Traditional antipsychotics can do all of the above, but this is a high price to pay to be free of hallucinations and delusions.

The ultimate antipsychotic agent might block dopamine receptors in the mesolimbic area (decreasing hallucinations and delusions) and liberate dopamine in the mesocortical area (treating negative and cognitive symptoms), while neither obstructing the function of the nigrostriatal tract

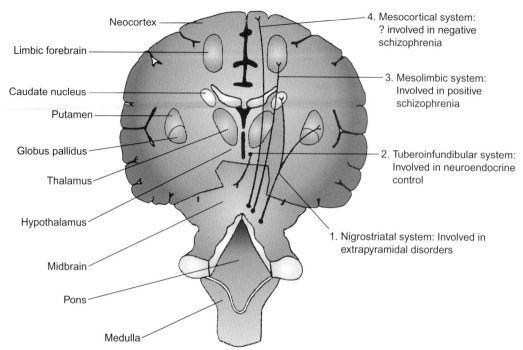

Neocortex

Limbic forebrain

Caudate nucleus

Putamen

Globus pallidus

Thalamus

Hypothalamus

Midbrain

Pons

Medulla

4. Mesocortical system:
? involved in negative
schizophrenia

3. Mesolimbic system:
Involved in positive
schizophrenia

2. Tuberoinfundibular system:
Involved in neuroendocrine
control

1. Nigrostriatal system: Involved in
extrapyramidal disorders

FIG 14-1 Four dopaminergic tracts are important for understanding the actions of antipsychotic drugs. *1, Nigrostriatal system:* When antipsychotic drugs antagonize this system, a pseudoparkinsonism effect, or extrapyramidal side effect, occurs. *2, Tuberoinfundibular system:* When antipsychotic drugs antagonize this system, the dopamine inhibition of the pituitary hormone prolactin is lifted and can lead to gynecomastia and galactorrhea. *3, Mesolimbic system:* When antipsychotic drugs antagonize this system, a decrease in the symptoms of schizophrenia occurs (primarily positive symptoms). This particular effect makes these drugs antipsychotic. *4, Mesocortical system:* When antipsychotic drugs antagonize this system, the disorder can worsen in some patients. Atypical antipsychotics are thought to antagonize serotonin receptors (5-HT$_{2A}$) in the cortex, which liberate dopamine there—that is, theories suggest that a mesocortical hypodopaminergic state might contribute to negative symptoms. Much remains to be understood about the role, if any, of the mesocortical dopaminergic tract in schizophrenia. (From Roberts, G.W., Leigh, P.N., & Weinberger, D.R. [1993]. *Neuropsychiatric disorders.* London: Wolfe.)

(i.e., not causing EPSEs) nor blocking receptors in the tuberoinfundibular tract (i.e., not elevating prolactin levels). Atypical antipsychotics *can* do this.

OVERVIEW

Pharmacologic Effects

Antipsychotic drugs are used primarily to treat psychotic disorders—specifically, schizophrenia, bipolar disorder, and other chronic mental illness. Tolerance to their antipsychotic effect is uncommon.

Central nervous system (CNS) effects include emotional quieting and sedation, which explains why these drugs previously were generally referred to as *major tranquilizers.* Emotional quieting enables the patient to take advantage of other forms of therapeutic intervention—for example, the therapeutic nurse-patient relationship and the well-managed milieu.

Sedation decreases insomnia, a frequent complaint of psychotic patients. Whether this is a result of the sedating effect itself or of being freed from disturbing thoughts (or a combination of the two) is not fully understood. Not all antipsychotic drugs are significantly sedating and yet are still therapeutic. The conclusion that the effectiveness of

antipsychotic agents results from more than their tranquilizing qualities alone is reasonable.

Psychiatric Symptoms Modified by Antipsychotic Drugs

A tranquilizing effect occurs within an hour or so after ingestion. Antipsychotic effects are often observed within a few weeks (Webster & Straley, 2014), with improvement continuing for 6 to 8 weeks or longer. D$_2$ blockade develops on the first dose. The lag time required for a clinical response surely indicates that neuronal adaptations must occur before a therapeutic response is seen (Nestler et al., 2009).

Antipsychotic drugs are most effective in treating the positive symptoms of schizophrenia (Box 14-4). Positive symptoms include hallucinations and delusions. Negative symptoms are less responsive to antipsychotic drugs, including the newer agents. Negative symptoms develop over an extended period and include flattened affect, verbal paucity, and a lack of drive or goal-directed activity. Referring again to Figure 14-1, the student can infer that positive symptoms arise from too much dopamine in the limbic area (hyperactive mesolimbic tract) and that negative symptoms arise from too little dopamine in the cortex (hypoactive mesocortical tract). It stands to reason that antipsychotic drugs that are strictly

BOX 14-4 POSITIVE AND NEGATIVE SYMPTOMS OF SCHIZOPHRENIA

Positive Symptoms: Caused by Excessive Dopamine in Mesolimbic Tract*

Abnormal thoughts
Agitation
Bizarre behavior
Delusions
Excitement
Feelings of persecution
Grandiosity
Hallucinations
Hostility
Illusions
Insomnia
Suspiciousness

Negative Symptoms: Caused by Too Little Dopamine in Mesocortical Tract*

Alogia
Anergia
Asocial behavior
Attention deficits
Avolition
Blunted affect
Communication difficulties
Difficulty with abstractions
Passive social withdrawal
Poor grooming and hygiene
Poor rapport
Poverty of speech

*This is an oversimplification of what is going on in the frontal and limbic lobes of the brain.

dopamine antagonists are better at decreasing the effect of dopamine in the limbic area than they are at increasing the effect of dopamine in the cerebral cortex. As discussed later in this chapter, atypical agents can increase the dopamine level in one area of the brain, while decreasing it in another.

Ultimately, improvement in positive and negative symptoms is the measurement of progress. Psychotic symptoms associated with other mental disorders also improve with these drugs.

Alterations of Perception

As a rule, the more bizarre the behavior of a person experiencing psychotic symptoms (more positive symptoms), the more likely that an antipsychotic drug will be beneficial. Hallucinations and illusions are reduced with these drugs. Even when the symptoms are not fully eradicated, antipsychotic drugs might enable the person to understand that hallucinations and illusions are not real, which is an improvement.

Alterations of Thought

Antipsychotic drugs improve reasoning, decrease ambivalence, and decrease delusions. Because clouded reasoning, ambivalence, and delusional thoughts are frustrating and sometimes

frightening, antipsychotic agents can free the patient to think more clearly and communicate better with others.

Alterations of Activity

Individuals with schizophrenia are often hyperactive because of their internal turmoil and, perhaps, their neurochemical state. Antipsychotic drugs slow psychomotor activity.

Alterations in Consciousness

Mental clouding and confusion are anxiety-producing symptoms associated with psychosis. Some mental health professionals believe that these disorders are the most disabling. Antipsychotic drugs are effective in decreasing confusion and clouding.

Alterations in Personal Relationships

Patients with schizophrenia often have histories of social withdrawal and might have few, if any, close personal relationships. If relationships with family members exist, they are often strained. Individuals with schizophrenia may invest little effort in their appearance and may not be particularly careful about their behavior. The combination of introspection, rumination, and self-focused speech produces ineffective communication patterns that reinforce isolation and alienation. In the give-and-take atmosphere of society, individuals with schizophrenia often have little to give and, as a result, are basically socially unattractive to most people. Antipsychotic drugs potentially can enable patients to become less focused on themselves and more focused on others. The socially damaging, self-absorbed thinking experienced by patients with schizophrenia might be a result of the considerable energy they must expend to maintain some degree of equilibrium in the face of psychological turmoil; this is similar to the way many people give less attention to their appearance or behavior during an acute illness. Antipsychotic drugs reduce the inner turmoil, freeing psychic energy for normal interpersonal relationships and for the therapeutic nurse-patient relationship.

? CRITICAL THINKING QUESTION

1. If the following are true …
   a. Excessive bioavailability of dopamine causes the positive symptoms of schizophrenia
   b. Atypical antipsychotic drugs are effective because they increase dopamine (5-HT$_{2A}$ antagonism and all that)
   … then why is it that patients who receive atypical antipsychotic drugs do not develop more symptoms of schizophrenia? (Hint: Reread my response to the student's question in this chapter.)

Alterations of Affect

Affective flattening, blunting, inappropriateness, and lability are affective symptoms sometimes associated with schizophrenia that often respond to antipsychotic drugs. However, a flat affect is a cardinal symptom of negative schizophrenia and might respond only to an atypical antipsychotic drug.

Pharmacokinetics

A detailed pharmacokinetic discussion of each antipsychotic agent is beyond the scope of this text. Rather, an overview of significant pharmacokinetic mechanisms is presented.

Absorption of these drugs is variable. Oral drugs are absorbed in 1 to 6 hours, whereas the newer disintegrating tablets are absorbed within 2 minutes. These newer, highly lipid-soluble drugs accumulate in fatty tissue and are released slowly, which might explain why patients who abruptly stop taking their medications continue to experience an antipsychotic effect for some time. This slow release from fatty stores might also account for nonadherence because the patient who stops taking this medication does not experience an immediate return of symptoms. The following clinical example probably represents this phenomenon.

Clinical Example

Bob, a 58-year-old military veteran with a long history of mental illness, has been taking haloperidol for 30 years. Over that time, the nursing staff at the Veterans' Administration hospital has gotten to know Bob well because he periodically requires hospital-based intervention. One day, Bob calls the nursing office on the psychiatric floor and tells the nurse that he believes that he can conquer his problems by using "mind over matter." He is going to stop all psychotropic medications. Bob appears to do quite well for a couple of weeks, causing some of the nursing staff to wonder about the new approach. At the end of 3 weeks, Bob is brought to the hospital in a highly disturbed psychotic state. His medication is reinstituted, and Bob's delusional thoughts subside.

Antipsychotics are highly bound (most between 90% and 99%) to plasma proteins. Physiologic changes that disrupt even slightly this level of protein-binding action might increase the percentage of free drug and potentially have a greater effect. As with most highly protein-bound drugs, a greater effect might occur in older adults (who more often experience a decline in serum protein levels).

Antipsychotics are metabolized in the liver by the cytochrome P-450 (CYP-450) enzyme system. The average half-life ranges from 10 to 30 hours. Impaired hepatic function extends the half-life and effect of these drugs. As noted in Chapter 24, a much higher percentage of people with schizophrenia smoke compared with the general population. Cigarette smoking (not the nicotine) causes an increase in the CYP-450 1A2 enzyme, which breaks down several antipsychotics including the following (Fankhauser, 2013):

SMOKING DECREASES THESE SERUM LEVELS	
MAJOR SUBSTRATES OF CYP-450 1A2	MINOR SUBSTRATES OF CYP-450 1A2
Clozapine	Asenapine
Olanzapine	Chlorpromazine
Thiothixene	Fluphenazine
Trifluoperazine	Haloperidol
	Perphenazine
	Ziprasidone

Many antipsychotic drugs are available in both oral and parenteral forms. Oral administration is the preferred route for various reasons, including the fact that patients generally prefer this route. However, tablets have consistently created a problem because they are so easy to "cheek." Cheeking occurs when patients place the tablet to one side of the mouth and pretend to swallow it. Nonadherence is thought to be the most important cause of symptom exacerbation and rehospitalization. Psychiatric patients might not want to take their medication for several reasons, including the admission of illness that taking oral medication might imply, paranoid fears of poisoning, or unpleasant reactions or side effects. A few oral versions of these agents dissolve instantly when placed in the mouth.

Parenteral drugs are usually used to treat acutely disturbed patients or patients who represent significant compliance risks. Long-acting injectable forms are also available and require injection only once every 2 to 4 weeks or less frequently (Kennedy, 2012). These long-acting injections prove beneficial for outpatients or for patients who are nonadherent. Some long-acting agents are as follows:

1. Fluphenazine decanoate
2. Haloperidol decanoate
3. Risperidone microspheres
4. Paliperidone palmitate (Invega Sustenna)
5. Olanzapine long-acting injectable
6. Aripiprazole microspheres (Abilify Maintena)

Table 14-3 lists the advantages of long-acting injectables.

When a patient does not respond to antipsychotic drug therapy, the nurse's assessment of the patient might be quite helpful to the prescriber. Two considerations should be kept in mind when assessing a patient's response:

1. Is the patient actually taking the drug?
2. Has the drug been given a fair trial?

? CRITICAL THINKING QUESTION

2. Refer to the clinical example about Bob. What pharmacokinetic process can explain a rationale for Bob doing fine without medication for a few weeks?

Side Effects

Antipsychotic drugs produce numerous side effects because of peripheral nervous system (PNS) and CNS actions (Box 14-5; see Table 14-1).

TABLE 14-3	ADVANTAGES OF LONG-ACTING INJECTABLE ANTIPSYCHOTIC DRUGS
1. Nonadherence can be distinguished from lack of efficacy.	
2. The nurse knows when nonadherence began.	
3. The patient does not need to take the antipsychotic on a daily basis.	
4. The drug avoids first-pass metabolism, and serum levels are more steady.	

> ### BOX 14-5 SUMMARY OF MAJOR ADVERSE RESPONSES TO ANTIPSYCHOTIC DRUGS
>
> **Anticholinergic Side Effects**
> *Cause:* Blockade of cholinergic receptors (muscarinic receptors)
> *Offending agents:* Anticholinergic drugs, such as low-potency antipsychotics and anticholinergic-antiparkinsonian drugs
> *Signs and symptoms:* Constipation, decreased sweating, dilated pupils, dry mouth, slowed bowels and bladder
>
> **Extrapyramidal Side Effects**
> *Cause:* Blockade of D_2 receptors
> *Offending agents:* Typically high-potency antipsychotics
> *Signs and symptoms:* Akathisia, akinesia, dystonia, parkinsonism, tardive dyskinesia
>
> **Neuroleptic Malignant Syndrome**
> *Cause:* Blockade of D_2 receptors
> *Offending agents:* Typically high-potency antipsychotics
> *Signs and symptoms:* High fever and rigidity—can be fatal

Anticholinergic Effects: Constipation, Decreased Sweating, Dilated Pupils, Dry Mouth, Slowed Bowel and Bladder

PNS anticholinergic effects are a result of the blocking of four cranial nerves that have parasympathetic components. The exception is decreased sweating, which is a sympathetic system function. The following illustrates these anticholinergic effects:

- Cranial nerve (CN) III: Oculomotor nerve blockade results in mydriasis (dilated pupils) and impaired accommodation. Blurred vision might result.
- CN VII: Facial nerve blockade results in dry mouth, decreased tearing, and dry nasal passages.
- CN IX: Glossopharyngeal nerve blockade results in dry mouth and dry nasal passages.
- CN X: Vagus nerve blockade results in tachycardia, constipation, and urinary hesitation.

  Nursing Alert: Anticholinergic Effects

1. Can increase intraocular pressure, aggravating narrow-angle glaucoma
2. Can intensify prostatic hypertrophy, making urination even more difficult
3. Can trigger arrhythmias and cause death

Antiadrenergic Effects: Decrease in Blood Pressure

Hypotension is the major antiadrenergic effect of antipsychotic drugs. The blocking of alpha-1 receptors is the primary cause of hypotension. Blocking these sympathetic receptors on peripheral blood vessels prevents these vessels from responding (constricting) automatically to changes in position. Hypotension occurs most often in older adults and when the individual stands or changes positions suddenly (orthostatic hypotension); precautions against falls must be instituted. In a healthy younger person, accommodation usually occurs within a few weeks; however, many patients cannot tolerate

orthostatic hypotension for that long. Hypotension also causes a reflex tachycardia that can cause general cardiovascular inefficiency. A reflex tachycardia is, by definition, tachycardia that automatically occurs as an adaptive function to compensate for lower extremity vasodilation. Antipsychotic drugs are prescribed cautiously for individuals with severe hypotension, heart failure, or a history of arrhythmias.

Cardiac Effects: Arrhythmias?

A concern among clinicians who prescribe antipsychotics is that these drugs have a potential for lengthening the QTc interval (a measure of ventricular depolarization and repolarization) (Washington et al., 2012). Although this concern is not as pronounced as it was previously, prudent practice dictates that attention be paid because lengthening the QTc interval can be associated with a fatal arrhythmia. A normal QTc interval is 330 to 440 msec. Drug-induced lengthening to greater than 450 msec for men and greater than 470 msec for women is considered QTc prolongation. Of the second-generation antipsychotics commonly prescribed, ziprasidone has the greatest risk of QTc lengthening (Washington et al., 2012). Electrocardiographic monitoring is important.

Extrapyramidal Side Effects: Akathisia, Akinesia, Dystonia, Parkinsonism, and Tardive Dyskinesia

The following formula traces the most familiar path leading to rehospitalization:

EPSEs → nonadherence → relapse → rehospitalization

Preventing or minimizing EPSEs whenever possible is important. It has been estimated that most patients who receive antipsychotic medications have EPSEs, and EPSEs account for many readmissions. High-potency traditional antipsychotics are most likely and atypical antipsychotics are least likely to cause EPSEs. Abnormal involuntary movement disorders develop because of drug-induced imbalances between dopamine and acetylcholine in a specific part of the brain. EPSEs can be grouped as follows: akathisia, akinesia, dystonia, TD, drug-induced parkinsonism, Pisa syndrome, and neuroleptic malignant syndrome (NMS). TD, a late-appearing dyskinesia, can be irreversible (Box 14-6).

Akathisia: Restlessness. Akathisia is a subjective feeling of restlessness exhibited by restless legs, jittery feelings, and nervous energy. Akathisia is the most common EPSE and responds poorly to treatment (Keller et al., 2013). It is a major reason why patients stop taking medications. Sometimes restless legs syndrome can be mistaken for akathisia and vice versa. It should be remembered that restless legs syndrome occurs specifically in the lower body and is exacerbated by caffeine, nicotine, and alcohol (Baker, 2012).

Akinesia and Bradykinesia: Slow Motion. Akinesia refers to an absence of movement; however, slowed movement, or bradykinesia, is more likely. Symptoms include weakness, fatigue, painful muscles, and anergia. Akinesia responds to anticholinergics.

Dystonia: Freezing. Dystonias are abnormal postures caused by involuntary muscle spasms. They elicit a sustained,

BOX 14-6 PROTOCOLS FOR CLOZAPINE THERAPY

1. Normal white blood cell count (WBC) is >3500/mm³, and normal absolute neutrophil count (ANC) is ≥2000/mm³.
2. If baseline WBC is <3500/mm³ and baseline ANC is <2000/mm³, do not start clozapine.
3. Once started, monitor WBC weekly.
4. If WBC and ANC are normal for 6 months (i.e., WBC ≥3500/mm³ and ANC 2000/mm³), monitor level every 2 weeks.
5. If WBC and ANC are normal for 1 year, monitor monthly.
6. If WBC becomes <3000/mm³ or ANC becomes <1500/mm³, discontinue clozapine. Monitor WBC and ANC daily.
7. If no sign of infection is present, clozapine therapy can be resumed when WBC is >3000/mm³ and ANC is >1500/mm³.
8. If WBC becomes <2000/mm³ and ANC becomes <1000/mm³, clozapine should be permanently discontinued.

twisted, and contracted positioning of the limbs, trunk, neck, or mouth. Dystonias tend to appear early in treatment. Types of dystonias include the following:

- Torticollis—contracted positioning of the neck
- Oculogyric crisis—contracted positioning of the eyes upward
- Laryngeal—pharyngeal constriction (potentially life-threatening)

Dystonias respond to anticholinergic drugs, which occasionally must be given parenterally because of the gravity of the situation.

Parkinsonism: Bradykinesia, Rigidity, Tremor. The cardinal symptoms of Parkinson's disease, which include tremors, bradykinesia, and rigidity, are present.

Tardive Dyskinesia: Irreversible? *Tardive* means "late appearing." TD is an EPSE that tends to develop after approximately 6 months or more of antipsychotic therapy and is not caused by the dopamine-acetylcholine imbalance per se; consequently, anticholinergics are ineffective. Anticholinergics typically worsen the symptoms of TD. Long-term use of antipsychotics is thought to cause dopamine receptors in the basal ganglia to become hypersensitive to dopamine. Symptoms are bothersome and can be embarrassing. Typical symptoms include tongue writhing, tongue protrusion, teeth grinding, and lip smacking. The symptoms stop with sleep. Although TD movements can be suppressed willfully for a short time, they eventually reappear. Often, TD is irreversible, but it can be reversed if the patient is closely monitored and the medication is stopped when symptoms first arise. Prevention is the best approach to dealing with TD.

Pisa Syndrome. Older individuals are particularly susceptible to this side effect of leaning to one side. Higher doses of antiparkinsonian drugs may be helpful.

Neuroleptic Malignant Syndrome. NMS is a potentially lethal side effect of antipsychotic agents. The incidence of NMS was formerly much greater than it is today, but with careful scrutiny of patients by nurses and physicians, a significant reduction in its incidence and mortality has occurred. NMS occurs most often when high-potency antipsychotic drugs are prescribed (e.g., haloperidol). NMS is not related to toxic drug levels and might occur after only a few doses. Typically, onset is within a week or so after initiation of an antipsychotic. The cardinal symptoms of NMS are high fever (temperature typically 101° F to 103° F but can increase to 108° F) and rigidity. Related and other symptoms include tremors, impaired ventilations, muteness, altered consciousness, and autonomic hyperactivity. Because an increased temperature is a chief sign of NMS, nurses should monitor temperatures closely.

Dantrolene (Dantrium), a skeletal muscle relaxant, and bromocriptine (Parlodel), a dopamine agonist, are drugs of choice for treating NMS. Antipsychotics should not be reinstituted for at least 2 weeks after complete resolution of NMS symptoms.

Endocrine Side Effects

Traditional antipsychotics elevate prolactin levels by blocking D_2 receptors (at about 70% occupancy). Dopamine inhibits prolactin, and when dopamine receptors are blocked, prolactin levels increase. Many bothersome side effects occur because of chronic elevation of prolactin levels (Table 14-4). Traditional agents are much more likely to cause hyperprolactinemia.

Metabolic Syndrome

Metabolic syndrome (or insulin resistance syndrome) manifests as reduced metabolism of glucose and resistance to insulin by insulin receptors on cells. Type 2 diabetes can result with the associated problems of hyperglycemia, obesity, elevated lipid levels, coagulation abnormalities, and hypertension. Atypical antipsychotics are more likely to cause metabolic syndrome (Table 14-5). The U.S. Food and Drug Administration (FDA) requires drug manufacturers to include a warning about this problem. Three or more of the following constitute metabolic syndrome (Keltner, 2006):

1. Abdominal girth greater than 40 inches in men and greater than 35 inches in women
2. Elevated triglycerides (≥150 mg/dL)
3. Reduced high-density lipoproteins (≤40 mg/dL in men or ≤50 mg/dL in women)
4. Elevated blood pressure or treatment for same
5. Elevated fasting glucose (≥100 mg/dL)

The atypical antipsychotics clozapine and olanzapine seem most likely to cause metabolic syndrome (Birkenaes & Andreassen, 2004).

TABLE 14-4 CONSEQUENCES OF CHRONIC PROLACTIN ELEVATION

WOMEN	MEN
Amenorrhea	Impotence
Loss of libido	Loss of libido
Galactorrhea	Gynecomastia
Long-term risk for osteoporosis	Lowered sperm count
Changes in menstrual cycle	Feminization

TABLE 14-5	COMPARISON OF METABOLIC EFFECTS OF ATYPICAL ANTIPSYCHOTICS		
DRUG	**WEIGHT GAIN**	**DYSLIPIDEMIA**	**HYPERGLYCEMIA**
Clozapine	+++	+++	+++
Olanzapine	+++	+++	+++
Risperidone	++	+	+
Quetiapine	++	++	++
Ziprasidone	+/0	+/0	+/0
Aripiprazole	+/0	+/0	+/0
Iloperidone	++	+/0	+/0
Paliperidone	+	+	+
Asenapine	+/0	+/0	+/0
Lurasidone	+/0	+/0	+/0

+++ = significant; ++ = intermediate; + = low; +/0 = low or neutral.
Adapted from Zeier, K., et al. (2013). Recommendations for lab monitoring of atypical antipsychotics. *Current Psychiatry, 12,* 51.

Sexual Side Effects

D_2 and alpha-2 blockade as well as the aforementioned elevated prolactin levels are thought to be responsible for sexual side effects. Sexual activity can be divided into three phases: desire, arousal, and orgasm. With a little imagination, one could verify that sexual activity pretty much follows that order of events. From a man's perspective, desire is step one. If there is no desire, it is very difficult to go to step two, arousal (i.e., an erection). If step two is accomplished, there is no guarantee that step three, orgasm, will occur.

Desire deficits are most likely caused by dopamine blockade. Because dopamine elevation is linked to schizophrenia, it is difficult to provide dopamine-enhancing agents without exacerbating symptoms. Arousal problems can be treated with sildenafil (Viagra). Invariably, in the authors' experience, the third phase of sexual behavior (orgasm) causes most of the problems. For many men, desire and arousal are not significant issues; however, having an orgasm is significant.

Gastrointestinal Effects

Weight gain can be significant, particularly for patients taking the newer agents. This phenomenon is probably related to blockade of histamine H_1, 5-hydroxytryptamine 2C (5-HT$_{2C}$), and other receptors. Insulin resistance is an outcome and a cause of excessive weight gain. Carbohydrate craving is a common feature.

Clinical Example

Bud, a 23-year-old patient with a diagnosis of schizophrenia, gained 105 pounds in less than 1 year on a particular atypical drug. He was finally switched to another agent and lost about 75 pounds of the extra weight.

Other Side Effects

Other side effects that might occur in patients taking antipsychotic drugs include jaundice, rare but serious blood dyscrasias, susceptibility to hyperthermia, sun-sensitive skin, nasal congestion, wheezing, and memory loss. Because the cholinergic system is implicated in memory and learning, low-potency antipsychotic drugs might play a role in the cognitive symptoms. Clozapine (Clozaril) causes agranulocytosis in 1% of patients and is potentially fatal. Agranulocytosis is discussed later in this chapter.

Nursing Implications
Therapeutic versus Toxic Levels

Overdoses of antipsychotic drugs are seldom fatal. An overdose can cause severe CNS depression, hypotension, and EPSEs. Restlessness or agitation, convulsions, hyperthermia, increased anticholinergic symptoms, and arrhythmias are other indicators of an overdose.

Use during Pregnancy

Antipsychotics pose few risks during pregnancy; nonetheless, they should be avoided during the first trimester (Richards et al., 1999). These drugs readily pass the placental barrier, reach significant levels in the fetus, and may cause EPSEs in some newborns. All atypical antipsychotic agents are FDA pregnancy category C, which means that in animal studies adverse effects have been demonstrated. Although a number of the atypicals have been given during pregnancy without problems arising, all of these drugs worsen or cause glucose intolerance, which can be potentially harmful (Robakis & Williams, 2013).

Use in Older Adults

Because older adults have decreased hepatic metabolism capability, reducing the dose in this age group is prudent. Age-related nigrostriatal and cholinergic degeneration cause pharmacodynamic responses that are more intense than pharmacodynamic responses experienced by younger individuals. Both extrapyramidal and anticholinergic effects can be heightened. Older adults are also at higher risk for TD. A black box warning for atypical agents was issued in 2005, indicating that older adults with dementia-related psychosis were at increased risk of dying from sudden death or pneumonia when treated with these drugs.

Side Effects

PNS anticholinergic and antiadrenergic effects of antipsychotic drugs are troublesome but not always as serious or as disturbing to the patient as are CNS EPSEs. The nurse can provide several specific interventions to ameliorate side effects or to prevent serious consequences (see the Peripheral Nervous System Effects and Nursing Interventions box and the Extrapyramidal Side Effects and Nursing Interventions box).

Interactions

Antipsychotic drugs interact with many other drugs. Because these interactions can be serious, the nurse must review offending agents and advise the family and patient accordingly. CNS depressants, such as alcohol, antihistamines, antianxiety drugs, antidepressants, barbiturates, meperidine, and morphine, have additive or pharmacodynamic effects that can cause profound CNS depression. A few of the most common adverse interactions are found in Table 14-6.

PERIPHERAL NERVOUS SYSTEM EFFECTS AND NURSING INTERVENTIONS

PNS EFFECT	NURSING INTERVENTIONS
Constipation	Encourage high dietary fiber and increased water intake; give laxatives as ordered.
Decreased sweating	Avoid exposure to extreme heat, if possible.
Dry mouth	Advise patient to take sips of water frequently; provide sugarless hard candies, sugarless gum, and mouth rinses.
Blurred vision	Advise patient to avoid potentially dangerous tasks. Reassure patient that normal vision typically returns in a few weeks, when tolerance to this side effect develops. Pilocarpine eye drops can be used on a short-term basis.
Mydriasis	Advise patient to report eye pain immediately.
Photophobia	Advise patient to wear sunglasses outdoors.
Orthostatic hypotension	Advise patient to get out of bed or chair slowly. If hypotension is a problem, measure blood pressure before each dose is given.
Tachycardia	Tachycardia is usually a reflex response to hypotension. When intervention for hypotension is effective, reflex tachycardia usually decreases.
Urinary retention	Encourage frequent voiding and voiding whenever the urge is present. Older men with benign prostatic hypertrophy are particularly susceptible to urinary retention.
Urinary hesitation	Provide privacy (some individuals struggle to urinate in front of others), run water in the sink, and so on.
Sedation	Help patient get up early and get the day started.
Weight gain	Help patient order an appropriate diet; diet pills should not be taken.

PNS, Peripheral nervous system.

EXTRAPYRAMIDAL SIDE EFFECTS AND NURSING INTERVENTIONS

EPSE	NURSING INTERVENTIONS
Akathisia	Be patient and reassure the patient who is jittery that you understand the need to move. Because akathisia is a major cause of nonadherence with antipsychotic regimens, a drug change is often necessary.
Dystonias	If a severe reaction such as oculogyric crisis or torticollis occurs, give benztropine (Cogentin) or diphenhydramine (Benadryl) immediately, as needed, and offer reassurance. For some situations, IM administration of benztropine is required because of the seriousness of the dystonic reaction.
Drug-induced parkinsonism	Antiparkinsonian drugs are probably indicated.
TD	Assess for signs and symptoms by using AIMS. Anticholinergic agents worsen TD.
NMS	Be alert for this potentially fatal side effect. Routinely take temperature and encourage adequate water intake for all patients on a regimen of antipsychotic drugs; routinely assess for rigidity, tremor, and similar symptoms.

AIMS, Abnormal involuntary movement scale; *EPSE,* extrapyramidal side effect; *IM,* intramuscular; *NMS,* neuroleptic malignant syndrome; *TD,* tardive dyskinesia.

CRITICAL THINKING QUESTION

3. In the Peripheral Nervous System Effects and Nursing Interventions box, pilocarpine eye drops are suggested for blurred vision. What category of drug does pilocarpine belong to, and how does it help blurred vision?

Prescription Drugs. The nurse should review prescriptions to serve as a safety net for the prescriber who might make an inadvertent error. This safety measure is also important because nurses often act as case managers or advocates for patients who are seeing many caregivers and receiving prescriptions from multiple providers.

Nonprescription Drugs. Many nonprescription drugs have potentially harmful interactive effects with antipsychotic drugs. CNS depressants such as alcohol, cold and influenza agents, and sleep aids can have additive effects. Other drugs decrease the effect of antipsychotics. For instance, antacids decrease absorption of antipsychotic drugs.

TABLE 14-6   ADVERSE INTERACTIONS OF ANTIPSYCHOTICS WITH SELECTED DRUGS

DRUG	EFFECT OF INTERACTION
Amphetamines	Decreased antipsychotic effect
Barbiturates	All cause respiratory depression and increase sedation; all decrease antipsychotic serum levels; hypotension
Benzodiazepines	Increased sedation; respiratory depression is possible
Cigarette smoking	Decreased serum levels of some antipsychotic drugs
Insulin, oral hypoglycemics	Control of diabetes is weakened
Levodopa	Decreased antiparkinsonian effect of levodopa; might exacerbate psychosis
Narcotics	Increased sedation; respiratory depression augmented

From Keltner, N.L., & Folks, D.G. (2005). *Psychotropic drugs* (4th ed.). St. Louis: Mosby.

Teaching Patients

Teaching patients is an important dimension of nursing care for patients who are taking antipsychotic drugs. The nurse should use discretion in selecting the content of educational sessions because some patients have a tendency to become anxious and paranoid about potential side effects. The nurse should focus on symptoms that can be seen or felt. The patient should be given a simply written description of drug benefits and side effects, with instructions on how to cope with the side effects. Having this information in a written format helps the patient and family be more in control and able to act as collaborators in treatment.

In addition to the education issues already mentioned, the patient and family should be taught the following:

- Avoid immersion in hot water because hypotension might occur, causing falls.
- Use a sunscreen to prevent sunburn, and use a maximum-strength sunscreen when sunbathing.
- Dress appropriately in hot weather, and drink plenty of water to avoid heat stroke.
- Avoid abrupt withdrawal of medication because EPSEs can occur.
- Take the drug as prescribed. Nonadherence is the leading cause of the return of symptoms and a leading cause of readmission.
- Immediately report signs of a sore throat, malaise, fever, or bleeding. These signs might indicate a blood dyscrasia.

CRITICAL THINKING QUESTIONS

4. The chapter states that low-potency antipsychotic drugs have fewer EPSEs than high-potency drugs. Why might this be true? (Hint: The answer is related to the type of effects that are more prominent with low-potency drugs and the kind of drugs that are used to treat EPSEs.)
5. It is easy to say that everyone who needs clozapine should have it. However, clozapine is an expensive drug and can cause fatal agranulocytosis. Focus on the patients who are most resistant to traditional drugs as well as on the compliance problems among these patients. Consider a delivery system for getting this drug to the patients who need it. How can this goal be accomplished? What role can nursing play in the solution to this problem?

TRADITIONAL (FIRST-GENERATION) DRUGS: INTRODUCED IN 1950

This section provides additional details about the traditional antipsychotics. Traditional antipsychotics account for only 3% of market sales but about 20% of prescriptions (IMS Health, 2002). These drugs are effective, but they have a higher risk for adverse effects. However, some patients do very well on these drugs. They remain viable options because they are effective and much cheaper for patients and payers. Because schizophrenia can be viewed as a lifelong illness, the difference in cost over many years dictates that traditional drugs at least be considered (Table 14-7). For example, a 1-month

TABLE 14-7 COST OF SELECTED ANTIPSYCHOTICS FOR 1 MONTH/YEAR: CHEAPEST TO MOST EXPENSIVE

ANTIPSYCHOTIC	DOSAGE (mg/day)	COST PER MONTH/YEAR
Haloperidol	1.5	$21/252
Chlorpromazine	200	$23/276
Perphenazine	24	$117/1404
Risperdal	2	$450/5400
Invega	6	$532/6384
Zyprexa	10	$546/6552
Seroquel	300	$549/6588
Abilify	10	$589/7068
Geodon	160	$622/7464

From Consumer Reports Best Buy Drugs. (2009). *Treating schizophrenia and bipolar disorder: the antipsychotics—comparing effectiveness, safety, and price.* Yonkers, NY: Consumer Reports Best Buy.

supply of haloperidol costs about $20, whereas a 1-month supply of paliperidone (Invega) costs more than $500.

Low-Potency Traditional Antipsychotics

Only the most prescribed traditional antipsychotics are discussed here. Also see Box 14-2.

Chlorpromazine

Chlorpromazine (Thorazine) was the first antipsychotic developed. When it became available to state hospitals in the United States, workers viewed it as a godsend. Some patients dramatically improved. Chlorpromazine is a low-potency agent and results in anticholinergic and antiadrenergic effects. It is also sedating and causes significant weight gain. EPSEs are moderately produced.

Thioridazine

Thioridazine is almost as old as chlorpromazine and was extensively prescribed. A few patients tend to respond to thioridazine better than to any other drug. However, cases of sudden death have been linked to thioridazine (Hennessy et al., 2004).

Moderate-Potency Traditional Antipsychotics

Some drugs do not fit into the high-potency versus low-potency conceptual framework. Loxapine and perphenazine are two significant moderate-potency drugs. Loxapine inhalation powder (Adasuve) was approved more recently to treat agitation in schizophrenia. Patients with both higher and lower levels of agitation have benefited from this new drug (Citrome, 2013). Evidence from the landmark Clinical Antipsychotic Trials and Intervention Effectiveness (CATIE) study (Lieberman et al., 2005) suggests that perphenazine, when compared with second-generation antipsychotics, was as effective as any of them with the exception of olanzapine. (Clozapine was not included in this trial.) Because perphenazine is so much less expensive, this can be an attractive alternative to the more expensive atypical agents.

High-Potency Traditional Antipsychotics
Fluphenazine

Fluphenazine (Prolixin), a high-potency antipsychotic, is commonly prescribed and considered to be an effective medication. Fluphenazine decanoate (Prolixin Decanoate), the long-acting form, is beneficial for patients who do not comply with a daily oral medication regimen. This injection can be given every 2 to 3 weeks.

Haloperidol

Haloperidol (Haldol) is a high-potency drug that tends to cause more EPSEs and fewer anticholinergic side effects than low-potency drugs. Dr. Henry Nasrallah (2013), a prominent psychiatrist from Ohio, has even questioned whether it should be banned owing to its adverse effects. Haloperidol accounts for about 7% of all antipsychotic drugs prescribed and is the most frequently prescribed traditional drug (IMS Health, 2002). It is used extensively in older adults (because of fewer anticholinergic effects) and in pediatric psychiatry.

A problem of ongoing concern to psychiatric nurses is the threat of aggressive behavior of psychiatric patients. Chemical restraint (an unfortunate choice of words for describing psychopharmacologic intervention of this type) is a means of relieving a patient of distressing symptoms that lead to aggressive behavior. Parenteral haloperidol alone or in combination with the benzodiazepine lorazepam (Ativan) is an excellent approach for helping patients stay in control. These two agents can be drawn up in the same syringe and administered as a single injection.

Haloperidol decanoate is a long-acting form and can be given at 2- to 4-week intervals (or longer). It is particularly beneficial for individuals who are nonadherent.

ATYPICAL ANTIPSYCHOTIC (SECOND-GENERATION) DRUGS: INTRODUCED IN 1990

Chlorpromazine, the first antipsychotic, was developed around 1950. Atypical agents were not marketed until 1990. During this 40-year period, hundreds of antipsychotic formulations were developed. Although the drugs were not terribly different, they were all traditional or typical. Atypical antipsychotics are atypical because they work differently (have a different mechanism of action) than the traditional drugs and have a greater effect on negative symptoms. There are two major mechanisms of action that make atypical agents different: (1) They block 5-HT_{2A} receptors (Figure 14-2). (2) They are faster "on-off" the D_2 receptor.

Serotonin (5-Hydroxytryptamine 2A) Antagonism

Because the 5-HT_{2A} receptor inhibits dopamine release, drugs that are 5-HT_{2A} receptor antagonists liberate dopamine. As previously noted and repeated here, these drugs have the following theoretical features that make them atypical:

1. Reduced risk for EPSEs: 5-HT_{2A} blockade modifies D_2 blockade.

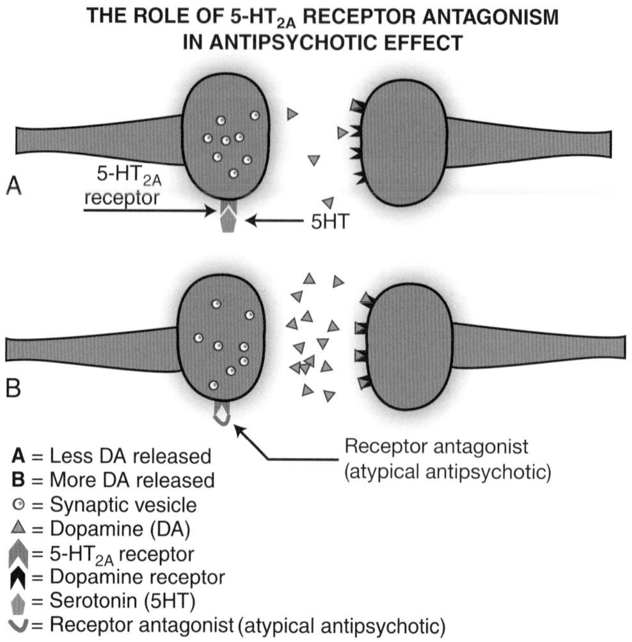

A = Less DA released
B = More DA released
⊙ = Synaptic vesicle
△ = Dopamine (DA)
⋀ = 5-HT_{2A} receptor
⋀ = Dopamine receptor
⬆ = Serotonin (5HT)
⌄ = Receptor antagonist (atypical antipsychotic)

FIG 14-2 Role of 5-HT_{2A} modulation of dopaminergic neurons and the role of atypical antipsychotics. **A,** The 5-HT_{2A} receptor inhibits the presynaptic dopamine neuron. When serotonin fits this receptor, it down-regulates dopamine release and can contribute to extrapyramidal side effects (EPSEs) (nigrostriatal tract), hyperprolactinemia (tuberoinfundibular tract), and negative and cognitive symptoms (mesocortical tract). **B,** An atypical antipsychotic has blocked the 5-HT_{2A} receptor. This antagonism increases release of dopamine into the synapse, decreasing EPSEs, stabilizing prolactin, and improving negative and cognitive symptoms. (From Keltner, N.L., & Folks, D.G. [2005]. *Psychotropic drugs* [4th ed.]. St. Louis: Mosby.)

2. Increased effectiveness in treating negative symptoms: Dopamine is increased in the frontal lobe.
3. Minimal risk of TD: Dopamine receptors do not become hypersensitive.
4. Reduced prolactin level elevation: Prolactin-inhibiting factor (i.e., dopamine) is still available.

Each of the four differences is produced by the blockade of 5-HT_{2A} receptors, which putatively liberates dopamine. The reasoning is as follows:

If EPSEs are caused by dopamine D_2 blockade, *atypicals* keep dopamine available and highly competitive for those receptors.

If negative symptoms are caused (at least partially) by decreased dopamine in the cortex, *atypicals* increase dopamine in the cortex.

If prolactin level elevation is caused by a deficiency in dopamine, *atypicals* increase dopamine in this tract.

If TD is caused by irritation of D_2 receptors being continually "grasped" by D_2 antagonists, *atypicals* prevent this from occurring.

In the years since their introduction, atypical drugs have totally dominated the market. However, they have not lived up to their initial promise. If cognitive symptoms are improved with these drugs, the improvement is not nearly as remarkable as hoped for (Nestler et al., 2009).

Generally, these agents have a broad affinity for several neurotransmitter systems thought to be implicated in schizophrenia. Additionally, they appear to demonstrate regionally specific activity in the brain. For example, they can modulate mesolimbic function without a significant effect on the nigrostriatal tract. Because of the complexity of these pharmacologic effects, a more refined receptor affinity profile could be developed for each of these drugs. However, this discussion is beyond the scope of this text.

Nursing Student: "Dr. Keltner, if atypical antipsychotics increase dopamine and if too much dopamine is the cause of schizophrenia, wouldn't atypicals make schizophrenia worse?"

Keltner: "That is a great question because it shows you are thinking. The answer is there is a paucity of 5-HT_{2A} receptors in the mesolimbic tract, so dopamine is not appreciably increased in that tract, and thus psychotic symptoms are not increased."

Fast-Off Theory

The fast-off theory states that how long a drug is on the D_2 receptor is significant. Dopamine antagonists have to "get on" the receptor to block dopamine from attaching to that same receptor. They eventually have to get off as well. This amount of time can be measured (i.e., how quickly a drug binds to and then dissociates from a receptor or its dissociation constant) (Steele et al., 2011). The smaller the dissociation constant, the more tightly the drug binds to the receptor. The larger the dissociation constant, the less affinity a drug has for the receptor. In a classic work, Kapur and Seeman (2001) theorized that differences in dissociation from the receptor is what really causes second-generation drugs to be atypical. For example, here are the binding affinities for a few selected antipsychotics and for dopamine itself (Steele et al., 2011):

Antipsychotic	Dissociation Constant
Aripiprazole	0.34
Clozapine	126
Dopamine	**1.75**
Haloperidol	0.7
Olanzapine	11
Quetiapine	160
Risperidone	4
Ziprasidone	5

Although mostly atypical antipsychotics are noted in this table, haloperidol has a significantly stronger binding to D_2 than does dopamine itself. One sees that risperidone binds more tightly to these receptors than either quetiapine or clozapine and would be predicted to cause a higher level of EPSEs than those two drugs. That is what we see in clinical practice. Risperidone can cause EPSEs at higher doses.

Potential Negative Effects of Second-Generation Antipsychotics

Although second-generation antipsychotics have numerous significant advantages, they are also known to cause several important adverse effects. These include metabolic dysregulation (see earlier discussion of metabolic syndrome) and its complications—obesity, diabetes, hyperlipidemia, and hypertension. The CATIE study found that 43% of outpatients with schizophrenia met the criteria for metabolic syndrome. Nasrallah (2012) pointed out that many psychiatrists and psychiatric nurse practitioners are not following guidelines to nip this problem in the bud.

Clozapine

Clozapine (Clozaril), released to the retail market in 1990, was the first truly new antipsychotic agent to be introduced into the United States in 40 years. Clozapine has been referred to as the "gold standard" in the management of schizophrenia. Although clozapine had been used in Europe and China for some time, it was not approved in the United States because of the seriousness of a major side effect called *agranulocytosis*. Because of this side effect, clozapine is indicated only after patients with severe schizophrenia have failed to respond to other antipsychotic drugs. The following summary underscores the severity of this adverse effect.

In Finland, during June and July 1975, 9 of 18 patients who developed clozapine-induced agranulocytosis died (Idanpaan-Heikkila et al., 1975). This alarming event sent shudders through the psychiatric community, and clozapine was not approved in the United States for another 15 years. By the mid-1980s, studies revealed a more optimistic picture of this drug and its effects. However, this picture was still tempered by an excessively high morbidity rate of 1% to 2% for agranulocytosis and a mortality rate of approximately 33% for patients developing this blood dyscrasia (Keltner, 1997). Current investigations have indicated a slightly lower morbidity rate of less than 1%; the mortality rate has also declined significantly. Side effects of clozapine result from its antagonism of cholinergic, alpha-1, alpha-2, and H_1 receptors. As demonstrated from comparing the receptor-antagonism profile of clozapine with the theoretical effects of receptor blockade shown in Table 14-2, clozapine causes significant anticholinergic effects—orthostasis, sedation, and weight gain. Sexual dysfunction also occurs and, with weight gain, is particularly troublesome and has social implications.

Clozapine is primarily metabolized by CYP-450 1A2. Most patients with schizophrenia smoke, and cigarette smoking induces CYP-450 1A2, causing a decreased level of clozapine (Keltner & Grant, 2006).

Clinical Example

During a group therapy session in a state public hospital, Bill continually stands up and cannot sit down for long. Bill sits down the moment the group leader instructs him to sit down, but he immediately stands up again. The group leader misinterprets Bill's behavior as defiance. This misinterpretation escalates into a confrontation that culminates when Bill is forcibly restrained and given an as-needed injection of an antipsychotic agent. Had the group leader been more aware of EPSEs, he would have suspected akathisia and would have further recognized that an antipsychotic would make the patient worse.

Agranulocytosis is clinically defined as an absolute neutrophil count less than 500/mm^3 and might be caused by bone marrow suppression. Because of its life-threatening potential, the manufacturer of Clozaril requires that its representative closely monitor patients. Box 14-6 outlines the protocols for clozapine therapy.

Clozapine is associated with several other important side effects, including dose-related seizures (5% at higher doses) and excessive salivation (about 30%). One would think that because clozapine is such a strong anticholinergic, dry mouth and not hypersalivation would be the problem, but that is not the case. Some patients carry paper cups to hold excessive saliva. It seems that although clozapine does block four of the five muscarinic subtypes, it is an agonist at M$_4$ (Hultfilz et al., 2012). This property accounts for the large amount of "extra" saliva produced in patients taking clozapine. Myocarditis is another significant side effect. Patients should be instructed to report dyspnea, fever, chest pain, palpitations, tachycardia, and other symptoms of heart failure immediately. Fatal overdoses have been associated with clozapine (Keck & McElroy, 2002).

Risperidone and Paliperidone

Risperidone (Risperdal), approved in 1994, is atypical but different from clozapine. Risperidone has a greater affinity for D$_2$ receptors and a similar antagonism of 5-HT$_{2A}$ receptors compared with clozapine; risperidone theoretically has a favorable receptor profile for both positive and negative schizophrenia. The lack of serious side effects associated with risperidone makes it a well-tolerated drug as well. Risperidone has little affinity for muscarinic (i.e., cholinergic) receptors, so anticholinergic side effects are minimized (see Table 14-1). In addition, risperidone does not appear to cause agranulocytosis, TD, or NMS. Risperidone appears to be a relatively safe drug. Nonetheless, risperidone significantly blocks alpha-1 and H$_1$ receptors, resulting in orthostatic hypotension, sedation, and appetite stimulation. At higher doses, patients taking risperidone have experienced EPSEs and hyperprolactinemia. Other side effects include insomnia (in some patients), agitation, headache, anxiety, and rhinitis. A long-acting intramuscular version is available.

Paliperidone (Invega) is part of the risperidone family and is manufactured by the same company that makes Risperdal. Similar to many drugs, a metabolite of risperidone has pharmacologic properties similar to the parent drug. In this case, paliperidone is that metabolite: 9-hydroxyrisperidone (risperidone with an additional hydroxyl [OH] group). It has a similar side effect profile as risperidone and presumably achieves its therapeutic effects by antagonism of D$_2$ and 5-HT$_{2A}$ receptors as does risperidone. Invega has the advantage of being an extended-release formulation. There is also a long-acting injectable form.

Olanzapine

Olanzapine (Zyprexa), which was released to the market in 1996, is comparable to risperidone in efficacy and side effect profile and does not cause agranulocytosis. Olanzapine blocks 5-HT$_{2A}$ and D$_2$ receptors significantly. It also has a high affinity for cholinergic, H$_1$, and alpha-1 receptors, resulting in anticholinergic effects of sedation, weight gain, and orthostasis. Olanzapine normalizes *N*-methyl-D-aspartate (NMDA) receptor function in the glutaminergic system, blocking some signs and symptoms associated with schizophrenia. It has a favorable side effect profile, with few incidents of EPSEs. Olanzapine causes considerable weight gain in some patients. In a 2005 study, 30% of patients who had been prescribed olanzapine gained at least 7% of their body weight during the trial (Lieberman et al., 2005). Olanzapine has proven effective in treating acute mania and is an FDA-approved drug for monotherapy for bipolar disorder. A long-acting injectable form is also available. The following clinical example illustrates how olanzapine made a significant difference in one man's life.

Quetiapine (Seroquel)

Scarecrow, scarecrow what's that you popping?
A powerful pill they call Oxy Contin
But it's so tiny, that it got you dragging
Haven't you heard big things come in small packages
I prefer the orange's with the black O-C
Take two and you cannot move up out ya seat
Some people melt 'em down in a needle and shoot 'em up
But I pop 'em with Seroquel like glue, I am stuck

Rap song by Lord Infamous

Quetiapine (Seroquel) was made available in 1997. Quetiapine, similar to clozapine, has a lower affinity for D_2 receptors than for 5-HT_{2A}. Quetiapine has little affinity for muscarinic cholinergic receptors; few anticholinergic side effects are expected. However, quetiapine antagonizes alpha-1 receptors, which leads to orthostatic hypotension, and antagonizes H_1 receptors, which leads to sedation and appetite stimulation. Clinically, quetiapine is effective for both positive and negative symptoms, provokes few EPSEs, does not significantly increase serum prolactin levels, and appears to improve elements of cognitive function. Current formulations must be titrated slowly over a 4- to 5-day period. Anecdotal reports suggest that the effective dose range is higher than manufacturer's recommendations. As the above-quoted lyrics might suggest, quetiapine is becoming a drug of choice for abuse in jails and prisons. The drug is taken orally, intranasally, and intravenously, and it provides both an anxiolytic and sedative effect.

Ziprasidone

Ziprasidone (Geodon) is effective for both positive and negative symptoms of schizophrenia. Ziprasidone acts on several neurotransmitter systems, has a high affinity for 5-HT_{2A} receptors and D_2 receptors, moderately blocks the reuptake of serotonin and norepinephrine, and is an agonist for the 5-HT_{1A} receptor. These pharmacologic properties suggest a drug that has the potential to ameliorate depression and anxiety, which are commonly associated with schizophrenia, and causes few EPSEs, few anticholinergic side effects, and mild antihistaminic effects. Common side effects include nausea, dyspepsia, abdominal pain, constipation, somnolence, insomnia, and coryzal symptoms. Ziprasidone appears to cause less weight gain than some other atypical agents. Ziprasidone has been linked to potential cardiac problems related to lengthening of the QTc interval. Studies have indicated a low potential for drug-drug interactions. An intramuscular form is available. Absorption is increased when ziprasidone is given with food.

Effects of 5-HT$_{1A}$ Agonism by Ziprasidone

• Decreased anxiety
• Decreased depressive symptoms
• Improvement in negative symptoms

CRITICAL THINKING QUESTION

6. Suppose that you are caring for a patient who needs medication but will not take it; for example, a patient with paranoid delusions might truly believe that you are poisoning her with the antipsychotic drug that has been prescribed for her. What are your legal and ethical grounds for nursing care in this situation?

Aripiprazole

Aripiprazole (Abilify) is also referred to as a dopamine system stabilizer. Dopamine system stabilizers are thought to balance the dopamine systems by increasing dopamine in brain areas in which dopamine is deficient and decreasing dopamine in brain areas in which dopamine is overactive. Figure 14-3 contrasts the blockade of D_2 receptors by traditional drugs (Figure 14-3, *A*) with the partial agonism of the same receptors by a drug such as aripiprazole (Figure 14-3, *B*). Aripiprazole accomplishes this because it is a partial dopamine agonist, producing activation where lower dopamine tone exists and inhibition at brain sites with high dopaminergic tone. Areas with too much dopamine begin to stabilize because the aripiprazole molecule is less potent than the dopamine molecule; this effect reduces positive symptoms. Mesocortical areas also begin to stabilize from the opposite direction. Patients begin to feel better, with more energy as negative symptoms subside. Aripiprazole also antagonizes 5-HT_{2A} receptors, as do other atypical drugs, and it is a partial agonist at the 5-HT_{1A} receptor. Clinical studies have suggested a very good side effect profile.

Asenapine

Asenapine (Saphris) is a newer atypical drug approved in 2009. It is available only as a sublingual tablet, so it is ineffective if swallowed. It is approved for the treatment of both acute schizophrenia and bipolar disorder. It has shown a low tendency to cause EPSEs in preclinical tests (Keltner et al., 2011), but anecdotal reports suggest that a slightly higher incidence may occur, particularly in the case of akathisia. Beyond giving patients, families, and clinicians another alternative, asenapine is marketed as being more effective in the treatment of cognitive and negative symptoms.

Iloperidone

Iloperidone (Fanapt) is also a newer atypical agent. It is an antagonist of both 5-HT_{2A} and D_2 receptors. It blocks histamine and alpha-1 receptors, and weight gain, sedation, and orthostasis are common effects. It is related to risperidone (it is a metabolite of risperidone) and can precipitate EPSEs, prolactin elevation, and hyperprolactinemia (Citrome, 2011).

Lurasidone

The last of the newer atypical agents is lurasidone (Latuda). It, too, blocks 5-HT_{2A} and D_2 receptors. It also blocks the

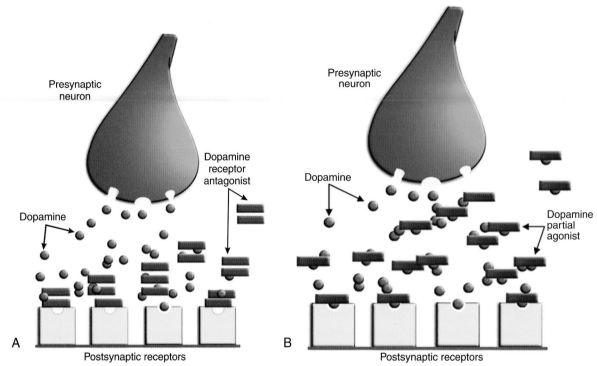

FIG 14-3 A, Dopamine receptor antagonism. **B,** Dopamine system stabilization. (From Keltner, N.L., & Johnson, V. [2002]. Biological perspectives. Aripiprazole: a third generation of antipsychotics begins? *Perspectives Psychiatric Care, 38,* 157.)

5-HT$_{1A}$ receptor, which is thought to account for antianxiety properties of this drug. Similar to ziprasidone, absorption is improved if taken with food. It has a good side effect profile with few instances of dizziness, orthostatic hypotension, cognitive problems, sedation, or weight gain reported (Keltner et al., 2011).

A NEW THEORY OF SCHIZOPHRENIA

> *… there is consensus that no antipsychotic has emerged as truly efficacious against the enduring cognitive and primary negative symptoms.*
>
> **Diana O. Perkins (2011)**

A new theory of schizophrenia and its treatment has captured a great deal of attention—the glutamate hypothesis (Steele et al., 2012). This newest biochemical model of schizophrenia is discussed in more detail in Chapter 24. But first, think about the quotation just given. A lot of ink has already been used explaining how the atypical antipsychotics are better for negative and cognitive symptoms of schizophrenia. They are, but better is not the same as "truly efficacious." This model states that the dopamine hypothesis is inadequate to explain the full range of symptoms we see in patients with schizophrenia. The dopamine hypothesis does a nice job of explaining hallucinations and delusions but a lousy job of explaining negative and cognitive symptoms. The argument goes something like this (Kantrowitz & Javitt, 2011):

1. Dopamine agonists such as levodopa do not cause negative and cognitive symptoms.
2. Dopamine antagonists do not "fix" negative and cognitive symptoms.
3. When the dopamine system is stabilized, these symptoms continue.

The glutamate system explains both positive and negative symptoms of schizophrenia. For example, when drug users overdose on phencyclidine (PCP) or ketamine a (K-hole), they demonstrate both positive and negative symptoms of schizophrenia. Because these drugs of abuse are known to block glutamate receptors (i.e., NMDA receptors), drugs that can increase glutamate might have antipsychotic possibilities. However, a fly in the ointment is the fact that glutamate does not pass the blood-brain barrier and that it requires an *obligate co-agonist* (i.e., glycine or a structurally related molecule). At the present time, the research on co-agonists seems to be going a little better, but this work is still under way. By the time this book is published, most likely a lot more will be known about these agents.

❓ CRITICAL THINKING QUESTION

7. Some clinicians believe that unless a patient has some level of EPSEs, the patient is not receiving enough medication. What might be the rationale for this view?

STUDY NOTES

1. The dopamine hypothesis of schizophrenia states that an excessive level of dopamine in the brain causes schizophrenia.
2. Antipsychotic drugs block dopamine receptors, reducing the effect of excessive dopamine in the brain, specifically in the mesolimbic tract.
3. Antipsychotic drugs are classified in two ways: traditional or first-generation antipsychotics and atypical or second-generation antipsychotics.
4. The traditional agents are divided further into high-potency and low-potency drugs.
5. Desired effects of antipsychotic drugs include sedation, emotional quieting, psychomotor slowing, and alleviation of major symptoms of schizophrenia (e.g., alterations in perceptions, thoughts, consciousness, interpersonal relationships, and affect).
6. Anticholinergic side effects (e.g., dry mouth, blurred vision, constipation) and EPSEs (e.g., akathisia, akinesia, dystonic reactions, drug-induced parkinsonism, Pisa syndrome, and TD) are the major categories of side effects associated with antipsychotic drugs.
7. High-potency antipsychotic drugs, such as haloperidol and fluphenazine, tend to cause more EPSEs. Low-potency antipsychotic drugs, such as chlorpromazine and thioridazine, tend to cause more anticholinergic and antiadrenergic side effects.
8. NMS is a serious adverse effect of antipsychotic drugs (primarily high-potency drugs).
9. Overdoses of antipsychotic drugs are seldom fatal.
10. Antipsychotic drugs interact with other CNS depressants, such as alcohol, meperidine, and morphine, increasing CNS depression.
11. Patient teaching should focus on recognizing side effects and on avoiding CNS depressants.
12. The nurse should routinely assess for NMS by taking the patient's temperature and evaluating for rigidity and tremors.
13. Clozapine, introduced into the United States in 1990, was the first truly new antipsychotic drug in 40 years.
14. Other atypical antipsychotics have a great affinity for D_2 and 5-HT_{2A} receptors, produce few EPSEs, and have had remarkable success in patients resistant to treatment.
15. The atypical antipsychotics go on and off the D_2 receptor much faster than traditional drugs.
16. Clozapine causes agranulocytosis, a potentially fatal illness.
17. Other atypical antipsychotics do not cause life-threatening agranulocytosis.
18. Metabolic syndrome can be a particularly troublesome and serious side effect of atypical agents.
19. Aripiprazole is called a dopamine system stabilizing antipsychotic. Its mechanism of action is unique—partial agonism of D_2 and 5-HT_{2A} receptors.
20. There are three newer antipsychotics—asenapine, iloperidone, and lurasidone. Time will tell if they are important additions to the treatment of schizophrenia.

REFERENCES

Baker, S. W. (2012). Differentiating restless legs syndrome from psychotropic side effects. *Current Psychiatry, 11*, 56.

Berkrot, B. (2010). *US prescription drug sales hit $300 bln in 2009.* Available from, http://www.reuters.com/article/2010/04/01/ims-uspharmaceuticals-idUSN3122364020100401, Accessed 02/17/2014.

Bezchlibnyk-Butler, K. Z., & Jeffries, J. J. (2007). *Clinical handbook of psychotropic drugs* (14th ed.). Seattle: Hogrefe & Huber.

Birkenaes, A. B., & Andreassen, O. A. (2004). The metabolic side effects of antipsychotic medications. *Psychiatry Review Series, 4*, 4.

Citrome, L. (2011). Iloperidone, asenapine, and lurasidone: A brief overview of 3 new second-generation antipsychotics. *Postgraduate Medicine, 123*, 153–162.

Citrome, L. (2013). Inhaled loxapine for agitation. *Current Psychiatry, 12*, 21.

Consumer Reports Best Buy Drugs. (2009). *Treating schizophrenia and bipolar disorder: The antipsychotics—comparing effectiveness, safety, and price.* Yonkers, NY: Consumer Reports Best Buy.

Fankhauser, M. P. (2013). Drug interactions with tobacco smoke: Implications for patient care. *Current Psychiatry, 12*, 12.

Hennessy, S., et al. (2004). Comparative cardiac safety of low-dose thioridazine and low-dose haloperidol. *British Journal of Clinical Pharmacology, 58*, 81.

Hultfilz, S., Garris, S., & Kennedy, M. L. (2012). Reducing hypersalivation. *Current Psychiatry, 11*, 6.

Idanpaan-Heikkila, J., et al. (1975). Clozapine and agranulocytosis [letter]. *Lancet, 2*, 611.

IMS Health. (2002). *Antipsychotic market sales.* Danbury, CT: IMS Health.

IMS Institute for Healthcare Informatics. (2011). *The use of medicines in the United States. Review of 2010.* Available from, http://www.imshealth.com/portal/site/imshealth/menuitem.a675781325ce246f7cf6bc429418c22a/?vgnextoid=16a34899b227f210VgnVCM100000ed152ca2RCRD&vgnextfmt=default, Accessed 12.09.13.

Jindal, R. D., & Keshavan, M. S. (2008). Classifying antipsychotic agents: Need for new terminology. *CNS Drugs, 22*, 1047.

Kantrowitz, J. T., & Javitt, D. C. (2011). Glutamate: New hope for schizophrenia treatment. *Current Psychiatry, 10*, 69.

Kapur, S., & Seeman, P. (2001). Does fast dissociation from the dopamine D_2 receptor explain the action of atypical antipsychotics? A new hypothesis. *American Journal of Psychiatry, 158*, 360–369.

Keck, P. E., & McElroy, S. L. (2002). Clinical pharmacodynamics and pharmacokinetics of antimanic and mood-stabilizing medications. *The Journal of Clinical Psychiatry, 63*, 3.

Keller, D. M., et al. (2013). Akathisia: Ants in your pants. *Perspectives in Psychiatric Care, 49*, 3.

Keltner, N. L. (1997). Catastrophic consequences secondary to psychotropic drugs. Part II. *Journal of Psychosocial Nursing and Mental Health Services, 35*, 48.

Keltner, N. L. (2000). Neuroreceptor function and psychopharmacologic response. *Issues in Mental Health Nursing, 21*, 31.

Keltner, N. L. (2006). Metabolic syndrome: Schizophrenia and atypical antipsychotics. *Perspectives in Psychiatric Care, 42,* 204.

Keltner, N. L., & Folks, D. G. (2005). *Psychotropic drugs* (4th ed.). St. Louis: Mosby.

Keltner, N. L., & Grant, J. S. (2006). Smoke, smoke, smoke that cigarette. *Perspectives in Psychiatric Care, 42,* 256.

Keltner, N. L., & Johnson, V. (2002). Biological perspectives. Aripiprazole: A third generation of antipsychotics begins? *Perspectives in Psychiatric Care, 38,* 157.

Keltner, N. L., Moore, R. L., & Grant, J. S. (2011). Update on newer antipsychotic drugs: Are they evidence based? *Perspectives in Psychiatric Care, 47,* 220.

Kennedy, W. K. (2012). When and how to use long acting injectable antipsychotics. *Current Psychiatry, 11,* 40.

Lieberman, J. A., et al. (2005). Effectiveness of antipsychotic drugs in patients with chronic schizophrenia. *New England Journal of Medicine, 353,* 1209.

Mark, T. L. (2010). For what diagnoses are psychotropic medications being prescribed? A nationally representative survey of physicians. *CNS Drugs, 24,* 319–326.

Mark, T. L., Levit, K. R., & Buck, J. A. (2009). Datapoints: Psychotropic drug prescriptions by medical specialty. *Psychiatric Services, 60,* 1167.

Nasrallah, H. A. (2012). Why are metabolic monitoring guidelines being ignored? *Current Psychiatry, 11,* 4.

Nasrallah, H. A. (2013). Haloperidol clearly is neurotoxic. Should it be banned? *Current Psychiatry, 12,* 7.

Nestler, E. J., Hyman, S. E., & Malenka, R. C. (2009). *Molecular neuropharmacology: A foundation for clinical neuroscience* (2nd ed.). New York: McGraw-Hill.

Perkins, D. O. (2011). Efficacy of available antipsychotics in schizophrenia. *Current Psychiatry, 10*(Suppl.), S15–S19.

Richards, S. S., Musser, W. S., & Gershon, S. (1999). *Maintenance pharmacotherapies for neuropsychiatric disorders.* Philadelphia: Brunner/Mazel.

Robakis, T., & Williams, K. E. (2013). Atypical antipsychotics during pregnancy. Make decisions based on available evidence, individualized risk/benefit analysis. *Current Psychiatry, 12,* 13.

Steele, D., et al. (2011). Antipsychotics and the "fast-off" theory. *Perspectives in Psychiatric Care, 47,* 160.

Steele, D., et al. (2012). The role of glutamate in schizophrenia and its treatment. *Perspectives in Psychiatric Care, 48,* 125.

Tripathi, A., & Macaluso, M. (2013). Antipsychotics for nonpsychiatric illness. Possible efficacy is based on receptor binding affinities. *Current Psychiatry, 12,* 23.

Washington, N. B., Brahm, N. C., & Kissack, J. (2012). Which psychotropics carry the greatest risk for QTc prolongation? *Current Psychiatry, 11,* 37.

Webster, A. J., & Straley, C. M. (2014). What is the relevance of a 2-week response to an antipsychotic? *Current Psychiatry, 13,* 52.

Zeier, K., et al. (2013). Recommendations for lab monitoring of atypical antipsychotics. *Current Psychiatry, 12,* 51.

BIBLIOGRAPHY

Ayd, F. J. (1991). The early history of modern psychopharmacology. *Neuropsychopharmacology, 5,* 71.

Bezchlibnyk-Butler, K. Z., & Jeffries, J. J. (2007). *Clinical handbook of psychotropic drugs* (14th ed.). Seattle: Hogrefe & Huber.

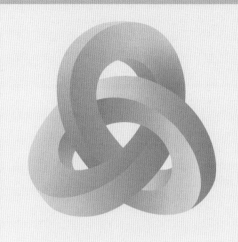

CHAPTER

15

Antidepressant Drugs

Norman L. Keltner

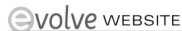 WEBSITE

http://evolve.elsevier.com/Keltner

LEARNING OBJECTIVES

- Understand the neurobiologic concepts of depression.
- Describe the differences among the classes of antidepressant drugs
- Discuss the side effects of antidepressant drugs.
- Identify the symptoms of toxicity for tricyclic antidepressants and monoamine oxidase inhibitors.

- Describe the potential interactions of antidepressant drugs.
- Discuss the implications of teaching patients about antidepressant drugs.
- Identify several nontraditional approaches to treating depression.

Antidepressants are used in the treatment of depression and other disorders. This chapter focuses on the psychopharmacologic classes of drugs used to treat depression (Box 15-1). Depressive disorders are discussed in detail in Chapter 25. Goals of antidepressant medications are as follows:
- Alleviate depressive symptoms
- Restore normal mood
- Prevent recurrence of depression
- Prevent a swing into mania for bipolar patients

BIOCHEMICAL THEORY OF DEPRESSION

Numerous theories exist concerning the cause of depression, but the efficacy of antidepressants is best understood from a neurochemical perspective that had its genesis more than 60 years ago. In the early 1950s, Bein isolated reserpine from *rauwolfia serpentina*, a naturally occurring medicinal agent that had been used to treat hypertension (Ayd, 1991). Reserpine was found to have additional value in the treatment of psychosis, but some patients developed profound depression and became suicidal. The researchers related this action of reserpine to norepinephrine depletion. From this early linking of neurotransmitter depletion to depression, scientists began conceptualizing pharmacologic interventions. The crucial step in the development of antidepressant drugs was the synthesizing of agents that would increase the intrasynaptic

availability of certain neurotransmitters, such as norepinephrine, serotonin, and dopamine. However, even this staple of common knowledge has is detractors. For example:

IS LOW SEROTONIN REALLY THE CULPRIT?

Not everyone thinks that a serotonin deficiency is the real problem in depression. Dr. Alan Gelenberg from Penn State University makes the memorable point, "There's really no evidence that depression is a serotonin-deficiency syndrome. It's like saying that a headache is an aspirin-deficiency syndrome." In other words, just because we can pop an aspirin and gain relief from a headache does not mean we are low on acetylsalicylic acid. It follows then, that just because SSRIs relieve depression does not mean that we have a serotonin deficiency (Swanson, 2013).

Beyond the notion of neurotransmitter deficiencies there are several interrelated biologic hypotheses concerning the etiology of depression, e.g., receptor dysregulation, altered genetic output, premature neuronal death, and lack of synaptogenesis.

The first complementary view suggests that changes in receptors and genes might be an important aspect of antidepressant activity. This suggestion is bolstered by the observation that antidepressants usually require 2 to 4 weeks for a

BOX 15-1 ANTIDEPRESSANT DRUGS BASED ON TRADITIONAL CLASSIFICATIONS

Selective Serotonin Reuptake Inhibitors
Citalopram (Celexa)
Escitalopram (Lexapro)
Fluoxetine (Prozac)
Fluvoxamine (Luvox)
Paroxetine (Paxil)
Sertraline (Zoloft)

Novel and Other Antidepressants
Bupropion (Wellbutrin, Aplenzin)
Desvenlafaxine (Pristiq)
Duloxetine (Cymbalta)
Mirtazapine (Remeron)
Venlafaxine (Effexor)
Vilazodone (Viibryd)

Tricyclic and Related Nonselective Cyclic Antidepressant Drugs
Amitriptyline (Elavil)
Desipramine (Norpramin)
Imipramine (Tofranil)
Nortriptyline (Aventyl, Pamelor)
Protriptyline (Vivactil)

Monoamine Oxidase Inhibitors
Seligiline (Emsam)—inhibits primarily MAO-B
Phenelzine (Nardil)
Tranylcypromine (Parnate)

---

clinical response. Elevations in these neurotransmitter levels occur within hours of treatment initiation, whereas receptor changes take approximately 2 to 4 weeks, and genetic changes take even longer.

NORM'S NOTES
These drugs are everywhere and probably are overprescribed. In fact, 3 of the top 13 drugs prescribed in the United States are antidepressants: Lexapro (#3), Effexor (#9), and Cymbalta (#13) (Drugs Topics Staff, 2010). I'd be very surprised if you didn't know someone taking one of the SSRIs (e.g., Prozac, Paxil, Zoloft). These are great drugs when really needed, but just numbing oneself to avoid some pain is not always best. So, even though I think highly of these drugs, I also think that they are overused. Often working through a problem can be the better option. Read this chapter carefully. I guarantee that you will need to be familiar with this information—it could help someone you know.

Antidepressant-mediated genetic modification might be the most important current hypothesis describing antidepressant action. This view states that reregulation of the complex workings of the second messenger system is the key to effectiveness of antidepressants. Figure 15-1 illustrates an important schematic of the second messenger system.

In depression, key genetic products are undersynthesized, and depression occurs. Of particular interest is a potential deficiency of brain-derived neurotrophic factor, which, at normal levels, would oppose cellular apoptotic forces (genetically programmed cell death). Left unopposed, apoptosis is accelerated. Depression might be caused by actual neuronal death, which is caused by dysregulated monoaminergic systems. A related concept is the notion that genetic dysregulation may cause a lack of synaptogenesis (the growth of new synapses) which, in turn, may be the final common pathway leading to depression (Swanson, 2013). The efficacy of antidepressants is probably related to regulation of the second messenger system and, by extension, the reregulation of genetic output (Stahl, 2000a).

Psychopharmacologic treatment is based on the restoration of normal levels of these neurotransmitters and the consequent neuronal changes (Figure 15-2). Available antidepressants achieve this goal in several distinct ways. Although the following list might appear complex, understanding these mechanisms provides a firm understanding of how antidepressants work (see Box 15-1). These categories of antidepressants are presented in roughly their order of popularity today (Box 15-2 presents statistics related to their "popularity").

1. *Selective serotonin reuptake inhibitors (SSRIs)*, such as sertraline
2. *Selective serotonin-norepinephrine reuptake inhibitors (SNRIs)*, such as venlafaxine
3. *Norepinephrine and dopamine reuptake inhibitors (NDRIs)*, such as bupropion
4. *Novel antidepressants*, such as mirtazapine and vilazodone
5. Nonselective inhibition of norepinephrine and serotonin, such as *tricyclic antidepressants (TCAs)*
6. Inhibition of enzymes, such as *monoamine oxidase inhibitors (MAOIs)*

Antidepressants are not always indicated when individuals report being depressed (e.g., grief); however, when antidepressants are indicated, most patients respond to treatment. Technically, treatment response means that the patient has experienced a 50% reduction in depression severity as measured by a standardized depression scale (Gumnick & Nemeroff, 2000). These drugs do not cure depression, but long-term use has been successful in reducing symptoms. Most relapses are associated with patient-initiated tapering off or discontinuance. However, after 2 years, about 20% of patients who are compliant with these medications experience antidepressant "poop out." It is unknown whether this loss of effectiveness is related to tolerance developing, worsening of the depression, or loss of a placebo effect (Dunlop, 2013).

TCAs have been available for some time and are still the first choice of some clinicians. For severe depression, TCAs appear to be more effective than SSRIs (Anderson, 1998). However, SSRIs and the novel antidepressants (see Box 15-2) are the first-line agents selected by most prescribers for several reasons (which are discussed later in the chapter). MAOIs are usually the last choice because of their serious side effects. Another effective treatment approach, electroconvulsive

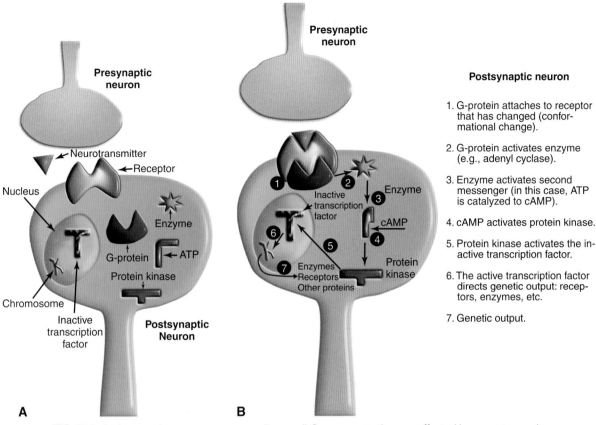

Postsynaptic neuron

1. G-protein attaches to receptor that has changed (conformational change).

2. G-protein activates enzyme (e.g., adenyl cyclase).

3. Enzyme activates second messenger (in this case, ATP is catalyzed to cAMP).

4. cAMP activates protein kinase.

5. Protein kinase activates the inactive transcription factor.

6. The active transcription factor directs genetic output: receptors, enzymes, etc.

7. Genetic output.

FIG 15-1 A, A second messenger system "at rest." Components that are affected by neurotransmitter activation of the second messenger system are labeled. **B,** Sequence of events that transpires with second messenger activation. Steps 1 to 7 indicate the sequence, with step 7 providing the genetic output: enzymes, receptors, and other proteins. It is thought that in depression, key genetic products are undersynthesized. Antidepressants "reregulate" the second messenger system.

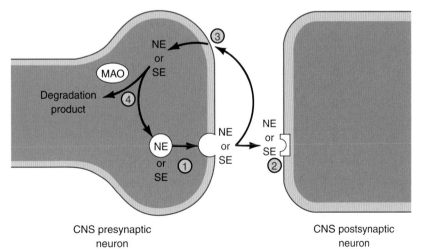

FIG 15-2 Depression results from an amine (e.g., norepinephrine, serotonin) concentration that is too low to activate sufficient receptors; mania results from overabundance of amines acting at receptors. The biogenic amine theory of depression is applied to actions of antidepressant drugs, tricyclic antidepressants (TCAs), selective serotonin reuptake inhibitors (SSRIs), and monoamine oxidase inhibitors (MAOIs), and to the action of lithium, which is used to treat mania. *1,* Lithium inhibits release of norepinephrine and serotonin; *2,* TCAs and MAOIs increase receptor sensitivity to norepinephrine and serotonin; *3,* TCAs block reuptake of norepinephrine and serotonin, SSRIs block reuptake of serotonin, and lithium enhances reuptake of norepinephrine and serotonin; *4,* MAOIs prevent degradation of norepinephrine and serotonin. *CNS,* Central nervous system; *MAO,* monoamine oxidase; *NE,* norepinephrine; *SE,* serotonin. (From Clark, J., Queener, S., & Karb, V. [1993]. *Pharmacologic basis of nursing practice* [4th ed.]. St. Louis: Mosby.)

BOX 15-2 **STATISTICS CONCERNING ANTIDEPRESSANTS**

- Antidepressants are the third most common type of prescription in U.S.
- Antidepressants are the number one medication prescribed for adults 18 to 44 years old.
- Between the years 1988-1994 and 2005-2008, antidepressant use increased 400%.
- Antidepressants are prescribed to 11% of all Americans >12 years old.
- Of Americans prescribed antidepressants, >65% have not seen a mental health professional within the last year.
- Women are 2.5 times more likely to take antidepressants than men.
- Antidepressants are prescribed to 23% of all women 40 to 59 years old.
- Whites are more likely than other ethnic groups to be prescribed antidepressants.
- Of patients prescribed antidepressants, 15% take more than one type.

From Pratt, L.A., Brody, D.J., & Qiuping, G. (2011). *Antidepressant use in persons aged 12 and over: United States, 2005-2008.* NCHS Data Brief No. 76. U.S. Department of Health and Human Services, Centers for Disease Control and Prevention, National Center for Health Statistics.

---

therapy, is discussed in Chapter 25. Consideration of various forms of psychotherapy and other psychotherapeutic interventions is always indicated.

SELECTIVE SEROTONIN REUPTAKE INHIBITORS

SSRIs are the most widely prescribed class of antidepressants (Gianoli & Petrakis, 2013). SSRIs are the first-line drugs for treatment of depression because they are effective antidepressants that have fewer side effects than TCAs and are far less dangerous than MAOIs (Table 15-1). SSRIs have fewer anticholinergic, cardiovascular, and sedating side effects. Fluoxetine (Prozac) was the first SSRI marketed in the United States. Stories of near-miraculous recoveries were followed by reports of major problems associated with this drug. Early anecdotal information, coupled with some research findings, associated fluoxetine with suicidal and homicidal behaviors. Antidepressants now carry a black box warning cautioning clinicians about the risk of suicidal thinking and behavior when these drugs are prescribed to children, adolescents, and young adults. Whether this increase in suicidal ideation is a product of the energizing effects of these drugs (e.g., fluoxetine is an *activating* drug) or is related to more basic mental processes has been debated by clinicians.

Another recognized phenomenon related to SSRIs is a high level of apathy that is apparently induced by these drugs. The antidepressant apathy syndrome manifests as lack of motivation, indifference, disinhibition, and poor attention. Lee and Keltner (2005) wondered whether some suicides and homicides that have occurred might be related to antidepressant-induced indifference and disinhibition. A website (www.ssristories.com) features summaries of violent behaviors purportedly driven by SSRIs or discontinuance of SSRIs. Following are some examples:

- January 2008: This story from Washington is titled, "Student takes loaded shotgun to school."
- February 2008: A school shooting in Illinois is reported in which five people were killed.
- March 2009: In Germany a young man killed 16 people in a school shooting.
- July 11, 2011: A 14-year-old boy killed a fellow student.
- October 26, 2011: A man in Nevada shot three people at his worksite.

It would be difficult to prove a cause-and-effect relationship between these antidepressants and aggressive acts; nonetheless, some individuals are convinced that a direct connection exists.

Pharmacologic Effect

The antidepressant effect of SSRIs is thought to be linked to their inhibition of serotonin reuptake into neurons. These drugs do not bind significantly to histaminic, cholinergic, dopaminergic, or adrenergic receptors, reducing many of the side effects that people who are taking TCAs experience.

Pharmacokinetics

SSRIs are absorbed in the gastrointestinal (GI) tract. Peak plasma levels are achieved for most of these drugs between 4 and 6 hours. SSRIs are metabolized in the liver and have relatively long serum half-lives. The long half-lives allow once-daily dosing schedules. Both fluoxetine and sertraline have active metabolites that significantly extend their half-lives. Abrupt cessation is associated with the development of specific signs and symptoms (Box 15-3).

Side Effects

As previously noted, SSRIs have few anticholinergic, antihistaminic, or antiadrenergic effects, and they do not cause the same intensity of side effects as those associated with TCAs. Dry mouth, blurred vision, sedation, and cardiovascular symptoms are not as common with these agents as with TCAs; however, these side effects do occur and can be very bothersome for some patients. However, GI symptoms, such as nausea, diarrhea, loose stools, and weight loss or gain, are common. It is believed that activation of 5-hydroxytryptamine 3 ($5\text{-}HT_3$) receptors by the elevated levels of serotonin causes these GI symptoms. Hyponatremia also has occurred with these drugs, mostly in older patients. Finally, in slightly more than 20% of patients, excessive sweating occurs (thermoregulation requires a "balance" between dopamine and serotonin neurons in the hypothalamus [Scarff, 2013]).

Central nervous system (CNS) effects include headache, dizziness, tremors, anxiety, insomnia, decreased libido, impotence, ejaculatory delay, and decreased orgasm. Of patients prescribed SSRIs, 50% or more may experience sexual dysfunction (Boxes 15-4, 15-5, and 15-6). Anxiety, insomnia,

TABLE 15-1   ANTIDEPRESSANTS

| | DOSAGES AND PHARMACOKINETICS | | | SPECIFICITY FOR NT REUPTAKE | | | ORTHOSTATIC HYPOTENSION | ANTICHOLINERGIC EFFECTS | INSOMNIA | SEDATION | SEXUAL DYSFUNCTION | GI EFFECTS |
	DAILY DOSAGE RANGE (mg)	HALF-LIFE (hr)*	PROTEIN BINDING (%)	NE	5-HT	DA						
Tricyclic Antidepressants (TCAs)												
Amitriptyline (Elavil)	75–300	31–46	97	1	3	1	XXXX	XXXX	X	XXXX	XX	X
Clomipramine (Anafranil)	75–300	15–37	97	1	4	1	XX	XXX	XX	XXX	XXX	XX
Desipramine (Norpramin)	75–300	12–24	90–95	5	1	1	X	X	X	X	X	X
Imipramine (Tofranil)	75–300	11–25	89–95	2	3	1	XX	XX	X	XXX	XXX	XX
Nortriptyline (Pamelor, Aventyl)	50–150	18–44	92	4	2	1	X	XX	X	XX	X	X
Selective Serotonin Reuptake Inhibitors (SSRIs)												
Citalopram (Celexa)	10–40	23–45	80	1	4	1	X	X	X	XX	XXXX	XXX
Escitalopram (Lexapro)	10–20	27–32	55	1	4	1	X	X	X	X	X	XXX
Fluoxetine (Prozac)	10–80	48–216	95	1	3	1	XX	X	XXXX	XX	XXXX	XXX
Fluvoxamine (Luvox)	50–300	15–19	80	1	4	1	X	X	XX	XX	XXXX	XXXX
Paroxetine (Paxil)	10–60	3–21	95	1	5	1	X	X	XX	XX	XXXX	XXX
Sertraline (Zoloft)	25–200	26–98	98	1	4	2	XX	XX	XX	XX	XXXX	XXX
Novel Antidepressants												
Bupropion (Wellbutrin)	150–450	8–15	80	1	0/1	2	X	X	XXXX	X	0	X
Desvenlafaxine (Pristiq)	50	10–11	30	2	4	1	X	X	X	XX	X	XX
Duloxetine (Cymbalta)	20–60	8–17	90	3	2	1	X	X	XX	X	XX	XXX
Mirtazapine (Remeron)	7.5–45	20–40	85	1	1	0	XX	XX	0	XXXX	X	X
Trazodone (Desyrel)	150–600	4–9	89–95	0	2	1	XX	XX	X	XXXX	X	XX
Venlafaxine (Effexor)	75–225	5–11	25	2	4	1	XX	XX	XX	X	XXX	XXX
Vilazodone (Viibryd)	10–40	25	96–99	0	4	0	X	X	X	X	X	X
Monoamine Oxidase Inhibitors (MAOIs)												
Phenelzine (Nardil)	30–90	2–3	?	—	—	—	XX	XX	X	XX	XXX	XX
Tranylcypromine (Parnate)	20–60	2–3	?	—	—	—	XX	XX	XXXX	X	XX	X
Seligiline (Emsam)	6–12	Continuous	90	—	—	—	X	X	X	XX	X	X

Scale for receptor antagonism specificity: 1, low; 5, high.
Severity of side effects: 0, none; X, low; XX, moderate; XXX, high; XXXX, very high.
5-HT, Serotonin; DA, dopamine; GI, gastrointestinal; NE, norepinephrine.
* With active metabolite.

Modified from Bezchlibnyk-Butler, K.Z., & Jeffries, J.J. (2007). Clinical handbook of psychotropic drugs. Seattle: Hogrefe & Huber; Crutchfield, D.B. (2004). Review of psychotropic drugs. CNS News Special Edition, 6, 51.

BOX 15-3 IS THERE A SELECTIVE SEROTONIN REUPTAKE INHIBITOR WITHDRAWAL SYNDROME?

A question many people have about selective serotonin reuptake inhibitors (SSRIs) is whether a withdrawal syndrome develops on abrupt cessation of these drugs. The answer to this question is yes. Abrupt discontinuation of SSRIs might cause the following symptoms.

Somatic symptoms: Dizziness, lethargy, nausea, vomiting, diarrhea, flulike symptoms (e.g., headache, fever, sweating, chills, malaise), insomnia, vivid dreams

Psychological symptoms: Anxiety, agitation, irritability, confusion, slowed thinking

Because of its long half-life, fluoxetine is less likely to cause a withdrawal syndrome. Paroxetine is most likely to cause a withdrawal syndrome.

From Lader, M. (2007). Pharmacotherapy of mood disorders and treatment discontinuation. *Drug, 67,* 1657.

BOX 15-4 SEXUAL DYSFUNCTIONS ASSOCIATED WITH SELECTIVE SEROTONIN REUPTAKE INHIBITORS

SEXUAL SEQUENCE	SELECTIVE SEROTONIN REUPTAKE INHIBITORS CAN CAUSE ANY OR ALL OF THE FOLLOWING
Desire	Decreased libido
Arousal	Erectile dysfunction or lack of vaginal lubrication
Orgasm	Inability to achieve orgasm (most common of these problems)

BOX 15-5 TREATMENT STRATEGIES FOR SEXUAL DYSFUNCTION RELATED TO SELECTIVE SEROTONIN REUPTAKE INHIBITORS

1. Wait and see if improvement in patient occurs naturally.
2. Decrease dosage of selective serotonin reuptake inhibitor (SSRI).
3. Time SSRI dose to maximize probability of sexual satisfaction.
4. Change antidepressants.
5. Augment with other drugs:
   Amantadine: Dopaminergic that inhibits prolactin
   Amphetamines: Increase dopamine
   Bupropion: Increases dopamine
   Buspirone: Binds to histamine, serotonin, and dopamine receptors
   Methylphenidate: Stimulant
   Sildenafil (Viagra): Enhances erections

Modified from Keltner, N.L., McAffee, K., & Taylor, C. (2002). Mechanisms and treatments for SSRI-induced sexual dysfunction. *Perspectives in Psychiatric Care, 38,* 111.

BOX 15-6 SELECTIVE SEROTONIN REUPTAKE INHIBITORS MOST LIKELY TO CAUSE SEXUAL DYSFUNCTION

Paroxetine (most likely)
Fluoxetine
Citalopram
Sertraline
Escitalopram (least likely)

and sexual dysfunction are thought to be related to serotonin 5-HT$_2$ receptor activation. Anecdotal reports from some practitioners suggest that 70% of patients experience some form of sexual dysfunction. For many individuals, sexual dysfunction is a major factor in decisions about compliance. Nonetheless, because of this overall side effect profile, SSRIs are frequently prescribed. Conversely, the incidence of premature ejaculation seems to be increasing in the general population, and some SSRIs are used to delay orgasm in these men. Although sildenafil (Viagra) has been used for years by men experiencing sexual dysfunction, including SSRI-induced sexual dysfunction, it has been demonstrated more recently that sildenafil is effective in treating anorgasmia in women taking serotonergic antidepressants as well (Burghardt & Gardner, 2013).

Interactions

SSRIs interact with several drugs (Table 15-2), and some of these interactions are related to SSRI inhibition of the cytochrome P-450 enzyme system. Combining SSRIs and MAOIs has proven to be fatal. This phenomenon is called *serotonin syndrome* or *serotonin toxicity* (Box 15-7).

Nursing Implications

Therapeutic versus Toxic Drug Levels

SSRIs have a low potential for overdose. Even high doses have not resulted in fatalities. Toxic symptoms include nausea,

TABLE 15-2 SIGNIFICANT DRUG INTERACTIONS WITH SELECTIVE SEROTONIN REUPTAKE INHIBITORS

DRUG	EFFECT OF INTERACTION
Irreversible MAOIs	*Avoid*; this combination can be fatal (i.e., serotonin syndrome)
Lithium	Increased lithium levels, increased serotonergic effect
Antipsychotics	Increased EPSEs
Benzodiazepines	Increased benzodiazepine half-life
TCAs	Increased TCA serum levels → toxicity Displacement of TCAs from serum proteins → toxicity

EPSEs, Extrapyramidal side effects; *MAOIs,* monoamine oxidase inhibitors; *TCAs,* tricyclic antidepressants.

BOX 15-7 SEROTONIN SYNDROME

- Serotonin syndrome can occur if a selective serotonin reuptake inhibitor is combined with the following:
  - Drugs that increase serotonin synthesis, such as tryptophan
  - Drugs that inhibit serotonin breakdown, such as monoamine oxidase inhibitors
  - Drugs that increase the release of serotonin, such as amphetamines, lithium, ecstasy
  - Drugs that inhibit serotonin reuptake, such as cocaine, dextromethorphan, some tricyclic antidepressants, venlafaxine
  - Drugs that are serotonin agonists, such as buspirone, lysergic acid diethylamide (LSD)
- Signs and symptoms of serotonin syndrome include the following:
  - *Cognitive effects:* Mental confusion, hypomania, hallucinations, agitation, headache, coma
  - *Autonomic effects:* Shivering, sweating, hyperthermia, hypertension, tachycardia, nausea, diarrhea
  - *Somatic effects:* Ataxia, myoclonus (muscle twitching), hyperreflexia, rigidity, tremor, ataxia

From Keltner, N.L., & Folks, D.G. (2005). *Psychotropic drugs* (4th ed.). St. Louis: Mosby; Utox Update. (2002). Serotonin syndrome. *Utah Poison Control Center, 4,* 1.

vomiting, tremor, myoclonus, and irritability. Treatment is symptomatic and supportive.

Use during Pregnancy

Most SSRIs are pregnancy category C drugs (meaning that they should be given only if the benefit justifies the potential risk to the fetus); only paroxetine (Paxil) has a category D rating (Friedman & Hall, 2013). However, these drugs should be avoided during the first trimester as a prudent precaution. The long half-lives of fluoxetine and sertraline might also be significant factors in treating a pregnant patient. In a thorough review of the literature, Malone and associates (2004) found that SSRIs were not associated with teratogenicity. Hence, these antidepressants are frequently continued during pregnancy. However, Keltner and Hall (2005) have reported on neonatal serotonin syndrome. Neonates who have been exposed to SSRIs in utero and are not breast-fed experience a withdrawal syndrome. This syndrome includes respiratory depression, hypoglycemia, tremor, and lower birth weight. These symptoms seem to have a short duration, and all affected neonates are typically symptom-free within 2 weeks. Nonetheless, pregnant women prescribed SSRIs should be well informed about this possibility.

Use in Older Adults

SSRIs are safe for use in older adults because of the good side effect profile of these drugs. As with most medications, SSRI dosage levels should be reduced in older adults. However, older adults' potential for weight loss must be monitored. The half-life of paroxetine increases two or three times in older adults, so extra precautions are warranted.

Individual Selective Serotonin Reuptake Inhibitors

Citalopram

Because of its pharmacologic profile (i.e., its weaker inhibition of P-450 enzymes compared with other SSRIs), citalopram (Celexa) has fewer serious drug-drug interactions. Citalopram is composed of stereoisomers that are mirror images of each other. To elaborate, your right hand and left hand are exactly alike but backward—that is, your left hand cannot fit into a right-handed glove. The two reverse-image isomers in citalopram are called *S* and *R*. It is believed that most side effects are caused by the R isomer, and most therapeutic benefits are derived from the S isomer. Figure 15-3 illustrates this concept.

A CASE OF SEROTONIN SYNDROME

Libby Zion was a freshman at Bennington College when she died at age 18 on March 5, 1984. Libby sought care in the emergency department at Cornell Medical Center in New York City. She presented with a temperature of 103.5° F and died 8 hours after being admitted. Other presenting symptoms were agitation, "strange jerking motions" of her body, and a bout of disorientation. Libby had a history of depression and had been prescribed the MAOI phenelzine. The emergency department physicians were unable to diagnose her condition definitively, but they admitted her for hydration and observation. Her death was caused by a combination of meperidine (Demerol) and the MAOI. The physician who prescribed meperidine was an intern. Because of this tragedy, graduate medical education was scrutinized and then criticized for the long hours intern and resident physicians were expected to work. In defense of these physicians, the concept of serotonin syndrome was very new, with the term not being coined until the early 1980s.

From Brody, J. (2007, February 27). A mix of medicines that can be lethal. *New York Times.* <www.nytimes.com/2007/02/27/health/27brody.html?n=Top/News/Health/Diseases,%20Conditions,%20and%20Health%20Topics/Antidepressants> Accessed February 5, 2010.

FIVE IMPORTANT ISSUES RELATED TO ANTIDEPRESSANT USE

1. *Serotonin syndrome:* Drugs that boost intrasynaptic serotonin can cause this syndrome, which comprises hyperthermia, rigidity, cognitive impairments, and autonomic symptoms.
2. *Antidepressant apathy syndrome:* Some people taking these drugs lose interest in life and the events around them.
3. *Antidepressant withdrawal syndrome:* Abrupt discontinuation of these drugs produces withdrawal symptoms.
4. *Antidepressant loss of effectiveness:* Sometimes these drugs just quit working (also known as drug "poop out").
5. *Antidepressant-induced suicide:* These drugs carry a black box warning about suicide, particularly in 18- to 24-year-old patients early in treatment.

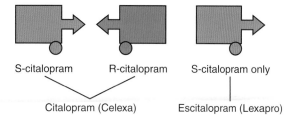

FIG 15-3 Model demonstrating the mirror image S and R isomers of citalopram and the S-only isomer of escitalopram.

Escitalopram

Escitalopram (Lexapro) is related to citalopram; the "es" stands for the S isomer. Theoretically, escitalopram should provide most of the therapeutic benefits of citalopram without all of its side effects. Escitalopram does have a better side effect profile and is prescribed at about half the dosage of citalopram. It has also been approved for treatment of generalized anxiety disorder.

Fluoxetine

Fluoxetine (Prozac) was the first SSRI developed and is frequently prescribed. Beyond the more typical uses of fluoxetine, it is approved for the treatment of bulimia and premenstrual dysphoric disorder (under the trade name Sarafem). Other uses include pain management and promoting smoking cessation. Fluoxetine has a long half-life of 10 days or longer (including its active metabolite). This feature makes it an ideal drug for individuals who forget to take their medications on time. A missed dose is not crucial. Drugs that have a high probability for serious interactions (e.g., MAOIs) need to be withheld for 6 weeks or more as fluoxetine is washing out of the system. Prozac is available in a once-weekly formulation for long-term treatment of depression; it is made with a special delayed-release coating. Lastly, fluoxetine is inexpensive compared with other SSRIs.

Fluvoxamine

Fluvoxamine (Luvox) is specifically approved for the treatment of obsessive-compulsive disorder (OCD). Fluvoxamine does not have an active metabolite and has a side effect profile similar to that of other SSRIs. This drug is not prescribed often for depression.

Paroxetine

Paroxetine (Paxil) is a potent serotonin reuptake blocker and is approved for the treatment of panic attacks. Because its metabolites are not active, paroxetine has a shorter half-life and poses fewer problems than other SSRIs if it needs to be discontinued. A common side effect is nausea, but this effect rarely leads to dose reduction or drug discontinuation. Paroxetine has also been shown to be effective for the prevention of depressive relapse. Similar to other SSRIs, paroxetine can be given on a once-daily basis and causes sexual side effects. It is approved for treatment of premenstrual dysphoric disorder.

A U.S. Food and Drug Administration (FDA) warning to physicians indicates that paroxetine may be teratogenic.

Apparently the risk of birth defects doubles for women taking this drug. The manufacturer has upgraded the pregnancy warning category to D.

Sertraline

Sertraline (Zoloft) is a widely marketed SSRI and was the second drug of this class to be used in the United States. Sertraline can also be given once daily (morning or evening) with or without food. Sertraline causes sexual dysfunction in men and women. Sexual function typically returns to normal 2 to 3 days after drug cessation.

Serotonin Norepinephrine Reuptake Inhibitors
Venlafaxine, Desvenlafaxine, Duloxetine

Venlafaxine (Effexor), desvenlafaxine (Pristiq), and duloxetine (Cymbalta) are structurally unrelated to other currently marketed antidepressants. These drugs are classified as SNRIs. At lower doses, venlafaxine causes serotonin to be enhanced; at medium to high doses, norepinephrine reuptake is inhibited; and at high doses, dopamine intrasynaptic levels are increased. These drugs appear to combine the best qualities of TCAs and SSRIs in that they inhibit the reuptake of both norepinephrine and serotonin, similar to TCAs, and, similar to SSRIs, do not bind significantly to muscarinic, histaminergic, or adrenergic receptors. Theoretically, few anticholinergic, antihistaminic, or antiadrenergic side effects should occur. However, venlafaxine has been documented to increase blood pressure, particularly at higher doses. Venlafaxine has a lower potential for drug interaction than other antidepressants and does not exaggerate the effects of alcohol. Venlafaxine is effective in treating generalized anxiety disorder, social phobias, SSRI-induced sexual dysfunction, OCD, and panic disorders. Desvenlafaxine is an active metabolite of venlafaxine. It appears to have the same good side effect profile, although nausea is a common complaint. Duloxetine has therapeutic and side effect profiles similar to those of venlafaxine. It is also approved for the treatment of diabetic neuropathy pain.

Norepinephrine Dopamine Reuptake Inhibitor
Bupropion

Bupropion (Wellbutrin, Zyban Alpenzin), an NDRI, is unique in two ways: (1) it is the only antidepressant with dopamine reuptake inhibition as a major mechanism of action, and (2) it does not affect serotonin systems. Bupropion has a good side effect profile. However, its ability to increase intrasynaptic dopamine is probably related to its inhibition of norepinephrine reuptake. Norepinephrine reuptake inactivates dopamine, so by blocking that reuptake, dopamine impact is greater.

Bupropion should not be given in combination with drugs that increase the dopamine level. Bupropion has proven to be an effective replacement for, or addition to, SSRIs when these drugs cause sexual dysfunction. Generally, it can be said that dopamine enhances sexuality and that serotonin inhibits sexual functioning. Because bupropion increases intrasynaptic dopamine, it offsets SSRI-mediated sexual inhibition and is prescribed in low doses along with SSRIs for this reason. Bupropion has a narrow therapeutic index but is far less lethal than TCAs or MAOIs.

Under the trade name Zyban, bupropion is marketed as a smoking cessation agent. Its effectiveness is probably related to two distinct mechanisms of action. First, it is a nicotinic antagonist preventing the nicotine from smoking to activate these receptors. Second, it is believed that its dopamine enhancement effect counters the cravings associated with nicotine withdrawal for smokers who have or who want to quit smoking.

Bupropion is contraindicated for individuals with seizure disorders. However, at typical dosages, it does not seem to be any more epileptogenic than other antidepressants in seizure-free individuals.

Novel Antidepressants
Mirtazapine

Mirtazapine (Remeron) is an *alpha-2 antagonist with 5-HT$_2$ and 5-HT$_3$ antagonism* that has been approved for major depression (Croom et al., 2009). Mirtazapine is thought to have a faster onset of action than the SSRIs. It is also used to reduce SSRI-induced sexual dysfunction. The pharmacologic effect of mirtazapine is different from that of other antidepressants: it selectively blocks alpha-2 autoreceptors, which increases norepinephrine and serotonin levels by using the presynaptic feedback system. When this system is blocked, it signals a need for more of these neurotransmitters. Related to its antihistaminic effects, sedation and weight gain are prominent side effects. Paradoxically, sedation decreases at higher dosage levels. An increase in serum cholesterol level occurs in some patients. Mirtazapine's uniqueness is attributable to its antagonism of both 5-HT$_2$ (i.e., reducing sexual dysfunction, anxiety, and insomnia) and 5-HT$_3$ (i.e., reducing GI distress). Remeron is available in an orally dissolvable form that dissolves on the tongue in approximately 30 seconds.

Vilazodone

Vilazodone (Viibryd) can be classified as a serotonin reuptake inhibitor. It is a newer drug (approved in 2011), but many clinicians and patients find it beneficial. It has a limited affinity for 5-HT$_{2A}$ receptors, and so theoretically it should not cause the level of sexual dysfunction associated with SSRIs. Vilazodone has a greater affinity for 5-HT$_{1A}$ receptors. Presynaptically, these receptors serve as autoreceptors and when inundated with serotonin "subsensitize," returning serotonin release to normal (Kalia et al., 2011).

Two New Antidepressants: Levomilnacipran and Vortioxetine

Levomilnacipran (Fetzima) and vortioxetine (Brintellix) are new antidepressants as of this writing. Levomilnacipran is an SNRI potently blocking the reuptake of serotonin and norepinephrine. Levomilnacipran has a half-life of 12 hours and a low protein binding of 22%. It is typically dosed at 40-120 mg/day. Vortioxetine is better thought of as an SRI having minimal effect on norepinephrine and dopamine transporters while significantly increasing the synaptic availability of serotonin (Lincoln & Wehler, 2014). Vortioxetine has a longer half-life (66 hours) and is highly bound (i.e. 98%) to proteins. The typical adult daily dosage is 10 to 20 mg.

Trazodone

Trazodone is now seldom prescribed as an antidepressant but is frequently prescribed for sleep in both depressed and nondepressed individuals. It is not addicting, and it does not produce a high, so it has advantages over benzodiazepines (e.g., diazepam, lorazepam).

Scopolamine

More recent studies at the National Institutes of Health indicate that the older drug scopolamine is an effective antidepressant (Drevets & Furey, 2010). Scopolamine has been available for more than 100 years and historically has been used to treat motion sickness and to dilate the pupil for ophthalmic examinations. According to Drevets and Furey (2010), scopolamine provided relief from depression within a few days—much faster than other antidepressants. Because scopolamine is a robust anticholinergic, it is assumed that this mechanism plays a major role in its relief of depression. Most theoretically troubling about this hypothesis is that a major impetus for finding newer drugs hinged on the annoying and sometimes dangerous anticholinergic effects of the TCAs. Adding to this dilemma, it may have been the anticholinergic property of TCAs that was responsible for their therapeutic effects and not the long-supposed elevations of norepinephrine and serotonin (see the next section).

TRICYCLIC ANTIDEPRESSANTS
Pharmacologic Effects

Theoretically, the serum level of monoamines (i.e., norepinephrine and serotonin) in a depressed person is so low that achieving a normal mood is impossible. TCAs block the reuptake of these released neurotransmitters, increasing the intrasynaptic levels and alleviating the symptoms of depression. In a large meta-analysis, Anderson (1998) concluded that TCAs were significantly more effective than SSRIs for severe depression.

Because reuptake terminates normal neurotransmitter activity, this blocking causes greater neurotransmitter availability and prolongs the stimulating action. Clinical studies have shown that this specific effect occurs quickly, yet there is a lag period of 2 to 4 weeks before an antidepressant effect is experienced.

TCAs can be categorized further as secondary amines or tertiary amines. Drugs that tend to increase the availability of norepinephrine more than serotonin are termed *secondary amines*, and drugs that tend to increase serotonin availability more than norepinephrine are called *tertiary amines*.

Secondary Amines (Enhance Norepinephrine More)	Tertiary Amines (Enhance Serotonin More)
Amoxapine	Amitriptyline
Desipramine	Clomipramine
Nortriptyline	Doxepin
Protriptyline	Imipramine

Although a strong potentiator of serotonin, clomipramine (Anafranil) is not typically prescribed for depression but is a drug of choice for OCD.

Other Therapeutic Effects of Tricyclic Antidepressants

Sedation is a therapeutic effect of some of these drugs because depressed patients commonly experience insomnia and agitation. Tolerance to sedation usually develops.

Lethargy is a common symptom of depression. Some TCAs, described as *activating antidepressants*, might alleviate lethargy.

Improved appetite is another effect of TCAs. Loss of appetite and a consequent loss of weight are symptoms of depression. This effect is probably related to the antihistaminic effect but might be related to improved mood. However, weight gain can be significant and might contribute to a new set of problems.

Anxiety reduction is another positive effect of TCAs.

Urinary hesitancy, although definitely problematic for many patients, can be used therapeutically for childhood enuresis.

Pharmacokinetics and Dosing

TCAs are absorbed well from the GI tract and are usually given orally. TCAs are metabolized in the liver, and some metabolites have antidepressant effects (e.g., desipramine is a metabolite of imipramine; nortriptyline is a metabolite of amitriptyline).

Peak plasma concentrations are reached in 2 to 4 hours, on average; however, because of a significant first pass through the liver, only about 30% to 70% of an oral dose reaches the bloodstream. TCAs are highly bound to plasma proteins, so their effects are produced by only a small fraction of free drug; even a small increase in free drug is potentially serious. Individuals with diminished liver function (e.g., older adults, children, alcoholics, individuals with a history of hepatitis) or individuals with decreased plasma protein levels (e.g., older adults) might be at special risk of elevated serum levels. Although serum levels are not routinely analyzed for these drugs, it has been found that levels of 50 to 300 ng/mL are therapeutic (Gillman, 2007).

The relatively long half-lives of these drugs usually allow once-daily dosing schedules. A steady state is typically reached in approximately 5 days. These drugs are initiated at low doses and increased every 3 to 5 days until the patient becomes intolerant of side effects. Older adults (>55 years old) are often started at half the regular adult dose.

All TCAs appear to be equally effective. Table 15-1 lists several important treatment parameters of antidepressants.

Side Effects

Patients taking TCAs experience undesirable side effects of both the peripheral nervous system (PNS) and the CNS. Tertiary amines (more serotonin enhancing) have more frequent and more severe side effects than secondary amines (more norepinephrine enhancing).

Peripheral Nervous System Effects

Anticholinergic effects. Anticholinergic effects on the peripheral autonomic nervous system range from annoying to dangerous and include the following:

- Dry mouth and anhidrosis (decreased sweating, which impairs cooling)
- Visual disturbances (e.g., mydriasis, blurred vision)
- Constipation
- Bladder dysfunction (e.g., urinary retention, urinary hesitancy)

Older adults are most susceptible to these side effects, and older men with benign prostatic hypertrophy are at special risk for bladder problems.

Cardiac effects. Anticholinergic effects on the cardiovascular system are common enough to warrant serious consideration. Essentially, the parasympathetic system serves as a brake for the heart; when this system is blocked by anticholinergics, the brake is released, and the heart speeds up. Tachycardias and arrhythmias can lead to myocardial infarction. TCAs can also have a quinidine-like effect that delays conduction. In susceptible patients, this effect can lead to heart block and deadly arrhythmias. These serious outcomes are primarily related to disruption of sodium channels when these agents are taken at very high doses (Stahl, 1998). Patients with a history of heart problems must be carefully evaluated. Amitriptyline is considered the most cardiotoxic antidepressant; with its high levels of sedation, anticholinergic activity, and orthostatic hypotension, amitriptyline is a less desirable drug for older adults (Gomez & Gomez, 1992).

Children have shown troublesome cardiovascular responses to TCAs (notably desipramine) that warrant serious consideration. Since these concerns were first noted, several deaths have occurred in children taking these drugs. In each case, sudden death, usually associated with physical activity, was the cause. The serum level might be almost 50% higher in children than in adults at the same dose (Bezchlibnyk-Butler & Jeffries, 2007).

Antiadrenergic effects (orthostasis). These drugs also block alpha-1-adrenergic receptors on peripheral blood vessels and inhibit the body's natural vasoconstricting reaction when a person stands. Blood pooling occurs in the lower extremities, leading to inadequate cerebral perfusion. The heart responds with a reflex tachycardia to help the body adapt. Dimming of vision, dizziness, and fainting cause a sense of loss of control and can lead to falls and serious injury. Healthy individuals frequently make cardiovascular accommodations, and this side effect diminishes within a few weeks. However, patients with a history of heart problems must be carefully evaluated and closely monitored.

Central Nervous System Effects

Sedation. Sedation is a common side effect and can be helpful because insomnia is a frequent symptom of depression. Sedation occurs because of histamine H_1 antagonism.

Cognitive or psychiatric effects. CNS effects include confusion, disorientation, delusions, agitation, anxiety, ataxia, insomnia, and nightmares. Blockade of cholinergic receptors accounts for some of these symptoms. These side effects might be found in a significant number of patients treated with TCAs. The effects usually occur when serum TCA levels are elevated and most often affect older adults. TCAs might aggravate existing dementia or mimic dementia.

Suicide

A clear association exists between suicide and depression. Most individuals who commit suicide are found to have demonstrated characteristics of depression. Consequently, considerable evidence exists to support treating depressed individuals who are suicidal with antidepressants. Paradoxically, however, antidepressants can *energize* patients who have been too depressed to act on their suicidal thoughts. Depressed individuals who are suicidal warrant special nursing consideration after antidepressant therapy has been initiated. Activating antidepressants such as desipramine and fluoxetine might increase the likelihood of energizing a patient in this manner. As discussed later, TCAs are generally highly toxic, which means that the actual drug a patient is taking to treat depression could be used to overdose and die. Only 21% of all suicide completers testing positive for antidepressants had taken TCAs; 44% tested positive for novel antidepressants and 35% tested positive for SSRIs (Jancin, 2005). Although it might appear as if TCAs are more effective at reducing suicide, many more individuals take novel antidepressants and SSRIs than take TCAs. Nonetheless, the statistics are interesting and worthy of discussion. Figure 15-4 provides a graphic example of the percentages of suicide victims who were taking antidepressants. Novel antidepressants have a lower potential for lethal overdose than TCAs and might be better suited for actively suicidal patients.

Interactions

TCAs are metabolized primarily by P-450 enzymes 2D6, 1A2, and 3A4. Several serious drug interactions occur with TCAs when drugs affecting these same enzymes are used. Other problematic interactions might also occur (Table 15-3).

Central Nervous System Depression

Increased CNS depression might occur when TCAs are taken with CNS depressants (e.g., alcohol, benzodiazepines).

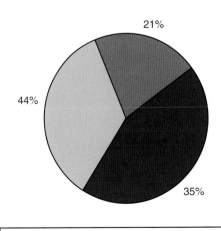

TCAs: amitriptyline, nortriptyline, doxepin
SSRIs: citalopram, sertraline, fluoxetine, paroxetine
Novel antidepressants: bupropion, mirtazapine, trazodone

FIG 15-4 Suicide completers testing positive for antidepressants: *SSRIs,* Selective serotonin reuptake inhibitors; *TCAs,* tricyclic antidepressants. (Modified from Jancin, B. [2005]. Toxicology shows antidepressants present in 21% of suicide completers. *Clinical Psychiatry News, 33,* 6.)

TABLE 15-3	SIGNIFICANT DRUG INTERACTIONS WITH TRICYCLIC ANTIDEPRESSANTS
DRUG	**EFFECT OF INTERACTION**
MAOIs	Hyperpyrexia, excitability, muscular rigidity, convulsions, fatal hypertensive crisis, mania
Sympathomimetics	Cardiac arrhythmias, hypertension
Warfarin	Increased bleeding
Barbiturates, carbamazepine, phenytoin	Decreased TCA effect
Antipsychotics	Increased EPSEs
Procainamide	Prolongation of cardiac conduction
Anticholinergics	Increased anticholinergic effect
Levodopa	Increased agitation, tremor, and rigidity
Alcohol, anticonvulsants, benzodiazepines	Increased sedation

EPSEs, Extrapyramidal side effects; *MAOIs,* monoamine oxidase inhibitors; *TCA,* tricyclic antidepressant.

Cardiovascular and Hypertensive Effects

Cardiovascular arrhythmias or hypertension can occur when sympathomimetic drugs are given with TCAs. Because TCAs block the reuptake of norepinephrine, sympathomimetic agents cause an increase in norepinephrine in the synaptic cleft. Interactants to avoid include norepinephrine, dopamine, ephedrine, and phenylpropanolamine (found in many over-the-counter stimulants). MAOI/TCA combinations are avoided by most clinicians, but others do combine the two antidepressants (and observe their patients carefully). Severe reactions, including high fever, seizures, and a fatal hypertensive crisis, can occur if MAOIs and TCAs are combined. MAOIs are not usually prescribed unless TCAs have failed. TCAs block alpha-adrenergic receptors, compromising the effectiveness of many antihypertensives to control hypertension.

Additive Anticholinergic Effects

Additive anticholinergic effects can occur when TCAs are given with other anticholinergic drugs, including antipsychotics, antiparkinsonian drugs, and antihistamines. Older adult patients are especially susceptible. All the PNS and CNS anticholinergic effects mentioned earlier in this chapter can be aggravated.

Nursing Implications
Therapeutic versus Toxic Blood Levels

TCAs do not produce euphoria and are not addicting, and the potential for abuse is not great. As noted earlier, therapeutic blood levels range up to 300 ng/mL with toxic reactions beginning at serum levels of 450 ng/mL (Gillman, 2007). Severe toxicity and death can occur at levels of 1000 ng/mL (Gillman, 2007). Overdose is an issue and accounts for a high number of intentional suicides. The difference between a therapeutic dose and a lethal dose is small. Outpatients who are at risk for suicide are frequently restricted to a 7-day supply.

Toxic blood levels can result in sedation, ataxia, agitation, stupor, coma, respiratory depression, and convulsions. Exaggeration of side effects previously mentioned can also occur. Cardiovascular reactions can occur suddenly and cause acute heart failure, even several days after the overdose. Cardiovascular reactions can be delayed; that is, they can occur after recovery from overdose. All antidepressant overdoses should be considered serious, and the patient should be admitted to a hospital for monitoring.

The nurse should be aware of several assessment and intervention strategies when a toxic level of TCAs is suspected (see the Key Nursing Interventions for TCA Overdose box).

KEY NURSING INTERVENTIONS
For Tricyclic Antidepressant Overdose

- Monitor blood pressure, heart rate and rhythm, and respirations.
- Maintain patent airway.
- An electrocardiogram is recommended.
- Use cathartics or gastric lavage with activated charcoal to *prevent further drug absorption* (for up to 24 hours).
- The antidote for severe tricyclic antidepressant poisoning (anticholinergic toxicity) is physostigmine (Antilirium), an acetylcholinesterase inhibitor (inhibits the breakdown of acetylcholine). Physostigmine should be given only to patients with life-threatening symptoms (e.g., coma, convulsions) because of the risk associated with its use.

Use during Pregnancy

These drugs have not been definitively found to cause teratogenic effects but should be avoided in the first trimester. Because depressive symptoms, such as loss of appetite, can interfere with fetal development by preventing adequate fetal weight gain, antidepressants should be prescribed cautiously to pregnant women. Antidepressants are typically placed in FDA pregnancy categories B or C. During pregnancy, TCAs with low anticholinergic effects (e.g., nortriptyline, desipramine) are preferred over drugs with high anticholinergic effects. TCAs must be tapered off before delivery to avoid transient perinatal toxicity (Cohen, 1989).

Depressive Symptoms Associated with Serotonin Deficiencies	Depressive Symptoms Associated with Norepinephrine Deficiencies
Anxiety	Fatigue
Panic	Apathy
Phobias	Cognitive disturbances
Posttraumatic stress disorder	Impaired concentration
Obsessions	Focusing attention
Compulsions	Slowed information processing
Eating disorders	Deficiencies in working memory

Although serotonin and norepinephrine deficiencies are both considered causative for depression, Stahl (2000b) noted that low levels of these two monoamines produce distinct depressive syndromes.

Use in Older Adults

TCAs should be given in reduced doses to older adult patients. The maxim "start low and go slow" is particularly true for these patients. The secondary amines (e.g., desipramine, nortriptyline, protriptyline) are preferred. Side effects previously mentioned (e.g., cardiovascular effects, orthostatic hypotension, cognitive impairment, and all peripheral anticholinergic effects) are more pronounced in this age group.

Side Effects

Selected side effects and appropriate nursing interventions are listed in the Side Effects and Nursing Interventions for Antidepressants box.

SIDE EFFECTS AND NURSING INTERVENTIONS FOR ANTIDEPRESSANTS

SIDE EFFECTS	INTERVENTIONS
Peripheral Nervous System	
Dry mouth	Advise frequent sips of water, hard candies, and sugarless gum.
Mydriasis	Advise wearing of sunglasses outdoors.
Diminished lacrimation	Suggest artificial tears.
Blurred vision	Caution patient about driving and potential for falls (usually subsides in 1 to 2 weeks).
Eye pain	Advise patient to report eye pain immediately because it might indicate an acute glaucoma attack.
Urinary hesitancy and retention	Monitor fluid intake. Patients should be told to avoid putting off urinating.
Constipation	Monitor fluid and food intake. Urge patients to heed the urge to defecate. A high-fiber diet and large amounts of water (2500 to 3000 mL/day) are helpful.
Anhidrosis	Decreased sweating can lead to an increase in body temperature. Adequate fluids, appropriate clothing, and sensible exercise should be stressed.
Cardiovascular effects	Tricyclic antidepressants are contraindicated during the recovery phase of myocardial infarction.
Orthostatic hypotension	Advise patient to rise slowly and dangle the legs before standing.
Central Nervous System	
Sedation	Caution patient about driving.
Delirium or mania	Discontinue the drug and call the physician.
Suicidal patients	Observe patients closely because antidepressants might increase motivation for suicide.

Interactions

The nurse should be aware of the drug interactants mentioned in Table 15-3. As a general rule, individuals who are taking TCAs should avoid certain types of drugs, both prescribed and over-the-counter, including the following:

- Drugs that depress the CNS
- Drugs that have anticholinergic properties

- Drugs that stimulate the CNS
- MAOIs (deaths have occurred)

Teaching Patients

The nurse should discuss the following side effects and important principles with patients and their families:

- A lag period of 2 to 4 weeks occurs before full therapeutic effects are experienced.
- Certain drugs must be avoided, including some over-the-counter preparations.
- Abrupt discontinuation can cause nausea, headache, and malaise.
- Eye pain must be reported immediately, particularly in older adults, in which undiagnosed narrow-angle glaucoma can lead to an emergency situation.
- Some side effects lessen after patients adjust to the medication.

Individual Tricyclic Antidepressants

The following brief descriptive statements about TCAs include only the unique features of usage and side effects. This chapter does not discuss the uses and side effects that are common to all the drugs.

Amitriptyline

Amitriptyline is highly anticholinergic and one of the most sedating and cardiotoxic antidepressants.

Desipramine

Desipramine is a secondary amine and a metabolite of imipramine. Desipramine is an *activating antidepressant* and might be advantageous for patients with apathy, lethargy, and hypersomnia. Because of its aforementioned effects on the cardiovascular system in children, desipramine should be used with care in this age group. It appears to be the most toxic TCA (Whyte et al., 2003).

Imipramine

Imipramine is the oldest TCA. None of the newer antidepressants have proven to be more effective. Because of its anticholinergic properties, imipramine has proven to be effective in the treatment of childhood enuresis. Imipramine should be used with care in children because of its cardiovascular effects.

Nortriptyline

Because nortriptyline, a secondary amine TCA, is sedating and has a good side effect profile, it is often prescribed for older adult patients who are depressed, agitated, and experiencing insomnia. It is the least toxic TCA (Whyte et al., 2003). Nortriptyline is a metabolite of the tertiary amine, amitriptyline.

MONOAMINE OXIDASE INHIBITORS

MAOIs were the first antidepressants "discovered" but are usually administered only to hospitalized patients or to individuals who can be closely supervised. In one study, 12% of psychiatrists had never prescribed an MAOI (Kosinski &

Rothschild, 2012). These drugs are not used much but warrant mention because they have potentially fatal interactions and can help the student conceptualize significant pharmacokinetic processes.

Two MAOIs that are occasionally used are phenelzine (Nardil) and tranylcypromine (Parnate). They are referred to as *irreversible nonselective inhibitors* because they inhibit both variants of monoamine oxidase: MAO-A and MAO-B (the nonselective part) and "stay on" the enzyme until it dies and is replaced (the irreversible part).

However, there are two selective MAOIs; one inhibits only MAO-A, and the other inhibits MAO-B. Moclobemide (Manerix) inhibits MAO-A (sometimes referred to as a reversible inhibitor of MAO-A) but is not available in the United States at the time of this writing and is not discussed further. More importantly, an irreversible selective inhibitor of MAO-B called selegiline has traditionally been used in the treatment of Parkinson's disease. It also has an antidepressant action, but at the higher doses required for this effect its selectivity is lost, and it also inhibits MAO-A. What makes seligiline special is its delivery mechanism. It is packaged in a novel vehicle—a transdermal patch that provides continuous release of medication over the day. It is marketed under the trade name Emsam (from the names of the children of the developer, Emily and Samuel). It causes fewer negative effects in the digestive system because it has limited MAO-A action and is absorbed through the skin rather than the intestinal tract. There is less need for dietary control compared with traditional MAOIs except when higher doses are prescribed (*Emsam package insert*, 2006).

Because of the serious adverse reactions to these drugs, especially life-threatening hypertension, the older irreversible MAOIs are almost always prescribed after other antidepressants have failed or for what is called *treatment-resistant depression*. Although some clinicians believe that MAOIs are particularly effective in treating atypical depression (e.g., hypersomnia, somatic anxiety, excessive hunger, extreme sensitivity to rejection), they are still seldom prescribed.

Pharmacologic Effects

MAOIs block monoamine oxidase, a major enzyme involved in the metabolic decomposition and inactivation of norepinephrine, serotonin, and dopamine. This enzyme inhibition lasts for 10 days with the irreversible MAOIs. The inhibition increases the levels of these neurotransmitters in the PNS and CNS. According to the neurochemical theory of depression, depressed individuals have lower than normal levels of these neurotransmitters available. MAOIs help to attain normal levels by slowing the deactivation of these amines. This action is in contrast to TCAs, which help attain normal levels by preventing the reuptake of amines by the neurons. Approximately 2 to 4 weeks is required for the antidepressant effect of MAOIs to occur, although, as is the case with TCAs, the inhibition of monoamine oxidase occurs immediately; this suggests that factors other than low levels of specific neurotransmitters are involved in depression.

Absorption, Distribution, and Administration

MAOIs are well absorbed from the GI tract and are given orally. They are metabolized in the liver. Because monoamine oxidase does not decline with age, MAOIs do not present the same age-related risks associated with other drugs.

Side Effects

MAOIs cause CNS, cardiovascular, and anticholinergic side effects. Serious life-threatening reactions can occur when irreversible MAOIs interact with certain drugs or foods (see the following discussion on interactions).

Because MAOIs increase the availability of biogenic amines in the brain, CNS hyperstimulation might occur, causing agitation, acute anxiety attacks, restlessness, insomnia, and euphoria. In individuals thought to have quiescent schizophrenia (an unrecognized, latent form), full schizophrenic episodes have erupted. Hypomania (which is less severe compared with full mania) is a more common effect.

Hypotension is a common cardiovascular effect, resulting from a slowdown in the release of norepinephrine. In contrast to the effect of TCAs, reflex tachycardia does not occur because other adrenergic nerves also experience the slowed release of norepinephrine, and the heart does not speed up reflexively. Hypotension, combined with the absence of a compensatory increased heart rate, can lead to heart failure.

MAOIs can cause anticholinergic effects such as dry mouth, blurred vision, urinary hesitancy, and constipation. Hepatic and hematologic dysfunctions can occur and, although rare, are potentially serious. Blood counts and liver function test results should be obtained before therapy begins.

Interactions

MAOIs have many serious interactions. Potentially lethal interactants include both drugs and foods.

Drug-Drug Interactions

The nurse should be aware of the following types of drug interactions (Table 15-4):

- Drug interactions that cause hypertension
- Drug interactions that cause severe anticholinergic responses
- Drug interactions that cause profound CNS depression

Sympathomimetic drugs are classified as direct-acting drugs, indirect-acting drugs, and mixed-acting drugs (having both direct and indirect properties). Indirect-acting and mixed-acting sympathomimetics cause serious and sometimes fatal hypertension. Direct-acting sympathomimetics add new norepinephrine to the body, whereas indirect-acting sympathomimetics release existing norepinephrine from the neurons. Because MAOIs increase the amount of stored norepinephrine in the PNS, a potential exists for indirect-acting and mixed-acting sympathomimetics to induce the release of large amounts of norepinephrine. Avoiding these interacting drugs is crucial. Even small amounts can trigger a hypertensive crisis. Typical indirect-acting and mixed-acting sympathomimetics include amphetamines, cocaine, methylphenidate (Ritalin), dopamine, and ephedrine. Over-the-counter weight

TABLE 15-4	SIGNIFICANT DRUG INTERACTIONS WITH IRREVERSIBLE NONSELECTIVE MONOAMINE OXIDASE INHIBITORS*
DRUGS	**EFFECT OF INTERACTION**
Anticholinergic drugs	Increase anticholinergic response
Anesthetics (general)	Deepen CNS depression
Antihypertensives (diuretics, beta blockers, hydralazine)	Cause hypotension
CNS depressants	Intensify CNS depression
Sympathomimetics (mixed-acting and indirect-acting): Amphetamines, methylphenidate, dopamine, phenylpropanolamine (in many over-the-counter hay fever, cold, and diet medications)	Precipitate hypertensive crisis, cardiac stimulation, arrhythmias, cerebrovascular hemorrhage
Sympathomimetics (direct-acting): Epinephrine, norepinephrine, isoproterenol; less likely to cause problems	Theoretically should not produce a reaction, but caution is recommended
Serotonergic drugs (e.g., SSRIs)	*Avoid*; this combination can be fatal

*Less severe interactions with these drugs also occur with the reversible selective inhibitors of monoamine oxidase, moclobemide and seligiline.

CNS, central nervous system; *SSRIs,* selective serotonin reuptake inhibitors.

loss and stimulant products contain phenylephrine, phenylpropanolamine, and pseudoephedrine, which are mixed-acting or indirect-acting sympathomimetics. Theoretically, direct-acting sympathomimetics such as norepinephrine, epinephrine, and isoproterenol should not trigger the release of existing norepinephrine. Finally, MAOIs should not be given in combination with TCAs except in unusually refractory cases and should never be given in combination with SSRIs.

The initial symptoms of hypertensive crisis are palpitation; tightness in the chest; stiff neck; and a throbbing, radiating headache. Extremely high blood pressure with elevation of the heart rate is common. Cardiovascular consequences have included myocardial infarction, cerebral hemorrhage, myocardial ischemia, and arrhythmias. Diaphoresis and pupillary dilation are also prominent signs.

Anticholinergic effects can be severe if other anticholinergic drugs are given with MAOIs. Typical anticholinergic side effects can be reviewed in the discussion of TCA side effects.

Finally, because MAOIs inhibit monoamine oxidase in the liver, some drugs, particularly CNS depressants, are not rapidly metabolized in the liver and result in serum levels high enough to cause serious depression of the CNS.

Meperidine (Demerol) is specifically contraindicated. A marked potentiation of this drug can occur, and deaths have been documented. Hypotensive drugs are also enhanced by MAOIs. The nurse should be aware that MAOI inhibition can continue for 10 days after tranylcypromine and phenelzine are discontinued. In other words, the potential for serious interactions continues for some time after MAOIs are discontinued.

Food-Drug Interactions

Food-drug interactions center on the amine tyramine, a decarboxylation product of tyrosine (the precursor to dopamine, norepinephrine, and epinephrine). Tyramine is found in many foods commonly consumed in the North American diet (Box 15-8). Only a few foods cause a severe reaction; these include aged cheese, bananas, salami, sauerkraut, soy sauce, all beers on tap, and coffee. However, some clinicians recommend that all high-protein foods that have undergone protein breakdown by aging, fermentation, pickling, or smoking be avoided. Hypertension and hypertensive crisis can develop from this food-drug combination. As noted, Emsam is less likely to have a reaction with food unless given at a high dosage.

BOX 15-8 TYRAMINE-RICH FOODS TO AVOID WITH MONOAMINE OXIDASE INHIBITORS

Alcoholic Beverages
Beer and ale
Chianti and sherry wine
Alcohol-free beer

Dairy Products
All mature cheese: Cheddar, blue, Brie, mozzarella
Sour cream
Yogurt

Fruits and Vegetables
Avocados
Bananas
Fava beans
Canned figs

Meats
Bologna
Chicken liver
Fish, dried
Liver
Meat tenderizer
Pickled herring
Salami
Sausage

Other Foods
Caffeinated coffee, colas, tea (large amounts)
Chocolate
Licorice
Sauerkraut
Soy sauce
Yeast

Nursing Implications

Therapeutic versus Toxic Drug Levels

An intensification of the effects already discussed occurs with overdose. A lethal dose of MAOIs is only 6 to 10 times the daily dose (see Table 15-1 for dosages). Careful monitoring when these medications are given is important. "Cheeking" and hoarding of these drugs can be disastrous. If MAOI overdose is indicated, the nurse should know the following:
- Emesis and gastric lavage might be helpful if performed early.
- Monitoring of vital signs is important.
- External cooling is warranted if high fever occurs.
- Hypotension should be treated in the standard manner.

Use during Pregnancy

MAOIs should be avoided during the first trimester of pregnancy. Later use is justified only when the anticipated benefit outweighs the potential risk to the fetus.

Use in Older Adults

MAOIs might be effective in older patients because monoamine oxidase activity increases with age. However, precautions for orthostatic hypotension should be observed in this age group.

Side Effects

The nurse should be familiar with the common side effects of MAOIs and the appropriate nursing interventions (see the Side Effects and Nursing Interventions for MAOIs box).

SIDE EFFECTS AND NURSING INTERVENTIONS FOR MONOAMINE OXIDASE INHIBITORS

SIDE EFFECTS	INTERVENTIONS
CNS hyperstimulation	Reassure the patient. Assess for developing psychosis, hypomania, or seizures. If symptoms warrant, withhold the drug and notify the physician.
Hypotension	Monitor blood pressure frequently and intervene to prevent falls and injuries; having patient lie down might help return blood pressure to normal.
Anticholinergic effects	See antidepressant side effects for appropriate nursing interventions.
Hepatic and hematologic dysfunction	Blood counts and liver function tests should be performed. If dysfunction is apparent, monoamine oxidase inhibitor should be discontinued.

Interactions and Contraindications

As noted earlier, the nurse must understand that drug-drug and food-drug interactions are serious and potentially fatal. MAOIs should not be given in combination with the following drugs:
- Other MAOIs
- TCAs or SSRIs

- Meperidine

Hypertensive crisis is a major concern. If it occurs, the nurse should do the following:

- Discontinue MAOIs and contact the physician.
- Know that therapy to reduce blood pressure is warranted (e.g., an alpha-1 blocker).
- Monitor vital signs.
- Have the patient walk (which decreases blood pressure slightly).
- Manage fever by external cooling.
- Institute supportive nursing care, as indicated.

Teaching Patients

The nurse must be persistent in teaching patients and their families about MAOIs and their side effects. Although most of these drugs are administered in a closely supervised setting, the nurse is nonetheless responsible for educating patients. Because patients taking MAOIs can experience serious reactions to some other drugs and foods, the nurse must clearly convey this information.

NONTRADITIONAL APPROACHES TO DEPRESSION

Supplementation with both vitamin D (Harris et al., 2013) and L-methylfolate (Fluitt, 2012) have been demonstrated to be helpful nonpsychotropic agents in depression. Vitamin D regulates tyrosine hydroxylase, which is needed to convert tyrosine to levodopa and subsequently dopamine and norepinephrine, whereas L-methylfolate modulates the tyrosine hydroxylase and tryptophan hydroxylase needed for dopamine and norepinephrine and serotonin synthesis. Many clinicians supplement antidepressant therapy with these agents.

> ### ? CRITICAL THINKING QUESTIONS
>
> 1. What is the supposed pharmacologic effect that causes SSRIs to result in sexual dysfunction?
> 2. Many older, experienced clinicians believe that TCAs are the best drugs for treating depression. Based on your reading about TCAs and the short paragraph on scopolamine, why may that be?

▮ STUDY NOTES

1. According to the neurochemical theory, depression is the result of a decreased availability of the neurotransmitters norepinephrine, serotonin, and possibly dopamine in the brain.
2. There are three classic classes of antidepressants: SSRIs, TCAs, and MAOIs. An additional major group of agents, some of which are quite popular, includes SNRIs, NDRIs, and mirtazapine. Sometimes drugs in this latter group are referred to as *novel* antidepressants.
3. SSRIs and TCAs block the reuptake of neurotransmitters back into nerve endings, increasing their availability.
4. MAOIs slow the breakdown of these neurotransmitters by inhibiting the enzyme monoamine oxidase, increasing the availability of these neurotransmitters.
5. SSRIs have fewer anticholinergic, antihistaminic, and antiadrenergic side effects than TCAs.
6. SSRIs are first-line drugs for the treatment of depression.
7. SSRIs are highly bound to serum proteins and can displace other protein-bound drugs.
8. All SSRIs affect cytochrome P-450 metabolizing enzymes and the metabolism of other drugs that are metabolized by this system.
9. Newer *novel* antidepressants include bupropion, venlafaxine, and mirtazapine. These agents are also first-line agents in the treatment of depression.
10. Common side effects of TCAs (e.g., dry mouth, blurred vision, constipation, tachycardia) are associated with their anticholinergic properties.
11. Because TCAs have a narrow therapeutic index, amounts even slightly higher than therapeutic doses can be fatal.
12. Patients should be taught about the lag time of 2 to 4 weeks that is required for a full therapeutic effect to be experienced with most antidepressants.
13. MAOIs can cause central (stimulation), cardiovascular (hypotension), and anticholinergic system side effects.
14. Traditional irreversible nonselective MAOIs interact with certain foods that contain tyramine (e.g., aged cheese, bananas, salami) and with indirect-acting and mixed-acting sympathomimetic drugs (e.g., amphetamines, methylphenidate [Ritalin]) to cause hypertensive crisis. Reversible inhibitors of MAO-A appear to have minimal interactions with foods containing tyramine.
15. MAOIs can also have a lag time of approximately 2 to 4 weeks.
16. Nontraditional agents such as vitamin D and L-methylfolate have been helpful in the treatment of depression.

REFERENCES

Anderson, I. M. (1998). SSRIs versus tricyclic antidepressants in depressed inpatients: A meta-analysis of efficacy and tolerability. *Depression and Anxiety, 7*(Suppl. 1), 11.

Ayd, F. J. (1991). The early history of modern psychopharmacology. *Neuropsychopharmacology, 5,* 71.

Bezchlibnyk-Butler, K. Z., & Jeffries, J. J. (2007). *Clinical handbook of psychotropic drugs.* Seattle: Hogrefe & Huber.

Burghardt, K. J., & Gardner, K. N. (2013). Sildenafil for SSRI-induced sexual dysfunction in women. *Current Psychiatry, 12,* 29.

Cohen, L. S. (1989). Psychotropic drug use in pregnancy. *Hospital and Community Psychiatry, 40,* 566.

Croom, K. F., Perry, C. M., & Plosker, G. L. (2009). Mirtazapine: A review of its use in major depression and other psychiatric disorders. *CNS Drugs, 23*, 427.

Drevets, W. C., & Furey, M. L. (2010). Replication of scopolamine's antidepressant efficacy in major depressive disorder: A randomized placebo-controlled trial. *Biological Psychiatry, 67*, 432.

Drugs Topics Staff. (2010). *Pharmacy facts and figures.* http://drugtopics.modernmedicine.com/Pharmacy+Facts+&+Figures, Accessed 8.01.10.

Dunlop, B. S. (2013). Depressive recurrence in antidepressant treatment (DRAT): 4 next-step options. *Current Psychiatry, 12*, 54.

Emsam package insert. (2006). Princeton: Bristol-Myers Squibb Company.

Fluitt, N. (2012). L-methylfolate: Another weapon against depression. *Current Psychiatry, 11*, P72.

Friedman, S. H., & Hall, R. C. W. (2013). Antidepressant use during pregnancy: How to avoid clinical and legal pitfalls. *Current Psychiatry, 12*, 10.

Gianoli, M. O., & Petrakis, I. L. (2013). Pharmacotherapy for comorbid depression and alcohol dependence. *Current Psychiatry, 12*, 24.

Gillman, P. K. (2007). Tricyclic antidepressant pharmacology and therapeutic drug interactions updated. *British Journal of Pharmacology, 151*, 737.

Gomez, G. E., & Gomez, E. A. (1992). The use of antidepressants with elderly patients. *Journal of Psychosocial Nursing and Mental Health Services, 30*, 21.

Gumnick, J. F., & Nemeroff, C. B. (2000). Problems with currently available antidepressants. *Journal of Clinical Psychiatry, 61*(Suppl. 6), 5.

Harris, H. W., et al. (2013). Vitamin D deficiency and psychiatric illness. *Current Psychiatry, 12*, 18.

Jancin, B. (2005). Toxicology shows antidepressants present in 21% of suicide completers. *Clinical Psychiatry News, 33*, 6.

Kalia, R., Mittal, M. S., & Preskorn, S. H. (2011). Vilazodone for major depressive disorder. *Current Psychiatry, 10*, 4.

Keltner, N. L., & Folks, D. G. (2005). *Psychotropic drugs.* St. Louis: Mosby.

Keltner, N. L., & Hall, S. (2005). Neonatal serotonin syndrome. *Perspectives in Psychiatric Care, 41*, 88.

Keltner, N. L., McAffee, K., & Taylor, C. (2002). Mechanisms and treatments for SSRI-induced sexual dysfunction. *Perspectives in Psychiatric Care, 38*, 111.

Kosinski, E. C., & Rothschild, A. J. (2012). Monoamine oxidase inhibitors: Forgotten treatment for depression. *Current Psychiatry, 11*, 21.

Lader, M. (2007). Pharmacotherapy of mood disorders and treatment discontinuation. *Drugs, 67*, 1657.

Lee, S. I., & Keltner, N. L. (2005). Antidepressant apathy syndrome. *Perspectives in Psychiatric Care, 41*, 188.

Malone, K. J., et al. (2004). Antidepressants, antipsychotics, benzodiazepines, and the breastfeeding dyad. *Perspectives in Psychiatric Care, 40*, 73.

Scarff, K. R. (2013). Options for treating antidepressant-induced sweating. *Current Psychiatry, 12*, 51.

Stahl, S. M. (1998). Basic pharmacology of antidepressants, part 1: Antidepressants have seven distinct mechanisms of action. *Journal of Clinical Psychiatry, 59*(Suppl. 4), 5.

Stahl, S. M. 2000a. Blue genes and the mechanism of action of antidepressants. *Journal of Clinical Psychiatry, 61*, 164.

Stahl, S. M. 2000b. *Essential psychopharmacology.* Cambridge, MA: Cambridge Press.

Swanson, J. (2013). *Serotonin deficiency may not cause depression after all. Scientific American,* . http://www.scientificamerican.com/article.cfm?id=unraveling-the-mystery-of-ssris-depression, Accessed 18.12.13.

Utox Update. (2002). Serotonin syndrome. *Utah Poison Control Center, 4*, 1.

Whyte, I. M., Dawson, A. H., & Buckley, N. A. (2003). Relative toxicity of venlafaxine and selective serotonin reuptake inhibitors in overdose compared to tricyclic antidepressants. *QJM, 96*, 369.

CHAPTER

16

Antimanic Drugs

Norman L. Keltner

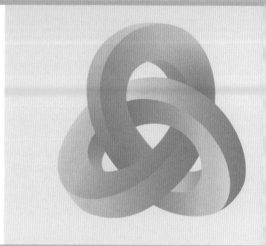

evolve WEBSITE

http://evolve.elsevier.com/Keltner

LEARNING OBJECTIVES

- Explain the mechanism of action of antimanic drugs.
- Discuss the side effects of antimanic drugs.
- Identify therapeutic versus toxic serum levels of lithium.

- Describe potential interactions of antimanic drugs.
- Discuss the implications of teaching patients about antimanic drugs.

Lithium has a unique and pivotal position in psychopharmacology. It preceded the introduction of chlorpromazine into psychiatry and in fact fired the first barrage that initiated the modern era of psychopharmacology.

Soares & Gershon (2000)

Antimanic drugs or mood stabilizers include lithium and several anticonvulsants. Antipsychotic drugs are also used to treat bipolar disorder. However, no single drug or combination of drugs is always effective. The two poles suggested in the term *bipolar* are dysphoria (or depression) and euphoria (or mania). Although these extremes in emotions are seemingly opposite, they are related. This chapter primarily focuses on the psychopharmacologic classes of drugs used to treat the euphoric end of the bipolar spectrum—the antimanic drugs (Table 16-1). These drug classes include lithium, anticonvulsants, and antipsychotic agents.

There are three overarching treatment issues in treating bipolar disorder:
1. Getting acute mania under control
2. Preventing relapse when remission occurs
3. Returning to the prior level of functioning (i.e., social, occupational, interpersonal)

TREATMENT GOALS FOR BIPOLAR DISORDER

1. Remission
2. Prevention
3. Return to premorbid function

The focus of treating acute symptoms is on helping the patient regain control. Box 16-1 lists the typical signs and symptoms associated with acute bipolar disorder (see Chapter 26 for a full discussion of bipolar disorders). *Maintenance therapy* attempts to prevent relapse, reduce suicide risks, improve functioning, and reduce what are called *subthreshold symptoms* (symptoms not quite reaching a level of clinical diagnostic significance).

LITHIUM

Lithium is considered the *gold standard* by many clinicians for the treatment of bipolar disorder (Gershon et al., 2009). Lithium, a naturally occurring element, is not much different from sodium. However, the differences are significant enough to make lithium useful in treating bipolar disorder. Lithium was discovered in 1817 and named after the Greek word for stone (*lithos*). It came to be touted as a cure for epilepsy, gout, and other problems. In 1949, Cade, an Australian, reported his research in the *Medical Journal of Australia*, showing lithium to be effective in the treatment of manic depression. Of the manic patients he treated, all demonstrated considerable improvement (Soares & Gershon, 2000). Lithium's effect was so pronounced that Cade (1949) called the illness a "lithium deficiency disease" (McIntyre et al., 2001). Also in 1949, the March 12th issue of the *Journal of the American Medical Association* reported two accounts of fatal lithium poisoning in cardiac patients who were given lithium chloride as a salt substitute. These deaths led to a 20-year hibernation for

TABLE 16-1	LITHIUM AND ANTICONVULSANTS USED FOR TREATMENT OF BIPOLAR DISORDER					
ANTIMANIC DRUG	USUAL ADULT DAILY DOSAGE	HALF-LIFE (HR)	THERAPEUTIC SERUM LEVEL	METABOLISM	COMMON SIDE EFFECTS	WARNINGS
Lithium	Acute: 600-1800 mg; maintenance: 900-1200 mg	~24	0.6-1.2 mEq/L	95% unchanged	N/V, diarrhea, polyuria, polydipsia, weight gain, tremor, fatigue	Lithium toxicity, teratogenicity
Carbamazepine	800-1000 mg and titrated upward until side effects or serum level reached	12-17; induces own metabolism	4-12 mcg/mL	P-450 enzymes	N/V, dizziness, sedation, rash, HA	Blood dyscrasias, teratogenicity
Divalproex	1000-1500 mg	6-16	50-115 mcg/mL	P-450 enzymes and direct conjugation with glucuronic acid	N/V, sedation, weight gain, hair loss	Hepatotoxicity, teratogenicity, pancreatitis
Lamotrigine	Begin at 25-50 mg and increase by 12.5-25 mg per week up to 250 mg bid	~24 with long-term use	NA*	Attaches to glucuronic acid by conjugation	HA, sedation, cognitive dulling, insomnia, ataxia, N/V, dizziness, diplopia	Serious rash (e.g., Stevens-Johnson), breast-feeding (?)
Oxcarbazepine	600-2400 mg in 2-3 divided doses	7-20 with active metabolites	15-35 mcg/mL	Metabolized to an active metabolite	Fatigue, N/V, dizziness, sedation, diplopia, hyponatremia	Teratogenicity, breast-feeding (?)
Gabapentin	900-4000 mg in 3 divided doses	5-7	NA*	Not metabolized	Sedation, fatigue, tremors, nausea, dry mouth, dizziness, diplopia, hyperthermia	Teratogenicity, breast-feeding (?)
Topiramate	Acute: 200-600 mg; maintenance: 50-400 mg	19-23	NA*	70% unchanged	Sedation, cognitive blunting, anxiety, tremors, weight loss, dizziness	Breast-feeding, cognitive dulling

HA, Headache; *NA,* not applicable; *N/V,* nausea and vomiting.
Modified from Bezchlibnyk-Butler, K.Z., & Jeffries, J.J. (2007). *Clinical handbook of psychotropic drugs.* Seattle: Hogrefe & Huber.
*Serum concentrations can be measured for these newer antiepileptics, but our understanding of how to utilize this information is limited.

lithium in the United States (Ayd, 1991). Fears of lithium were compounded by a lack of interest on the part of drug companies. As a natural element, lithium is not patentable; consequently, a drug company might invest research funds only to have another pharmaceutical company legally use the findings (Ayd, 1991). Lithium was not made available in the United States until 1970.

Lithium is now used for the treatment and prophylaxis of the manic phase of manic-depressive illness. About 70% to 80% of individuals who take lithium for long-term prophylaxis and about 50% who are treated for the more acute phase have a therapeutic response to this drug (U.S. Surgeon General, 1999). Additionally, a growing body of clinical research supports its use as an antidepressant, for augmentation of other antidepressants in refractory depression, and for other disorders. Finally, for reasons not yet understood, lithium seems to have a greater antisuicide effect than the other antimanic drugs (Kovacsics et al., 2009).

NORM'S NOTES

These drugs are a little more challenging. We have the gold standard (lithium), but antiepileptic drugs are typically first-choice agents, particularly divalproex. The trick for knowing the reason for antimanic treatment is to find the similarities in action of both antiepileptics and lithium. How do these drugs slow down manic thinking? If you can nail that down, then you are really beginning to learn about psychotropic drugs.

Pharmacologic Effects

Exactly how lithium achieves its normalizing effect on mania is unknown. Its similarity to calcium, sodium, and potassium may be related to its therapeutic effects. For instance, by substituting for sodium, lithium compromises the ability to release, activate, and respond to neurotransmitters. When taken in therapeutic amounts, lithium inhibits the release of norepinephrine, serotonin, and dopamine, while facilitating their reuptake into presynaptic terminals (Lehne, 2007). The net effect of this action is to decrease the synaptic levels of these neurotransmitters—the very action that one would surmise needs to occur in the hyperactive state of mania. Lithium also normalizes a dysfunctional second messenger system (Nestler et al., 2009). This multistep system eventuates in activation of transcription factors that instruct genes on what proteins to synthesize (e.g., enzymes, receptors, neurotrophic factors). In bipolar disorder, the second messenger system is too active. Lithium and other antimanic agents are thought to reset this system. Lithium specifically prevents the full expression of inositol, a second messenger that increases the release of calcium. Calcium triggers the expulsion of neurotransmitters into the synapse. Lithium reduces neurotransmitter release by modulating the second messenger system.

Using El-Mallakh's (1996) model as an explanatory guide, we can expand this information. Lithium can substitute for sodium, normalizing Na^+,K^+-ATPase pump activity, and it increases the number of sodium pumps. The net effect is a decrease in the intracellular sodium level, which creates a higher threshold for cell depolarization. Apparently, lithium also accelerates calcium removal from the neuronal terminal, normalizing calcium-dependent neurotransmitter release and synthesis, cytoskeletal remodeling, and neuronal excitability (Manji & Lenox, 2000). The overall effect is a reduction in neurotransmitter release. Function of gamma-aminobutyric acid (GABA), an inhibitory neurotransmitter system, is also enhanced.

It is unclear exactly how lithium is effective. At least four hypotheses have been advanced (El-Mallakh, 1996; Lehne, 2007; Nestler et al., 2009):

1. Lithium substitutes for sodium and regulates calcium.
2. Lithium inhibits the release and facilitates the reuptake of norepinephrine, serotonin, and dopamine.
3. Lithium regulates the Na^+,K^+-ATPase pump.
4. Lithium stabilizes the second messenger system, regulating intracellular signaling.

Pharmacokinetics

Lithium is well absorbed from the gastrointestinal tract and is given orally in tablets, capsules, or concentrate. Peak blood levels are reached in 1 to 3 hours. The kidneys excrete more than 95% of the amount ingested unchanged. Lithium is not metabolized. Renal disease lengthens the half-life, necessitating a reduction in dose. Lithium's typical plasma half-life is about 24 hours. The absorption and excretion of lithium and sodium are closely linked. Lithium is reabsorbed with sodium in the proximal tubule. Diuretics, particularly diuretics affecting the loop of Henle and the distal tubule (e.g., thiazides), lead to increased retention of lithium, and the dosage may need to be reduced 25% to 50% (Andreasen & Ellingrod, 2013; Katzung et al., 2009). If dietary sodium intake increases, plasma lithium levels are likely to decrease because lithium is excreted more rapidly. Conversely, if sodium in the diet decreases, or if sodium is lost in ways other than through the kidneys (e.g., sweating,

WHAT GOES WRONG IN BIPOLAR DISORDER

What is known about bipolar disorder is that affected individuals have specific signs and symptoms (e.g., elevated mood, grandiosity, irritability, insomnia, anorexia). What is not known is exactly what causes this disorder to happen. The question remains: "What goes wrong in bipolar disorder?" El-Mallakh (1996) has proposed a convincing model for the pathology of bipolar disorder, suggesting that a disruption in ion regulation is the cause. Ion regulation is important for normal mood. A key part of ion regulation is the sodium (Na^+) and potassium (K^+)–activated adenosine triphosphatase (ATPase) pump. Bipolar depression and mania are related, and this model proposes a biochemical explanation.

WHAT GOES WRONG IN BIPOLAR DISORDER—CONT'D

According to this model, both bipolar depression and mania result from a decrease in Na+,K+-ATPase activity. As activity declines, neuronal membranes become irritable, requiring fewer stimuli to provoke cell firing. As sodium accumulates intracellularly because of this faulty pumping action, hyperpolarizing functions of inhibitory neurotransmitters (e.g., GABA) are diminished. Additionally, because neurotransmitter release is calcium dependent, the presynaptic terminals might release more neurotransmitter because of a related deficiency in sodium-dependent calcium efflux. All these factors contribute to increased neurotransmitter release and firing—or mania.

However, the term *bipolar* means two poles—the pole of mania and the pole of depression. These two poles are related. As the Na+,K+-ATPase pump continues to decrease in activity, neuronal irritability reaches a point whereby less stimulation triggers depolarization. The neuron fires more easily, but the action potential loses amplitude. This loss of amplitude causes calcium channels to decrease their activity and results in a subsequent reduction in neurotransmitter release. Mania is the first disorder to occur when ion dysregulation occurs, but as the Na+,K+-ATPase pump becomes more dysfunctional, the depressive side of bipolar disorder develops. Catatonia might be the ultimate expression of ionic dysregulation (El-Mallakh, 1996).

diarrhea), lithium levels increase. These considerations are important; therapeutic serum levels need to be stable because therapeutic levels of lithium are not much lower than toxic levels. Diet and activity levels should not change abruptly.

Lithium is effective in about 50% of cases; however, 7 to 10 days is required to achieve a clinical response. Lithium dosage is based on both clinical response and serum lithium levels. The typical dosage for acute mania is 600 mg three times per day, which usually produces a serum level of 1 to 1.5 mEq/L. Desirable maintenance blood levels are 0.6 to 1.2 mEq/L, which can be maintained on a dosage of 900 to 1200 mg/day. Blood levels greater than 1.5 mEq/L can be toxic, but moderate to severe toxicity typically develops only after blood levels exceed 2 mEq/L.

Figure 16-1 presents an explanation of how lithium works using the biogenic amine theory.

Side Effects

Side effects of lithium are linked to serum blood levels. Blood levels greater than 1.5 mEq/L can be considered toxic. Common side effects are nausea, dry mouth, diarrhea, and thirst. Drowsiness, mild hand tremor, polyuria, weight gain, a bloated feeling, sleeplessness, and

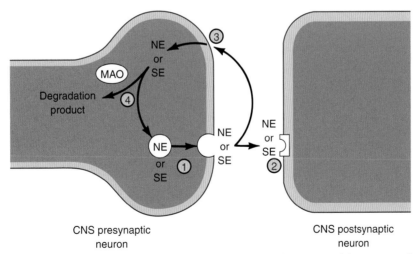

CNS presynaptic neuron

CNS postsynaptic neuron

FIG 16-1 Depression results from an amine (e.g., norepinephrine, serotonin) concentration that is too low to activate sufficient receptors; mania results from overabundance of amines acting at receptors. The biogenic amine theory of depression is applied to actions of antidepressant drugs—tricyclic antidepressants (TCAs), selective serotonin reuptake inhibitors (SSRIs), and monoamine oxidase inhibitors (MAOIs)—and to the action of lithium, which is used to treat mania. *1,* Lithium inhibits release of norepinephrine and serotonin; *2,* TCAs and MAOIs increase receptor sensitivity to norepinephrine and serotonin; *3,* TCAs block reuptake of norepinephrine and serotonin, SSRIs block reuptake of serotonin, and lithium enhances reuptake of norepinephrine and serotonin; *4,* MAOIs prevent degradation of norepinephrine and serotonin. *CNS,* Central nervous system; *MAO,* monoamine oxidase; *NE,* norepinephrine; *SE,* serotonin. (From Clark, J., Queener, S., & Karb, V. [1993]. *Pharmacologic basis of nursing practice* (4th ed.). St. Louis: Mosby.)

lightheadedness are other common side effects. Polyuria and polydipsia occur in about 70% of patients taking lithium (Maxmen & Ward, 2002). Side effects occur at therapeutic levels but usually decrease or cease after 3 to 6 weeks. However, these same side effects increase in severity at toxic serum levels.

Side effects unrelated to serum levels include weight gain, a metallic taste, headache, edema of the hands and ankles, and pruritus. Even at therapeutic levels, lithium can affect thyroid gland function. Approximately 30% of patients develop clinical hypothyroidism, with some needing levothyroxine (Bezchlibnyk-Butler & Jeffries, 2007). Lithium can also impair mental or physical abilities required for driving.

Lithium is generally contraindicated in patients with cardiovascular disease. Lithium might also harm the fetus and is a U.S. Food and Drug Administration (FDA) category D drug (evidence of fetal risk has been established). Adverse reactions to toxic blood levels are discussed later in the chapter.

Lithium negatively affects the kidneys. Lithium therapy is contraindicated for patients with renal disease; if lithium is necessary, close supervision of these patients is recommended. Lithium-induced renal insufficiency (creatinine level consistently >2 mg/100 mL) is apparently uncommon. However, nephrogenic diabetes insipidus (NDI) develops in a significant number of patients taking lithium. NDI is caused by inhibition of the action of antidiuretic hormone (ADH), or vasopressin, on the kidneys, specifically, the distal tubule and collecting duct cells (Andreasen & Ellingrod, 2013). When ADH is blocked, the patient experiences polyuria (defined as urinating >3 L/day). If a patient experiences NDI, often lithium is discontinued, or the dosage is reduced (Andreasen & Ellingrod, 2013).

Keltner and Grant (2008) discussed another major concern with lithium therapy—neuropathy. In their article, they cited two case studies in which individuals developed what appeared to be irreversible neuropathy. It is clear from the literature that lithium can cause life-threatening conditions (Alexander et al., 2008; Aral & Vecchio-Sadus, 2008) and irreversible neurotoxicity (Adityanjee et al., 2005). One case follows.

CASE EXAMPLE

Bill, a 38-year-old white man, is now confined to a wheelchair. He was diagnosed with bipolar disorder in his early twenties. Bill was arrested and placed in jail. While there, he was given his prescribed amounts of lithium. Bill had apparently misled his prescriber, and the clinician had increased the dosage of the lithium Bill was receiving. In essence, Bill said that he was taking his lithium as prescribed, but in reality he was not. The clinician was aware of therapeutic lithium levels and continued to increase the lithium dosage in an attempt to achieve a therapeutic serum level (0.6 to 1.2 mEq/L). When incarcerated, Bill's daily dosage was 2100 mg/day—definitely on the high end. Once jailed, the officers made sure Bill took the correct amount of lithium. In a short while, Bill became sick and then comatose. He was taken to a hospital where he remained for 6 weeks. He came close to dying and now cannot walk.

❓ CRITICAL THINKING QUESTION

1. If a person taking lithium experiences serious diarrhea, what will happen to the person's serum level?

Interactions

Familiarity with the drugs that can elevate lithium serum levels is essential. Diuretics (except acetazolamide [Diamox]) decrease lithium excretion and elevate serum lithium levels. Indomethacin and other nonsteroidal antiinflammatory drugs (NSAIDs) reduce renal elimination of lithium by preventing the natural antagonism of ADH by prostaglandin (Andreasen & Ellingrod, 2013), increasing serum lithium levels. Switching to a low-salt diet after treatment commences also elevates serum lithium levels.

Some drugs and other agents decrease serum lithium levels and pose the problem of inadequate treatment and symptom exacerbation. Agents that increase lithium excretion decrease lithium levels. Acetazolamide (Diamox), caffeine, and alcohol are included in this group.

Combining lithium with antipsychotic drugs or benzodiazepines is common. These drugs are ordered with lithium because of lithium's clinical response lag time of 1 to 2 weeks. Antipsychotic agents are prescribed to produce a tranquilizing effect until lithium produces a clinical response as well as for their antimanic properties.

THERAPEUTIC SERUM LEVELS (0.6-1.2 MEQ/L)	MILD TO MODERATE TOXICITY (1.5-2 MEQ/L)	MODERATE TO SEVERE TOXICITY (2-3 MEQ/L)	SEVERE TOXICITY (>3 MEQ/L)
Hand tremor (fine)	Diarrhea	Previous symptoms *and*	Previous symptoms *and*
Memory problems	Vomiting	Ataxia	Seizures
Goiter	Drowsiness	Giddiness	Organ failure
Hypothyroidism	Dizziness	Tinnitus	Renal failure
Mild diarrhea	Hand tremor (coarse)	Blurred vision	Coma
Anorexia	Muscular weakness	Large output of dilute urine	Death
Nausea	Lack of coordination	Delirium	
Edema	Dry mouth	Nystagmus	
Weight gain			
Polydipsia, polyuria			

Diuretics and NSAIDs increase lithium serum levels, and toxicity can result. A few other drugs and agents decrease lithium levels, and symptom breakthrough can occur.

Nursing Implications

Therapeutic versus Toxic Drug Levels

Therapeutic serum lithium levels are 0.6 to 1.2 mEq/L. The optimal maintenance level is approximately 0.8 mEq/L. Serum levels greater than 1.5 mEq/L can cause adverse reactions. Typically, higher serum levels correspond directly to the severity of the reaction. Mild to moderate toxic reactions occur at 1.5 to 2 mEq/L, and moderate to severe reactions occur at 2 to 3 mEq/L. At serum levels greater than 3 mEq/L, multiple organs and organ systems might be involved, leading to coma and death (Alexander et al., 2008). Serum levels should be monitored and should not exceed 2 mEq/L.

No antidote is available for lithium poisoning. Discontinuing the drug might be enough when supportive nursing care is available. Gastric lavage has been used successfully. Parenteral normal saline might provide enough volume and sodium to prevent major problems for serum levels less than 2.5 mEq/L. For more severe lithium poisoning, forced diuresis or hemodialysis might be needed.

Use during Pregnancy

Treating bipolar disorder during pregnancy is difficult. Cessation of lithium during pregnancy is suggested because of fetal cardiovascular malformation when lithium is taken in the first trimester and neonatal toxicity if taken thereafter. However, whether this toxicity is as common as previously thought is now debated (Katzung et al., 2009). The occurrence of major congenital abnormalities for fetuses of mothers taking lithium is 4% to 12%, and for fetuses of mothers taking the anticonvulsant alternatives, it is 2% to 4% (Bezchlibnyk-Butler & Jeffries, 2007). The risk of congenital abnormalities in the general population is 2% to 4% (Fact Sheet, 1998). Postnatal treatment also poses problems because lithium is present in breast milk at 30% to 100% of the mother's serum level.

HIGHLIGHTING THE EVIDENCE

The pregnancy category of divalproex (Depakote) and other valproates (i.e., valproate sodium [Depacon] and valproic acid [Depakene and Stavzor]) has been changed from D (*the potential benefit of the drug in pregnant women may be acceptable despite its potential risks*) to X (*risks outweigh any benefit*) for pregnant women using these medications for migraine headaches. This prohibition does not extend to other uses of divalproex such as for epilepsy or bipolar treatment; however, caution and vigilance are warranted (valproates remain category D drugs for these conditions). Children 6 years of age born to women who took divalproex or other valproates throughout their pregnancy had lower IQ scores than children of women treated with other antiepileptics. More information can be obtained at http://1.usa.gov/16caQrJ.

From Aschenbrenner, D.S. (2013). Drug watch: two drugs receive pregnancy category changes. *The American Journal of Nursing, 113,* 27.

KEY NURSING INTERVENTIONS
for Patients Taking Lithium

- Prepare the patient for expected side effects without instilling anxiety.
- Discuss the side effects that should subside (e.g., nausea, dry mouth, diarrhea, thirst, mild hand tremor, weight gain, bloatedness, insomnia, lightheadedness).
- Identify the side effects that require immediate notification of the physician (e.g., vomiting, severe tremor, sedation, muscle weakness, vertigo).
- Suggest taking lithium with meals to reduce nausea.
- Suggest drinking 10 to 12 glasses of water per day to reduce thirst and maintain normal fluid balance.
- Advise the patient to elevate the feet to relieve ankle edema.
- Advise the patient to maintain a consistent dietary sodium intake but to increase sodium if a major increase in perspiration occurs.

Use in Older Adults

Older adult patients can benefit from lithium, but because of the severity of side effects and adverse reactions, these patients must be assessed for renal function and dietary history. Lithium-induced reactions are more likely in this age group. Serum levels of 0.4 to 0.8 mEq/L are appropriate for older patients.

Side Effects

Because lithium has a narrow therapeutic index, serum lithium levels should be determined frequently. After the patient is stabilized, monthly or less frequent serum level determinations are usually adequate. Blood levels are usually drawn before the first dose in the morning. However, the nurse should not rely on laboratory tests alone and should continue clinical evaluation of the patient. (See the Key Nursing Interventions for Patients Taking Lithium box.)

Interactions

The nurse should help patients understand the basic mechanisms affecting serum lithium levels. Drug interactions that increase or decrease serum levels should be reviewed. The nurse must impress on all patients, even if they are reluctant to do so, the necessity for alerting all other health care providers that they are receiving lithium treatment.

Teaching Patients

The nurse should teach patients and their families the following precautions:

- Symptoms of minor toxicity, which include vomiting, diarrhea, drowsiness, muscular weakness, and lack of coordination
- Symptoms of major toxicity, which include giddiness, tinnitus, blurred vision, and dilute urine
- Side effects associated with lithium and the proper time to notify the physician

BOX 16-2   PATIENT GUIDELINES FOR TAKING LITHIUM

To achieve a therapeutic effect and prevent lithium toxicity, patients taking lithium should be advised of the following:
1. Lithium must be taken on a regular basis, preferably at the same time daily. For example, a patient who is taking lithium on a three-times-daily schedule and forgets a dose should wait until the next scheduled time to take the lithium but should not take twice the amount at that time because lithium toxicity could occur.
2. When lithium treatment is initiated, mild side effects such as a fine hand tremor, increased thirst and urination, nausea, anorexia, and diarrhea or constipation might develop. Most of the mild side effects are transient and do not indicate lithium toxicity. Additionally, in some patients taking lithium, some foods such as celery and butterfat have an unappealing taste.
3. Serious side effects of lithium that necessitate its discontinuance include vomiting, extreme hand tremor, sedation,

muscle weakness, and vertigo. The prescribing physician should be notified immediately if any of these side effects occur.
4. Lithium and sodium are eliminated from the body through the kidneys. An increase in salt intake increases lithium elimination, and a decrease in salt intake decreases lithium elimination. The patient must maintain a balanced diet and salt intake. The patient should consult with the prescribing physician before making any dietary alterations.
5. Various situations can require an adjustment in the amount of lithium administered to a patient; examples are the addition of a new medication to the patient's drug regimen, a new diet, or an illness with fever or excessive sweating.
6. For determination of lithium levels, blood should be drawn in the morning approximately 8 to 12 hours after the last dose was taken.

- Avoidance of conception because lithium might harm the fetus
- Avoidance of driving until stabilized on lithium

Box 16-2 provides a complete list of patient guidelines for taking lithium.

? CRITICAL THINKING QUESTION

2. Johnny is a good basketball player. He is 23 years old and is taking lithium. Because Johnny sweats a lot on the days he plays (approximately four times per week), his nurse is concerned about his serum levels being consistent. What is this nurse considering? (See item number 4 in Box 16-2 for a hint to this question.)

ANTICONVULSANTS

Although lithium is the gold standard for bipolar disorder, many patients do not respond. Most patients with a diagnosis of bipolar disorder have one or more subsequent bouts with the disorder. Because of the seriousness of bipolar disorder, researchers have diligently sought alternatives for patients who do not respond to lithium. An anticonvulsant is often the first drug prescribed. The drug most frequently prescribed is divalproex (Depakote), a valproate. Other anticonvulsant alternatives include carbamazepine, gabapentin, lamotrigine, oxcarbazepine, and topiramate. Table 16-2 provides a summary of the evidence for the effectiveness of these drugs for mania, depression, and maintenance therapy. As can be readily identified, not all of these agents are effective for all three dimensions of bipolar disorder.

Divalproex and Other Valproates

Divalproex (Depakote, a tablet) and other valproates (e.g., valproic acid [Depakene, a syrup], valproate sodium [Depacon, an injection]) have been used since the 1960s as antiepileptic agents. In 1995, these drugs were approved for the treatment of mania and are considered first-line agents.

TABLE 16-2   EVIDENCE SUPPORTING ANTIEPILEPTIC DRUGS FOR MOOD DISORDERS

MEDICATION	MANIA	DEPRESSION	MAINTENANCE
Divalproex	XXX	X	XX
Carbamazepine	XXX	X	XX
Lamotrigine	0	0	XXX
Gabapentin	0	0	X
Oxcarbazepine	X	X	X
Topiramate	0	0	X

XXX = Strong evidence; XX = moderate evidence; X = weak evidence; 0 = no evidence.
Adapted from Gerst, T.M., Smith, T.L., & Patel, N.C. (2010). Antiepileptics for psychiatric illness: find the right match. *Current Psychiatry, 9,* 51.

Valproates appear to be particularly effective for patients with acute mania and for patients with mania secondary to a general medical condition (Haddad et al., 2009). The effectiveness of the valproates (and all anticonvulsants) might be related to their inhibition of kindling activity in the brain. The concept of kindling can be explained as follows: Just as kindling in the fireplace is the first step in building a fire, some abnormal brain activities might begin as kindling and then spread. A little water can douse the fire when it first starts but is ineffective in the control of a raging fire. The mechanisms of action listed in the following box normalize and stabilize neuronal activity; this increases the threshold of stimulation needed for cell firing.

HOW VALPROATES WORK

Although the precise nature of the action of valproates is unknown, three mechanisms might be responsible for their antimanic effect:
1. Increase in the inhibitory role of GABA
2. Suppression of sodium influx into the neuron
3. Suppression of calcium influx through specific calcium channels

Advantages of the valproates are that they have a rapid onset, can be used initially without attempting lithium, and are well tolerated with little effect on cognition. Disadvantages include transient hair loss, weight gain, tremors, gastrointestinal upset, and dose-related thrombocytopenia. Polycystic ovary syndrome in women and reduction in intelligence in children exposed to valproates in utero are major concerns that should be considered (Pontius, 2012).

Bioavailability is approximately 100%, with up to 95% protein binding. The drug can be replaced at binding sites by other drugs such as carbamazepine or warfarin, causing toxic effects. Valproates have a half-life of 6 to 16 hours and reach a steady state in 2 to 5 days. Therapeutic serum levels are 50 to 115 mcg/mL or levels consistent with their antiepileptic effects.

Other Anticonvulsants Used to Treat Bipolar Disorder

Carbamazepine

Carbamazepine (Tegretol) is effective for most patients who do not respond to lithium or to the valproates; it also has a faster onset of action compared with lithium. Patients with a rapidly cycling bipolar episode are more likely to be unresponsive to lithium and to respond to carbamazepine. Carbamazepine sometimes might be given in combination with lithium. Carbamazepine's therapeutic antimanic serum levels are 4 to 12 mcg/mL. Although generally well tolerated, side effects include nausea, anorexia, and occasional vomiting. Sedation and drowsiness are other common side effects. The most serious potential side effect of carbamazepine is agranulocytosis. Complete blood counts should be obtained weekly when this drug treatment is initiated. Drugs that inhibit the cytochrome P-450 3A4 enzyme, such as selective serotonin reuptake inhibitors, can cause toxic effects (Cozza et al., 2003).

Lamotrigine

Lamotrigine (Lamictal) is approved for the treatment of bipolar disorder, including bipolar depression. This drug works by manipulating the GABA system, inhibiting neuronal firing. Other mechanisms of action include blocking of voltage-gated sodium and calcium channels, further inhibiting neuronal conduction. Finally, lamotrigine is believed to inhibit the excitatory neurotransmitter glutamate. Similar to the effects of most drugs, lamotrigine causes numerous side effects; one particular adverse reaction that is especially noteworthy is lamotrigine-induced rash. Lamotrigine can cause moderate skin rashes (about 10% of patients) and potentially fatal Stevens-Johnson syndrome (1% to 2% of children). Predictors of rash include high initial dose, rapid increase in dosage, and young age (Gerst et al., 2010).

Oxcarbazepine

Oxcarbazepine (Trileptal) is becoming a commonly prescribed agent for bipolar disorder. Oxcarbazepine is structurally related to carbamazepine and has similar pharmacologic activity. However, it does not cause some of the more serious adverse reactions associated with carbamazepine.

Gabapentin

Gabapentin (Neurontin) tends to be used in an adjunctive role and not as monotherapy. As an adjunctive agent, it is believed to be particularly effective if the patient also experiences anxiety. Similar to lamotrigine, gabapentin up-regulates the GABA system, blocks sodium and calcium voltage-gated channels, and inhibits glutamate (glutamate increases cell firing).

Topiramate

Topiramate (Topamax) has a mechanism of action similar to that of gabapentin. It increases GABA activity, blocks voltage-gated sodium and calcium channels, and inhibits the excitatory neurotransmitter glutamate. Many patients report weight loss with this drug (the only anticonvulsant known to have this effect). However, whatever positive response this effect has among clinicians and patients is tempered by a cognitive dulling that some patients have reported.

ANTIPSYCHOTICS

Antipsychotics are discussed in detail in Chapter 14. All atypical antipsychotics except clozapine (although it is effective) have been approved for the treatment of mania. The traditional antipsychotic haloperidol is also effective and may have a more rapid onset of action than either lithium or the atypical agents (Tohen & Vieta, 2009). These agents have proven to be effective for the treatment of bipolar disorder both as monotherapy and as an adjunct to mood stabilizers. Antipsychotics are particularly beneficial for control of acute mania. A brief description of these drugs is given here.

Aripiprazole: Aripiprazole (Abilify) was previously referred to as a third-generation agent because of some unique properties. Today it is referred to as a second-generation antipsychotic. It has been shown to be effective in the treatment of bipolar disorder.

Asenapine: Asenapine (Saphris) is the newest antipsychotic approved for bipolar disorder. It is given sublingually, providing rapid absorption. It is approved by the FDA for treating acute mania and mixed episodes (Foster et al., 2011).

Clozapine: Clozapine (Clozaril) is very effective for the treatment and prophylaxis of acute mania; however, the same concern associated with its more conventional antipsychotic use remains problematic—that is, agranulocytosis. Hematologic monitoring is required.

Olanzapine: Olanzapine (Zyprexa) is approved as monotherapy for acute and maintenance treatment of bipolar disorder. Its particular pharmacologic profile might reduce the risk of precipitating a depression after treatment for acute mania. Olanzapine is associated with significant weight gain in some patients.

Quetiapine: Quetiapine (Seroquel) is used to treat bipolar disorder. It can control acute mania and rapidly cycling mania and is used prophylactically.

Risperidone: Risperidone (Risperdal) has been established as an effective agent for acute bipolar disorder. It does not cause as much weight gain as other mood stabilizers.

Ziprasidone: Ziprasidone (Geodon) has also received approval to be used for treatment of acute bipolar disorder. It causes little or no weight gain and is reported to be well tolerated.

OTHER TREATMENTS FOR BIPOLAR DISORDER

Several benzodiazepines (e.g., clonazepam [Klonopin], lorazepam [Ativan]) and calcium channel blockers (e.g., nimodipine, verapamil) have been used with some success in treating bipolar disorder. Agitation, insomnia, and anxiety are probably treatable by the benzodiazepines. Finally, electroconvulsive therapy has proven useful for bipolar disorder and was used effectively before the discovery of lithium and these other drugs (Geoghegan & Stevenson, 1949). Electroconvulsive therapy is particularly valuable for pregnant patients, who should avoid medication that is teratogenic (American Psychiatric Association, 2002).

WHAT YOU CAN EXPECT TO SEE PRESCRIBED FOR BIPOLAR DISORDER

The first issue is whether the prescriber will attempt to treat bipolar disorder with one medication (monotherapy) or with a combination of antimanic agents. The more common of each follows (American Psychiatric Association, 2002; Stahl, 2004):

1. **Monotherapy**

First-line approaches	Either lithium or a valproate
Second-line approach	Atypical antipsychotic
Third-line approach	Carbamazepine or lamotrigine or gabapentin or topiramate

2. **Combination Therapy**

Atypical approach	Atypical antipsychotic (e.g., olanzapine) *plus* lithium or a valproate
Benzodiazepine approach	Benzodiazepine *plus* lithium or a valproate
Typical approach	Typical antipsychotic (e.g., haloperidol) *plus* lithium or a valproate
Mood stabilizers	*Two or more* mood stabilizers

3. **For Severe Acute Mania**
Lithium or a valproate *plus* an atypical antipsychotic

4. **For Bipolar Depression**

First-line approaches	Lithium *or* lamotrigine *or* electroconvulsive therapy

STUDY NOTES

1. Antimanic or mood stabilizers are used to treat bipolar disorder (i.e., manic depression).
2. There are two overarching treatment concerns: (a) controlling the symptoms of acute mania and (b) maintenance treatment.
3. Goals of *maintenance treatment* are as follows:
   a. Prevention of relapse
   b. Reduction of suicides
   c. Improvement of functioning
   d. Reduction of subthreshold symptoms
4. Lithium is a naturally occurring element that has been a mainstay of bipolar disorder treatment for more than 50 years.
5. Other first-line agents used to treat bipolar disorder are anticonvulsants and antipsychotics.
6. Lithium alters intracellular conductance; anticonvulsants act on the GABA system and sodium and calcium voltage-gated channels.
7. Clinically therapeutic serum levels of lithium are 0.6 to 1.2 mEq/L; at higher serum levels, serious or fatal reactions can occur.
8. Common side effects of lithium include nausea, dry mouth, diarrhea, thirst, and mild hand tremor.
9. Lithium has a narrow therapeutic index and a lag time of 7 to 10 days.
10. Divalproex and other valproates are effective, have rapid onset of action, and are relatively well tolerated.
11. Carbamazepine has a more rapid onset compared with lithium and is generally well tolerated.
12. Other anticonvulsants, such as lamotrigine, oxcarbazepine, gabapentin, and topiramate, have been proven to be effective in treating bipolar disorder.
13. Use of lamotrigine must be accompanied by close assessment for skin rashes. Some of these rashes, such as Stevens-Johnson syndrome, have proven fatal.
14. Topiramate causes weight loss and is associated with cognitive dulling.
15. Antipsychotic drugs control the symptoms of acute mania and act as mood stabilizers.

REFERENCES

Adityanjee, Munshi, K.R., & Thampy, A. (2005). The syndrome of irreversible lithium-effectuated neurotoxicity. *Clinical Neuropharmacology, 28*, 38.

Alexander, M. P., et al. (2008). Lithium toxicity: A double-edged sword. *Kidney International, 73*, 233.

American Psychiatric Association. (2002). Practice guidelines for the treatment of patients with bipolar disorder. *American Journal of Psychiatry, 159*(Suppl. 4), 16.

Andreasen, A., & Ellingrod, V. L. (2013). Lithium-induced diabetes insipidus: Prevention and management. *Current Psychiatry, 12*, 42.

Aral, H., & Vecchio-Sadus, A. (2008). Toxicity of lithium to humans and the environment—a literature review. *Ecotoxicology and Environmental Safety, 70*, 349.

Aschenbrenner, D. S. (2013). Drug watch: Two drugs receive pregnancy category changes. *The American Journal of Nursing, 113*, 27.

Ayd, F. J. (1991). The early history of modern psychopharmacology. *Neuropsychopharmacology, 5*, 71.

Bezchlibnyk-Butler, K. Z., & Jeffries, J. J. (2007). *Clinical handbook of psychotropic drugs*. Seattle: Hogrefe & Huber.

Cade, J. F. (1949). Lithium salts in the treatment of psychotic excitement. *The Medical Journal of Australia, 36*, 349.

Cozza, K. L., Armstrong, S. C., & Oesterheld, J. R. (2003). *Drug interaction principles for medical practice*. Washington, DC: American Psychiatric Publishing.

El-Mallakh, R. S. (1996). *Lithium: Actions and mechanisms*. Washington, DC: American Psychiatric Press.

Fact sheet: Taking mood stabilizers during childbearing years. *NAMI Advocate, 19*, (1998). 16.

Foster, A., Sheehan, L., & Johns, L. (2011). Promoting treatment adherence in patients with bipolar disorder. *Current Psychiatry, 10*(7), 45–52.

Geoghegan, J. J., & Stevenson, G. H. (1949). Prophylactic electroshock. *American Journal of Psychiatry, 105*, 494.

Gershon, S., Chengappa, K. N., & Malhi, G. S. (2009). Lithium specificity in bipolar illness: A classic agent for the classic disorder. *Bipolar Disorders, 11*(Suppl. 2), 34.

Gerst, T. M., Smith, T. L., & Patel, N. C. (2010). Antiepileptics for psychiatric illness: Find the right match. *Current Psychiatry, 9*, 51.

Haddad, P. M., et al. (2009). A review of valproate in psychiatric practice. *Expert Opinion on Drug Metabolism & Toxicology, 5*, 539.

Katzung, B. G., Masters, S. B., & Trevor, A. J. (2009). *Basic and clinical pharmacology* (11th ed.). New York: Lange.

Keltner, N. L., & Grant, J. S. (2008). Irreversible lithium-induced neuropathy: Two cases. *Perspectives in Psychiatric Care, 44*, 290.

Kovacsics, C. E., Gottesman, I. I., & Gould, T. D. (2009). Lithium's antisuicidal efficacy: Elucidation of neurobiological targets using endophenotype strategies. *Annual Review of Pharmacology and Toxicology, 49*, 175.

Lehne, R. A. (2007). *Pharmacology for nursing care*. St. Louis: Saunders.

Manji, H. K., & Lenox, R. H. (2000). The nature of bipolar disorder. *Journal of Clinical Psychiatry, 61*(Suppl. 13), 42.

Maxmen, J. S., & Ward, N. G. (2002). *Psychotropic drugs: Fast facts* (3rd ed.). New York: WW Norton.

McIntyre, R. S., et al. (2001). Lithium revisited. *Canadian Journal of Psychiatry, 46*, 322.

Nestler, E. J., Hyman, S. E., & Malenka, R. C. (2009). *Molecular neuropharmacology* (2nd ed.). New York: McGraw-Hill.

Pontius, E. (2012). Concerns about valproate (Letter). *Current Psychiatry, 11*, 5.

Soares, J. C., & Gershon, S. (2000). The psychopharmacologic specificity of the lithium ion: Origins and trajectory. *Journal of Clinical Psychiatry, 61*(Suppl. 9), 16.

Stahl, S. M. (2004). Drug combinations for bipolar spectrum disorders: Evidence-based prescribing or prescribing-based evidence? *Journal of Clinical Psychiatry, 65*, 1298.

Tohen, M., & Vieta, E. (2009). Antipsychotic agents in the treatment of bipolar mania. *Bipolar Disorders, 11*(Suppl. 2), L45.

U.S. Surgeon General. (1999). *Mental health: A report from the Surgeon General*. Washington, DC: Department of Health and Human Services.

Antianxiety Drugs

Norman L. Keltner

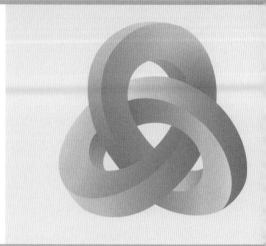

e*volve* WEBSITE

http://evolve.elsevier.com/Keltner

LEARNING OBJECTIVES

- Describe the differences between benzodiazepines and buspirone.
- Identify when benzodiazepines are indicated.
- Discuss the side effects of benzodiazepines.
- Identify benzodiazepines that are appropriate for older adults.
- Identify the specific antidote for benzodiazepine overdose.
- Describe potential drug interactions with benzodiazepines.
- Discuss the implications for teaching patients about antianxiety drugs.

CASE EXAMPLE

Annie dreaded what would happen next—she had been down this road many times before. There she was, minding her own business, just wanting to watch a movie, like any normal person, but then she noticed her breathing was off. Immediately she began to monitor her breathing, and soon it seemed as if she just could not get enough air. She remembered a recent visit to the emergency department when the nurse patiently showed her that her oxygen saturation levels were good. She remembered, but it didn't help. It wasn't that she believed that this time was different, that this time she was going to suffocate. No, that might be a textbook explanation, but it wasn't her explanation. She could not breathe, and knowing that "it was all in her head" did not seem to help. Soon she would be spiraling into symptoms that, like an Old Testament prophet, would beget more apprehension, which would beget more symptoms—palpitations, dizziness, a fear of fainting, trembling, feeling that things around her were unreal, fear of going crazy—which would beget more dread. Worst of all, she feared looking foolish. What if she lost control and started gulping big chunks of air down? What if she …? What would they think of her? (Keltner et al., 2003).

People have been seeking relief from anxiety since the beginning of recorded history. Alcohol is the oldest drug used to reduce anxiety, and it has been used by countless millions to self-medicate fears, phobias, and nerves. In more recent times, other drugs have been developed to alleviate anxiety. In the early 1900s, bromo seltzers were advertised as having anxiolytic properties but had to be withdrawn from the market because of their addictive qualities. In the 1930s and 1940s, barbiturates were heralded as having potential to treat anxiety, but they too were found to have many adverse effects, including seizures, dependence, addiction, and withdrawal.

The first drug that was specific for treating anxiety was meprobamate (Miltown, Equanil), which was developed in 1955 (Ayd, 1991). This drug, with its ability to calm nerves, to blur the reality of stressors, and to make people feel better in general, was a national sensation. How it was received probably says far more about the American psyche than about the efficacy of meprobamate. The United States was ready for a drug to buffer the stressors of a busy society. For several years, meprobamate was a widely prescribed medication but, similar to alcohol, bromo seltzer, and barbiturates, problems surfaced. Individuals using meprobamate were subject to abusing it, developed tolerance, and experienced lethal overdose. Its appeal as an antianxiety agent began to diminish. Fortunately, new agents to calm the trembling hands of a nation besieged with anxiety were waiting in the wings.

Before the end of the 1950s, another class of antianxiety drugs was developed—the benzodiazepines. These drugs had advantages over barbiturates in that they were less likely to be abused and were safer when overdoses occurred. Although first synthesized in the 1930s, benzodiazepines were not discovered to have a psychiatric effect until the late 1950s. Eventually, several thousand benzodiazepine derivatives would be synthesized, including familiar drugs such as diazepam (Valium), lorazepam (Ativan), alprazolam (Xanax), oxazepam (Serax), and clonazepam (Klonopin). All of these agents manipulate the gamma-aminobutyric acid (GABA) system. However, these drugs were also linked to significant problems. Benzodiazepines were abused, induced tolerance, and were implicated in lethal overdoses (although always when combined with other drugs). Many American adults use or have used benzodiazepines.

Clinical researchers and drug manufacturers continue to search for the perfect antianxiety drug—a drug that ameliorates anxiety without significant adverse effects. A nonbenzodiazepine antianxiety agent that has been widely marketed is buspirone (BuSpar). Buspirone does not have the potential for abuse, dependency, and withdrawal associated with benzodiazepines. The selective serotonin reuptake inhibitors (SSRIs) were developed in the late 1980s. These agents have emerged as a first-line treatment choice for anxiety. Because they are discussed in detail in Chapter 15, this chapter presents only a brief review.

A large group of unrelated drugs appear to have antianxiety properties or at least have been found useful in the treatment of specific anxiety-like syndromes. Examples of drugs with antianxiety properties include some beta blockers (e.g., propranolol [Inderal]), antihistamines, monoamine oxidase inhibitors, tricyclic antidepressants (TCAs), clonidine (Catapres), phenothiazines, hydroxyzine (Vistaril), and opioids. A few of these agents are discussed briefly at the end of the chapter.

MODELS OF ANXIETY

Anxiety and its causes are discussed in Chapter 27. Basically, there are three areas involving causative factors:
1. Autonomic nervous system dysregulation
   a. Dysregulation of beta-adrenergic receptors
   b. Inhibition of GABA
2. Neuroendocrine overactivity
3. Faulty thinking

The autonomic nervous system overperforms when a person is anxious (Box 17-1, Figure 17-1). Studies have found that beta agonists, such as isoproterenol, cause anxiety. Adrenergic autoreceptors (alpha-2 receptors) also produce anxiety when blocked by drugs. However, alpha-2 agonists, such as the antihypertensive clonidine, have antianxiety properties. The extension of this thinking suggests that individuals with anxiety are believed to experience alpha-2 autoreceptor underfunctioning, which causes the

BOX 17-1	AUTONOMIC (ADRENERGIC SYSTEM) SYMPTOMS OF ANXIETY

Tachycardia
Dilated pupils
Tremor
Sweating

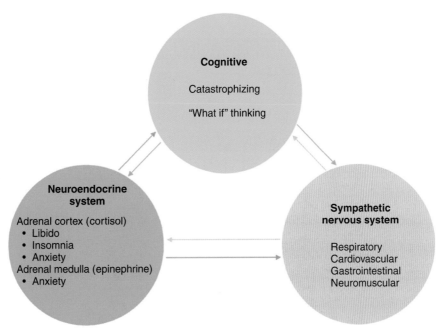

FIG 17-1 Interacting systems of panic attacks. (From Keltner, N.L., Perry, B.A., & Williams, A.R. [2003]. Panic disorder: a tightening vortex of misery. *Perspectives in Psychiatric Care, 39,* 38.)

locus ceruleus, the site of norepinephrine synthesis in the brain, to overproduce norepinephrine. As we discuss later, serotonin-enhancing agents play a major role in the treatment of anxiety, which is probably related to modulation of adrenergic neurons by serotonin.

GABA inhibition might play a role in anxiety because these neurons synapse with adrenergic neurons in the brain. As GABA inhibition is lifted, there is greater inhibition of the adrenergic system. This view is supported by the fact that GABAergic drugs such as benzodiazepines decrease anxiety, whereas GABA receptor blockers such as flumazenil cause anxiety.

Increased levels of the hormone cortisol, which is secreted by the adrenal cortex in response to increased hypothalamic release of corticotropin-releasing hormone or increased anterior pituitary release of adrenocorticotropic hormone, are related to increased anxiety and insomnia.

People who have anxiety, particularly people who experience panic attacks, tend to engage in negative thinking. These negative thoughts (also known as *what if* or *catastrophic*

thinking) can trigger anxiety. Box 17-2 lists the symptoms of panic attack.

BENZODIAZEPINES

Although benzodiazepines are not considered first-line agents by psychiatric professionals, these drugs are still frequently prescribed by clinicians and so are extensively discussed in this chapter. Many benzodiazepines are on the market. Table 17-1 presents information on benzodiazepines, including duration of effect, the usual adult daily dose, equivalent dose, elimination half-life, anxiolytic effect, and sedative effect. Historically, antianxiety agents have been referred to as *anxiolytics* or *minor tranquilizers*. Benzodiazepines are widely used by both psychiatric and general medicine patients (and might be prescribed more often by nonpsychiatric clinicians). Major indications for benzodiazepines include chronic anxiety, time-limited treatment for crisis, presurgery jitters, acute mania, and panic disorder (Dunlop et al., 2012).

Anxiety is a subjective experience but can be observed by others (Box 17-3). The anxious person feels excessively alert, is easily startled, is restless, might talk too much, visually scans the environment, has tremors, and might have dilated pupils. Although many people use these drugs, as needed, benzodiazepines generally should not be taken for the stresses of everyday life. Benzodiazepines have no therapeutic value in the treatment of psychosis. Box 17-4 outlines mental health and related issues amenable to benzodiazepines. Box 17-5 summarizes acceptable parameters for using these agents.

How Benzodiazepines Work

Benzodiazepines enhance the effects of the inhibitory neurotransmitter GABA. GABA is the major inhibitory neurotransmitter in the brain and is found in roughly 40% of all neurons. GABA attaches to GABA receptors, which trigger

---

BOX 17-2	SYMPTOMS ASSOCIATED WITH PANIC ATTACKS

Palpitations
Sweating
Trembling or shaking
Shortness of breath
Feeling of choking
Chest pain
Nausea and abdominal distress
Feeling dizzy, unsteady, lightheaded, faint
Derealization
Fear of losing control or going crazy
Fear of dying
Tingling sensations
Chills or hot flashes

TABLE 17-1 FREQUENTLY PRESCRIBED BENZODIAZEPINES AND BUSPIRONE

USUAL DAILY ANXIETY DRUG DOSAGE (mg/day)	EQUIVALENT DOSE (mg)	HALF-LIFE (hr)	ANXIOLYTIC EFFECT	SEDATIVE EFFECT
Benzodiazepine (Shorter Acting)				
Alprazolam (Xanax), 0.75-4*	0.50	12-15	XX	X
Lorazepam (Ativan), 2-6* (P)	1	10-20	XXX	XX
Oxazepam (Serax), 30-60	30	5-20	XX	X
Temazepam (Restoril), 10-60	30	10-15	X	XXX
Benzodiazepine (Longer Acting)				
Chlordiazepoxide (Librium), 15-100* (P)	10	5-30†	XX	—
Clonazepam (Klonopin), 0.5-10*	0.25-0.5	18-60†	XX	X
Diazepam (Valium), 4-40* (P)	5	20-80†	XXX	XX
Nonbenzodiazepine				
Buspirone (BuSpar), 15-40*	NA	2-11†	XX	—

*Given in divided doses.
†With active metabolites.
N/A, not applicable; *P,* parenteral form available; *X,* mild effect; *XX,* moderate effect; *XXX,* strong effect.
Modified from Bezchlibnyk-Butler, K.Z., & Jeffries, J.J. (2007). *Clinical handbook of psychotropic drugs* (17th ed.). Seattle: Hogrefe & Huber; Bostwick, J.R., Cahser, M.I., & Yasugi, S. (2012). Benzodiazepines: a versatile clinical tool. *Current Psychiatry, 11,* 54.

BOX 17-3 SUBJECTIVE SYMPTOMS OF ANXIETY OBSERVABLE BY OTHERS

Patient might be:
- Anxious
- Apprehensive
- Compulsive
- Fearful
- Experiencing feelings of dread
- Irritable
- Intolerant
- Nervous
- Overconcerned
- Panicky
- Phobic
- Preoccupied
- Experiencing repetition in motor activities
- Feeling threatened
- Wound up
- Sensitive to shame
- Worried

BOX 17-4 CONDITIONS AMENABLE TO BENZODIAZEPINE TREATMENT

Acute agitation
Alcohol withdrawal
Antipsychotic-induced akathisia and tremor
Catatonia
Generalized anxiety disorder
Insomnia
Panic disorder
Social anxiety

BOX 17-5 WHEN BENZODIAZEPINES ARE APPROPRIATE FOR TREATING ANXIETY

1. Coadministration for 2 to 4 weeks when initially treating with SSRIs or venlafaxine
2. Patients wanting to avoid sexual side effects of antidepressants
3. Patients taking aspirin or NSAIDs on a long-term basis
4. Patients with comorbid epilepsy or bipolar disorder

NSAIDs, Nonsteroidal antiinflammatory drugs; *SSRIs,* selective serotonin reuptake inhibitors.
Adapted from Dunlop, B.W., Schneider, R., & Gerardi, M. (2012). Panic disorder: break the fear circuit. *Current Psychiatry, 11,* 36.

the opening of chloride channels. Chloride has a hyperpolarizing effect on the neuron, which makes the neuron less responsive to excitatory neurons. Benzodiazepines have the pharmacodynamic property of causing the GABA receptor to respond more robustly to GABA. Specifically, benzodiazepines activate the $GABA_A$ receptor subtype. The overall effect is one of slowing down or halting neuronal firing. Neuronal inhibition is important—as important to brain function as

the brake is to the operation of a car. Driving a car without a brake risks being involved in an accident. A brain without the inhibition of GABA can produce thought acceleration, autonomic dysfunction, excessive anxiety, panic, or even seizure activity—or, to stretch the analogy, a runaway brain. Benzodiazepines help GABA tone down or inhibit the anxiety response to stressors.

GABA is a product of the Krebs cycle. It is synthesized by the decarboxylation of glutamate (i.e., the acid group of the amino acid glutamate is taken off), an amino acid produced from the Krebs cycle.

GABA receptors are located on approximately 40% of all neurons (Sugerman, 2005). GABA receptors are composed of five subunits on a particular receptor complex; these subunits can be arranged in any number of configurations (Seighart, 1995). The composition of these subunits determines the functional characteristics of the receptor (Löw et al., 2000). Because of these unique configurations, some GABA receptors are selective for specific ligands (molecules that bind to and evoke a response from the receptor). Specific subunit configurations exist for benzodiazepines—a benzodiazepine receptor site. Because the place where benzodiazepines attach to the receptor is different from where GABA attaches, it is said to be an *allosteric* site (Nestler et al., 2009). When attaching to these sites, benzodiazepines enhance the effects of GABA. Because benzodiazepines do not connect directly to the GABA site, the effect created by benzodiazepines is dependent on endogenous GABA. In other words, benzodiazepines would be inactive in the absence of GABA. Other allosteric sites on GABA receptors include sites for barbiturates and alcohol. It is no wonder then that an overdose of any of these three categories of drugs can cause a kind of "drunkenness." Barbiturates are particularly interesting because they both enhance GABA and mimic GABA. They do this by opening chloride channels directly (the GABA site "thinks" the barbiturates are GABA). Barbiturates can cause profound central nervous system (CNS) depression and even death from overdose, whereas the level of CNS depression caused by benzodiazepines is limited (Lehne, 2007).

Pharmacologic Effects

Benzodiazepines have a generally depressive effect on the CNS, including the limbic system, the thalamus, the hypothalamus, and the reticular activating system (through which incoming sensory information is funneled). Benzodiazepines have the following major therapeutic effects (Ashton, 2000; Devlin & Roberts, 2009):

1. They reduce anxiety (at 20% binding to GABA receptors).
2. They promote sleep (at 30% to 50% binding to GABA receptors).
3. They produce hypnosis and amnesia (at 60% binding to GABA receptors).

Because benzodiazepines depress the reticular activating system, incoming stimuli are muted and evoke less reaction. To illustrate the concept of *muting,* two symptoms are highlighted: hyperalertness and environmental scanning. An anxious person uses these defensive reactions to guard against an environment perceived to be threatening. A stressed out person might overreact to being startled because the body's system is on alert. As the antianxiety agent decreases environmental input, a general relaxing of the anxious posture takes place. The body's reactor is toned down, and the environmental stressors are tuned out.

These drugs can cause several levels of CNS depression, from sedation to anesthesia. Benzodiazepines accomplish this CNS depression by sedating the patient and depressing the inhibitory neurons that affect arousal. The latter effect causes a state of disinhibition, or loosening, of inner impediments to conduct. Disinhibition results in feelings of euphoria and excitement, which can lead to poor judgment. The natural restraint that minimizes social blunders is depressed.

To visualize the potential allure of benzodiazepines, one might imagine a tension continuum, with anxiety at one end and a carefree sense of being at the other. Benzodiazepines have the potential to move an anxious person from the agony of the anxiety end to the relaxed feeling of the carefree end. In therapeutic doses, this degree of shift from anxiety to disinhibition is not gained or sought, but because of the possibility of reaching a carefree zone, benzodiazepines have become drugs of abuse. In addition, many polysubstance abusers use benzodiazepines because of their ability to increase the high of other drugs.

The inhibiting effect of benzodiazepines also accounts for their anticonvulsive activity. Intravenous diazepam and lorazepam are first-line agents for status epilepticus, and clonazepam is regularly prescribed orally as an anticonvulsant.

Paradoxical Reactions to Benzodiazepines

A few people have a paradoxical reaction to benzodiazepines (Mancuso et al., 2004). Symptoms include agitation, emotional lability, talkativeness, and occasionally rage. Spiegel and colleagues (2012) suggest the disinhibiting effects on processing in the prefrontal cortex (the area that monitors inhibition and socially acceptable behaviors) are at the root of these untoward responses. Children, older adults, patients with poor impulse control, and individuals with organic brain syndrome are most at risk.

Pharmacokinetics

Benzodiazepines are readily absorbed after oral ingestion; however, intramuscular administration produces slow and inconsistent absorption for most of these drugs (lorazepam is an exception). Benzodiazepines are highly lipid-soluble and readily cross the blood-brain barrier. Benzodiazepines are metabolized by the liver but do not significantly induce their own hepatic metabolism (compared with barbiturates), and they are excreted in the urine. The active metabolites can exert an effect for 10 days. A convenient way of categorizing benzodiazepines is to divide them into drugs with shorter half-lives (≤20 hours) and drugs with longer half-lives (>20 hours). Of the selected benzodiazepines with shorter half-lives listed in Table 17-1, lorazepam, oxazepam, and temazepam (Restoril) are preferable

for use in older adults. Chlordiazepoxide (Librium) and diazepam have longer half-lives and have an extended duration of action. These drugs are unsuitable for use in older patients. A benzodiazepine-induced delirium has been associated with the longer acting drugs in this class (Spiegel et al., 2012).

Considering only the half-life is misleading. An important factor in half-life determination is the metabolic process that each benzodiazepine undergoes. Most benzodiazepines are oxidized in the liver to active metabolites, but the liver becomes less efficient at metabolizing these drugs over a lifetime because hepatic function and hepatic volume change with age. The half-life of diazepam is approximately 20 hours in a young man but stretches to 80 hours in an 80-year-old man. A few benzodiazepines (e.g., lorazepam, oxazepam, temazepam) rely on conjugation with glucuronic acid to form inactive metabolites. This process is not significantly affected by the aging process. Because the half-lives of these drugs remain stable throughout life, and because these drugs have no active metabolites, they are better suited for use in older adults.

Hepatic metabolism is the primary mechanism for drug disposition. Drugs that interfere with liver metabolism (e.g., alcohol) dangerously compound the effect of benzodiazepines.

Side Effects

CNS side effects such as drowsiness, fatigue, and decreased coordination are commonly exhibited. Some mental impairment and slowing of reflexes also occur. Less frequently, confusion, depression, and headache might be present. Peripheral nervous system effects include occasional constipation, double vision, hypotension, incontinence, and urinary retention. Benzodiazepines can exacerbate narrow-angle glaucoma. Older adults with impaired liver or renal function and debilitated individuals experience increased side effects and consequently should receive a decreased amount of these drugs (see Common Side Effects of Benzodiazepines box [Charlson et al., 2009] and the discussion of pharmacokinetics earlier in the chapter).

COMMON SIDE EFFECTS OF BENZODIAZEPINES

Anterograde amnesia (no new memories)
Ataxia
Confusion
Depression
Drowsiness
Dysarthria
Headache
Impairment of mental functions
Increased reaction time
Lassitude
Lightheadedness
Motor incoordination
Sexual dysfunction
Skin reactions
Weight gain

Charlson, R., et al. (2009). A systematic review of research examining benzodiazepine-related mortality. *Pharmacoepidemiology and Drug Safety, 18,* 93.

TABLE 17-2 SYMPTOMS EMERGING AFTER WITHDRAWAL FROM BENZODIAZEPINES			
NEUROLOGIC	**GASTROINTESTINAL**	**PSYCHIATRIC**	**OTHER**
Convulsions	Nausea	Anxiety	Tachycardia
Insomnia	Vomiting	Irritability	Sweating
Lightheadedness	Diarrhea	Cognitive	
Involuntary movements	Weight loss	Memory impairment	
Headache	Decreased appetite	Depression	
Weakness		Confusion	

Dependence, Withdrawal, and Tolerance

In addition to the undesired effects already listed are the triple problems of dependence, withdrawal, and tolerance.

Dependence

Dependence is a state in which the body functions normally when the drug is present and functions abnormally when the drug is absent. Dependence can develop within a few weeks or months of regular use. When a benzodiazepine is withdrawn from a dependent person, symptoms such as agitation, tremor, irritability, insomnia, vomiting, sweating, and convulsions might be experienced. Ashton (2000) described three types of benzodiazepine dependence:

1. *Therapeutic dose dependence.* Individuals take the drug as prescribed but develop a need for the drug; they have outgrown the original reason for taking the drug but now need it to get through the day.
2. *Prescribed high-dose dependence.* Individuals are still taking prescribed benzodiazepines but have talked their physician into escalating the dose. Sometimes individuals are receiving prescriptions from more than one clinician.
3. *Recreational benzodiazepine abuse.* Individuals use benzodiazepines outside the traditional medical system. Benzodiazepines are often used to enhance the effects of other abused substances. Typically, the amount of drug used is significantly greater than the amount prescribed for medicinal purposes. For example, a high-end dose of diazepam is 40 mg/day, but recreational abusers often ingest 100 mg daily. Some abusers take benzodiazepines intravenously.

Withdrawal

Abrupt withdrawal from benzodiazepines can cause troublesome to serious effects. Agitation, tremor, irritability, insomnia, vomiting, sweating, convulsions, and psychotic episodes have occurred. Gradual tapering of the dose is imperative. Because GABA is an inhibitory neurotransmitter, releasing its inhibition results in the *"taking off the brake"* phenomenon. Because long-term use of benzodiazepines reduces the number of GABA receptors, an abrupt discontinuation of these drugs leaves the brain unable to fulfill inhibitory functions (Ashton, 2000; Ashton, 2004). The adverse effects previously mentioned occur. The tapering or withdrawal process is highly individual (usually over about 7 weeks) but can take 1 year or longer in some heavily dependent individuals. Table 17-2 provides a more complete list of withdrawal symptoms.

Tolerance

Tolerance to the effects of benzodiazepines occurs, so individuals need an increasing amount of the drug to achieve the same effect. Tolerance to sedation develops quickly (within weeks), whereas tolerance to antianxiety effects occurs slowly (over a few months). Anticonvulsive tolerance also develops slowly, so the use of benzodiazepines for epilepsy is probably ill advised for most patients. Cognitive and memory effects appear to continue as long as these agents are used (Ashton, 2000, 2004). Tolerance develops to some of the desired effects of benzodiazepines (i.e., hypnotic, anxiolytic, anticonvulsive effects), although tolerance does not appear to develop to the unwanted effects of cognitive and memory deficits. According to several news sources, Michael Jackson was taking 40 Xanax per night. Although the pill strength was not mentioned, this is a large dosage of this benzodiazepine.

Interactions

Benzodiazepines are CNS depressants and interact *additively* with other CNS depressants. Alcohol, TCAs, opioids, antipsychotics, and antihistamines increase the sedative effects of benzodiazepines. In addition, grapefruit juice can cause problems because it inhibits the cytochrome P-450 3A4 enzyme, extending the life of several benzodiazepines. Table 17-3 lists major interactants for benzodiazepines.

TABLE 17-3 MAJOR INTERACTIONS WITH BENZODIAZEPINES	
INTERACTANT	**INTERACTION**
Alcohol and other CNS depressants	Increased sedation, CNS depression
Antacids	Impaired absorption rate of benzodiazepine
Disulfiram (Antabuse) and cimetidine (Tagamet)	Increased plasma level of benzodiazepines that are oxidized (e.g., diazepam)
Phenytoin	Increased anticonvulsant serum level
TCAs	Increased sedation, confusion, impaired motor function
MAOIs	CNS depression
Succinylcholine	Decreased neuromuscular blockage

CNS, Central nervous system; *MAOIs*, monoamine oxidase inhibitors; *TCAs*, tricyclic antidepressants.

Nursing Implications

Therapeutic versus Toxic Drug Levels. Benzodiazepines taken alone are relatively safe drugs (Charlson et al., 2009). Overdoses hundreds of times higher than a therapeutic dose have been reported without resulting in death. However, if benzodiazepines are combined with other drugs, such as alcohol, the effect can be fatal. Signs and symptoms of overdose include somnolence, confusion, coma, diminished reflexes, and hypotension. Effective treatment begins with emptying the stomach by induced vomiting and gastric lavage, followed by activated charcoal. The nurse should monitor blood pressure, pulse, and respirations and provide supportive care as indicated.

Benzodiazepine Receptor Antagonist. Flumazenil (Romazicon) blocks the benzodiazepine-binding site on the GABA receptor. It selectively blocks benzodiazepine receptors but does not block adrenergic or cholinergic receptors. Because flumazenil does not stimulate the CNS and does not block other receptors, it usually can be given when benzodiazepine overdose is suspected without fear of unexpected interactions. A response to flumazenil typically occurs within 30 to 60 seconds. Two important considerations when giving flumazenil are that (1) it does not speed up the metabolism or excretion of benzodiazepines and (2) it has a short duration of action. These considerations present a clinical management problem. If the patient responds to flumazenil, benzodiazepines are present, but because flumazenil does not speed up metabolism and has a short duration of action, the patient might recover only to return to the same state as before flumazenil. This problem requires constant vigilance by the nurse and repeated doses of flumazenil as the body eliminates the benzodiazepine from the system. Flumazenil might not reverse benzodiazepine-induced respiratory depression and can precipitate seizures (Lehne, 2007).

Use during Pregnancy. The association of benzodiazepine use and fetal abnormalities has not been supported (Maxmen & Ward, 2002). Some concern exists that benzodiazepines might be associated with cleft lip and cleft palate in the first trimester, but the evidence has been inconclusive. However, these findings might warrant discontinuance during pregnancy. Additionally, floppy infant syndrome has been associated with benzodiazepine use during labor (Malone et al., 2004). Benzodiazepines are also known to be found in breast milk, so nursing mothers must be cautious about their use (Hale, 2002). If the drug cannot be discontinued without exacerbation of symptoms, tapering to the lowest possible dose is desirable, as is the use of shorter acting agents, such as alprazolam or lorazepam (Malone et al., 2004).

Use in Older Adults. As mentioned in the discussion on pharmacokinetics, specific benzodiazepines are acceptable for use in older adults, but most are not recommended. This dichotomy is based on metabolic processes. Lorazepam and oxazepam are considered to be the best benzodiazepines for older individuals. Temazepam and occasionally alprazolam are also used in this age group. The other benzodiazepines, including diazepam and chlordiazepoxide, have extended half-lives and active metabolites and should not be routinely prescribed for older patients.

Side Effects. The most common side effects are related to sedation and mental alertness. The patient should be cautioned about driving or operating hazardous machinery. Tolerance to sedation develops quickly. Blood pressure should be monitored routinely. A decrease in systolic blood pressure of 20 mm Hg while the patient is standing warrants withholding the drug and notifying the physician.

Interactions. Benzodiazepines interact with many CNS depressants. The nurse should explain this carefully to patients who are taking benzodiazepines. A high percentage of psychiatric patients abuse drugs, so a real potential exists for deadly combinations to be taken. These patients also are likely to develop a cross-tolerance to drugs metabolized in the liver. For example, individuals who develop a tolerance to alcohol have an increased tolerance to diazepam but not when alcohol and diazepam are taken together. Hearing a patient who is experienced in taking diazepam speak with disdain about typical doses is not uncommon—for example, "Ten milligrams of Valium doesn't even touch me!" Although diazepam alone might not touch these patients, diazepam combined with alcohol *will*. The nurse should remind these patients that if they mix diazepam with enough alcohol, they might die.

Teaching Patients. Patient education is important because benzodiazepines have tremendous potential for abuse or misuse. Consequently, teaching patients and their families about these drugs is important. The nurse should teach the following precautions:

- Benzodiazepines are not intended for the minor stresses of everyday life.
- Over-the-counter drugs might enhance the actions of benzodiazepines.
- Certain herbal preparations such as kava and valerian cause an additive effect.
- Driving should be avoided until tolerance develops.
- The prescribed dose should not be exceeded.
- Alcohol and other CNS depressants exacerbate the effects of benzodiazepines.
- Hypersensitivity to one benzodiazepine might mean hypersensitivity to another.
- These drugs should not be stopped abruptly.

Selected Benzodiazepines

Alprazolam. Alprazolam (Xanax) is particularly useful for generalized anxiety, adjustment disorders, panic disorder, and anxiety associated with depression. It is also prescribed as an antitremor agent. Alprazolam has been criticized for its potential to cause addiction and dependence, and there have been reports of alprazolam-induced violent or aggressive behavior. Little risk exists of accumulation of alprazolam during repeated dosing.

Chlordiazepoxide. Chlordiazepoxide (Librium) is prescribed for anxiety disorders, the relief of the symptoms of anxiety, and acute alcohol withdrawal. Chlordiazepoxide is absorbed well orally. Additionally, chlordiazepoxide can be used as an antitremor agent. Parenteral chlordiazepoxide is used as an antipanic agent. Accumulation occurs with this drug.

Clonazepam. Clonazepam (Klonopin) is used most often as an anticonvulsant but also has clinical use in the treatment of panic disorder. Clonazepam is weakly lipophilic (i.e., does not sequester readily in adipose tissue), and it has a small volume of distribution. It does not produce as much drug accumulation as one might expect (Freeman, 2012). Patients taking clonazepam over the long term should be slowly tapered off this drug because evidence suggests that abrupt withdrawal can precipitate status epilepticus. Clonazepam is also used for benzodiazepine withdrawal (Keltner & Folks, 2005).

Diazepam. Diazepam (Valium) is an often prescribed antianxiety agent that has multiple uses related to its CNS depressive effect. In addition to treating anxiety disorders and providing short-term relief from symptoms of anxiety, diazepam is used preoperatively to relieve presurgery jitters, for skeletal muscle spasms (e.g., lower back pain), as a drug of choice (intravenously) for status epilepticus, and as an adjunct for endoscopic procedures. Additionally, diazepam might be useful for symptomatic relief of alcohol withdrawal.

Lorazepam. Lorazepam (Ativan) is used to treat anxiety disorders and can be used as an antitremor agent, antipanic agent, anticonvulsant (parenteral only), and antiemetic for patients with cancer undergoing chemotherapy. Lorazepam plus haloperidol injections are often used in the emergency department for very agitated or combative patients. The metabolites of lorazepam are inactive, so the effects of this drug do not persist. Patients with impaired liver function can handle this drug better than most other benzodiazepines because lorazepam is metabolized by a conjugative process to inactive metabolites. Lorazepam is recommended for use in older patients when a benzodiazepine is indicated.

Oxazepam. Oxazepam (Serax) is similar to lorazepam in that its metabolite is inactive and it is metabolized by a conjugative reaction. The drug is effective for a relatively short time (24 hours) and is suitable for patients with liver disorders and for older adults. Oxazepam is used for anxiety associated with depression and for relief from acute alcohol withdrawal.

NONBENZODIAZEPINE: BUSPIRONE

Buspirone (BuSpar) is a first-line agent for anxiety. It is not a benzodiazepine and does not bind to benzodiazepine recognition sites but probably acts as an agonist at the presynaptic serotonin 1A receptor. Considerable interest exists in buspirone because it differs from benzodiazepines in several important ways. Advantages of buspirone are as follows:

- It is not sedating.
- It does not cause a high, so it has almost *no abuse potential*.
- It has no cross-tolerance with sedatives or alcohol.
- It does not produce dependence, withdrawal, or tolerance.
  Buspirone has one disadvantage:
- It has a delayed onset of antianxiety effect compared with benzodiazepines (1 to 6 weeks).

Buspirone's effects help distinguish anxiety control from the sedative and euphoric actions of older benzodiazepines. Buspirone is particularly effective in reducing symptoms of worry, apprehension, difficulties with concentration and

cognition, and irritability. These subjective symptoms are probably more serotonin-based than the more physical symptoms of anxiety (Stahl, 2000). Buspirone does not depress the CNS, and its lack of a sedative effect makes it less attractive for abuse. Because it has no abuse potential, buspirone is not a controlled substance.

Buspirone provides relief from anxiety within 7 to 10 days, but *maximal* therapeutic gain is not achieved until 3 to 6 weeks after treatment is initiated. Buspirone has a relatively short half-life, so it is usually given in divided doses. Buspirone is extensively metabolized after the first pass; 1% to 4% becomes bioavailable. Foods increase its bioavailability by decreasing first-pass metabolism. Side effects include dizziness, nausea, headache, nervousness, lightheadedness, and excitement. Buspirone is a remarkably safe drug and has few drug interactions.

The benzodiazepine should not be stopped immediately when switching from a benzodiazepine to buspirone. Because of dissimilarities in their pharmacologic properties, benzodiazepines must be tapered (to prevent withdrawal effects) while buspirone is initiated.

SELECTIVE SEROTONIN REUPTAKE INHIBITORS

SSRIs are first-line agents for anxiety spectrum disorders and are discussed in detail in Chapter 15 (Dunlop et al., 2012). The fact that these drugs work so well in treating anxiety underscores the overlapping nature of depression and anxiety. They are mentioned only briefly here. Box 17-6 summarizes the typical approach to treating anxiety.

SSRIs are prescribed for generalized anxiety disorder (GAD), obsessive-compulsive disorder (OCD), panic attacks,

---

BOX 17-6 TYPICAL APPROACH TO TREATING ANXIETY: STAYING THE COURSE

People who seek professional help for anxiety are hurting. Although it has been noted in the text that selective serotonin reuptake inhibitors (SSRIs) are the first-line treatment choice, they do not act rapidly. Although it is debated in professional meetings and in scholarly journals, often the anxious individual is prescribed an SSRI and a benzodiazepine. Because the SSRI will take some time to "work," the patient would be too miserable without some extra help. Benzodiazepines provide that immediate help the patient is seeking. After several weeks or so, the hope is that the patient can be weaned off the benzodiazepine and then rely on the SSRI for relief. As noted in Chapter 15, SSRIs act through the second messenger system. Within weeks, the actual genetic output of the neuron begins to change. In some ways, benzodiazepines are similar to *aspirin*, and SSRIs are similar to *antibiotics*. One medication first treats the symptoms, while the other treats the real problem. It is very important to stay the course with the SSRIs. If there is no improvement in 4 weeks, the dose should be increased every 2 to 4 weeks until remission of symptoms or until side effects are so troublesome that a dosage increase would be unwise (Dunlop et al., 2012).

TABLE 17-4   ANTIDEPRESSANTS INDICATED FOR ANXIETY

AGENT	DOSAGE CLASS	DOSAGE RANGE (mg/day)	COMMENT (FDA APPROVAL)
Clomipramine (Anafranil)	SRI	100-250	Approved for OCD; 250 mg is the maximum dose because of increased risk of seizures
Escitalopram (Lexapro)	SSRI	10-30	Approved for GAD
Fluoxetine (Prozac)	SSRI	20-80	Approved for OCD, panic disorder (maximum 60 mg/day)
Fluvoxamine (Luvox)	SSRI	100-300	Approved for OCD
Paroxetine (Paxil)	SSRI	40-60	Approved for panic, OCD, social anxiety, GAD (maximum 50 mg/day), PTSD (maximum 50 mg/day)
Sertraline (Zoloft)	SSRI	50-200	Approved for panic, OCD, PTSD
Venlafaxine (Effexor XR)	SNRI	75-225	Approved for GAD
Duloxetine (Cymbalta)	SNRI	60-120	Approved for GAD

FDA, U.S. Food and Drug Administration; GAD, generalized anxiety disorder; OCD, obsessive-compulsive disorder; PTSD, posttraumatic stress disorder; SNRI, selective serotonin-norepinephrine reuptake inhibitor; SRI, serotonin reuptake inhibitor; SSRI, selective serotonin reuptake inhibitor.
From Keltner, N.L., & Folks, D.G. (2005). *Psychotropic drugs* (4th ed.). St. Louis: Mosby.

posttraumatic stress disorder (PTSD), and social phobias. OCD is perhaps the most difficult mental disorder to treat satisfactorily. Several SSRIs are considered first-line approaches to the treatment of OCD (Table 17-4). Specifically, fluoxetine (Prozac), fluvoxamine (Luvox), paroxetine (Paxil), and sertraline (Zoloft) are approved for treatment of this disorder. SSRIs are probably the most effective as well as the safest agents for prophylaxis and long-term treatment of panic attacks. GABA receptors are thought to be involved in the pathophysiology of panic disorders. It has been theorized that the overwhelming anxiety associated with panic might stem from abnormal serotonin transmission. Effectiveness of SSRIs in panic and other anxiety disorders can be partially explained by serotonin's role in up-regulating GABA transmission in the prefrontal cortex. By up-regulating inhibitory neurons, a more inhibitory effect can be expected. This hypothesis agrees with what we know about symptoms of anxiety.

Venlafaxine and Duloxetine. Venlafaxine (Effexor, Effexor XR) and duloxetine (Cymbalta) are selective serotonin-norepinephrine reuptake inhibitors and are approved for GAD. Venlafaxine was the first drug approved for both GAD and major depression. This agent offers a dual approach to treatment because it blocks the reuptake of both serotonin (at lower doses) and norepinephrine (at medium to higher doses). Doses at the higher ranges are believed to be more effective, possibly because of the increased norepinephrine reuptake inhibition at these ranges (Lee & Keltner, 2006). Table 17-5 outlines pharmacologic interventions for specific anxiety disorders.

OTHER DRUGS WITH ANTIANXIETY PROPERTIES

Clomipramine and Other Tricyclic Antidepressants

Clomipramine (Anafranil) is one of two drugs considered most effective for OCD (the other is the SSRI fluvoxamine). Clomipramine is a serotonin reuptake inhibitor, although it is not as potent as the more traditional SSRIs. The major central side effects of clomipramine include headache, reduced libido, nervousness, myoclonus, and increased appetite. Peripheral effects include dry mouth, constipation, ejaculation failure (42%), erectile dysfunction (20%), and weight gain (Keltner & Folks, 2005). Imipramine (Tofranil) and desipramine (Norpramin) have proven to be effective for panic-anxiety attacks. Trazodone (Desyrel) has a highly sedative quality and is often prescribed for individuals who are experiencing anxiety (particularly older adults) to facilitate sleep.

Clonidine

Clonidine (Catapres) is an alpha-2 agonist. Because agonistic stimulation of autoreceptors such as alpha-2 causes a decrease in neurotransmitter production, it follows that this drug typically indicated for hypertension could have antianxiety effects, and it does.

Gabapentin

Gabapentin (Neurontin) is a commonly used anticonvulsant with antianxiety properties. It has been found to be effective in the treatment of social phobia and moderately effective in the treatment of OCD. It also has been used to augment the antidepressant treatment of PTSD (Dowben, et al., 2011).

Hydroxyzine

Hydroxyzine (Vistaril, Atarax) has also been used successfully with anxious patients. It is an older agent and was used infrequently for many years but has experienced a "comeback" of sorts. It is an antihistamine (first generation); thus it blocks histamine and cholinergic receptors. However, it also blocks serotonin receptors and this mechanism is thought to be responsible for its anxiolytic properties (Dowben, et al., 2013). It has few significant side effects when given in appropriate doses, is inexpensive, is not typically habit forming, and has many dosage forms.

TABLE 17-5 PHARMACOLOGIC INTERVENTIONS FOR SPECIFIC ANXIETY DISORDERS

DISORDER	PHARMACOLOGIC TREATMENT
Panic Disorder Exhibited as discrete and intense period of anxiety, apprehension, and distress Associated symptoms include palpitations, sweating, trembling, and dyspnea	SSRIs: Perhaps the safest for long-term and prophylactic doses; gradual titration to sertraline 50 mg qd or paroxetine 40 mg qd (minimum effective dosages) Benzodiazepines: Clonazepam (average dosage 1.5 mg/day) and alprazolam (average dosage 3 mg/day) can provide more immediate relief TCAs: Same dosage as that used in treating depressive syndromes, but dose level should be carefully titrated because of risk of a paradoxical effect
Phobic Disorder *Agoraphobia* Fear of being away from home or in situations in which escape is inhibited	Alprazolam at the relatively high dosage of 3-6 mg/day has proven effective TCAs: Dosage typically 150-200 mg/day SSRIs and highly serotonergic TCAs (e.g., clomipramine, amitriptyline, trazodone) are effective for agoraphobia
Social Phobia Persistent fears of situations in which the person is exposed to the scrutiny of others (e.g., stage fright)	Beta blockers: Often taken in combination with antidepressants or benzodiazepine; propranolol 10-20 mg tid or qid Benzodiazepines alone or in combination with antidepressants Clonazepam: 0.5 mg bid SSRIs: Low doses initially
Obsessive-Compulsive Disorder Obsessions, compulsions, or both	Clomipramine: 100-200 mg/day Fluvoxamine: 200-300 mg/day Other SSRIs or gabapentin (Neurontin): Titrated to 1800-2400 mg/day
Posttraumatic Stress Disorder* Reexperiencing of trauma, avoidance, hyperarousal	SSRIs: Treatment of choice Antipsychotics: Appropriate if psychotic or subsyndromal symptoms occur Mood stabilizers: Appropriate for mood vacillations and irritability

bid, Twice a day; *qd,* every day; *qid,* four times a day; *SSRIs,* selective serotonin reuptake inhibitors; *TCAs,* tricyclic antidepressants; *tid,* three times a day.
*Dowben, J.S., Grant, J.S., & Keltner, N.L. (2007). Psychobiological substrates of posttraumatic stress disorder: part II. *Perspectives in Psychiatric Care, 43,* 146.

Pregabalin

Pregabalin (Lyrica) is used for the treatment of anxiety spectrum disorders, neuropathic pain, and seizures. It is related to gabapentin in that it inhibits neuronal excitability. It is a second-line agent but has been found to be effective (Westenberg, 2009).

Propranolol

Propranolol (Inderal) is a beta blocker that effectively interrupts the physiologic responses of anxiety related to social phobia. As noted earlier, autonomic dysregulation is a factor in anxiety. It makes sense that a drug that blocks these receptors could be effective. Propranolol is less effective than benzodiazepines but is safe and has little abuse

potential. Most side effects are transient and mild. However, bradycardia, lightheadedness, and heart block have been reported.

? CRITICAL THINKING QUESTIONS

1. Although barbiturates and benzodiazepines both affect GABA receptors, why can an overdose of barbiturates (without coadministration of other drugs) be fatal, whereas an overdose of benzodiazepines (without coadministration of other drugs) is apparently not fatal?
2. Flumazenil (Romazicon) is given for benzodiazepine overdose. Why doesn't it serve to reverse the effects of other GABA agonists?

STUDY NOTES

1. Antianxiety agents are commonly prescribed psychotropic drugs.
2. SSRIs are first-line agents used to treat anxiety. They are discussed in detail in Chapter 15.
3. The nonbenzodiazepine buspirone is also a first-line agent that is relatively safe and interacts with few other drugs.
4. Benzodiazepines are also commonly used.
5. Diazepam (Valium) is the prototype benzodiazepine; however, other benzodiazepines, particularly alprazolam (Xanax) and lorazepam (Ativan), are used extensively.
6. Benzodiazepines have four basic clinical uses: (a) for chronic anxiety, (b) for time-limited periods in people going through crises, (c) for presurgery nervousness, and (d) for the treatment of panic disorder.
7. The ability to mute incoming stimuli gives benzodiazepines a great potential for abuse.
8. Benzodiazepines can cause a physical dependence and produce a withdrawal syndrome. Discontinuance should be tapered gradually.
9. Side effects of benzodiazepines include drowsiness, fatigue, ataxia, and other peripheral and central effects; however, tolerance to side effects occurs.
10. Benzodiazepines are safe drugs when taken alone but can be deadly if mixed with other CNS depressants (e.g., alcohol).
11. Benzodiazepines that ultimately rely on conjugation with glucuronic acid to inactive metabolites are more appropriate for older adults (e.g., lorazepam [Ativan], oxazepam [Serax]).
12. Buspirone (BuSpar) is a nonbenzodiazepine and is used extensively for the treatment of anxiety. Buspirone differs from the benzodiazepines in the following ways:
    a. It is not sedating.
    b. It does not cause a high, so it has almost *no abuse potential.*
    c. It has no cross-tolerance with sedatives or alcohol.
    d. It takes 1 to 6 weeks to be effective.
    e. It does not produce dependence, withdrawal, or tolerance.
    f. It does not cause muscle relaxation.

REFERENCES

Ashton, C. H. (2000). *Benzodiazepines: How they work and how to withdraw.* Newcastle, England: University of Newcastle.

Ashton, H. (2004). Benzodiazepine dependence. In P. Haddad, S. Dursun, & B. Deakin (Eds.), *Adverse syndromes and psychiatric drugs: A clinical guide* (pp. 239). Oxford: Oxford University Press.

Ayd, F. J. (1991). The early history of modern psychopharmacology. *Neuropsychopharmacology, 5,* 71.

Bezchlibnyk-Butler, K. Z., & Jeffries, J. J. (2007). *Clinical handbook of psychotropic drugs* (17th ed). Seattle: Hogrefe & Huber.

Bostwick, J. R., Cahser, M. I., & Yasugi, S. (2012). Benzodiazepines: A versatile clinical tool. *Current Psychiatry, 11,* 54.

Charlson, R., et al. (2009). A systematic review of research examining benzodiazepine-related mortality. *Pharmacoepidemiology and Drug Safety, 18,* 93.

Devlin, J. W., & Roberts, R. J. (2009). Pharmacology of commonly used analgesics and sedatives in the ICU: Benzodiazepines, propofol, and opioids. *Critical Care Clinics, 25,* 431.

Dowben, J. S., Grant, J. S., & Keltner, N. L. (2007). Psychobiological substrates of posttraumatic stress disorder: Part II. *Perspectives in Psychiatric Care, 43,* 146.

Dowben, J. S., Grant, J. S., & Keltner, N. L. (2011). Clonidine: Diverse use in pharmacologic management. *Perspectives in Psychiatric Care, 47*(2), 105–108.

Dowben, J. S., Grant, J. S., Froelich, K. D., & Keltner, N. L. (2013). Hyroxyzine for anxiety: Another look at an old drug. *Perspectives in Psychiatric Care, 49*(2), 75–77.

Dunlop, B. W., Schneider, R., & Gerardi, M. (2012). Panic disorder: Break the fear circuit. *Current Psychiatry, 11,* 36.

Freeman, S. A. (2012). Clonazepam dosing. (Letter) *Current Psychiatry, 11,* 19.

Hale, T. W. (2002). *Medications and mothers' milk* (10th ed.). Amarillo, TX: Pharmasoft.

Keltner, N. L., & Folks, D. G. (2005). *Psychotropic drugs* (4th ed.). St. Louis: Mosby.

Keltner, N. L., Perry, B. A., & Williams, A. R. (2003). Panic disorder: A tightening vortex of misery. *Perspectives in Psychiatric Care, 39,* 38.

Lee, S. I., & Keltner, N. L. (2006). Serotonin and norepinephrine reuptake inhibitors (SNRIs): Venlafaxine and duloxetine. *Perspectives in Psychiatric Care, 42,* 144.

Lehne, R. A. (2007). *Pharmacology for nursing care.* Philadelphia: Saunders.

Löw, K., et al. (2000). Molecular and neuronal substrate for the selective attenuation of anxiety. *Science, 290,* 131.

Malone, K., et al. (2004). Antidepressants, antipsychotics, benzodiazepines, and the breastfeeding dyad. *Perspectives in Psychiatric Care, 40,* 73.

Mancuso, C. E., Tanzi, M. G., & Gabay, M. (2004). Paradoxical reactions to benzodiazepines: Literature review and treatment options. *Pharmacotherapy, 24*(1177), 2004.

Maxmen, J. S., & Ward, N. G. (2002). *Psychotropic drugs: Fast facts* (3rd ed.). New York: WW Norton.

Nestler, E. J., Hyman, S. E., & Malenka, R. C. (2009). *Molecular neuropharmacology: A foundation for clinical neuroscience.* New York: McGraw-Hill.

Seighart, W. (1995). Structure and pharmacology of gamma-aminobutyric acid-A receptor subtypes. *Pharmacological Reviews, 47,* 181.

Spiegel, D. R., Kumari, N., & Petri, J. D. (2012). Safer use of benzodiazepines for alcohol detoxification. *Current Psychiatry, 11,* 10.

Stahl, S. M. (2000). *Essential psychopharmacology* (2nd ed). New York: Cambridge University Press.

Sugerman, R. A. (2005). Functional neuroanatomy. In N. L. Keltner & D. G. Folks (Eds.), *Psychotropic drugs* (pp. 12–38) (4th ed.). St. Louis: Mosby.

Westenberg, H. G. (2009). Recent advances in understanding and treating social anxiety disorder. *CNS Spectrums, 14*(2 Suppl. 3), 24.

Antidementia Drugs

Norman L. Keltner

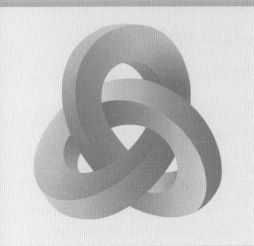

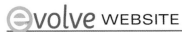 WEBSITE

http://evolve.elsevier.com/Keltner

LEARNING OBJECTIVE

- Identify the drugs used in the treatment of Alzheimer's disease and other dementias.

Drugs used for Alzheimer's disease (AD) can be roughly categorized as drugs used for treatment and drugs used for prevention. Neither treatment nor preventive drugs provide the definitive approach that patients and families seek. Nevertheless, the available agents provide some relief and might help prevent AD. In addition to the drugs used to treat or prevent AD, there are a few experimental agents that show promise. Although significant limitations exist, current approaches target specific physiologic mechanisms; this hardly resembles the serendipitous approach that dominated drug discovery during the early years of psychopharmacology.

DRUGS USED TO TREAT DEMENTIAS

AD is a degenerative disease that is progressive and brutal. Patients with AD lose memory-making ability, experience memory loss, cannot find the right words to express themselves, and have generalized cognitive impairment. The neurobiologic reasons for this are neuronal death and neurotransmitter deficiency. At this point, the most common approach to treatment attempts to restore neurotransmitter loss. The less common drug approach attempts to and might halt neuronal dying. Chapter 28 provides greater detail, but, simply, neuronal loss occurs in many places in the brain; however, the hippocampus, where memories are made, is never spared. Neurotransmitter restoration focuses on one primary neurotransmitter, acetylcholine (ACh), but other systems degenerate as well—the dopamine system and the norepinephrine system.

AGENTS THAT RESTORE ACETYLCHOLINE

Background

To understand the agents used to restore acetylcholine losses completely, it is important to review related concepts. Cholinergic pathways, enzymes, enzyme inhibition, types of ACh receptors, and types of cholinesterases (ChE) are discussed to facilitate the understanding of how these drugs work.

Cholinergic Pathways

Cholinergic pathways, although just one of several neurotransmitter systems affected, are selectively destroyed in AD. Most cholinergic fibers (about 90%) arise from one area, the nucleus basalis of Meynert. As might be suspected, the hippocampus is particularly rich in cholinergic receptors, and loss of ACh in this area causes the aforementioned memory-making loss. The amygdala, the locus of human emotion, is in front of the hippocampus and plays a role in memorization selection (Miller, 2005). Stated another way, many of our memories are linked to emotional events, so we often remember embarrassing or frightening moments. The amygdala apparently drives this type of memory-making selection. The amygdala is depends heavily on ACh for this function and suffers significantly as ACh pathways decline.

Enzymes

Enzymes are large molecules that are produced according to specific genetic coding. Enzymes provide the catalytic force that drives production of energy and the material required for the building blocks of life itself.

Enzyme configuration is such that certain molecules, including neurotransmitters and drugs, fit onto the enzyme and then undergo metabolic change. The enzyme is a catalyst of the metabolic change but not a participant. It is not changed itself, but repeats its catalytic activity many times. In the case of ChE, a single molecule can metabolize 5000 molecules of ACh every second (Figure 18-1) (Purves et al., 1997).

ChE breaks down ACh into the inactive metabolites choline and acetate. Once fragmented, these inactive remnants of ACh can no longer activate cholinergic receptors. Because a loss of ACh is the primary neurotransmitter loss in AD, attempting to prevent the breakdown of ACh has proven to be the most effective means for restoring this neurotransmitter.

Enzyme Inhibition

The approach to inhibiting ACh metabolism centers around blocking the enzyme ChE; this is accomplished by introducing molecules into the system that preferentially attach to ChE. When this blocking is accomplished, ACh cannot be metabolized, increasing the availability of this neurotransmitter to postsynaptic cholinergic receptors.

Types of Acetylcholine Receptors

Two types of ACh receptors have been identified in humans: muscarinic receptors and nicotinic receptors. *Muscarinic receptors* are divided into five subtypes; however, for the purpose of this discussion, they are grouped simply as

muscarinic receptors. Muscarinic receptors are the primary targets in treating AD. Muscarinic receptors are better known than nicotinic receptors because a blockade of these receptors (i.e., an antimuscarinic or anticholinergic effect) causes many of the side effects frequently encountered by nurses. For instance, dry mouth, dry eyes, blurred vision, urinary hesitancy, and constipation are caused by blockade of these receptors. An interesting effect of anticholinergic drugs (e.g., diphenhydramine [Benadryl], benztropine mesylate [Cogentin]) that cause these effects is that such drugs can compromise cognition as well. As people age, they become more susceptible to these effects. Stimulating these same receptors improves cognition. That is the therapeutic "bang" that ACh-enhancing agents provide.

The *nicotinic receptor* is best understood as two subtypes: (1) subtypes on the cell bodies of the postganglionic neurons in the autonomic nervous system (N_N) and (2) subtypes on skeletal muscles (N_M). However, there are also central nervous system nicotinic receptors that play a role in mental behaviors. When nicotinic receptors are activated, an up-regulation of norepinephrine, glutamate, gamma-aminobutyric acid, and dopamine occurs, all of which improve attention, memory, mood, and cognition. Down-regulation of nicotinic receptors is linked to poor attention, sensory gating dysfunction, memory problems, and impaired cognition. As is widely known, nicotinic receptors are stimulated by smoking. However, what is less well known is that smoking and the boosting of brain nicotine is a putatively therapeutic contribution to schizophrenia, attention-deficit/hyperactivity disorder, and presumably cognitive disorders (Keltner & Lillie, 2009). A very specific nicotinic receptor, $\alpha 4\beta 2$, has a role in attention and memory (Miller, 2008; Kuehn, 2006). When stimulated by nicotine, this receptor improves those functions. If one cannot concentrate, one cannot remember; if one cannot remember, one cannot learn. Attention, memory, and learning are cognitive skills enhanced by nicotine stimulation of a specific nicotinic receptor subtype (Keltner & Lillie, 2009). A greater appreciation for the potential of nicotinic receptor enhancers and their possible contribution to cognitive improvements has evolved over the last few years.

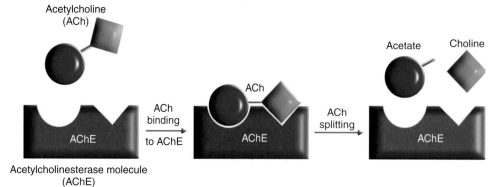

FIG 18-1 An acetylcholine (ACh) molecule and an acetylcholinesterase (AChE) molecule *(left panel)*. AChE binds the ACh molecule *(center panel)*. The products of AChE's metabolic activity, acetate and choline *(right panel)*. (Courtesy of Vicki Johnson. Modified from Lehne, R.A. [2003]. *Pharmacology for Nursing Care*. St. Louis: Saunders.)

Types of Cholinesterase

Just as there are two types of monoamine oxidase enzymes, so there are two types of ChE. Acetylcholinesterase (AChE) is more common in the brain. The other ChE, butyrylcholinesterase (BChE), is more common in the periphery (Box 18-1). Because a central nervous system effect is required to treat AD, drugs that inhibit both ChEs have greater potential for causing unnecessary and often adverse effects. For example, inhibiting BChE produces nausea and vomiting, diarrhea, facial flushing, sweating, rhinitis, bradycardia, and leg cramps. The ideal drug might selectively inhibit AChE, while not inhibiting BChE.

Cholinesterase Inhibitors

Three drugs known as *cholinesterase inhibitors* target ACh deficiency (Table 18-1). By attaching to and blocking ChE, these drugs substantially increase the amount of intrasynaptic ACh available to cholinergic receptors. A fourth drug, tacrine, is mentioned for heuristic and ethical reasons. Tacrine is discussed first.

BOX 18-1	CHOLINESTERASES: PRIMARY SITE OF ACTION
ACETYLCHOLINES-TERASE	**BUTYRYLCHOLINESTERASE**
Brain	Periphery
	Plasma
	Skeletal muscles
	Placenta
	Liver

Tacrine

Tacrine (Cognex) has been discontinued in the United States but it is still worth reading about because there is a lesson to be learned. Tacrine was the first cholinesterase inhibitor (both AChE and BChE) available for use. It was widely heralded because before tacrine, there was little hope for patients with AD. In an article in the *New England Journal of Medicine* published in 1986, it was reported that a patient returned to work, while another took up golf after being prescribed tacrine (Keltner, 1994). It was soon revealed that the *research was misrepresented*, and the authors received an unprecedented rebuke by the U.S. Food and Drug Administration (FDA). Tacrine may cause severe hepatotoxicity owing to exhaustion of enzymatic resources (Robles, 2009). This adverse effect led to its withdrawal from the market.

Donepezil

Donepezil (Aricept) was approved in 1996 and is a reversible inhibitor of ChE. Tacrine inhibited both AChE and BChE, whereas donepezil is much more selective for AChE (1200 to 1 times more selective for AChE), so theoretically its use should cause fewer peripheral side effects (Geldmacher, 1997). Other advantages include absence of hepatotoxicity, once-daily dosing related to a longer half-life, and 100% bioavailability whether taken with or without food. Some peripheral effects have been reported, including gastrointestinal problems and bradycardia, suggesting that selectivity for brain AChE is incomplete (Figure 18-2). Until more recently the highest dosage of donepezil was 10 mg/day. However, more recent studies show that donepezil at higher

TABLE 18-1	ANTIDEMENTIA DRUGS				
DRUG	**TYPICAL DAILY DOSAGE**	**HALF-LIFE (hr)**	**PROTEIN BINDING (%)**	**CYTOCHROME P-450 ENZYMES**	**MECHANISM OF ACTION**
Donepezil (Aricept)	5-10 mg at bedtime	~70	~95	2D6, 3A4	ChE inhibitor
Rivastigmine (Exelon)	6-12 mg in 2 divided doses	~2	~40	Not metabolized	ChE inhibitor
Galantamine (Razadyne)	8-16 mg twice a day	~6	Insignificant	2D6	ChE inhibitor
Memantine (Namenda)	20 mg in 2 divided doses	~60-80	~45	Not extensively metabolized	NMDA antagonist

ChE, Cholinesterase; *NMDA*, N-methyl-D-aspartate.

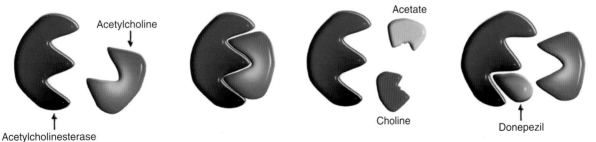

FIG 18-2 The same process as shown in Figure 18-1 is illustrated. However, AChE is inhibited from its metabolic activity by the AChE inhibitor donepezil *(last panel)*. ACh survives and builds up in the synapse. (Courtesy of Vicki Johnson. Modified from Lehne, R.A. [2003]. *Pharmacology for Nursing Care.* St. Louis: Saunders.)

doses has proven helpful to patients with moderate to severe AD (Singh & Grossberg, 2012). What is interesting is the dosage of the new tablet: 23 mg. See Box 18-2 for a view of this unusual formulation.

Rivastigmine

Rivastigmine (Exelon) was approved for treatment of AD in 2000. It also inhibits ChE but does so in a slightly different way than the previously described ChE inhibitors. Donepezil is a reversible inhibitor of ChE, whereas rivastigmine is said to be irreversible. Stated another way, donepezil slips off and on ChE continuously, whereas rivastigmine remains attached and forms a covalent bond with the enzyme. Rivastigmine remains effective until the life cycle of the enzyme is complete. Rivastigmine has a relatively short plasma half-life (about 2 hours) but has an inhibition half-life of 10 hours. Essentially, while attached irreversibly to ChE, rivastigmine is not factored into the plasma level.

Rivastigmine is not metabolized by cytochrome P-450 enzymes, so it does not interact with drugs metabolized by this system. In regard to this aspect of drug administration, rivastigmine has an advantage over tacrine and donepezil. Rivastigmine prefers AChE over BChE but still produces peripheral side effects (Alagiakrishnan et al., 2000).

Galantamine

Galantamine (Razadyne) is the last ChE inhibitor we discuss. It also demonstrates preference for AChE over BChE; however, the ability of galantamine to stimulate presynaptic muscarinic receptors to release more ACh sets it apart (Birks, 2006). As a result of this latter mechanism, galantamine produces a few more cholinergic side effects, such as gastrointestinal symptoms. An added feature with galantamine is its ability to modulate nicotinic receptors in the brain. As noted previously, nicotinic receptors are thought to play a role in cognitive activities. There is some evidence that galantamine might also provide neuroprotection by up-regulating neurotrophic factors such as bcl-2 via nicotinic receptors (Geerts, 2005; Robles, 2009). Such findings, if replicable, may give galantamine an advantage over other drugs in this class.

Galantamine is readily absorbed; it has a bioavailability of about 85% and a half-life of about 6 hours. It has a high volume of distribution and insignificant protein binding. It is metabolized by the cytochrome P-450 enzyme system, so it can interact with drugs catalyzed by this system.

Summary of Cholinesterase Inhibitors

Elevating ACh levels does not slow the disease process of AD or the other irreversible dementias. If one of these drugs is discontinued, the patient's cognitive abilities are what they would have been had the drug never been administered. These drugs, all approved for mild to moderate AD, help the patient preserve cognitive performance longer than if he or she had not taken the medication. Eventually, the underlying neurodegeneration becomes so profound that these efforts to bolster ACh no longer mask the devastation of the brain. If the observation that galantamine increases neuroprotective factors is correct, it would be the exception; however, there is little evidence at this time to suggest that non–ACh-enhancing mechanisms of these drugs have a significant impact on AD (Pepeu & Giovannini, 2009).

AGENTS THAT MAY RETARD NEURODEGENERATION

AD progressively marches through the brain, leaving dead neurons in its path. Although the analogy of a destroyer marching through the brain does not reflect exactly what occurs, it does come close.

Neurons probably die in several ways. One of these is what has been identified as *neuronal excitotoxicity*. Excitotoxicity, or very rapid firing of the neuron, is caused by aberrant (i.e., sustained) depolarization of the glutamate–N-methyl-D-aspartate receptor (NDMA) complex. Glutamate is an excitatory neurotransmitter, and NDMA is a glutamate receptor. Whenever this coupling causes too many neuronal firings, the neuron can die. One approach to preventing excitotoxicity is to give a drug that blocks NDMA receptors.

Memantine

Memantine (Namenda) is an NDMA antagonist (Figure 18-3). Although it is not completely understood, glutamate in a patient with AD becomes overactive and kills neurons (Singh & Grossberg, 2012). By blocking the NDMA receptor, memantine prevents glutamate from overstimulating it. This blockade results in a reduction in the number of depolarizations. However, in some cases, the neuron is permanently depolarized (rendering the neuron useless), and memantine restarts normal cell activity (Johnson & Kotermanski, 2006). Although the manufacturer of Namenda clearly states on the package insert that it (the manufacturer) does not claim the drug can slow neuronal degeneration, the implication is that it can (Keltner & Williams, 2004).

NDMA receptor antagonists are familiar to nurses in the emergency department because of the use of the drug phencyclidine (PCP). PCP is an NDMA antagonist. Users of the drug exhibit behaviors similar to those of paranoid schizophrenia. They are often violent and then, just as quickly, become nonviolent. The conundrum for the clinician is this: too much NDMA stimulation (i.e., excitotoxicity) can cause neuronal death, whereas too little (i.e., NDMA antagonism) can lead to psychotic behavior. Memantine is formulated so

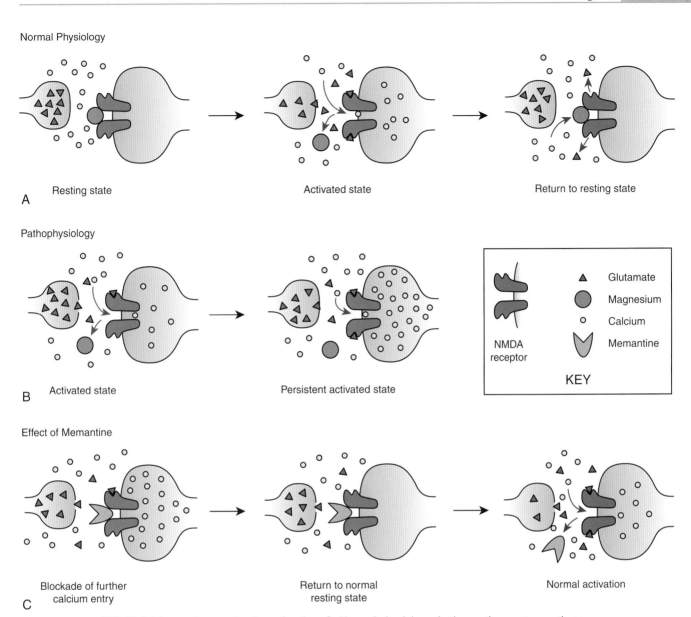

Normal Physiology

A   Resting state   Activated state   Return to resting state

Pathophysiology

B   Activated state   Persistent activated state

KEY

▲ Glutamate
● Magnesium
○ Calcium
▽ Memantine

NMDA receptor

Effect of Memantine

C   Blockade of further calcium entry   Return to normal resting state   Normal activation

FIG 18-3 Memantine mechanism of action. **A,** Normal physiology. In the resting postsynaptic neuron, magnesium occupies the *N*-methyl-ᴅ-aspartate (NMDA) receptor channel, blocking calcium entry. Binding of glutamate to the receptor displaces magnesium, allowing calcium to enter. When glutamate dissociates from the receptor, magnesium returns to the channel and blocks further calcium inflow. The brief period of calcium entry constitutes a "signal" in the learning and memory process. **B,** Pathophysiology. Slow but steady leakage of glutamate from the presynaptic neuron keeps the NMDA receptor in a constantly activated state, allowing excessive influx of calcium, which can impair memory and learning and can eventually cause neuronal death. **C,** Effect of memantine. Memantine blocks calcium entry when extracellular glutamate is low and stops further calcium entry, which allows intracellular calcium levels to normalize. When a burst of glutamate is released in response to an action potential, the resulting high level of glutamate is able to displace memantine, causing a brief period of calcium entry. When glutamate diffuses away, memantine reblocks the channel and stops further calcium entry, despite continuing low levels of glutamate in the synapse (not shown). (From Lehne, R.A. [2010]. *Pharmacology for Nursing Care.* St. Louis: Elsevier.)

that NDMA stimulation does not occur, and severe behavioral effects do not develop. This is a fine line for prescribers to walk. It is hoped that this explanation allows you to appreciate the risks and benefits involved in treating this devastating illness.

Memantine has a long half-life (60 to 80 hours), but it is not metabolized to a great degree. Most memantine is excreted unchanged. The latter property (i.e., not being metabolized) accounts for few drug interactions. Memantine is often co-prescribed with donepezil or other cholinesterase inhibitors (Singh & Grossberg, 2012). Studies indicate significantly slower rates of deterioration with this combination (Atri et al., 2008).

Memantine has few side effects of significance and few, if any, drug interactions. In contrast to the ChE inhibitors, it is approved by the FDA for moderate to severe AD.

Secretase Inhibitors

One of the explanations for neurodegeneration in AD is the festering of snipped off pieces of amyloid precursor proteins, which lead to neuronal death. This cutting is achieved by enzymes known as *secretases*. Secretase inhibition research is an evolving story; however, there is hope associated with these drugs because they get at the core of AD treatment: preventing neurodestruction (Pissarnitski, 2007; Rafii & Aisen, 2009). At the present time, many serious side effects are associated with these drugs. Chapter 28 provides greater detail about this pathologic process.

Dihydropyridine Calcium Channel Blockers

Dihydropyridine calcium channel blockers have recently been viewed as a possible new tool in the fight to treat Alzheimer's disease. (Motiwala, Ojike, & Lippmann, 2013). These drugs, including amlodipine (Norvasc), nilvadipine (Escor and others), and nitrendipine (Baypress), are antihypertensives. Hypertension causes small vessel changes, inflammation, and a compromise of the blood-brain barrier. In turn, these conditions may precede cognitive decline. Collectively dihydropyridines are thought to be able to reduce amyloid formation, reduce secretase activity, and reduce amyloid precursor proteins. Motiwala et al (2013) note that patients under the age of 75 taking antihypertensives decrease the probability of developing dementia by 8% each year.

DRUGS TO PREVENT ALZHEIMER'S DISEASE

Drugs used to treat AD are useful and widely prescribed, but they do not stop the destructive onslaught of the disorder (Sapra & Kim, 2009). That being the case, it is even more important to find means of preventing AD, if that is possible. Although no one knows with certainty whether the following drugs do prevent or forestall AD, evidence has suggested that they might. Because these drugs are benign in regard to severe consequences, they might be worth promoting in the hope that they might be preventive.

Nonsteroidal Antiinflammatory Drugs

Cyclooxygenase (COX) is an enzyme that synthesizes prostaglandins, which protect the stomach, promote platelet aggregation, and increase renal blood flow but also cause inflammation, pain, and fever. The positive effects mentioned are attributed to the enzymatic action of COX-1, whereas the negative effects are attributed to the enzymatic action of COX-2. COX-2 inhibitors have the potential to decrease inflammation and fever. Some researchers believe that one of the ways in which neurons die is related to a *low-burner*

inflammatory process. Studies have suggested a significant decline in the incidence of AD if these nonsteroidal antiinflammatory drugs (NSAIDs) are used on a regular basis. Other researchers are not convinced (Pasqualetti et al., 2009). There is some evidence that long-term use (>2 years) can play a preventive role if initiated 2 years before neurodegeneration begins (whether or not noticed by the family or patient). NSAIDs are of no value after the disease passes this critical point.

Statins

In the last 20 years or so, the use of statin drugs to reduce elevated cholesterol levels has skyrocketed. Some clinicians believe that there is a relationship between high cholesterol levels and AD. If their theory is correct, statins, with their cholesterol-lowering potential, might provide dual benefits.

Estrogen

Some researchers believe that the decrease in the estrogen level after menopause increases the risk of women developing AD. Studies have suggested that women taking estrogen reduce their risk of developing AD. However, more recent studies confirm that estrogen does not reduce the risk of AD. Decreased estrogen levels have also been associated with increased risk of heart attacks and other cardiovascular complications.

B, D, and E Vitamins

An elevated serum level of homocysteine, an amino acid, is thought to be associated with AD (Selley, 2004). The higher the blood level of homocysteine, the greater the association. Because deficiency of three B vitamins (B_6, B_{12}, and folic acid [a form of B_9]) is linked to an elevated homocysteine level, some clinicians have attempted to prevent AD by prescribing these vitamins. B vitamins are required for monoamine production, DNA synthesis, and maintenance of phospholipids (Ramsey & Muskin, 2013). Logic suggests that adequate levels of B vitamins could be restorative. However, at this time, there is no conclusive evidence that taking these B vitamins slows or prevents AD. Vitamin D deficiency has been linked to cognitive dysfunction. Foods high in vitamin D (e.g., salmon, tuna, beef, liver, milk) are thought to be helpful in stopping cognitive decline (LaFerney, 2012). Vitamin E has also been promoted as effective in treating AD. However, more recent evidence has refuted that assertion (Lehne, 2010).

? CRITICAL THINKING QUESTIONS

1. Why can a large dose of Benadryl cause fuzzy thinking in an older adult?
2. If someone you know has been diagnosed with Alzheimer's disease, would it be a good idea for them to start taking an NSAID?

STUDY NOTES

1. Drugs used to treat dementias can be categorized as (a) drugs for treatment of dementia and (b) drugs for prevention of dementia.

2. The causes of AD can be broadly grouped as (a) neuronal death and (b) neurotransmitter deficiency.

3. The most common drug interventions restore deficient neurotransmitters.

4. The primary neurotransmitter deficiency is ACh.

5. Agents that restore ACh levels do so by blocking the enzyme that metabolizes ACh.

6. ChEs break down ACh. The two types are (a) AChe and (b) BChE.

7. Antidementia drugs attach to ChEs and prevent them from bonding to and subsequently metabolizing ACh.

8. Three drugs are available that are identified as ChE (or AChE or BChE) inhibitors: donepezil, rivastigmine, and galantamine.

9. Memantine is an NMDA receptor inhibitor and has a different mechanism of action.

10. Theoretically, memantine could prevent neuronal death.

11. Other drugs are used to prevent dementias.

12. NSAIDs; statins; estrogen; and B, D, and E vitamins are used to prevent AD. However, much research remains to be carried out before such claims can be broadly accepted.

REFERENCES

Alagiakrishnan, K., Wong, W., & Blanchette, P. L. (2000). Use of donepezil in elderly patients with Alzheimer's disease—A Hawaii-based study. *Hawaii Medical Journal, 59,* 57.

Atri, A., et al. (2008). Long-term course and effectiveness of combination therapy in Alzheimer disease. *Alzheimer Disease and Associated Disorders, 22,* 209.

Birks, J. (2006). Cholinesterase inhibitors for Alzheimer's disease. *Cochrane Database of Systematic Reviews, 1,* CD005593.

Geerts, H. (2005). Indicators of neuroprotection with galantamine. *Brain Research Bulletin, 64,* 519.

Geldmacher, D. S. (1997). Donepezil (Aricept) therapy for Alzheimer's disease. *Comprehensive Therapy, 23,* 492.

Johnson, J. W., & Kotermanski, S. E. (2006). Mechanisms of action of memantine. *Current Opinion in Pharmacology, 6,* 61.

Keltner, N. L. (1994). Tacrine: A pharmacological approach to Alzheimer's disease. *Journal of Psychosocial and Mental Health Nursing Services, 32*(3), 37.

Keltner, N. L., & Lillie, K. (2009). Nicotinic receptors: Implications for psychiatric care. *Perspectives in Psychiatric Care, 45,* 151.

Keltner, N. L., & Williams, B. (2004). Memantine: A new approach to Alzheimer's disease. *Perspectives in Psychiatric Care, 40,* 123.

Kuehn, B. M. (2006). Link between smoking and mental illness may lead to treatments. *JAMA, 295,* 483.

LaFerney, M. C. (2012). Vitamin D deficiency in older adults. *Current Psychiatry, 11,* 63.

Lehne, R. A. (2010). *Pharmacology for nursing care.* St. Louis: Saunders.

Miller, M. C. (2005). What is the amygdala and what are its functions? *The Harvard Mental Health Letter, 21,* 8.

Miller, M. C. (2008). Helping psychiatric patients to stop smoking. *The Harvard Mental Health Letter, 25,* 4.

Motiwala, F., Ojike, N., & Lippmann, S. (2013). Dihydropyridine calcium channel blockers in dementia and hypertension. *Current Psychiatry, 12,* 41.

Pasqualetti, P., et al. (2009). A randomized controlled study on effects of ibuprofen on cognitive progression of Alzheimer's disease. *Aging Clinical and Experimental Research, 21,* 102.

Pepeu, G., & Giovannini, M. G. (2009). Cholinesterase inhibitors and beyond. *Current Alzheimer Research, 6,* 86.

Pissarnitski, D. (2007). Advances in gamma-secretase modulation. *Current Opinion in Drug Discovery & Development, 10,* 392.

Purves, D., et al. (1997). *Neuroscience.* Sunderland, MA: Sinauer Associates.

Rafii, M. S., & Aisen, P. S. (2009). Recent developments in Alzheimer's disease therapeutics. *BMC Medicine, 7,* 7.

Ramsey, D., & Muskin, P. R. (2013). Vitamin deficiencies and mental health: How are they linked? *Current Psychiatry, 12,* 37.

Robles, A. (2009). Pharmacological treatment of Alzheimer's disease: Is it progressing adequately? *The Open Neurology Journal, 3,* 27.

Sapra, M., & Kim, K. Y. (2009). Anti-amyloid treatments in Alzheimer's disease. *Recent Patents on CNS Drug Discovery, 4,* 143.

Schwartz, L. M., & Woloshin, S. (2012). How the FDA forgot the evidence: The case of donepezil 23 mg. *BMJ, 344,* e1086.

Selley, M. L. (2004). Increased homocysteine and decreased adenosine formation in Alzheimer's disease. *Neurological Research, 26,* 554.

Singh, I., & Grossberg, G. T. (2012). High-dose donepezil or memantine: Next step for Alzheimer's disease? *Current Psychiatry, 11,* 20.

Over-the-Counter Drugs

Aida J. Sapp*

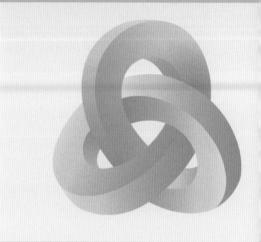

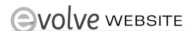 WEBSITE

http://evolve.elsevier.com/Keltner

LEARNING OBJECTIVES

- Define alternative therapy.
- Trace the historical use of alternative therapies and over-the-counter drugs to their current state of use.
- Name common natural products, herbs, and dietary supplements used for psychiatric symptoms, and discuss current research conclusions regarding their efficacy.

- Describe how natural products, herbs, and dietary supplements are regulated.
- Name three dangerous interactions with over-the-counter drugs or herbal medicines.
- Explain the role of the nurse in assessment and intervention with patients using natural products, herbs, and dietary supplements.

Over 100,000 over-the-counter drugs (OTC) and drug products are available today (U.S. Food and Drug Administration, 2012a). A comprehensive survey on use by Americans of alternative and complementary therapies has continued to provide data from which other studies have emerged (Table 19-1) (Barnes et al., 2004; Barnes, et al., 2008). In addition to herbal medicines and food supplements, the wide range of nonpharmacologic options includes acupuncture, aromatherapy, yoga, biofeedback, relaxation, meditation, and hypnosis (Werneke, 2009). Each year, $27 billion is spent on alternative therapies (Barnes et al., 2004; Institute of Medicine, 2005). This figure is remarkable, considering that most of this money is an out-of-pocket expense, not usually reimbursed by health insurance (Snyder & Lindquist, 2001). According to Nahin and colleagues (2009), expenditures have continued to increase slightly as noted in a 2007 National Health Interview Survey, which reported approximately $34 billion spent on complementary and alternative medicine (CAM), of which approximately $14.8 billion accounted for nonvitamin, nonmineral natural products (typically herbs). Of the world's population, 80% rely on therapies called *alternative* in the United States (Folks & Gabel, 2001) but that are mainstream in other countries (Yarnell & Abascal, 2004). Estimates have suggested that one of three consumers

in the United States uses alternative therapies in one form or another. Kaufman and associates (2002) found that 16% of users of prescription medication also took at least one herb or supplement, with the incidence (22%) being highest among users of fluoxetine. Reasons Americans choose to use natural products, herbs, and dietary supplements include the belief that improved health can be attained in combination with conventional medical treatments, the desire to try an interesting therapy, the belief that conventional medical treatment will not help, taking the suggestion of a conventional health care professional to try a complementary or alternative therapy, and the expense of conventional medical treatments (National Center for Complementary and Alternative Medicine, 2007).

Among people using alternative therapies along with traditional medicine, fewer than 50% disclose this use to their health care provider (Robinson & McGrail, 2004). Because alternative therapies might interact with traditional therapies and might have their own side effects, it is important for the health care provider to know whether a patient is using these therapies. Equally important is the knowledge of the health care provider regarding the use of OTCs by the patient. Interestingly, older adults are the largest consumers of OTC medications according to Qato and colleagues (2008).

*This chapter is a revision of the text originally written by Beverly Hogan and previously rewritten by Teena M. McGuinness.

TABLE 19-1	**SUMMARY OF STUDIES CITED IN CHAPTER**
Herbals	
St. John's wort	Beaubrun & Gray, 2000
	Knuppel & Linde, 2004
	Linde & Knuppel, 2005
	Sarris & Kavanagh, 2009
Kava	Anke & Ramzan, 2004a
	Sarris & Kavanagh, 2009
Valerian	Agins & Lehne, 2004
	Glass et al., 2003
	Hallam et al., 2003
	Malva et al., 2004
Ginkgo	Abascal & Yarnell, 2004b
	Beaubrun & Gray, 2000
Omega-3 fatty acids	Cronin, 2004
	Fenton et al., 2001
	Hallahan & Garland, 2004
	Harris et al., 2004
	Joy et al., 2000
	Meletis & Barker, 2004
	Silvers et al., 2005

Models of enhanced communication regarding working with patients who use traditional medicine and CAM have been proposed (National Center for Complementary and Alternative Medicine, 2012; Shelley et al., 2009). From the patient perspective, necessary attributes to be demonstrated by the health care professional include openness, respect, and interest. Characteristically, the use of these treatments is motivated by cultural identity, family history, and proximity to home. In addition, there is a need for the health care professional to initiate the discussion about alternative treatments and have awareness that these treatments can still be clinical and evidence-based. Lastly, the health care professional need not be a content expert (Shelley et al., 2009). Nurses need to know about these therapies to provide culturally competent care and obtain essential information (Hsu et al., 2009; McDowell & Burman, 2004; Snyder & Lindquist, 2001).

NORM'S NOTES
This is a hot topic and presents a moving target. It is almost impossible to keep up with the various claims being made on late night or early morning television. Some of these agents or remedies really work. As for the others, you can hardly tell what works. Maybe they work for some people and not for others. I think the author of this chapter has done a good job of selecting the therapies that have some support. Nurses should know something about them.

Consumers of mental health services are also seeking alternative treatments (Parslow & Jorm, 2004; Simon et al., 2004; Werneke, 2009). The most commonly used herbs are for mental health–related symptoms (Beaubrun & Gray, 2000). Most people in the United States with self-defined anxiety attacks or severe depression use some form of natural products, herbs, and dietary supplements to treat these conditions.

Most users of CAM do not report their use, suggesting that herbals are being used to augment prescribed psychotropic medicine (Kessler et al., 2001; Parslow & Jorm, 2004).

This chapter uses the term *alternative* to refer to therapies that are not generally accepted by conventional Western medicine. The term *complementary therapy* is used to refer to treatments used in conjunction with conventional Western medicine. These therapies are referred to together as *CAM therapies* (Box 19-1).

BACKGROUND

The alternative health movement arose from concerns about the effects of stress on health. A proliferation of research and the development of the new field of psychoneuroimmunology resulted. These scientifically based findings brought about a renewed interest in mind-body interactions. A dissatisfied yet receptive consumer waited.

The growing popularity of alternative treatments attracted the attention of many special-interest groups and eventually resulted in the creation by the federal government of the Office of Alternative Medicine. The mission of the Office of Alternative Medicine was to provide the public with information regarding the safety and efficacy of these therapies. The U.S. Food and Drug Administration (FDA) was unable to regulate herbals because herbs were classified as dietary and nutritional supplements. In 1994, the FDA, as a result of the Dietary Supplement and Health Education Act (DSHEA), was able to require labeling on herbals, stating that there was "no proof of efficacy, safety, or standards for quality control" (Dietary Supplement Health and Education Act of 1994, 2005). As herbals and other alternative therapies continued to gain popularity in the United States, the Office of Alternative Medicine, as a division of the National Institutes of Health (NIH), broadened its scope to include research as an objective and was renamed the National Center for Complementary and Alternative Medicine (NCCAM). One directive of the NCCAM is to fund research into the efficacy and safety of alternative treatments.

BOX 19-1	**RESOURCES FOR LEARNING MORE ABOUT COMPLEMENTARY AND ALTERNATIVE MEDICINE AND THERAPIES**

- American Botanical Council. <www.herbalgram.org>
- Herb Research Foundation. <www.herbs.org>
- U.S. Food and Drug Administration. <www.fda.gov>
- National Center for Complementary and Alternative Medicine, National Institutes of Health. <www.nccam.nih/gov>
- Cochrane Collaboration.* <http://www.cochrane.org>
- Kush, R.D., et al. (2007). *Physician's desk reference for herbal medicines* (4th ed.). Montvale, NJ: Thomson PDR.
- Skidmore-Roth, L. (2009). *Mosby's handbook of herbs and natural supplements* (4th ed.). St. Louis: Mosby.

*Ongoing registry of randomized controlled trials related to complementary and alternative medicine.

The remainder of this chapter focuses on biologically based therapies and general concerns related to CAM.

HERBAL THERAPIES

Herbs include plant roots, tree barks, berries, leaves, resins, and flowers. Herbal therapy has been used for centuries and was referred to in the writings of Hippocrates. Although 30% of all modern drugs are derived from plants, only 1% of plants have been analyzed for their potential medicinal uses. Other cultures have known the value of various herbs for treating particular conditions, and some have developed a wide knowledge base, although it would not be considered scientific by our standards (Mikhail et al., 2004). However, whether or not scientifically supported, herbal medicine use is an important part of the health beliefs of many people.

In the United States, 20% of people use herbs for chronic conditions. Most herbs are generally not recommended for use in pregnancy, and some are known abortifacients (Folks & Gabel, 2001). A common misconception associated with herbals is that "natural" equals not harmful. There are numerous reports in medical and scientific journals of severe reactions to herbs, including liver failure, renal failure, gastrointestinal tract obstruction, cardiac arrhythmias, seizure exacerbation, development of psychiatric symptoms, and fatalities (Clough et al., 2004; Ernst, 2004). The variability of herbal preparations and their impurities make adverse reactions possible and unpredictable. Although many people in other parts of the world have used herbals safely for thousands of years, commercial preparations in the United States might not be equivalent. Some authors have suggested that the time has come for a new way to report reactions, such as reliable online information and a feedback system (Peters et al., 2003). In particular, reports and investigations should focus on the responses of sensitive subpopulations, such as pregnant women, young individuals, and older adults (Chui et al., 2013; NTP Herbal Medicine Fact Sheet, 2003).

Four of the 12 most common herbs are used to treat or prevent psychiatric symptoms (Beaubrun & Gray, 2000). Herbals are among the most frequently tried alternative therapies for depression (Ernst, 1998; Linde et al., 2005; Parslow & Jorm, 2004). Table 19-2 summarizes herbals used for psychiatric symptoms. The use of herbal preparations for mental health–related symptoms is apparently so common that it has been called part of the hidden mental health network (Simon et al., 2004).

A noteworthy caveat from a study examining the lay public's preference for treatment of mental health–related

TABLE 19-2   COMMON HERBS USED TO TREAT PSYCHIATRIC SYMPTOMS

HERBAL PRODUCT	CONTRAINDICATIONS	ADVERSE SIDE EFFECTS	DRUG INTERACTIONS
Angelica	Diabetes Peptic ulcer disase Bleeding disorders Pregnancy Breast-feeding	CV: Decreased BP GI: Anorexia, flatulence, spasms, dyspepsia Integumentary: Photosensitivity, phototoxicity, dermatitis	Increased PTT with anticoagulants
Chamomile	Known abortifacient Cross-sensitivity to sunflowers, ragweed, and members of aster family (Echinacea)	Hypersensitivity—allergic reactions Burning of face, mouth, eyes, and mucous membranes	Anticoagulants Increases effects of CNS drugs
Ginkgo biloba	Pregnancy Breast-feeding Peptic ulcer disease and other bleeding problems	Headache, anxiety, restlessness	Trazodone
Kava (Piper methysticum)	Hepatotoxicity (?) Liver failure (?)	Scaling, yellowing of skin Overdose	Antiparkinsonian agents Benzodiazepines CNS depressants
Melatonin			More data needed
St. John's wort (Hypericum perforatum)	Pregnancy Breast-feeding	Dizziness, insomnia, restlessness, constipation, abdominal cramps, photosensitivity	Protease inhibitors Olanzapine (Zyprexa) Oral contraceptives
Valerian (Valeriana officinalis)	Pregnancy Breast-feeding	Dependence	MAOIs, Warfarin, Phenytoin

BP, Blood pressure; CNS, central nervous system; CV, cardiovascular; GI, gastrointestinal; MAOIs, monoamine oxidase inhibitors; PTT, prothrombin time.
From Keltner, N., & Folks, D. (2005). Drugs used in alternative and complementary medicine.

symptoms did *not* identify treatment with psychotropic medication or visiting a psychiatrist as the first choice (except in the case of schizophrenia). Instead, alternative therapies or psychotherapy were more likely to be recommended (Riedel-Heller et al., 2005). This is a topic of importance in a psychiatric mental health nursing course.

HERBALS TO TREAT ANXIETY AND DEPRESSION

St. John's Wort

St. John's wort (*Hypericum perforatum*) is a popular treatment for mild to moderate depression; it is also used to treat anxiety, seasonal affective disorder, and sleep disorders. The herb is available in capsule, tea, or tincture form. St. John's wort is among the top-selling botanical products in the United States. Because its efficacy is firmly established, it is expected to continue to be in even greater demand because of having fewer and less severe side effects compared with traditional antidepressant drugs (Linde et al., 2005; National Center for Complementary and Alternative Medicine, 2013; Sarris et al., 2011).

Although no consensus exists regarding the mechanism of action for St. John's wort, it is thought to have an affinity for many neurotransmitters (Keltner & Folks, 2005). Several mechanisms of action have been proposed, including the following:

- Inhibition of monoamine (serotonin, dopamine, and norepinephrine) reuptake
- Modulation of interleukin-6 activity

Increases in the levels of interleukin-6, a protein involved in intercellular communication in the immune system, might lead to increases in adrenal regulatory hormones such as cortisol (elevated cortisol is associated with depression; see Chapter 25) (Folks & Gable, 2001).

An analysis of 23 European clinical studies of St. John's wort concluded that it has antidepressive effects in cases of mild to moderate depression (the dose varied considerably among the studies) (Linde & Knuppel, 2005). These studies compared St. John's wort with tricyclic antidepressants but not the newer antidepressants. More recent studies have shown inconsistent and mixed results with regard to its effectiveness (Hicks et al., 2004; Knuppel & Linde, 2004; Linde & Knuppel, 2005). Studies compared St. John's wort with selective serotonin reuptake inhibitors (SSRIs), showing similarity in effectiveness (Szegedi et al., 2005; vanGurp et al., 2002). Given the number of prescriptions written annually for SSRIs, St. John's wort is a potential contender for treating less severe forms of depression.

St. John's wort is generally safe, with most side effects emerging at dose ranges exceeding those recommended for depression. There have been case reports of St. John's wort exacerbating mania. It might increase the risk for serotonin syndrome and should not be taken with other antidepressants, particularly SSRIs (Beaubrun & Gray, 2000; Zhou et al., 2004).

St. John's wort is thought to induce an increase in cytochrome P450 3A4 levels, potentially speeding the metabolism of many drugs. For example, it decreases blood levels of protease inhibitors, such as those used in treatment of HIV infection (Folks & Gabel, 2001; Skidmore-Roth, 2009). The mechanisms for many other interactions have not been clearly elucidated, intensifying the need for health care providers to be aware of patients taking this herbal (Hoblyn & Brooks, 2005; Zhou et al., 2004). Some reports have suggested that St. John's wort might reduce the effectiveness of oral contraceptives, increasing the risk of pregnancy (Ayd, 2000; Zhou et al., 2004).

St. John's wort appears to be efficacious in the treatment of mild to moderate depression (Saeed et al., 2009; Sarris et al., 2011); its use in severe depression *cannot* be recommended (Beaubrun & Gray, 2000; Knuppel & Linde, 2004; Linde & Knuppel, 2005). There is a high potential for interactions with conventional and herbal medicines. It was not shown to improve symptoms of attention-deficit/hyperactivity disorder in a randomized controlled trial (Weber et al., 2008).

S-Adenosyl-ʟ-methionine

S-Adenosyl-ʟ-methionine (SAM-e) has been shown to be effective for depression associated with HIV infection (Shippy et al., 2004). SAM-e is widely used in Europe and is popular in the United States. Numerous studies have suggested SAM-e to be useful as an adjunct or sole therapy for depression (Brown et al., 1999). One study from Harvard University found that SAM-e augmented antidepressant response in nonresponders to conventional antidepressants (Alpert et al., 2004). SAM-e received support in 2005 when the U.S. Agency for Healthcare Research and Quality concluded that it worked as well as antidepressant drugs in providing partial relief of symptoms (Agency for Healthcare Research and Quality, 2002). In addition to a having a faster onset of antidepressant effect than standard SSRIs or selective serotonin-norepinephrine reuptake inhibitors (Saeed et al., 2009), SAM-e is safe, with no evidence of hepatotoxicity or adverse drug interactions (Michoulon as quoted in Schardt, 2009). Clinical data for SAM-e are strongly suggestive of antidepressant efficacy, but until more rigorously generated data become available, it is impossible to reach a definitive conclusion (Carpenter, 2011).

Kava

Kava is part of traditional religious and social ceremonies in Polynesia and other Pacific islands. Kava is prized for its ability to soothe the worried mind. The active ingredients are kava-kava pyrones, which are thought to inhibit monoamine oxidase B (Uebelhack et al., 1998). Kava has also been assumed to have an affinity for benzodiazepine receptors (Folks & Gabel, 2001), explaining its effectiveness in reducing anxiety.

However, kava interacts with antiparkinsonian drugs, benzodiazepines, and other drugs that act on the central nervous system (Skidmore-Roth, 2009). Long-term or heavy use may result in scaly, yellowed skin (Keltner & Folks, 2005; McEnany, 2001; National Center for Complementary and Alternative Medicine, 2013). There was widespread panic when reports of kava causing liver failure were publicized in the media, but these reports have not resulted in fewer sales (Mills et al., 2004). As a result of concern regarding hepatotoxicity, sales of kava have been banned in Germany, Canada, Switzerland, and France but not in the United States (Agins & Lehne, 2004). There are some indications that hepatotoxicity was secondary to kava's potent inhibition of the cytochrome P-450 enzyme systems, increasing the likelihood of interactions with other herbals or conventional medications, which were the real culprits (Anke & Ramzan, 2004a, 2004b; Clouatre, 2004; Hoblyn & Brooks, 2005). Other reports have indicated that liver problems are rare when kava is used alone and that liver enzyme levels return to baseline after discontinuation of kava (Clough et al., 2003). However, reports of sudden death (Clough et al., 2004) and acute hepatotoxicity (hepatitis and liver failure) indicate the need for caution (Estes et al., 2003; National Center for Complementary and Alternative Medicine, 2013). In a comprehensive review of kava for evidence of efficacy, the treatment of generalized anxiety was supported (Sarris & Kavanagh, 2009).

Kava has been used for many years by people around the world with apparent safety. However, care is urged because NCCAM-funded studies on kava were suspended after the FDA issued a warning that using kava supplements had been linked to a risk of hepatotoxicity.

Clinical Example

Sherry S., a 26-year-old African-American woman, was admitted to the psychiatric unit for depression with psychotic features. Sherry received a 1-mg injection of lorazepam (Ativan) in the emergency department. On admission to the unit, Sherry was noted to have slurred speech, poor coordination, and slow responses. Sherry has not been on any scheduled or prescribed medications, but the nurse found a bottle of kava among Sherry's belongings. Sherry's excessive response to the lorazepam was most likely a result of her concomitant use of the herbal preparation kava.

Valerian

More than 250 different species of valerian are native to Europe and Asia. The variety used for anxiety comes from the plant *Valeriana officinalis*. Considerable difference exists in the potency of valerian, depending on the manufacturing process. It has been shown to be effective in decreasing sleep latency, nocturnal awakening, and a subjective sense of good sleep (Beaubrun & Gray, 2000). There is some indication that the sedative effect develops slowly over a period of weeks (Agins & Lehne, 2004). Valerian has an affinity for gamma-aminobutyric acid (GABA) A and serotonin 1A receptors (Keltner & Folks, 2005). Valerian has been studied extensively for its effectiveness in relieving anxiety. In a direct

comparison with triazolam (Halcion), temazepam (Restoril), and diphenhydramine (Benadryl), valerian provided equivalent anxiolytic benefit with a slightly better side effect profile (Glass et al., 2003; Hallam et al., 2003). There are also preliminary reports of a possible neuroprotective function for valerian (Malva et al., 2004; Taibi et al., 2004).

Possible adverse effects of valerian include enhancing the effects of other central nervous system–acting drugs and negating the effects of other drugs, including monoamine oxidase inhibitors, warfarin, and phenytoin (Skidmore-Roth, 2009). There have been some indications that the valepotriate content of valerian has possible carcinogenic effects. *V. officinalis*, the most commonly purchased form of valerian, has the lowest concentration of valepotriate (Taibi et al., 2004). Valerian must be protected from light and moisture, or its effectiveness is altered (Keltner & Folks, 2005).

Valerian appears to be useful for anxiety and insomnia; however, some clinicians urge caution regarding potential dependence and withdrawal. Studies suggest that it is generally safe to use for short periods, such as 4 to 6 weeks; no information is available regarding its long-term safety (National Center for Complementary and Alternative Medicine, 2012). Based on the notion that valerian effects are mediated by GABA, caution is indicated with regard to preanesthetic use as well (Yuan et al., 2004).

ANXIOLYTIC HERBALS WITHOUT SUFFICIENT EVIDENCE OF EFFICACY AND SAFETY

Multiple studies have demonstrated the ability of chamomile to promote relaxation and sleep and decrease anxiety (Skidmore-Roth, 2009). In a study of the effect of 300 mg/kg of chamomile administered to laboratory rats, a decreased sleep latency was observed (Shinomiya et al., 2005), suggesting that the reported effects of chamomile as a hypnotic are probably valid. However, there is no clear scientific evidence to support the use of chamomile at this time.

Several studies have shown angelica to cause significant muscle relaxation without changes in level of consciousness. At the present time, studies on the use of angelica for specific psychiatric disorders are insufficient, but it remains a promising herb for treating anxiety because of its potential to facilitate relaxation without also impairing cognition and motor behavior. In laboratory testing, angelica essential oils decreased aggressive behavior and increased social interaction in mice (Min et al., 2005). There is insufficient evidence of efficacy and safety for the use of angelica at the present time.

HERBALS FOR MEMORY AND DEMENTIA

Ginkgo

As one of the top-selling herbs in the United States, *Ginkgo biloba* showed initial promise in improving memory, concentration, and mood in patients with dementia. However, an NIH-funded study of the ginkgo product EGb-761 found that it did not produce a significant decrease in the incidence of dementia and Alzheimer's disease in elderly adults. A large study called the Ginkgo Evaluation of Memory evaluated 3000 volunteers 75 years old and older who took 240 mg of ginkgo daily; they were evaluated on a regular basis for about 6 years (National Center for Complementary and Alternative Medicine, 2008). Ginkgo did not slow cognitive decline.

Ginkgo has also been used as an antidote to treat erectile dysfunction caused by antidepressants. Ginkgo helps modulate vascular tone and decreases thrombosis by antagonizing the platelet-activating factor; it might increase the effects of anticoagulants and should be used with caution in patients with potential bleeding problems, such as peptic ulcer disease (Folks & Gabel, 2001; Skidmore-Roth, 2009). Of particular concern with regard to interactions is the fact that older adults often take multiple drugs, increasing the risk of an interaction if they are also taking ginkgo. For example, ginkgo interacts with several psychotropic drugs, aspirin, ibuprofen, some antihypertensives, and cardiovascular drugs (Bressler, 2005). Close monitoring is required for patients taking other medications because of the potential for interaction.

HERBALS THAT MIGHT CAUSE PROBLEMS FOR PATIENTS RECEIVING PSYCHIATRIC CARE

- Ginseng can exacerbate mania and precipitate acute anxiety and insomnia.
- Evening primrose can exacerbate mania.
- Yohimbine (often taken for its ability to stimulate sexual excitation) can cause nervousness, irritability, and insomnia.
- Reports have suggested that severe extrapyramidal symptoms have been seen after heavy betel nut consumption in patients on neuroleptics (Ayd, 2000).
- Herbals are known to interact with certain drugs and raise a concern for patients taking drugs with a narrow therapeutic window, such as tricyclic antidepressants and lithium (Hatcher, 2001).

Clinical Example

Thomas J. is a 76-year-old African-American man who has been on a maintenance dosage of warfarin (Coumadin) since he underwent open heart surgery 6 months ago. Thomas was admitted to the general medical unit with an abnormal prothrombin time. During assessment of his medication adherence practices, Thomas tells the nurse practitioner that he takes ginkgo for his memory. The treatment team was able to make appropriate dosage adjustments for the warfarin and further evaluated his complaints about his memory.

VITAMIN, MINERAL, AND NUTRITIONAL SUPPLEMENT THERAPIES

Melatonin

Several studies have demonstrated the efficacy of melatonin in reducing sleep onset latency and the number of nocturnal awakenings. Some promising studies have been conducted on the use of melatonin in resynchronizing the biologic clock and preventing what has been called *ICU syndrome* (i.e., delirium, psychosis) (Arendt, 2005; McEnany, 2001).

Some authors have attributed some depressive symptoms to an excessive avoidance of the sun, an extreme no more helpful than overexposure (Horowitz, 2004). Sunlight is essential for the body's production of vitamin D and affects levels of melatonin, which are important for regulating circadian rhythms. Seasonal affective disorder, thought to be related to altered sunlight and melatonin levels, has been effectively treated by sunlight or full-spectrum lighting. Melatonin might have some role in the treatment of seasonal affective disorder as well as sleep disorders (Arendt, 2005).

Vitamins C and E

Although neither vitamin C nor vitamin E alone shows a protective benefit in preventing Alzheimer's disease, there might be a synergistic effect if the two are taken together (Zandi & Anthony, 2004). Vitamin E is frequently recommended for patients with tardive dyskinesia.

Folate, Niacin, Pyridoxine, and Zinc

Numerous psychiatric disorders have been associated with vitamin and mineral deficiencies. Decreased folate levels have been associated with lowered response rates to standard antidepressant pharmacotherapy. Studies have shown that augmentation with a folate supplement increases medication response in both treatment-naïve and treatment-resistant depressed patients regardless of whether or not they have folate deficiency (Morris et al., 2008). However, a challenge in research methodology with folate is the impact of routine fortification in diets on the effects observed in studies of supplementation (Freeman et al., 2010). Vitamin B deficiency (particularly niacin and pyroxidine) has been associated with anxiety, and zinc deficiency is linked to attention-deficit/hyperactivity disorder (Coppen & Bolander-Gouaille, 2005; Meletis & Barker, 2004; Sachdev et al., 2005; Tiemeier et al., 2003).

Omega-3 Fatty Acids

The interest in essential fatty acids (EFAs) began when the observation was made that people living in areas where fish constitutes a large portion of their diet have a lower incidence of disease. Omega-3 and omega-6 EFAs have now been well established as essential for normal functioning of the nervous system. Research has shown that the ratio of these EFAs is important for proper neurotransmitter function and other brain neuronal activity. Although the exact ratio has not been agreed on, it is generally accepted that a typical Western diet contains far greater amounts of omega-6 EFAs and smaller amounts of omega-3 EFAs, disrupting the balance considered optimal for neuronal and brain function. Apparently, omega-6 EFAs, in the absence of at least an equivalent amount of omega-3 EFAs, can promote an inflammatory response, with oxidative damage to cell membranes, increasing the likelihood of several diseases. The FDA has already endorsed fish oil supplementation, a source of omega-3 EFAs, for its cardiovascular benefits (U.S. Food and Drug Administration, 2004).

Four studies have demonstrated positive results in ameliorating depression after 2 or more weeks of omega-3 supplementation. A potentially beneficial antidepressant effect may occur, especially for individuals with low serum EFA. In addition, omega-3 may aid patients with comorbid cardiovascular disease, which has increased risk in depression. However, precautions must be taken with high dosages, which may increase international normalized ratio values and create significant implications for individuals taking warfarin (Sarris et al., 2010).

Problems with lipid metabolism have been suggested in both bipolar disorder and schizophrenia (Cronin, 2004). Clinical studies with psychiatric patients have shown decreased levels of omega-3 EFAs and some improvement in symptoms with supplementation (Harris et al., 2004). Early results from a few trials also suggested a positive effect of omega-3 EFAs over placebo for clinical outcomes in patients with schizophrenia (Fenton et al., 2001; Joy et al., 2000, 2003). The benefit of this type of supplementation in patients with schizophrenia continues to be promising (Meletis & Barker, 2004). Patients with subacute mania treated with omega-3 EFAs had significantly longer periods of remission compared with a placebo group (Stoll et al., 1999). Beneficial effects for depression and schizophrenia have also been observed (Stoll, 2001). Some studies failed to find a significant improvement with supplemental fish oil compared with antidepressant therapy alone (Silvers et al., 2005). Questions remain regarding dosing; however, there is a benign side effect profile with occasional reports of diarrhea or gastrointestinal upset (Saeed et al., 2009).

The psychiatric conditions of attention-deficit/hyperactivity disorder and borderline personality disorder as well as the phenomena of deliberate self-harm and violence have been ameliorated by the supplementation of EFAs in numerous clinical trials (Hallahan & Garland, 2004). Also, what these disorders share in common is impulsivity, a behavior known to be associated with low cerebrospinal fluid levels of serotonin. Supplementation with fish oil, which is high in omega-3 EFAs, is thought to increase available serotonin and reduce impulsivity, particularly aggression (Hallahan & Garland, 2004).

GENERAL CONCERNS REGARDING HERBS AND SUPPLEMENTS

Safety and Efficacy of Herbals

The method of manufacture of herbals determines the potency of an herb. Herbal concentration and dose potency are highly dependent on several factors, for which there can be great variability (St. John's wort and the Treatment of Depression, 2007). Although the American Herbal Association and the American Botanical Council have attempted to regulate safety, there is currently no guarantee of purity or standardization of herbal products. A *Los Angeles Times* survey indicated that 3 of 10 herbal products contained only half the potency listed on the product label (Beaubrun & Gray, 2000; Hatcher, 2001; Snyder & Lindquist, 2001).

Although safety and purity of herbal preparations should be standardized for consistency, one has only to watch television or see billboards along the highway advertising FDA-approved medicines that have been recalled, removed from the market, or studied with excess industry bias. Some authors believe that there are inconsistent standards applied to herbals (Kirsch, 2003). Strong feelings abound regarding the need for conventional medicine to have control of herbal medicines; for example, Agins and Lehne (2004) emphatically stated:

> It's time for the scientific community to stop giving alternative therapy a free ride. There cannot be two kinds of medicine—conventional and alternative. There is only medicine that has been adequately tested and medicine that may or may not work …. If it is found to be reasonably safe and effective, it will be accepted. (p. 1139)

It might be useful to remember that it was the medical community who rejected these remedies in the first place, and whether or not medical practitioners believe them useful, people will take them anyway. Apparently, the solution to this threat is regulation. A lack of control and a feeling of powerlessness led many consumers to look outside conventional medicine in the first place. Previously grandfathered in the DSHEA, the use of herbs is now threatened by efforts to restrict the sale of herbs as part of consumer safety. Referred to as the CODEX rules, these rules represent an international effort to restrict health claims for herbals and would require a physician's prescription, defeating one of the primary reasons why people turn to herbals. There is no recommendation that the prescribing of herbals be left to certified herbalists or Naturopathic Doctors. There is a fine line between the rights of individuals and responsibilities of the government. Because herbs have become popular and profitable, some regulation may be necessary for consumer safety. Standardization of doses enables greater consistency by people who self-administer herbals.

Another potential problem includes findings that many people who use alternative remedies are doing so without any type of supervision (Benotsch et al., 2013; Eisenberg et al., 1998). Potentially, this self-medicating might lead to a dangerous delay in seeking more efficacious care. For example, if the treatment does not work, the patient might become more symptomatic during the trial of herbals and become less able to seek other medical care. Anxiety is a good example. Overreliance on herbals can present some of the same problems as benzodiazepine dependence or abuse. Individuals who had misused OTC medications reported more symptoms of depression, anxiety, and somatic distress in a recent research study, which highlights the need for additional research to elucidate more knowledge regarding the misuse of OTC medications (Benotsch et al., 2013; Cooper, 2013). Delaying more effective treatments such as cognitive-behavioral psychotherapy might make it more difficult to achieve the maximum benefit offered by this approach. Patients who use both conventional and alternative medicines without informing their prescriber place

BOX 19-2 GENERAL PRECAUTIONS FOR CONSUMERS AND HEALTH CARE PROFESSIONALS REGARDING HERBALS

- Avoid products with multiple herbs. Check the active and inactive ingredients for possible combinations and additives.
- Avoid imported herbs because of differences in dose effects.
- Buy only from reputable, established companies and with the *United States Pharmacopeia* (USP) seal of approval.
- Always inform the health care provider of any use of herbal products, including topicals, and any complementary health practices used.
- Health care providers need a full picture of what is done to manage health; communication can be facilitated by using NCCAM Time to Talk campaign tips (available at http://www.nccam.nih.gov/timetotalk).
- Discontinue if any unusual side effects occur, and report negative side effects or adverse reactions to the FDA at www.fda.gov/medwatch, or call 1-800-332-1088.
- Avoid herbals during pregnancy, when attempting to get pregnant, and during breast-feeding.
- Avoid self-medicating with herbals before a medical illness has been ruled out.

themselves at risk for herb-drug interaction, overmedication or undermedication, and difficulty in appropriate management of their health (Dasgupta & Hammett-Stabler, 2011). Nondisclosure, as opposed to talking about one's values and beliefs with the health care provider, interferes with a collaborative relationship between the patient and the health care provider. Box 19-2 summarizes general precautions regarding herbals.

 CRITICAL THINKING QUESTION

1. What are the implications of patients who self-medicate with over-the-counter drugs? Are there any dangers? What are the possible benefits?

FUTURE DIRECTIONS OF INTEGRATIVE HEALTH CARE

As conventional health care has advanced technologically and diagnostically, it makes sense that a focus be shifted to the biologic aspects of health. Western medicine has been called "broken" by some and amazingly "miraculous" by others. One thing is clear: the public wants the opportunity to be empowered in their health care. The mind-body connection is a powerful one, as has been revealed by 3 decades of research. There is a call for all health care practitioners to incorporate the core concepts of CAM therapies into the care of patients. Health care practitioners in a newly evolving health care system must have interpersonal competencies that promote respect, empathy, and concern for the patients they are treating (Gilbert, 2003).

The term *integrative health care* connotes blending the best practices from both conventional and alternative medicine

(National Center for Complementary and Alternative Medicine, 2013). Health care practitioners are entering the health care environment at one of the most opportune moments in the history of medicine. Conventional health care has become a comprehensive science, with the capability to diagnose all types of disease states of the body and mind. Barrett and colleagues (2003) noted that the definition of health adopted by the World Health Organization, "a state of complete physical, mental, and social well-being," is not easily reconciled with the general disease-treating framework of conventional medicine. At the same time, some alternative health care practitioners can provide such an excellent healing environment that a treatment effect occurs, independent of the curative method used. The move toward alternative therapies is a natural occurrence in a system of health care that has become fragmented and focused on cost, disease, and overreliance on medication (U.S. Food and Drug Administration, 2012b). A combined approach offers the patient the absolute best care.

The direction of alternative, complementary, or integrative medicine depends greatly on economic and political powers (Barrett et al., 2003). Some health care practitioners are vehemently opposed to the alternative and complementary health movement. Clash exists as practitioners and researchers seek to answer questions regarding the use of alternative medicines and therapies (Engdahl, 2012; Zott, 2012). Ernst (2004) called for an open mind in regard to CAM therapies, pointing out that dissenters often are using circular reasoning—that is, alternative therapies are considered a waste of research funds because there is no scientific proof of their efficacy. Consumer empowerment and choice can be a threatening concept for health care practitioners who are used to a more authoritarian approach.

The alternative health care movement has implications for psychiatry and nursing. Although previously little was known about biologic markers for mental illness, much is now known. Research has revealed a plethora of knowledge about neurotransmitters, hormonal influences, and structural abnormalities of the brain. Intrapsychic and environmental influences on this system were ignored along the way to the current state of focusing almost exclusively on the biologic aspects of mental illness (Riedel-Heller et al., 2005).

In addition, there is a growing abundance of preclinical and clinical studies that reveal a range of complex psychotropic activity from herbal medicines potentially beneficial for treating depression, anxiety, and sleep disorders (Sarris et al., 2011). However, before becoming too enthusiastic, it is important to approach the use of herbals with caution. At the present time, there are only three herbal medicines that have replicated randomized controlled trials (via meta-analysis). These include St. John's wort for major depression (*H. perforatum*), kava for anxiety disorders (*Piper methysticum*), and valerian for insomnia (*V. officinalis*).

Many herbal medicines have not been thoroughly tested using large sample sizes. A significant consideration in evaluating herbals is that metabolism and the resultant biotransformation, both in context of enzymatic and hepatic processes, create new chemical structures. In vitro evidence does not calculate into clinical efficacy in humans (Sarris et al., 2011).

Varied outcomes of studies conducted in Europe and the United States further complicate an already complex picture in the use of herbals. Mixed outcomes ranging from positive to modest to weak also create a moving target both in replicated studies and in newer meta-analyses (Fournier et al., 2010; Linde et al., 2008; Sarris & Kavanagh, 2009; Werneke et al., 2004).

NORM'S NOTES
The use of alternative and complementary therapies is widespread and still growing. Traditional medicine has been unable to meet the needs of a public that believes good health is a right. The statistical table of prevalence of mental disorders in Chapter 2 and in all psychopathology chapters reflects data that have not changed much for about 30 years. However, during that time, many new, supposedly wonderful medications have been discovered. The conventional psychotropic drug industry is a multibillion dollar concern, but the actual number of people with a drug-treatable disorder has increased. Consequently, many Americans now look outside the traditional psychiatric drug manufacturing complex to see whether they can "fix" themselves. The alternative and complementary approach to mental health care derives, in part, from this disillusionment and disappointment.

The values of alternative medicine run the risk of falling prey to the same problems affecting conventional medicine if conflict over its use becomes too intense. When considering alternative therapies, it is important to keep an open mind—some are helpful; some cause harm; and some, although harmless, probably offer no more than a placebo effect. The alternative therapy movement holds a valuable lesson if we can learn it: patients want to be treated holistically. If, instead of learning this lesson, health care determines how to profit from controlling a patient's access to alternative treatments, the opportunity to defragment the health care system will be lost. Many people consider integrative approaches both an opportunity to transform medicine and a sign that the next major transformation is unfolding before us. It is hoped that we will continue listening and responding to this message.

? CRITICAL THINKING QUESTION

2. What do you think about patients taking health into their own hands and engaging in practices that have not been supported by scientific research and are not endorsed by the health care community?

▌ STUDY NOTES

1. The NIH has created an office of complementary and alternative medicine, NCCAM (http://nccam.nih/gov).

2. The FDA does not regulate herbal products but does require labeling that indicates lack of proven efficacy and quality control standards.

3. St. John's wort is the most widely used herbal for depression. Studies have generally demonstrated the effectiveness of St. John's wort for mild to moderate depression. It should not be taken with other antidepressants, especially SSRIs, and generally has a high potential for interaction with other drugs. In particular, St. John's wort might interfere with the protease inhibitors often prescribed for HIV-positive patients.

4. Kava is an herbal anxiolytic without the problems of altered coordination and alertness associated with normal doses of benzodiazepines. Problems can occur if taken with central nervous system–acting drugs, and overdose is possible. Concerns about liver toxicity have decreased but have not eliminated sales in the United States. It is unclear what mechanism is involved in altering liver function in certain individuals.

5. Valerian is an herbal anxiolytic useful for anxiety and insomnia. Withdrawal syndromes similar to benzodiazepine discontinuation can occur. Valerian might increase the effects of other centrally acting drugs and might reduce the effectiveness of anticoagulants and anticonvulsant drugs.

6. Chamomile and angelica have been used for anxiety, but there are fewer supporting studies compared with kava and valerian.

7. Ginkgo is one of the top-selling herbals in the United States for brain trauma, memory impairment, and cerebral insufficiency. Ginkgo should not be taken by anyone with a history of bleeding problems.

8. Melatonin has been suggested as possibly useful for ICU syndrome and for sleep.

9. Omega-3 fatty acids, found in fish oils, show promise for improving clinical outcomes in many conditions, including mania and schizophrenia.

10. Some herbals are known to be problematic for patients with psychiatric disorders, particularly evening primrose, yohimbine, ginseng, chaste tree, and betel nut.

11. One concern about patients taking herbals and/or over-the-counter medications without supervision is that patients might delay seeking essential treatment.

12. Health care professionals should routinely question patients about the use of herbals or other alternative therapies. It is essential for the health care professional to examine his or her own attitude and manner so that patients feel comfortable disclosing their use.

13. Nurses demonstrating the ability to integrate CAM into their clinical practice can be certified through examination and adherence to standards of practice by the American Holistic Nurses Association, with the designation of HNC located at www.ahncc.org. Nurses possessing HNC credentials might also have been trained in alternative therapies through special education or credentialing.

REFERENCES

Abascal, K., & Yarnell, E. (2004b). Alzheimer's disease, part 2: A botanical treatment plan. *Journal of Alternative and Complementary Medicine (New York, N.Y.)*, *10*, 67.

Agency for Healthcare Research and Quality. (2002). http://archive.ahrq.gov/clinic/tp/sametp.htm, Accessed 14.02.14.

Agins, A., & Lehne, R. (2004). Herbal supplements. In R. Lehne (Ed.), *Pharmacology for nursing care* (pp. 1171–1174). St. Louis: Saunders.

Alpert, J. E., et al. (2004). S-Adenosyl-l-methionine (SAMe) as an adjunct for resistant major depressive disorder: An open trial following partial or nonresponse to selective serotonin reuptake inhibitors or venlafaxine. *Journal of Clinical Psychopharmacology*, *24*, 661.

American Holistic Nurses Association. http://www.ahna.org/Education/Certification, Accessed 04.05.14.

Anke, J., & Ramzan, I. 2004a. Kava hepatotoxicity: Are we any closer to the truth? *Planta Medica*, *70*, 193.

Anke, J., & Ramzan, I. 2004b. Pharmacokinetic and pharmacodynamic drug interactions with kava (Piper methysticum Forst. f.). *Journal of Ethnopharmacology*, *93*, 153.

Arendt, J. (2005). Melatonin: Characteristics, concerns, prospects. *Journal of Biological Rhythms*, *20*, 291.

Ayd, F. (2000). Evaluating interactions between herbal and psychoactive medications. *Psychiatric Times*, *17*, 45.

Barnes, P. M., Bloom, B., & Nahin, R. L. (2008). Complementary and alternative medicine use among adults and children: United States. 2007. *National Health Statistics Reports*, *12*, 1.

Barnes, P., et al. (2004). Complementary and alternative medicine use among adults: United States. 2002. *Advance Data*, *343*, 1.

Barrett, B., et al. (2003). Themes of holism, empowerment, access, and legitimacy define complementary, alternative, and integrative medicine in relation to conventional biomedicine. *Journal of Alternative and Complementary Medicine (New York, NY)*, *9*, 937.

Beaubrun, G., & Gray, G. (2000). A review of herbal medicines for psychiatric disorders. *Psychiatric Services*, *51*, 1130.

Benotsch, E. G., Koester, S., Martin, A. M., Cejka, A., Luckman, D., & Jeffers, A. J. (December 17, 2013). Intentional misuse of over-the-counter medications, mental health, and polysubstance use in young adults. *Journal of Community Health*, doi:10.1007/s10900-013-9811-9.

Bressler, R. (2005). Herb-drug interactions: Interactions between Ginkgo biloba and prescription medications. *Geriatrics*, *60*, 30.

Brown, R., Bottiglieri, T., & Colman, C. (1999). *Stop depression now: SAM-e: The breakthrough supplement that works as well as prescription drugs in half the time with no side effects*. New York: G.P. Putnam's Sons.

Carpenter, D. J. (2011). St. John's wort and S-adenosyl methionine as "natural" alternatives to conventional antidepressants in the era of the suicidality boxed warning: What is the evidence for clinically relevant benefit? *Alternative Medicine Review*, *16*, 17.

Chui, J. A., Stone, J. A., Martin, B. A., Croes, K. D., & Thorpe, J. M. (November 6, 2013). Safeguarding older adults from inappropriate over-the-counter medications: The role of community pharmacists. *The Gerontologist*, doi:10.1093/geront/gnt130.

Clouatre, D. L. (2004). Kava kava: Examining new reports of toxicity. *Toxicology Letters*, *150*, 85.

Clough, A. R., Bailie, R. S., & Currie, B. (2003). Liver function test abnormalities in users of aqueous kava extracts. *Journal of Toxicology Clinical Toxicology*, *41*, 821.

Clough, A. R., Rowley, K., & O'Dea, K. (2004). Kava use, dyslipidaemia and biomarkers of dietary quality in aboriginal people in Arnhem Land in the Northern Territory (NT), Australia. *European Journal of Clinical Nutrition*, *58*, 1090.

Cooper, R. J. (2013). Over-the-counter medicine abuse – A review of the literature. *Journal of Substance Use*, *18*(2), 82–107.

Coppen, A., & Bolander-Gouaille, C. (2005). Treatment of depression: Time to consider folic acid and vitamin B12. *Journal of Psychopharmacology*, *19*, 59.

Cronin, D. (2004). Supporting mental health with polyunsaturated fatty acids. *Journal of Alternative and Complementary Medicine (New York, N.Y.)*, *10*, 95.

Dasgupta, A. & Hammett-Stabler, C. A. (Eds.), (2011). *Herbal supplements: Efficacy, toxicity, interactions with western drugs and effects on clinical laboratory tests*. Hoboken, NJ: Wiley.

Dietary Supplement Health and Education Act of 1994. (2005). http://www.fda.gov/RegulatoryInformation/Legislation/FederalFoodDrugandCosmeticActFDCAct/SignificantAmendmentstotheFDCAct/ucm148003.htm, Accessed 14.06.06.

Eisenberg, D., et al. (1998). Trends in alternative medicine use in the United States, 1990–1997: Results of a follow-up national survey. *JAMA, the Journal of the American Medical Association*, *280*, 1569.

Engdahl, S. (Ed.), (2012). *Current controversies: Alternative therapies*. New York: Greenhaven Press.

Ernst, E. (1998). Harmless herbs? A review of the recent literature. *American Journal of Medicine*, *104*, 170.

Ernst, E. (2004). The "improbability" of complementary and alternative medicine. *Archives of Internal Medicine*, *164*, 914.

Estes, J. D., et al. (2003). High prevalence of potentially hepatotoxic herbal supplement use in patients with fulminant hepatic failure. *Archives of Surgery*, *138*, 852.

Fenton, W. S., et al. (2001). A placebo-controlled trial of omega-3 fatty acid (ethyl eicosapentaenoic acid) supplementation for residual symptoms and cognitive impairment in schizophrenia. *American Journal of Psychiatry*, *158*, 207101.

Folks, D., & Gabel, T. (2001). Herbaceuticals in psychiatry. In N. Keltner & D. Folks (Eds.), *Psychotropic drugs* (pp. 513–539) (3rd ed.). St. Louis: Mosby.

Fournier, J., et al. (2010). Antidepressant drug effects and depression severity: A patient-level meta-analysis. *JAMA, the Journal of the American Medical Association*, *303*, 47.

Freeman, M. P., et al. (2010). Complementary and alternative medicine in major depressive disorder: The American Psychiatric Association Task Force report. *Journal of Clinical Psychiatry*, *71*, 6.

Gilbert, M. (2003). Weaving medicine back together: Mind-body medicine in the twenty-first century. *Journal of Alternative and Complementary Medicine (New York, N.Y.)*, *9*, 563.

Glass, J. R., et al. (2003). Acute pharmacological effects of temazepam, diphenhydramine, and valerian in healthy elderly subjects. *Journal of Clinical Psychopharmacology*, *23*, 260.

Hallahan, B., & Garland, M. (2004). Essential fatty acids and their role in the treatment of impulsivity disorders. *Prostaglandins, Leukotrienes, and Essential Fatty Acids*, *71*, 211.

Hallam, K. T., et al. (2003). Comparative cognitive and psychomotor effects of single doses of Valeriana officianalis and triazolam in healthy volunteers. *Human Psychopharmacology*, *18*, 619.

Harris, J., et al. (2004). Statin treatment alters serum n-3 and n-6 fatty acids in hypercholesterolemia patients. *Prostaglandins, Leukotrienes, and Essential Fatty Acids*, *71*, 263.

Hatcher, T. (2001). The proverbial herb. *American Journal of Nursing, 101,* 36.

Hicks, S. M., et al. (2004). The significance of nonsignificance in randomized controlled studies: A discussion inspired by a double-blinded study on St. John's wort (Hypericum perforatum L.) for premenstrual symptoms. *Journal of Alternative and Complementary Medicine (New York, N.Y.), 10,* 925.

Hoblyn, J. C., & Brooks, J. O., 3rd. (2005). Herbal supplements in older adults. Consider interactions and adverse events that may result from supplement use. *Geriatrics, 60,* 22.

Horowitz, S. (2004). The brighter aspects of ultraviolet light. *Journal of Alternative and Complementary Medicine (New York, N.Y), 10,* 304.

Hsu, M., et al. (2009). Use of antidepressants and complementary and alternative medicine among outpatients with depression in Taiwan. *Archives of Psychiatric Nursing, 23,* 75.

Institute of Medicine. (2005). *Complementary and alternative medicine in the US.* Washington, DC: National Academy of Sciences.

Joy, C. B., Mumby-Croft, R., & Joy, L. A. (2000). Polyunsaturated fatty acid (fish or evening primrose oil) for schizophrenia. *Cochrane Database of Systematic Reviews, 2,* CD001257.

Joy, C. B., Mumby-Croft, R., & Joy, L. A. (2003). Polyunsaturated fatty acid supplementation for schizophrenia. *Cochrane Database of Systematic Reviews, 2,* CD001257.

Kaufman, D. W., et al. (2002). Recent patterns of medication use in the ambulatory adult population of the United States: The Slone survey. *JAMA, the Journal of the American Medical Association, 287,* 337.

Keltner, N. & Folks, D. (2005). Drugs used in alternative and complementary medicine. St. Louis: Mosby.

Kessler, R., et al. (2001). The use of complementary and alternative therapies to treat anxiety and depression in the United States. *American Journal of Psychiatry, 158,* 289.

Kirsch, I. (2003). St John's wort, conventional medication, and placebo: An egregious double standard. *Complementary Therapies in Medicine, 11,* 193.

Knuppel, L., & Linde, K. (2004). Adverse effects of St. John's wort: A systematic review. *Journal of Clinical Psychiatry, 65,* 1470.

Linde, K., Berner, M., & Kriston, L. (2008). St. John's wort for major depression. *Cochrane Database of Systematic Reviews, 18,* CD000448.

Linde, K., & Knuppel, L. (2005). Large-scale observational studies of hypericum extracts in patients with depressive disorders—A systematic review. *Phytomedicine, 12,* 148.

Linde, K., et al. (2005). St John's wort for depression. *Cochrane Database of Systematic Reviews, 18,* CD000448.

Malva, J. O., Santos, S., & Macedo, T. (2004). Neuroprotective properties of Valeriana officinalis extracts. *Neurotoxicity Research, 6,* 131.

McDowell, J., & Burman, M. (2004). Complementary and alternative medicine: A qualitative study of beliefs of a small sample of Rocky Mountain area nurses. *Medsurg Nursing, 13,* 383.

McEnany, G. (2001). Herbal psychotropics, part 3: Focus on kava, valerian, and melatonin. *Journal of the American Psychiatric Nurses Association, 6,* 126.

Meletis, C., & Barker, J. (2004). Mental health not all in the mind—Really a matter of cellular biochemistry. *Journal of Alternative and Complementary Medicine (New York, NY), 10,* 28.

Mikhail, N., Wali, S., & Ziment, I. (2004). Use of alternative medicine among Hispanics. *Journal of Alternative and Complementary Medicine (New York, N.Y.), 10,* 851.

Mills, E., et al. (2004). Impact of federal safety advisories on health food store advice. *Journal of General Internal Medicine, 19,* 269.

Min, L., et al. (2005). The effects of angelica essential oil in social interaction and hole-board tests. *Pharmacology, Biochemistry, and Behavior, 81,* 838.

Morris, D. W., Trivedi, M. H., & Rush, A. J. (2008). Folate and unipolar depression. *Journal of Alternative and Complementary Medicine (New York, NY), 14,* 277.

Nahin, R. L., et al. (2009). *Costs of complementary and alternative medicine (CAM) and frequency of visits to CAM practitioners: United States 2007.* National Health Statistics Reports, No. 18, Hyattsville, MD: National Center for Health Statistics.

National Center for Complementary and Alternative Medicine. (2007). *The use of complementary and alternative medicine in the United States.* http://nccam.nih.gov/news/camstats/2007/camsurvey_fs1.htm, Accessed 13.02.14.

National Center for Complementary and Alternative Medicine. (2008). *Ginkgo.* http://nccam.nih.gov/health/ginkgo, Accessed 13.02.14.

National Center for Complementary and Alternative Medicine. (2012). *Time to talk campaign.* http://nccam.nih.gov/timetotalk, Accessed 18.03.13.

National Center for Complementary and Alternative Medicine (2013). *Mind-body medicine: An overview.* http://nccam.nih.gov/health/backgrounds/mindbody.htm, Accessed 13.02.14.

NTP herbal medicine fact sheet. (2003). http://www.micromedex.com/products/herbalmed/herbalmed_brochure.pdf, Accessed 11.11.09.

Parslow, R., & Jorm, A. (2004). Individuals prescribed antidepressants or anxiolytics might replace or augment such medications with complementary and alternative medicines (CAMs). *Journal of Affective Disorders, 82,* 77.

Peters, D., et al. (2003). Time for a new approach for reporting herbal medicine adverse events? *Journal of Alternative and Complementary Medicine (New York, N.Y.), 9,* 607.

Qato, D. M., Alexander, G. C., Conti, R. M., Johnson, M., Schumm, P., & Lindau, S. T. (2008). Use of prescription and over-the-counter medications and dietary supplements among older adults in the United States. *JAMA: the Journal of the American Medical Association, 300,* 2867–2878. doi:10.1001/jama.2008.892.

Riedel-Heller, S., Matschinger, H., & Angermeyer, M. (2005). Mental disorders—Who and what might help? Help-seeking and treatment preferences of the lay public. *Social Psychiatry and Psychiatric Epidemiology, 40,* 167.

Robinson, A., & McGrail, M. (2004). Disclosure of CAM use to medical practitioners: A review of qualitative and quantitative studies. *Complementary Therapies in Medicine, 12,* 90.

Sachdev, P. S., et al. (2005). Relationship of homocysteine, folic acid and vitamin B12 with depression in a middle-aged community sample. *Psychological Medicine, 35,* 529.

Saeed, S. A., et al. (2009). CAM for your depressed patient: 6 recommended options. *Current Psychiatry, 8,* 39.

Sarris, J., & Kavanagh, D. J. (2009). Kava and St John's wort: Current evidence for use in mood and anxiety disorders. *Journal of Alternative and Complementary Medicine (New York, N.Y.), 15,* 827.

Sarris, J., Kavanagh, D. J., & Byrne, G. (2010). Adjuvant use of nutritional and herbal medicines with antidepressants, mood stabilizers and benzodiazepines. *Journal of Psychiatric Research, 44,* 32.

Sarris, J., et al. (2011). Herbal medicine for depression, anxiety and insomnia: A review of psychopharmacology and clinical evidence. *European Neuropsychopharmacology, 21,* 841.

Schardt, D. (2009). Worth the cost? The lowdown on three expensive supplements. *Nutrition Action Healthletter, 36,* 9.

Shelley, B. M., et al. (2009). "They don't ask me so I don't tell them": Patient-clinician communication about traditional, complementary, and alternative medicine. *Annals of Family Medicine, 7,* 139.

Shinomiya, K., et al. (2005). Hypnotic activities of chamomile and passiflora extracts in sleep-disturbed rats. *Biological & Pharmaceutical Bulletin, 28,* 808.

Shippy, R. A., et al. (2004). S-Adenosylmethionine (SAM-e) for the treatment of depression in people living with HIV/AIDS. *BMC Psychiatry, 4,* 38.

Silvers, K., et al. (2005). Randomised double-blind placebo-controlled trial of fish oil in the treatment of depression. *Prostaglandins, Leukotrienes, and Essential Fatty Acids, 72,* 211.

Simon, G., et al. (2004). Mental health visits to complementary and alternative medicine providers. *General Hospital Psychiatry, 26,* 171.

Skidmore-Roth, L. (2009). *Handbook of herbs and natural supplements.* St. Louis: Mosby.

Snyder, M., & Lindquist, R. (2001). Issues in complementary therapies: How we got to where we are. *Online Journal of Issues in Nursing, 6,* 1.

St. John's wort and the treatment of depression. (2007). NCCAM Publication No. D005. http://nccam.nih.gov/health/stjohnswort/index.htm, Accessed 13.02.14.

Stoll, A. L., Severus, W. E., Freeman, M. P., et al. (1999). Omega-3 fatty acids in bipolar disorder: A preliminary double-blind, placebo-controlled trial. *Archives of General Psychiatry, 56,* 407.

Stoll, A. L. (2001). *The omega-3 connection: The groundbreaking anti-depression diet and brain program.* New York: Simon and Schuster.

Szegedi, A., et al. (2005). Acute treatment of moderate to severe depression with hypericum extract WS5570 (St. John's wort): Randomised controlled double-blind non-inferiority trial versus paroxetine. *BMJ (Clinical Research Ed.), 330,* 503.

Taibi, D., Bourguignon, Z. C., & Taylor, A. (2004). Valerian use for sleep disorders related to rheumatoid arthritis. *Holistic Nursing Practice, 18,* 120.

Tiemeier, H., et al. (2003). Plasma fatty acid composition and depression are associated in the elderly: The Rotterdam study. *The American Journal of Clinical Nutrition, 78,* 40.

U.S. Food and Drug Administration. (2004). *FDA announces qualified health claims for omega-3 fatty acids.* Created September 8, 2004, Updated April 2, 2013, http://www.fda.gov/SiteIndex/ucm108351.htm, Accessed 13.02.14.

U.S. Food and Drug Administration. (2012a.). *Over-the-counter (OTC) drug product review process.* Retrieved February 14, 2014 from http://www.fda.gov/drugs/developmentapprovalprocess/smallbusinessassistance/ucm052786.htm.

U.S. Food and Drug Administration. (2012b.). *Drug applications for over-the-counter (OTC) drugs.* Retrieved February 14, 2014 from http://www.fda.gov/drugs/developmentapprovalprocess/howdrugsaredevelopedandapproved/approvalapplications/over-the-counterdrugs/default.htm.

Uebelhack, R., Franke, L., & Schewe, H. J. (1998). Inhibition of platelet MAO-B by kava pyrone-enriched extract from Piper methysticum Forster (kava-kava). *Pharmacopsychiatry, 31,* 187.

vanGurp, G., et al. (2002). St John's wort or sertraline? Randomized controlled trial in primary care. *Canadian Family Physician Médecin de Famille Canadien, 48,* 905.

Weber, W., et al. (2008). Hypericum perforatum (St. John's wort) for attention-deficit/hyperactivity disorder in children and adolescents: A randomized controlled trial. *JAMA, the Journal of the American Medical Association, 299,* 2633.

Werneke, U. (2009). Complementary medicines in mental health. *Evidence-Based Mental Health, 12,* 1.

Werneke, U., Horn, O., & Taylor, D. (2004). How effective is St. John's wort? The evidence revisited. *Journal of Clinical Psychiatry, 65,* 611.

Yarnell, E., & Abascal, K. (2004). Herbal medicine in Korea: Alternative is mainstream. *Alternative and Complementary Therapies, 10,* 161.

Yuan, C. S., Mehendale, S., Xiao, Y., et al. (2004). The gamma-aminobutyric acidergic effects of valerian and valerenic acid on rat brainstem neuronal activity. *Anesthesia and Analgesia, 98,* 353.

Zandi, P., & Anthony, J. (2004). Reduced risk of Alzheimer disease in users of antioxidant vitamin supplements: The Cache County Study. *Archives of Neurology, 61,* 82.

Zhou, S., et al. (2004). Pharmacokinetic interactions of drugs with St John's wort. *Journal of Psychopharmacology, 18,* 262.

Zott, L. M. (Ed.), (2012). *Opposing viewpoints series: Alternative medicine.* New York: Greenhaven Press.

CHAPTER

20

Introduction to Milieu Management

Debbie Steele

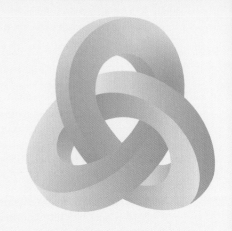

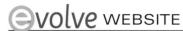 WEBSITE

http://evolve.elsevier.com/Keltner

LEARNING OBJECTIVES

- Define the terms *therapeutic milieu, therapeutic environment,* and *therapeutic community*.
- Describe the goal of managing the therapeutic environment in the care of psychiatric patients.

- Identify the elements of the therapeutic environment.
- Discuss several ways in which nurses can influence the therapeutic environment.

Note to Students: *Political, social, economic, and other forces have resulted in a health care system that changes quickly. These forces dictate the setting in which care takes place. For example, managed care insurance plans favor the use of less expensive forms of treatment than the inpatient unit. Although hospitals used to employ most psychiatric nurses, a great number of psychiatric nurses currently practice in community settings. Despite the rapidly changing mental health system, treatment principles remain the same when the nurse is guided by the professional definition of nursing—that is, attention to the range of human experiences and responses to health and illness within the physical and social environments (American Nurses Association, 2003). The treatment environment is affected by many variables, but it is the nurse's involvement in creating a therapeutic environment that ultimately determines the overall atmosphere of the treatment setting. This role is true in any specialty area, but it is the focus of psychiatric nursing and therefore the purpose for including these chapters.*

There is an international initiative to integrate recovery-oriented practices into the delivery of all mental health services.

For example, the President's New Freedom Commission on Mental Health reported that recovery is the most important goal for the mental health system (SAMHSA, 2006). The most recent definition of *recovery* is "a process of change through which individuals improve their health and wellness, live a self-directed life, and strive to reach their full potential" (SAMHSA, 2011). In keeping with national policy initiatives, psychiatric nurses are being challenged to integrate recovery into all of their practices (McLoughlin et al., 2013). A therapeutic environment is a vital ingredient in facilitating the journey of recovery for patients within health care settings. Attention to the therapeutic environment ensures protection of patients from potentially harmful effects and maximizes opportunities for patients to learn something about themselves and their difficulties in everyday living. The terms *therapeutic environment* and *therapeutic milieu* are sometimes used interchangeably to describe the atmosphere of a psychiatric setting. Strictly speaking, a therapeutic milieu refers to a formalized treatment modality called *milieu therapy*. Regardless of the term used, all treatment environments have an impact on patient outcomes. This is also true in nonpsychiatric patient care environments (e.g., medical surgical, intensive care, postpartum units), even when the environment is not avowed the primacy given in a psychiatric setting. A significant responsibility of psychiatric nurses is the management of the environment, one of the three tools of the psychotherapeutic management model described in Chapter 1.

Patients cannot be in an inpatient setting without being affected by the environment. When you really understand this, it will change a lot of things about your understanding of nursing. Here's the question: How can you shape an environment to make it more therapeutic? This chapter presents a history of the concept of milieu therapy, followed by a discussion of components that are essential for creating a therapeutic environment.

HISTORICAL OVERVIEW

The discussion in this section focuses on *milieu therapy* as it applies to hospital inpatient settings. It is assumed that similar principles could be applied in most treatment settings.

For many years, custodial care was the norm in inpatient settings. Custodial care referred to a *mindset* in which patient care focused exclusively on the patient's activities of daily living, such as hygiene, nutrition, elimination, and safety needs. Custodial care was a paternalistic system in which the staff knew what was best for the patient. Few attempts were made to allow the patient to participate in his or her own treatment, and beyond basic needs, there were no efforts to provide structured treatment activities. After World War II, some professionals were concerned that many opportunities to enhance treatment were being missed. Schwartz and Stanton (1954) noted the discrepancy between "what could be and what was" in the hospital. They believed that a better result from hospitalization might be realized if *all* dimensions of care were focused on their potential for therapeutic benefit.

The most notable figure of this time was Maxwell Jones. In 1953, Jones wrote his landmark book, *The Therapeutic Community*, in which he described the benefits of an environment that was therapeutic in and of itself. Jones (1953) proposed patient involvement in decision making through daily group meetings, termed *therapeutic community meetings*. In these daily meetings, patients participated in planning ward activities. Patient self-responsibility was an important concept in the therapeutic community, whereby patients were expected to take an active role in their treatment. Increasingly, the importance of the patients' contribution to their own treatment was recognized, and this approach replaced the paternalistic system of the professional treatment team knowing best. Milieu therapy and therapeutic community came to reflect the idea of comprehensive use of the environment as a tool to facilitate the recovery of patients experiencing psychiatric and mental health problems.

The environment of the acute inpatient psychiatric facility of today is significantly different from that of the 1960s and 1970s. In particular, the number of units or beds is much fewer. The patients' average length of stay is greatly reduced. The acuity of psychotic and detained patients is higher, as is the increased risk of violence. The U.S. Department of Health and Human Services (1999) reported that contemporary psychiatric units have become short-term intensive care settings to contain and resolve crises. Staff members are presented with the challenge of applying therapeutic milieu principles in an environment in which the primary directive is rapid stabilization of symptoms and return of the patient to a less expensive community-based treatment program. All of these factors pose a great challenge to staff members who are expected, and who themselves expect, to create a therapeutic as well as a safe environment for the patients in their charge (Norton, 2004). The constant change and demands associated with a rapid turnover of patients requires nurses to reevaluate the environment continuously in tandem and in coordination with the entire multidisciplinary team.

THE JOINT COMMISSION: ENVIRONMENT OF CARE ISSUES

The Joint Commission, formerly known as the Joint Commission on the Accreditation of Healthcare Organizations, requires that institutions routinely evaluate the environment for its ongoing effectiveness to provide care. Additionally, the facility must establish a social environment supporting its basic philosophy. Box 20-1 lists the The Joint Commission environment of care

---

BOX 20-1 THE JOINT COMMISSION ENVIRONMENT OF CARE STANDARDS

Environmental safety is attained through:
- Ongoing assessment and maintenance of all equipment
- Hazard surveillance
- Reporting and investigation of safety issues
- Monitoring of safety management techniques and procedures
- Orientation programs that address safety issues

A health care facility ensures the security of all people through:
- Mechanisms for addressing security issues
- Provision of appropriate identification for all staff, patients, and visitors
- Security orientation programs
- Mechanisms for handling emergencies
- Mechanisms for interacting with the media

The social environment must provide:
- Space for storage of grooming and hygiene articles
- Closet and drawer space for personal property
- Clothing that is suitable for clinical conditions

The physical setting must provide:
- Adequate privacy to ensure respect for patients
- Door locks consistent with program goals
- Availability of telephones that allow for private conversations
- Sleeping rooms with doors for privacy unless clinically contraindicated
- Furnishings suitable to the population served
- Access to the outdoors unless contraindicated for therapeutic reasons

From Joint Commission on Accreditation of Healthcare Organizations (2001). *Comprehensive accreditation manual for hospitals* (EC-1). Chicago: JCAHO.

standards for inpatient psychiatric units. These standards also apply to outpatient clinics and counseling centers.

Clinical Example

A day treatment program for patients with chronic mental illness is housed in a large rustic building in a rural county in a southeastern state in the United States. Within easy walking distance of the day treatment program are two group homes. Many of the residents from the group home are also patients at the day treatment center. The therapeutic environment for the day treatment program includes a range of structured treatment activities, such as educational classes; group and individual therapy; and basic living skills such as making a budget, riding the bus, reading food labels for nutrition, planning meals, and washing clothes. For the patients living in the group home, many of these activities are enhanced and reinforced by trained staff members who structure the days and evenings at the group home. Both treatment settings manage the environment to make it therapeutic for patients.

NURSING AND THE THERAPEUTIC ENVIRONMENT

Florence Nightingale recognized the importance of the environment on the patient's recovery. Nurses have traditionally been responsible for activities that involve management of the unit environment.

Patients benefit from a therapeutic environment because it provides opportunities to try new behaviors and solve problems in real-life situations with others. Nurses draw on their therapeutic relationship with patients to create corrective learning experiences in the treatment environment. Interactions with patients are opportunities to help them learn and adapt to their problems in daily living. Distortions, conflicts, and inappropriate behavior are dealt with in the here and now of each interaction and relate back to the patient's treatment plan.

Psychiatric nurses must take an active role to ensure that the environment is therapeutic. Paying attention to one's personal values, reactions, and preconceptions is one aspect of keeping the environment therapeutic. Other important elements involve altering the environment through a careful, active, and coordinated process of providing structured therapeutic activities and interactions. For example, inpatient education groups have been found to have a positive effect on patients' well-being and ability to cope with their illness (Hatonen et al., 2008). Ensuring that patients have information related to their disease process and participation in decision making concerning their own care is facilitated by effective communication skills of the nurse and positive nurse-patient interactions. Nonformal education has also been found to be valued by patients. Thomas and associates (2002) found that patients expressed a desire to examine their perceptions of care received through more interaction and deeper connections with nurses. Research has shown that a therapeutic environment also benefits nurses because positive nurse-patient relationships contribute to professional satisfaction and the knowledge that the nurse has made a difference (Thomas et al., 2005).

HIGHLIGHTING THE EVIDENCE
Evidence-Based Practice

Thomas and associates (2002) wanted to know how patients experienced the inpatient acute care psychiatric environment. In their study, eight inpatients ranging in age from 23 to 58 years old on the acute psychiatric unit of a metropolitan general hospital participated in interviews about their experience of the environment.

The essential purpose of the hospital was to provide a refuge from self-destructiveness. Prominent aspects of patients' experience within the place of refuge fit into three interrelated themes: (1) like me/not like me, (2) possibilities/no possibilities, and (3) connection/disconnection.

Refuge from Self-Destructiveness
In contrast to the chaotic outside world, the hospital was portrayed as a safe house, neutral territory, and a cooling-down place. Hospitalization provided a calming respite from the daily struggle against self-destructive impulses.

Like Me/Not Like Me
In the psychiatric unit, identity was affirmed amid kindred souls. There was solidarity among the patients, often referred to as *bonding*, which most patients did not experience in the outside world—that is, when not in the hospital.

Possibilities/No Possibilities
Hospitalization opened possibilities for the future. Participants described feeling more level-headed, straightened out, and back in balance again. Despite goals and determination to follow up with aftercare plans, patients feared being released from the safe hospital environment.

Connection/Disconnection
The connection/disconnection theme refers to patients' experiences within the milieu of connecting—or failing to connect—with other people. Socialization with other patients was valued by patients. Interactions with professional staff tended to be superficial.

Universally, patients perceived peer-administered therapy as the most beneficial aspect of their hospitalization. They expressed longing for a deeper connection with staff and more insight-oriented therapies.

ELEMENTS OF THE TREATMENT ENVIRONMENT

The environment provides a context in which patients can move forward toward their goal of optimal health. The following interrelated elements provide the foundation necessary for the nurse to manage the environment effectively:

- Safety
- Structure
- Norms
- Limit setting
- Balance

Safety

Safety is primary to all other aspects of the environment. Safety involves both physical and psychological protection. In acute mental health units, safety is always the priority. Nurses working with severely depressed patients in inpatient settings have 24-hour responsibility for caring for people at risk for suicide. Nurses and other team members endeavor to provide patients with a safe hospital environment to prevent harm. Environmental interventions include removing harmful items (e.g., belts, shoelaces, keys) and placing them in a locked container. Patients are placed on 24-hour-a-day observations on a one-to-one basis. To minimize the distress caused by the process, the patient should be informed of the plan of care, including the level of observations. Additionally, nurses should strive to form a human-to-human connection with the patient. The provision of a therapeutic relationship helps patients address their suicidal feelings and allows the nurse to convey to the patient that his or her life has value. The nurse creates and provides an environment where the patient can begin to explore and discuss painful emotions. The nurse understands the importance of demonstrating unconditional acceptance, tolerance, and understanding as an integral part of a safe and caring environment. The role of the nurse is primarily to address the patient's need for emotional and physical security (Cutcliffe & Barker, 2002).

Management of the unit environment also includes protection from physical harm as a result of patients' verbal and physical aggression. Aggression is defined as an expression of hostility or intent to do harm (Duxbury, 2002). Nurses should create and adhere closely to the nursing policies and procedures developed for control of aggression. These policies usually involve intervening before an aggressive event occurs by such actions as sending a patient to his or her room, talking one to one with a patient, assisting with problem solving in conflicts between patients, administering as needed (prn) medications, and using seclusion or restraints to control behavior as a last resort. Intervening before situations escalate requires that the nurse be aware of the unit environment at all times, either by direct observation or through the reports of psychiatric technicians and aides. The relationship between the nurse and psychiatric technicians or other unlicensed assistive personnel needs to involve an active, team-oriented approach for mutual understanding of goals for the patient. Most psychiatric units require the documentation of safety observations (often termed *rounds*) on patients, at a frequency ranging from hourly checks to constant observation. The routine and prescribed safety observations on a psychiatric unit are done with the safety of both staff and patients in mind and are essential for maintaining the safety of the environment.

Environmental care is focused on protecting patients from all threatening events. To this end, it might be necessary to restrict visitors known to disparage patients. Intrusive behaviors such as getting in other people's private space or bullying others about personal characteristics need to be dealt with by staff to protect patients from this destructive behavior in the treatment environment. Safety cannot be fully accomplished unless the nurses are regularly out among the patients in the environment.

Psychiatric patients are a vulnerable population because of the ease with which their illness can be blamed for any allegations they might make; it is essential to be attentive to complaints of abuse made by patients. Patients with paranoia, delusions, or personality disorders might distort events as abuse; however, all allegations require the attention of the treatment team. Incident reports, follow-up by management, and notification of patient representatives or advocates might be necessary when allegations of abuse are made. Complaints against staff members are especially difficult for staff committed to the care of their patients, but it is important to be attentive to patterns suggestive of patients being exploited by staff members and to take action when suspicious or confirmed patterns are discovered. Patients need to know that staff members will not harm them and will not permit anyone else to do so. Posting patient rights, including telephone numbers to access assistance for violations of these rights, creates feelings of safety by empowering patients in an environment that can leave them feeling vulnerable.

Clinical Example

John is angry with another patient and is threatening him with bodily harm. The nurse intervenes by firmly directing John to go to his room. The nurse stays with John and encourages him to talk about what he is feeling as an alternative action, rather than acting aggressively toward others.

Structure

Structure refers to the physical environment, daily schedules of treatment activities, and informal rules of interacting between patients and staff. Structure is an essential component of a therapeutic milieu. Nurses lead activities such as patient education and social skills training groups. Teaching about medications, side effects, and aftercare support for both patients and families is an important function of the psychiatric nurse in inpatient settings.

Psychosocial groups led by social workers or trained therapists are incorporated into the daily schedule of patient events. Patients also may be offered individual or family therapy depending on available resources.

Recreation and art are an important aspect of the structured treatment environment. Occupational or recreational therapists ideally fulfill this function. Recreation and art therapy provide an opportunity for patients to socialize and interact with others. They also serve as a welcome distraction from painful feelings and distressing perceptions. The goal of recreation therapy is to use leisure, recreation, and sport activities to treat, improve, or maintain the physical, mental, and emotional well-being of patients served. Interventions include structured activities that enhance specific functional skills, organized sports, and fitness activities. A few examples of recreational activities include bingo, basketball, Ping-Pong, cards, and games.

Art therapy has been found to facilitate the creation of new ways of coping. Spandler and colleagues (2007) noted how participating in creative activities helped a patient cope more effectively with the distress of hearing voices, which in the past had been dealt with through self-harm. Self-expression through art therapy can be a productive means of recreating painful memories or images. Through art therapy, patients are able to make their difficulties more visible to themselves and others. As patients are provided a means of relating to their experiences in new and different ways, they feel a sense of validation and normalcy.

Nurses and the various therapists work together as a team in determining which scheduled activities are in accord with the current level of functioning and within the ability of each patient on the unit. For example, a depressed inpatient may be at a higher level of functioning than a patient experiencing perceptual disturbances associated with psychosis.

The physical design of the unit is also an aspect of structure. Adequate space, areas for socializing and receiving visitors, telephones, and areas for privacy all are required elements of a therapeutic environment. Additionally, patients need a central location to interact with each other; often, this is the day room. Research has shown that patients believe that they are truly able to connect with others and work on problems in their inner sanctuary during these informal gatherings (Thomas et al., 2002).

Norms

Norms are specific expectations of behavior that permeate the treatment environment; they are intended to promote safety and trust in the environment through the sanctioning of socially acceptable behaviors and consistency about what to expect. Norms create an environment that is predictable and applicable to all patients. Many people admitted for acute inpatient psychiatric care do not know why they are in the hospital, how long they will be there, what will be provided, and what is required of them. The communication of expectations related to norms enables respect and protection of the patients' integrity. Many of the behavioral norms are related to activities of daily living. For example, patients are expected to bathe, brush their hair and teeth, and dress appropriately to the environment. Other types of norms are focused on personal responsibility, such as the expectations that (1) patients will not harm themselves or others, (2) patients will attend and participate in group meetings and other unit activities, and (3) patients will focus on their personal treatment plan. How norms are communicated is of particular importance in an inpatient setting where some of the patients may be there involuntarily. Whenever possible, patients should be offered a sense of control, and staff should avert power struggles with patients whose tolerance and resilience is tenuous. Norms related to unit rules and activities were clearly articulated by a patient as follows, "You might not like some of the things you have to do and you might not agree with the rules, but you can kinda see how it's best in the long run cause you have so many different people and problems to deal with; I guess it keeps it smooth."

Clinical Example

The nurse and the patient together develop mutual relational interventions via open dialogue, negotiation, and collaboration. For example, instead of the nurse passively ignoring an unkempt patient who is disoriented and easily agitated, the nurse can say, "I am wondering what would happen if you took a shower?" or "When would you like to take a shower?"

Limit Setting

Limit setting is an important therapeutic method extensively applied in mental health practice. Setting limits includes approaches for regulating patients' behavior through the use of verbal and nonverbal nurse communications, fast-acting sedating medications, and environmental modalities such as restraints and seclusion. The purpose of limit setting is to (1) maintain or create security for patients and health care personnel and (2) facilitate patients' growth and development. In practice, limit setting is largely employed to prevent or limit inappropriate, aggressive, or unsafe behavior of patients. It is also sometimes necessary to set limits or regulate behaviors such as excessive requests, overt and covert sexual advances, and refusal to participate in treatment activities. Limit-setting strategies such as persuasion are a frequently used method to get patients to adapt to the unit rules.

HIGHLIGHTING THE EVIDENCE
Current Research

Aiming to improve nursing practice, Vatne and Fagermoen (2007) explored the characteristics of nurses' limit-setting interventions. In this study, psychiatric nurses said that respecting patients' integrity and autonomy was highly valued. However, because of the importance of safety and security, the nurses also acknowledged the value of therapeutic limit-setting interventions. This schism reflects the conflicting norms, beliefs, and feelings of psychiatric nurses about their own practice. These findings point to the significance of developing professional therapeutic skills for limit setting, built on ongoing dialogue and collaboration with patients.

Specific means of decreasing the use of limit setting (which patients may perceive as intrusive) involves an attitude of making unit rules and expectations clear as well as encouraging patients to take responsibility for self. Key concepts that support this strategy involve patients being advised of unit rules on admission and at frequent intervals, depending on their capacity to comprehend and attend to these rules. Written copies of unit rules should be provided to each patient and posted on the unit in a highly visible location. Although limits are a natural part of daily living, patients who are new to a unit cannot be expected to understand all the rules. Unit expectations should be communicated impartially and with a nonjudgmental attitude.

CRITICAL THINKING QUESTION

1. How can limit setting be viewed as coercive by patients in acute psychiatric units?

Balance

Balance, perhaps more than any other element of managing the therapeutic environment, represents the value of developing expertise in nursing. Balance involves the process of gradually allowing independent behaviors in a dependent situation. It might be necessary to make specific judgments about a patient's readiness to assume certain responsibilities for his or her care versus providing assistance when the patient might be unable to act on his or her own behalf. Making this decision requires the nurse to weigh the multiple and competing needs of the patient involved as well as the needs of other patients and staff on the unit. How aggressive incidents are perceived and managed by nurses illustrates the importance of a balanced approach. For example, although deescalation is the expected method for dealing with patients' verbal outbursts, Duxbury (2002) emphasized the importance of nurses seeking to intervene before the escalation. Being deliberate in spending time with patients and seeking their perspective can prove beneficial in preventing misunderstandings and subsequent aggression. However, exploration of the patients' perspective is essential not just in relation to aggressive incidents. Patients who are depressed and anxious can also benefit from the development of this practice. Instead of focusing on the behavior of a patient, nurses are encouraged to seek to understand the nature of the patient's problem within the context of the unit. An overall proactive stance can be accomplished as nurses approach patient deficits and needs based on an accurate, comprehensive evaluation. Consistency in responding to patients' behaviors and requests is essential in providing a safe, therapeutic environment.

CRITICAL THINKING QUESTION

2. How can consistency and follow-through by nurses contribute to a therapeutic environment?

THE NURSE AS MANAGER OF THE TREATMENT ENVIRONMENT

Environmental modification is an important intervention of the psychiatric nurse (Baker, 2000; Norton, 2004) and entails using the elements of safety, structure, norms, limit setting, and balance to achieve patients' treatment goals. Through environmental modification, the nurse can enhance the therapeutic environment for the patient. Physical arrangements, safety issues, and other features can create an atmosphere in which patients can learn new behaviors or become aware of their personal strengths. Responsiveness to the needs of patients necessitates that nursing staff continually review environmental norms, rules, and regulations as an important aspect of managing and modifying the environment. Flexibility in maintaining a therapeutic environment is accomplished by this ongoing evaluation of effectiveness. The care plan illustrates how environmental modification is used as a tool for meeting the patients' treatment goals. One of the most challenging and rewarding aspects of psychiatric nursing is the ability to affect the experience of patients in the hospital in a positive, therapeutic, and creative way. Nurses have published both research and anecdotal details of their successes in implementing an improved therapeutic environment in psychiatric care settings (Baker, 2000; Baker et al., 2002).

From the patient's perspective, being forced into treatment activities by nursing staff may interfere with the development of a therapeutic nurse-patient relationship. Occasionally, disagreement over rules is the precipitating factor leading to patient aggression. Rules on a psychiatric unit are intended for safety, but they can turn into a battle for control. A high level of skill is required of nurses as they enforce rules and norms in the treatment environment. A delicate balance exists between enhancement of the nurse-patient relationship and expectations related to unit rules. Excessive focus on rules and efficiency may become the tendency of some nursing staff members, whereas the priority of maintaining the therapeutic relationship is paramount for others. An experienced nurse instinctively relates to the uniqueness of each patient, based on his or her previous experience and skills. Awareness of the patient's perspective, coupled with consistency and creativity among the nursing staff, can go a long way in creating a therapeutic yet safe milieu.

CRITICAL THINKING QUESTION

3. A 32-year-old man with a diagnosis of schizophrenia, undifferentiated type, has been admitted to a psychiatric hospital because of recent thoughts related to self-mutilation. The patient lives with his mother, who does not feel comfortable in her ability to keep her son from harming himself. How might the use of a therapeutic environment assist this patient and family?

CARE PLAN

Assessment	**Problems:** A 23-year-old man has been unable to manage the auditory hallucinations (voices) telling him to cut (self-mutilate).
	1. Patient states that he thinks God wants him to cut, admitting to auditory hallucinations.
	2. Patient's mood is anxious with constricted affect.
	3. Patient tends to isolate in his room.
	4. Patient expresses negative symptoms such as avolition.
	5. Patient has gained 40 lb in the past year (on antipsychotics).
	6. Patient is religiously preoccupied.
Diagnosis	Risk for self-mutilation related to command hallucinations telling him to cut.

(Continued)

⊚ CARE PLAN—CONT'D

Outcomes	Short-term goals
Date met: _____	Patient will explore thoughts related to anxious feelings with staff.
Date met: _____	Patient will report a decrease in anxiety based on a scale of 1 to 10.
Date met: _____	Patient will participate in groups and recreation and art therapy every day.
Date met: _____	Patient will contract for safety with nurse every shift.
	Long-term goals
Date met: _____	Patient will report confidence in ability to manage command hallucinations.
Date met: _____	Patient will participate in follow-up individual and family psychotherapy.

Planning and Interventions   **Nurse-patient relationship:** Assist patient to identify and explore feelings of anxiety related to thoughts of self-mutilation; encourage patient to participate in all psychoeducational and therapy groups; encourage patient to participate in recreational and art programs to divert thoughts away from command hallucinations; assess for presence and content of auditory hallucinations; and contract for safety every shift.

Psychopharmacology: Aripiprazole (Abilify) 10 mg PO every day; discuss role of medications and related side effects.

Milieu management: Support patient's efforts to decrease anxiety level by managing disruptive patients on the unit. Encourage patient to spend time in the day room interacting with other patients. Monitor progress in using the diversion techniques and their effectiveness. Involve patient in ongoing treatment plan.

▌ STUDY NOTES

1. Environmental modification is the purposeful use of all interpersonal and environmental forces to enhance the mental health of psychiatric patients through the development of a therapeutic environment.

2. Because nurses use environmental modification as a tool for assisting patients, nurses have a significant part of the responsibility for shaping the therapeutic environment.

3. The Joint Commission has very clear standards regarding the effects of the environment of care on inpatient psychiatric settings. Safety and a functional environment conducive to patient care are major priorities of the environment of care.

4. Historically, nurses provided only custodial care, but after World War II, Jones (1953) and others conceptualized an environment in which all aspects of the psychiatric patient's day would be used to promote mental health; this was termed *milieu therapy*.

5. The therapeutic environment in inpatient settings has diminished as biologically based treatments have gained prominence and community care has become the preferred setting for treatment. In inpatient settings, safety is a priority goal.

6. Principles of milieu therapy can also be applied to community settings.

7. All treatment environments can be therapeutic or nontherapeutic.

8. Psychiatric nurses manage the treatment environment by modification of five elements: safety, structure, norms, limit setting, and balance.

9. Creating and managing a therapeutic environment requires the psychiatric nurse to be active.

REFERENCES

American Nurses Association, (2003). *Nursing's social policy statement.* Washington, DC: Author.

Baker, J. A. (2000). Developing psychosocial care for acute psychiatric wards. *Journal of Psychiatric and Mental Health Nursing, 7,* 95.

Baker, J. A., et al. (2002). The construction and implementation of a psychosocial interventions care pathway within a low secure environment: A pilot study. *Journal of Psychiatric and Mental Health Nursing, 9,* 737.

Cutcliffe, J., & Barker, P. (2002). Considering the care of the suicidal client and the case for 'engagement and inspiring hope' or 'observations.' *Journal of Psychiatric and Mental Health Nursing, 9,* 611.

Duxbury, J. (2002). An evaluation of staff and patient views of and strategies employed to manage inpatient aggression and violence on one mental health unit: A pluralistic design. *Journal of Psychiatric and Mental Health Nursing, 9,* 325.

Hatonen, H., et al. (2008). Mental health: Patients' experiences of patient education during inpatient care. *Journal of Clinical Nursing, 17,* 752.

Joint Commission on Accreditation of Healthcare Organizations. (2001). *Comprehensive accreditation manual for hospitals.* Chicago: JCAHO.

Jones, M. (1953). *The therapeutic community.* New York: Basic Books.

McLoughlin, K. A., et al. (2013). Recovery-oriented practices of psychiatric-mental health nursing staff in an acute hospital setting. *Journal of the American Psychiatric Nurses Association, 19,* 1.

Norton, K. (2004). Re-thinking acute psychiatric inpatient care. *The International Journal of Social Psychiatry, 50,* 274.

SAMHSA. (2006). *National consensus statement on mental health recovery.* http://www.samhsa.gov/samhsa_news/volumexiv_2/article4.htm, Accessed 27.10.12.

SAMHSA. (2011). *Recovery defined—A unified working definition and set of principles.* http://blog.samhsa.gov/2011/05/20/recovery-defined-a-unified-working-definition-and-set-of-principles/, Accessed 27.10.12.

Schwartz, A., & Stanton, M. (1954). *The mental hospital.* New York: Basic Books.

Spandler, H., et al. (2007). Catching life: The contribution of arts initiatives to recovery approaches in mental health. *Journal of Psychiatric and Mental Health Nursing, 14,* 791.

Thomas, S., Martin, T., & Shattell, M. (2005, February 3). *Longing to make a difference: Nurses' experience of the acute psychiatric inpatient environment.* Presented at the 19th Annual Convention of the Southern Nursing Research Society, Atlanta, GA.

Thomas, S., Shattell, M., & Martin, T. (2002). What's therapeutic about the therapeutic milieu? *Archives of Psychiatric Nursing, 16,* 99.

U.S. Department of Health and Human Services. (1999). *Mental health: A report of the surgeon general.* Rockville, MD: U.S. Department of Health and Human Services, Substance Abuse and Mental Health Services Administration, Center for Mental Health Services, National Institutes of Health, National Institute of Mental Health. http://www.surgeongeneral.gov/library/mentalhealth/home.html, Accessed 09.09.09.

Vatne, S., & Fagermoen, M. (2007). To correct and to acknowledge: Two simultaneous and conflicting perspectives of limit-setting in mental health nursing. *Journal of Psychiatric and Mental Health Nursing, 14,* 14.

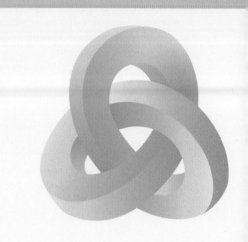

Variables Affecting the Therapeutic Environment: Violence and Suicide

Debbie Steele

evolve WEBSITE

http://evolve.elsevier.com/Keltner

LEARNING OBJECTIVES

- Discuss the impact of recovery-oriented care on the inpatient psychiatric milieu.
- Describe the five stages of the assault cycle.
- Explain the nursing interventions appropriate to the escalation and crisis phases of the assault cycle.
- Describe the nursing care of patients in seclusion and restraints.

- Differentiate between suicidal ideation, threats, gestures, attempts, and completion.
- Discuss nursing interventions related to suicidality.
- Describe the impact that aggressive and suicidal patients have on nursing staff.

In Chapter 20, management of the treatment environment was presented as a process whereby the nurse modifies elements of the treatment environment, including safety, structure, norms, limit setting, and balance. The psychiatric nurse must be aware of each of these essential elements while making decisions about how to modify various aspects of the environment to meet the treatment needs of patients. In this chapter, the focus is on the issues of violence and suicidality, particularly in the inpatient setting.

CURRENT TRENDS

Psychiatric inpatient and outpatient settings have changed significantly over the past 20 years. In 1990, the average inpatient psychiatric stay was 1 month, whereas the average stay in 2009 was 1 week. As a result of insurance and managed care restrictions, patients must meet stringent criteria to be admitted for a psychiatric hospitalization (i.e., imminent danger to self or others or grave disability). The cost-efficient managed care approach forces inpatient units into a rapid return of the patient to the community for less expensive treatment options. This trend has resulted in high turnover and even higher patient acuity rates.

Patients hospitalized in psychiatric hospitals are among the sickest, with seemingly limitless needs, poor insight, frequent readmissions, few placement alternatives, and bouts of unpredictable behavior. Despite the increased acuity

of these patients, there has been a continual push by the federal government, Substance Abuse and Mental Health Services Administration, American Psychiatric Association, American Psychiatric Nurses Association, and National Association of Psychiatric Health Systems to eliminate the use of seclusion and restraint in psychiatric treatment (Goetz & Taylor-Trujillo, 2012). As part of this mandate, nurses are required to use less restrictive measures before using the more restrictive interventions of seclusion and restraints. In response, new nursing practices have been initiated in psychiatric facilities related to the management of aggression and violence.

> **NORM'S NOTES**
> If there is one aspect of psychiatric nursing that most students (and many practicing nurses) fear, it is confrontation with an angry, aggressive, or violent mentally ill person. I don't blame you for feeling that way—in some ways this fear is good because it can motivate you to learn the material in this chapter. Aggressive outbursts, both verbal and physical, do happen, but the good news is that they do not occur nearly as often as you might imagine. This chapter provides important concepts on how to prevent (i.e., deescalate) aggressiveness and how to deal with aggression when it occurs.

AGGRESSION AND VIOLENCE

The potential for violence on hospital psychiatric units is a well-known environmental hazard. In addition to the physical danger that violent inpatients present to themselves, peers, and hospital staff, their actions are frightening and disrupt the therapeutic environment. At its worst, violent behavior can result in serious injury or death.

Violence on an inpatient psychiatric unit cannot always be predicted. It is important to be able to intervene when clear warning signs are evident. Nurses cannot know what is occurring on the unit unless they spend time interacting with their patients at frequent, regular intervals. Expert nurses use their assessment skills as well as their previous experiences to interpret inappropriate behavior within the context and knowledge of a patient's pathology. Understanding the patient's experience is considered a crucial factor in anticipating aggressive behavior. Carlsson and colleagues (2004) found that the nurse's presence and ability to be with the patient as a unique person in a stressful situation was considered essential for dealing with potentially violent patients. The necessity of staff-patient interaction cannot be overemphasized.

Although there are no guarantees against the occurrence of violence toward nursing staff, one variable affecting the risk of aggression is staff attitude. Violence on psychiatric units results from the complex interactions among patients, nursing personnel, and the culture of the specific unit. Strategies for decreasing the potential for violence focus on enhancing the nurse-patient relationship by way of improving communication skills, advocating for clients, being available, using continual clinical assessment skills, providing patient education in an open dialog, and collaborating with patients in treatment planning. The culture of the unit can be improved by providing meaningful patient activities and appropriate levels of stimulation and unit staffing (Janner & Delaney, 2012).

HIGHLIGHTING THE EVIDENCE

Research

Hospital policies focused on decreasing patient violence have been provided by McKinnon and Cross (2008). The authors identified the following priorities:
- Risk management: To identify high-risk patients
- Training: To ensure that all staff members are suitably prepared in the management of patient violence and that they feel confident and competent to deal with issues as they arise
- Sanctioning patients who assault staff and other patients: To make them accountable for their actions
- Incident reporting systems: To ensure that there are adequate and well-functioning processes to manage incidents and their sequelae, including rectifying any problems
- Comprehensive orientation package: To inform patients about the role of the treatment team, including expectations pertaining to therapeutic interactions and that violence is unacceptable

Working with psychiatric patients who may become violent requires nurses to be aware of their own aggressive impulses, the way in which they deal with their anger, and the methods they use to channel their anger into constructive and productive actions. Knowing how nurses respond to patients who show anger, anxiety, fear, panic, and assaultive behaviors is important (O'Donovan, 2007). Nurses cannot defuse patients' anger or aggression when they are in a similar state, and their anger might intensify patients' emotions; additionally, nurses are ineffective if they withdraw from hostile or demanding patients.

When patients become aggressive, nurses might experience frustration, a feeling of professional inadequacy, or a sense of failure. They might become overly controlling and engage in power struggles with patients. A nurse's participation in physically controlling violent patients can damage the chances of developing or continuing a therapeutic relationship. However, when nurses view patients' aggressive behaviors as a form of communication and focus on assisting patients with their own unique coping skills, the therapeutic relationship is strengthened. Nurses have the opportunity to convey to patients that help is available so they can deal more constructively with the environmental stresses that caused the initial problems and hospitalization (Lindsey, 2009).

? CRITICAL THINKING QUESTION

1. A visitor to the unit begins to hit a patient. How would you handle this situation?

MANAGEMENT OF INPATIENT AGGRESSION

Restraints and seclusion have traditionally been known to be indispensable interventions used to regulate potentially dangerous patient behavior or to prevent injuries and to diminish agitation (Hoekstra et al., 2004). However, the accumulating evidence against use of restraints and seclusion has led to new state and federal regulations designed to reduce and ultimately to prevent their use (Huckshorn, 2006). Taylor and associates (2012) described how a new seclusion and restraint program initiated at an acute psychiatric hospital required a significant culture change for nursing staff. The authors found that a 75% reduction in seclusion and restraint events occurred as a result of the following strategies: more complete assessment at admission, greater communication, staff education, and building relationships with patients. For example, the individualized plan of care included admission information such as what has worked in the past to control patient outbursts, what worsens outbursts, and what appears to reduce the risk of outbursts. A history of trauma was assessed to determine vulnerabilities or triggers that may be exacerbated during hospitalization. Trauma-informed care recognizes the importance of avoiding revictimization or recurrent traumatization on the unit. This admission information is used to create individualized care plans that are preventive in nature and emphasize self-management and patient responsibility (Goetz & Taylor-Trujillo, 2012).

NURSING INTERVENTIONS BASED ON THE ASSAULT CYCLE

The assault cycle can be used as a framework for nursing interventions that aim to prevent aggression and violence. On the most basic level, the goal of all interventions is to avoid physical and emotional harm to patients and staff. Smith's stress model (1981) describes the assault cycle with five stages of a predictable pattern or chain of aggressive responses to emotional or physical stress. Patients who are repeatedly assaultive exhibit behavior patterns that are ritualistic, stereotypical, and automatic. As the acuity of the aggressive response increases, a comparable decrease occurs in patients' problem-solving abilities, creativity, spontaneity, and behavioral options. The five-phase assault cycle includes the following:

1. *Triggering phase.* The stress-producing event occurs, initiating the stress responses.
2. *Escalation phase.* Responses represent escalating behaviors that indicate a movement toward the loss of control.
3. *Crisis phase.* During this period of emotional and physical crisis, loss of control occurs.
4. *Recovery phase.* In this period of cooling down, the person slows down and returns to normal responses.
5. *Postcrisis depression phase.* In this period, the person attempts reconciliation with others.

An overview of the assault cycle follows, interspersed with nursing interventions based on deescalation techniques. Deescalation is defined by Cowin and coworkers (2003) as a "gradual resolution of a potentially violent and/or aggressive situation through the use of verbal and physical expression of empathy, alliance and non-confrontational limit setting that is based on respect" (p. 65). Simply put, deescalation is defusing or "talking down" the agitated patient into a calmer state with the goal of preventing aggressive or violent behavior. Deescalation comprises a specific set of learned skills as explained next (Table 21-1).

Triggering Phase

The triggering phase is characterized by the automatic, negative emotional response patients have to stressful events that may occur while they are on the unit. Initially, as patients' negative emotions are aroused, their responses are nonviolent and present no danger to others. The behavior reflects

TABLE 21-1 INTERVENTIONS BASED ON ASSAULT CYCLE

PHASE	BEHAVIORS	NURSING INTERVENTIONS
Triggering phase: +1 to +2 level of anxiety	Muscle tension, changes in voice quality, tapping of fingers, pacing, repeated verbalizations, restlessness, irritability, anxiety, suspiciousness, perspiration, tremors, glaring, changes in breathing	Convey empathic support. Encourage ventilation. Use clear, calm, simple statements. Ask patient to maintain control. Facilitate problem solving by discussing alternative solutions. If needed, ask patient to go to a quiet area. Offer safe tension reduction measures. If needed, offer oral medications (prn).
Escalation phase: +2 to +3 level of anxiety	Pale or flushed face, screaming, anger, swearing, agitation, hypersensitivity, threats, demands, readiness to retaliate, tautness, loss of reasoning ability, provocative behaviors, clenched fists	Take charge with calm, firm directions. Direct patient to a quiet room for "time out." Offer oral medications (prn), if ordered. Ask the staff to be on standby at a distance. Prepare for a "show of concern."
Crisis phase: +3 to +4 level of anxiety	Loss of self-control, fighting, hitting, rage, kicking, scratching, throwing things	Use involuntary seclusion, restraints, or IM medications (prn), if ordered. Initiate intensive nursing care.
Recovery phase: +3 to +2 level of anxiety	Accusations, recriminations, lowering of voice, decreased body tension, change in conversational content, more normal responses, relaxation	Continue intensive nursing care. Process the incident with staff and other patients. Assess patient and staff injuries. Evaluate patient's progress toward self-control.
Postcrisis depression phase: +2 to +1 level of anxiety	Crying, apologies, reconciliatory interactions, repression of assaultive feelings (which might later appear as hostility, passive aggression)	Process incident with patient. Discuss alternative solutions to the situation and feelings. Progressively reduce the degree of restraint and seclusion. Facilitate reentry to unit.

IM, Intramuscular; *prn,* as needed.
Data from Maier, G.J. (1996). Managing threatening behavior: the role of talk up and talk down. *Journal of Psychosocial Nursing and Mental Health Services, 34,* 25; Smith, P. (1981). Empirically based models for viewing the dynamics of violence. In K. Babich (Ed.), *Assessing patient violence in the health care setting.* Boulder, CO: Western Interstate Commission for Higher Education; Stevenson, S. (1991). Heading off violence with verbal de-escalation. *Journal of Psychosocial Nursing and Mental Health Services, 29,* 6.

patients' usual coping and defense mechanisms. The nurse must assess how patients have coped with negative emotions in the past so that when they are triggered, the nurse becomes proactive and assists patients in behaving appropriately with their emotions. For example, if a patient's stressor is another individual in the immediate environment, the two patients can be separated, and nurses can talk with each patient individually to promote safe ventilation of emotions.

To facilitate ventilation of negative emotions such as anger, emphasis is on being supportive by using empathic, nondirective, yet concerned techniques. The nurse speaks softly in calm, clear, simple statements, avoiding any challenge to the patient. Aggressive, confrontational, or threatening approaches at this time usually result in escalation. Although ventilation is encouraged, other techniques found to be useful include relaxation techniques such as deep breathing. Patients' display of anger is socially embarrassing for them and counterproductive, leaving them with feelings of vulnerability and loss of autonomy. To protect the dignity of patients and the rights and safety of others, patients can be asked to take a "time out" in their rooms or at least move to a quieter area; other patients might be asked to leave the scene (Kozob & Skidmore, 2001a). It is important for nurses to compliment patients for their use of positive solutions.

Additional nursing interventions include helping patients identify productive coping skills that have worked in the past. Common suggestions may include journal writing, exercising, punching pillows, pounding clay, or walking up and down the hall. Oral antianxiety or antipsychotic medications can also be offered (Kozob & Skidmore, 2001b). A focus on the patients' strengths and self-responsibility needs to be integrated into the approach of nursing staff to patients through this process.

Clinical Example

John Henderson has been a patient on the unit for 3 days. While talking to his wife on the telephone, he becomes upset and raises his voice to her. The nurse calmly suggests that he tell his wife that he will continue their conversation later. He hangs up the telephone and starts pacing in the hallway. The nurse says, "Tell me what you are upset about." For 15 minutes, he describes the telephone conversation in detail, expresses anger toward his wife, and says he is afraid she will divorce him. As he visibly calms down, the nurse asks, "What would be most helpful in handling the situation with your wife?"

Escalation Phase

The escalation phase is characterized by an escalation of inappropriate or irrational behaviors such as swearing, screaming, and threatening. Deescalation techniques in this phase include allowing the patient whatever time is necessary to reduce his or her anxiety, fear, or anger. Telling aggressive patients that nurses are there to "support" them helps to reframe the situation from a confrontational to a collaborative encounter (Goetz & Taylor-Trujillo, 2012). For example, at a safe distance, the nurse calls the patient by name and states in a calm, firm manner that the nurse is there to assist the patient in

working through his or her feelings. The nurse avoids sudden movements and loud tones so as not to appear to be attacking.

If the patient has orders for as needed (prn) antianxiety or antipsychotic medications, an oral dose can be offered early in the escalation phase. If the oral dose is refused or if the escalation is rapid, an intramuscular (IM) medication might be preferred. Among the oral antianxiety medications, lorazepam (Ativan) and alprazolam (Xanax) are often the drugs of choice because they take effect rapidly and have relatively few side effects. Lorazepam might be given via the IM route. Among the antipsychotics, the medications that can be given orally (quetiapine [Seroquel]) or orally or intramuscularly (haloperidol [Haldol] and ziprasidone [Geodon]) have lower sedating effects but help decrease agitation.

Given the principle of the least restrictive environment, a time out in a quiet room is first offered by the nurse in a kind but firm manner. If this measure is ineffective, more restrictive measures might be instituted when the patient's behavior compromises the culture of safety. Other staff members might be called to be on standby, but they should initially try to remain out of the patient's view. When patients are potentially violent, their physical proximity to others is perceived as being much closer than it actually is, and they might feel threatened.

If the patient is unable to use his or her coping skills effectively and safety is threatened, the nurse asks for staff assistance for a stronger "show of concern" (Goetz & Taylor-Trujillo, 2012). This action involves having four to six staff members within sight of the patient but at a greater distance from the patient than the primary nurse so that they do not appear ready to attack the patient. Frequently, when the patient becomes aware of the other staff members and is informed that the staff will help the patient control his or her behavior, the patient can gain reasonable composure, cooperate with the nurse's request, take the medications, and go to a quieter room with or without staff escort (Lindsey, 2009). If these interventions do not work, the patient is usually close to entering the crisis phase.

Crisis Phase

The crisis phase is reached when the patient is approaching an attack on the environment, self, other patients, or staff. Verbal limits are ineffective, and external control by the staff is essential. In these emergency or crisis situations, immediate seclusion, restraint, or the administration of stat. medications becomes necessary. The patient has the right to refuse medication, but staff might give it in the presence of an *immediate* physical threat to others. These actions should be supported by emergency protocols that have been approved by the physicians and hospital, and any actions taken should be carefully and thoroughly documented in the patient's records.

Psychiatric emergencies must be dealt with in coordinated and organized ways, and the staff must have the opportunity to role-play their approach in advance of a crisis. All staff members should master self-protection techniques against behaviors such as kicking, hitting, and biting. Facilities must provide deescalation programs for all staff members; they are required to update these skills yearly. Staff members who are well trained in deescalation techniques are less likely to be victims of patient assaults.

Seclusion

Seclusion is the process of placing the patient alone in a specially designed, lockable room equipped with a security window or a camera for observation. Nurses make the decision to initiate and terminate the seclusion of patients according to established protocols and are almost always involved in the care of patients during seclusion. The principle of seclusion is *containment*: restricting patients so that they do not hurt themselves or others, decreasing stimulation, and increasing intensive nursing care. Agitation and disruptive or inappropriate sexual behaviors are other reasons for seclusion. Seclusion is viewed as a preventive strategy to *avoid* aggressive assaults as well as a responsive action. Time out, closer supervision, quiet interactions, and medication are therapeutically effective when used appropriately for brief periods.

The degree of seclusion depends on the patient's current status. The patient who is able to choose time out voluntarily might stay willingly in his or her room without a locked door. Others may be escorted by two staff members, without bodily contact, to a seclusion room that contains only a bed (bolted to the floor) and a mattress or just a mattress on the floor. This type of room decreases stimuli, protects the patient from injury, prevents destruction of property, and provides for the patient's privacy. The door, lockable from the outside, keeps the patient from leaving the room, if needed. Dangerous articles (e.g., belts, sharp objects such as pens and keys, shoes, eyeglasses) are taken away from the patient.

Restraint

The staff must take immediate action when assaults occur. Six to eight staff members (including hospital security officers if insufficient unit staff members are available) are needed to control a patient *safely* and ensure that no injuries to the staff, patient, or other patients on the unit occur. The number of staff needed should not be underestimated because of the size, age, or gender of the patient. Some agencies include information about patients' previous athletic interests and accomplishments (e.g., weight lifting or a black belt in karate) on the admission form.

Details of restraint procedures, including therapeutic holds for children, are not described here, but a general outline is presented. To prepare for control of a patient, staff members remove their own glasses, rings, earrings, pens, watches, keys, and anything else that might cause injury to the patient or staff. Furniture and objects that can be used as weapons are removed from the area. One staff member becomes the team leader to organize and direct the planned, coordinated approach, while the original staff member continues talking with the patient. At least one staff member takes the other patients to a safe place and stays with them.

The team approaches the patient calmly, in a "show of concern." The patient is told that the team is here to help, will not hurt the patient, and will not allow the patient to hurt anyone else. The nurse should inform the patient that although physical contact is employed as a last resort, the minimum amount of force will be used to ensure everyone is safe. During physical contact, the team should continue to interact with the aggressive patient in such a manner to cease physical contact at the first available opportunity. As two team members approach from each side and take control of the patient's arms, three other staff members quickly take control of the patient's legs and head so that the patient can be carried to the room or held on the floor until a bed is brought to the patient. Physical contact is protective and defensive, not aggressive. One staff member brings the restraint cuffs, opens doors, and moves obstacles. A nurse prepares the IM medication (or calls to get an order if no routine prn order exists).

In the seclusion room, the patient is usually placed on the bed on his or her back. Four or more staff members hold the patient's extremities and head securely, without hyperextending the patient's joints. Wrist and ankle restraints are applied to all four extremities and secured to the frame of the bed. The patient's arms are tied in a position at the side, not above the head. The restraints are tight enough to inhibit slipping out of them but not tight enough to interfere with circulation. The patient should be free of all belongings that might be used to cause harm to self or others. Medications might be administered at this time. A waist restraint, a restraint between the ankles, or a restraint blanket (or any combination of these) is applied *only* if the patient is at risk of injury because of fighting the restraints. Before staff members leave, the patient is checked for injuries and observed for the ability to move safely in the restraints.

Within 1 hour, an order to restrain the patient must be obtained, and a physician must perform a face-to-face evaluation of the patient. Federal, state, and hospital regulations or policies govern the extent to which the patient must be evaluated by the nurse and physician for the need to continue the restraints, by the physician in a face-to-face examination, and in the progress notes by the nurse and physician (Huckshorn, 2004).

Care of Patients in Seclusion or Restraints

When a patient is placed in seclusion or restraints, intensive nursing care is instituted. The patient is continuously observed directly or by video monitor. Other patients are not allowed to be near a restrained patient. The patient's mental status, response to and side effects of medications, hydration, nutrition, elimination, range of motion, vital signs, and hygiene are monitored. Immediate attention to any injuries resulting from the incident or from the restraints is critical and requires documentation. Every 2 hours, with two staff members present, the restraints are removed one at a time, for 10 minutes each, to allow range-of-motion activities. Change of position and skin care are also important. Restricting visitors, telephone calls, and diversional materials, such as radios and magazines, reduces stimuli; however, regular staff contact decreases the patient's sense of isolation and loneliness.

Recovery and Postcrisis Depression Phase

In this phase, patients are assured that they are not being punished while in seclusion and that they will be allowed back in the milieu as soon as possible. Patients must be assisted in relaxing, sleeping, and benefiting from this phase of cooling down and reconciliation. The time that patients are in restraints or seclusion should be a supportive, restorative time. Otherwise, patients remain afraid, frustrated, and angry, possibly leading to future aggression. After patients are calm, they are encouraged to discuss the circumstances during which they lost control and alternatives for handling similar situations in the future (Kozob & Skidmore, 2001a).

Patients are ready to be released from restraints when they can verbalize feeling less anxious and agitated and have an increased attention span, reality orientation, and sound judgment. Patients might be kept in the seclusion room briefly to assess their reaction to release from the restraints. Patients need assistance to reenter the unit with as little fear and embarrassment as possible. The nurse's role is to help other patients accept these patients back into the unit.

Immediately after a patient has been secluded and restrained, a code event review is initiated to ensure that no staff injuries have occurred, evaluate the way the situation was handled, and give mutual support and feedback. This debriefing by staff involves focusing on the specifics of the event as well as the success of techniques used or not used. Data are collected such as the patient's aggression level, response effectiveness, safety issues, and future recommendations. This review of events serves to reinforce safety education and identify areas for improvement (Goetz & Taylor-Trujillo, 2012). In addition, careful documentation must be recorded in the patient's chart to include the patient's behaviors before, during, and after the incident and a rationale for why physical control interventions, seclusion, and restraint were used. Staff perceptions are compared for accuracy. Documentation is descriptive, sequential, organized, and specific about what was seen, heard, and felt; what was said and by whom; who was notified; and what actions were taken and will be taken. The request for and granting of a physician's order for seclusion or restraint are also recorded (Huckshorn, 2004).

Other patients' reactions to restraint and seclusion situations should be discussed openly and explored in a unit meeting with staff. The reasons for and the purpose of seclusion and restraint need to be discussed in a matter-of-fact and honest manner. Patients must have the opportunity to share their concerns, reactions, and fears of losing control and be reminded to approach staff if they begin feeling upset and angry. It is important for patients on the unit to know that the safety of all patients is the primary concern, not punishment or mere control of a patient's behavior. Although restraints and seclusion are sometimes necessary, they still remain a method of last resort.

In light of these new philosophical changes, nurses often express concern and negativity when the topic of restraint reduction arises (Curran, 2007). Some preliminary evidence has suggested that efforts to decrease the use of restraints might be accompanied by an increased risk of harm to psychiatric patients and staff (Khadivi et al., 2004). Because staff and patient safety is perceived to be at risk, the idea of staff being discouraged from placing the patient in restraints may lead to nursing staff having a decreased sense of security in their environment. Curran (2007) reported that the barriers to restraint reduction are complex, involving knowledge deficits, fear, and traditional cultural practices.

Making a change in the culture of safety on inpatient psychiatric units has been the subject of more recent research. McLoughlin and associates (2013) noted the need for more formal education in the recovery model for nurses and patients. As would be expected, seasoned nurses are reluctant to incorporate recovery-oriented practices such as self-management and personal responsibility into acute psychiatric settings because of safety concerns. It may be more difficult to integrate recovery principles with children and adults who are displaying psychosis. Modification becomes necessary based on the individual's needs and circumstances. With patients who are unable to make sound decisions related to their safety and well-being, it becomes the nurses' responsibility to do more for these individuals when they can do less and to do less for the individuals when they can do more for themselves. Nurses must assess the situation continually and seek to empower individuals in their own decision making as they move toward enhanced self-direction.

Although this chapter has focused on nursing interventions related to aggression and violence in acute psychiatric hospitals, aggressive behavior may occur in any setting, including medical and surgical units, nursing homes, community health settings, clinics, and especially emergency departments. One survey of emergency department nurses found that 25% of those surveyed had been physically assaulted within the last year (Gacki-Smith et al., 2009). Nonpsychiatric staff might be less familiar with anticipating, preventing, and managing aggression compared with psychiatric nursing staff members, who are trained in assessing and defusing anger and in safely deescalating aggressive behaviors.

SUICIDE

All human beings periodically experience psychological burdens, pain, and stress during their lifetime, and having transient thoughts of wanting to die may be a natural response to emotional pain. Although most people develop nonsuicidal strategies for coping with the inevitable suffering in life, for some people, suicide becomes a solution to these overwhelming feelings. In the midst of the psychological pain, suicide can become a gripping and viable means of escape. Suicide

> **? CRITICAL THINKING QUESTION**
>
> 2. Why is it important for other patients to share their opinions and reactions about the seclusion and restraint of another patient?

may be considered as both a coping mechanism and a failure to cope (Cutcliffe & Links, 2008; Lakeman & FitzGerald, 2008; Paterson et al., 2008).

Suicidal behavior can be considered a problem-solving behavior reflecting a person's way of relating to the world. For example, an individual with HIV may choose suicidal behavior as a means of enhancing a sense of control over life. Fantasizing about the time, place, and method of one's own death allows a person to feel a sense of escape from the suffering. Having the possibility of an escape may make it easier for the individual to carry on and endure emotional pain. Contemplation of suicide and suicidal gestures or attempts, once relinquished, often are met with a sense of relief (Lakeman & FitzGerald, 2008). Suicide may serve several functions: (1) an escape, (2) a means of ensuring control, (3) a solution, and (4) a cry for help.

Shneidman, a suicidologist, coined the term *psychache* to describe the agony associated with suicidality. "Psychache is the hurt, anguish, or ache that takes hold in the mind. It is intrinsically psychological—the pain of excessively felt shame, guilt, fear, anxiety, loneliness, angst, dread of growing old or of dying badly …. Suicide happens when the psychache is deemed unbearable and death is actively sought to stop the unceasing flow of painful consciousness" (Shneidman, 1996). When suicidal individuals can no longer bear their pain and suffering, crisis intervention becomes necessary. For some individuals, hospitalization becomes the best choice for providing safety from harm.

RISK FACTORS

Chronic mental disorders most closely associated with risk for suicide include major depressive disorder, schizophrenia, and substance abuse. The relationship between suicide and mental illness is complex, with higher rates of completed and attempted suicide in people diagnosed with mental disorders compared with the general population. A psychiatric diagnosis is considered to be the most reliable risk factor for committed suicides. Suicide is the cause of death in 10% to 15% of all patients with depression, schizophrenia, or alcoholism.

Schizophrenic patients with frequent bouts of suicidal ideation have a greater number of hospital admissions and a longer duration of illness. Approximately 50% of suicidal patients who had auditory hallucinations stated they were told to self-harm by the voices. Simms and colleagues (2007) determined that suicidal attempts by these patients were primarily made on impulse and were not well thought out. These findings stress the importance of assessing suicidality in all psychiatric hospitalized patients (Box 21-1).

Suicide is the leading cause of death in psychiatric hospitals and is reportedly the most distressing event on an inpatient unit. Environmental factors known to influence the occurrence of inpatient suicide include inadequate patient intake assessments, inadequate staffing levels, insufficient staff orientation and training, infrequent patient observations, inadequate communication, and patient assignment to inappropriate units (Lynch et al., 2008). Hanging, suffocation,

---

HIGHLIGHTING THE EVIDENCE
Research

In a qualitative study, Carlen and Bengtsson (2007) offered insight into the suffering experienced by patients with suicidal ideation. The authors found three prominent themes: hopelessness, meaninglessness, and being out of control. A brief description of each theme follows:

Hopelessness: Feelings of hopelessness dominate their perception of their life situation. These feelings include a conviction that their feelings would never change. Hopelessness prevents suicidal patients from finding solutions to painful problems.

Meaninglessness: Suicidal patients disclose feelings of not having something to live for. They believe they hold no significance for others and nobody cares about them or would miss them if they died. They also believe it would be a relief for relatives and friends if they were to take their own life.

Being out of control: Being out of control encompasses exaggerated thoughts and catastrophic feelings. Thoughts related to committing suicide can become like an obsession, as if suicide forces itself on the patient. Patients try to brush it away, but it returns as an involuntary thought.

From Carlen, P., & Bengtsson, A. (2007). Suicidal patients as experienced by psychiatric nurses in inpatient care. *International Journal of Mental Health Nursing, 16,* 257.

BOX 21-1 RISK FACTORS ASSOCIATED WITH SUICIDE

- Recent losses
- History of prior suicide attempts
- Substance abuse
- Family history of psychiatric disorders
- Having a family member who has committed suicide
- Hopelessness
- Poor impulse control
- Lack of social support
- Recent release from inpatient psychiatric hospitalization

---

and jumping are known to be the most frequent methods of suicide in inpatient settings (The Joint Commission, 2007). Exposed pipes, fire safety sprinkler heads, and curtain rods all are high-risk environmental hazards. Patient items such as belts, shoelaces, and drawstring pants are also potentially dangerous. Additional precautions to be employed on inpatient units to decrease the possibility of suicidal attempts are provided by The Joint Commission (Box 21-2).

ASSESSMENT OF SUICIDAL PATIENTS

Critical interdisciplinary activities associated with suicide precautions include frequent suicide assessments. The Joint Commission (2007) recommends that suicide assessments be performed on admission; during any changes in precaution or privilege level, mental status, medication, or treatment protocol; and before hospital discharge. A suicide risk assessment addresses suicidal thoughts, intent, plan, and lethality of suicide plan.

BOX 21-2   **THE JOINT COMMISSION TIPS FOR PREVENTING INPATIENT SUICIDES**

Environmental factors that mitigate inpatient suicides include the following:

- Breakaway bars, rods, showerheads
- Low-flushing toilets, weight-tested for safety
- Adequate visualization of high-risk areas
- Use of monitoring equipment
- Suicide risk assessments, with psychometric properties
- Checking for contraband on admission
- Observation at frequency prescribed by risk
- Engagement of family and friends
- Identification of high-risk populations
- Prescribed observation checklist
- Consideration of staff assignment, including consideration of circadian rhythms, workloads, and time pressures
- Staff performance reviews and quality improvement protocols
- Provisions for shift change
- Using medications to treat conditions that contribute to risk

From Joint Commission on Accreditation of Healthcare Organizations (2001). *Comprehensive accreditation manual for hospitals.* Chicago: JCAHO.

The issue of suicidality can be viewed on a continuum ranging from suicidal ideation to completed suicide. *Suicidal ideation* involves a person's thoughts and wishes related to wanting to die. Suicidal ideas may vary from quite nonspecific thoughts that life is not worth living to specific thoughts of death, including intent and a plan. Suicidal ideation may be accompanied by threats, gestures, and attempts. *Suicidal threats* involve an individual's declaration of intent to end his or her life. *Suicidal gestures* are coping strategies used by suicidal individuals; these nonlethal self-injury acts include cutting or burning of the skin and ingesting small amounts of drugs. *Suicide attempts* are the actual implementation of a self-injurious act with the express purpose of ending one's life. Suicide attempts are considered self-destructive behavior serious enough to warrant medical contact. *Completed suicide* is the term used exclusively when individuals have successfully ended their lives.

A suicidal patient is fraught with conflicting feelings, particularly ambiguity about the future. The more depressed and hopeless the patient, the more detailed the plan, the more lethal and accessible the method, the greater the likelihood that a suicidal effort will be successful. In some cases, the impulsive behaviors of suicidal individuals experiencing ambiguous feelings about taking their own life can prove to be fatal. Intended and unintended death is more likely to occur when a more lethal method is contemplated.

SUICIDE INTERVENTIONS

The following general guidelines are useful for nurses who work with suicidal patients:

1. Developing the nurse-patient relationship, which is built on trust and understanding, is the most important component of positive patient outcomes. As trust is developed, the patient is more apt to reveal information vital to determining the likelihood of an imminent crisis related to suicidal ideation.

2. The first step in the assessment of potential suicidality is asking the patient about suicidal thoughts. Screening for suicidal ideation is essential in determining a patient's level of suicidality. Nurses ask directly about thoughts of suicide as part of the screening. Sample screening questions include: Have you been having any thoughts about wanting to harm yourself? Have you been feeling like you don't want to live anymore? Identification of suicidal ideation allows nurses to focus on ensuring patient safety in light of the presence of self-harming cognitions.

3. If a patient is positive for suicidal ideation, the nurse should ask about the plan (i.e., how the patient intends to accomplish the suicide). Patients who have a well-developed plan are considered at increased risk for suicide attempt and suicide completion.

    a. Lethality associated with suicidality is related to accessibility—the means to commit suicide.

    b. If a patient mentions the use of a gun, family members should be notified either to remove any firearms from the home entirely or to lock guns and ammunition securely in separate locations.

    c. If the patient mentions overdosing on drugs, the same recommendations are applied to restricting access to potentially lethal prescriptions, over-the-counter medications, and alcohol.

4. When asking a patient about a suicidal plan, it is important for the nurse to understand the following:

    a. Talking to patients about their suicidal intentions does not drive them to suicide. Asking patients direct questions elicits useful information and may provide patients with a sense of relief (e.g., "Finally, someone hears me").

    b. Many people who have died as a result of suicide did not mean to die; they tragically miscalculated. Many people who die as a result of suicide do so accidentally.

5. Previous attempts are known to be a risk factor associated with suicide. It is essential to ask the patient about previous suicide attempts.

    a. The nurse should ask about the method of previous attempt.

    b. The nurse should ask how the patient was rescued.

    c. The nurse should ask about the patient's response to treatment and follow-up care.

6. Patients should be evaluated for major depressive symptoms, recent losses, alcohol or drug abuse, and command hallucinations, all of which place individuals at an increased risk for suicide.

7. The nurse should communicate openness and acceptance of the suicidal patient's feelings and life situation. The nurse should encourage exploration and open expression

of suicidal feelings, allowing patients to understand their problems better within an emotionally safe nurse-patient relationship.

8. Close observation, also called *one-to-one observation*, is the standard of care for patients experiencing suicidal thoughts, severe anxiety, and agitation. Suicidal patients on inpatient psychiatric units are regularly assessed using one of two levels of suicide prevention:

   a. Frequent observation (sometimes referred to as *level 1*) is used for patients who are not considered to be at immediate risk of suicide. The nursing staff provides periodic observation (every 15 minutes) and monitors drug taking, eating utensils, shaving gear, and other potentially dangerous devices in the environment. The staff communicates concern and control with this close observation of patients and their environment. Patients are asked to sign a no-suicide contract with the nurse stating that they will not harm themselves during hospitalization and will seek out a staff member should they begin to contemplate self-injurious behavior. Although not legally binding, no-suicide contracts can serve to deter the acting out of harmful and potentially fatal behavior. Suicidal patients who are admitted to an inpatient unit commonly start to feel better almost immediately. As a result of the safe environment provided, patients may deny having suicidal thoughts shortly after admission. Simply having a structured, safe environment can elicit feelings of hopefulness and a brighter future. As patients are removed from their stressful situations and have the opportunity to interact with objective mental health professionals, they have the opportunity to think more clearly and recognize potential options for their future. However, the nurse must understand that it is the maintenance of the safe environment that is the primary cause of the patient's more positive feelings and thinking. Frequent observation as well as other safety measures should be continued even when a patient no longer admits to suicidal ideation while hospitalized.

   b. Continuous observation (sometimes referred to as *level 2*) is used for patients who present an immediate and serious threat of suicidal behavior. Level 2 also might be initiated for patients who refuse to sign a no-suicide contract. Uninterrupted observation is typically required. This approach is an expensive use of human resources but provides the needed control and human interaction. Patients at serious risk are usually confined to the unit and have restrictions on visitors and where meals are taken and have bathroom supervision.

Patients who experience bouts of suicidality eventually are discharged from the inpatient setting to community

---

⊚ CARE PLAN

A 23-year-old man with a diagnosis of schizophrenia, paranoid type, has been admitted to a psychiatric hospital because of command hallucinations telling him to kill himself. The patient lives with his mother, who does not feel comfortable in her ability to keep her son from harming himself. How might nursing care assist this patient and family?

Assessment

Problems:
1. Patient admits to auditory hallucinations telling him to kill himself.
2. Patient is easily agitated and increasingly paranoid.
3. Patient tends to isolate in his room.
4. Patient is religiously preoccupied.
5. Patient is logical, linear, organized, and coherent.
6. Patient is able to contract for suicide while hospitalized but not after discharge.
7. Patient denies substance abuse and dependence.

Diagnosis
Risk for self-directed violence related to command hallucinations telling him to kill himself.

Outcomes

Short-term goals

Date met: _____ Patient will explore suicidal thoughts with staff.

Date met: _____ Patient will contract for safety with nurse every shift.

Date met: _____ Patient will connect suicidal thoughts to current stressors.

Long-term goals:

Date met: _____ Patient will report confidence in ability to manage suicidal thoughts.

Date met: _____ Patient will participate in follow-up individual and family psychotherapy.

Planning and Interventions

Nurse-patient relationship: Assess for presence of suicidal ideation. Assess severity of suicidality, asking patient about intent and plan related to suicidal thoughts. Contract for safety every shift. Allow patient to share feelings such as hopelessness, helplessness, shame, and despair. Assist patient in connecting suicidal thoughts to current stressors.

Psychopharmacology: Paliperidone (Invega) 12 mg PO every morning; discuss role of medications and related side effects.

Milieu management: Continuous observation with restrictions, such as confinement on the unit. Keep environment free of harmful objects. Encourage patient to spend time in day room interacting with other patients. Collaborate with patient in ongoing treatment plan.

resources. Continuity of care is best provided through careful and thoughtful patient and family discharge planning. The Joint Commission (2007) recommends the following discharge instructions:

- Explain the uneven recovery path from their illness, especially depression (e.g., "There are likely to be times when you feel worse and times when you will feel better. Contact our health care clinician if you start having difficulty dealing with your depressive thoughts").
- Inform family and friends (if indicated) about the signs of increased suicide risk, especially sleep disturbance, anxiety, agitation, and suicidal expressions and behaviors.
- Document if the patient does not wish to permit contact with family.
- Provide information for a follow-up appointment, which may include contacting the current provider or scheduling an appointment.
- If the presence of firearms has been identified, document instructions given to patient and significant other.
- Provide prescriptions that allow for a reasonable supply of medication to last until the first follow-up appointment (when indicated).
- Provide information about local resources available, such as emergency contact numbers (local and national numbers, such as 1-800-273-TALK) and instructions.

? CRITICAL THINKING QUESTION

3. What positive and negative effects can an inpatient hospitalization have on a patient's emotional recovery?

BURNOUT AND SECONDARY TRAUMATIZATION

The daily stress of dealing with patients with emotional and behavioral problems can be taxing for nursing staff caring for patients in acute psychiatric hospitals. Psychiatric nurses must manage violent and suicidal patients, yet they are charged with keeping the environment safe for all patients and staff. This negative workplace experience results in negative feelings, such as fear and anxiety. Stressors such as these take their toll on the nurse in the form of burnout (also known as *emotional exhaustion*), secondary traumatization, and posttraumatic stress disorder (PTSD).

Burnout is a psychological experience caused by long-term involvement in emotionally demanding situations. Although a subjective phenomenon, burnout has a clear relationship with the organizational setting in which it occurs. It is a process that involves intense emotional labor leading to symptoms such as emotional exhaustion, depersonalization, and reduced personal achievement. Burnout is associated with nurses' tendency to evaluate themselves negatively, particularly in relation to their work with patients (Dickinson & Wright, 2008). Younger and less experienced mental health care providers have a tendency to be at greater risk for burnout.

Burned-out staff members score high on scales measuring feelings of being emotionally burdened, and they tend to overinterpret patient care failures as their own fault (Thomas et al., 2005). This tendency leads to a spiraling process of decreased effectiveness in nurse-patient interactions at all levels, so assistance may be required (Box 21-3). Some manifestations of burnout on a psychiatric unit are low morale; passivity; avoidance; disinterest; chronic complaining; and negative, hostile reactions to others (Schreiber & Lutzen, 2000). Caring for patients on a psychiatric unit involves emotional work that requires nurses to suppress their usual human reactions to others in the name of social acceptability—that is, professionalism (Mann & Cowburn, 2005).

In recent decades, increased attention has been given to the effects of trauma on individuals. The professional literature related to working with trauma revealed the phenomenon of vicarious traumatization, also called *secondary traumatization*, *helper stress*, or *compassion fatigue* (Thomas & Wilson, 2004). Vicarious traumatization refers to the transformation that occurs in the health care worker who empathically engages with patients' traumatic experiences and their sequelae (Pearlman & Mac Ian, 1995). Nurses who continually hear patients' distressing and traumatic stories are at increased risk for secondary traumatization. These frequent encounters influence the nurses' personal sense of safety and their views of others' trustworthiness. As nurses are confronted with the poor prognoses associated with many hospitalized patients, they may experience disillusionment, cynicism, and despair (Robinson et al., 2003).

Being injured by a patient is similar emotionally to being a victim of crime and can lead to PTSD. Experiencing physical and emotional harm at the workplace can destroy the staff member's sense of trust in others and sense of control of his or her life. The staff member often expresses feelings of guilt, vulnerability, irritability, depression, anxiety, nightmares, grief, and fear of the patient who caused the injury. The assault might be minimized, and feelings might even be denied if emotional support and debriefing are not provided after the medical examination and treatment have been completed. If the injured staff member is away from work for a while, the rest of the staff might be unaware that their emotions have subsided much more than the emotions of their injured colleague. To ensure that the staff victim achieves emotional resolution of the incident, supportive interventions should be available (Richter & Berger, 2006). Peer support programs that understand the dynamics of assault and the common responses of victims is important. The needs of the victim determine the type of support and counseling initiated and

BOX 21-3   RESOURCES FOR BURNOUT

It is important that nurses seek out assistance for preventing and recovering from burnout. Examples of potential professional resources are professionals with experience in burnout and nursing literature, such as Dr. Marion Conti-O'Hare, author of *The Nurse as Wounded Healer: From Trauma to Transcendence* (Sudbury, MA: Jones & Bartlett, 2002) and the American Nurses Association (http://www.nursingworld.org). Involvement in one's professional association can be a great resource for new and experienced nurses.

maintained. In addition, victims are encouraged to share their feelings with family or significant others. The goal of this process is to facilitate emotional resolution, help the person remain productive, and decrease the chance of resignation and development of PTSD (Poster, 1996). More research is needed that focuses on the cumulative effects of vicarious traumatization, coupled with direct trauma and violence, on inpatient psychiatric nursing staff.

CLINICAL SUPERVISION FOR PSYCHIATRIC NURSES

Clinical supervision is one intervention known to assist psychiatric nurses who experience high levels of stress associated with the overwhelming responsibility of caring for patients and families with complex and difficult mental health care needs. This stress management strategy helps nurses to avoid burnout and job-related stress (Edwards et al., 2006). Clinical supervision provides a structured mechanism of allowing nurses to reflect on their day-to-day practices as well as validate their complex and challenging clinical decisions. As staff nurses are provided an opportunity to examine their attitudes, reactions, and conflicts with patients, they are led to find new ways of approaching patient problems. Activities such as clinical supervision also help nurses develop sensitivity to the patient.

Clinical supervision is recognized as a vital component of modern, effective psychiatric care. Traditionally, mental health care professions have an established culture of clinical supervision. For example, clinical social workers consider supervision to be essential for sustaining reflective practice. Clinical supervision is defined as a formal relationship-based education and training that is work-focused. Supervisors aim to manage, support, develop, and evaluate the work of supervisees through corrective feedback. Supervision differs from related activities such as mentoring and coaching (Milne, 2007). Although psychiatric nursing employs a form of clinical supervision, the manner practiced by other mental health professions remains more of an aspiration than a reality. Clinical supervision within the nursing arena is most frequently seen as part of management, rather than properly regarded as something nonhierarchical, nonjudgmental, and focused on the nurse (supervisee) rather than the organization. Benefits of supervision serve to clarify values, promote self-awareness, provide a role model, evaluate best practices in health care, and protect against burnout. There is evidence that good supervision contributes to general well-being, knowledge, confidence, morale, understanding, and job satisfaction (Launer, 2007).

Clinical supervision is used not only to address the emotional impact of patient encounters but also to examine issues within the team and the broader workplace setting. Two approaches to supervision are equally effective: one-to-one sessions and group meetings. Clinical supervision, done properly, provides a checks-and-balances system built to promote professional development that ultimately benefits the nurse, the patients, and the rest of the nursing staff. Research shows that this type of organizational support to nurses translates into improved patient outcomes.

EFFECTIVE FUNCTIONING IN THE ACUTE PSYCHIATRIC SETTING

At the close of this chapter, discussing solutions is in order. Norton (2004) has indicated that one way to reduce frustration is for inpatient units to define how the different parts fit together into a functioning whole; this applies to other aspects of psychiatric care as well. Clearly articulating the real purpose of the unit, as opposed to holding to standards of care that cannot be met in this new era of psychiatric care, allows all parties to be more realistic about the intent of the inpatient unit or other treatment settings.

Compulsory mental health treatment is a controversial issue, particularly in the area of involuntary hospitalization and forced medication. In light of the patient acuity seen in psychiatric hospitals, current practices continue to rely on the use of medications and other biologically based interventions as the solution. As previously mentioned, recovery-oriented care is a patient-led and family-led initiative that emphasizes collaboration between patients and providers to ensure that treatment respects patients' preferences and perspectives. This increasingly influential movement is expected to continue to play a pivotal role in the restructuring of mental health services in the future. Because nurses are educated to provide holistic patient-centered care, they may find themselves trapped between the medical model and recovery principles. Psychiatric nurses are weighed down by administrative, technical, and crisis tasks that take them away from collaborating with and empowering patients. This conflict can lead to burnout for nurses and other hospital staff. More recently, efforts have taken place to reconcile the divergent approaches of mental health care personnel and consumers. Young and colleagues (2005) reported on the effectiveness of inviting, and even mandating, that consumers (individuals diagnosed with mental disorders) serve on boards of mental health care facilities in order to be a part of the review process for agencies receiving state funds.

▌ STUDY NOTES

1. An increase in patient acuity as well as a more rapid turnover in patient admissions and discharges in psychiatric hospitals creates stress for staff members and patients.
2. The assault cycle describes the predictable phases of aggression: triggering, escalation, crisis, recovery, and depression.
3. Verbal and physical aggression requires safe, immediate interventions based on the principle of the least restrictive alternative.
4. Tension reduction, medications, physical control, seclusion, and restraints are to be used judiciously in the escalation and crisis phases of the assault cycle.

5. Patients in seclusion and restraints require intensive physical and emotional nursing care.

6. Suicide is a complex issue—a spectrum ranging from ideation to completed suicide.

7. Suicide may be seen as both a coping mechanism and a failure to cope.

8. Identifying patients who are at imminent risk for suicide in the inpatient setting is a critical clinical challenge.

9. It is important for the nurse to communicate openness and acceptance of the suicidal patient's feelings and life situation.

10. Open expression of suicidal feelings allows patients to understand their problems better within an emotionally safe nurse-patient relationship.

11. Hopelessness, meaninglessness, and feeling out of control are common emotions associated with suicidal ideation.

12. Caring for aggressive and suicidal patients on a continuous basis can lead to burnout and secondary traumatization.

13. Clinical supervision for nursing staff can be a tool to facilitate improved staff cohesion, morale, and the ability to maintain therapeutic relationships with patients.

14. Recovery-oriented care has influenced treatment settings by providing feedback to staff about the patient's perspective of the treatment environment.

REFERENCES

Carlen, P., & Bengtsson, A. (2007). Suicidal patients as experienced by psychiatric nurses in inpatient care. *International Journal of Mental Health Nursing, 16*, 257.

Carlsson, G., et al. (2004). Violent encounters in psychiatric care: A phenomenological study of embodied caring knowledge. *Issues in Mental Health Nursing, 25*, 191.

Cowin, L. S., et al. (2003). De-escalating aggression and violence in the mental health setting. *International Journal of Mental Health Nursing, 12*, 64.

Curran, S. S. (2007). Staff resistance to restraint reduction: Identifying and overcoming barriers. *Journal of Psychosocial Nursing and Mental Health Services, 45*, 45.

Cutcliffe, J., & Links, P. (2008). Whose life is it anyway? An exploration of five contemporary ethical issues that pertain to the psychiatric nursing care of the person who is suicidal: Part two. *International Journal of Mental Health Nursing, 17*, 246.

Dickinson, T., & Wright, K. (2008). Stress and burnout in forensic mental health nursing: A literature review. *British Journal of Nursing, 17*, 82.

Edwards, D., et al. (2006). Clinical supervision and burnout: The influence of clinical supervision for community mental health nurses. *Journal of Clinical Nursing, 15*, 1007.

Gacki-Smith, J., et al. (2009). Violence against nurses working in US emergency departments. *The Journal of Nursing Administration, 39*, 340.

Goetz, S. B., & Taylor-Trujillo, A. (2012). A change in culture: Violence prevention in an acute behavioral health setting. *Journal of the American Psychiatric Nurses Association, 18*, 96.

Hoekstra, T., Lendemeijer, H., & Jansen, M. (2004). Seclusion: The inside story. *Journal of Psychiatric and Mental Health Nursing, 11*, 276.

Huckshorn, K. A. (2004). Reducing seclusion and restraint use in mental health settings: Core strategies for prevention. *Journal of Psychosocial Nursing and Mental Health Services, 42*, 22.

Huckshorn, K. A. (2006). Re-designing state mental health policy to prevent the use of seclusion and restraint. *Administration and Policy in Mental Health, 33*, 482.

Janner, M., & Delaney, K. R. (2012). Safety issues on British mental health wards. *Journal of the American Psychiatric Nurses Association, 18*, 104.

Joint Commission on Accreditation of Healthcare Organizations, (2001). *Comprehensive accreditation manual for hospitals.* Chicago: JCAHO.

Khadivi, A. N., et al. (2004). Association between seclusion and restraint and patient-related violence. *Psychiatric Services (Washington, D.C.), 55*, 1311.

Kozob, M. L., & Skidmore, R. (2001a). Seclusion and restraint: Understanding recent changes. *Journal of Psychosocial Nursing and Mental Health Services, 39*, 25.

Kozob, M. L., & Skidmore, R. (2001b). Least to most restrictive interventions. *Journal of Psychosocial Nursing and Mental Health Services, 39*, 32.

Lakeman, R., & FitzGerald, M. (2008). How people live with or get over being suicidal: A review of qualitative studies. *Journal of Advanced Nursing, 64*, 114.

Launer, J. (2007). Moving on from Balint: Embracing clinical supervision. *British Journal of General Practice, 57*, 182.

Lindsey, P. L. (2009). Psychiatric nurses' decision to restrain. *Journal of Psychosocial Nursing and Mental Health Services, 47*, 41.

Lynch, M. A., et al. (2008). Assessment and management of hospitalized suicidal patients. *Journal of Psychosocial Nursing and Mental Health Services, 46*, 45.

Maier, G. J. (1996). Managing threatening behavior: The role of talk up and talk down. *Journal of Psychosocial Nursing and Mental Health Services, 34*, 25.

Mann, S., & Cowburn, J. (2005). Emotional labour and stress within mental health nursing. *Journal of Psychiatric and Mental Health Nursing, 12*, 154.

McKinnon, B., & Cross, W. (2008). Occupational violence and assault in mental health nursing: A scoping project for a Victorian Mental Health Service. *International Journal of Mental Health Nursing, 17*, 19.

McLoughlin, K. A., et al. (2013). Recovery-oriented practices of psychiatric-mental health nursing staff in an acute hospital setting. *Journal of the American Psychiatric Nurses Association, 19*, 1.

Milne, D. (2007). An empirical definition of clinical supervision. *British Journal of Clinical Psychology, 46*, 437.

Norton, K. (2004). Re-thinking acute psychiatric inpatient care. *International Journal of Social Psychiatry, 50*, 274.

O'Donovan, A. (2007). Patient-centred care in acute psychiatric admission units: Reality or rhetoric? *Journal of Psychiatric and Mental Health Nursing, 14*, 542.

Paterson, B., et al. (2008). Managing the risk of suicide in acute psychiatric inpatients: A clinical judgment analysis of staff predictions of imminent suicide risk. *Journal of Mental Health, 17*, 410.

Pearlman, L., & Mac Ian, P. (1995). Vicarious traumatization: An empirical study of the effects of trauma work on trauma therapists. *Professional Psychology, Research and Practice, 26*, 558.

Poster, E. C. (1996). A multinational study of psychiatric nursing staffs' beliefs and concerns about work safety and patient assault. *Archives of Psychiatric Nursing, 10*, 365.

Richter, D., & Berger, K. (2006). Post-traumatic stress disorder following patient assaults among staff members of mental health hospitals: A prospective longitudinal study. *BMC Psychiatry, 6*, 15.

Robinson, J., Clements, K., & Lands, C. (2003). Stress among psychiatric nurses: Prevalence, distribution, correlates, and predictors. *Journal of Psychosocial Nursing and Mental Health Services, 41*, 33.

Schreiber, R., & Lutzen, K. (2000). Revisiting nursing in a nontherapeutic environment. *Issues in Mental Health Nursing, 21*, 257.

Shneidman, E. (1996). *The suicidal mind*. Oxford: Oxford University Press.

Simms, J., et al. (2007). Correlates of self-harm behavior in acutely ill patients with schizophrenia. *Psychology and Psychotherapy, 80*, 39.

Smith, P. (1981). Empirically based models for viewing the dynamics of violence. In K. Babich (Ed.), *Assessing patient violence in the health care setting*. Boulder, CO: Western Interstate Commission for Higher Education.

Stevenson, S. (1991). Heading off violence with verbal de-escalation. *Journal of Psychosocial Nursing and Mental Health Services, 29*, 6.

Taylor, K., et al. (2012). Characteristics of patients with histories of multiple seclusion and restraint events during a single psychiatric hospitalization. *Journal of the American Psychiatric Nurses Association, 18*, 160.

The Joint Commission, (2007). *A resource guide for implementing the Joint Commission on Accreditation of Healthcare Organizations (JCAHO) 2007 patient safety goals in suicide*. http://www.naphs.org/Teleconference/documents/ResourceGuide_JCAHOSafetyGoals2007_final.pdf, Accessed 01.10.09.

Thomas, R. B., & Wilson, J. P. (2004). Issues and controversies in the understanding and diagnosis of compassion fatigue, vicarious traumatization, and secondary traumatic stress disorder. *International Journal of Emergency Mental Health, 6*, 81.

Thomas, S., Martin, T., & Shattell, M. (2005, February 3). *Longing to make a difference: Nurses' experience of the acute psychiatric inpatient environment*. Presented at the 19th Annual Convention of the Southern Nursing Research Society, Atlanta, GA.

Young, A., et al. (2005). Use of a consumer-led intervention to improve provider competencies. *Psychiatric Services, 56*, 967.

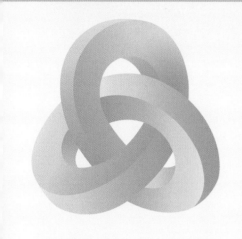

Therapeutic Environment in Various Treatment Settings

Debbie Steele

⊖volve WEBSITE

http://evolve.elsevier.com/Keltner

LEARNING OBJECTIVES

- Describe the various treatment activities used in the following inpatient psychiatric settings:
  - Intensive care or acute psychiatric units (locked units)
  - Child-adolescent psychiatric units
  - Acute substance abuse units
  - Co-occurring disorders units
  - Medical-psychiatric units
  - Geropsychiatric units
  - State psychiatric hospitals
  - State forensic hospitals
- Describe the treatment environment of community psychiatric settings, including:
  - Group homes
  - Partial hospitalization
  - Day treatment centers

Inpatient and outpatient psychiatric treatment centers serve a multitude of unique needs of patients with mental health disorders. The therapeutic environment is enhanced through the use of various structured activities arranged by a multidisciplinary team. In this chapter, key activities are described, along with an explanation of the various inpatient and outpatient treatment settings.

INPATIENT SETTINGS

Treatment Activities

The following types of therapeutic activities are offered in psychiatric settings in both inpatient and outpatient environments: (1) occupational therapy, (2) recreational therapy, (3) psychoeducation, (4) group therapy, (5) spirituality groups, and (6) community meetings. Many different disciplines are involved in enhancing the effectiveness of the therapeutic modalities offered to patients in the recovery process.

Occupational Therapy

Occupational therapists are trained professionals concerned with the functional abilities of patients as these abilities affect their capacity to work and perform tasks of daily living. Occupational therapists assist patients in mastering skills needed for self-care, work, and play. Activities of daily living are used by the occupational therapist to help people with mental disabilities achieve maximal functioning and independence at home and in the workplace. Arts and crafts classes are carefully selected based on the functional assessment of the occupational therapist of patients' deficits and strengths. For example, certain arts and crafts might be selected for their value in improving the patient's attention span and concentration. Other activities, such as games, can be fun and promote socialization with others. Learning to make time for pleasure and fun can be therapeutic for individuals dealing with the

NORM'S NOTES
I have mentioned the importance of the environment, but, as I noted in Chapter 1, one size does not fit all. How can you apply these concepts to different types of settings? Does it even matter? Both answers are "yes." You can't get away from your environment, and the people under your care can't get away from their environment. This chapter provides some ideas about how the concept of environmental manipulation can foster a therapeutic atmosphere in many diverse settings. And, as you might guess, what might be therapeutic in one setting might not be therapeutic in another.

stressors of life complicated by a mental illness. Specific therapy approaches are selected by occupational therapists and patients based on joint decisions in treatment team meetings.

Recreational Therapy

Leisure time is important for all individuals and is useful in promoting mental health. For the psychiatric patient, recreational activities are an important intervention in meeting treatment outcomes. Recreational therapists and occupational therapists assist patients in finding activities that help them learn to balance work and play. Individualized plans of care may involve exercise groups, such as aerobics or strength training. The level and type of exercise are determined based on the abilities of the patient. The benefits of exercise in modulating depression and anxiety have been well documented. Exercise therapy is also a therapeutic outlet for agitation and aggression.

HIGHLIGHTING THE EVIDENCE

The Wellness Recovery Action Plan (WRAP) is an evidence-based approach to group therapy that is consistent with recovery-oriented care. WRAP can be used in various mental health settings by certified peer specialists or other staff. The WRAP approach is designed to help patients create their own plan of care for staying well through a process of (1) decreasing and preventing intrusive or troubling behaviors and thoughts, (2) increasing personal empowerment, (3) improving quality of life, and (4) assisting individuals in achieving their own life goals and dreams (Copeland, n.d.). Pratt and associates (2013) conducted a study on the WRAP approach in Scotland. The authors found that WRAP groups offered participants information about the concept of recovery that most had not heard before, leading some participants to develop a useful, powerful new perspective of their experience. Participants described feeling they were capable of taking ownership of their own well-being for the first time. As stated by one participant, "WRAP offers a reminder of what you are like when you are well, and that offered hope and uncovered strategies for overcoming challenges when encountering an episode of illness" (p. 7).

Psychoeducation

Psychoeducation involves educating patients and families regarding symptom recognition and management. The goal of psychoeducation is to provide social support and share information relevant to the mental disorder so that patients can adapt to living with a chronic illness and find ways to remain stable. Empirical evidence has shown that understanding mental illness helps patients and their families cope more positively with the illness. Numerous studies have demonstrated the value of psychoeducation groups in improving quality of life, preventing relapse, and altering negative family reactions (Bond & Campbell, 2008; Dixon et al., 2000; Herz et al., 2000; Motlova, 2000; Pekkala & Merinder, 2000; Schimmel-Spreeuw et al., 2000).

Researchers have found psychoeducation to be very effective for improving treatment adherence rates (Colom et al., 2004; Keller, 2004; Sajatovic et al., 2004). Because families often assume much of the care burden for patients with chronic mental illness, inclusion of family members

---

BOX 22-1 EXAMPLES OF TOPICS FOR PSYCHOEDUCATIONAL GROUPS

- Recognizing signs of relapse
- Using public transportation
- Talking with your therapist, case worker, and psychiatrist
- Coping with stress
- Managing your medications
- Coping with symptoms
- Knowing when to call your physician
- Getting along with family members
- Returning to work
- Anger management
- Interpersonal skills
- Living skills

---

in psychoeducational groups is essential. Box 22-1 lists examples of topics appropriate for psychoeducational groups. Theoretically, any member of the treatment team could offer psychoeducational groups, and in many cases the psychiatric nurse uses this format for patient and family teaching, particularly in preparation for discharge.

Group Therapy

Group therapy is a beneficial and effective treatment option employed in many psychiatric settings. Groups are an economical way of working with a large number of patients. The many benefits associated with group therapy include (1) an opportunity to address issues with input from others (gain new insight, knowledge, and perspective), (2) feeling of acceptance and a sense of belonging, and (3) being accountable to a group of people with similar struggles (Keats & Sabharwal, 2008). Group therapy is a type of therapeutic environment of its own because it uses many of the important principles known to benefit patients with psychiatric disorders, including openness, giving and receiving feedback, respect, privacy, acceptance, independence, and individual responsibility. Group therapy can be particularly effective when members are in the group over a long period of time, allowing some of the unique curative factors of group work to develop.

Groups can be formatted in many ways—open or closed, process-oriented or psychoeducational, time-limited or ongoing. The type of group therapy depends on the purpose intended. For example, process-oriented groups may address such issues as self-esteem and anxiety. Box 22-2 lists the various types of group therapy practiced in psychiatric settings. Group therapy is applicable to the full spectrum of mental disorders, including child, adult, and elderly populations.

BOX 22-2 TYPES OF GROUP THERAPY

- Cognitive-behavioral
- Psychodynamic
- Gestalt
- Systems
- Interpersonal
- Family systems

HIGHLIGHTING THE EVIDENCE

Current Research

In an attempt to improve patient collaboration and satisfaction, Lim and colleagues (2007) interviewed patients in an acute mental health setting seeking to evaluate occupational services. Half of the patients indicated that occupational therapy assisted them by improving their concentration, focusing their minds, giving structure to their day, providing opportunities to socialize and interact with others, relieving boredom, and aiding in their recovery. Activities found to be most beneficial, useful, and enjoyable included cookery groups and sports and gym sessions. The researchers emphasized the need for occupational therapists to explain the purpose of occupational therapy to new patients and provide more individualized interventions in consultation with them.

Spirituality Groups

Spirituality groups help to instill hope and encourage patients to begin looking at their faith and spirituality as potential resources in their recovery. Although spirituality groups are not consistently offered in psychiatric treatment settings, The Joint Commission (formerly the Joint Commission on Accreditation of Healthcare Organizations) has standards requiring the assessment and interdisciplinary planning for the spiritual concerns and needs of patients. A chaplain or other mental health treatment team professional conducts these groups; the focus of these groups is usually on topics such as forgiveness, grieving, and finding meaning in life. During the group meetings, the group leader encourages the patients to discuss spiritual thoughts and feelings they have been experiencing—both uplifting thoughts and spiritual challenges and struggles. An important overall goal of the spirituality group is to help patients in their personal quest for spiritual, emotional, and relational growth and healing. As patients grow spiritually, they find increased strength and power to help them cope with and overcome the problems and challenges in their life. Patients vary in their response to these groups in the inpatient setting, faring better in the community setting when they are higher functioning both physically and emotionally (Richards et al., 2007). The topic of religion and spirituality must be discussed cautiously, particularly if there are patients in the group having religious preoccupations.

Community Meetings

Community meetings provide a forum for addressing the daily needs associated with community living and may take place in an inpatient or community setting. For example, a halfway house may have daily morning meetings to welcome new patients, review program rules, and make general announcements about the day's activities. Community meetings also allow patients to initiate discussions of community or individual concern and receive feedback from staff and other patients. Patient-patient and patient-staff conflicts may occur, requiring a skilled group leader to assist the involved individuals in handling the situation in a positive fashion. Common patient-patient concerns involve control of the television, the radio being played too loudly, and personal hygiene (e.g., someone is not bathing regularly). Community meetings are not forums for discussing the individual treatment needs and issues of patients; rather, they serve to address daily aspects of being in the treatment environment.

Inpatient Psychiatric Environments

This section provides an overview of the various inpatient treatment environments available to patients with mental health disorders. Each of these therapeutic settings focuses on a particular population with unique needs. The various activities described earlier in the chapter play an integral role in the structure of these therapeutic environments.

Intensive Care or Acute Psychiatric Units (Locked Units)

Acute psychiatric units provide 24-hour structured inpatient treatment within a locked setting. Treatment emphasis is on short-term, intense therapeutic interventions designed to provide the patient with rapid evaluation and stabilization of symptoms. Criteria for admission to an acute psychiatric unit include danger to self, danger to others, and gravely disabled. Patients may be admitted on either a voluntary or an involuntary basis. The severity of patients' illnesses tends to be quite high, requiring close supervision and intervention by nursing staff. Presenting problems include acute and severe or persistent mental illnesses, organic brain syndrome, detoxification from alcohol or drugs, acute situational or emotional distress, suicide threats or attempts, and medication adjustments. Staff includes psychiatrists, social workers, registered nurses, licensed practical nurses, certified nursing assistants, psychologists, marriage and family therapists, and occupational or recreational therapists.

Child-Adolescent Inpatient Units

Child-adolescent inpatient units offer comprehensive psychiatric assessment, stabilization, and short-stay intensive treatment to children and adolescents 2 to 17 years old who have complex psychiatric conditions. Common conditions that are treated on these units include severe depression, bipolar disorders, impulse-control disorders, phobias and other anxiety disorders, schizophrenia and other psychotic disorders, and eating disorders. Staff consists of an extensive interdisciplinary team (Box 22-3).

BOX 22-3 INTERDISCIPLINARY TEAM ON A CHILD-ADOLESCENT INPATIENT UNIT

- Dietitians
- Educators
- Nurses
- Occupational therapists
- Pediatric mental health specialists
- Physicians
- Psychologists
- Social workers
- Speech and language disorders specialists

The child-adolescent unit must meet specific age-appropriate criteria in terms of the physical environment and the treatment activities offered. Patients' schedules include time for individual, group, and family therapy; psychopharmacology consultation; and schoolwork. Time is also included for patients to play with their peers. Behavior management is a priority for some of these children and adolescents. Time-out, level or step programs, skills training groups, and seclusion all are approaches used to protect patients from harming themselves or others. Gullick and colleagues (2005) studied the factors associated with use of seclusion in children and adolescents in an eight-bed inpatient child and adolescent psychiatric unit in Australia. These researchers found that patients with greater psychopathology and family problems had a higher incidence of seclusion. See Chapter 34 for further discussion of the child and adolescent population.

Child and family–centered care is increasingly being perceived as an essential element in the care of children admitted to psychiatric inpatient units. Interventions include individual and group parent education sessions and family evaluations and treatment (Regan et al., 2006). Treatment focus is on the patient and family working together to address the issues that led to the hospitalization. In addition to working with staff to design a treatment plan and set shared goals, parents are expected to spend significant time with their children at the hospital. Parental participation is critical to all aspects of care and vital to the successful return of the child to his or her home, school, and community. Essential elements of the child and family–centered care approach need to be modified to take into account the special circumstances associated with adolescents and children who have grown up entirely in foster care or group home settings.

Acute Substance Abuse Treatment Centers

Substance abuse treatment centers provide detoxification and acute inpatient medical and psychiatric stabilization and treatment to individuals who are seeking help with an identified drug or alcohol problem. Admission criteria are based on the need for an inpatient level of care that may include detoxification from alcohol or opioids, including prescription narcotics, and detoxification and stabilization for patients in pain management programs. Therapeutic activities on substance abuse units include rigorous patient education, sensitization groups, and confrontational feedback sessions. See Chapter 31 for further discussion of patients with substance-related problems.

Clinical Example
Mary is a 37-year-old white woman who has experienced episodes of depression since her early twenties. Mary takes Paxil CR, 25 mg daily, for depression. A recent series of stressors involving her work and marriage precipitated an inpatient admission. Mary is married to a man with an alcohol problem and a pattern of irresponsibility related to family finances. Mary's husband recently informed her that he has a girlfriend and wants a divorce. Yesterday, she took an overdose of Paxil and called her husband in despair.

Her husband called the police who brought her to a local emergency department. Mary was treated and later that day admitted to an acute psychiatric unit. During group therapy, Mary is encouraged to journal, writing down her feelings. In recreation therapy, Mary uses a stationary bicycle to help elevate her mood. The occupational therapist assists Mary in creating a ceramic cup. While participating in individual therapy with the social worker, Mary becomes aware of the effect of her actions on her children. The nurse works with Mary to reinforce all these therapeutic activities and identifies problem areas to explore with her in their one-to-one therapeutic interactions.

Clinical Example
Sara is a 42-year-old white woman who has been drinking alcohol excessively and taking alprazolam (Xanax) for the past 3 years. Sara's withdrawal symptoms were managed on the inpatient substance abuse unit. Sara attends educational sessions about addiction, alcoholism, and dealing with unhealthy relationships. Sara also attends group therapy, in which she talks about many underlying unaddressed feelings of grief about her mother's death. As Sara progresses through treatment, she will participate in numerous therapy groups aimed at helping her avoid relapse after discharge.

Co-occurring Disorders Inpatient Units

Inpatient units for patients with co-occurring disorders focus on the treatment of substance abuse and mental illness in a psychiatric hospital setting. The goals of treatment are twofold: simultaneous resolution of the medical and psychological crises. These units provide detoxification services and psychotherapy and group activities. Treatment plans address the patients' substance abuse or dependence, psychiatric illness, and the relationship between the co-occurring disorders. Psychopharmacology for these patients can be particularly challenging because of the nature of the dual diagnoses. During hospitalization, patients begin to build the skills, knowledge, and motivation to abstain from substance misuse and to maintain gains achieved toward positive outcomes. These patients are at increased risk of suicide, violence, and discharge against medical advice. After patients are stabilized medically and psychologically, they are referred to co-occurring disorder programs in the community setting.

HIGHLIGHTING THE EVIDENCE
Co-occurring Disorders

A comparison of hospital-based inpatient treatment and community residential care for patients with co-occurring disorders was conducted by Timko and colleagues (2006). They found that patients in the community setting achieved better substance use and psychiatric outcomes compared with hospitalized patients. Results of the study emphasize the need for ongoing community treatment after individuals with co-occurring disorders are discharged from an inpatient setting.

MEDICAL-PSYCHIATRIC HOSPITAL UNITS

Medical-psychiatric units are specially designed for mentally ill patients with coexisting medical problems in need of hospitalization. These specialized units are equipped to address the comorbid conditions simultaneously, improving outcomes. Nurses working on these units must have knowledge of psychological disorders, psychotropic drugs, medical diseases, and medications. The focus of therapeutic activities depends on the nature of the psychological and medical infirmity. Some geriatric psychiatric units have been reclassified as medical-psychiatric units because of the large number of medical problems in this population (Inventor et al., 2005).

Clinical Example

Marvin is a 47-year-old African-American man with a history of bipolar disorder, diabetes, and congestive heart failure. He was brought to the emergency department with a blood sugar level of 643 mg/dL and severe dehydration. Marvin stopped taking his medications recently because he believed he was able to handle his problems on his own. He has been walking the streets and preaching to people in fast-food restaurants. Last night, the McDonald's store manager found Marvin babbling and acting "drunk." The manager called the police, who then escorted Marvin to the local emergency department. Typically, Marvin's diabetes is difficult to control. After Marvin was rehydrated and his blood sugar level restabilized, Marvin was admitted to the integrated medical-psychiatric unit for close observation of his medical status and simultaneous participation in treatment activities for his mental illness. Marvin attends a psychoeducational group with several other patients who also have problems with substance abuse and exacerbation of serious medical problems. When Marvin is stabilized medically, he will participate in other treatment activities.

Geropsychiatric Units

Population demographics reflect an increasingly aging population with medically complex conditions. Patients on geropsychiatric units have a psychiatric disorder, one or more acute or chronic health conditions, and an array of normal age-related physical changes. The most commonly occurring mental disorders include Alzheimer's disease, depression, bipolar disorder, anxiety disorder, delirium, and schizophrenia (Smith et al., 2005). Additionally, older patients are at increased risk for medical complications related to hypertension, kidney disease, Parkinson's disease, heart disease, and numerous other chronic physical problems (Inventor et al., 2005).

Specific considerations related to the treatment environment are dictated by the unique needs of this medically compromised older adult population with psychiatric problems. The physical structure of geropsychiatric units must be designed with the frail, elderly, cognitively impaired patient in mind. For example, the unit should be free of unnecessary noise to counter the vulnerability of older patients to sensory overstimulation. A smaller unit with fewer patients has been shown to improve interaction not only among patients but also between patients and staff (Day et al., 2000; Teresi et al., 2000).

Older patients with dementia may experience confusion and disorientation leading to difficulty navigating the hospital environment. Interventions such as environmental cues have been found to be helpful in geropsychiatric settings. Environmental cues may include (1) large orientation boards on which the date, time, and location of daily events are posted; (2) clearly marked names or graphic images (e.g., bathrooms, bedrooms with patients' names on the doors); and (3) color coding of different locations.

Falls are of great concern on the geropsychiatric unit. Inventor and colleagues (2005) reported that 22% of the older adult population in this setting take more than four prescribed drugs, increasing their susceptibility to drug interactions and falls. Because older patients are likely to have impairment in mobility, balance, and vision, increased lighting and simple, uncluttered rooms facilitate comfort and safety.

The importance of the environment for patients in a geropsychiatric unit is evident by the increasing number of studies on facility design and planning. These studies have shown an association between the environmental design of the unit and patients' level of improvement in regard to variables such as self-care, agitation, and mood. Group therapy, for patients able to participate, might involve issues such as grief and loss. For less cognitively functional patients, group therapy might involve orientation, memory enhancement, and reminiscence activities in a more structured format. See Chapters 28 and 35 for discussion of the unique care needs of the geriatric patient.

State Psychiatric Hospitals

Traditionally, state psychiatric hospitals provided long-term treatment to individuals with intellectual and developmental disabilities, chronic psychiatric disorders, and forensic cases. In 1999, there was an aggressive movement toward deinstitutionalization as a result of the Olmstead decision making "unjustified isolation" of individuals with cognitive disabilities in institutions a violation of the Americans with Disabilities Act. Population characteristics in state psychiatric hospitals have changed, reflecting an increase in forensic patients who are more severely psychotic (Salzer et al., 2006).

The environment at state psychiatric hospitals is highly restrictive. In some facilities, *treatment malls* are built and used to provide programs focused on rehabilitation and recovery. The rehabilitative focused approach employs (1) skills-based relapse prevention programs to decrease recidivism rates, (2) cognitive-behavioral programs to decrease symptom severity, and (3) psychoeducation to improve patients' knowledge of their illness (Birkmann et al., 2006). Daily and weekly activities, such as community meetings, anger management, gardening, and computer skills groups, are geared toward the goal of community reintegration (Citrome et al., 2008).

State Forensic Hospitals

Patients confined to state forensic facilities have a diagnosable mental illness and have been convicted by a court of a criminal offense. State forensic hospitals are the most restrictive of all treatment environments. Patients residing in forensic psychiatric facilities have been charged with criminal offenses and are deemed too dangerous to reside in the community. State forensic hospitals are a secure environment with strict rules and regulations to ensure safety for the general population. Buildings are designed with maximum security to prevent patients from escaping. Guard-controlled doors, metal detectors, and strategically placed checkpoints throughout the facility are common features of state forensic facilities.

Patients in forensic psychiatric settings are guilty of committing a crime believed to be associated with their mental illness. Notorious individuals who exemplify the types of patients cared for by forensic psychiatric nurses include Andrea Yates, the Texas woman who drowned her five children, and Lee Malvo, the teenager who participated in the Washington, DC, sniper shootings with his father figure, John Muhammad. Psychiatric nurses in forensic settings must possess a unique set of skills and competencies.

Nurses working in forensic psychiatric settings must be aware of their feelings toward patients. Nurses are expected to demonstrate respect for the humanity of the patient regardless of the person's background or diagnosis. Patients often have been detached from society's norms because of the way they think and behave (Bowring-Lossock, 2006). Nurses must interact with these offenders in an ethical manner, cognizant of the fact that they are mentally ill.

HIGHLIGHTING THE EVIDENCE

Evidence-Based Practice

Centering on the importance of a caring relationship, Rask and Brunt (2007) developed a conceptual model using verbal and social interactions in nurse-patient communications in forensic psychiatric settings. Based on their research, the following six categories were identified:

Building and sustaining relationships. Supports the ability of patients to develop healthy trust in another person. As patients feel more secure, it may help them to open up and share their thoughts and feelings. To maintain this sense of trust, nurses need to act and communicate in clear, respectful ways with their patients.

Supportive and encouraging interactions. Encouraging patients when they do something good; helping patients seize opportunities to make progress; assisting patients to cope with their problems by talking to them when they are having difficulty; giving patients space to reflect on their difficulties, enabling them to develop new coping skills.

Social skills training. Helps develop and improve patients' skills in relating to others; increases the ability of patients to decode, interpret, and act on social signals to develop healthier interpersonal relationships; provides feedback to patients related to their behavioral and communication skills.

Reality orientation. Confronting interventions designed to help patients work through or gain insight into the content, meaning, and effects of the criminal behavior that led to incarceration; develops the patient's awareness of limited attitudes or behavior of which they are unaware; explains consequences of behavior.

Reflective interactions. Talking to patients about their feelings and thoughts in relation to other people; talking to patients about their inner world, memories, and experiences; helping patients reflect on earlier experiences, such as childhood abuse, and change how they perceive themselves and their problems.

Practical skills training. Reinforces positive behavioral patterns of everyday living, such as maintaining personal hygiene, eating regular meals, and sleeping regular hours; encourages patients to learn new skills to participate in a broader social context.

❓ CRITICAL THINKING QUESTION

1. How has the trend for hospitalized psychiatric patients to be more acutely ill now than they were in the past affected the nursing profession?

❓ CRITICAL THINKING QUESTION

2. Should society be investing resources into the treatment of patients who have committed heinous crimes? How would it be determined that a patient was rehabilitated?

COMMUNITY TREATMENT SETTINGS

As the focus of psychiatric care has shifted away from inpatient and state psychiatric hospitals, community treatment programs have increased. At the present time, much psychiatric care takes place in group homes, in day programs, or through support offered to patients and their family members via home health visits. Psychiatric patients in these community settings are more acutely ill than ever before. This section focuses on the unique aspects of community psychiatric treatment.

Group Homes

A group home is a moderately sized, approximately 6- to 12-bed program located in a neighborhood setting that is staffed with nonclinical paraprofessionals who provide specialized services offered within the context of a "24/7" homelike milieu. It is a structured service program that creates a physically, emotionally, and psychologically safe environment for children, adolescents, or adults with moderate psychological needs who either are too young or lack the skills necessary to function in an independent living situation. A group home is designed to serve as an alternative living arrangement to the family home. Staff members are expected to support the residents in life skills development. Residents are expected to abide by the house rules, which are clearly communicated during community group meetings. Therapeutic activities such as psychoeducation, individual and group therapy, and medication management may be offered in-house or accessed through community providers as needed. Nursing staff are not always employed in these settings but rather serve as consultants.

Group homes for children or adolescents require a 24-hour structured supportive and educational milieu. Residents may have a history of suicidal or homicidal thoughts or impulses but no immediate plan of intent and no recent exacerbation of symptoms. Children may be having moderate to severe functional problems in school or community settings (e.g., school suspension, involvement with the law) because of the inability to accept age-appropriate direction or supervision from the parent or guardian. Typically, the poor impulse control experienced by the child or adolescent is expressed through periodic verbal aggression directed toward self and others, interfering with the development of successful interpersonal relationships. For some older children and adolescents convicted of sexually aggressive behavior, a specialized group home setting may be an option over a locked juvenile detention facility.

Partial Hospitalization

Partial hospitalization is a short-term, ambulatory treatment program for patients transitioning from an acute psychiatric inpatient facility. As a result of brief inpatient hospital stays, psychiatric patients with severe and enduring symptoms are often poorly stabilized before their hospital discharge and so require ongoing intensive treatment. The goal of the partial hospitalization approach is to reduce the likelihood of rehospitalization and to facilitate successful integration into a community setting (Yanos et al., 2009). The partial hospitalization facility is usually connected with a hospital. The program provides full-day psychiatric rehabilitation services, including psychoeducation, nursing services, psychiatric medication evaluation and monitoring, case management services, and individual psychotherapy. Regulatory agencies and third-party payers require a registered nurse in these facilities to attend, at the minimum, to urgent care matters that might arise and to assist with medication administration and management. Treatment is structured similarly to the inpatient environment, but patients are considered safe enough to be able to return to their residence in the evening. After completing a partial hospitalization program, patients are stepped down to a community mental health center for day treatment or outpatient care.

Day Treatment

Day treatment programs focus on patient stabilization, rehabilitation, and recovery in a community outpatient setting. The programs are designed to (1) maintain or enhance current levels of functioning, (2) maintain community living, and (3) develop self-awareness through the exploration and development of intrapersonal strengths and interpersonal relationships. Day treatment is similar to the partial hospitalization program in that patients attend the scheduled activities for a prescribed number of hours and specified frequency. Day treatment programs represent a midpoint between hospitalization and outpatient clinic visits.

Handa and colleagues (2009) reported on a continuous day treatment program for patients with a diagnosis of schizophrenia. The treatment program employed a recovery model, whereby patients are treated for mental illness with the goal of living, working, learning, and participating fully in the community. Characteristically, recovery is not viewed as a cure but rather as a process; it is viewed as an attitude of hope and a sense of control over one's life. The recovery model is gaining prominence in the mental health field as consumers and families are advocating for a recovery-oriented approach that is person-centered rather than illness-focused.

Clinical Example

Peter is a 25-year-old single, white man with schizophrenia. He has a history of multiple hospitalizations. Typical symptoms include paranoid delusions, acute agitation, impulsiveness, and verbally threatening behavior. The staff day treatment center is collaborating with Peter to plan an individualized treatment program. His counselor has daily interactions with Peter to teach and promote more socially appropriate behavior through modeling and mentoring. Peter has repeated opportunities to rehearse new interpersonal skills, which are reinforced by his mother at home.

Day Treatment Center for Patients with Co-occurring Disorders

The term *co-occurring disorders* refers to the comorbidity of a mental disorder and a substance addiction disorder. More than 50% of patients in mental health treatment settings have a coexisting substance-related disorder. Similarly, more than 50% of patients in substance abuse treatment settings have a coexisting psychiatric disorder (Minkoff, 2001). The prevalence of co-occurring disorders has been found to be even higher among the veteran population (Pray & Watson, 2008). Patients with co-occurring disorders are more difficult to treat successfully than patients with either substance abuse diagnosis or a mental disorder. Rather than parallel treatment for mental health and addictions, patients receive intensive, coordinated community-based mental health and substance abuse treatment provided by a team of professionals.

Interventions found to be successful at day treatment centers are extensive and comprehensive. Group sessions are useful in motivating patients with co-occurring disorders to set goals. (See Box 22-4 for examples of co-occurring disorder groups.) Day treatment centers offer an integrated approach that focuses on patients developing coping skills to manage the anxiety, frustration, and problems of daily living. Lectures, videos, and discussions on relapse prevention are crucial aspects of the program and assist patients in identifying their high-risk situations and practicing alternative

---

BOX 22-4 CO-OCCURRING DISORDER GROUPS

- Medication management
- Community meetings
- Wellness classes
- Vocational classes
- Family psychoeducation

coping strategies. These patients are also encouraged to attend Alcoholics Anonymous or Narcotics Anonymous groups and to secure a sponsor.

SUMMARY

This chapter has provided an overview of the various psychotherapeutic environments in inpatient and outpatient settings. There is a continuum of care ranging from intensive care psychiatric inpatient hospitalization to day treatment centers for patients with psychiatric disorders. Nurses fill a wide variety of health care roles depending on the treatment setting. In most settings, nurses are responsible for providing psychoeducation related to mental disorders and medication regimens. Additionally, nurses are responsible for managing the therapeutic milieu and coordinating the various interdisciplinary activities. In settings where paraprofessionals are responsible for the various activities, such as group homes, nurses may serve as consultants. Regardless of the settings, the goal of treatment is the stabilization, rehabilitation, and recovery of patients with psychiatric disorders.

STUDY NOTES

1. A variety of health care professionals are involved in the treatment milieu of a psychiatric facility, including physicians, nurses, psychologists, social workers, chaplains, and occupational and recreational therapists.
2. Members of the treatment team and patients attend therapeutic community meetings to welcome new patients, review milieu rules, and make general announcements about the day's activities. (*Note:* Not all units have therapeutic community meetings.)
3. Various treatment activities are employed within psychiatric settings, such as group therapy, recreational therapy, exercise therapy, spirituality groups, and psychoeducation.
4. Patients in intensive care or acute, locked psychiatric units are often admitted involuntarily and usually need close supervision and intervention by nursing staff.
5. A special focus of the child-adolescent psychiatric unit is the inclusion of parents in the treatment program.
6. Medical-psychiatric units are specialty psychiatric environments that address the needs of patients with a chronic medical illness and coexisting psychiatric problems.
7. Therapeutic activities on a substance abuse unit tend to employ confrontation because of the extensive use of denial by patients with substance abuse problems.
8. Patients with both a substance abuse problem and a psychiatric diagnosis can be treated on co-occurring disorder units, which balance confrontational and supportive approaches.
9. Geropsychiatric units address specialized needs of older adults, including environmental modifications necessary because of sensory losses and other safety factors.
10. A forensic hospital is the most restrictive of all treatment environments.
11. Significant levels of psychiatric care are provided in group homes, partial hospitalization programs, and other community settings.
12. Preparing patients to live in the community requires an emphasis on social skills, independent living skills, and prevention of relapse and rehospitalization.

REFERENCES

Birkmann, J., et al. (2006). A collaborative rehabilitation approach to the improvement of inpatient treatment for persons with a psychiatric disability. *Psychiatric Rehabilitation Journal, 29,* 157.

Bond, G., & Campbell, K. (2008). Evidence-based practices for individuals with severe mental illness. *Journal of Rehabilitation, 74,* 33.

Bowring-Lossock, E. (2006). The forensic mental health nurse. A literature review. *Journal of Psychiatric and Mental Health Nursing, 13,* 780.

Citrome, L., et al. (2008). Integrating state psychiatric hospital treatment and clinical research. *Psychiatric Services, 59,* 958.

Colom, F., et al. (2004). Psychoeducation in bipolar patients with comorbid personality disorders. *Bipolar Disorders, 6,* 294.

Copeland, M. (n.d.). *The wellness recovery action plan (WRAP).* Retrieved on January 12, 2014 from: http://copelandcenter.com/wellness-recovery-action-plan-wrap.

Day, K., Carreon, D., & Stump, C. (2000). The therapeutic design of environments for patients with dementia: A review of the empirical research. *Gerontologist, 40,* 397.

Dixon, L., Adams, C., & Lucksted, A. (2000). Update on family psychoeducation for schizophrenia. *Schizophrenia Bulletin, 26,* 5.

Gullick, K., et al. (2005). Seclusion of children and adolescents: psychopathological and family factors. *International Journal of Mental Health Nursing, 14,* 37.

Handa, K., et al. (2009). Continuous day treatment programs promote recovery in schizophrenia. A case-based study. *Psychiatry, 6,* 32.

Herz, M. I., et al. (2000). A program for relapse prevention in schizophrenia: A controlled study. *Archives of General Psychiatry, 57,* 277.

Inventor, B., et al. (2005). The impact of medical issues in inpatient geriatric psychiatry. *Issues in Mental Health Nursing, 26,* 23.

Keats, P., & Sabharwal, V. (2008). Time-limited service alternatives: Using therapeutic enactment in open group therapy. *The Journal for Specialists in Group Work, 33,* 297.

Keller, M. B. (2004). Improving the course of illness and promoting continuation of treatment of bipolar disorder. *Journal of Clinical Psychiatry, 65*(Suppl. 15), 10.

Lim, K., Morris, J., & Craik, C. (2007). Inpatients' perspectives of occupational therapy in acute mental health. *Australian Occupational Therapy Journal, 54,* 22.

Minkoff, K. (2001). Best practices. Developing standards of care for individuals with co-occurring psychiatric and substance use disorders. *Psychiatric Services, 52,* 597.

Motlova, L. (2000). Psychoeducation as an indispensable complement to pharmacotherapy in schizophrenia. *Pharmacopsychiatry, 33*(Suppl. 1), 47.

Pratt, R., et al. (2013). Experience of wellness recovery action planning in self-help and mutual support groups for people with lived experience of mental health difficulties. *The Scientific World Journal.* Retrieved January 12, 2014 from, http:dx.doi.org/10.1155/2013/180587.

Pray, M., & Watson, L. (2008). Effectiveness of day treatment for dual diagnosis patients with severe chronic mental illness. *Journal of Addictions Nursing, 19,* 141.

Pekkala, E., & Merinder, L. (2000). Psychoeducation for schizophrenia. *Cochrane Database of Systematic Reviews,* (4), CD002831.

Rask, M., & Brunt, D. (2007). Verbal and social interactions in the nurse-patient relationship in forensic psychiatric nursing care. A model and its philosophical and theoretical foundation. *Nursing Inquiry, 14,* 169.

Regan, K., Curtin, C., & Vorderer, L. (2006). Paradigm shifts in inpatient psychiatric care of children. Approaching child- and family-centered care. *Journal of Child and Adolescent Psychiatric Nursing, 19,* 29.

Richards, P., Hardman, R., & Berrett, M. (2007). *Spiritual approaches in the treatment of women with eating disorders.* Washington, DC: American Psychological Association.

Sajatovic, M., Davies, M., & Hrouda, D. R. (2004). Enhancement of treatment adherence among patients with bipolar disorder. *Psychiatric Services, 55,* 264.

Salzer, M., Kaplan, K., & Atay, J. (2006). State psychiatric hospital census after the 1999 Olmstead decision. Evidence of decelerating deinstitutionalization. *Psychiatric Services, 57,* 1501.

Schimmel-Spreeuw, A., Linssen, A. C., & Heeren, T. J. (2000). Coping with depression and anxiety: Preliminary results of a standardized course for elderly depressed women. *International Psychogeriatrics/IPA, 12,* 77.

Smith, M., Specht, J., & Buckwalter, K. (2005). Geropsychiatric inpatient care: What is the state of the art? *Issues in Mental Health Nursing, 26,* 11.

Teresi, J., Holmes, D., & Ory, M. (2000). The therapeutic design of environments for people with dementia: Further reflections and recent findings from the National Institute on Aging Collaborative Studies of Dementia special care units. *Gerontologist, 40,* 417.

Timko, C., et al. (2006). Dual disgnosis patients in community or hospital care: One year outcomes and health care utilization and costs. *Journal of Mental Health, 15,* 163.

Yanos, P., et al. (2009). Partial hospitalization. Compatible with evidence-based and recovery-oriented treatment? *Journal of Psychosocial Nursing and Mental Health Services, 47,* 41.

CHAPTER

23

Introduction to Psychopathology

Norman L. Keltner

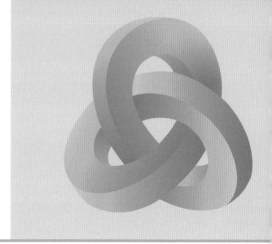

evolve WEBSITE

http://evolve.elsevier.com/Keltner

LEARNING OBJECTIVES

- Describe the extent of mental illness in the United States.
- Identify the most common mental disorders in the United States.
- List the three requirements for understanding psychopathology.
- Describe several guidelines applicable to all aspects of psychotherapeutic management.

Old paradigm: *Caring teachers urged caring students to be more caring. (Yawn!)*

New paradigm: *Caring is not enough. Psychiatric nurses must understand psychobiology and psychopharmacology.*

According to Reeves and colleagues (2013), 25% of the U.S. adult population is affected by mental disorders during a given year. As noted in Table 23-1, anxiety disorders are the most prevalent, followed by mood, impulse-control, and substance abuse disorders. This table, which is also found in Chapter 2 and in most chapters in this unit, lists prevalence rates for a 12-month period. Among specific disorders, major depression (one type of mood disorder) and phobias are most common. Lifetime incidence of these disorders is slightly higher (Kessler et al., 2005b, National Institute of Mental Health, 2005; U.S. Surgeon General, 1999). Table 23-2 provides the data for lifetime prevalence rates for the most common mental and chemical abuse disorders. Many individuals have a comorbid status; for example, an individual may be depressed and anxious and abuse a chemical or have some other combination of disorders. Psychiatric morbidity is concentrated, with approximately 23%

of the population having a history of three or more comorbid disorders (Kessler et al., 2005a). Most of these individuals do not seek professional help, suggesting a great reservoir of unmet mental health needs in the United States.

The incidence of psychopathology is high, and the nurse's understanding of psychopathology is basic for effective psychotherapeutic management of mental disorders. Understanding psychopathology requires the following standards:

1. Knowledge should be organized.
2. Operational definitions should be formed.
3. Criteria for diagnosis should be developed.

Several diagnostic systems have been developed, but this text relies on criteria from the *Diagnostic and Statistical Manual of Mental Disorders (DSM)*, which is published by the American Psychiatric Association and is the official diagnostic manual in use in the United States. The current version, *DSM-5* (American Psychiatric Association, 2013), is the seventh version since the *DSM* was first published in 1952 (*DSM-I, DSM-II, DSM-III, DSM-III-R, DSM-IV,* and *DSM-IV-TR*). Because diagnostic consistency among clinicians is so important, psychiatric experts are constantly evaluating and

TABLE 23-1	12-MONTH PREVALENCE RATE OF MENTAL DISORDERS IN THE UNITED STATES*	
DISORDERS	**APPROXIMATE PERCENTAGE >17 YEARS OLD (%)* (UNLESS NOTED FOR CHILDREN)**	**GENDER OVERREPRESENTATION**
Anxiety disorders	18.1 overall	
Agoraphobia	1.7	Female
Panic disorder	2.4	Female
Panic attacks	11.2	Female
Social anxiety	7	Female
Specific phobia	7-9	Female
Separation anxiety	1.2	Equal
Generalized anxiety disorder	2	Female
Posttraumatic stress disorder	3.4	Female
Obsessive-compulsive disorder	1.2	Equal
Major depression	8.6	Female
Bipolar disorder I and II	1.8	BD I: ~Equal
		BD II: Female
Autism spectrum disorders	1 in children	Males
Disruptive, impulse control, and conduct disorders	8.9 overall	
Conduct disorders*	4 in children	Males
Attention-deficit/hyperactivity disorder*	5 in children; 2.5 in adults	Males
Substance use disorders	8.9 overall	
Alcohol use disorder	8.5 in adults; 2.5 in 12- to 17-year-olds	Males
Drug use disorders	1.4	Males
Schizophrenia	1.1	~Equal

*Not one source has all of this information. This information has been derived from the following sources: Kessler, R.C., et al. (2012). Twelve-month and lifetime prevalence and lifetime morbid risk of anxiety and mood disorders in the United States. *International Journal of Methods of Psychiatric Research, 21,* 169; Substance Abuse and Mental Health Services Administration (2009). *Results from the 2008 national survey on drug use and health: national findings.* <http://www.samhsa.gov/data/nsduh/2k8nsduh/2k8Results.htm> Accessed November 13, 2013; American Psychiatric Association. (2013). *Diagnostic and statistical manual of mental disorders* (5th ed.). Arlington, VA: APA.

TABLE 23-2	LIFETIME PREVALENCE RATES FOR MENTAL DISORDERS IN THE UNITED STATES*
DISORDERS	**LIFETIME PREVALENCE RATE (%)**
Anxiety disorders (all)	28.8
Panic disorder	6.8
Agoraphobia disorder	3.7
Social phobia	13
Separation anxiety	8.7
Specific phobia	18.4
Generalized anxiety disorder	9
Posttraumatic stress disorder	10.1
Obsessive-compulsive disorder	2.7
Mood disorders (all)	20.8
Major depressive disorder	29.9
Bipolar disorders I and II	4.1
Dysthymia	2.5
Cyclothymia	0.4-1
Schizophrenia	0.3-0.7
Schizoaffective	0.34
Substance abuse disorder (all)	14.6
Alcohol use disorder	13.2
Drug use disorder	7.9
Attention-deficit/hyperactivity disorder	8.1
Any mental or chemical abuse disorder	46.4

*Not one source has all of this information. This information has been derived from the following sources: Kessler, R.C., et al. (2005b). Lifetime prevalence and age-of-onset distributions of DSM-IV disorders in the national comorbidity survey replication. *Archives of General Psychiatry, 62,* 593; Kessler, R.C., et al. (2012). Twelve-month and lifetime prevalence and lifetime morbid risk of anxiety and mood disorders in the United States. *International Journal of Methods of Psychiatric Research, 21,* 169; Substance Abuse and Mental Health Services Administration (2009). *Results from the 2008 national survey on drug use and health: national findings.* <http://www.samhsa.gov/data/nsduh/2k8nsduh/2k8Results.htm> Accessed November 13, 2013; American Psychiatric Association (2013). *Diagnostic and statistical manual of mental disorders (DSM-5).* Arlington, VA: APA.

updating criteria for this manual. All chapters in this unit are developed around *DSM* criteria. Not all psychiatric professionals, including some at the National Institute of Mental Health, have endorsed this newest version. However, this text follows the basic diagnostic reasoning as set forth in *DSM-5. DSM-IV-TR* and previous editions used a multiaxial system to capture more than symptoms. These axes looked at contributing factors such as medical condition and environmental problems. *DSM-5* does not use this approach, although these issues are not completely ignored. Following is a list of the former five axes.

Axis I: Clinical disorders (e.g., schizophrenia, bipolar disorder, depression)

Axis II: Personality or developmental disorders (e.g., paranoid or borderline personality disorders, mental retardation)

Axis III: General medical conditions (that are potentially relevant to understanding the mental disorder) (e.g., neoplasms, endocrine disorders)

Axis IV: Psychosocial and environmental problems (e.g., divorce, education, housing)

Axis V: Global assessment of functioning (e.g., rating of psychological, social, and occupational functioning on a mental health scale [0 to 100])

These five axes provide a holistic approach to assessing the patient. *DSM-5* collapses the first three axes into one category. Environmental stressors (previously Axis IV) are captured by a coding system in the new manual. Finally, the Global Assessment of Functioning (commonly referred to as the GAF) was deemed too arbitrary or unspecific to merit continuation. The American Psychiatric Association

NORM'S NOTES

This chapter provides an overview of some statistics about mental illness and a rationale for the nurse's need to know psychopathologic concepts. A disturbing point that you cannot detect from Table 23-1 is that things are not getting better. I can see it because I've been around a long time and know the older stats. Even though billions of dollars have been spent, actually more people have mental disorders today than they did 30 years ago. I must admit I'm a little discouraged.

recommends the more reliable World Health Organization Disability Assessment Schedule (WHODAS), which is available at http://www.who.int/classifications/icf/whodasii/en/.

BEHAVIOR

Patients' behaviors are described to help the student identify behavioral phenomena. Some behaviors can be observed directly (objective assessment or signs), whereas the patient must report other behaviors (subjective assessment or symptoms). Knowledge of these signs and symptoms helps the nurse anticipate and plan appropriate interventions.

ETIOLOGY

For many years, psychiatric clinicians have typically fallen into one of two camps in regard to what causes mental disorders: those who subscribe to the nature argument and believe that mental disorders arise from *nature* (e.g., organic, biologic, genetic) and those who subscribe to the nurture argument and believe that mental disorders arise from *nurture* (e.g., psychodynamic, functional, environmental stressors, early life experiences). In recent years, most clinicians have come to recognize that both views provide valuable insights into the complexities of the human mind. Research has suggested that some life experiences (i.e., nurture) change biology (i.e.,

nature), underscoring a more holistic view of mental illness. Threads of the "nature versus nurture" argument (or the "biologic versus psychodynamic" argument) are presented in discussions of etiologies; however, the overriding theme of this unit is the recognition of the unifying symptoms that point to the contributions of each etiologic factor.

PSYCHOTHERAPEUTIC MANAGEMENT

Sections on psychotherapeutic management in each chapter draw on the general intervention strategies presented in Units II to IV to develop appropriate interventions for each disorder. In addition, a case study and a related nursing care plan are presented for each disorder. A sample nursing care plan is found at the end of this chapter. The following rules provide relevant guidelines for all aspects of psychotherapeutic management:

- Provide support for patients.
- Strengthen patients' self-esteem.
- Treat adult patients as adults.
- Prevent failure or embarrassment.
- Treat patients as individuals.
- Provide reality testing.
- Handle hostility therapeutically.
- Be calm and matter-of-fact about norms and limits.

NURSES NEED TO UNDERSTAND PSYCHOPATHOLOGY

Nurses cannot gain a true understanding of patients with mental disorders until they understand mental disorders. Psychiatric nursing is more than warm, caring feelings about patients. Although being affirming and kind are wonderful attributes in daily life, more is required of an effective psychiatric nurse. This "more" is based on an understanding of psychopathology.

A psychiatric nurse can no more effectively plan and provide psychiatric care without an understanding of psychopathology than a medical-surgical nurse can plan and provide care without an understanding of pathophysiology. In this unit, authors provide a discussion of psychopathology for each disorder. We have included chapters on the following mental disorders: schizophrenia, depression, bipolar disorders, anxiety-related disorders, cognitive disorders, personality disorders, sexual disorders, substance-related disorders, and eating disorders.

> **? CRITICAL THINKING QUESTION**
>
> 1. The biologic versus psychodynamic argument has gone on for a long time. Why is it important to be open to both points of view? Although you might not have used the same words, you probably had a bias one way or the other before you started nursing school. What was your bias?

◎ CARE PLAN

Name: _____   *Admission Date:* _____

DSM-5 Diagnosis: _____

Assessment   Areas of strength: _____

                        Problems: _____

Diagnoses
                        _____

                        _____

                        _____

Outcomes   **Short-term goals**

Date met: _____

Date met: _____

Date met: _____

                        Long-term goals

Date met: _____

Date met: _____

Planning and Interventions   Nurse-patient relationship: _____

                        _____

                        Psychopharmacology: _____

                        _____

                        Milieu management: _____

                        _____

Evaluation   _____

                        _____

Referrals   _____

                        _____

▌ STUDY NOTES

1. According to Reeves and colleagues, about 25% or more of Americans have some type of mental or addictive disorder in any given 12-month period.

2. Anxiety disorders are the most common category of mental disorders, followed by mood disorders, impulse-control disorders, and substance use disorders.

3. Understanding psychopathology is fundamental for effective psychotherapeutic management; it requires organizing knowledge, defining terms operationally, and developing criteria for diagnosis.

4. *DSM-5* (American Psychiatric Association, 2013) is the official diagnostic system for psychiatry used in the United States.

5. Etiologic explanations of mental disorders can be broadly placed in one of two categories: biologic (natural or organic causes) and psychological (nurturing, psychodynamic, or functional causes).

6. Guidelines appropriate for all aspects of psychiatric care include supportive care, strengthening self-esteem, preventing failure or embarrassment, treating patients as individuals, reinforcing reality, and handling patients' hostility calmly and matter-of-factly.

REFERENCES

American Psychiatric Association, (2013). *Diagnostic and statistical manual of mental disorders* (5th ed.). Arlington, VA: APA.

Kessler, R. C., et al. (2012). Twelve-month and lifetime prevalence and lifetime morbid risk of anxiety and mood disorders in the United States. *International Journal of Methods of Psychiatric Research, 21,* 169.

Kessler, R. C., et al. (2005a). Prevalence, severity, and comorbidity of 12-month DSM-IV disorders in the national comorbidity survey replication. *Archives of General Psychiatry, 62,* 617.

Kessler, R. C., et al. (2005b). Lifetime prevalence and age-of-onset distributions of DSM-IV disorders in the national comorbidity survey replication. *Archives of General Psychiatry, 62,* 593.

National Institute of Mental Health, (2005). *Statistics.* www.nimh.nih.gov/health/topics/statistics/index.shtml, Accessed 10.02.10.

Reeves, W. C., et al. (2013). *Mental illness surveillance among adults in the United States.* Atlanta: Centers for Disease Control.

Substance Abuse and Mental Health Services Administration, (2009). *Results from the 2008 national survey on drug use and health: National findings.* http://www.samhsa.gov/data/nsduh/2k8nsduh/2k8Results.htm, Accessed November 13, 2013.

U.S. Surgeon General. (1999). *Mental health: A report from the Surgeon General.* Washington, DC: Department of Health and Human Services.

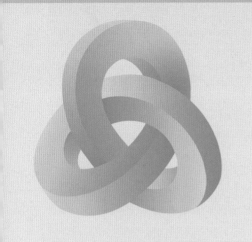

Schizophrenia Spectrum and Other Psychotic Disorders

Norman L. Keltner

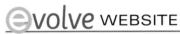 WEBSITE

http://evolve.elsevier.com/Keltner

LEARNING OBJECTIVES

- Define the term *schizophrenia*.
- Describe the major historic figures, events, and theories that have contributed to the current understanding of schizophrenia.
- Identify Bleuler's "four A's."
- Recognize the *DSM-5* criteria and terminology for schizophrenia.
- Differentiate and describe type I (positive) and type II (negative) subtypes.
- Recognize and describe objective and subjective symptoms of schizophrenia.

- Identify biologic explanations for schizophrenia.
- Describe two theoretical psychodynamic explanations for schizophrenia.
- Develop a nursing care plan for patients with schizophrenia.
- Identify the major drugs used in the treatment of schizophrenia, their mechanisms of action, their target symptoms, and their major side effects.
- Evaluate the effectiveness of nursing interventions for patients with schizophrenia.

There are three inescapable "facts" about schizophrenia (Weinberger, 1987):

1. Age at onset: Onset is almost always during late adolescence or early adulthood.
2. Role of stress: Onset and relapse are almost always related to stress.
3. Efficacy of dopamine antagonists: Drugs that block dopamine receptors are therapeutic.

Psychosis is a "... disorder in which the highest mental functions, such as thought, language, emotions, conation, and cognition, are drastically disrupted" (Nasrallah, 2012). An impaired ability to relate to others makes it worse. Common symptoms of psychosis include hallucinations, delusions, and difficulty with thought organization. Psychosis can be present in schizophrenia, acute mania, depression, drug intoxication, dementia, and delirium and can be caused by brain trauma. Schizophrenia is one of the most common causes of psychosis.

SCHIZOPHRENIA

Although many laypeople are quite sophisticated medically, it is common to hear the word *schizophrenia* defined as

split personality. Split personality refers to something like a Jekyll and Hyde experience or a multiple personality disorder. This popular depiction does not begin to portray schizophrenia. Schizophrenia is not characterized by a changing personality; it is characterized by a deteriorating personality. This popular notion of a dramatic personality change comes far short of capturing the devastating effect that schizophrenia has on the life of a person and the person's family. Simply stated, schizophrenia is one of the most profoundly disabling mental or physical illnesses that the nurse will ever encounter.

NORM'S NOTES
This might be the most important chapter in this book. Although schizophrenia affects only about 1% of the adult population (Table 24-1), it is a devastating disorder because it has ripple effects that have a disproportionate impact on society. These are the people that you might walk by (or around) in our cities, not wanting to interact with them at all. They might scare you at times or offend in other ways. After reading this chapter and after having a good clinical experience, I think your attitude about these individuals will change.

TABLE 24-1   12-MONTH PREVALENCE RATE OF MENTAL DISORDERS IN THE UNITED STATES*

DISORDERS	APPROXIMATE PERCENTAGE >17 YEARS OLD (%)* (unless noted for children)	GENDER OVERREPRESENTATION
Anxiety disorders	18.1 overall	
Agoraphobia	1.7	Female
Panic disorder	2.4	Female
Panic attacks	11.2	Female
Social anxiety	7	Female
Specific phobia	7-9	Female
Separation anxiety	1.2	Equal
Generalized anxiety disorder	2	Female
Posttraumatic stress disorder	3.4	Female
Obsessive-compulsive disorder	1.2	Equal
Major depression	8.6	Female
Bipolar disorder I and II	1.8	BD I: ~Equal BD II: Female
Autism spectrum disorders	1 in children	Male
Disruptive, impulse control, and conduct disorders	8.9 overall	
Conduct disorders*	4 in children	Male
Attention-deficit/hyperactivity disorder*	5 in children; 2.5 in adults	Male
Substance use disorders	8.9 overall	
Alcohol use disorder	8.5 in adults; 2.5 in 12- to 17-year-olds	Male
Drug use disorders	1.4	Male
Schizophrenia	1.1	~Equal

*No one source has all of this information. This information has been derived from the following sources: Kessler, R.C., et al. (2012). Twelve-month and lifetime prevalence and lifetime morbid risk of anxiety and mood disorders in the United States. *International Journal of Methods of Psychiatric Research, 21,* 169; Substance Abuse and Mental Health Services Administration (2009). *Results from the 2008 national survey on drug use and health: national findings.* <http://www.samhsa.gov/data/nsduh/2k8nsduh/2k8Results.htm> Accessed November 13, 2013; American Psychiatric Association (2013). *Diagnostic and statistical manual of mental disorders* (5th ed.). Arlington, VA: APA.

Schizophrenia is a diagnostic term used to describe a major psychotic disorder characterized by disturbances in the following areas:

- Perception (e.g., hallucinations)
- Thought processes (e.g., thought derailment)
- Reality testing (e.g., delusions)
- Feeling (e.g., flat or inappropriate affect)
- Behavior (e.g., social withdrawal)
- Attention (e.g., inability to concentrate)
- Motivation (e.g., cannot initiate or persist in goal-directed activities)

Contributing to overall deterioration is a decline in psychosocial functioning. Schizophrenia typically first appears in late adolescence or early adulthood. Schizophrenia affects men and women almost equally; however, gender differences do exist (Seeman, 2010). Box 24-1 highlights some of the gender differences in expression of this disorder.

Studies have shown that approximately 1% of the population experiences schizophrenia during their lifetime. Although the prevalence rate and symptom presentation for schizophrenia are fairly constant worldwide, inner-city residents, people from lower socioeconomic classes, and individuals who experience prenatal difficulties are more likely to be affected (Box 24-2) (American Psychiatric Association, 2013). Economic costs are in the tens of billions of dollars each year. The cost in human suffering is incalculable.

BOX 24-1   TYPICAL GENDER-BASED DIFFERENCES IN SCHIZOPHRENIA

- Age of onset is typically 4 to 6 years earlier in men.
- Men have a more severe course.
- Women have more positive symptoms (e.g., hallucinations).
- Estrogen modulates dopamine function and presumably plays a protective role for women.
- Women are more compliant with medications.
- Women tend to have lower blood levels and longer half-lives of medications.

BOX 24-2   PRENATAL AND PERINATAL EVENTS ASSOCIATED WITH SCHIZOPHRENIA

- Maternal influenza
- Birth during late winter or early spring
- Obstetric complications
- Prenatal exposure to lead
- Maternal starvation
- Perinatal exposure to cats (i.e., viral zoonosis)

Data from Bachmann et al. (2008), Opler et al. (2004), and APA (2013).

BOX 24-3   EVOLUTION OF SCHIZOPHRENIC SUBTYPING

1860	Morel coins the term *dementia praecox.*
1871	Kahlbaum uses the term *catatonia* to describe patients immobilized by psychological factors.
1874	Hecker uses the term *hebephrenia* to describe patients with silly, bizarre, and regressed behaviors.
1878	Kraepelin adds the term *paranoia* to describe highly suspicious patients.
1899	Kraepelin groups all three patient categories under the heading *dementia praecox.*
1900s	Bleuler introduces the term *schizophrenia* to describe these mental disorders.
1952	*DSM-I:* Includes 9 subtypes for schizophrenia.
1968	*DSM-II:* Includes 11 subtypes.
1980	*DSM-III:* Reduced to 5 subtypes: disorganized, catatonic, paranoid, undifferentiated, and residual.
1982	Andreasen and Olsen (1982), Crow (1982), and others categorize schizophrenia based on symptoms: positive (type I) and negative (type II).
1994	*DSM-IV:* Includes same subtypes as *DSM-III.*
1997	American Psychiatric Association recognizes the addition of the subtype "disorganized" to the positive and negative subtyping concept.
2000	*DSM-IV-TR:* Includes same subtypes.
2013	*DSM-5:* Removes subtypes.

DSM, Diagnostic and Statistical Manual of Mental Disorders.

Box 24-3 outlines the statistical epidemiologic realities of schizophrenia.

Morel was the first to name the psychiatric symptoms of schizophrenia. In 1860, while treating an adolescent boy, Morel used the phrase *dementia praecox* (precocious senility) to describe the group of symptoms he observed (Kolb & Brodie, 1982). Kahlbaum (in 1871) and Hecker (in 1874) added to the diagnostic nomenclature with their categories *catatonia* and *hebephrenia* (Sadock & Sadock, 2003). In 1878, Kraepelin added the term *paranoia* and engaged in a rigorous study of what is now called *schizophrenia.* Kraepelin found commonalities among the three mental disorders (catatonia, hebephrenia, and paranoia) and grouped them in 1899 under the diagnostic term that Morel had coined 40 years before— *dementia praecox* (Sadock & Sadock, 2003). Kraepelin believed that schizophrenia was the result of neuropathologic factors; he envisioned a progressive deteriorating course, resulting in disabling mental impairment with little hope of recovery.

It was left to Bleuler in the early 1900s to coin the term *schizophrenia* in a book subtitled *The Group of Schizophrenias.* Bleuler believed that schizophrenia does not always follow a course of deterioration (making the term *dementia* inappropriate), and it does not always occur early in life (making the term *praecox* also inappropriate). Bleuler broadened Kraepelin's concept by focusing on symptoms and identified four primary symptoms that he believed were present in all individuals with schizophrenia. All four of these classic symptoms begin with the letter "A" (Bleuler's "four A's"), which facilitates memorization: *a*ffect disturbance, *a*utism, *a*ssociative looseness, and *a*mbivalence.

Kraepelin and Bleuler, two historical giants of psychiatry, founded two divergent views of schizophrenia. In using the diagnostic category of dementia praecox, Kraepelin revealed a conceptual alignment between schizophrenia and disorders such as Alzheimer's disease, which have a less optimistic prognosis. Bleuler developed a school of thought that was much broader and more optimistic than that of Kraepelin. Based on Bleuler's wider grouping, pessimism eased, and some clinicians began to see improvements in their patients. Although Kraepelin based his views on biology, Bleuler, influenced by the master analyst Freud and other psychodynamic theorists, sought psychological explanations for schizophrenia. For most of the twentieth century, Freud's psychoanalytic explanations and, by extension, Bleuler's thinking dominated the understanding of schizophrenia. However, as the limitations of "talking" cures became more evident, mental health professionals became less interested in the psychodynamic approach. In the past 30 years or so, a resurgence of interest in biologic research has resulted in renewed respect for Kraepelin's work.

Course of Illness

Schizophrenia typically first occurs in adolescence or early adulthood, a time during which brain maturation is almost complete. There are three overlapping phases of the disorder, as follows:

- *Acute phase:* The patient experiences severe psychotic symptoms.
- *Stabilizing phase:* The patient is getting better.
- *Stable phase:* In this phase, the patient might still experience hallucinations and delusions, but the hallucinations and delusions are not as severe or disabling as they were during the acute phase.

Most patients alternate between acute and stable phases.

Clinical Example- Hallucinating but Stable

Billy is a 39-year-old man living in a psychiatric residential facility who attends a day treatment program Monday through Friday. Although Billy experiences hallucinations frequently, most often visual hallucinations, he is stabilized. All staff members agree that Billy is not a danger to himself or others and that the day treatment program is more appropriate for him than a state hospital would be.

❓ CRITICAL THINKING QUESTION

1. Why do you think Kraepelin was so pessimistic about the patients he saw with dementia praecox?

DSM-5 Terminology and Criteria

Since the inception of schizophrenia as a diagnostic entity, attempts have been made to divide it into subtypes. However, *DSM-5* has abandoned the subtyping of schizophrenia because the American Psychiatric Association (2013) found it unhelpful and limiting (see Box 24-3 and *DSM-5* Criteria box). Although *DSM-5* criteria have been thoughtfully deliberated, we find the subtyping approach based on type I (or positive) versus type II (or negative) symptoms clinically helpful because it can be predictive of medication response. The student should realize that most patients are not "either/or" but have a mixture of positive and negative symptoms.

Positive versus Negative Schizophrenia

Positive (type I) schizophrenia has a different constellation of symptoms than negative (type II) schizophrenia (Box 24-4). Type I is positive in the sense that symptoms are an embellishment of normal cognition and perception. The symptoms are additional. Positive symptoms are believed to be the result of elevated dopamine levels affecting the limbic areas of the brain.

DSM-5 CRITERIA

Schizophrenia

Diagnostic Criteria

A. Two (or more) of the following, each present for a significant portion of time during a 1-month period (or less if successfully treated). At least one of these must be (1), (2), or (3):
   1. Delusions.
   2. Hallucinations.
   3. Disorganized speech (e.g., frequent derailment or incoherence).
   4. Grossly disorganized or catatonic behavior.
   5. Negative symptoms (i.e., diminished emotional expression or avolition).

B. For a significant portion of the time since the onset of the disturbance, level of functioning in one or more major areas, such as work, interpersonal relations, or self-care, is markedly below the level achieved before the onset (or when the onset is in childhood or adolescence, there is failure to achieve expected level of interpersonal, academic, or occupational functioning).

C. Continuous signs of the disturbance persist for at least 6 months. This 6-month period must include at least 1 month of symptoms (or less if successfully treated) that meet criterion A (i.e., active-phase symptoms) and may include periods of prodromal or residual symptoms. During these prodromal or residual periods, the signs of the disturbance may be manifested by only negative symptoms or by two or more symptoms listed in criterion A present in an attenuated form (e.g., odd beliefs, unusual perceptual experiences).

D. Schizoaffective disorder and depressive or bipolar disorder with psychotic features have been ruled out because either (1) no major depressive or manic episodes have occurred concurrently with the active-phase symptoms or (2) if mood episodes have occurred during active-phase symptoms, they have been present for a minority of the total duration of the active and residual periods of the illness.

E. The disturbance is not attributable to the physiological effects of a substance (e.g., a drug of abuse, a medication) or another medical condition.

F. If there is a history of autism spectrum disorder or a communication disorder of childhood onset, the additional diagnosis of schizophrenia is made only if prominent delusions or hallucinations, in addition to the other required symptoms of schizophrenia, are also present for at least 1 month (or less if successfully treated).

Specify if:

The following course specifiers are only to be used after a 1-year duration of the disorder and if they are not in contradiction to the diagnostic course criteria.

First episode, currently in acute episode: First manifestation of the disorder meeting the defining diagnostic symptom and time criteria. An acute episode is a time period in which the symptom criteria are fulfilled.

First episode, currently in partial remission: Partial remission is a period of time during which an improvement after a previous episode is maintained and in which the defining criteria of the disorder are only partially fulfilled.

First episode, currently in full remission: Full remission is a period of time after a previous episode during which no disorder-specific symptoms are present.

Multiple episodes, currently in acute episode: Multiple episodes may be determined after a minimum of two episodes (i.e., after a first episode, a remission and a minimum of one relapse).

Multiple episodes, currently in partial remission

Multiple episodes, currently in full remission

Continuous: Symptoms fulfilling the diagnostic symptom criteria of the disorder are remaining for the majority of the illness course, with subthreshold symptom periods being very brief relative to the overall course.

Unspecified

Specify if:

With catatonia (refer to the criteria for catatonia associated with another mental disorder, pp 119-120, for definition).

Coding note: Use additional code 293.89 (F06.1) catatonia associated with schizophrenia to indicate the presence of comorbid catatonia.

Specify Current Severity

Severity is rated by a quantitative assessment of the primary symptoms of psychosis, including delusions, hallucinations, disorganized speech, abnormal psychomotor behavior, and negative symptoms. Each of these symptoms may be rated for its current severity (most severe in the last 7 days) on a 5-point scale ranging from 0 (not present) to 4 (present and severe). (See Clinical-Rated Dimensions of Psychosis Symptom Severity in the chapter "Assessment Measure.")

Note: Diagnosis of schizophrenia can be made without using this severity specifier.

From the American Psychiatric Association. (2013). *Diagnostic and statistical manual of mental disorders* (5th ed.). Washington, DC: APA.

*This is an oversimplification of what occurs in the limbic and frontal lobes of the brain.

Clinical Example: Positive Symptoms

John is sitting in the day room on the psychiatric unit when his eyes begin to dart back and forth, and he becomes increasingly anxious. You ask, "John, are you hearing something that I cannot hear?" "Can't you hear them?" he replies. "They are going to get me." John's auditory hallucination is a positive symptom because it is an exaggeration of a normal perception (he is "hearing" without an auditory stimulus).

Type II is labeled negative because symptoms are essentially an absence or diminution of normal cognition and perception (e.g., lack of affect, lack of energy). Type II is related, at least in part, to a hypodopaminergic process. These symptoms also can be caused by cortical structural changes. Pathoanatomy consistently mentioned in the literature includes decreased cerebral blood flow and increased ventricular brain ratios. Decreased frontal blood flow is most pronounced in the dorsolateral prefrontal cortex. Ventricular enlargement can be detected on computed tomography (CT) and magnetic resonance imaging (MRI) with the naked eye. Other pathoanatomic features observed that might contribute to negative symptoms include a modest reduction in brain weight and cerebral atrophy.

Clinical Example: Negative Symptoms

Philip Wilson has a long history of mental problems. Mr. Wilson is a patient in the state hospital system. The summary note written by the nursing team leader includes the following observation: "Mr. Wilson is isolative and, for the most part, expressionless. He spends long hours sitting and staring out of the window. Attempts to engage Mr. Wilson in unit activities have not been successful."

One consequence of the positive versus negative subtyping approach has been the tendency by a few professionals to be too pessimistic about the prognosis of patients with type II schizophrenia. Kopelowicz and Bidder (1992), who cautioned nurses and others against such rash and uninformed thinking, divided negative symptoms into primary and secondary. The secondary symptoms are therapeutically accessible, particularly early in the course of the illness. Secondary symptoms include symptoms caused by the following:
- Medications
- Hospitalizations
- Loss of social supports
- Socioeconomic decline

If assessed early, secondary negative symptoms can be arrested.

Clinical Example: Lack of Connectedness

Merritt is a homeless man with a long history of mental illness. He has not seen his family in many years. Although his family was supportive at one time, they simply grew tired of trying to cope with him. At this point, even modest improvements in his mental health are compromised by his lack of social support.

According to biologic theory, typical antipsychotic drugs (drugs that antagonize primarily dopamine D_2 receptors) are likely to be beneficial for positive symptoms because positive schizophrenia is a hyperdopaminergic process. In contrast, negative schizophrenia is thought to be more structurally related and a hypodopaminergic process. Traditional antipsychotics have relatively less effect and might cause negative symptoms to worsen. The more excessive the symptoms are (as in positive schizophrenia), the greater the likelihood of a favorable response to antipsychotics. As noted in Chapter 14, atypical antipsychotic drugs, such as clozapine (Clozaril), risperidone (Risperdal), olanzapine (Zyprexa), quetiapine (Seroquel), ziprasidone (Geodon), and aripiprazole (Abilify), benefit negative symptoms because they affect dopamine receptors and antagonize serotonin 5-hydroxytryptamine 2A receptors, which liberate dopamine in cortical areas. The dopamine corrects the hypodopaminergic state. Most of these newer drugs are expensive. For example, a 30-day supply of Zyprexa could cost more than $500, whereas the same amount of Haldol might cost about $20 (see Table 14-7).

Behavior

People who are treated for mental problems come to the attention of mental health professionals in one of two ways.

The first is when people seek help. They do so because they have experienced such troubling subjective symptoms that they want professional intervention. However, professional help often is not sought until people have exhausted self-help aids, friends, and family, leading to the second way in which people come to the attention of the mental health system, which is by drawing attention to themselves through behaviors that bother, concern, or frighten other people. These indicators of a mental disorder are apparent to others and are called *objective signs*. As discussed in Chapter 3, help is sometimes resisted, and the person must be treated on an involuntary basis.

Subjective and objective categories are not as discrete as they might appear at first. For example, hallucinations are subjective phenomena but might easily cause objective signs that get the attention of others (e.g., a person who talks back to an auditory hallucination). Nonetheless, dividing the expressions of schizophrenia into subjective symptoms and objective signs is a rational and convenient approach for understanding this mental disorder. Several rating scales for severity of schizophrenia have been developed, and it is important that all psychiatric nurses be familiar with them. Six significant alterations occur in schizophrenia and can be grouped into objective signs or subjective symptoms (Box 24-5). Alterations in personal relationships and alterations of activity are highly visible to others (objective signs), whereas altered perception, alterations of thought, altered consciousness, and alterations of affect are more subjective in nature.

Objective Signs

Alterations in Personal Relationships. Patients with schizophrenia have troubled interpersonal relationships.

Often, these problems develop over a long period, well before schizophrenia is diagnosed, and become more pronounced as the illness progresses. It is common to hear that a person was asocial, a loner, or a social misfit before being diagnosed.

Frequently, patients become less concerned with their appearance and might not bathe without persistent prodding. Table manners and other social skills might diminish to the point at which patients are disgusting to others. These behaviors are related to introspection (autism) and apathy. Patients are focused on internal processes to the extent that their external social world collapses. Schizophrenia can cause a diminished energy level (anergia), which also complicates social interactions.

Interpersonal communication becomes inadequate and might be inappropriate. Again, internal processes are at work. Hostility, a common theme, also distances patients from others. Finally, patients with schizophrenia withdraw, further compromising their ability to engage in meaningful social interactions.

Clinical Example: Loneliness and Schizophrenia
William is a white man in his early forties with schizophrenia. He can be seen walking near the university where I work. He nearly always wears the same clothes. He arrives early at Starbuck's almost every morning. He never buys anything, but the young women working there give him a glass of water. He doesn't talk. He sits and sips. He is obese and typically smelly. He has nowhere to go, no one to see, and no friends.

Alterations of Activity. Patients with schizophrenia also display alterations of activity. Patients might be too active (psychomotor agitation)—they are unable to sit still and continually pace—or they might be inactive or catatonic. These signs respond to antipsychotic drugs but can also be caused by them. The following clinical example illustrates this point.

BOX 24-5 OBJECTIVE AND SUBJECTIVE BEHAVIORAL DISORDERS IN SCHIZOPHRENIA

Objective Signs
Alterations in Personal Relationships
- Decreased attention to appearance and social amenities related to introspection and autism
- Inadequate or inappropriate communication
- Hostility
- Withdrawal

Alterations of Activity
- Psychomotor agitation
- Catatonic rigidity
- Echopraxia (repetitive movements)
- Stereotypy (repetitive acts or words)

Subjective Symptoms
Altered Perception
- Hallucinations
- Illusions
- Paranoid thinking

Alterations of Thought
- Loose associations

- Retardation
- Blocking
- Autism
- Ambivalence
- Delusions
- Poverty of speech
- Ideas of reference
- Mutism

Altered Consciousness
- Confusion
- Incoherent speech
- Clouding
- Sense of "going crazy"

Alterations of Affect
- Inappropriate, blunted, flattened, or labile affect
- Apathy
- Ambivalence
- Overreaction
- Anhedonia

Clinical Example: Symptoms or Side Effects?

The nurse must be careful in assessing alterations in activity. Restlessness might be caused by akathisia (an extrapyramidal side effect [EPSE] of antipsychotic drugs) or might be a manifestation of schizophrenia. However, rigidity might be a warning sign of neuroleptic malignant syndrome (NMS), not catatonia. Both EPSEs and NMS are side effects of antipsychotic drugs. Accurate assessment is critical. Although it is appropriate to administer an as needed (prn) dose of haloperidol for psychomotor agitation or catatonia, haloperidol intensifies akathisia and might prove fatal for patients with NMS.

Subjective Symptoms

Subjective symptoms, by definition, are experienced by patients in a personal way. Patients might hide these symptoms from others. For example, if a patient experiences the delusion that he is a famous person, he might be able to keep it to himself. Some clinicians advise patients who resist psychiatric care to "keep your symptoms to yourself, and no one will ever know." Presumably, there are individuals in society who are not reporting their subjective symptoms to anyone and are avoiding psychiatric intervention. For the most part, however, subjective symptoms of schizophrenia spill over into behavior in public view. Subjective symptoms can be grouped into four categories.

Altered Perception. Altered perception includes hallucinations, illusions, and paranoid thinking. Hallucinations are false sensory perceptions and can be auditory, visual, olfactory, tactile, gustatory, or somatic (strange body sensations). Auditory hallucinations are the most common in schizophrenia and often take the form of accusations ("You slut," "Hey, queer") or commands ("Get away from these people"). (Interestingly, about 10% to 15% of the adult population report auditory hallucinations [Crowner, 2014].) Visual hallucinations are not as common in schizophrenia. (The nurse might suspect a toxic process such as drugs or fever if visual hallucinations are present.) Hallucinations are probably caused by a hyperdopaminergic state in the limbic areas.

Illusions are misinterpretations of real external stimuli. For example, a tree might be mistaken for a threatening person. Illusions are often associated with physical illness as well as schizophrenia.

Clinical Example: Delirium versus Schizophrenia

Delirium: While lying in bed with a low-grade fever, Gladys, a 68-year-old woman, asks, "Are those cobwebs on the wall?" Her son responds, "No, Mama, those are just shadows from your bedside lamp." Gladys laughs and says, "I guess my mind is going."
Schizophrenia: Tim, a patient in a day treatment program, mistakes a tennis shoe on the porch for a rat.

Paranoid thinking is characterized by a persistent interpretation of the actions of others as threatening or demeaning. Paranoid themes can color delusions and hallucinations as well as the ordinary behavior of others. It is important for the student to differentiate paranoid thinking associated with

a paranoid personality disorder from paranoid delusions. Paranoid thinking is less severe than paranoid delusions. Paranoid thinking might be corrected with facts, whereas paranoid delusions cannot. The phenomenon of paranoia is increasing in our society (Keltner & Davidson, 2009).

Clinical Example: Paranoid Personality versus Paranoid Schizophrenia

Paranoid personality: Bill, a voluntary patient on the adult unit, has sought help because of trouble on the job and at home. His ability to get along with people has deteriorated to the point that he has no friends. Bill's wife has started divorce proceedings, and he has sought treatment, hoping that she will change her mind. Over the last few years, Bill has been obsessed with the thought that his wife is cheating on him. He follows her when she leaves the house, sometimes listens to her telephone calls, and has confronted her with accusations of infidelity. Whenever he finds he is mistaken, he is relieved for a while and apologizes for not trusting her, but soon he begins to have the same paranoid thoughts. His paranoid thinking has caused alterations in his personal relationships.
Paranoid schizophrenia: Fred is a 28-year-old unemployed laborer. The police recently brought Fred to the emergency department. Fred had been at the downtown bus station preaching loudly to all who passed. He spoke of a conspiracy of African-Americans and Jews who plan to take over America. Fred tells the emergency department nurse that he feared for his life. He adds that he has proof that the FBI was behind President Kennedy's assassination.

A final example of altered perception is based on the observation that the ability to adapt perceptually (or attend selectively) is altered in patients with schizophrenia.

Clinical Example: Altered Perception

A patient is looking out of a seventh-floor window. The nurse approaches to look and notices activity in the yard below. The nurse assumes that the patient is observing the same activity and comments. However, the patient is not looking beyond the wire mesh screen in the window. He is unable to filter out what would not be a distraction for most people. The inability to filter out extraneous stimuli (ability to attend selectively) is a perceptual problem for some patients.

Alterations of Thought. Alterations of thought are common in schizophrenia and are sometimes disturbing and frightening. Antipsychotic drugs are often beneficial. Common thought disorders include thought retardation, blocking, autism, ambivalence, loose associations, delusions, poverty of speech, and concrete thinking.

Thought retardation is a slowing of mental activity. A patient might state, "I just can't think." Blocking is the interruption of a thought and the inability to recall it. This disorder is very disturbing to patients and sometimes frightening. Blocking might be caused by the intrusion of hallucinations, delusions, or emotional factors. The following is a common example of blocking that could happen to anyone.

Clinical Example: Blocking

Joe, a 49-year-old teacher, is in the middle of a lecture when he loses his "train of thought." He cannot remember what point he is developing or where to go next. He stalls for time, realizing that he is in a potentially embarrassing situation. Finally, he finds his notes and proceeds, a little shaken and distracted but able to continue.

Autism occurs when patients are introspective to the extent that they are distracted from external events. Patients are preoccupied with themselves and might be oblivious to the reality around them, which results in a personalized view of reality.

Ambivalence is a state in which two opposite, strong feelings exist simultaneously. Patients might be both attracted to and repelled by a person, object, or goal. Ambivalence (e.g., love/hate) toward a domineering parent is common. Another common example is the simultaneous need for and fear of people, resulting in immobilization. Schizophrenic patients might be immobilized by their ambivalence regarding a simple matter, such as deciding whether to drink orange juice or apple juice for breakfast. In these cases, it is therapeutic for the nurse to make decisions for patients, if patients will allow this. The following clinical example illustrates ambivalence that occurs in some families, and it is not meant to depict schizophrenic ambivalence.

Clinical Example: Ambivalence Toward Dear Old Dad

Joyce, a 38-year-old librarian, has ambivalent feelings toward her father. He still tells her what to do, and she has a hard time standing up for herself. Joyce realizes that her periodic need for financial assistance is partially responsible for her predicament. Joyce also finds that she avoids calling her father, and because he calls her excessively to find out what she is doing, she cringes when the telephone rings. Although Joyce does not have schizophrenia, she does experience ambivalence. She loves her father, but, in her words, "He is driving me crazy."

Loose association is a pattern of speech in which a person's ideas slip off one track onto another that is completely unrelated or only slightly related. An occasional change of topic without obvious connection does not indicate loose associations.

EXAMPLE OF LOOSE ASSOCIATIONS

The following example of loose associations is based on a conversation with Bill, a 46-year-old patient attending day treatment. Because of the severity of his disorder, he was admitted to a state hospital shortly after this interaction.
Nurse: "How are you doing today, Bill?"
Bill: "Do it. Get it on with monster woman. Do it. Sure Bill sure. Do it. Prevented. There goes the doctor. Kills a woman to have a baby. Fish woman. Purple bologna. That was good. Was that a 38, 25, or 44-45 magnum? White hair. A pig. Ham social security. USDA. USGI grocery store. Paycheck. Money. Funny. Money. Meat. Charles Atlas. Arnold. Hercules. Destroyed Bill. Destroyed Charles Atlas. Charley. Charles Manson. Manchild Part I of Bill. Charley Manson Bill. Helter Skelter. White people. Bride of Frankenstein blood drinkers." As is readily apparent, Bill's communication pattern at this time is incoherent. With effort, one can see some of the underlying connections of these disconnected words and phrases, but, overall, Bill's dialogue cannot be followed.

Delusions are fixed, false beliefs and can take many forms. Delusions are described as fixed beliefs because they cannot be changed by logical persuasion. Delusions are described as false because they are not based in reality. Delusional content often relates to life experiences and can include erotomanic, somatic, grandiose, religious, nihilistic, referential, and paranoid content. An example of each type follows:

- *Erotomanic*: A patient believes that Sandra Bullock is in love with him.
- *Somatic delusions*: After medical tests confirm otherwise, a patient still insists, "I have cancer in my stomach."
- *Grandiose delusions*: A patient states, "I am the president."
- *Religious delusions*: A woman attempts to kill her children because she believes the devil wants her to do so: "The devil told me to kill my children."
- *Nihilistic delusions*: A patient states, "I am dead." In response to saying, "If you are dead, how can you talk?" The patient says, "I don't know, but I'm dead."
- *Delusions of reference*: "The TV is talking about me. The guests on *Oprah* are making fun of me."
- *Delusions of influence*: "I can control her with my thoughts."
- *Paranoid delusions*: "They all think that I am a homosexual."

Related phenomena sometimes encountered are the schizophrenic delusions that thoughts can be inserted or withdrawn by others: "Other people can read my mind"; "My thoughts are being broadcast so that everyone can hear."

Poverty of speech is manifested by the inability to formulate and articulate thoughts that are relevant to the discussion at hand. Vocabulary is markedly limited in individuals who experience poverty of speech.

Concrete thinking is the inability to conceptualize the meanings of words and phrases. For example, a concrete response to the proverb "People who live in glass houses should not throw stones" might be "The glass would break." These individuals are likely to misinterpret jokes or similes. For example, the meaning of "a diamond in the rough" or "cool as a cucumber" might be lost completely on a person exhibiting concrete thinking.

Altered Consciousness. Altered consciousness is perhaps the symptom that is most troubling to patients; however, it is also responsive to antipsychotic drugs. Manifestations of altered consciousness include confusion, incoherent speech, clouding, and a sense of going crazy. The last manifestation of altered consciousness—going crazy—deserves special mention. Many students are surprised when they enter a psychiatric facility to find that patients are not crazy. Although psychiatric patients by definition are struggling with mental disorders, psychiatric units are not wild, bizarre environments. Patients can readily differentiate between the normal struggle of dealing with a mental disorder and the feeling of going crazy (loss of control). The student will observe that patients on the psychiatric unit define a fellow patient who has become wild or who is loudly talking to himself or herself as "crazy." In other words, this behavior is unusual— even on a psychiatric unit. Referring to the discussion of incompetence in Chapter 3, the student can appreciate why the designation of incompetence is reserved for only a few individuals.

Alterations of Affect. Alterations of affect are varied and include inappropriate, flattened, blunted, or labile affects; apathy; ambivalence; and overreaction. For example, responding to bad news with laughter is an affective response that does not match the circumstances and is *inappropriate*. If a patient is unable to generate much affect, and the response to the bad news is weakly appropriate, the affect is *blunted* or *dull*. The inability to generate any affective response is referred to as a *flattened affect*. Labile affect is a condition in which emotional tone changes quickly. A patient might be telling a happy story, suddenly begin to cry, and then quickly return to a happy disposition.

Apathy, which can be defined as a lack of concern or interest, is the inability to generate a normal response to people, situations, or the environment.

Another alteration of affect is the tendency to overreact to events. An analogy is a small child who must put so much energy into closing a car door that the door slams shut, offending the ears and nerves of adults nearby. Because of physical limitations, the child has to push as hard as possible to overcome inertia. Because of emotional limitations, schizophrenic patients overreact to normal events to overcome mental and social inertia, and, similar to the child, these patients might offend the sensitivities of people nearby.

Etiology

Many authorities suggest that multiple factors must cause schizophrenia because no single theory satisfactorily explains the disorder. Explanations can be categorized broadly into biologic or psychological (psychodynamic) causes. These two categories parallel the nature versus nurture debate discussed in Chapter 23. Biologic theories and psychodynamic theories are discussed here, followed by a vulnerability-stress model, an eclectic approach that seems to describe the major forces at work in the genesis and outcomes of schizophrenia.

Biologic Theories: Biochemical, Neurostructural, Genetic, and Perinatal Factors

People don't cause schizophrenia, they merely blame each other for doing so.
    E. Fuller Torrey (quoted in BCSS, 2008a).

Biologic theorists posit that schizophrenia is caused by anatomic or physiologic abnormalities. Biologic explanations include biochemical, neurostructural, genetic, and perinatal

risk factors and other theories. Biologic explanations have driven the development of biologic interventions such as psychotropic drugs.

Some clinicians have been reluctant to endorse biologic theories because the exclusive use of biologic approaches, such as psychotropic drugs, excludes interpersonal factors. However, the psychotherapeutic management model recognizes the importance of both biologic and interpersonal interventions.

A positive result of biologic theories has been the minimization of the blaming that is inherent in other explanations. Just as viewing alcoholism as an illness has helped clinicians, families, and patients to get beyond blaming and on to treatment, biologic theories have facilitated the treatment of schizophrenia. To illustrate, just as diabetic patients must learn to cope with their illness (e.g., a change in lifestyle), psychiatric patients must learn to cope with the limitations of their illness.

Biochemical Theories. Biochemical theory can be traced to 1952, when Delay and Deniker reported the antipsychotic effects of the dopamine receptor antagonist, chlorpromazine. The prevailing biochemical explanation is referred to as the *dopamine hypothesis*. According to this hypothesis, excessive dopaminergic activity in limbic areas causes acute positive (type I) symptoms of schizophrenia (hallucinations, delusions, and thought disorders). Excessive dopamine might be a result of increased dopamine synthesis, increased dopamine release, or an increase in the number and activity of dopamine receptors. It is also known that drugs that increase dopamine, such as levodopa, varenicline (Chantix), and amphetamines, can cause a psychotic state (see the box entitled Cigarette Smoking and Schizophrenia). This hypothesis is attractive because it is easy to grasp and because drugs that block dopamine seem to be extremely effective in the treatment of schizophrenia. However, it takes days, weeks, or months to establish the clinical effectiveness of these drugs, whereas the central nervous system dopamine receptors are blocked within a few minutes. Therefore, it seems that the dopamine hypothesis is too simplistic and that other factors are involved in explaining the effectiveness of antipsychotic drugs.

Keltner and Grant (2006) outlined the following apparent positive effects of smoking on schizophrenia caused by stimulation of nicotinic receptors in the brain:

1. Improved cognition
2. Improved negative symptoms
3. Protective effects against extrapyramidal side effects (EPSEs)
4. Improved auditory gating
5. Improved memory and attention

Sepe and colleagues (2012) developed a mnemonic to help patients stop smoking, "*QUIT*":

Question each patient to understand the pros and cons of quitting.

Understand the nature of the addiction.

Identify risk factors and triggers.

Talk with—not to—your patient.

CIGARETTE SMOKING AND SCHIZOPHRENIA

People with schizophrenia tend to smoke a lot. Although approximately 23.9% of the general public smokes, studies have indicated that 85% of individuals with schizophrenia smoke (Anonymous, 2008; Goldberg, 2010; National Cancer Institute, 2006). The difference in cigarette use between this population and the general population is significant, but there are noticeably fewer attempts at smoking cessation. Some researchers have argued that to deprive the schizophrenic person of the joys of smoking would be unduly cruel—smoking presumably being one of the few pleasures that they have (Dalack et al., 1998).

Why do people with schizophrenia smoke so much? The answer to this question probably lies in the biochemical changes produced by nicotine. All drugs of abuse cause changes in brain dopamine levels. Dopamine axons from the ventral tegmental area are afferents through the reward pathway, including the putative pleasure nucleus, the nucleus accumbens. Nicotine increases the release of dopamine in the nucleus accumbens. This occurs because nicotinic receptors synapse on dopamine afferents in the reward pathway—that is, nicotine modulates dopamine release. Nicotine also modulates dopamine afferents to the prefrontal cortex (mesocortical tract). When coupled with the supposition that negative symptoms are related to a hypodopaminergic process, nicotinic stimulation of dopamine in prefrontal areas might produce a therapeutic effect. In other words, the answer to the question, "Why do patients with schizophrenia smoke so much?" is simply this: It makes them feel better.

SELECTED STRUCTURAL BRAIN IMAGING FINDINGS IN SCHIZOPHRENIA

1. Cerebral ventricular enlargement
2. Smaller cerebral and cranial size
3. Hypoplasia of the medial (limbic) temporal structures, especially the hippocampus

From Nasrallah, H.A. (1993). Neurodevelopmental pathogenesis of schizophrenia. *Psychiatric Clinics of North America, 16,* 269.

Neurostructural Theories. Neurostructural theorists have proposed that schizophrenia, particularly negative (type II) schizophrenia, is a result of pathoanatomy. The three specific neurostructural changes mentioned most often are increased ventricular brain ratios, brain atrophy, and decreased cerebral blood flow. CT, MRI, positron emission tomography (PET), and single-photon emission computed tomography (SPECT) are techniques used for visualizing the brain. CT and MRI provide images of brain structure (e.g., for ventricular brain ratios and brain atrophy). PET and SPECT provide information on both brain structure and brain activity.

Ventricular Brain Ratios. The finding that a significant subgroup of individuals with schizophrenia has enlarged ventricles was first reported by Johnstone and colleagues in 1976. Individuals with enlarged ventricles have a poor prognosis and exhibit negative symptoms.

Although ventricular enlargement is not peculiar to schizophrenia, anatomic findings are substantially different from findings for neurodegenerative disorders, such as Alzheimer's disease. Ventricular enlargement in schizophrenia is not associated with a neurodegenerative process (Bogerts et al., 1993; Marsh et al., 1994); that is, one would not expect to find a gradual increase in ventricular volume over time in a patient with schizophrenia. However, in a patient with Alzheimer's disease, ventricles continue to increase in volume as brain cells die. Not all patients with schizophrenia have abnormally enlarged ventricles. About 50% of these patients fall within the range of control or normal subjects (Cannon & Marco, 1994). This overlapping effect has led researchers to study monozygotic twins when one twin has schizophrenia. In documented cases in which the affected twin had ventricles falling within the normal range, pathoanatomic deviance can be demonstrated only when contrasted with the ventricles of the unaffected (i.e., nonschizophrenic) twin. Roberts and colleagues (1993) demonstrated that an otherwise normal-appearing ventricle is enlarged compared with the perfect control—the ventricles of the monozygotic twin.

Brain Atrophy. More than 100 years ago, Alzheimer described brain cell loss in schizophrenia. Anatomic pathology in cortical and subcortical areas has been suggested by brain imaging techniques and confirmed by postmortem examinations of individuals with schizophrenia. Limbic, hippocampal, and thalamic structures; temporal lobes; the amygdala; and the substantia nigra are specific lobes and nuclei found to have undergone neuropathologic changes.

The dopamine hypothesis, although limited in explanatory power, continues to have great educational value for the following reasons:

1. Drugs that increase dopamine (i.e., dopaminergics such as levodopa, Chantix, and amphetamine) can cause psychotic symptoms.
2. Drugs that block dopamine (i.e., antipsychotics) alleviate psychotic symptoms.

Other proposed neurotransmitter contributors to schizophrenia include serotonin and glutamate. Serotonin inhibits dopamine synthesis and release; serotonin antagonists potentially increase dopamine levels. This characteristic is one of the neurophysiologic properties presumed to cause atypical antipsychotics to be effective. These agents are referred to as *serotonin-dopamine antagonists* by some clinicians and manufacturers.

Glutamate, a product of the Krebs cycle, also has been proposed as a factor in schizophrenia. Glutamate contributes to the regulation of N-methyl-D-aspartate (NMDA) receptors, which are necessary for cognitive processes. Too little glutamate can lead to hallucinations. For example, the street drug phencyclidine (PCP) antagonizes NMDA receptors and can cause a psychotic state. Excessive levels of glutamate lead to overstimulation of the NMDA receptors, increasing intracellular levels of calcium and causing increased neuronal firing. This cellular excess is referred to as *excitotoxicity* and causes neuronal death. Cell death plays a role in schizophrenia (Keltner & Lillie, 2009). Treatment with glutamate has not been particularly promising at this point.

Cerebral Blood Flow. Individuals with atrophic changes also have decreased cortical blood flow, particularly in the prefrontal cortex, with a consequent decrease in metabolic activity (British Columbia Schizophrenia Society, 2008a). Cognitive demands, such as organizing, planning, learning from experience, problem solving, introspection, and critical judgment, are compromised.

Genetic Theories. The estimated heritability of schizophrenia is 70% to 90% (Zhang & Malhotra, 2013). The relatives of patients with schizophrenia have a greater incidence of the disorder than chance alone would allow. Although a huge amount of resources have been directed at finding the genetic cause of schizophrenia, the results are not specific. Almost every chromosome has been linked to schizophrenia (Williams, 2003). Genetic studies may hold great promise, but much remains to be discovered about this illness. At this point, it is probably safe to say that multiple genetic deficits converge to give rise to schizophrenia.

The genetic risk for schizophrenia is shown in Box 24-6. Of particular interest to clinicians is the risk associated with having a parent with schizophrenia. Although the risk reaches 35% if both parents have schizophrenia, this higher incidence alone does not adequately address the debate of nature (genetics) versus nurture (upbringing). For instance, a parent with a mental disorder might rear children inadequately to the extent that the children are predisposed to schizophrenia based on the parenting skills, not genetics.

To control the nurture variable, researchers have studied monozygotic (identical) and dizygotic (fraternal) twins. Monozygotic twins have consistently shown a higher concordancy rate (meaning both twins do or do not have symptoms of schizophrenia). Concordancy rates are 50% for monozygotic twins. This rate is 50 times higher than the risk for the general population, and it is 3 times higher than the risk for dizygotic twins.

These findings seem to establish the genetic or nature basis of schizophrenia; however, there are still extraneous variables that cannot be explained. For example, many monozygotic twins are dressed alike and often are misidentified; their upbringing might be identical, too. Some experts argue that it is no wonder that monozygotic twins have a high concordancy rate. Unless researchers can control the environmental variable, the relative impact of nature and nurture cannot be reported with confidence.

BOX 24-6	HERITABLE RISK FOR SCHIZOPHRENIA	
Identical twin affected		50%
Fraternal twin affected		15%
Brother or sister affected		10%
One parent affected		15%
Both parents affected		35%
Second-degree relative affected		2%-3%
No affected relative		1%

Modified from Roberts, G.W., Leigh, P.N., & Weinberger, D.R. (1993). *Neuropsychiatric disorders*. London: Mosby Europe.

To control for the variable of environment, studies have been conducted of monozygotic twins who were separated at birth and reared apart. Monozygotic concordancy rates remained significantly higher in these studies.

> **? CRITICAL THINKING QUESTION**
>
> 2. Why does type I schizophrenia often evolve into type II schizophrenia?

Perinatal Risk Factors. Multiple nongenetic factors influence the development of schizophrenia. Some researchers believe that schizophrenia can be linked to prenatal exposure to influenza; birth during the winter; prenatal exposure to lead; minor malformations developing during early gestation; exposure to viruses from house cats; and complications of pregnancy, particularly during labor and delivery (Andreasen, 1999; Torrey & Yolken, 1995). The research about influenza epidemics is inconclusive, but there is evidence that individuals with schizophrenia are more likely to have been born in the winter months (American Psychiatric Association, 2013). Research of cohorts conceived during devastating influenza epidemics has revealed a meaningfully higher incidence of schizophrenia in products of conception (i.e., children) during this time. Other researchers have suggested a high incidence of birth trauma and injury among individuals with schizophrenia. These studies suggest a relationship between schizophrenia and birth problems, particularly when adverse events occur during the second trimester of pregnancy (Roberts et al., 1993).

Psychodynamic Theories

Psychodynamic theories of schizophrenia are not given much weight today, but at one time they held sway in psychiatric circles. These theories focus on the individual's responses to life events. The common theme of these theories is the internal reaction to life stressors or conflicts. These explanations include developmental and family theories.

Developmental Theories of Schizophrenia. During the early part of the twentieth century, Meyer and Freud emphasized the significance of developmental psychiatry. They believed that the seeds of mental health and illness are sown in childhood. An extension of their arguments is that events in early life can cause severe problems such as schizophrenia. Freudian concepts are still used meaningfully in discussions of schizophrenia. These concepts include poor ego boundaries, fragile ego, ego disintegration, inadequate ego development, regressed or id behavior, and love/hate (ambivalent) relationships.

The work of two later developmental theorists, Erikson (1968) and Sullivan (1953), more directly explains schizophrenia. Erikson, who theorized an eight-stage model of human development, saw the first step, trust or mistrust, as crucial to later interpersonal relationships. A child who is deprived of a nurturing, loving environment or is neglected or rejected is vulnerable to mental disturbances. Inadequate passage through this stage predisposes the person to mistrust, isolative behaviors, and other asocial behaviors—the very behaviors found in schizophrenia. Therapeutic intervention focuses on the reestablishment of trust through consistent, anxiety-free relationships.

Sullivan, using different terms, expressed essentially the same ideas. The absence of warm, nurturing attention during the early years blocks the expression of these same affective responses in later years. Without this capacity, a person exhibits disordered social interactions and other disturbances. These individuals learn to avoid interpersonal interactions because these interactions are painful.

Family Theories of Schizophrenia. Family theories of schizophrenia are linked naturally to developmental theories. If early life experiences are crucial in development, the argument is made that the family—the environment in which most people grow—is significant to the development of mental health or illness. Lack of a loving and nurturing primary caregiver, inconsistent family behaviors, and faulty communication patterns are thought to be responsible for mental problems in later life.

Outdated and harmful theories specifically tailored to the families of schizophrenic individuals were the schizophrenogenic mother theory and the double-bind theory. The word *schizophrenogenic* literally means "to cause schizophrenia." Perhaps this definition has been the greatest disservice of psychodynamic theories. Essentially, this notion states that the blame for schizophrenia can be placed on the mother. The double-bind theory described family practices in which the child was damned if he did and damned if he didn't. An example often used was the child who was expected to do well in school but was criticized for taking time away from the family to study. Acocella (2000) captured some of the ideology behind these assertions:

> Psychoanalysis took a while to conquer the United States, but once it did, after the Second World War, its dominance was unquestioned, and its arrogance breathtaking. Schizophrenia, autism, and numerous other disorders were blamed on the mother, with no evidence, just utter certainty (p. 11).

Geiser and associates (1988) noted that family theories were actually blame theories. Families have been viewed as causative agents, saboteurs of treatment, toxic influences, and as patients themselves. Sometimes families have been treated with hostility and distrust. Because families bear the brunt of preprofessional and postprofessional care of these patients, it is important to work with families without alienating them.

Although most professionals have abandoned these harmful notions, many laypeople still labor under these misconceptions. Hence, they are mentioned in this textbook.

Clinical Example: Unbelievable but True

Many of us think back to our childhood and remember birthday parties and games, such as hide-and-seek and baseball games. Al thinks back to his past and remembers molestation, cruelty, and punishment. Al has been diagnosed with schizophrenia since the age of 20.

Al is the next-to-youngest of eight children. According to Al, more than half of his siblings have a major mental illness. Al states, "My mama had schizophrenia for 10 years, then God saved her." When asked about his relationship with his mother now, Al states that she left the rest of the family after "daddy" died. When questioned about his father, Al speaks of the way his father used to beat his mother and the children. Al recalls seeing his father beat one brother so severely he thought the boy might die. Al further described a beating he received from his father that left him bleeding. When asked why he thought his father beat him, Al responded, "He got mad a lot. I forgot to get firewood like he asked me to."

In discussing his illness, Al was asked to describe when he first started hearing voices. He replies, "When I was little, after those boys did that to me. I was out fixing my bicycle and I heard the devil talk to me over and over." Al reports numerous incidents of abuse during his life. At one point during the interview, Al states his belief that his schizophrenia is God's punishment for what he had done.

Al's first documented psychiatric episode occurred in the early 1980s. In the psychological evaluation emanating from this experience, the psychiatrist noted the presence of hallucinations and delusions; Al described spaceships and command hallucinations, and he stated that he had killed Christ. His condition deteriorated further, and he was committed to a public hospital. During his hospitalization, Al was given a diagnosis of schizophrenia.

Today, Al lives in a residential group home and attends day treatment. He continues to manifest both auditory and visual hallucinations. Although prescribed two atypical antipsychotic drugs, symptom control varies from day to day (Keltner et al., 2001).

Vulnerability-Stress Model of Schizophrenia

It is generally believed by most clinicians and researchers that schizophrenia has multifactorial causes, with many susceptibility genes interacting with numerous environmental factors to yield what is called schizophrenia. Insel (2004), Director of the National Institute of Mental Health, referred to schizophrenia as a "perfect storm" of events. Suspected environmental influences have been previously discussed.

As previously stated, no single theory adequately answers the questions about the genesis of schizophrenia. The vulnerability-stress model addresses the various forces that cause schizophrenia in some cases and in other cases cause the broader schizophrenia spectrum problems of schizoaffective disorders and schizophrenia-related personality disorders. This model recognizes that both biologic (including genetic) and psychodynamic predispositions to schizophrenia, when coupled with stressful life events, can precipitate a schizophrenic process. According to this model, people with a predisposition to schizophrenia might (but not always) avoid serious psychiatric disease if they are protected from the stresses of life. Individuals with a similar vulnerability might develop schizophrenia if exposed to stressors. To illustrate the point, a wealthy person might be spared the brunt of some stressors because of wealth, whereas a poor person, struggling to meet basic needs, confronts stressors on a daily basis. According to this model, the poor person is more likely to display symptoms of schizophrenia.

As noted earlier, schizophrenia is overrepresented among poor people. Individuals with schizophrenia tend to drift downward socioeconomically. This unenviable status enhances their vulnerability by exposing them to constant stressors.

Student Example: The Straw That Broke The...

This situation is easily applied to you and your peers. Students who need to deal only with the stress of nursing school have it hard enough. Students who must deal with the stress of nursing school plus significant financial and family responsibilities have a heavier load to manage. When a surprise assignment or change in schedule comes along, the student who already has multiple stressors often has a more difficult time adjusting to school demands.

SPECIAL ISSUES RELATED TO SCHIZOPHRENIA

Many special issues need to be clarified to help the student focus on the breadth of concerns involved in the psychiatric nursing care of patients with schizophrenia. Box 24-7 lists key objectives when working with patients and families.

Comorbid Medical Illnesses

There are many special issues related to schizophrenia, but the issue of most concern currently is the high concordancy rate of other medical problems superimposed on schizophrenia. This is referred to as *comorbidity*. About 50% to 60% of patients with schizophrenia have a comorbid condition (Batki et al., 2009). Specifically, there is a higher incidence of hypertension, diabetes, cardiovascular disease, and metabolic syndrome in patients with schizophrenia (Cohn, 2012; Newcomer, 2008). An overall life expectancy decrease of about 20% has been consistently found in mortality studies among this diagnostic group (Allison et al., 2009). This situation (i.e., poor health, premature death) is confounded and perpetuated by poor lifestyle choices. For example, it is clear from both the literature and personal experience that patients with schizophrenia tend to be more sedentary, make poorer food choices (high fat, high carbohydrates), abuse substances at higher rates, and smoke more cigarettes than the general public (Vreeland, 2007). The metabolic syndrome is a very serious issue among patients taking antipsychotic drugs. Chapter 14 addresses this issue in greater depth.

BOX 24-7	**KEY OBJECTIVES FOR TREATING PATIENTS WITH SCHIZOPHRENIA**

- Work with the family.
- Treat depression.
- Minimize stressful interactions.
- Treat substance abuse.
- Avoid lengthy, intense verbal interactions.

Families of Schizophrenic Individuals

Families have often been blamed for the problems of individuals with schizophrenia. It is no wonder that some families are suspicious of professionals who might view the family as the villain. It is also not surprising that many of these families have little desire to be studied.

Although research has substantiated the state of turmoil in these families, many clinicians argue that dysfunctional families are not the cause of schizophrenia, but rather the result of having a family member with this illness (Ghosh & Greenberg, 2009). Nevertheless, when a family becomes destabilized, there is a high probability that the dysfunctional family will have a negative effect on the schizophrenic member.

Individuals with schizophrenia can be a disruptive influence on the family, particularly when they are noncompliant with prescribed medications or when they use mind-altering drugs. Although there is a consensus that negative features (e.g., emotionally overinvolved, hostile, critical) are present in many families of schizophrenic patients, these families are studied after schizophrenia has been identified—years after the family might have been disrupted by the illness. This observation leads to the "chicken or egg" question raised previously: Do disruptive families cause individuals to have schizophrenia, or do individuals with schizophrenia cause families to become disruptive?

Although blame might be warranted in some family situations, in most cases it is not. Blaming the family leads to a sense of alienation between the family and treatment team. Nurses should remember that families bear the brunt of care outside the hospital. Most discharged psychiatric patients are sent home to live with their families; the family's stake in the patient's care is obvious. As time goes on, these families tend to become increasingly isolated and feel more frustrated, helpless, and hopeless, even though they care very much about the patient.

Clinical Example: A Burned-out Family

Pete is 24 years old. At age 19, he began having symptoms that eventually led to a diagnosis of schizophrenia. Through several hospitalizations and outpatient treatment programs, he continued to live at home with his parents. Pete started having delusions that people were watching him. His paranoid thinking reached such levels that his presence in the home completely disrupted family life. Pete would barricade himself in his room, believed that his parents were part of a conspiracy to spy on him, and occasionally became physically violent. After a fourth hospitalization 2 years earlier, Pete's parents informed the treatment team that he was no longer welcome in their home. They verbalized fear of Pete and worried about how he was affecting his younger siblings in the home. Although his parents live within 50 miles of Pete, they seldom visit.

Depression and Suicide in Schizophrenia

Depressive symptoms are frequently a part of the psychopathology of schizophrenia, with some studies suggesting that approximately 25% of schizophrenic patients experience depression (Siris, 2012). These symptoms can occur at any time during the illness, including years after the acute phase, but they do respond to antidepressants. A related phenomenon is the high incidence of suicide attempts (20%) and deaths (5% to 10%) among schizophrenic patients (American Psychiatric Association, 2013). Suicide is the leading cause of premature death in patients with schizophrenia. There are several risk factors for the high prevalence of suicide (American Psychiatric Association, 2013):

1. Depression related to schizophrenia
2. Hopelessness related to schizophrenia
3. Being unemployed
4. Comorbid substance use

Cognitive Dysfunction

It is well established that patients with schizophrenia have cognitive impairment. For example, memory, attention, and executive function are affected. Research has shown that cognitive deficits are a better predictor of declining abilities to engage in basic activities of daily living than positive or negative symptoms. Because cognitive ability directly influences so many aspects of successful living, it is important to discuss this aspect of schizophrenia. Traditional antipsychotics do not reduce cognitive symptoms and might exacerbate them. For example, EPSEs such as akinesia cause cognitive slowdown. Atypical agents are known to improve performance of some aspects of cognitive ability.

Relapse

Nonadherence to medications and exposure to significant stressors are the most common causes of relapse. Psychoeducation aimed at these issues is important.

Stress

Earl is a 36-year-old African-American man who lives in a board and care home in a suburb of Birmingham, Alabama. He receives a monthly check for $700 that goes to his board and care home operator; $655 is deducted for his room and board. He theoretically has $45 per month to spend on sodas, cigarettes, clothes, snacks, or for a trip to McDonald's. However, he does not get to "hold" his money and, according to Earl, he does not always get the full amount. This level of poverty is a stressor for Earl.

One of the three inescapable facts noted at the beginning of this chapter is the role of stress in onset and relapse. According to the vulnerability-stress model, people with schizophrenia are vulnerable to stress. Common stressors can be categorized as follows:

1. Biologic (e.g., medical illness)
2. Psychosocial (e.g., loss of a relationship)
3. Sociocultural (e.g., homelessness)
4. Emotional (e.g., persistent criticism)

The therapeutic mandate is to minimize the impact of stress on vulnerable individuals. The following two basic strategies are used:

1. Reducing stress and stressor accumulation
2. Developing coping skills

Because of their economic and social status, many individuals with schizophrenia face major stressors routinely. Stated another way, some individuals most vulnerable to stress have more stress to handle. Helping patients learn to identify and avoid stressful events is an important task for the psychiatric nurse.

Substance Abuse in People with Schizophrenia

Substance abuse is the most common comorbid psychiatric condition associated with schizophrenia, and it seems to be increasing. A high percentage of people with schizophrenia abuse alcohol, drugs, or both. Alcohol, marijuana, and cocaine account for most of the drugs abused. In contrast to the general population, individuals with schizophrenia have little chance of using alcohol in a social manner. This abuse might be related to an underdeveloped reward pathway in the brain (Anonymous, 2003).

Drug abuse has a negative effect on the treatment of patients with schizophrenia and is associated with poor outcomes. When substance abuse begins, the individual is less likely to take medications and accept other treatments and more likely to become hostile, violent, and suicidal (Anonymous, 2003). Substance abuse probably accounts for the overrepresentation of schizophrenic individuals who are jailed. For example, alcohol causes disinhibition, aggressiveness, and poor judgment. These symptoms are already present in patients with severe mental illness. These same symptoms and related lack of social skills hinder patients with schizophrenia from fully benefiting from treatment programs such as Alcoholics Anonymous and Narcotics Anonymous.

> **? CRITICAL THINKING QUESTION**
>
> 3. Why do you think the rate of substance abuse is so high among individuals with schizophrenia?

Work

The lack of work, the inability to work, and the lack of a desire to work all are features of schizophrenia. Because work, or what one does for a living, is a major defining characteristic in this society, the fact that many people with schizophrenia do not work adds to their inability to fit in. The major problem confronting these individuals is not so much a lack of skill but an inability to cope on the job socially. Routine behaviors such as joking, inviting someone out, or having insight into the way one is affecting others are the major obstacles to a productive work life for people with schizophrenia.

Psychosis-Induced Polydipsia

Psychosis-induced polydipsia, or compulsive water drinking (4 to 10 L/day), is seen in 6% to 20% of patients with psychosis (American Psychiatric Association, 1997). The desire to drink probably occurs because of thirst and osmotic dysregulation; it is characterized by a compulsive approach to water ingestion. The major concern associated with polydipsia is hyponatremia. Hyponatremia causes lightheadedness, weakness, lethargy, muscle cramps, nausea and vomiting, confusion, convulsions, and coma. Treatment includes frequent weighings, restricted fluid intake, sodium replacement, and positive reinforcement.

CONTINUUM OF CARE FOR PEOPLE WITH SCHIZOPHRENIA

Rather than starting to release patients in a few locales and measuring the outcome, officials implemented the policy in cities and counties across the United States virtually simultaneously, based on widespread hope that the new drugs would cure people and the widespread belief in state legislatures that the policy would save taxpayers money.

E. Fuller Torrey (1997, p. B4)

By "policy," Torrey means deinstitutionalization, and, driven by this policy, an array of services, or a continuum of care, has developed. Most clinicians agree that a community setting is good for some patients and an institutional setting is better for others (Keltner, 2008). The continuum of care for patients with schizophrenia includes the following (American Psychiatric Association, 1997):

- Acute symptoms—short-term hospitalization
- Treatment-resistant—long-term hospitalization
- Stable but chronic—day treatment
- Some level of supervision needed—if family is unable, supportive housing including foster care, a board and care home, or a nursing home

PSYCHOTHERAPEUTIC MANAGEMENT

Most schizophrenics go on for years struggling alone without anyone to help them become stronger than their symptoms.

P.J. Ruocchio (1989, p. 188)

Think about Ruocchio's statement, specifically "... struggling alone without anyone to help them become stronger than their symptoms." What an utterly profound insight. Remember it whenever you care for a patient with schizophrenia. Psychotherapeutic management is aimed at helping patients become stronger than their symptoms. The nursing interventions used in the treatment of patients with schizophrenia are derived from the appropriate development of the nursing care plan.

Psychotherapeutic Nurse-Patient Relationship

Pharmacotherapy can improve some of the symptoms of schizophrenia but has limited effect on social impairments that characterize the disorder and limit functioning and quality of life.

N.A. Huxley et al. (2000, p. 187)

Huxley has it right. Drugs can do a lot, but there is more to it than the old "diagnose and adios" mentality in some agencies. The objective of the psychotherapeutic nurse-patient relationship is to build a therapeutic alliance with patients. A long-term relationship in which trust has developed is probably more significant and therapeutic than a particular theory of care. Insight therapy has limited usefulness with this population, whereas less invasive modalities, such as supportive therapy, problem solving, and social skills training that focus

on behavior and not meaning, are more helpful. Long-term, trusting relationships yield better compliance with medications and better outcomes with psychological resources.

The objective of this section is to provide basic concepts for working with patients with schizophrenia. General principles for developing a therapeutic nurse-patient relationship are presented. In addition, the Key Nursing Interventions for Developing the Therapeutic Nurse-Patient Relationship box lists some of these specific principles as well as some patient comments that the student might encounter. Examples of therapeutic responses by the nurse are also given.

General principles for developing a therapeutic nurse-patient relationship include the following:

- Be calm when talking to patients. *Rationale:* Anxiety is contagious and counterproductive when working with patients who have schizophrenia.
- Accept patients as they are, but do not accept all behaviors. *Rationale:* Everyone wants to be accepted. The focus is on behaviors, which communicates very directly that behaviors can change.
- Keep promises. *Rationale:* Dependability builds trust.
- Be consistent. *Rationale:* Consistency increases trust.
- Be honest. *Rationale:* Honesty strengthens trust.
- Do not reinforce hallucinations or delusions. *Rationale:* The nurse should simply state his or her perception of reality, voice doubt about the patient's perceptions, and move on to discuss real people or events.
- Orient patients to time, person, and place, if indicated. *Rationale:* Orientation reinforces reality. However, use good judgment. To be continually reminded that you are disoriented takes an emotional toll.
- Do not touch patients without warning them. *Rationale:* Patients who are suspicious might perceive a touch as a threat and retaliate.
- Avoid whispering or laughing when patients are unable to hear all of a conversation. *Rationale:* Have you ever wondered whether you were the subject of discussion when you were around people who whispered or giggled? Suspicious patients interpret these actions as a personal affront.
- Reinforce positive behaviors. *Rationale:* Appropriate reinforcement can increase positive behaviors.
- Avoid competitive activities with some patients. *Rationale:* Competition is threatening and can lead to decreased self-esteem.
- Do not embarrass patients. *Rationale:* Patients with schizophrenia often avoid social contact because they fear embarrassment.
- For withdrawn patients, start with one-to-one interactions. *Rationale:* Even in group situations, it is probably most therapeutic for interactions to be a series of nurse-patient interactions rather than patient-patient interactions. Nurse-patient interactions are less threatening to patients and can evolve into a wider circle of social interaction.
- Allow and encourage verbalization of feelings. *Rationale:* Patients are helped if they can say what they think without the nurse becoming defensive.

PATIENT AND FAMILY EDUCATION

Schizophrenia

Illness

Schizophrenia is a brain disease that disrupts perceptions, thinking, feelings, and behaviors. It can cause distortions of reality; false beliefs; hallucinations; and changes in speech patterns, moods, and behaviors. It disrupts the person's ability to function, socialize, and work.

Medications

1. Some medications for schizophrenia might cause uncomfortable, but typically temporary, side effects. Some of these side effects can be lessened with other medications, nondrug interventions, or both.

2. As a result of these side effects, the patient might not want to take the prescribed medications. The physician needs to know this immediately.

3. It is crucial for the patient to continue taking the medications, even after the patient feels better or the symptoms of illness are no longer evident.

Other Issues

Discuss early symptoms with the patient, which might indicate the beginning of a relapse. Make an agreement with the patient about the actions that family, friends, or both will take to get the patient appropriate help.

KEY NURSING INTERVENTIONS

For Developing the Therapeutic Nurse-Patient Relationship

The following are specific interventions and examples for developing a therapeutic nurse-patient relationship, including examples of appropriate responses. These examples are meant to illustrate some of the common situations described in the text. Each patient is unique, and that uniqueness might necessitate a variation of the suggested response.

INTERVENTION	RATIONALE
Do not argue about delusions.	Arguing tends to reinforce delusions and can make patients angry. Reflect reality, and attempt to distract patients in a matter-of-fact manner.
	Patient: The FBI and the Mafia are both after me.
	Nurse: I know your thoughts seem real to you; however, it does not seem reasonable to me. I also want you to know that you are safe here. Let's go into the day room and talk.
	Proceed to talk about occupational therapy efforts (or a similar topic) that focus on the patient's real world.
Do not reinforce hallucinations.	*Patient:* The voices are calling me terrible names.
	Nurse: I do not hear anything but your voice and mine.
	Patient looks around the room, eyes darting to the corners of the room.
	Nurse: It looks like you might be listening to something. Are you hearing voices?
	This effort might lead to identifying and avoiding triggering events.
	Patient: I started hearing the voices last night right after I went to bed.
	Nurse: Tell me about your evening last night. There might be a link between something that happened and your hearing voices again.
Focus on real people and real events.	This helps patients stay in touch with reality.
	Patient: I keep hearing the voices.
	Nurse: I understand, but I want to help you focus away from those voices. Let's go to the day room and talk.
	Proceed to bring patients closer to reality by talking about daily life.
Be diligent in attempting to understand patients.	It is therapeutic to help patients communicate what they want to say; however, use good judgment. Pushing too hard to understand can be frustrating for the patient.
	Patient: I could have been bitten. It was never a dog's day.
	Nurse: I am not sure what you are saying, but I want to understand. Are you talking about almost being hurt?
Attempt to balance siding with inappropriate behavior and crushing a fragile ego.	Time and effort help the nurse learn to negotiate artfully between these potentially negative outcomes.
	Patient: I am going to hit that bastard if he says another word to me.
	Nurse: I know you are upset with him. Let's talk about other ways you can deal with this situation.
	If a patient is acting odd and the nurse suspects he or she is hallucinating, the patient should be asked about it.
	Help patients to identify the stressors that might precipitate hallucinations or delusions.

Psychopharmacology

Lieberman (1997) compared the discovery of antipsychotic drugs to the discovery of insulin. The development of this class of medications revolutionized mental health treatment. The student is encouraged to review Chapter 14, which provides a complete discussion of antipsychotic drugs.

Schizophrenic patients need to take their antipsychotic drugs as prescribed, but many do not. Box 24-8 lists some strategies to promote adherence to drug therapy. Box 24-9 reviews major side effects. (For a full review of these side effects, see Chapter 14.) Because of racial and ethnic variation, Asians and Hispanics with schizophrenia might need a lower dosage of antipsychotic medications than white patients to achieve the same blood levels (U.S. Surgeon General, 1999). As many experienced clinicians have thought, more recent

findings imply that how a patient responds to an antipsychotic initially (first 2 to 4 weeks) is a good predictor of how well a patient will respond to that particular medication (Webster & Straley, 2014).

Milieu Management

Milieu management is an important dimension of the psychiatric nursing care of patients with schizophrenia. With the dramatic introduction of psychotropic drugs in the 1950s, other forms of treatment such as milieu therapy were abandoned. Now that psychopharmacologists have had free reign for decades, it is clear that drugs alone are not enough. A therapeutic treatment approach is best developed with all three components of psychotherapeutic management in place.

Therapeutic manipulation of the environment can occur at both the inpatient and the outpatient levels and helps patients function better. As a rule of thumb, low-intensity, calm environments benefit patients with schizophrenia. General principles that specifically address the environment of schizophrenic patients follow.

For disruptive patients:
- Set limits on disruptive behavior.
- Decrease environmental stimuli. For example, many nurses find that soft or classical music calms an environment, whereas hard rock or rap music creates agitation.
- Observe escalating patients frequently to intervene. Intervention (e.g., medication) before acting out occurs protects patients and others physically and prevents embarrassment for escalating patients.
- Modify the environment to minimize objects that can be used as weapons. Some units use furniture so heavy that it cannot be lifted by most people.
- Be careful in stating what the staff will do if a patient acts out; however, follow through once a violation occurs (e.g., "If you break the window, we will place you in restraints").
- When using restraints, provide for safety by evaluating the patient's status of hydration, nutrition, elimination, and circulation.

For withdrawn patients:
- Arrange nonthreatening activities that involve patients in doing something (e.g., a walking tour of a park, painting).
- Arrange furniture in a semicircle or around a table, which forces patients to sit with someone. Interactions are permitted in this situation but should not be demanded. Sit in silence with patients who are not ready to respond. Some may move the chair away despite the nurse's efforts.
- Help patients to participate in decision making as appropriate.
- Reinforce appropriate grooming and hygiene.
- Provide psychosocial rehabilitation—training in community living, social skills, and health care skills.

For suspicious patients:
- Be matter-of-fact when interacting with these patients.

BOX 24-8 NURSING INTERVENTIONS TO INCREASE DRUG ADHERENCE

- Observe patients for side effects and intervene accordingly. Akathisia is a troubling side effect that patients cannot tolerate.
- When giving tablets or pills, make sure patients do not "cheek" the medications (hide the medication in cheeks or mouth) to spit them out or hoard them for later.
- At discharge, teach patients and their families about drugs, including side effects, potential interactions, and dosage schedules.
- Long-acting injectable drugs are effective for patients who do not adhere to drug therapy.

BOX 24-9 REVIEW OF MAJOR SIDE EFFECTS OF ANTIPSYCHOTIC DRUGS

Dopamine D_2 blockade in nigrostriatal tract, causing *EPSEs*
  Parkinsonism
  Akathisia
  Dystonias
  Neuroleptic malignant syndrome
  Pisa syndrome
Muscarinic blockade in parasympathetic systems, causing *anticholinergic effects*
  Dry mouth
  Blurred vision
  Constipation
  Urinary hesitation
  Tachycardia
Hypersensitivity to dopamine in nigrostriatal tract, causing *tardive dyskinesia*
Elevated prolactin related to dopamine blockade in tuberoinfundibular tract, causing *amenorrhea*, *galactorrhea*, *impotency*, and *decreased libido*
Histamine blockade, causing *sedation*
Alpha-1 blockade, causing *orthostatic hypotension*

EPSEs, Extrapyramidal side effects.

- Staff members should not laugh or whisper around patients unless the patients can hear what is being said. The nurse should clarify any misperceptions that patients have.
- Do not touch suspicious patients without warning. Avoid close physical contact.
- Be consistent in activities (time, staff, approach).
- Maintain eye contact.

For patients with impaired communication:
- Be patient and do not pressure patients to make sense.
- Do not place patients in group activities that would frustrate them, damage their self-esteem, or overtax their abilities.
- Provide opportunities for purposeful psychomotor activity.

For patients with hallucinations:
- Attempt to provide distracting activities.
- Discourage situations in which patients talk to others about their disordered perceptions.
- Monitor television selections. Some programs seem to cause more perceptual problems than others (e.g., horror movies).
- Monitor for command hallucinations that might increase the potential for patients to become dangerous (Scott & Resnick, 2013).
- Have staff members available in the day room so that patients can talk to real people about real people or real events.

For disorganized patients:
- Remove disorganized patients to a less stimulating environment.
- Provide a calm environment; the staff should appear calm.
- Provide safe and relatively simple activities for these patients.

CASE STUDY

The police bring Bill Wilson, a 25-year-old man, to the hospital. He was in a downtown bus station preaching loudly. He states in the emergency department that he had spoken to God and that God had told him to save San Francisco. He admits to hearing both God and Satan arguing and is terrified at times. In talking with his family, staff members discover that Bill was a solid student until about a year ago. He began to struggle in school but continued to pass his course work. He dropped out of school 3 months ago. His family believes his problem started when his girlfriend of 4 years broke off their engagement.

Bill began hearing voices a couple of weeks ago, according to his family, but the family lost contact with him until they were notified of this hospitalization. Bill's family is committed to helping him. On admission to the unit, Bill is oriented to time, place, and person but states, "God has chosen me to be his special angel. I must save the sinners of San Francisco." Bill then stands up and turns his head rapidly from side to side. When asked why he is turning his head, he says, "God and Satan are arguing about what I should do."

See the nursing care plan for Bill Wilson on p. 266.

OTHER SCHIZOPHRENIA SPECTRUM DISORDERS

In addition to schizophrenia, several other psychotic disorders are described in *DSM-5* with which the student should be familiar. Interventions for these disorders are directed at prominent symptoms and are the same as the interventions used for the symptoms of patients with schizophrenia.

CASE STUDY

Emma Rice, a 40-year-old woman with a history of multiple admissions, is admitted to the psychiatric unit. She was found wandering downtown incoherent and disheveled. During the assessment interview, Emma is noted to have a flat affect and is withdrawn. She reports not seeing her family for 5 years and cannot remember when she last held a job. There is no history of hallucinatory or delusional thought content in this recent occurrence. The staff knows Emma and knows that, during past admissions, she has responded to the less expensive haloperidol. After admission, Emma says, "Let me go. Go on, onward, backward. (pause) Emma hide, died." When asked where she lives, Emma slowly responds, "Over there, somewhere, anywhere, nowhere." Emma's board and care operator knows her well and has indicated that a bed is being held for Emma.

See the nursing care plan for Emma Rice on p. 266.

Clinical Example- A Life Gone to Hell

Patty is a 42-year-old white woman who was referred to the county mental health department by her sister after attempting suicide by combining a large number of benzodiazepines with a six-pack of beer. Patty states that most of her "mental" problems began when she became pregnant at age 18. At the time, she was unmarried and alienated from her parents. Patty raised her daughter, Billie, alone until she eventually married another man. At age 25, Patty became pregnant again and gave birth to a son. Her husband, an alcoholic, had abused Patty to some extent, but the abusive behavior became more frequent and more severe as Patty entered her early thirties. There had been suspicion that he had sexually abused Billie, but nothing conclusive was documented. Patty and her husband divorced when the boy was 7 years old. The court awarded the child to the husband. Today, Patty has little contact with her daughter, son, ex-husband, or parents. She frequently has auditory hallucinations telling her to kill herself and has nightmares about killing her son and ex-husband. She attends a day treatment program 5 days a week and lives in a one-bedroom apartment alone. Patty is very sad and always looks at the floor. She is consumed with guilt. She does not initiate conversation with others at the day treatment program. She states that she continues to hear voices and thinks about suicide all the time.

Delusional Disorder

People with delusional disorder display symptoms similar to symptoms seen in patients with schizophrenia. However, substantial differences exist and necessitate a diagnostic differentiation. The following symptoms differentiate delusional disorders from schizophrenic disorders (American Psychiatric Association, 2013):

- Delusion persists for at least 1 month.
- The patients have never met the criteria for schizophrenia.
- The behavior of these patients is relatively normal except in relation to their delusions.
- If mood episodes have occurred concurrently with delusions, their total duration has been relatively brief.
- The symptoms are *not* the direct result of a substance-induced or medical condition.
- If hallucinations are present, they are not prominent.

Brief Psychotic Disorder

The category of brief psychotic disorder includes all psychotic disturbances that last less than 1 month and are not related to a mood disorder, a general medical condition, or a substance-induced disorder (American Psychiatric Association, 2013). At least one of the following psychotic disturbances must be present: delusions, hallucinations, disorganized speech, or grossly disorganized or catatonic behavior. *DSM-5* cautions against applying these standards to people from a culture in which they are exhibiting acceptable behavior.

Schizophreniform Disorder

Patients with schizophreniform disorder display symptoms that are typical of schizophrenia and last at least 1 month but no longer than 6 months. This cautious approach spares an individual the lifelong diagnosis of schizophrenia until professionals are absolutely sure of the diagnosis.

Schizoaffective Disorder

Schizoaffective disorder is a psychosis characterized by both affective (mood disorder) and schizophrenic (thought disorder) symptoms, with substantial loss of occupational and social functioning. It is about one third as common as schizophrenia (American Psychiatric Association, 2013). Because this disorder is a hybrid of two disorders believed to have different biochemical origins, schizoaffective disorder is a puzzle to many clinicians. Affective disorders cause people to be extremely depressed or elated, and schizophrenia is expressed as positive, negative, or disorganized symptoms. The fact that patients with affective disorders can experience positive and negative symptoms as well as the fact that patients with schizophrenia experience mood changes partially explains the difficulty in diagnosis. The diagnosis of schizoaffective psychosis helps bridge the gap between the affective disorders and schizophrenia.

In this disorder, schizophrenic symptoms are dominant but are accompanied by major depressive or manic symptoms. Patients with schizoaffective disorder will have experienced delusions or hallucinations in the absence of a prominent mood disturbance, but symptoms of a mood disorder are present for most of the total disorder's duration (American Psychiatric Association, 2013). The prognosis for schizoaffective disorder is better than the prognosis for schizophrenia but significantly less optimistic than the prognosis for mood disorders (American Psychiatric Association, 1997).

? CRITICAL THINKING QUESTION

4. If a first-degree relative of yours had schizophrenia, what behavior might cause you to refuse to live with that person?

FUTURE DIRECTIONS

An evolving area of research focuses on early identification and intervention in schizophrenia. The National Institute of Mental Health, the primary source of funding for neuroscientific studies of mental illness, has made this area of research a funding priority. It has long been known that early treatment of schizophrenia symptoms results in better outcomes. Similarly, there is some indication that identifying the prodromal manifestations of schizophrenia might alter the course of illness. The ability to offer screening tests, such as blood tests, brain imaging, and checking for simple but often overlooked signs such as impaired smell and eye tracking, offers the hope of reducing the disabling effects of schizophrenia. Box 24-10 lists some behavioral early warning signs of schizophrenia. If several of these signs are present in a young person, it behooves the nurse, even if just a neighbor, to suggest professional evaluation. As stated, the earlier the better.

BOX 24-10 EARLY WARNING SIGNS OF SCHIZOPHRENIA

- Deterioration of personal hygiene
- Bizarre behavior
- Irrational statements
- Social withdrawal, isolation, and reclusiveness
- Shift in basic personality
- Deterioration of social relationships
- Inability to concentrate or to cope with minor problems
- Extreme preoccupation with religion or with the occult
- Excessive writing without meaning
- Indifference
- Dropping out of activities or out of life
- Decline in academic or athletic interests

From British Columbia Schizophrenia Society (2008b). *Schizophrenia: early warning signs* (9th ed.). <www.bcss.org/2008/07/resources/early-warning-signs> Accessed January 22, 2014.

◎ CARE PLAN

Name: *Bill Wilson*
DSM-5 Diagnosis: Schizophrenia

Admission Date: _____

Assessment

Areas of strength: Past accomplishments; past good heterosexual interpersonal relationships; alert, oriented to time, place, person; acute symptoms respond to medications; family support.

Problems: Religious hallucinations, religious delusions, thought disorder; broken engagement; dropped out of school.

Diagnoses

Disturbed sensory perception (auditory) related to thought disturbance, as evidenced by hallucinations.

Anxiety related to disturbed perceptions, as evidenced by fear and extraneous movements.

Outcomes
Date met: _____
Date met: _____
Date met: _____

Short-term goals
Patient will voice freedom from hallucinations.
Patient will report lack of fear of others.
Patient will discuss feelings about loss of girlfriend.

Date met: _____
Date met: _____
Date met: _____

Long-term goals
Patient will verbalize need for medication and counseling.
Patient will make appointment for outpatient program assessment in mid-July.
Patient will return to school in September.

Planning and Interventions

Nurse-patient relationship: Do not reinforce hallucinations and delusions; voice doubt; encourage identification of strengths and accomplishments; encourage expression of feelings about broken engagement; discuss plans for immediate future.

Psychopharmacology: Olanzapine (Zyprexa) 10 mg qd.

Milieu management: Provide distracting activities; monitor television, particularly religious programming and movies with satanic themes; encourage participation in self-esteem and anger management groups.

Evaluation
Patient responding to Zyprexa.

Referrals
Will see Ms. White, RN, CS, once a week as outpatient. Appointment in 3 weeks with R. Jones for education counseling.

◎ CARE PLAN

Name: *Emma Rice*
DSM-5 Diagnosis: Schizophrenia

Admission Date: _____

Assessment

Areas of strength: Board and care operator knows Emma well and wants her back. Staff knows and understands Emma.

Problems: Affective flattening, loose associations, withdrawn, chronic course of illness, no family support.

Diagnoses

Impaired verbal communication related to thought disturbance, as evidenced by impaired articulation and loose association of ideas.

Bathing and hygiene self-care deficit related to thought disturbance, as evidenced by inability to maintain appearance at satisfactory level.

Social isolation related to lack of trust, as evidenced by absence of supportive significant other.

Outcomes
Date met: _____
Date met: _____
Date met: _____

Short-term goals
Patient will talk in a coherent manner.
Patient will carry out activities of daily living.
Patient will participate in nonthreatening activities.

Date met: _____
Date met: _____
Date met: _____

Long-term goals
Patient will maintain outpatient program.
Patient will return to board and care.
Patient will comply with medication regimen.

Planning and Interventions

Nurse-patient relationship: Be patient; treat as adult; encourage hygiene and appropriate dress; reinforce positive social behaviors; start with one-to-one interactions with nurse and then encourage independent social behaviors.

Psychopharmacology: Haloperidol (Haldol) 5 mg bid PO (concentrate). Long-acting form may be needed on discharge.

◎ CARE PLAN—CONT'D

	Milieu management: Start patient in occupational therapy by the end of the week; invite patient to sit with staff and other patients; encourage her to make decisions about meals or some other simple tasks; provide resocialization group experience and community living education.
Evaluation	Patient stabilized on medications.
Referrals	Will see Ms. Brown, RN, CS, once a week and will attend outpatient resocialization group five times a week. Board and care operator will monitor drugs and arrange transportation.

PRINCIPLES OF PSYCHOTHERAPEUTIC MANAGEMENT

Nurse-Patient Relationship Principles
Focus on behavior, not meaning
A long-term relationship is most therapeutic
Accept patient but not all behaviors
Be consistent
Do not reinforce hallucinations and delusions
Avoid whispering or laughing if patient cannot hear all of conversation

Psychotropic Drugs
Traditional Antipsychotics
Haloperidol (Haldol)
Fluphenazine (Prolixin)
Chlorpromazine (Thorazine)

Atypical Antipsychotics
Aripriprazole (Abilify)

Asenapine (Saphris)
Clozapine (Clozaril)
Iloperidone (Fanapt)
Lurasidone (Latuda)
Olanzapine (Zyprexa)
Paliperidone (Invega)
Quetiapine (Seroquel)
Risperidone (Risperdal)
Ziprasidone (Geodon)

Milieu Management Principles
Modify environment to decrease stimulation and for safety
Staff consistency is crucial
Arrange environment to reduce withdrawn behavior
Monitor television watching
Protect patient's self-esteem

▌ STUDY NOTES

1. The concept of schizophrenia has evolved over the last 100 years as a result of the contributions of early theorists, such as Kraepelin and Bleuler, and modern theorists, such as Andreasen, Insel, Weinberger, and Torrey.

2. *DSM-5* is the major source for diagnostic criteria for schizophrenia.

3. Bleuler identified what he thought to be the four primary symptoms of schizophrenia (also known as Bleuler's "four A's"): (1) *a*ffective disturbances, (2) loose *a*ssociations, (3) *a*mbivalence, and (4) *a*utism.

4. Andreasen, Crow, and others have conceptualized schizophrenia as having only two subtypes: type I (positive symptoms and usually treatable with traditional antipsychotic drugs) and type II (negative symptoms). Some researchers have added another subtype labeled *disorganized*.

5. Objective signs of schizophrenia include alterations in personal relationships and activity.

6. Subjective symptoms of schizophrenia include alterations in perception, thought, consciousness, and affect.

7. Causative theories for schizophrenia are numerous and include both biologic theories (dopamine hypothesis, pathoanatomy, and genetic theories) and psychodynamic theories (developmental and family theories).

8. The dopamine hypothesis—that schizophrenia is a result of increased bioavailability of dopamine in the brain—is a widely held theory of the cause of schizophrenia.

9. Antipsychotic drugs block dopamine receptors and relieve acute symptoms of schizophrenia.

10. Nursing interventions include developing a therapeutic nurse-patient relationship. Several general principles underlie the nurse's interactions with patients who have schizophrenia, including being calm, accepting, dependable, consistent, and honest.

11. In addition to these basic principles, several basic interventions are therapeutic for most patients with schizophrenia. These basic interventions include what *the nurse should not do* (do not reinforce hallucinations and delusions, do not touch patients without warning, do not whisper or laugh when patients cannot hear the conversation, do not compete with patients, and do not embarrass patients) and what *the nurse should do* (provide reality testing, assist with orientation when appropriate, reinforce positive behaviors, and encourage verbalization of feelings).

(Continued)

STUDY NOTES—CONT'D

12. Psychopharmacology is an important part of the nurse's role in caring for patients with schizophrenia. Understanding the importance of adherence to the medication regimen is critical.

13. Nurses are typically responsible for the environment. Strategies for working with disruptive, withdrawn, suspicious, and disorganized patients are crucial for developing a therapeutic environment.

14. Other psychoses listed in *DSM-5* include schizoaffective disorder, delusional disorder, brief psychotic disorder, and schizophreniform disorder.

REFERENCES

Acocella, J. (2000). The empty couch. *The New Yorker, 8*(11), 200.

Allison, D. B., et al. (2009). Obesity among those with mental disorders: A National Institute of Mental Health meeting report. *American Journal of Preventive Medicine, 36,* 341.

American Psychiatric Association, (1997). Practice guidelines for the treatment of patients with schizophrenia. *American Journal of Psychiatry, 154*(Suppl. 4), 1.

American Psychiatric Association, (2013). *Diagnostic and statistical manual of mental disorders* (5th ed.). Arlington, VA: APA.

Andreasen, N. C. (1999). Understanding the causes of schizophrenia. *New England Journal of Medicine, 340,* 645.

Andreasen, N. C., & Olsen, S. (1982). Negative vs. positive schizophrenia. *Archives of General Psychiatry, 39,* 789.

Anonymous, (2003). Schizophrenia and drug abuse. *Harvard Mental Health Letter, 20,* 4.

Anonymous, (2008). Helping psychiatric patients to stop smoking. *Harvard Mental Health Letter, 25,* 4.

Bachmann, S., et al. (2008). Psychopathology in first-episode schizophrenia and antibodies to toxoplasma gondii. *Psychopathology, 38,* 87.

Batki, S. L., et al. (2009). Medical comorbidity in patients with schizophrenia and alcohol dependence. *Schizophrenia Research, 107,* 139.

Bogerts, B., et al. (1993). Hippocampus-amygdala volume and psychopathology in chronic schizophrenia. *Biological Psychiatry, 33,* 236.

British Columbia Schizophrenia Society, (2008a). *Schizophrenia: Basic facts about schizophrenia.* www.bcss.org/wp-content/uploads/2008/02/basic-facts-14/pdf, Accessed 22.01.14.

British Columbia Schizophrenia Society, (2008b). *Schizophrenia: Early warning signs* (9th ed.). www.bcss.org/2008/07/resources/early-warning-signs, Accessed 22.01.14.

Cannon, T. D., & Marco, E. (1994). Structural brain abnormalities as indicators of vulnerability to schizophrenia. *Schizophrenia Bulletin, 20,* 89.

Cohn, T. (2012). The link between schizophrenia and diabetes. *Current Psychiatry, 11,* 29.

Crow, T. J. (1982). Two dimensions of pathology in schizophrenia: Dopaminergic and nondopaminergic. *Psychopharmacology Bulletin, 18,* 22.

Crowner, M. (2014). Hearing voices, time traveling, and being hit with a high-heeled shoe. *Current Psychiatry, 13,* 57.

Dalack, G. W., Healy, D. J., & Meador-Woodruff, J. H. (1998). Nicotine dependence in schizophrenia: Clinical phenomena and laboratory findings. *American Journal of Psychiatry, 155,* 1490.

Erikson, E. (1968). *Childhood and society.* New York: W.W. Norton.

Geiser, R., Hoche, L., & King, J. (1988). Respite care for the mentally ill patients and their families. *Hospital & Community Psychiatry, 39,* 291.

Ghosh, S., & Greenberg, J. (2009). Aging fathers of adult children with schizophrenia: The toll of caregiving on their mental and physical health. *Psychiatric Services, 60,* 982.

Goldberg, J. O. (2010). Successful change in tobacco use in schizophrenia. *Journal of the American Psychiatric Nurses Association, 16,* 30.

Huxley, N. A., Rendall, M., & Sederer, L. (2000). Psychosocial treatments in schizophrenia: A review of the past 20 years. *The Journal of Nervous and Mental Disease, 199,* 187.

Insel, T. (2004, July). *Lecture "Mental Health and Genetics" presented at the Summer Genetics Institute.* Bethesda, MD: National Institutes of Health.

Johnstone, E. C., et al. (1976). Cerebral ventricular size and cognitive impairment in chronic schizophrenia. *Lancet, 2,* 924.

Keltner, N. L. (2008). Looking back at state hospitals: A biological advantage? *Perspectives in Psychiatric Care, 44,* 124.

Keltner, N. L., & Davidson, G. (2009). The normalization of paranoia. *Perspectives in Psychiatric Care, 45,* 228.

Keltner, N. L., & Grant, J. S. (2006). Smoke, smoke, smoke that cigarette. *Perspectives in Psychiatric Care, 42,* 256.

Keltner, N. L., & Lillie, K. (2009). Nicotinic receptors: Implications for psychiatric care. *Perspectives in Psychiatric Care, 45,* 151.

Keltner, N. L., et al. (2001). Nature vs nurture: Two brothers with schizophrenia. *Perspectives in Psychiatric Care, 37,* 88.

Kessler, R. C., et al. (2012). Twelve-month and lifetime prevalence and lifetime morbid risk of anxiety and mood disorders in the United States. *International Journal of Methods of Psychiatric Research, 21,* 169.

Kolb, L. C., & Brodie, H. K. H. (1982). *Modern clinical psychiatry.* Philadelphia: Saunders.

Kopelowicz, A., & Bidder, T. G. (1992). Dementia praecox: Inescapable fate or psychiatric oversight? *Hospital & Community Psychiatry, 43,* 940.

Lieberman, J. A. (1997). Atypical antipsychotic drugs: The next generation of therapy. *Decade of the Brain, 8,* 1.

Marsh, L., et al. (1994). Medial temporal lobe structure in schizophrenia: Relationship of size to duration of illness. *Schizophrenia Bulletin, 11,* 225.

Nasrallah, H. A. (1993). Neurodevelopmental pathogenesis of schizophrenia. *Psychiatric Clinics of North America, 16,* 269.

Nasrallah, H. A. (2012). Impaired mental proprioception in schizophrenia. *Current Psychiatry, 11,* 5.

National Cancer Institute, (2006). *Cigarette smoking and cancer: Questions and answers.* www.cancer.gov/cancertopics/factsheet/Tobacco/cancer, Accessed 22.01.14.

Newcomer, J.W. (2008). Antipsychotic medications: metabolic and cardiovascular risk. *Journal of Clinical Psychiatry, 68*(Suppl. 4), 8.

Opler, M. G., et al. (2004). Prenatal lead exposure, delta-aminolevulinic acid, and schizophrenia. *Environmental Health Perspectives, 112,* 548.

Roberts, G. W., Leigh, P. N., & Weinberger, D. R. (1993). *Neuropsychiatric disorders.* London: Mosby Europe.

Ruocchio, P. J. (1989). How psychotherapy can help the schizophrenic patient. *Hospital & Community Psychiatry, 40,* 188.

Sadock, B. J., & Sadock, V. A. (2003). *Synopsis of psychiatry* (9th ed.). Philadelphia: Lippincott Williams & Wilkins.

Scott, C. L., & Resnick, P. J. (2013). Evaluating psychotic patients' risk of violence: A practical guide. *Current Psychiatry, 12,* 29.

Seeman, M. V. (2010). Schizophrenia: Women bear a disproportionate toll of antipsychotic side effects. *Journal of the American Psychiatric Nurses Association, 16,* 21.

Sepe, P., Kay, A., & Stober, K. (2012). QUIT: A mnemonic to help patients stop smoking. *Current Psychiatry, 11,* 41.

Siris, S. G. (2012). Treating 'depression' in patients with schizophrenia. *Current Psychiatry, 11,* 35.

Substance Abuse and Mental Health Services Administration, (2009). *Results from the 2008 national survey on drug use and health: National findings.* http://www.samhsa.gov/data/nsduh/2k8nsduh/2k8Results.htm, Accessed 13.11.13.

Sullivan, H. S. (1953). *The interpersonal theory of psychiatry.* New York: W.W. Norton.

Torrey, E. F. (1997). The release of the mentally ill from institutions: A well-intentioned disaster. *The Chronicle of Higher Education, 43,* B4.

Torrey, E. F., & Yolken, R. H. (1995). Could schizophrenia be a viral zoonosis transmitted from house cats? *Schizophrenia Bulletin, 21,* 167.

U.S. Surgeon General, (1999). *Mental health: A report of the Surgeon General.* Washington, DC: Department of Health and Human Services.

Vreeland, B. (2007). Bridging the gap between mental and physical health: A multidisciplinary approach. *Journal of Clinical Psychiatry, 68*(Suppl. 4), 26.

Webster, A. J., & Straley, C. M. (2014). What is the relevance of a 2-week response to an antipsychotic? *Current Psychiatry, 13,* 52.

Weinberger, D. R. (1987). Implications of normal brain development for the pathogenesis of schizophrenia. *Archives of General Psychiatry, 44,* 660.

Williams, M. (2003). Genome-based drug discovery: Prioritizing disease-susceptibility/disease-associated genes as novel drug targets for schizophrenia. *Current Opinion in Investigational Drugs (London, England: 2000), 41,* 31.

Zhang, J.-P., & Malhotra, A. K. (2013). Genetics of schizophrenia: What do we know? *Current Psychiatry, 12,* 25.

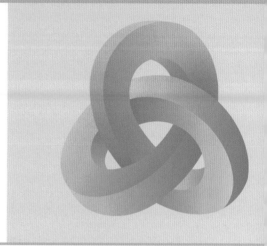

evolve WEBSITE

http://evolve.elsevier.com/Keltner

LEARNING OBJECTIVES

- Recognize the *DSM-5* criteria for depressive disorders.
- Compare and contrast the following depressive disorders: major depressive disorder, disruptive mood dysregulation disorder, persistent depressive disorder (dysthymia), and premenstrual dysphoric disorder.
- Describe the biologic and psychodynamic explanations for depressive disorders.
- Describe effective nursing interventions for depressed patients.

- Identify the major indications for electroconvulsive therapy (ECT).
- Describe the nurse's role in caring for patients before and after ECT.
- Recognize warning signs of suicide.
- Describe interventions to prevent suicide.
- Describe family issues related to depressive disorder.

Most people are about as happy as they make up their minds to be.

Abraham Lincoln

Depression is the oldest and most frequently described psychiatric illness (Belcher & Holdcraft, 2001). The existence of depression has been documented since biblical times. Historically, many important individuals have experienced the devastating symptoms of depression, including King Saul, Job, Elijah, Jeremiah, Mary and Abraham Lincoln, Ernest Hemingway, Eugene O'Neill, and Winston Churchill. More recently, newscaster Mike Wallace, actresses Brooke Shields and Ashley Judd, and actors Drew Carey and Heath Ledger are known to have had this disorder. Normal feelings of sadness are appropriate in many situations. It would be abnormal not to feel sad in certain situations, such as when a loved one dies or when other losses occur in a person's life. However, these feelings are usually short-lived and do not persist in altering the person's ability to function. When an individual's mood causes clinically significant distress or impairment in social or occupational functioning, a diagnosis of depressive disorder is warranted. Because there is a notable

connection between major depressive disorder (MDD) and suicide, early diagnosis and intervention may increase the chances of a favorable outcome. A discussion of suicide and depression is presented at the end of the chapter. Demographic factors and prevalence rates of depressive disorders are shown in Table 25-1A and B.

DEPRESSIVE DISORDERS

The American Psychological Association recognizes eight major types of depressive disorders (American Psychiatric Association, 2013): MDD, disruptive mood dysregulation disorder, persistent depressive disorder (dysthymia), premenstrual dysphoric disorder, substance-induced or medication-induced depressive disorder, depressive disorder secondary to a medical condition or treatment of a medical condition, other known depressive disorders, and unknown etiology of depressive disorder. All of the depressive disorders share the common features of sadness, feeling empty, irritable mood, and somatic and cognitive changes that significantly affect the person's ability to function. This chapter focuses on the four most common types of depressive disorders.

NORM'S NOTES

The content of depressive disorders in *DSM-5*, although written by physicians and psychologists, is used by psychiatric nurses. Advance practice nurses use the language of *DSM-5* in their practice as they diagnose, plan care for, and treat individuals with depression. *DSM-5* provides a common language necessary for the interdisciplinary team approach to patient care. Nursing rhetoric regarding depressive disorders can be difficult for individuals outside the nursing profession. However, particular nursing terms have been accepted as standard medical terms. For example, *activities of daily living* is a common term used to evaluate the functioning of depressed patients. As psychiatric nurses continue to develop theories and research useful in understanding the responses of depressed patients, they incorporate language found in *DSM-5* as well as nursing rhetoric.

MAJOR DEPRESSIVE DISORDER

Major depressive disorder is characterized by one or more major depressive episodes, which are defined by at least 2 weeks of depressed mood or loss of interest accompanied by at least four additional symptoms. Individuals may describe their mood as depressed, sad, hopeless, discouraged, or "down in the dumps." Loss of interest or pleasure may be portrayed as feeling "blah," having no feelings, not caring anymore, and social withdrawal. Individuals may present with physical complaints such as insomnia and fatigue. The presentation of psychomotor agitation (inability to sit still, pacing, handwringing, and rubbing the skin) or retardation (slowed speech, thinking, and body movements) is associated with greater severity of the disorder, as is the presence of excessive or inappropriate guilt. Weight gain and suicidality are more evident when

TABLE 25-1 12-MONTH PREVALENCE RATES OF MENTAL DISORDERS AND DEPRESSIVE DISORDERS IN THE UNITED STATES

A. 12-Month Prevalence Rate of Mental Disorders in the United States*

DISORDERS	APPROXIMATE PERCENTAGE >17 YEARS OLD (%)* (unless noted for children)	GENDER OVERREPRESENTATION
Anxiety disorders	18.1 overall	
Agoraphobia	1.7	Female
Panic disorder	2.4	Female
Panic attacks	11.2	Female
Social anxiety	7	Female
Specific phobia	7-9	Female
Separation anxiety	1.2	Equal
Generalized anxiety disorder	2	Female
Posttraumatic stress disorder	3.4	Female
Obsessive-compulsive disorder	1.2	Equal
Major depression	8.6	Female
Bipolar disorder I and II	1.8	BD I: ~Equal
		BD II: Female
Autism spectrum disorders	1 in children	Male
Disruptive, impulse control, and conduct disorders	8.9 overall	
Conduct disorders*	4 in children	Male
Attention-deficit/hyperactivity disorder*	5 in children; 2.5 in adults	Male
Substance use disorders	8.9 overall	
Alcohol use disorder	8.5 in adults; 2.5 in 12- to 17-year-olds	Male
Drug use disorders	1.4	Male
Schizophrenia	1.1	~Equal

B. 12-Month Prevalence Rate of Depressive Disorders in the United States†

DISORDERS	APPROXIMATE PERCENTAGE >17 YEARS (%)	GENDER OVERREPRESENTATION
Major depressive disorder	7	Female
Disruptive mood dysregulation disorder	2-5‡	Male
Persistent depressive disorder	0.5-1.5	Unknown
Premenstrual dysphoric disorder	1.8	Female only

*No one source has all of this information. This information has been derived from the following sources: Kessler, R.C., et al. (2012). Twelve-month and lifetime prevalence and lifetime morbid risk of anxiety and mood disorders in the United States. *International Journal of Methods of Psychiatric Research, 21,* 169; Substance Abuse and Mental Health Services Administration (2009). *Results from the 2008 national survey on drug use and health: national findings.*
<http://www.samhsa.gov/data/nsduh/2k8nsduh/2k8Results.htm> Accessed November 13, 2013; American Psychiatric Association (2013). *Diagnostic and statistical manual of mental disorders* (5th ed.). Arlington, VA: APA.
†From American Psychiatric Association (2013). *Diagnostic and statistical manual of mental disorders* (5th ed.). Arlington, VA: APA.
‡Ages 6 to 18.

recurrent depressive episodes occur. In children and adolescents, an irritable or cranky mood may be the prevalent symptom. Major depression is a disorder of *severity* and is treatable, with 80% of individuals able to resume normal activities within a few weeks (National Institute of Mental Health, 2011). *DSM-5* criteria for MDD are presented in the *DSM-5* Criteria box (American Psychiatric Association, 2013).

DISRUPTIVE MOOD DYSREGULATION DISORDER

Disruptive mood dysregulation disorder typically is applied to children and adolescents 6 to 18 years old. The prominent feature is severe, chronic irritability interspersed with an angry mood. The severe irritability is manifested as frequent temper outbursts in response to frustration at least three times a week. These outbursts appear in the form of verbal rages or physical aggression or both toward people or property. The onset of disruptive mood dysregulation disorders must be before 10 years of age. Because of their severe irritability and low frustration tolerance, affected children generally experience marked disruption in family and peer relationships as well as school performance.

PERSISTENT DEPRESSIVE DISORDER (DYSTHYMIA)

Persistent depressive disorder, also known as *dysthymia*, is diagnosed when a person has a depressed mood that occurs for most of the day for at least 2 years (at least 1 year for children and adolescents). The criteria for dysthymia are almost identical to the criteria of MDD; however, the symptoms are more subtle and nonremittent. Individuals describe their mood as sad or "down in the dumps." Because of the chronicity of the disorder, the depressive symptoms become a part of the individual's day-to-day experience (i.e., "I've always been this way"). In addition, the individual may complain of sleeping and eating disturbances, fatigue, low self-esteem, difficulty making decisions, and feelings of hopelessness.

PREMENSTRUAL DYSPHORIC DISORDER

Premenstrual dysphoric disorder is characterized by mood swings, irritability or anger, dysphoria, and anxiety symptoms that occur before and during menstruation. Other symptoms include lethargy, fatigue, sleep disturbances, difficulty concentrating, changes in appetite, and a sense of being

---

DSM-5 CRITERIA

Major Depressive Disorder

Diagnostic Criteria

A. Five (or more) of the following symptoms have been present during the same 2-week period and represent a change from previous functioning; at least one of the symptoms is either (1) depressed mood or (2) loss of interest or pleasure.

Note: Do not include symptoms that are clearly attributable to another medical condition.

1. Depressed mood most of the day, nearly every day, as indicated by either subjective report (e.g., feels sad, empty, hopeless) or observation made by others (e.g., appears tearful). (Note: In children and adolescents, can be irritable mood.)
2. Markedly diminished interest or pleasure in all, or almost all, activities most of the day, nearly every day (as indicated by either subjective account or observation).
3. Significant weight loss when not dieting or weight gain (e.g., a change of more than 5% of body weight in a month) or decrease or increase in appetite nearly every day. (Note: In children, consider failure to make expected weight gain.)
4. Insomnia or hypersomnia nearly every day.
5. Psychomotor agitation or retardation nearly every day (observable by others, not merely subjective feelings of restlessness or being slowed down).
6. Fatigue or loss of energy nearly every day.
7. Feelings of worthlessness or excessive or inappropriate guilt (which may be delusional) nearly every day (not merely self-reproach or guilt about being sick).
8. Diminished ability to think or concentrate, or indecisiveness, nearly every day (either by subjective account or as observed by others).

9. Recurrent thoughts of death (not just fear of dying), recurrent suicidal ideation without a specific plan, or a suicide attempt or a specific plan for committing suicide.

B. The symptoms cause clinically significant distress or impairment in social, occupational, or other important areas of functioning.

C. The episode is not attributable to the physiological effects of a substance or to another medical condition.

Note: Criteria A-C represent a major depressive episode.

Note: Responses to a significant loss (e.g., bereavement, financial ruin, losses from a natural disaster, a serious medical illness or disability) may include the feelings of intense sadness, rumination about the loss, insomnia, poor appetite, and weight loss noted by criterion A, which may resemble a depressive episode. Although such symptoms may be understandable or considered appropriate to the loss, the presence of a major depressive episode in addition to the normal response to a significant loss should also be carefully considered. This decision inevitably requires the exercise of clinical judgment based on the individual's history and the cultural norms for the expression of distress in the context of loss.

D. The occurrence of the major depressive episode is not better explained by schizoaffective disorder, schizophrenia, schizophreniform disorder, delusional disorder, or other specific and unspecified schizophrenia spectrum and other psychotic disorders.

E. There has never been a manic episode or a hypomanic episode.

Note: This exclusion does not apply if all the manic-like or hypomanic-like episodes are substance-induced or are attributable to the physiological effects of another medical condition.

From the American Psychiatric Association (2013). *Diagnostic and statistical manual of mental disorders* (5th ed.). Washington, DC: APA.

overwhelmed or out of control. Physical symptoms such as breast tenderness or swelling, pain, and a sensation of bloating or weight gain may be present. Typically, symptoms peak around the onset of menses and remit after the menstrual period begins. The intensity and expression of symptoms vary based on social and cultural background, family perspective, and religious beliefs.

Depressive Disorder Specifiers

Each of the above-described depressive disorders can be categorized further into subtypes, also called *specifiers*. These specifiers provide more clarity to the presentation of the depressive disorders, such as with atypical features, anxious features, mixed features, melancholic features, catatonic features, peripartum onset, psychotic features, or seasonal pattern. Overarching symptoms are the same across these subgroups, but variances in expression occur.

Atypical depression is characterized by symptoms that typically do not appear in MDD. For example, the individual's mood brightens considerably in response to actual or potential positive events. Other symptoms include increased appetite or weight gain, hypersomnia, leaden paralysis (heavy feelings in arms and legs), and extreme sensitivity to interpersonal rejection. Atypical depression might be the one type of depression in which monoamine oxidase inhibitors (MAOIs) are first-choice drugs (Anonymous, 2005).

Anxious depression is characterized by anxious distress during a depressive episode. Prominent symptoms may include feeling keyed up, tense, unusually restless, loss of control, difficulty concentrating, or fear that something awful may happen. Higher levels of anxiety are associated with higher suicide risk.

Mixed depression is characterized by manic or hypomanic symptoms occurring within a major depressive episode. Manic or hypomanic symptoms appear as an elevated, expansive mood; inflated self-esteem; grandiosity; more talkative than normal; flight of ideas; racing thoughts; or increased energy or goal-directed behavior. This type of MDD is associated with increased or excessive involvement in activities that have a high potential for painful consequences (e.g., buying sprees, sexual indiscretions, foolish business investments). During these periods, the individual has a decreased need for sleep, feeling rested despite sleeping less than usual.

Melancholic depression is characterized by anhedonia (loss of pleasure in activities) and an inability to be cheered up. At least three of the following depressive symptoms are found in melancholic patients: profound despondency, despair, or moroseness; depression worse in the morning; early morning awakening; marked psychomotor retardation or agitation; significant anorexia or weight loss; and excessive or inappropriate guilt. This diagnosis is more likely to be associated with dexamethasone nonsuppression and elevated cortisol levels.

Catatonic features are marked by significant psychomotor alterations, including immobility, excessive motor activity, mutism, echolalia (parrot-like repetition of words), and inappropriate posturing. Although this symptom is more often associated with schizophrenia, more cases actually occur in patients with mood disorders.

Peripartum depression or "baby blues," which occurs during pregnancy or in the first 30 days postpartum, is one of the most common medical complications of childbearing (Sit & Wisner, 2009). Severe anxiety and panic attacks can occur. Each year in the United States, 500,000 pregnancies occur in women with psychiatric disorders, half of which are thought to be unplanned, so it is little wonder that many of these women might experience postpartum depression (Brand & Brennan, 2009). Many women without a history of mental health issues also experience postpartum depression. In worst-case scenarios, infanticide is known to occur during a peripartum-onset episode, most often associated with psychosis involving command hallucinations to kill the infant or delusions that the infant is possessed. The risk of peripartum depression reoccurring with each subsequent delivery is 30% to 50%.

In *psychotic depression*, a person has delusions and hallucinations in conjunction with mood disturbance. These perceptual problems can be differentiated between mood-congruent and mood-incongruent psychosis. With mood-congruent psychosis, the content of the delusions and hallucinations is consistent with the depressive themes of personal inadequacy, guilt, disease, death, personal destruction, or deserved punishment. With mood-incongruent psychosis, the delusions or hallucinations involve bizarre content. Psychotic depression is associated with a poorer prognosis compared with other forms of depression. Antidepressants and antipsychotics are usually required for satisfactory treatment (Schwartz, 2005).

Seasonal depression occurs in conjunction with a seasonal change most often beginning in fall or winter and remitting in spring (in the Northern Hemisphere). Less commonly, there may be summer depressive episodes. As might be expected, the higher the latitude, the more likely this type of depression will occur. Prominent symptoms include decreased energy, hypersomnia, overeating, weight gain, and a craving for carbohydrates.

Occurrence in Specific Populations
Adults

Depression (all types) is one of the most prevalent mental health problems in the United States, with about 30 million people affected at any given time (Kessler et al., 2003). Depression is predicted to become the leading cause of disability in the future. Lifetime risk for depression in women is 10% to 20% compared with lifetime risk for men of about 5% to 10% (American Psychiatric Association, 2010). By later life, the risk becomes about 50:50 (Anonymous, 2003b). Although depression can occur at any age, the average age of adult onset is in the middle to late twenties. Some individuals have a single episode of major depression, recover, and never experience another depressive episode. However, about 80% of individuals who experience a single episode eventually have recurrent episodes. Manic phases in addition to depressive episodes are experienced by 5% to 10% of individuals (Nemeroff, 1998). The prevalence rates appear to be unrelated to ethnicity; however, low-income groups and individuals with a positive family history of depression are at increased risk (up to three times greater risk).

Maternal mental health can affect the mother's child. Brand and Brennan (2009) noted that more than 500,000 pregnancies each year in the United States involve women who have a diagnosed mental illness. Because half of all pregnancies are unplanned, they deduce that 250,000 pregnant women are coping with both a psychiatric disorder and an unplanned pregnancy. They specifically followed the children of perinatally depressed women and found significant reduction in cognitive ability. Hays et al. (2008) reported that the average IQ in young boys raised by mothers who had not been depressed was 22 points higher compared with boys raised by mothers who were depressed. If these observations reflect reality, the implications for mental health nurses are huge.

Children and Adolescents

The occurrence of depression in children and adolescents can be more devastating than in adults. Children with depressed parents are at greater risk of developing the disorder than children with parents who are not clinically depressed, and the onset of childhood depression predisposes a child to develop depression as an adult. Nurses need to be able to assess children and their families for possible symptoms of depression and develop appropriate interventions for them. Certain events might predispose children and adolescents to develop MDD, including the following:

1. Loss of parents through divorce, separation, or death
2. Death of other individuals close to the child
3. Death of a loved pet
4. Move to another neighborhood or town
5. Academic problems or failure
6. Significant physical illness or injury

Culture, Age, and Gender

Individuals from certain ethnic, racial, or cultural groups might express depressive symptoms differently than European Americans. For example, people from Hispanic, Latino, and Mediterranean groups might describe their sadness or guilt in terms of being nervous or having headaches or stomachaches. Individuals from Asian cultures might describe themselves as being out of balance or feeling weak and nervous. Native American and Asian-American groups withdraw for meditation and personal growth as part of their culture to cope with symptoms of depression. Chapter 5 presents more specific information on expression of emotional states in different ethnic, racial, and cultural groups.

Nurses and other health care providers can misinterpret symptoms of depression in children, adolescents, women, and older adults. For example, depressive symptoms in children and adolescents might mimic normal developmental changes. Reports of depression by women might be dismissed as symptoms of conditions expressed in ways similar to depression. The gender disparity for depression is puzzling. Finally, recognizing symptoms of depression in older adults is particularly challenging because many symptoms of depression are similar to symptoms of dementia, diabetes, and cardiac conditions.

FACTS ABOUT DEPRESSION

1. About 7% of the adult population of the United States will experience major depression in the next 12 months.
2. Over an entire lifetime, about 16.5% of Americans will experience major depression.
3. The first onset of major depression typically occurs between the ages of 25 and 30 years.
4. On average, an episode of depression lasts about 20 weeks, 12 weeks if treated, and up to 52 weeks if untreated.
5. Most individuals with a first episode of major depression have another episode (the average is five or six episodes over a lifetime).
6. Some patients never recover from the first episode.
7. Stress plays a role in the onset and exacerbation of depression.
8. Early life stress can change brain structure and function, lowering the threshold for adult depressive episodes.

Modified from Kessler, R.C., et al. (2005a). Lifetime prevalence and age-of-onset distributions of DSM-IV disorders in the National Comorbidity Survey Replication. *Archives of General Psychiatry, 62,* 593; Kessler, R.C., et al. (2005b). Prevalence, severity, and comorbidity of 12-month DSM-IV disorders in the National Comorbidity Survey Replication. *Archives of General Psychiatry, 62,* 617; Sadock, B.J., & Sadock, V.A. (2003). *Synopsis of psychiatry* (9th ed.). Philadelphia: Lippincott Williams & Wilkins

CRITICAL THINKING QUESTION

1. What factors do you think contribute to the high levels of depression in the United States?

BEHAVIORIAL SYMPTOMS OF DEPRESSION

Depression results in both objective and subjective behaviors. Objective signs, such as agitation, can be observed by the nurse. Painful subjective symptoms, such as hopelessness, might be hidden by depressed individuals. Objective and subjective symptoms in depression are difficult to differentiate, perhaps more than in schizophrenia. Objective signs are typically extensions of a subjective state. The nurse is encouraged to observe for visible signs of depression and to be aware of, assess for, and expect subjective anguish and anger.

Clinical Example

Mrs. Lewis is a 50-year-old woman who presents with dysphoria, tearfulness, suicidal ideation, loss of energy and sexual interest, and insomnia. Although she feels hopeless about the future and worries that she will never get better, she denies that she is really depressed. Mrs. Lewis is an extremely devout woman and believes that someone truly walking with the Lord would not find himself or herself in her situation. Mrs. Lewis believes that she is a burden to her family; she also has fears related to her physical health. Mrs. Lewis also feels guilty for not being able to handle her situation. Her husband, also a religious person, has been dutifully patient throughout all this turmoil but is growing tired of her pessimism, crying, and lack of interest in sex. The nurse fears that a breakup of this 25-year marriage might occur if Mrs. Lewis does not respond to treatment.

Objective Signs

Depressed patients often demonstrate behavior that is noticeable to others, but these patients might not want to talk to anyone and might seek to be alone. If someone intrudes into the obsessive thinking of their inner world, depressed patients might become irritable and strike out at the intruder. Two general areas of objective signs are alterations of activity and altered social interactions.

Alterations of Activity

Patients might exhibit psychomotor agitation or retardation. Psychomotor agitation appears as pacing, engaging in hand-wringing, and the inability to sit still. These patients might pull or rub their hair, skin, clothing, or other objects. Tying and re-tying shoes and buttoning and unbuttoning a shirt or blouse are common behaviors. Psychomotor retardation is marked by a slowing of speech, increased pauses before answering, soft or monotonous speech, decreased frequency of speech (poverty of speech), and muteness. In addition, a general slowing of body movements occurs. Patients might state that they are "tired all the time," even when they are not physically active. For example, a patient might have difficulty getting up from a chair to turn off the television. Even the smallest task might seem unbearable.

Involvement in activities of daily living declines as well. Depressed individuals often neglect performing basic personal hygiene measures, such as bathing, shaving, putting on clean clothes, or wiping their mouths after eating. However, these latter objective signs are probably a result of more than a lack of energy. Apathy—a lack of feeling, absence of emotion, or an inability to be motivated—plays an important role in these behaviors as well. An extreme extension of these anergic symptoms is seen in cases in which depressed people lie in bed and become incontinent or constipated because of the inability to muster the energy (both physical and psychological) to walk to the bathroom.

Depressed people usually experience a change in eating behaviors that results in either weight loss or gain. Sleeping patterns change as well. Depressed individuals might experience insomnia (difficulty falling asleep), middle insomnia (difficulty remaining asleep), or terminal insomnia (early morning awakening). Hypersomnia (increased or prolonged sleeping or both) is an atypical symptom of depression. Depressed people might deny that they are depressed, yet spend hours by themselves. In this case, the nurse should not confuse a request to "go to my room and lie down" with hypersomnia. Many depressed people want to lie down but do not sleep. There, in the solitude of an empty room, these individuals descend into uninterrupted, self-defeating ruminations.

Clinical Example

Jan Treback is a 60-year-old white woman who has been successful in business for many years. She recently became very upset at work when her boss confronted her about her work. Jan had not been happy about the company CEO assigning her a new boss 6 months ago. The new boss was overbearing, and Jan didn't feel like she was trusted even though she had worked at the business for 25 years.

Jan had left work because she felt too upset to stay and basically was told by the Human Resources Department to take some time off. She decided to see a psychiatrist and a therapist. The psychiatrist started Jan on citalopram. The therapist diagnosed dysthymia based on Jan's reported symptoms of feeling blue most days for most of her adult life. She had a tendency to overeat, felt fatigued most days, never felt like she got enough sleep, and isolated herself at times. She did not have a history of suicidal ideation. She lived with her daughter and granddaughter and had been divorced for more than 30 years.

Altered Social Interactions

Depressed individuals often have poor social skills that are linked directly to other symptoms of depression. Underachievement causes a lack of productivity on the job and at home. The self-absorbing nature of depression causes these individuals to be easily distracted and reduces their interest in people, their ideas, or their problems. Depression causes problems with thinking, idea development, and problem solving. In addition, conversations are difficult to maintain, and only with great effort can a depressed person sustain a facial expression of interest and concern. Depressed individuals are also withdrawn and often prefer social isolation over social interaction with others. Hobbies and vocations that were once actively pursued become unimportant and might be abandoned or engaged in halfheartedly. Finally, the body language of depression (e.g., saddened facial expression, drooping posture) serves as a social barrier.

Subjective Symptoms
Alterations of Affect

Alterations of affect are the symptoms primarily associated with depression, which is reasonable, because these disturbances dominate the internal world of a depressed person. Affect describes the emotional range that is outwardly reflecting one's feelings, mood, and emotional tone. Some of the terms used to describe affect include *flat*, *blunted*, and *labile*. Congruency of affect and mood is demonstrated when there is consistency between the two (flat affect congruent with depressed mood). For depressed individuals, affect and mood may also be incongruent, observed as labile affect incongruent with depressed mood.

Anxiety, doom and gloom, fear, self-destructive thoughts, and panic attacks all are products of the depressed mind. Because of this anguish, depressed individuals vacillate between sadness and apathy. When the pain becomes too great, patients shut down and become apathetic. Finally, although most laypeople consider sadness to be the universal symptom of distress, apathy actually comes closer to being continually present in depressed individuals.

Inappropriate guilt is often associated with depression. Guilt may manifest as an overreaction to some current failing or might be associated with an indiscretion in the distant past that cannot be forgiven. Guilt can also take the form of accepting responsibility for occurrences in which the person had little impact or take the form of obsessional preoccupation with such thoughts as "What if I had only …?" The person becomes immobilized with "should haves" and "could haves." An even more morbid extension of guilt is the psychotic delusion of guilt for calamities that happened far away, even on the other side of the world.

Anxiety is a companion of depression. Depressed individuals are filled with anxiousness and dread. A ringing telephone holds the potential for catastrophic news. A siren might mean a loved one has been injured. A child at school might not return. Although these terrible things do happen, most people go on with life comforted by the knowledge that they will probably not happen if inappropriate risks are minimized. However, for many depressed individuals, the telephone causes the same anxious reaction each and every time it rings.

Worthlessness can range from a feeling of inadequacy to total devaluation. Depressed individuals might scan the environment for clues to their inadequacy. As one person remarked, "I knew I wasn't any good; it just took a while to figure out why." Some individuals have a hypersensitivity to how they are perceived by others, always assuming the worst.

Alterations of Cognition

Alterations of cognition include ambivalence and indecision, inability to concentrate, confusion, loss of interest and motivation, memory problems, pessimism, self-blame, self-deprecation, self-destructive thoughts, thoughts of death and dying, and uncertainty. The inability of depressed individuals to make a decision is particularly difficult for others to understand. Faced with even a simple decision, much vacillation is expressed. Once a decision is made, depressed individuals might be obsessed with "what if" questions. Major decisions can be immobilizing.

Alterations of a Physical Nature

Alterations of a physical nature are common in depressed individuals. Almost all parts of the body can be affected. Common physiologic symptoms include abdominal pain, anorexia, chest pain, constipation, dizziness, fatigue, headache, indigestion, insomnia, menstrual changes, nausea and vomiting, and sexual dysfunction. Additionally, as mentioned in the previous discussion of cultural aspects, cultural practices of some ethnic and racial groups might mimic depressive symptoms, or depression might be expressed somatically.

These subjective symptoms come to the attention of the nurse because of the numerous somatic complaints of depressed individuals. Some people become preoccupied with their bodies to the extent that every twinge and body change is greeted with great alarm and dread. One recovering depressed patient joked, "I have had a hundred heart attacks." Monitoring of body functions is common in the general population and is no doubt related to various factors, including perhaps this society's obsession with fitness. However, overinvestment in self-assessment by depressed individuals is pathologic; the degree of this thinking sets apart persons who are depressed. Chest pain, an unusual spot on the face or abdomen, and stomach pain all can precipitate a panic attack in some people. Panic attacks occur in 15% to 30% of individuals with MDD (American Psychiatric Association, 1993).

Alterations of Perception

Some depressed individuals have altered perceptions. Delusions and hallucinations are typically congruent with the depressed mood (e.g., a delusion of persecution because of a moral or ethical mistake). Somatic delusions (e.g., "My body is full of cancer") and nihilistic delusions (e.g., "My brain is dying") are common forms of psychotic delusions in depressed individuals. Hallucinations tend to be less elaborate than the hallucinations of schizophrenics and tend to focus on personal faults—for example, "You are no good. You don't deserve your family."

ETIOLOGY OF DEPRESSION

Biologic Theories of Depression

The etiology of depression has been biologically attributed to alterations in neurochemical, genetic, endocrine, and circadian rhythm functions and changes in brain anatomy. These alterations produce physical and psychological changes expressed as depression.

Neurochemical Theories

Research findings suggest that neurochemical depression results when levels of certain neurotransmitters are altered. The biogenic amines norepinephrine and serotonin are most often mentioned, but dopamine, another biogenic amine, is involved as well. Figure 25-1 illustrates the proposed roles of the three key monoamines. Dysregulation of acetylcholine

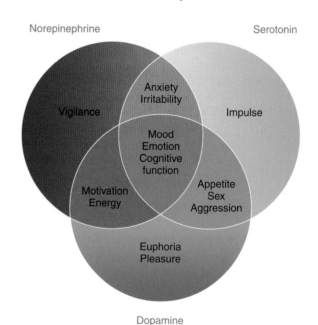

Proposed Roles for the Three Key Monoamine Systems

FIG 25-1 Proposed roles for the three key monoamine systems. (From Healy, D., & McMonagle, T. [1997]. The enhancement of social functioning as a therapeutic principle in the management of depression. *Journal of Psychopharmacology, 11* (Suppl.), S25.)

and gamma-aminobutyric acid (GABA) might contribute to the development of biochemical depression as well. More specifically, when the levels of these neurotransmitters are altered at receptor sites, or when receptor sensitivity changes, a neurochemical depression might result. For example, the serotonergic receptors originate in the raphe nuclei of the brainstem and are located near the midline for most of the length of the brainstem. The more rostral neurons (toward the head) project throughout the cortex. Each serotonergic neuron sends more than 500,000 terminals to the limbic system and to the cortex, contributing to the regulation of many psychological functions (Dubovsky, 1994). Norepinephrine or noradrenergic pathways originate in the locus ceruleus and innervate all areas of the cortex, the hypothalamus, and the hippocampus (Keltner et al., 2001b). As is the case with serotonin, norepinephrine neurons innervate and contribute to regulation of brain areas with various functions.

It might be appealing to conceptualize depression as a decreased level of serotonin and norepinephrine or to suggest that depression can be successfully treated by increasing the bioavailability of these amines. However, doing so oversimplifies both the problem and the solution. A more informed way of looking at depression is to think of it as a monoaminergic dysregulation. It is not so much that monoamines are lacking, but that the cells they activate have lost the capacity to respond in a healthy manner; intracellular processes no longer effectively produce the transcription factors necessary for neuronal development. When the receptor is occupied with serotonin (or norepinephrine), a cascade of intracellular events is initiated (i.e., the second messenger system). This cascade results in the production of proteins such as enzymes, receptors, and neuroprotective proteins. When some part of this process is dysfunctional, the end products needed for cell sustenance are compromised. Antidepressants probably stabilize this intraneuronal environment.

Other hypotheses include the sensitivity of both presynaptic and postsynaptic receptors and the modulating effects of acetylcholine and GABA on aminergic systems (Keltner et al., 2001a). For example, it is believed that beta autoreceptors, which normally inhibit the release of norepinephrine, are down-regulated by antidepressants, disinhibiting norepinephrine release (i.e., increasing synaptic norepinephrine). Too many norepinephrine or serotonin receptors might be thought of as a positive situation. However, excessive (up-regulation of) receptors indicate insufficient levels of these neurotransmitters. This action is an example of the body compensating for decreased monoamine availability. However, all the up-regulation and down-regulation of receptors might be a result of the intracellular response to antidepressants mentioned earlier. Finally, peptides, dietary practices, and nutritional status are being examined for their biochemical roles in the development of depression because food intake affects the development of the precursor amino acids required for neurotransmitter synthesis. There is still much to learn about the biochemistry of depression.

Genetic Theories

Other researchers have contended that depression might be genetically based and that heredity might predispose individuals to develop depression. Several studies have examined the incidence of depression in twins. Research has indicated that two thirds of twins are concordant for MDD if one or both of the biologic parents has been diagnosed with MDD (Shucter et al., 1996). Another view proposes that mothers who are depressed tend to rear children who are more susceptible to depression. Discerning the genetic, inherited, and psychosocial influences is a difficult task.

Endocrine Theories

Endocrine changes related to depression have also been investigated. Normally, the hypothalamic-pituitary-adrenal (HPA) axis is a system that mediates the stress response. However, in some depressed people, this system malfunctions and creates cortisol, thyroid, and hormonal abnormalities. Dysregulation of the HPA axis results in hypercortisolemia (in about 40% to 60% of depressed patients), nonsuppression by dexamethasone, and elevated levels of corticotropin-releasing factor (CRF) (Keltner et al., 2001b; Michelson, 2009). The hypersecretion of cortisol is the result of an overexpression of the CRF gene (leading to increased CRF synthesis) and an increase in CRF-producing neurons in the hypothalamus. This action leads to increased pituitary release of adrenocorticotropic hormone (ACTH) and subsequent hypersecretion of cortisol by the adrenal glands. Nemeroff (1998) noted that early life exposure to overwhelming trauma literally changes the expression of CRF neurons in the hypothalamus. Events such as early loss of parents, inadequate parenting, or childhood sexual and physical abuse (Tomoda et al., 2009) create an adult who is overly responsive to stressors and vulnerable to depression. Essentially, a physical change brought about by childhood stressors causes a long-term or even permanent hyperactivity of central corticotropin-releasing hormones, leaving the adult highly vulnerable to stress. Nemeroff (1998) called this phenomenon the "stress-diathesis model of depression."

The dexamethasone suppression test (DST) fails to suppress cortisol in about 40% of depressed patients. In nondepressed individuals, an elevated serum cortisol level sends a message to the hypothalamus and the anterior pituitary to decrease the release of CRF and ACTH, respectively, slowing cortisol release. Dexamethasone acts only on the anterior pituitary gland, and it suppresses the release of ACTH in nondepressed individuals. In some, but not all, depressed persons, an injection of dexamethasone does not cause cortisol suppression, indicating that the person's stress response mode overrides his or her negative feedback system. This malfunctioning and its results are more pronounced in severely depressed patients (Michelson, 2009). The presence of endocrine disease, caused by disease in any component of the HPA axis, has also been associated with the development of depressive symptoms (Maes et al., 1994). Controversy exists regarding the role of genetics and hormonal explanations of depression in women; some researchers have contended that women have a predisposition to develop depressive symptoms and MDD because of fluctuations in hormone levels. Other researchers have contended that these fluctuations influence the development of MDD through their interaction with neurotransmitters, psychosocial factors, and the stress system.

Circadian Rhythm Theories

Individuals experiencing circadian rhythm changes are at increased risk for developing depressive symptoms and MDD. These changes might be caused by medications, nutritional deficiencies, physical or psychological illnesses, hormonal fluctuations associated with a woman's reproductive system, or aging (McEnany, 1995a, 1995b; Warren, 1997). Circadian rhythms are responsible for the daily regulation of wake-sleep cycles, arousal and activity patterns, and hormonal secretions associated with these regulatory mechanisms. In depressed individuals, these regulatory mechanisms are altered, which leads to shortened latency in rapid eye movement (REM) sleep and sleep disturbances such as insomnia, frequent waking, and increasingly intensified dreaming (Anonymous, 2005).

Changes in Brain Anatomy

Evidence exists indicating that depression might result from or cause atrophy of specific brain locations. For example, loss of neurons and white matter in the frontal lobes, cerebellum, and basal ganglia has been identified by many scientists (Soares & Mann, 1997a, 1997b; Teodorczuk et al., 2010; Tomoda et al., 2009). Other findings include a reduction in brain-derived neurotrophic factor, a protein that helps neurons develop (Duman et al., 1997). Stahl (2000) suggested that a deficiency in brain-derived neurotrophic factor allows the apoptosis proteins (apoptosis is the cell's self-regulated function of cell extinction) to dominate, leading to premature neuronal death and atrophy in specific brain areas. The hippocampus is particularly susceptible to premature apoptotic processes. Although the notion of identifiable areas of brain atrophy has not been widely embraced, many believe that this hypothesis will become well accepted as diagnostic tools become more advanced.

Psychological Theories of Depression

The psychological explanations for depression flow from psychoanalytic, cognitive, interpersonal, and behavioral perspectives. In addition, related psychosocial-psychodynamic views explain depression from three general themes, individually or combined: (1) adverse early life experiences, (2) intrapsychic conflicts, and (3) reactions to life events (i.e., stressors).

Psychoanalytic theorists have contended that depression occurs as a result of an early life loss (Freud, 1957). Freud viewed depression as the aggressive instinct inappropriately directed at the self, often triggered by the loss of a loved person or object (object loss). This loss predisposes the adult to depression when adult losses trigger the memory of the childhood loss. By understanding (i.e., gaining insight into) one's thoughts, feelings, and motives, one can heal. Many clinicians believe that this approach is not in the patient's best interest because it focuses on problems in the past and often creates more issues than it solves.

Cognitive theorists have contended that depression results when a person perceives all stressful situations as being negative (Beck, 1976, 1991). In addition, a depressed person reacts to all situations as if they are stressful and sees himself or herself, others, and daily events in a negative light. This reaction to stress is grounded in early childhood losses (e.g., often the loss of a parent through death, leaving the home, or divorce) and serves as the basis for how the depressed person makes decisions and sees himself or herself in relationship to other persons and occurrences. Cognitive therapy aims at symptom removal by identifying and correcting distorted, negative, moment-by-moment maladaptive thinking and seeks to prevent recurrence by correcting dysfunctional assumptions. Most clinicians, including clinicians heavily steeped in a biologic framework, believe that medications serve the purpose of preparing the mind to work on faulty thinking. Cognitive approaches are ideal when used in conjunction with antidepressants.

Interpersonal theorists believe that when a person has interpersonal difficulties, coping with individuals, life events, and life changes can be inordinately stressful and lead to depression (Klerman, 1989). Role issues, social isolation, prolonged grief reaction, and role transition are major interpersonal themes. Interpersonal difficulties are viewed as causal, concomitant, or exacerbating in maintaining factors for depression (Depression Guideline Panel, 1993).

Behavioral theorists propose that a person develops depression when he or she develops feelings of helplessness and unworthiness and then learns to use these attitudes to evaluate life outcomes (Abramson et al., 1978).

Debilitating Early Life Experiences

According to traditional psychiatric thought, events in early life can lay the foundation for adult depression. Developmental theorists view the early years of life as the foundation of lifelong mental health. Although these theorists use different words to designate life stages, their views of the importance of a solid, nurturing early life environment are similar. Early losses, maternal inconsistency, the giving and withholding of love by the caregiver, and various types of abuse all are given as causative agents for depression. Even prebirth experiences may affect the child (Pearson et al., 2010).

Intrapsychic Conflict

Intrapsychic conflict refers to the conflicts people have when they have mixed emotions about a behavior, event, or situation. For instance, an individual who has been brought up to refrain from sexual activity but who also has strong urges to experience sex has a conflict. To refrain from sexual activity increases sexual frustration and to engage in sexual activity might cause anxiety, guilt, and fear. People are faced with intrapsychic conflicts all the time. Persistent and unsuccessful resolution of these conflicts can lead to depression.

Reactions to Life Events (Stress)

Most people view depression as a reaction to life stress. Loss is a major theme, including loss of a loved one, of a job, of self-esteem, or of familiar surroundings. Reacting to loss with grief and sadness is normal; overreacting is abnormal. Probably half of all depressive events are jump-started by stress. However, exactly when normal becomes abnormal is unclear.

Clinical Example

Elle is a 45-year-old, well-educated, intelligent white woman who has been in and out of therapy over the course of 15 to 20 years. Elle grew up in northern Mississippi with two brothers and a very physically and emotionally abusive father. Elle reports that when she was quite young, her mother left home and did not return for several years. Elle left home at age 17 and was married twice and divorced shortly after each marriage. She has a history of depression, and she attempted suicide 20 years ago. After many turbulent years, she started going to bars in hopes "that I might get killed." She refers to this period as her "death hunt days." After emotional and financial collapse, Elle has recently returned to her father's home. He continues to control her life in every way. She has commented that her life is so futile that she would rather be dead.

ASSESSMENT OF DEPRESSION

Assessment of depression may be accomplished through both nonbiologic and biologic assessment methods. For accurate assessment of depression, the following should be addressed:

1. History of onset of symptoms
2. Presence of comorbid substance, alcohol, and medication use
3. Physical examination to rule out the presence of medical conditions (Box 25-1)
4. Presence of non–mood-related psychiatric disorders
5. Patient resources and social support systems
6. Interpersonal and coping abilities
7. Level of stressors
8. Presence of suicidal ideation

Nurses can be instrumental in collecting all of this information because they are often the health care professionals who initially assess patients and develop the database for use in the general diagnostic and nursing processes.

Cultural Issues and Assessing Depression

Selection of an assessment instrument is based on the nurse's clinical knowledge and experience as well as on the age and mental capability of the person being assessed. Only limited measures have been developed and normed for use in different ethnic, racial, and cultural groups. The lack of measurement specificity for these populations can lead to misdiagnosis or underdiagnosis. Because some researchers have contended that culturally competent measures predict

---

DYSFUNCTIONAL GRIEF

If you live long enough, you will experience grief—an intense but normal response to loss—typically the loss of someone very close to you. Typically, we think of grief as a reaction to death, but it can also be a reaction to divorce, relocation to another part of the country, terminal illness (e.g., anticipatory grief), or natural disaster. As noted, grief is normal. To lose someone close—for example, a mother, father, brother, sister, wife, husband, or child—and not experience grief is abnormal.

Typically, the grief response lasts about 6 months. People experiencing grief report a choking sensation, emptiness, shortness of breath, weakness, and sighing. They also use the term *waves* to verbalize how these feelings roll over them. After about 6 months, the grieving person begins to return to normal, but waves of grief can continue to occur for some time.

During my teenage years (i.e., the early 1960s), I was acquainted with an older woman in my hometown of Manteca, California. She had lost her only son in World War II, and his photograph was displayed on her piano. Not often, but on occasion, she would pick up his photograph and begin to cry; 20 years later, she still experienced a wave of grief from time to time.

Dysfunctional grief is said to occur when these symptoms extend beyond 6 months. Zeitlin (2001) outlined the risk factors for dysfunctional grieving, as follows:

1. History of psychiatric disorders
2. Ambivalent, overly close, or intense relationship with deceased
3. History of multiple recent losses
4. Loss of a parent or a significant person during childhood
5. Lack of social support
6. Deaths by suicide, AIDS, murder, or other unexpected means

Differentiating grief and depression is not always simple, but the following guidelines can be useful (Anonymous, 2002):

GRIEF	DEPRESSION
Natural response to death	An illness
Self-limited and improves	Persistent and can worsen with time
Responsive to social contacts	Burdened by social contacts
Rarely suicidal	Suicidal ideations common
Typically does not need antidepressants	Responsive to antidepressants

BOX 25-1 MEDICAL CONDITIONS COMMONLY ASSOCIATED WITH DEPRESSION

Central Nervous System Disorders
Alzheimer's disease
Amyotrophic lateral sclerosis
Brain tumor
Cerebrovascular accident (stroke)
Chronic subdural hematoma
Multiple sclerosis
Normal-pressure hydrocephalus
Parkinson's disease
Subarachnoid hemorrhage

Collagen Vascular Diseases
Polymyalgia rheumatica
Rheumatoid arthritis
Systemic lupus erythematosus
Temporal arteritis

Toxic-Metabolic Disturbances and Endocrinopathies
Addison's disease
Cushing's disease
Diabetes mellitus
Electrolyte disorders
Hypercortisolemia
Hypoglycemia
Hypothyroidism

Metal intoxication
Parathyroid disorders
Uremia

Infections
AIDS
Encephalitis
Hepatitis
Infectious mononucleosis
Influenza
Syphilis
Tuberculosis
Viral pneumonia

Neoplastic Disorders
Carcinoma of head of pancreas
Chronic myelogenous leukemia
Lymphoma
Other malignant disease
Small cell carcinoma of lung

Other
Chronic fatigue syndrome
Chronic obstructive pulmonary disease
Decreased bone density

Modified from Ford, C.V., & Folks, D.G. (1985). Psychiatric disorders in geriatric medical/surgical patients: II. review of clinical experience in consultation. *Southern Medical Journal, 78,* 397; Michelson, D. (2009). Depression: body and brain. *Biological Psychiatry, 66,* 405.

relevant criteria more accurately than non–culturally competent measures, this assessment deficiency should be viewed as clinically significant. Routine review of cultural competence issues facilitates accurate and valid assessment for all patients.

Assessment of Depression
Depression in Older Adults
Depression in older adults is a major health concern. The prevalence of MDD declines with age, but symptoms of depression increase. Depressive symptoms are common, but because of the overlapping symptoms of physical illness and the depressive side effects of many medications, diagnosis is complex. To acquaint the nurse with potential confounding variables, depression-causing illnesses that share symptoms with depression are listed in Box 25-1.

If depression is related to a treatable medical illness, elimination of the illness often returns the depressed mood to normal. However, MDD and medical illness can coexist, and treatment needs to be instituted in these cases. The nurse should also be aware that some people who are given a diagnosis of dementia are actually depressed (referred to as *pseudodementia*). It is important to differentiate between depression and dementia. Depression and dementia can occur comorbidly, in which case both disorders must be treated. Comorbid MDD and dementia tend to occur early in the course of Alzheimer's disease.

Depression manifesting in later life may be related to grief issues confronted by older adults, including loss of spouse, family members, children, jobs, housing, income, mobility, and health. As a result of these inevitable losses, older adults are at increased risk of suicide. Men have an increased risk over women. Older white men have the highest risk of suicide in the United States. Suicide is discussed at the end of this chapter.

Nonbiologic Assessment Measures
Nonbiologic assessments comprise standardized verbal and written measurement scales. Obtained data can be used in conjunction with *DSM-5* criteria and biologic assessments to give a more accurate diagnosis regarding MDD. Various instruments might be used for assessment purposes. The Hamilton Depression Scale and the Geriatric Depression Scale are important examples of these assessment tools.

Biologic Assessment Measures
Dexamethasone suppression test. Although not frequently ordered, the DST is a diagnostic test for MDD in adults that measures the function of the HPA axis. Urine and blood samples are collected before the test to determine baseline levels of cortisol. A single injection of the drug dexamethasone is given to the patient. Urine and blood cortisol levels are monitored for 24 hours. A positive result

occurs when cortisol levels do not decrease (i.e., are not suppressed) or return to 5 μg/dL or greater within 24 hours (Fountoulakis et al., 2008). Failure of cortisol suppression occurs in 40% of severely depressed patients. The DST is not specific for depression because cortisol levels are not suppressed in individuals with dementia, alcohol withdrawal, and bulimia.

Growth hormone assessment. Growth hormone secretion is often used as a biologic assessment measure in childhood depression. Past research has indicated that some depressed children might have decreased secretion of growth hormone during the day and increased secretion while asleep. This test is not useful in adolescents and adults.

Polysomnographic measurements. Polysomnographic findings (i.e., examination of sleep patterns) are used to assess depression in adults. The REM stage usually begins within 70 to 100 minutes of a person falling asleep and increases in length throughout the night. However, in depressed adults, the REM latency phase is shortened, which results in frequent night and early morning wakening. Antidepressants can restore the normal pattern of REM sleep.

PUTTING IT ALL TOGETHER

PSYCHOTHERAPEUTIC MANAGEMENT

The nurse uses the nursing process to develop appropriate nursing interventions and strategies, expected outcomes, and evaluation of the outcomes for depressed patients. The intervention strategy described in this book, psychotherapeutic management, emphasizes the nurse-patient relationship, psychopharmacology, and milieu management. The case study and care plan presented in this section are geared toward the nursing management of the depressed patient who is being treated in a psychiatric outpatient environment. Indeed, in the current managed care environment, most psychiatric patients are rarely hospitalized and if they are hospitalized, it is for short periods of time (3 to 5 days). Consequently, the nursing management of depressed individuals primarily occurs in medical settings or outpatient clinics. In addition, it is imperative that nurses in any setting be familiar with the *DSM-5* criteria of MDD and with the information regarding mood disorders presented in this chapter.

Nurse-Patient Relationship

The objective of this section is to provide specific principles of therapeutic communication for nurses who work with depressed patients.

1. Depressed individuals have low self-esteem. The most effective approach to bolster self-esteem is to accept patients as they are (negative attitude and all), help them focus on the positive (accomplishments, good points), provide successful experiences with positive feedback, keep self-help strategies simple, and help patients avoid embarrassing social blunders (e.g., smelly clothes, unkempt appearance).

2. Development of a meaningful relationship in which depressed individuals are valued as human beings is important to their sense of personal worth. It is important for the nurse to be honest and to work on developing trust. Doing specific things that are in the best interest of each patient develops the trusting relationship. For example, a patient might wish to tell the nurse something of clinical significance but does not want the nurse to share the information with other staff members. The nurse builds trust by telling the patient that significant information will be shared only with staff members who have a need to know. The patient learns to trust the nurse as a professional whose primary concern is the patient's best interest.

3. The nurse who works effectively with depressed patients must have sincere concern for patients and be empathic. The nurse acknowledges the emotional pain and suffering conveyed by patients and offers to help patients work through the pain. Empathy, when added to an adequate dosage of antidepressant, can bolster treatment success.

4. It is usually ineffective to outline logically why a patient is a worthwhile human being. However, the nurse can point out small visible accomplishments and strengths—for example, "I'm glad you combed your hair today." A patient might agree with everything the nurse says but remain just as depressed. Intellectual understanding does not help severely depressed patients. However, cognitive-behavioral therapists have been successful in helping some depressed individuals learn to reprogram negative thoughts—for example, to progress from "I can't do anything right" to "I can learn from my mistakes."

5. Depressed individuals are typically dependent. The nurse might notice that he or she (i.e., the nurse) is taking on responsibility for the depression of patients. The nurse should recognize, but not resent, this tendency in depressed individuals to become dependent. The nurse should reward small decisions and independent actions.

6. The nurse should not attempt to embarrass patients out of being depressed. For example, pointing out less fortunate people in the hope that such an action might bring depressed individuals to their senses provides, at best, short-lived relief based on the misfortune of others.

7. The nurse should never reinforce hallucinations, delusions, or irrational beliefs. The nurse cannot agree with the delusions, and arguing seems to reinforce them. The nurse should state his or her perception of reality, voice doubt about the patient's perceptions, and move on to discuss real people and events.

8. Depressed individuals tend to be angry (Figure 25-2). Sometimes, they surprise even themselves with the hateful or hostile things that they say. It is important for the nurse to learn to handle hostility therapeutically by recognizing the anger, not taking it personally,

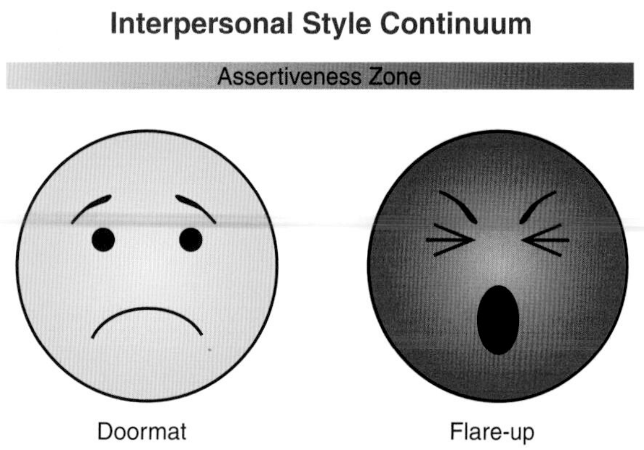

Interpersonal Style Continuum

Assertiveness Zone

Doormat   Flare-up

FIG 25-2 Depressed individuals often adopt an interpersonal style that causes them to be "doormats"—that is, they allow people to walk all over them. Sometimes the individual with a "doormat" personality explodes when he or she has had too much. These outbursts are typically followed by more recrimination and regret. The nurse can help patients learn to avoid these extremes of interpersonal behavior by teaching them to use assertiveness techniques.

and not retaliating in word, deed, or some passive-aggressive form. Encouraging verbal expressions of anger helps release patients' tension.

9. The nurse can help withdrawn patients emerge from their social isolation by spending time with them (even without speaking), providing a nonthreatening one-to-one relationship, practicing assertive interactions, and being accepting.
10. Depressed individuals can have difficulty making simple decisions. It is not therapeutic to badger patients into making a decision, but it is therapeutic to provide decision-making opportunities as patients are able to comply. Initially, the nurse might need to make decisions for patients—for example, "It is time for your bath" or "Here is your apple juice." When possible, the nurse

helps guide patients to appropriate decisions by using problem-solving techniques—that is, identifying options, the advantages and disadvantages of each option, and the potential consequences of each decision. (See Key Nursing Interventions for Depressed Patients box.)

Psychopharmacology

To understand the range of information required for effective psychopharmacologic intervention, the student is encouraged to review Chapter 15, which provides a complete discussion of antidepressant drugs. A brief review of critical parameters of antidepressant drug administration is given in Box 25-2 and in the Side Effects of Antidepressant Drugs box.

SIDE EFFECTS OF ANTIDEPRESSANT DRUGS

Antidepressants (TCAs, SSRIs)
Sexual dysfunction (depressed libido, arousal, or orgasm)
Dry mouth
Nasal congestion
Urinary hesitancy
Urinary retention
Blurred vision
Constipation
Sedation, ataxia
Confusion
Orthostatic hypotension
Arrhythmias, tachycardia, palpitations
Decreased sweating

MAOIs
Overstimulation (e.g., agitation, hypomania)
Blurred vision, hypotension, dry mouth, constipation
Hypertensive crisis related to food-drug or drug-drug interactions

MAOIs, Monoamine oxidase inhibitors; *SSRIs,* selective serotonin reuptake inhibitors; *TCAs,* tricyclic antidepressants.

KEY NURSING INTERVENTIONS
for Depressed Patients

The psychiatric nurse should consider the following intervention principles when working with depressed patients.

INTERVENTION	RATIONALE
Accept patients where they are and focus on their strengths.	Depressed persons have low self-esteem, and this is the best approach to recapturing some sense of value.
Reinforce decision making by patients.	Depressed patients struggle to make simple decisions. By reinforcing patients' efforts to make simple decisions, the nurse helps patients move toward health.
Respond to anger therapeutically.	Depressed persons are typically angry. By understanding that anger is a symptom of depression, the nurse can focus on the issue at hand and help patients move toward a more acceptable style of interaction.
Spend time with withdrawn patients.	Withdrawn patients are aware of their surroundings. By spending time (frequent but brief contact) with these patients, the nurse communicates patients' worth and, consequently, might be available during a time when patients feel comfortable with initiating dialog. Make decisions for patients that they are not ready to make for themselves. Some patients cannot make a decision. Simply present situations to these patients that do not require decision making (e.g., "It's time to go for a walk").
Involve patients in activities in which they can experience success.	People can feel good about themselves in several ways. One way to develop self-worth is through accomplishment.

BOX 25-2   IMPORTANT POINTS FOR ADMINISTERING ANTIDEPRESSANT DRUGS

- Most antidepressants have a lag time of 2 to 4 weeks before a full clinical effect occurs.
- Many reports suggest that these drugs might provoke suicidal ideation and behavior.
- Suicidal patients may "cheek" these drugs to build up a supply for an overdose. Tricyclic antidepressants (TCAs) have a narrow therapeutic index.
- Monitor vital signs of patients who take TCAs and monoamine oxidase inhibitors (MAOIs):
  1. TCAs can cause orthostatic hypotension, reflex tachycardia, and arrhythmias.
  2. MAOIs have the potential for triggering a hypertensive crisis.
- Monitor sexual side effects of selective serotonin reuptake inhibitors (SSRIs) because they occur frequently and lead to noncompliance.
- Be aware of the drug-drug and food-drug interactions associated with MAOIs.
- Observe for early signs of toxicity:
  1. TCAs: Drowsiness, tachycardia, mydriasis, hypotension, agitation, vomiting, confusion, fever, restlessness, sweating
  2. MAOIs: Dizziness, vertigo, fatigue
  3. SSRIs: Have a low probability for causing toxicity

Milieu Management

Milieu management is an important dimension of the psychiatric nursing care of depressed patients. The student is referred to Unit IV for a discussion of milieu management. General principles that specifically address the environment of depressed patients are presented here.

For Patients with Low Self-Esteem

- Encourage patients with low self-esteem to participate in activities, including group activities, in which they can experience accomplishment and receive positive feedback. Most people develop a sense of self-worth through mastery or accomplishment. Simply telling patients that they are okay is not convincing. Provide successful experiences, however small.
- Provide assertiveness training. Many depressed individuals feel like "doormats" because of their interactional problems; their communication history is typically a lifetime of being taken advantage of, punctuated by periodic outbursts of anger when they become fed up. Assertiveness training helps these patients learn to take care of their needs and to express their feelings along the way; the extremes of "doormat" and "flare-up" are avoided.
- Help patients avoid embarrassing themselves through socially unacceptable appearance or behavior. Many appearance problems are related directly to depressed individuals' preoccupation, apathy, and decreased energy level. For example, food stains on clothes, food in a beard, an unattended runny nose, uncombed hair, urine on trousers, and an unzipped fly might be seen in depressed individuals

who cannot pay attention to these hygienic concerns. Help patients shower and dress appropriately. Remind patients to go to the bathroom. In some cases, it is better to encourage patients to walk with the nurse (e.g., to the bathroom area or to the shower).

For Withdrawn Patients

- Keep contacts with withdrawn patients brief but frequent. Depressed patients often do not want anyone around or, at least, anyone to talk to them. Their wishes are not a good indicator of what should be done. Spending time with patients is constructive; allowing patients to isolate themselves is not constructive. Patients might need to increase physical activity before they are able to verbalize issues.
- Many patients are insistent about going to their rooms to lie down. They might stay there all day if the nurse does not intervene. Locking a patient's room during the day might be required to keep a withdrawn or isolative patient from disappearing for hours at a time. Sitting in silence during an activity is better than ruminating in isolation.

For Anorectic Patients

- The nursing staff must take responsibility for ensuring that depressed patients eat. It is irresponsible to set a tray down in front of a depressed person, particularly in his or her room, and then leave. The nurse must encourage patients to eat and might even spoon-feed them, if required.
- Allow patients to participate in selecting preferred foods from the menu.
- Promote a proper diet, adequate fluids, and exercise. Provide small, frequent meals. Record intake.
- Constipation is a side effect not only of antidepressants but also of depression. A diet with adequate fiber content and sufficient fluids is important. Monitoring and recording bowel elimination is also important.
- If patients will eat food brought from home, permit them to do so.

For Patients with Sleep Disturbances

- Depressed individuals want to sleep, but many have insomnia. Tremendous fatigue is real to these patients because the sleep they manage to get is usually not restful. Patients often wake up looking and feeling exhausted. The nursing staff should record the amount and quality of patients' actual sleep. Patients who lie down during the day might be isolating themselves and not sleeping. An accurate understanding of the amount of sleep being obtained helps the nurse formulate an intervention strategy.
- People with insomnia often engage in self-defeating behaviors, such as daytime napping and drinking stimulants (e.g., coffee, colas). Eliminating these behaviors increases the likelihood of nighttime sleep.
- Chronic insomnia in depressed persons appears to blunt their response to antidepressants (Jancin, 2005), so successfully dealing with insomnia offers the possibility of a twofold benefit.

❓ **CRITICAL THINKING QUESTION**

2. Do you think physicians have the right to help terminally ill patients end their lives? Should adults in their right minds be allowed to commit suicide?

SOMATIC THERAPIES

Somatic therapies are treatment approaches that use physiologic or physical interventions to effect behavioral change. The most common form of somatic therapy is electroconvulsive therapy (ECT), which is discussed in detail. Box 25-3 outlines early efforts in somatic therapy, summarizing the history of insulin-coma therapy and initial convulsive therapies. Other somatic therapies used to treat depression include transcranial magnetic stimulation (TMS), bright light therapy (BLT), and vagus nerve stimulation (VNS).

ECT and psychosurgery emerged as treatment forms in the 1930s. The roots of ECT lie in the misconception of early twentieth-century psychiatrists that epilepsy and schizophrenia were incompatible (Abrams, 1997). Advocates of ECT and psychosurgery envisioned and promised dramatic relief from the curse of mental illness. Over time, inappropriate use and disappointing results, coupled with the development of psychotropic drugs and a growing general distrust of psychiatric hospitals, created a climate of hostility toward these therapies and their practitioners. In the 1960s and early 1970s, the use of both therapies came to a virtual standstill. However, in about the last 20 years, ECT has emerged again as a useful treatment alternative when more traditional approaches have failed. With rigid treatment criteria and careful pretreatment evaluation, many psychiatric patients respond to these somatic therapies.

NORM'S NOTES
Somatic therapies, especially ECT, are terribly misunderstood. If antidepressants are not working for someone with severe depression, ECT usually helps them. If you know someone who just cannot seem to improve with the various antidepressant medications available, particularly if that person has entertained thoughts of suicide, please talk to someone in his or her family about this option. The kind of procedure you see in older movies has not been used in most hospitals (in industrialized countries) since the 1960s. Modern ECT is safe and effective, and it saves lives.

ELECTROCONVULSIVE THERAPY

Cerletti and Bini (Cerletti's assistant), two Italian psychiatrists, introduced ECT in 1938. The first patient had schizophrenia and, after 11 treatments, experienced a full recovery. The first ECT treatment in the United States was in 1940. ECT was previously commonly referred to as *electroshock therapy* (EST) or simply *shock therapy*. Both terms are considered pejorative today.

During ECT, an electric current is passed through the brain, causing a seizure. Historically, this seizure resulted in a full grand mal convulsion accompanied by the various complications of these convulsions—muscle soreness, fractures, dislocations, sprains, and tongue lacerations. These seizures and the resulting grotesque facial grimaces have been dramatically captured on film and graphically detailed in literature. In films and novels, ECT has been portrayed as a devious tool used by psychiatrists and psychiatric nurses who are themselves demented. The novel, *One Flew Over the Cuckoo's Nest*, by Ken Kesey, and the 1975 movie of the same name created a firestorm of hostility against the use of ECT. In his book, Kesey portrayed ECT as an agent used to maintain control over sane but highly individualistic patients. This public attack on ECT, linked with reports of inappropriate use, virtually stopped the use of ECT in the United States. Inappropriate use of ECT included administering ECT for almost all conditions and, from the accounts of former patients, using it as punishment for noncompliant behavior.

However, despite the negative perceptions, ECT remains a viable treatment approach because many mental health professionals know it to be an effective treatment. In the process of waiting to evaluate the efficacy of other treatments, many patients have suffered needlessly. Many clinicians now argue that ECT should be considered earlier in the treatment process because it is the most effective antidepressant. About 100,000 patients receive ECT treatments annually in the United States (Smith, 2001).

BOX 25-3 EARLY SOMATIC THERAPIES

Insulin-Coma Therapy: 1933
Insulin-coma therapy was introduced in 1933 by Sakel, a Viennese physician, after he accidentally discovered that giving too much insulin to a psychotic diabetic patient produced a reduction in the patient's symptoms. Insulin shock therapy gained a wide following for some time in hopes of alleviating the debilitating symptoms of psychosis (Colaizzi, 1996; Dorman, 1995).

First Convulsive Therapies: 1934
Meduna, a Hungarian, was the originator of convulsive therapy. In 1934, Meduna introduced camphor oil–induced and then Metrazol-induced convulsion therapy based on his pathologic observation that the glial cells of patients with schizophrenia were different from the glial cells of patients with epilepsy. Meduna erroneously concluded that schizophrenia and epilepsy were mutually exclusive disorders (Abrams, 1997). Fink (1999) chronicled one of Meduna's first patients, a 33-year-old man who had been psychotic, mute, and withdrawn for 4 years:

"Two days after the fifth (camphor oil) injection, on February 10 in the morning, for the first time in four years, he got out of his bed, began to talk, requested breakfast, dressed himself without help, was interested in everything around him, and asked about his disease and how long he had been in the hospital. When the patient was told he had been in the hospital for 4 years he did not believe it!" (p. 88).

Modern Electroconvulsive Therapy

ECT is the most effective antidepressant remedy available (Scott, 2008). During ECT, an electric current is passed through the brain for 0.2 to 8.0 seconds, causing a seizure (Fink, 1999). Induction of a seizure is necessary for a therapeutic outcome (Krystal et al., 2000). The seizure resulting from ECT must be of sufficient quality to produce the best effect. Seizures are timed and subdivided into motor convulsions (at least 20 seconds required), increased heart rate (for 30 to 50 seconds), and a brain seizure as monitored by an electroencephalogram (for 30 to 150 seconds) (Fink, 1999). The patient is given an oximeter-monitored anesthetic to ensure optimal oxygenation.

Three basic medications are typically used for ECT. These medications are used to prevent aspiration of body secretions, for anesthesia, and for body paralysis to prevent seizure-related injuries. The medications are as follows:

1. Atropine, the prototype anticholinergic, to reduce secretions
2. Methohexital (Brevital) intravenously to cause immediate anesthesia
3. Succinylcholine (Anectine) intravenously for its neuromuscular blocking effect

Nursing Responsibilities after Electroconvulsive Therapy

1. The nurse or anesthesiologist mechanically ventilates the patient with 100% oxygen until the patient can breathe unassisted.
2. The nurse monitors for respiratory problems.
3. ECT causes confusion and disorientation; it is important to help with reorientation (time, place, person) as the patient emerges from this groggy state.
4. Because approximately 5% to 10% of patients awake in an agitated state, the nurse might need to administer a benzodiazepine, as needed (Fitzsimons, 1995).
5. Observation is necessary until the patient is oriented and steady, particularly when the patient first attempts to stand.
6. All aspects of the treatment should be carefully documented for the patient's record.

An electroencephalogram monitors seizure activity. Blood pressure, oxygen saturation, and heart rate are also monitored. Oxygen is administered immediately before and after treatment because of interruption of breathing caused by the succinylcholine and the electrically induced seizure.

? CRITICAL THINKING QUESTIONS

3. ECT has been considered a political issue. Do you think opponents of ECT tend to be more on the left or the right of the political spectrum?
4. ECT is more effective than antidepressants in the treatment of severe depression. Nonetheless, there is reluctance to use ECT. If you or a member of your family were severely depressed, which of these two treatment forms would you want? Carefully consider the stigma of ECT as well as the effects of anesthesia and memory loss.

How Does It Work—Rebooting, Rebalancing, Rebuilding?

Although more than 100 theories have been advanced to explain ECT, no one knows for sure how it works. Several theorists have advanced promising explanations (Bezchlibnyk-Butler & Jeffries, 2007; Esel et al., 2008; Fink, 1999; Miller, 2007; Pierce et al., 2008; Sadock & Sadock, 2003). Keltner and Boschini (2009) capture the most convincing of these explanations: *rebooting*, *rebalancing*, and *rebuilding*:

1. As ECT treatment progresses, the brain waves are slowed; this might be likened to *rebooting* a computer by first shutting down the system.
2. The *rebalancing* of neurotransmitters:
   a. Second messenger system changes, such as changes in G-protein coupling, changes in adenyl cyclase and phospholipase C (i.e., the second messengers), and regulation of calcium entry into neurons
   b. Down-regulation of beta-adrenergic postsynaptic receptors
   c. Possible changes in serotonergic receptors
   d. Changes in dopaminergic, GABAergic, and cholinergic systems
3. The brain *rebuilding* effect of induced seizures (e.g., increased neuronal sprouting, more brain-derived neurotrophic factor); this might be compared with going to the weight room. Just as weak muscles can be strengthened by lifting heavy weights, perhaps the brain, in its fight against depression or psychosis, is strengthened by induced seizures.

Number of Treatments Needed for Effectiveness

Typically, patients are given ECT two to three times a week, up to a total of 6 to 12 treatments (or until the patient improves or is obviously not going to improve). Patients often experience relief after 2 or 3 treatments, but occasionally 20 treatments may be needed. If improvement is not observed after about 12 treatments, continuing ECT is usually not helpful. Although ECT is generally effective, relapse occurs frequently. Many patients require continuation or maintenance ECT treatments to function at their best (see later discussion).

Indications for Electroconvulsive Therapy: Major Depression

Although ECT was originally developed for schizophrenia, its primary indication soon shifted to patients who were severely depressed, particularly patients manifesting delusions and psychomotor retardation. Severely depressed patients account for about 85% to 90% of all patients receiving ECT. These patients respond better and more rapidly to ECT than to antidepressants (Scott, 2008). Potter and Rudorfer (1993) suggested a hierarchy of patients who should receive ECT, as follows:

1. Patients who require a rapid response (e.g., suicidal or catatonic patients)

2. Patients who cannot tolerate or be exposed to pharmacotherapy (e.g., pregnant women)
3. Patients who are depressed but have not responded to multiple and adequate trials of medication

Clinical Example

Penny Jones is a 48-year-old woman who worked for the postal service until 3 weeks ago. She was admitted to an acute psychiatric facility accompanied by her daughter, who indicated that her mother had lost 30 lb during the last 4 months. The daughter further described her mother as having a poor appetite, being isolative, awakening early in the morning with the inability to fall back to sleep, and verbalizing thoughts with suicidal overtones. The daughter stated that her mother's actions scare her.

Ms. Jones states that life is intolerable, and she does not want to live anymore without Jerry. The daughter explains that Jerry was the patient's husband, who died 5 months ago.

Ms. Jones sought psychiatric help immediately and was prescribed sertraline 25 mg/day for 1 week and then 50 mg/day. She improved slightly but has relapsed into a deeper depression and has lately begun to verbalize suicidal thoughts. Based on her poor response to antidepressants and her suicidal thoughts, a course of six ECT treatments was prescribed. Ms. Jones tolerated the procedures well. Her suicidal ideations ceased, she began interacting with others spontaneously, and she regained her appetite. She was discharged during the third week of her hospitalization.

Disorders, depressive symptoms, and conditions that respond to ECT are listed in Table 25-2 (Swartz, 1993). Box 25-4 lists conditions that do not respond to ECT.

Contraindications to Electroconvulsive Therapy

Lisanby (2007) noted that ECT is a potentially life-saving procedure. As such, there should be few contraindications to its use. However, most clinicians are still reluctant to prescribe ECT if any of the conditions listed in Box 25-5 are present.

Advantages of Electroconvulsive Therapy

Historically, ECT has been viewed as providing the fastest relief for depression (Roose & Nobler, 2001). ECT is a safe procedure; only a few ECT-related deaths have been reported (Nuttall et al., 2004; Sackeim et al., 1993). ECT has about the same risk as that associated with general anesthesia: 1 death

---

BOX 25-4 CONDITIONS NONRESPONSIVE TO ELECTROCONVULSIVE THERAPY

Anxiety disorders
Behavioral disorders
Mild depressions
Personality disorders
Phobic disorders
Somatoform disorders

BOX 25-5 CONDITIONS THAT CAUSE INCREASED RISK FOR PATIENTS RECEIVING ELECTROCONVULSIVE THERAPY

Very High Risk
Recent myocardial infarction
Recent cerebrovascular accident
Intracranial mass
Increased intracranial pressure

High Risk
Angina pectoris
Congestive heart failure
Extremely loose teeth (aspiration)
Severe pulmonary disease
Severe osteoporosis
Major bone fractures
Glaucoma
Retinal detachment
Thrombophlebitis
High-risk pregnancy
Use of monoamine oxidase inhibitors (MAOIs) (severe hypertension)*
Use of clozapine (seizures, delirium)

*Some studies indicate that MAOIs given in conjunction with electroconvulsive therapy do not cause a serious interaction. Modified from Bezchlibnyk-Butler, K.Z., & Jeffries, J.J. (2007). *Clinical handbook of psychotropic drugs* (7th ed.). Seattle: Hogrefe & Huber; Ziring, B. (1993). Issues in the perioperative care of the patient with psychiatric illness. *Medical Clinics of North America, 77,* 443.

TABLE 25-2 DISORDERS, DEPRESSIVE SYMPTOMS, AND CONDITIONS THAT RESPOND TO ELECTROCONVULSIVE THERAPY

DISORDERS	DEPRESSIVE SYMPTOMS	CONDITIONS
Severe depression	Anhedonia	Tardive dystonia
Refractory depression	Anorexia	Tardive dyskinesia
Catatonia	Delusions	Akathisia
Mania	Insomnia	Parkinsonian symptoms
Some types of schizophrenia	Muteness	Neuroleptic malignant syndrome
	Psychomotor retardation	
	Suicidal ideations	

Data from Swartz, C.M. (1993). Seizure benefit: grand mal or grand bene? *Neurologic Clinics, 11,* 151.

per 50,000 patients (Gitlin et al., 1993). ECT is not only safe, but it is also more effective than antidepressants for certain groups of patients. Finally, ECT can be used safely and effectively in older patients, including the old-old (>85 years old), and in adolescents (Cohen et al., 2000; Tomac et al., 1997).

Disadvantages of Electroconvulsive Therapy
Provision of Only Temporary Relief

The major disadvantage of ECT is that treatment provides only temporary relief; it does not provide a permanent cure (Lisanby et al., 2008). Many patients are able to remain free of depression for long periods, and others might never need treatment again. However, some patients receiving ECT might need another series of treatments within a few months. Some psychiatrists order maintenance or continuation ECT (about once a month for 6 to 12 months or longer); however, there is still much to learn about the benefits of this approach. Studies have suggested that continued periodic treatments of ECT plus an antidepressant significantly reduce relapse rates (Gagne et al., 2000).

Memory Loss

Memory impairment, both retrograde (memory before treatment) and anterograde (memory and the ability to learn new things after treatment), has been frequently cited as a side effect of ECT. Events closest in time to ECT are most frequently affected. Although memory is impaired for events both before and after each treatment, and confusion occurs immediately after each treatment, there does not seem to be any substantial loss of mental function for most patients after the treatment series has been completed. Because depression can cause memory loss as well, it is not always clear whether memory impairment is related to ECT or to depression. Unilateral placement of the electrodes—that is, both electrodes placed on the nondominant side of the head (for right-handed individuals, this would be the right side)—minimizes treatment impact on memory and learning but might not be as effective. Bifrontal placement (placed a few inches apart on the front of the head) also causes fewer problems with memory and learning (Bailine et al., 2000). Preexisting cognitive problems increase the risk of treatment-related memory issues (Pierce et al., 2008).

Adverse Physiologic Effects

Adverse physiologic effects of ECT include cardiac effects, such as hypertension, arrhythmias, alterations of cardiac output, and changes in cerebrovascular dynamics. Hemodynamic changes, in combination with increased muscle tone, have been postulated to result in a generalized increase in oxygen consumption. Increases in myocardial oxygen consumption might result in ischemia (Ziring, 1993). ECT does not cause brain damage (Abrams, 1997).

OTHER SOMATIC THERAPIES
Vagus Nerve Stimulation

VNS has been approved by the U.S. Food and Drug Administration to treat depression. This procedure has demonstrated efficacy in severe, treatment-resistant depression.

Specifically, a pacemaker-like device stimulates the vagus nerve. VNS has demonstrated an ability to reduce depression symptoms in more than half the patients studied (Splete, 2005).

Bright Light Therapy

BLT, formerly called *phototherapy*, exposes patients to intense light (5000 lux-hours) each day. The rationale for this treatment comes from several studies plus anecdotal reports indicating that environmental factors play a role in mood disorders. Seasonal affective disorder results from decreased exposure to sunlight and usually occurs in and around the winter season. BLT used for individuals with seasonal affective disorder relieves symptoms of depression. Apparently, morning administration is most beneficial.

BLT works in just a few days. The precise mechanism of action of how exposure to intense light produces an antidepressant effect is unclear; however, it is believed that its therapeutic effect is mediated by the eyes, not the skin. Other conditions thought to respond to BLT include bulimia, sleep maintenance insomnia, and nonseasonal depression. Because phototherapy produces few, if any, significant adverse effects (e.g., nausea, eye irritation), the risk-to-benefit ratio favors its use. Contraindications include glaucoma, cataracts, and use of photosensitizing medications.

> **? CRITICAL THINKING QUESTION**
>
> 5. Does it make common sense that a bright light could improve a person's mental health? Does a sunny day help your mood?

Repetitive Transcranial Magnetic Stimulation

TMS or repetitive TMS produces a magnetic field over the brain, influencing brain activity. TMS apparently increases the release of neurotransmitters or down-regulates beta-adrenergic receptors (or both), ameliorating depressive symptoms and possibly other disorders. Because TMS does not require anesthesia, it is an attractive alternative to ECT if conclusive evidence of its efficacy can be demonstrated. Some studies have suggested that it is as effective as ECT in nonpsychotic patients (Fitzgerald, 2004). Adverse effects include seizures in previously seizure-free individuals, headache, and transient hearing loss. Patients with metal implanted in their bodies (e.g., plates), pacemakers, heart disease, or increased intracranial pressure should be carefully evaluated before receiving TMS.

SUICIDE AND DEPRESSION

> *Most people who commit suicide die accidentally.*
>
> *Anonymous*

The death by suicide of psychiatric patients is of particular importance to the nurse because of opportunities for assessment and intervention. Suicide is a complex phenomenon influenced by a person's cultural beliefs, values, and norms. Suicide can occur in children, adolescents, and adults. Because suicide is such an important topic, it is addressed separately in Chapter 21. Nurses should be aware that suicide is not exclusively committed by people with the diagnosis of major depression. The psychiatric nurse must continually assess for suicide potential among all patients, especially patients with schizophrenia and alcoholism. However, even when individuals with a "nondepression" background kill themselves, they are typically experiencing a period of despair. Specifically, a significant number of people (approximately 10%) with the diagnosis of schizophrenia commit suicide, and the number is even greater for people with alcoholism. Alcoholics typically kill themselves in response to loss (e.g., divorce, separation, being fired) and when they have been drinking. The following topics are worth reiterating in case the reader has not had time to review Chapter 21: the nomenclature of suicide, suicide risk assessment, and most likely victims of suicide.

Suicide Nomenclature

Following is a brief description of suicide nomenclature:

Suicidal ideation level: Suicidal ideation includes a person's thoughts regarding suicide as well as suicidal gestures and threats.

Suicidal gestures: Suicidal gestures are a person's nonlethal self-injury acts, including cutting or burning of skin areas or ingesting small amounts of drugs. Others often see these gestures as attention-getting measures and do not consider them to be serious problems that might lead to a suicide attempt or completion.

Suicidal threats: Suicidal threats are a person's verbal statements that might declare their intent to commit suicide. Threats often precede an actual suicidal attempt.

Suicidal attempts: Suicidal attempts are the actual implementation of a self-injurious act with the express purpose of ending one's life.

Suicide Risk Assessment

It is important for the nurse to assess the suicidal potential of psychiatric patients because these patients are at an increased risk of suicide. Most facilities provide the nurse with a format for evaluating suicidal lethality. The crucial variables are the plan, the method, and the provision for rescue.

Plan

A more developed plan is associated with a higher risk of suicide. People who have carefully developed a suicidal plan are more serious about suicide and present a higher risk compared with people who have no plan. Although impulsive suicide attempts can result in death, generally they are less often lethal because the lack of planning sometimes foils the effort.

Method

Some methods of attempting suicide are more lethal than others. Accessibility of the means to commit suicide is important as well. Having three bottles of pills on hand is more lethal compared with having to make an appointment with a physician

to ask for a prescription. A crucial factor in determining the lethality of a particular method is the amount of time between initiation of the suicide method and delivery of the lethal impact of that method. For instance, a person using a gun has no opportunity to avoid the bullet once the trigger is pulled. However, sitting in the garage with the motor running affords some time to choose an alternative to self-destruction, as does taking an overdose of certain drugs. Lethal methods of suicide include the use of guns (91% lethal), jumping from high places, drowning (84%), hanging (82%), carbon monoxide poisoning and other gases (64%), and overdose with certain drugs (e.g., barbiturates, alcohol, several central nervous system depressants) (Miller et al., 2004). Methods that are less likely to be lethal include wrist cutting and overdosing on aspirin or diazepam (Valium).

Rescue

The person who deliberately attempts to deceive would-be rescuers has an increased lethality potential. For instance, a woman who says she is going to the ocean for the weekend and then drives to the mountains makes it difficult for family and friends to intervene. A person who leaves a note or makes a telephone call before making an attempt is more likely to be rescued.

Summary

The more detailed the plan, the more lethal and accessible the method, and the more effort exerted to block rescue, the greater the likelihood will be of the suicidal effort being successful. However, impulsive efforts of suicidal individuals with rescuers in sight have proved fatal, particularly when a lethal method (e.g., a gun) has been selected.

Suicide Victims

The prototypical suicide victim is an unemployed white man, living alone, who has made a serious suicide attempt in the past. Men are four times as likely as women and whites are twice as likely as African-Americans to complete a suicide attempt successfully (Anonymous, 2003a). Greater than 70% of all suicides are committed by white men (Pearson, 1998).

Although the overall suicide rate for the general adult population in the United States is high, it is considerably lower than the suicide rate for people with psychiatric disorders. Psychiatric diagnosis is the most reliable risk factor for suicide. Approximately 90% of all suicides are committed by individuals with a diagnosable mental or substance abuse disorder. It is estimated that over a period of 10 to 15 years, 10% to 15% of all patients with depression, schizophrenia, or alcoholism will die by suicide. Table 25-3 compares the suicide rates by diagnostic entity of the general population with the suicide rates of individuals with a mental disorder (Clark et al., 1987). Box 25-6 lists other risk factors that have been related empirically to completed suicide.

? CRITICAL THINKING QUESTION

6. How would you differentiate between a suicidal gesture and a suicidal threat when assessing a depressed patient?

TABLE 25-3	CLINICAL RISK FACTORS FOR SUICIDE IN THE UNITED STATES	
POPULATION	**SUICIDES PER 100,000**	
Adult general public	<20	
Schizophrenic	140	
Depressed	230	
Alcoholic	270	

BOX 25-6 RISK FACTORS FOR COMPLETED SUICIDE

Male
White or Native American
Age 60 years or older
Hopelessness
General medical illness
Severe anhedonia
Living alone
Prior suicide attempts
Unemployed or financial problems

CASE STUDY

Will S. is a 35-year-old African-American man who has been in and out of mental health facilities for several years. Before his formal entrance into the mental health system, he had had several brushes with the law, primarily related to driving under the influence (DUI) of alcohol. It is thought that Will was self-medicating with alcohol and with other substances long before he was able to admit that he had a problem. Will developed hepatitis B through sexual activity 1 year after being diagnosed with major depression. Following this diagnosis, Will attempted to kill himself on at least five occasions. During a brief period of his depression, he developed auditory hallucinations accusing him of being gay. Although this was a relatively brief episode and did not recur, Will is very troubled by it, believing that these hallucinations make him "certifiably crazy." Will now lives with his widowed father who seems to be very pleased to have Will "back home again." Will continues to attend an outpatient program 3 days per week. He verbalizes wanting to go back to work but cannot seem to get moving. A long-standing fear of crowds and people remains. As Will says, "I'm not out of the woods, but I am a lot better than I was."

◎ CARE PLAN

Name: Will S.   ***Admission Date:*** _____
DSM-V Diagnosis: Major depression

Assessment	**Areas of strength:** Will understands his disease, has a good relationship with his father, is financially stable, is willing to acknowledge his problems and work on them, and is motivated to go back to work. **Problems:** Will verbalizes motivation but seems "stuck"; he enjoys living with his father, but he is too dependent for a 35-year-old man; he continues to be intimidated by crowds and people and has a suicidal history.
Diagnoses	Risk for self-injury related to depression as evidenced by history of suicide attempts. Social isolation related to anxiety, as evidenced by withdrawal from people and uncommunicative behavior.
Outcomes Date met: _____ Date met: _____ Date met: _____ Date met: _____ Date met: _____ Date met: _____ Date met: _____	**Short-term goals** Learn and develop coping skills for dealing with other patients at mental health treatment center. Participate in class activities at mental health treatment center. Develop socialization skills. Continue to comply with medication regimen. **Long-term goals** Seek out information about jobs at his skill level. Practice coping skills learned at mental health treatment center in public areas. Make steps to return to a more independent lifestyle.
Planning and Interventions	**Nurse-patient relationship:** Develop a trusting relationship based on honesty and genuine concern for the patient. Spend time with him, and reinforce his strengths and accomplishments. Help patient develop coping skills, and work with him to obtain job information. **Psychopharmacology:** Risperidone 3 mg qd; sertraline 50 mg qd; alprazolam 1 mg prn. **Milieu management:** Minimize patient's tendency to isolate himself by encouraging social interaction. As tolerated, draw patient into group situations. Keep patient's environment safe to prevent self-injury.
Evaluation	Patient is doing better but still tends to avoid large groups of people. He is consistently taking his medications, and no psychotic behavior has been observed or reported.
Referrals	Refer patient to a therapist for individual therapy. Patient is a candidate for a mental health system–sponsored apartment in the near future.

PATIENT AND FAMILY EDUCATION

Depression

Illness

Depression is a life-altering process or state. Depression might be precipitated by overwhelming life stresses, including loss (e.g., death, divorce, job), medications, medical illnesses, and specific chemical deficiencies in the brain. These precipitating factors are not mutually exclusive and might interact to produce depression. For example, it is believed that chronic exposure to intense stress can alter brain chemistry. Support for the chemical deficiency view has increased over the last 2 decades because medications known to relieve depressive states correct the chemical deficiencies previously noted. Nine cardinal symptoms define depression: (1) depressed mood, (2) apathy, (3) changes in weight, (4) sleep disturbances, (5) movement disturbances, (6) lack of energy, (7) sense of worthlessness, (8) inability to concentrate, and (9) thoughts of death. An individual with most of these symptoms (depressed mood or apathy must always be present) should be given a diagnosis of depression.

Medications

1. The most popular antidepressants are the selective serotonin reuptake inhibitors (SSRIs). Well-known drugs in this category include fluoxetine (Prozac), sertraline (Zoloft), paroxetine (Paxil), escitalopram (Lexapro), and citalopram (Celexa). These drugs are effective and have few side effects. However, sexual dysfunction, defined as a loss of interest in sex or the inability to perform sexually, is common and disturbing to many patients. This side effect motivates some patients to stop taking their SSRI. Other medications can be added that might restore sexual vitality (e.g., bupropion [Wellbutrin], sildenafil [Viagra]).

2. An older group of medications, referred to as tricyclic antidepressants (TCAs), is still commonly prescribed (e.g., amitriptyline [Elavil], nortriptyline [Pamelor], desipramine [Norpramin]). Although they have a higher rate of side effects than SSRIs, TCAs are equally effective and are considerably less expensive. The most common side effects are a decrease in blood pressure when standing, dry mouth, constipation, and a racing heart (at times).

3. Numerous other agents are also available (e.g., Wellbutrin, venlafaxine [Effexor], mirtazapine [Remeron], desvenlafaxine [Pristiq]). All these drugs seem to be effective and cause fewer side effects for most people.

Other Issues

It is easy to be angry with a depressed person—to wonder why that person simply cannot snap out of it. If a family member feels this way, it might help to compare the situation with someone with diabetes. Individuals with diabetes have a reduced level of insulin; they cannot just snap out of it. The same is true of a depressed person with changed levels of brain chemicals. However, just as the person with diabetes is not powerless, the person who is depressed also is not powerless. For example, individuals with diabetes who do not adhere to a diabetic diet or take medications as prescribed can make their condition become worse. An individual with depression might need to avoid certain substances, associations, and situations.

STUDY NOTES

1. MDD, disruptive mood dysregulation disorder, dysthymia, and premenstrual dysphoric disorder are significant depressive disorders.

2. *DSM-5* defines major depression as an episode of depression without a history of manic episodes.

3. Disruptive mood dysregulation disorder is diagnosed primarily in children and adolescents who experience frequent outbursts of rage and physical aggression.

4. Dysthymia is characterized by its chronicity.

5. Reacting to a disappointment or loss with sadness, guilt, or depression is normal; however, if any of these reactions persists too long, a diagnosable depression exists.

6. A high correlation exists between depression and suicide.

7. There are several subtypes of depression, including atypical depression, melancholic depression, catatonic depression, peripartum depression, psychotic depression, and seasonal depression.

8. Depression is common in the United States. Women have a lifetime risk of 10% to 20%, and men have a lifetime risk of about 5% to 10%.

9. Many early-life traumas are associated with depression in children.

10. People from different ethnic and cultural groups might experience depression differently.

11. Objective signs of depression include alterations in activity and social interactions.

12. Subjective symptoms of depression include alterations in affect, cognition, physical nature (somatic concerns), and perception.

13. Biologic explanations for depression include neurotransmitter, genetic, endocrine, and circadian rhythm dysfunctions. Psychological explanations include debilitating early-life experiences, intrapsychic conflicts, and reaction to life events.

14. Assessment of depression includes consideration of cultural influences, age (older adults are particularly vulnerable), nonbiologic standardized tests, and biologic indices (DST, growth hormone tests, and polysomnography).

15. Psychotherapeutic management includes developing a therapeutic nurse-patient relationship, administering antidepressant drugs when appropriate, and providing a well-managed milieu with a particular emphasis on safety.

16. Somatic therapies are treatment approaches that use physiologic or physical interventions to effect behavioral change.
17. The most common form of somatic therapy is ECT.
18. During ECT, an electric current is passed through the brain, causing a grand mal seizure.
19. Modern ECT uses anesthesia and muscle relaxants to prevent convulsive jerks that previously caused broken bones; oxygen is given to guard against brain damage.
20. ECT is indicated for the treatment of severe depression, depression that is unresponsive to other treatments, mania, catatonia, and some types of schizophrenia.

21. The psychiatric nurse should suspect suicidal ideation in most depressed patients because suicide is a prevalent theme among this patient population.
22. The prototypical suicide victim is an unemployed white man living alone. Greater than 70% of all suicides are committed by white men. Elderly men are at particularly high risk.
23. In assessing the lethality of suicide, the psychiatric nurse should consider the plan, the method, and the prevention of rescue.

REFERENCES

Abrams, R. (1997). *Electroconvulsive therapy.* New York: Oxford University Press.

Abramson, L. Y., Seligman, M. E., & Teasdale, J. D. (1978). Learned helplessness in humans: Critique and reformulation. *Journal of Abnormal Psychology, 87,* 48.

American Psychiatric Association. (1993). Practice guidelines for major depressive disorder in adults. *American Journal of Psychiatry, 150*(Suppl.), 1.

American Psychiatric Association. (2010). *Diagnostic and statistical manual of mental disorders, text revision* (4th ed.). Arlington, Virginia: APA.

American Psychiatric Association. (2013). *Diagnostic and statistical manual of mental disorders* (5th ed.). Arlington, Virginia: APA.

Anonymous. (2002). Coping with grief. *Psychiatric Services (Washington, D.C.), 53,* 19.

Anonymous. (2003a). Confronting suicide: Part I. *The Harvard Mental Health Letter, 19,* 1.

Anonymous. (2003b). Depression in old age. *The Harvard Mental Health Letter, 20,* 5.

Anonymous. (2005). Atypical depression. *The Harvard Mental Health Letter, 22,* 1.

Bailine, S. H., et al. (2000). Comparison of bifrontal and bitemporal ECT for major depression. *American Journal of Psychiatry, 157,* 121.

Beck, A. T. (1976). *Cognitive therapies and the emotional disorders.* New York: International Universities Press.

Beck, A. T. (1991). *Depression: Causes and treatment.* Philadelphia: University of Pennsylvania Press.

Belcher, J. V., & Holdcraft, C. (2001). Web-based information for depression: Helpful or hazardous? *Journal of the American Psychiatric Nurses Association, 7,* 61.

Bezchlibnyk-Butler, K. Z., & Jeffries, J. J. (2007). *Clinical handbook of psychotropic drugs* (7th ed.). Seattle: Hogrefe & Huber.

Brand, S. R., & Brennan, P. A. (2009). Impact of antenatal and postpartum maternal mental illness: How are the children? *Clinical Obstetrics and Gynecology, 52,* 441.

Clark, D. C., et al. (1987). A field test of Motto's risk estimator for suicide. *American Journal of Psychiatry, 144,* 923.

Cohen, D., et al. (2000). Absence of cognitive impairment at long-term follow-up in adolescents treated with ECT for severe mood disorder. *American Journal of Psychiatry, 157,* 460.

Colaizzi, J. (1996). Transorbital lobotomy at Eastern State Hospital (1951–1954). *Journal of Psychosocial Nursing and Mental Health Services, 34,* 16.

Depression Guideline Panel. *Depression in primary care, detection and diagnosis.* (Vol. 1) (1993). In Washington, DC: US Government Printing Office, DHHS Pub No 93-0550.

Dorman, J. (1995). The history of psychosurgery. *Texas Medicine, 91,* 54.

Dubovsky, S. L. (1994). Beyond the serotonin reuptake inhibitors: Rationales for the development of new serotonergic agents. *Journal of Clinical Psychiatry, 55*(Suppl. 2), 34.

Duman, R. F., Heninger, C. R., & Nestler, E. J. (1997). A molecular and cellular theory of depression. *Archives of General Psychiatry, 54,* 597.

Esel, E., et al. (2008). The effects of electroconvulsive therapy on GABAergic function in major depressive patients. *The Journal of ECT, 24,* 224.

Fink, M. (1999). *Electroshock.* New York: Oxford University Press.

Fitzgerald, P. (2004). Repetitive transcranial magnetic stimulation and electroconvulsive therapy: Complementary or competitive therapeutic options in depression? *Australasian Psychiatry, 12,* 234.

Fitzsimons, L. (1995). Electroconvulsive therapy: What nurses need to know. *Journal of Psychosocial Nursing and Mental Health Services, 33,* 14.

Fountoulakis, K. N., et al. (2008). Revisiting the Dexamethasone Suppression Test in unipolar major depression: An exploratory study. *Annals of General Psychiatry, 7,* 22.

Freud, S. *Mourning and melancholia.* (Vol. 14). (1957). In London: Hogarth Press.

Gagne, G. G., Jr., et al. (2000). Efficacy of continuation ECT and antidepressant drugs compared to long-term antidepressants alone in depressed patients. *American Journal of Psychiatry, 157,* 1960.

Gitlin, M. C., et al. (1993). Splenic rupture after electroconvulsive therapy. *Anesthesia and Analgesia, 76,* 1363.

Hays, D. F., et al. (2008). Antepartum and postpartum exposure to maternal depression: Different effects on different adolescent outcomes. *Journal of Child Psychology and Psychiatry, and Allied Disciplines, 49,* 1079.

Jancin, B. (2005). Insomnia might blunt response to antidepressants. *Clinical Psychiatry News, 33,* 53.

Keltner, N. L., & Boschini, D. (2009). Electroconvulsive therapy. *Perspectives in Psychiatric Care, 45,* 79.

Keltner, N. L., Hogan, B., & Guy, D. M. (2001a). Dopaminergic and serotonergic receptor function in the CNS. *Perspectives in Psychiatric Care, 37,* 65.

Keltner, N. L., et al. (2001b). Adrenergic, cholinergic, GABAergic, and glutaminergic receptor function in the CNS. *Perspectives in Psychiatric Care, 37,* 140.

Kessler, R. C., et al. (2003). The epidemiology of major depressive disorder: Results from the National Comorbidity Survey Replication. *Journal of the American Medical Association, 289,* 3095.

Klerman, G. L. (1989). The interpersonal model. In J. J. Mann (Ed.), *Models of depressive disorders.* New York: Plenum Press.

Krystal, A. D., et al. (2000). ECT stimulus intensity: Are present ECT devices too limited? *American Journal of Psychiatry, 157,* 963.

Lisanby, S. H. (2007). Electroconvulsive therapy for depression. *New England Journal of Medicine, 357,* 1939.

Lisanby, S. H., et al. (2008). Toward individualized post-electroconvulsive therapy care: Piloting the Symptom-Titrated, Algorithm-Based Longitudinal ECT (STABLE) intervention. *The Journal of ECT, 24,* 179.

Maes, M., et al. (1994). A further investigation of basal HPT axis function in unipolar depression: Effects of diagnosis, hospitalization, and dexamethasone administration. *Psychiatry Research, 51,* 185.

McEnany, G. W. (1995a). *Neuropsychiatric disorders: Dementia versus depression versus drug intoxication.* Presented at the Contemporary Forum's Tenth Anniversary Conference on Psychiatric Nursing, Boston.

McEnany, G. W. (1995b). *Restless nights: Understanding and treating sleep disturbances.* Presented at the Contemporary Forum's Tenth Anniversary Conference on Psychiatric Nursing, Boston.

Michelson, D. (2009). Depression: Body and brain. *Biological Psychiatry, 66,* 405.

Miller, M. C. (2007). Electroconvulsive therapy. *The Harvard Mental Health Letter, 23,* 14.

Miller, M., Azrael, D., & Hemenway, D. (2004). The epidemiology of case fatality rates for suicide in the northeast. *Annals of Emergency Medicine, 43,* 723.

National Institute of Mental Health. (2011). *Depression.* http://www.nimh.nih.gov/health/publications/depression/complete-index.shtml, Accessed November 11, 2013.

Nemeroff, C. B. (1998). The neurobiology of depression. *Scientific American, 278,* 42.

Nuttall, G. A., et al. (2004). Morbidity and mortality in the use of electroconvulsive therapy. *The Journal of ECT, 20,* 237.

Pearson, J. (1998). *Suicide in the United States. The decade of the brain.* Arlington, VA: National Alliance on Mental Illness.

Pearson, R. M., et al. (2010). Depressive symptoms in early pregnancy disrupt attentional processing of infant emotion. *Psychological Medicine, 40,* 621.

Pierce, K., et al. (2008). Electroconvulsive review: Current clinical standards. *Psychopharmacology Review, 43,* 35.

Potter, W., & Rudorfer, M. (1993). Electroconvulsive therapy: A modern medical procedure. *New England Journal of Medicine, 328,* 12.

Roose, S. P., & Nobler, M. (2001). ECT and onset of action. *Journal of Clinical Psychiatry, 62*(Suppl. 4), 24.

Sackeim, H. A., et al. (1993). Effects of stimulus intensity and electrode placement on the efficacy and cognitive effects of electroconvulsive therapy. *New England Journal of Medicine, 328,* 839.

Sadock, B. J., & Sadock, V. A. (2003). *Synopsis of psychiatry* (9th ed.). Philadelphia: Lippincott Williams & Wilkins.

Schwartz, T. L. (2005). Unipolar, bipolar, and psychotic depression. *Clinical Psychiatry News, 33*(Suppl.), 1.

Scott, A. I. (2008). Decreased usage of electroconvulsive therapy: Implications. *British Journal of Psychiatry, 192,* 476.

Shucter, S. R., Downs, N., & Zisook, S. (1996). *Biologically informed psychotherapy for depression.* New York: Guilford Press.

Sit, D. K., & Wisner, K. L. (2009). Identification of postpartum depression. *Clinical Obstetrics and Gynecology, 52,* 456.

Smith, D. (2001). Shock and disbelief. *Atlantic Monthly, 287,* 79.

Soares, J. C., & Mann, J. J. (1997a). The anatomy of mood disorders: Review of structural neuroimaging studies. *Biological Psychiatry, 41,* 86.

Soares, J. C., & Mann, J. J. (1997b). The functional neuroanatomy of mood disorders. *Journal of Psychiatric Research, 31,* 397.

Splete, H. (2005). VNS therapy is approved for severe depression. *Clinical Psychiatry News, 33,* 1.

Stahl, S. M. (2000). Blue genes and the monoamine hypothesis of depression. *Journal of Clinical Psychiatry, 61,* 77.

Swartz, C. M. (1993). Seizure benefit: Grand mal or grand bene? *Neurologic Clinics, 11,* 151.

Teodorczuk, A., et al. (2010). Relationship between baseline white-matter changes and development of late-life depressive symptoms: 3-year results from the LADIS study. *Psychological Medicine, 40,* 603.

Tomac, T. A., Rummans, T. A., & Pileggi, T. S. (1997). Safety and efficacy of electroconvulsive therapy in patients over age 85. *American Journal of Geriatric Psychiatry, 5,* 126.

Tomoda, A., et al. (2009). Reduced prefrontal cortical gray matter volume in young adults exposed to harsh corporal punishment. *NeuroImage, 47*(Suppl. 2), T66.

Warren, B. J. (1997). Depression, stressful life events, social support, and self-esteem in middle class African American women. *Archives of Psychiatric Nursing, 11,* 107.

Zeitlin, S. V. (2001). Grief and bereavement. *Primary Care, 28,* 415.

Ziring, B. (1993). Issues in the perioperative care of the patient with psychiatric illness. *Medical Clinics of North America, 77,* 443.

Bipolar Disorders

Norman L. Keltner

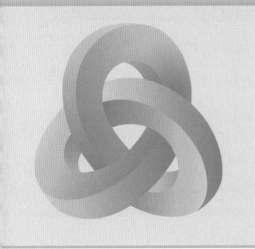

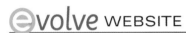

http://evolve.elsevier.com/Keltner

LEARNING OBJECTIVES

- Recognize the *DSM-5* criteria and terminology for bipolar disorder.
- Describe the objective and subjective symptoms of bipolar disorder.
- Explain the biologic and psychosocial hypotheses for bipolar disorder.

- Describe the psychotherapeutic management issues related to bipolar disorder.
- Formulate a nursing care plan for bipolar disorder using the psychotherapeutic management model.

Nothing is more addictive than the high of a manic euphoria. Once you have tasted that soaring, exhilarating, invincible, phantasmagorical feeling of, "It's great to be me! I can do anything!," once you've experienced the rush of your mind in overdrive, the creativity pouring through it, the connectivity of burgeoning lateral thinking, the ridiculous ease of witty repartee, the unutterable knowledge of your own immensity, your own infinity, then life without another mania is a dreary prospect indeed.

M. Orum

GENERAL DESCRIPTION OF BIPOLAR DISORDER

Bipolar disorders are disorders in which individuals experience the extremes of mood polarity. Individuals might feel very euphoric or very depressed. A depressive episode is not required for this diagnosis, but a manic episode is required. Bipolar disorder has been deemed the most expensive mental health disorder (Centers for Disease Control, 2013).

Box 26-1 lists the symptoms likely to occur in either a manic episode or a depressive episode. Bipolar disorder can be traced from earliest recorded history to the present day. Thousands of years ago, the Greeks recognized the vacillation between extremes of elation and depression. Other people have also observed and recorded wide mood swings for the historic record. Although the term *bipolar disorder (BD)* is

the accepted diagnostic terminology, many professionals as well as much professional literature still use the terms *manic-depressive* or *bipolar affective disorder*. These terms are used interchangeably in this chapter.

Epidemiologic research has indicated that about 5 million women and men in the United States (about 1.8% of the adult population) experience bipolar disorders (BD I, BD II, and cyclothymic disorder) yearly (American Psychiatric Association, 2013). The median age of onset is 25 years with men having an earlier age onset (Centers for Disease Control, 2013). Slightly more than 0.6% of the U.S. population has the more debilitating BD I. Approximately 4.1% of the U.S. population have major bipolar disorders at some point during their lifetime (American Psychiatric Association, 2013; Kessler et al., 2005b). Another 2% have what has been referred to as *subthreshold bipolar disorder*, or a bipolar spectrum disorder; this simply means that a large number of people do not meet the criteria for a diagnosis but nonetheless experience distressing symptoms (Paris, 2009; Zoler, 2005a). Because statistics can be mind numbing, they are repeated for clarity as follows (American Psychiatric Association, 2013; Centers for Disease Control, 2013):

1. 0.6% have BD I over the course of 1 year
2. 1.8% have BD I or BD II over the course of 1 year
3. 1% may experience cyclothymic disorder over their lifetime
4. 4.1% develop BD I or BD II in their lifetime
5. Median age of onset is 25

BOX 26-1 SYMPTOMS OCCURRING DURING MANIC AND DEPRESSIVE EPISODES

Manic Episode
Elevated mood
Grandiosity, inflated self-esteem
Irritability
Anger
Insomnia
Anorexia
Flamboyant gestures
Flight of ideas, racing thoughts
Distractibility
Hyperactivity
Involvement in pleasurable activities
Loud, rapid speech; talkative
High energy
Increased interest in sex
High rate of suicide
Excessive makeup

Other Symptoms
Labile mood
Delusions
Hallucinations

Depressed mood
Low self-esteem

Depressive Episode
Withdrawal
Passivity
Insomnia, daytime sleepiness
Anorexia
Sluggish thinking
Difficulty concentrating, distractibility
Inertia
Diminished interest in activities, inappropriate or excessive guilt
Decrease in speech
Fatigue
Decreased interest in sex
High rate of suicide

Other Symptoms
Memory loss
Abnormal thoughts about death
Weight loss

BOX 26-2 FACTS ABOUT BIPOLAR DISORDER

1. Average age of onset is early twenties for both men and women.
2. BD I occurs about equally in men and women.
3. Up to 50% of patients with bipolar disorders are nonadherent with medications.
4. In a given year, BD I affects more than 0.6% of the adult population.
5. In a given year, all bipolar disorders affect more than 1.8% of the adult population.
6. People with bipolar disorders account for about one fourth (25%) of all completed suicides.
7. About 37% of patients with bipolar disorders relapse in the first year, and only 24% regain a "normal" life.
8. Untreated, a person with a bipolar disorder might experience 10 or more episodes over a lifetime.
9. Bipolar disorder runs in families.
10. Chronic interpersonal and occupational difficulties are experienced by 60% of people with bipolar disorders.

Modified from American Psychiatric Association (2002, 2013); Anonymous (2008).

Similar to schizophrenia, onset tends to be in the early twenties, and for 90% of affected individuals, symptoms are recurrent (Box 26-2). The few individuals who have a later onset typically experience a less severe course (Moon, 2005). BD I appears to be almost equally common among men and women but with evidence of a difference in order of expression. If the first episode is a manic episode, it more likely occurred in a man, but for both women and men, depression is more likely to be experienced first (American Psychiatric Association, 2002). There is also evidence to support the belief that pregnancy often causes relapse in women with a history of bipolar

disorder (Zoler, 2005b). There are no reports of differential incidence based on ethnic or racial groups. Some individuals are often given a misdiagnosis of schizophrenia when a diagnosis of bipolar disorder would be more appropriate. This misdiagnosis is understandable because these two disorders share common characteristics (Anonymous, 2009; Sherman, 2005). Table 26-1 compares the 12-month prevalence rate of bipolar disorders with other mental disorders. Table 26-2 outlines the similarities between BD I and schizophrenia.

NORM'S NOTES
This is a fascinating subject. Note Ms. Orum's quote at the beginning of the chapter. She is honest—she was addicted to the euphoric highs of manic depression. When you meet people with this condition, you might be intimidated because they are moving so fast mentally. Their thoughts can fly so quickly that you cannot keep up, but you are there to be therapeutic. This is where your instructor really needs to give you guidance. Talking to a person in a manic state is one of the most challenging situations in psychiatric nursing.

DSM-5 TERMINOLOGY AND CRITERIA

DSM-5 defines several variations under the category of bipolar disorders, as previously noted. To understand *DSM-5* diagnostic categories, the student must be able to distinguish the basic syndromes presented, such as the manic episode and the hypomanic episode.

 CRITICAL THINKING QUESTION

1. Can a person fall within the bipolar spectrum but not meet the *DSM-5* criteria for bipolar disorder?

TABLE 26-1 12-MONTH PREVALENCE RATE OF MENTAL DISORDERS IN THE UNITED STATES*

DISORDERS	APPROXIMATE PERCENTAGE >17 YEARS OLD (%)* (unless noted for children)	GENDER OVERREPRE-SENTATION
Anxiety disorders	18.1 overall	
Agoraphobia	1.7	Female
Panic disorder	2.4	Female
Panic attacks	11.2	Female
Social anxiety	7	Female
Specific phobia	7-9	Female
Separation anxiety	1.2	Equal
Generalized anxiety disorder	2	Female
Posttraumatic stress disorder	3.4	Female
Obsessive-compulsive disorder	1.2	Equal
Major depression	8.6	Female
Bipolar disorder I and II	1.8	BD I: ~Equal
		BD II: Female
Autism spectrum disorders	1 in children	Male
Disruptive, impulse control, and conduct disorders	8.9 overall	
Conduct disorders*	4 in children	Male
Attention-deficit/ hyperactivity disorder*	5 in children; 2.5 in adults	Male
Substance use disorders	8.9 overall	
Alcohol use disorder	8.5 in adults; 2.5 in 12- to 17-year-olds	Male
Drug use disorders	1.4	Male
Schizophrenia	1.1	~Equal

*No one source has all of this information. This information has been derived from the following sources: Kessler, R.C., et al. (2012). Twelve-month and lifetime prevalence and lifetime morbid risk of anxiety and mood disorders in the United States. *International Journal of Methods of Psychiatric Research, 21,* 169; Substance Abuse and Mental Health Services Administration (2009). *Results from the 2008 national survey on drug use and health: national findings.* <http://www.samhsa.gov/data/nsduh/2k8nsduh/2k8Results.htm> Accessed November 13, 2013; American Psychiatric Association (2013). *Diagnostic and statistical manual of mental disorders* (5th ed.). Arlington, VA: APA.

Manic Episodes

Manic episodes are characterized by an elevated, expansive, or irritable mood and are fundamental to the diagnosis of BD I. To meet diagnostic criteria, the symptoms must persist for at least 1 week (or less time if hospitalization is required).

TABLE 26-2 SIMILARITIES BETWEEN BIPOLAR I DISORDER AND SCHIZOPHRENIA

	BIPOLAR I	SCHIZOPHRENIA
Gender affected	Equal	Equal
Mean age of onset	20s	20s
Genetic factors	Yes	Yes
One affected parent	25% risk	15% risk
Two affected parents	50% risk	35% risk
Identical twin	40%-80%	50%
Course	Chronic	Chronic
Suicide	15%	10%
Cigarette smoking	Increased	Increased
Substance abuse	Increased	Increased
Ventricular enlargement	Yes	Yes
Hippocampal volume	Reduced	Reduced
Very sensitive to stress	Yes	Yes

Modified from Sherman, C. (2005). Schizophrenia-bipolar I theory gains traction. *Clinical Psychiatry News, 33,* 27.

Symptoms are listed in Box 26-1. Manic episodes usually begin suddenly, escalate rapidly, and last a few days to several months. Judgment is impaired, social blunders occur, and involvement with alcohol and drugs is common. Onset is usually in the early twenties. Individuals experiencing a manic episode have an inflated view of their importance, sometimes reaching grandiosity (e.g., "I'm so important that the president needs my advice on international affairs"). The impairment is sufficiently serious that functioning deteriorates at home, work, school, or in social contexts. Other symptoms include a decreased need for sleep, talkativeness, racing thoughts, and distractibility. The mind seems to go faster and faster. Individuals experiencing a manic episode might engage in risky behavior, such as sexual relationships that are not in keeping with their normal conduct. People might speculate on a risky business venture because they understand the big picture of business. People have lost everything in these periods of manic thinking. Excess is common: spending sprees, sexual indiscretions, loud clothing, and excessive makeup are often seen in individuals in a manic state. Hospitalization is frequently required to prevent harm to the person or to others. Manic episodes can also be part of other mental disorders or a general medical condition (Box 26-3), or they might be substance-induced (Box 26-4).

Relapse: Relapse is a fact of life with mania. Research suggests that 37% of patients relapse in 1 year, 60% relapse within 2 years, and 73% relapse within 5 years (Anonymous, 2008).

Famous people with bipolar disorder: Many famous people have had bipolar disorder. Although there are many historical figures that could be mentioned, perhaps more meaningful to nursing students would be contemporary figures from American culture (*List of people believed to have been affected by bipolar disorder;* n.d.):

Kurt Cobain (singer)
Patricia Cornwell (author)
DMX (rapper)
Patty Duke (actress)

BOX 26-3 MEDICAL CONDITIONS THAT CAUSE MANIA

Anoxia
Hyperthyroidism
Hemodialysis
Lyme disease
Hypercalcemia
AIDS
Stroke
Brain tumor
Multiple sclerosis
Normal-pressure hydrocephalus
Other neurologic disorders

From Keltner, N.L., & Folks, D.G. (2005). *Psychotropic drugs* (4th ed). St. Louis: Mosby.

BOX 26-4 DRUGS THAT CAN CAUSE MANIA

Antidepressants
Steroids
Anticholinergics
Stimulants
Levodopa

Mel Gibson (actor)
Jesse Jackson, Jr. (politician)
Margot Kidder (actress)
Amy Winehouse (singer)

The following clinical example outlines the success and then the failure of a successful businessman.

Clinical Example

Bill is a 50-year-old former chief executive officer of a computer software company. Bill built the company from scratch into a multimillion dollar–a–year endeavor. It was his second time to develop a profitable business from the ground up. In the late 1980s, while in his early thirties, Bill left a nationally recognized computer company and went into business on his own. Within 3 years, his company was remarkably profitable with what seemed an unlimited potential. However, 4 years later, the business was bankrupt. He started a second business in 1998 and experienced even more success with it. Eventually, the new business became insolvent as well. The reason that both businesses failed is directly linked to Bill's bipolar disorder. Although he credits the energy and goal-directed drive associated with the illness for helping him achieve great success, grandiose (e.g., unwarranted expansion, excessive spending) and unrealistic (e.g., he believed the government could not function without his computer applications) thinking eventually drove his business into the ground. As he puts it, "I also lost two businesses, two wives, and three children because of this illness." Both episodes of bipolar disorder required hospitalization.

Bill has never really recovered from the financial and personal setbacks of his last nervous breakdown. He now lives in a county-operated apartment complex with other people who have a persistent mental disorder. Bill has a limited income and, although significantly improved, continues to display mood lability and other residual symptoms. He volunteers at a community mental health center and acknowledges that he most likely will never be a wheeler-dealer again. He is able to laugh about the good old days, when he would drive into a Cadillac dealership and buy two cars, one for himself and one for his girlfriend of the moment.

DSM-5 CRITERIA

Bipolar I Disorder

Diagnostic Criteria

For a diagnosis of bipolar I disorder, it is necessary to meet the following criteria for a manic episode. The manic episode may have been preceded by and may be followed by hypomanic or major depressive episodes.

Manic Episode

A. A distinct period of abnormally and persistently elevated, expansive, or irritable mood and abnormally and persistently increased goal-directed activity or energy, lasting at least 1 week and present most of the day, nearly every day (or any duration if hospitalization is necessary).

B. During the period of mood disturbance and increased energy or activity, three (or more) of the following symptoms (four if the mood is only irritable) are present to a significant degree and represent a noticeable change from usual behavior:
   1. Inflated self-esteem or grandiosity
   2. Decreased need for sleep (e.g., feels rested after only 3 hours of sleep)
   3. More talkative than usual or pressure to keep talking
   4. Flight of ideas or subjective experience that thoughts are racing
   5. Distractibility (i.e., attention too easily drawn to unimportant or irrelevant external stimuli), as reported or observed
   6. Increase in goal-directed activity (either socially, at work or school, or sexually) or psychomotor agitation (i.e., purposeless non–goal-directed activity)
   7. Excessive involvement in activities that have a high potential for painful consequences (e.g., engaging in unrestrained buying sprees, sexual indiscretions, or foolish business investments)

C. The mood disturbance is sufficiently severe to cause marked impairment in social or occupational functioning or to necessitate hospitalization to prevent harm to self or others, or there are psychotic features.

D. The episode is not attributable to the physiological effects of a substance (e.g., a drug of abuse, a medication, other treatment) or to another medical condition.

Note: A full manic episode that emerges during antidepressant treatment (e.g., medication, electroconvulsive therapy) but persists at a fully syndromal level beyond the physiological effect of that treatment is sufficient evidence for a manic episode and, therefore, a bipolar I diagnosis.

Note: Criteria A-D constitute a manic episode. At least one lifetime manic episode is required for the diagnosis of bipolar I disorder.

From American Psychiatric Association (2013). *Diagnostic and statistical manual of mental disorders* (5th ed.). Arlington, Virginia: APA.

Hypomanic Episodes

My manias, at least in their early and mild forms, were absolutely intoxicating states that gave rise to great personal pleasure, an incomparable flow of thoughts, and a ceaseless energy that allowed the translation of new ideas into papers and projects.

Dr. Kay Redfield Jamison (1997, pp. 5-6)

The hypomanic episode is similar to the manic episode but denotes a less severe level of impairment. Because patients feel good about themselves and their life, hypomania is perceived as normal. Both BD II and cyclothymia diagnoses require evidence of a hypomanic episode. Because the level of severity is subjective, *DSM-5* attempts to differentiate hypomanic from manic episodes with more objective criteria. For a hypomanic episode to be diagnosed, the length of the episode must be at *least 4 days* in duration but not severe enough to warrant hospitalization. Additionally, the episode is not severe enough to cause "marked impairment" at home, work, school, or in the social milieu but is observable by others and is distinct from the person's typical behavior. The episode is characterized by an abnormal period of persistent elevated, expansive, or irritable mood. Additionally, the individual must experience at least three of the following symptoms:

- Increased self-esteem or grandiosity
- Decreased need for sleep
- Increased talkativeness
- Subjective sense that thoughts are racing
- Distractibility
- Increase in goal-directed activity (usually social, occupational, educational, or sexual) or motor agitation
- Excessive involvement in pleasurable activities that have a high potential for painful consequences

Wilf (2012) questioned whether the threshold of 4 days causes us to miss some individuals who are headed for trouble. He suggested that consideration be given to treating individuals manifesting hypomanic symptoms even when they do not meet the full 4-day criterion.

Depressive Episodes

Bipolar depression causes more suffering than the manic state (Anonymous, 2008). Bipolar depression differs from unipolar (regular major depression) in some significant ways and tends to be more debilitating. First, depressive symptoms tend to be atypical. Atypical depressions cause hypersomnia not insomnia, hyperphagia not anorexia, and weight gain not weight loss. The person might develop an intense craving for carbohydrates and might experience a leaden paralysis, with little energy to propel himself or herself around. Bipolar depression typically develops at a younger age than unipolar depression, and the patient is more likely to express paranoid thoughts, be irritable, and experience hallucinations.

BIPOLAR DISORDERS

DSM-5 bipolar diagnoses are based on an understanding of manic episodes, hypomanic episodes, and major depression.

As noted, *DSM-5* divides bipolar diagnoses into BD I, BD II, cyclothymic disorders, and substance- or medication-induced bipolar disorder.

Bipolar Diagnoses
Bipolar I Disorder

BD I is the most significant of the bipolar disorders. In BD I, the patient experiences swings between manic episodes (defined earlier) and major depression (defined in Chapter 25). Figure 26-1 illustrates the subtle differences in the bipolar disorders. *DSM-5* provides numerous *specifiers*. These specifiers include:

With anxious distress
With mixed features

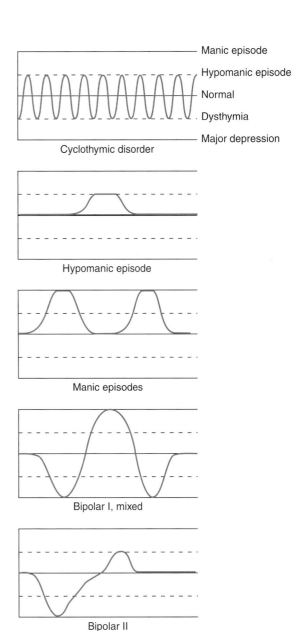

FIG 26-1 Differences in the bipolar disorders on the mood continuum. By understanding this figure, the student can conceptualize the differences among these bipolar disorders.

With rapid cycling
With melancholic features
With atypical features
With psychotic features
With catatonia
With peripartum onset
With seasonal pattern

Bipolar II Disorder

BD II is similar to BD I, with the major exception being that the person has never experienced a manic episode but only a hypomanic episode. In this disorder, the person has experienced major depression (lasting at least 2 weeks) but has experienced a hypomanic episode (lasting at least 4 days), rather than a full manic episode. There seems to be a higher incidence of this disorder among women. Over the course of a few years, 5% to 15% of individuals with BD II go on to develop a full manic episode (American Psychiatric Association, 2013).

> **? CRITICAL THINKING QUESTION**
>
> 2. What do you think of the following statement? "There are many people in American society who could be diagnosed as hypomanic. Many high-level, workaholic executives are hypomanic and just don't know it."

Cyclothymic Disorder

Cyclothymic disorder is defined as a swing between a hypomanic episode and dysthymia. The swings in either direction are not severe enough to warrant the ultimate diagnoses of manic episode and major depression. Using a pendulum as a metaphor, the person experiencing cyclothymic disorder swings from one side to the other but never reaches the extremes of the arc. The person is elated and expansive but does not meet the criteria for manic episode. Cyclothymic disorder is characterized by symptoms that have occurred for at least 2 years, without symptom remission for more than 2 months. The person experiences numerous hypomanic episodes and numerous dysthymic-level episodes. Cyclothymic disorder is equally distributed between men and women, with a lifetime risk of 0.4% to 1%. About 15% to 50% of these individuals go on to develop full-blown bipolar disorder (American Psychiatric Association, 2013).

Behavior

Objective Behavior

The person experiencing a manic episode appears enthusiastic and euphoric. Other people around the person recognize these behaviors as excessive. Objective behaviors include disturbances of speech; of the individual's social, interpersonal, and occupational relationships; and of activity and appearance. Violent behavior, divorce, spousal and child abuse, job loss, and academic failure are common features of this illness.

Clinical Example

Sue is a 45-year-old Jewish woman who is admitted for bipolar disorder. Police were called to the Greyhound bus station, where they found Sue annoying customers. She claimed to be a Messianic Jew and was preaching to anyone who would politely listen. She resisted the officers and repeatedly stated that she was the "woman at the well" and had married Christ. On arriving on the unit, it was noted that Sue had excessive bright-red lipstick on, dramatically enhanced eyebrows, and turquoise eye shadow. The rest of her clothing appeared unattended to, and she was dirty and smelly. She is known to the hospital staff and, after her initial physical assessment, was prescribed and received lithium. This particular drug had been quite effective in the past.

Disturbed Speech Patterns. The following are examples of disturbed speech patterns of manic individuals:
- Rapid speech
- Pressured speech
- Loud speech
- Easily distracted

Manic patients might speak loudly in a rapid-fire fashion; they monopolize the dialogue and deflect attempts by others to contribute to the dialogue. Conversations are filled with jokes and puns. Sarcastic and biting remarks are common. Even though mental health professionals are aware of this tendency, the ability of manic patients to find a weak spot often frustrates, embarrasses, and angers mental health professionals. The tendency to complain often and loudly is also present. Manic patients have the ability to engage staff members in debate and place them on the defensive. Speech is often dramatic, and it is common for manic individuals to burst into song. Speech is often pressured (i.e., they have a compulsion or strong need to talk).

These patients also are easily distracted. For example, while in the middle of an apparently meaningful discussion, a patient might be distracted by a bird flying outside the window and change the topic of the conversation to flying. This phenomenon, in which patients jump from topic to topic, is referred to as *flight of ideas*.

Altered Social, Interpersonal, and Occupational Relationships. Manic individuals often have changes in their relationship patterns, such as the following:
- Failed relationships
- Job loss and job failure
- Overbearing behavior
- Increased sex drive
- Alienation of family

Clinical Example

Demographics: A young man (Bob, age 30) and a young woman (Mary, age 26), are engaged, with a wedding date planned for the near future.

Background: Both are college-educated, with particularly promising careers.

The setting: Mary flies into a rage and breaks off the engagement when Bob asks her if she will let the pets out. Mary leaves for 3 weeks, then returns the day before a relative's funeral. Bob attends with her, and she introduces him as her fiancé.

The crisis: After the funeral, she tells Bob: "I got married to my old boyfriend while I was gone. It was a mistake. I went to see my doctor. He thinks I have bipolar disorder."

As this clinical example suggests (Shattell & Keltner, 2004), a manic episode can cause chaos in the life of an individual and the people close to that individual.

Manic patients irritate others with their impulsive behaviors, fault finding, anger, and blaming. This disorder destroys relationships. In a classic article, Janowsky et al. (1970) list five tendencies that cause social, interpersonal, and occupational problems for bipolar patients:

1. *Manipulation of the self-esteem of others.* Patients use coercive techniques to increase or decrease another's self-esteem. It is easy to fall prey to the manipulation of praise (e.g., "No one here really understands me but you"). It is just as easy to feel the ego-deflating wrath when plans are thwarted. Some insightful nurses have remarked about feeling like "having been played like a yo-yo."
2. *Ability to find vulnerability in others.* Manic patients can exploit weakness in others or create conflicts among staff members.
3. *Ability to shift responsibility.* Through the technique mentioned earlier, patients shift personal responsibility (e.g., being late) to someone else. Nurses are particularly vulnerable in this area because they are trained to take responsibility for many concerns of their patients.
4. *Limit testing.* Manic patients keep pushing the limits established by the treatment setting. If a limit is relaxed, these patients push it even more.
5. *Alienation of family.* Manic patients can drive away their families with their behavior. The cyclic nature of the disorder at first inspires hope in the family. After numerous cycles, families often sink into a demoralized state. Divorce related to child and spousal abuse is common during severe manic episodes.

NORM'S NOTES

Each semester, many of my students question why a patient's family is distant or even out of the picture altogether. In other words, some students suspect that the family has abandoned the patient. My advice is something you have heard all your life: There are two sides to every story. Some families give up too easily, and others have exhausted all avenues to make things work—and they didn't work. Right or wrong, many tired and demoralized families have flown a white flag and retreated.

The same behaviors that drive away family also drive away friends, lovers, bosses, coworkers, ministers, and nonpsychiatric health care providers.

Several trends have been noted among individuals with bipolar disorder:

1. Failed relationships are common for individuals who do not receive adequate treatment.
2. Most individuals report difficulties maintaining long-term friendships.
3. Job loss and job change are common.
4. A need to engage people, even strangers, in conversation characterizes bipolar disorder. Although at first behavior such as this attracts others, soon the overbearing and intrusive nature of the conversation alienates and even frightens people.
5. Mood lability can cause these individuals to fall in and out of love rapidly, with all the associated problems for themselves and others.

The effects of bipolar illness permeate all types of relationships. The expansive mood overflows into excesses as well. The otherwise faithful spouse might become sexually promiscuous, the otherwise thrifty homemaker might go on a shopping or spending spree, and the conservative investor might make a dangerously speculative investment. Divorce rates are two to three times higher than for comparable couples (American Psychiatric Association, 2002).

Alterations in Activity and Appearance. Manic patients are often hyperactive and agitated. Overt manifestations, such as pacing, flamboyant gestures, colorful dress, singing, and excessive use of makeup, are common. Patients also might dress sloppily and omit personal grooming; they might not need sleep or perhaps need only a few hours per night. Some patients have gone for days without sleep, and reports of manic patients dropping from exhaustion previously were common. Many manic patients have poor nutrition because they stop eating; they simply do not have the patience, the ability to sit still long enough, or the desire to eat.

Subjective Behavior

Alterations of Affect. Manic patients experience euphoria and a high regard for self. The inflated self-image can reach levels of grandiosity. Subjectively, the person going through a manic episode experiences an elevated mood, a feeling of joy, and a sense of greatness. A certain sense of invincibility leads to the social, interpersonal, and occupational problems already discussed.

Another significant symptom is a labile or quickly changing affect. Rapid mood swings are exhibited as changing from elation to irritability or from happiness to anger. For example, a 64-year-old woman was laughing and talking about her personal acquaintance with former President Bush. "You know, my husband's name was George." She abruptly began to cry. "He is dead, you know." She quickly returned to the topic of her importance, becoming very excited, with an elevated mood.

Alterations of Perception. Delusions and hallucinations occur, and their content is typically consistent with mood. For example, if a patient is grandiose about his or her importance to the government, a mood-congruent delusion might include paranoid thinking related to being pursued by enemy forces.

Etiology

Psychosocial Theories. At one time, most psychiatric professionals believed that bipolar illness or manic-depressive illness was caused by psychological difficulties. Developmental theorists have hypothesized that faulty family dynamics during early life are responsible for manic behaviors in later life. According to this view, the mother (or primary caregiver) enjoys being the giver of life and resents autonomy. As the child grows more independent, the mother becomes unhappy, so to please the mother, the child becomes more dependent; that is, to gain affection, the child at an early age learns to deny his or her own natural tendencies. According to this view, the unnatural tension between dependence and independence and the inherent ambivalence in this family environment can be a causative factor in bipolar illness. Others have suggested that the polar events (e.g., approval or disapproval) of childhood are so significant for some people that an adult emotional counterpart to the emotional roller coaster results—for example, receiving approval (elation) and disapproval (depression). Although some psychosocial explanations seem more credible than others, many professionals believe that family dynamics play an important role in the genesis of manic-depressive illness.

Another psychosocial hypothesis explains manic episodes as a defense against or massive denial of depression. According to this view, manic-depressive individuals go through life appearing to be independent and excessive to others (e.g., too pushy, too talkative, and too manipulative), only to be eventually blocked by someone who no longer tolerates being pushed, talked to, or manipulated. When this happens, the manic individual (who is actually overdependent) can become psychotic.

Neurotransmitter and Structural Hypotheses

Although some professionals still believe in the importance of psychological influences, most are aware of the role of biology. Just as depression seems to be caused by neurotransmitter deficiency, manic episodes also seem to be related to excessive levels of norepinephrine and dopamine, an imbalance between cholinergic and noradrenergic systems, or a deficiency in serotonin. El-Mallakh (1996) proposed that bipolar disorder, including both manic and depressive symptoms, arises from ion dysregulation. Box 26-5 summarizes this interesting hypothesis. *If* the ion view is correct, *then* differences between normal depression (or unipolar depression) and the depression associated with bipolar disorder can be more clearly appreciated. A common diagnostic mistake is making an incorrect diagnosis of major depression in someone who is actually experiencing the depressive aspect of bipolar disorder. Prescribing an antidepressant would be appropriate for unipolar depression, but such a treatment strategy is controversial when a patient has bipolar depression. Giving an antidepressant to a patient with bipolar depression often pushes the individual into a manic state (American Psychiatric Association, 2013). Nonetheless, treating bipolar depression with antidepressants is common but usually is tried only after several other options have failed.

A more compelling view of altered biochemistry in bipolar disorder has been advanced by Manji and Lenox (2000). They outlined the evidence for a breakdown in the complicated second messenger systems of neurons. In the multistep second messenger system, when a neurotransmitter binds to a receptor, intracellular processes are triggered. First, a protein (called a *G-protein*) attaches to the underbelly of the receptor complex, which triggers the attachment of an enzyme. This enzyme stimulates another intracellular entity (often either cyclic adenosine monophosphate or inositol), which causes the activation of protein kinases that turn on transcription factors in the nucleus. At this point, the

---

BOX 26-5   WHAT GOES WRONG IN BIPOLAR DISORDER

It is known that individuals with bipolar disorder have specific signs and symptoms (e.g., elevated mood, grandiosity, irritability, insomnia, anorexia). What is not known is exactly what causes this disorder to happen. The question remains: "What goes wrong in bipolar disorder?" El-Mallakh (1996) has proposed a convincing model for the pathology of bipolar disorder, suggesting that a disruption in ion regulation is the cause. Ion regulation is important for normal mood. A key part of ion regulation is the sodium (Na^+) and potassium (K^+)–activated adenosine triphosphatase (ATPase) pump. As this chapter explores, bipolar depression and mania are related, and this model proposes a biochemical explanation.

According to this model, both bipolar depression and mania result from a decrease in Na^+,K^+-ATPase activity. As activity declines, neuronal membranes become irritable, requiring fewer stimuli to provoke cell firing. As Na^+ accumulates intracellularly because of this faulty pumping action, hyperpolarizing functions of inhibitory neurotransmitters (e.g., gamma-aminobutyric acid) are diminished. Additionally, because neurotransmitter release is calcium dependent, the presynaptic terminals might release more neurotransmitter because of a related deficiency in Na^+-dependent calcium efflux. All of these factors contribute to increased neurotransmitter release and firing—or mania.

However, the term *bipolar* means "two poles"—the pole of mania and the pole of depression. These two poles are related. As the Na^+,K^+-ATPase pump continues to decrease in activity, neuronal irritability reaches a point whereby less stimulation triggers depolarization. The neuron fires more easily, but the action potential loses amplitude. This loss of amplitude causes calcium channels to decrease their activity and results in a subsequent reduction in neurotransmitter release. Mania is the first disorder to occur when ion dysregulation occurs, but as the Na^+,K^+-ATPase pump becomes more dysfunctional, the depressive side of bipolar disorder develops. Catatonia might be the ultimate expression of ionic dysregulation.

transcription factors can instruct genes to synthesize factors such as enzymes, receptors, or reuptake proteins or, in other words, the proteins that cause the neuron to function. Manji and Lenox (2000) showed that in bipolar disorder there is greater activity than normal with G-proteins and protein kinases and with other steps in the second messenger system. (See Figure 15-1 for a summary of the second messenger system.)

Biologic findings also suggest that brain lesions, white matter changes, and loss of periventricular gray matter are more common in people with bipolar disorder (Moore et al., 2000; Sherman, 2005; Wessa et al., 2009). Knowing what to make of these structural findings is difficult, but the neurotransmitter hypotheses are consistent with explanations of the putative mechanisms of some antimanic drugs.

Genetic Considerations

It seems clear that genetics has a role in bipolar disorder (American Psychiatric Association, 2013). Monozygotic (identical) twins have a very high concordance rate (up to 80%), whereas dizygotic (fraternal) twins have a slightly higher rate than normal siblings and other close relatives. Siblings and close relatives have a higher incidence of manic-depressive illness than the general population, and cyclothymic characteristics are common among family members of bipolar patients. The following risks have been established for developing bipolar disorder (Craddock et al., 2009):

1. First-degree relative—5% to 10%
2. Identical twin with bipolar disorder—40% to 80%

Significant issues arise surrounding family planning counseling for women with bipolar illness, including the heritability of the disease, the stress of parenthood, and the effect an ill parent has on a child. The teratogenicity of lithium, carbamazepine, and valproic acid is a concern when treating a pregnant woman with bipolar disorder. Consequently, pregnant women with bipolar disorder should be prescribed these drugs only when the risk of not doing so is greater than the risk of fetal insult. Because of these teratogenic effects, atypical antipsychotics are more likely to be prescribed to a pregnant woman.

Comorbidity

About 87% of individuals with a manic-hypomanic disorder have a comorbid mental health disorder (Kessler et al., 2005a). Comorbid mental disorders that occur in up to 50% of patients with bipolar disorders include borderline personality disorder, attention-deficit/hyperactivity disorder, generalized anxiety disorder, panic disorder, social phobias, obsessive-compulsive disorder, and posttraumatic stress disorder (Klassen et al., 2010; Marsee & Gross, 2013).

Abuse of alcohol and other substances is more common among individuals with bipolar disorder than in individuals with any other *DSM-5* diagnosis (Suppes et al., 2000). More than half of individuals with a diagnosis of bipolar disorder abuse alcohol (American Psychiatric Association, 2013), and 60% of patients with BD I have a lifetime

---

> ### BOX 26-6 PROBLEMS WITH ALCOHOL AND DRUG ABUSE IN PATIENTS WITH BIPOLAR DISORDER
>
> 1. Decreased compliance with antimanic medications
> 2. Compromised treatment results
> 3. Increased hospitalizations
> 4. Poorer treatment outcomes
> 5. Earlier onset of mood symptoms
> 6. Higher rates of anxiety
> 7. More suicide attempts
> 8. More accidents
> 9. More hospitalizations

Modified from Kosten & Kosten (2004); Nery & Soares (2011).

diagnosis of a substance abuse disorder (Nery & Soares, 2011). Additionally, individuals known to abuse drugs are five to eight times more likely to have bipolar disorder than the general public (Kessler et al., 1997). Patients with bipolar disorder who abuse drugs have higher hospitalization rates and poorer chances of recovery than their peers who do not abuse drugs (Nejtek et al., 2008). When alcohol use is superimposed on co-occurring bipolar disorder and substance abuse, early depression is a frequent outcome (Jaffee et al., 2009). Some clinicians believe that most first-time diagnoses of bipolar disorder are made in the emergency department related to the consequences of alcohol or other substance abuse. Strakowski and DelBello (2000) advanced the following four hypotheses to account for the high rate of substance abuse in patients with bipolar disorder:

1. Substance abuse occurs as a symptom of bipolar disorder.
2. Substance abuse is an attempt by patients with bipolar disorder to self-medicate.
3. Substance abuse causes bipolar disorders.
4. Substance use and bipolar disorders share a common risk factor.

The use and abuse of alcohol and other substances cause several problems for the patient with bipolar disorder: relapse rates increase, response to lithium decreases, remission is delayed, poor treatment compliance occurs, and poor treatment outcomes are common (Nery & Soares, 2011; Suppes et al., 2000). Box 26-6 outlines problems with substance use disorder in regard to patients with bipolar disorders (Kosten & Kosten, 2004).

PUTTING IT ALL TOGETHER

PSYCHOTHERAPEUTIC MANAGEMENT

There are three treatment goals when working with patients with bipolar disorder, as follows:

1. Getting acute mania under control
2. Preventing relapse when remission occurs

3. Returning to the prior level of functioning (i.e., social, occupational, interpersonal)

Nurse-Patient Relationship

The Key Nursing Interventions for a Manic Episode box lists specific interventions to be used with patients who experience manic episodes.

- *Matter-of-fact tone.* A matter-of-fact tone minimizes the need for the patient to respond defensively and avoids power struggles. By providing emotional support and responding to patients in a matter-of-fact manner, the nurse conveys both control of the situation and empathy.
- *Clear, concise directions and comments.* Working with hyperactive patients who are highly talkative, easily distracted, experience flight of ideas, and have poor judgment and a labile affect is difficult. When the nurse is confronted with talkative patients, it is not unusual for the nurse to attempt to use familiar skills. For example, most people learn not to interrupt another person until a pause. The pause might never come with manic patients. To be effective, the nurse might need to raise his or her hand and say, "Wait just a minute. I do not want to be rude, but I would like to say something." As a patient starts improving, the nurse might be able to work out a nonverbal signal to indicate when the patient needs to stop and let someone else speak. Although manic patients are talkative, there is a tendency for the talk to be superficial. When talking to hyperactive patients, the nurse should keep remarks brief and simple. Many patients literally cannot tolerate a lengthy discussion of any subject.
- *Limit setting.* When the nurse is leading a group, a talkative patient can be disruptive because of the following tendencies:
  - Manipulation of the self-esteem of others
  - Ability to find vulnerability of others
  - Ability to shift responsibility to others
  - Limit testing

These patients have the ability to damage the self-esteem of other patients, ridicule the nurse, blame others, pick fights, create problems between patients, and manipulate others. The nurse needs to protect vulnerable patients and keep them from being drawn into the anger that manic patients feel. When the nurse is able to remain calm instead of becoming angry, it helps manic patients and the other patients in the group. This calmness should be based on an understanding of psychopathology; otherwise, it might be simply an unhealthy defense by the nurse (e.g., "You cannot bother me; you are not important enough"). The nurse absolutely does not want to convey that he or she is engaged in an adult version of the childish behavior of plugging the ears and saying, "I can't hear you." It is also important to avoid arguing with patients about unit rules and limits. Do not debate these issues with patients. Simply state the unit policy and move on. Debating and arguing reinforces the tendencies mentioned earlier.

Psychopharmacology

Medication adherence in BD is a priority because of the potential neurodegeneration in BD and the neuroprotective effects of mood stabilizers and some atypical antipsychotics.
Foster et al., 2011

The efficacy of lithium and other mood stabilizers in the treatment of bipolar disorder has been recognized for years. Checking blood levels of lithium is crucial because this drug has a narrow therapeutic index. Maintenance blood levels between 0.6 and 1.2 mEq/L are standard and can usually be maintained on a dosage of 900 to 1200 mg/day. There are several alternatives to lithium. Anticonvulsants and atypical antipsychotics are very valuable drugs. The most beneficial anticonvulsants are the valproates, particularly divalproex sodium (Depakote). It is the *most prescribed* drug for bipolar disorder now with at least twice the prescriptions of lithium. Other effective anticonvulsants include carbamazepine (Tegretol) and lamotrigine (Lamictal). Lamotrigine has a

---

KEY NURSING INTERVENTIONS

for a Manic Episode

Patients Too Busy to Eat
The nurse should use the following interventions to maintain the patient's body weight:
1. Provide patients with foods that can be eaten on the run (sometimes referred to as *finger foods*) because some patients cannot sit long enough to eat.
2. Provide high-protein, high-calorie snacks for patients. A vitamin supplement might be indicated.
3. Weigh patients regularly (sometimes weighing daily is needed).

Patients Who Cannot Sleep
Manic patients experience insomnia. The nurse can help patients maximize the opportunity for sleep by doing the following:
1. Provide a quiet place to sleep.
2. Structure patient's days so that there are fewer stimulating activities toward bedtime.

3. Do not allow caffeinated drinks before bedtime.
4. Assess the amount of rest that patients are receiving. Manic patients are not capable of judging the need for rest, and exhaustion and death have resulted from lack of rest.

Other Nursing Interventions
- Reinforce reality. Manic patients also experience disturbances in perception. The intervention strategies outlined for other patients with disturbed perceptions are recommended for manic patients as well.
- Respond to legitimate complaints. Although many frivolous complaints arise, the nurse must respond to legitimate complaints to defuse irritability and develop trust.
- Redirect patients into more healthy activity. The bipolar patient's distractibility serves as an intervention tool when the patient engages in nonproductive behavior.

PATIENT AND FAMILY EDUCATION

Bipolar Disorder

Illness

Bipolar disorder is a brain disorder that disrupts mood. The patient might experience extreme moods—bouncing from depression to euphoria (or mania)—or might primarily exhibit symptoms of mania. About 0.6% of the adult population has BD I. Manic episodes are characterized by an elevated mood, irritability, inflated self-esteem, decreased need for sleep, talkativeness, distractibility, and excessive involvement in pleasurable activities. The disorder is typically diagnosed first in the early twenties and occurs about equally in men and women. Because of the pursuit of pleasurable activities, many patients with bipolar disorder overspend, become sexually involved in situations that they would normally avoid, and invest in unwise business dealings. Both dress and language can become loud and excessive. Involvement with drugs and alcohol is common.

Medications

Lithium has been the mainstay of treatment for patients with bipolar disorders; however, it is not prescribed as much as it previously was. It has some troubling side effects, so the physician or nurse practitioner may prescribe divalproex sodium (Depakote) instead. Lithium is a naturally occurring element and is located on the periodic table in the same column as sodium and potassium. Lithium is so similar to sodium that the nervous system mistakes it for sodium. However, because lithium reacts more slowly than sodium, it can be given to slow down the nervous system. Lithium works but causes some predictable side effects (e.g., fine tremor, thirst, frequent urination). Although lithium is effective for most patients, it can also cause problems because the difference is slight between a therapeutic dose and a harmful dose (or toxic dose). Because of this concern, patients with a diagnosis of bipolar disorder must have their blood tested frequently for lithium content. After long-term and stable use of lithium, blood draws become less frequent.

Antiepileptic drugs such as divalproex sodium are also used to treat bipolar disorder. Divalproex sodium is an excellent drug and the most often prescribed drug for bipolar disorder. It has fewer side effects than lithium and is safer all around. Although safer than lithium, divalproex sodium and other antiepileptic drugs also produce some significant serious side effects.

Atypical antipsychotic agents have been approved to treat bipolar disorder as well. These drugs are effective but have been known to cause substantial weight gain.

Other Issues

Patients with bipolar disorder can be very difficult to live with. Their self-importance, nonstop behavior, talkativeness, style of dress, and irritability can overwhelm a family member. However, these individuals can be remarkably creative and productive. It is important when living or dealing with individuals with this diagnosis to be matter-of-fact, clear, and concise in communication; to set limits; and to redirect critical negativism into healthier activities. Although difficult at times, it is important for the psychiatric nurse to avoid personalizing the negative, sarcastic, and rude comments that these individuals might direct toward the nurse. Solid research supports family therapy over individual therapy. Working within the context of family has been found to reduce relapse dramatically.

---

special niche because it has been found to be particularly effective in treating the depressive phase of bipolar disorder. Newer anticonvulsants such as gabapentin (Neurontin), oxcarbazepine (Trileptal), and topiramate (Topamax) are also used occasionally. Atypical antipsychotics are also approved for the treatment of acute manic episodes. The use of antidepressants to treat bipolar depression is debatable because these drugs can trigger mania (American Psychiatric Association, 2002). These drugs are discussed in detail in Chapters 14 and 15.

Milieu Management

Milieu management is an important dimension of the nursing care of manic patients because these patients test the unit or day treatment program perhaps more than any other group of patients.

1. *Safety.* It is important for the nurse to prevent manic patients from hurting themselves or others. Manic patients can become angry when things do not go their way. This pathologic irritability leads to arguments, fights, self-injury (e.g., hitting the wall, not paying attention to the environment), and hurting others. It is reassuring to patients to realize that the staff will not let them harm themselves or others.

2. *Consistency among staff.* Because manic patients tend to create conflict, pick on vulnerable individuals (patients and staff), blame others, test limits, and shift responsibility to others, the nurse must carefully develop a plan of care. Nursing and

CASE STUDY

Mr. Casey Bates, a 50-year-old attorney, was admitted to the unit with the diagnosis of bipolar I disorder, manic type. The police arrested him after he started a fight with three Hispanic men in a bar. He had been drinking heavily. He was hyperactive, distractible, irritable, talkative, and demanding on admission. He demonstrated flight of ideas and was verbally hostile concerning a Hispanic coworker, whom he accused of sleeping with his wife. Mr. Bates has vowed to get even. He made several comments about Hispanics in general while looking at Mr. Lopez, a Hispanic nurse.

This is Mr. Bates' third hospitalization. The first occurred 12 years ago when he contracted a *Candida* infection after having sexual intercourse with his wife. The second hospitalization occurred in 2008. No precipitating event was recorded, and Mr. Bates does not recollect anything unusual about the second admission.

Mr. Bates has responded well to lithium in the past; during his last hospitalization, he was also given olanzapine because of his agitation. Between hospitalizations, Mr. Bates has functioned well and is considered a good attorney. His partners appreciate his perfectionist tendencies. Mrs. Bates states that Mr. Bates has not slept in 3 days and has not stopped to eat for some time (the actual length of time is unclear). She reports a good marriage until Mr. Bates stopped taking his lithium, which he says he will no longer take. She wants him to "get better and come home." The head nurse decides to streamline the admission process because of Mr. Bates' agitated state. He is taken to a quiet area and given peanut butter crackers and milk.

other staff members should meet often to defuse conflict and clarify communication. All staff members should be aware of intervention strategies and agree to abide consistently by team decisions. Inexperienced staff members must guard against falling prey to esteem-building statements that tend to split the staff (e.g., "You're the only one who understands").

3. *Reduction of environmental stimuli.* Because manic patients are hyperactive, talkative, irritable, and angry, it is important to decrease environmental stimuli. Patients are distractible and respond to all sorts of environmental cues; it is important to modify the environment as much as possible. Helpful environmental modifications include limited activities with others, gross motor activities (e.g., walking, sweeping, aerobics) to discharge some of the need to be active, and a public room with no television or compact disc player.

4. *Dealing with patients who are escalating.* Manic patients can become hostile and aggressive. It is important for the staff to deal with this aggressiveness in a calm, confident manner. For patients who are escalating, an antipsychotic drug, such as haloperidol, can be administered to prevent physical aggressiveness, and potential weapons (e.g., chairs, pool cues) can be removed. Limits and the consequences of violating these limits should be reviewed. Do not include limits that are not significant. It is countertherapeutic to defend a poor policy, and it is also countertherapeutic to allow patients to debate a unit issue. It is therapeutic to follow through with appropriate action should a patient violate a unit norm.

5. *Reinforcement of appropriate hygiene and dress.* Patients with bipolar disorder often forget hygiene behaviors, appearing disheveled and unclean at times. Simple reminders to shower, brush teeth, and wear clean clothes can correct some problems. The nurse should also monitor for flamboyant and suggestive dress that might ultimately embarrass the patient.

6. *Nutrition and sleep issues.* Both inadequate nutrition and inadequate sleep patterns plague patients with bipolar disorder.

7. *Routines.* One of the most important contributions the nurse can make is the establishment of routines. A routine bedtime, mealtime, and wake-up time can be immensely therapeutic to patients with bipolar disorder.

YOUNG MANIA RATING SCALE

The Young Mania Rating Scale (YMRS), a popular scale for assessing the severity of mania, is summarized in Box 26-7. The YMRS is an 11-item scale with a maximum score of 60 possible (Young et al., 1978). Each of the 11 items has a 5-item gradient. For example, item 3, sexual interest, can be scored from 0 to 4:

0 = Normal; not increased
1 = Mildly or possibly increased
2 = Definite subjective increase on questioning
3 = Spontaneous sexual content; elaborates on sexual matters; hypersexual by self-report
4 = Overt sexual acts (toward patients, staff, or interviewer)

The typical minimum score for inclusion in a drug study is 20. Improvement is usually defined as a decrease in a person's YMRS score of 50%. In other studies, improvement might be defined as a specific score, such as 15. It is important to take note of how *success* is being defined in any particular study.

BOX 26-7   YOUNG MANIA RATING SCALE (YMRS)

Guide for Scoring Items

The purpose of each item is to rate the severity of that abnormality in the patient. When several keys are given for a particular grade of severity, the presence of only one is required to qualify for that rating.

The keys provided are guides. One can ignore the keys if that is necessary to indicate severity, although this should be the exception rather than the rule.

Scoring between the points given (whole points or half-points) is possible and encouraged after experience with the scale is acquired. Scoring between points is particularly useful when the severity of a particular item in a patient does not follow the progression indicated by the keys.

1. Elevated mood
   0 = Absent
   1 = Mildly or possibly increased on questioning
   2 = Definite subjective elevation; optimistic, self-confident; cheerful; appropriate to content
   3 = Elevated, inappropriate to content; humorous
   4 = Euphoric; inappropriate laughter; singing
2. Increased motor activity/energy
   0 = Absent
   1 = Subjectively increased
   2 = Animated; gestures increased
   3 = Excessive energy; hyperactive at times; restless (can be calmed)

4 = Motor excitement; continuous hyperactivity (cannot be calmed)
3. Sexual interest
   0 = Normal; not increased
   1 = Mildly or possibly increased
   2 = Definite subjective increase on questioning
   3 = Spontaneous sexual content; elaborates on sexual matters; hypersexual by self-report
   4 = Overt sexual acts (toward patients, staff, or interviewer)
4. Sleep
   0 = Reports no decrease in sleep
   1 = Sleeping less than normal amount by up to 1 hour
   2 = Sleeping less than normal by more than 1 hour
   3 = Reports decreased need for sleep
   4 = Denies need for sleep
5. Irritability
   0 = Absent
   2 = Subjectively increased
   4 = Irritable at times during interview; recent episodes of anger or annoyance on ward
   6 = Frequently irritable during interview; short or curt throughout
   8 = Hostile, uncooperative; interview impossible
6. Speech (rate and amount)
   0 = No increase
   2 = Feels talkative

BOX 26-7 YOUNG MANIA RATING SCALE (YMRS)—CONT'D

4 = Increased rate or amount at times, verbose at times
6 = Push; consistently increased rate and amount; difficult
to interrupt
8 = Pressured; uninterruptible, continuous speech
7. Language/thought disorder
0 = Absent
2 = Circumstantial; mild distractibility; quick thoughts
4 = Distractible; loses goal of thought; changes topics frequently; racing thoughts
6 = Flight of ideas; tangentiality; difficult to follow; rhyming, echolalia
8 = Incoherent; communication impossible
8. Content
0 = Normal
2 = Questionable plans; new interests
4 = Special project(s); hyperreligious
6 = Grandiose or paranoid ideas; ideas of reference
8 = Delusions; hallucinations

9. Disruptive/aggressive behavior
0 = Absent, cooperative
2 = Sarcastic; loud at times, guarded
4 = Demanding; threats on ward
6 = Threatens interviewer; shouting; interview difficult
8 = Assaultive; destructive; interview impossible
10. Appearance
0 = Appropriate dress and grooming
1 = Minimally unkempt
2 = Poorly groomed; moderately disheveled; overdressed
3 = Disheveled; partly clothed; garish makeup
4 = Completely unkempt; decorated; bizarre garb
11. Insight
0 = Present; admits illness; agrees with need for treatment
1 = Possibly ill
2 = Admits behavior change but denies illness
3 = Admits possible change in behavior but denies illness
4 = Denies any behavior change

From Young, R.C., et al. (1978). A rating scale for mania: reliability, validity and sensitivity. *British Journal of Psychiatry, 133,* 429. © 1978, The Royal College of Psychiatrists.

CARE PLAN

Name: Casey Bates   Admission Date: _____

DSM-5 Diagnosis: Bipolar I Disorder

Assessment	**Areas of strength:** Patient's marriage is solid between hospitalizations. Patient's partners like him and are eager for him to return to work. Patient has good adjustment between hospitalizations. He has responded well to lithium in the past.
	Problems: Patient is threatening and irritating others. Patient has legal problems from bar fight. Patient is threatening to get even with his wife's alleged lover. Patient has not complied with medication regimen recently and states that he will not take lithium.
Diagnoses	Risk for other directed violence related to mania, delusions, irritability, and verbal hostility.
	Fatigue related to insomnia, as evidenced by lack of sleep for 3 days.
	Nutrition, altered: less than body requirements related to anorexia and hyperactivity, as evidenced by lack of interest in food.
Outcomes	*Short-term goals*
Date met: _____	Patient will not hurt anyone while in hospital.
Date met: _____	Patient will comply with medication regimen.
Date met: _____	Patient will become less agitated.
Date met: _____	Patient will comply with unit norms and limits.
	Long-term goals
Date met: _____	Patient will remain free of manic episodes.
Date met: _____	Patient will continue to take lithium on outpatient basis.
Date met: _____	Patient will resolve legal problems.
Date met: _____	Patient will join manic-depressive support group.
Planning and Interventions	**Nurse-patient relationship:** Talk to patient in a matter-of-fact tone, and clearly indicate that aggressive behaviors are unacceptable. Set firm, clear limits. Do not engage in debates over unit policy or limits. Keep comments brief and simple. Do not respond to sarcastic remarks with anger. Reinforce good behavior and confront (carefully) unacceptable behavior.
	Psychopharmacology: Lithium carbonate 600 mg tid PO (concentrate); olanzapine 15 mg HS.
	Milieu management: Provide quiet room and decrease stimuli. Do not include in group activities for a few days. Provide opportunities for rest, and monitor sleep. Provide finger foods and weigh daily. Set limits.
Evaluation	Mr. Bates is less agitated and is taking lithium on schedule. He is beginning to talk less about his wife's alleged infidelity. He has not lost weight. He continues to test limits.
Referrals	Schedule outpatient appointment, and give patient and wife telephone number for manic-depressive support group.

STUDY NOTES

1. Bipolar disorders (e.g., BD I and BD II) occur in about 1.8% of the adult population in any given 12-month period. About 4.1% of Americans are affected by these disorders in their lifetime.

2. Manic episodes are characterized by a distinct period (1 week at least or shorter if hospitalized) during which there is an abnormal and persistent elevated, expansive, or irritable mood. These symptoms tend to occur suddenly and escalate rapidly, lasting a few days to several months. At least three other symptoms are required (see Box 26-1).

3. Hypomanic episodes are characterized by the set of symptoms that occur in manic episodes except that the symptoms are not as severe; occur over a 4-day period; do not cause significant social, occupational, or interpersonal problems; and do not require hospitalization.

4. BD I is described as a swing in mood from a manic episode to major depression.

5. BD II is described as a swing in mood from a hypomanic episode to major depression.

6. Cyclothymic disorder is described as a swing in mood from a hypomanic episode to dysthymia (depressive episode not as severe as episodes with major depression).

7. Objective signs of bipolar illness include altered speech patterns; altered social, interpersonal, and occupational relationships; and altered activity and appearance.

8. Subjective symptoms of bipolar illness include alterations in affect and perception.

9. Psychosocial theories of bipolar illness include theories about family dynamics and psychoanalytic explanations that view manic behavior as a defense against overwhelming feelings of depression.

10. Biologic explanations of bipolar disorder include excessive levels of neurotransmitters (norepinephrine and dopamine) and genetics (up to 80% concordancy rates among identical twins in some studies).

11. Lithium is a drug of choice for the treatment of bipolar disorders; however, the valproates (e.g., valproic acid [Depakene], divalproex sodium [Depakote]) are prescribed more often. Atypical antipsychotics are also approved for bipolar disorder.

REFERENCES

American Psychiatric Association. (2002). Practice guidelines for the treatment of patients with bipolar disorder. *American Journal of Psychiatry*, 159(Suppl. 4), 16.

American Psychiatric Association. (2010). Diagnostic and statistical manual of mental disorders, text revision (4th ed.). Arlington, VA: APA.

American Psychiatric Association. (2013). Diagnostic and statistical manual of mental disorders (5th ed.). Arlington, VA: APA.

Anonymous. (2008). Improving outcomes in bipolar disorder. Psychosocial therapies augment medication, but challenges remain. *Harvard Mental Health Letter*, 24(1).

Anonymous. (2009). Schizophrenia and bipolar disorder may share genetic origins. *Harvard Mental Health Letter*, 25, 7.

Centers for Disease Control and Prevention. (2013). Burden of mental illness. www.cdc.gov/mentalhealth/basics/burden.htm, Accessed 02.03.14.

Craddock, N., O'Donovan, M. C., & Owen, M. J. (2009). Psychosis genetics: Modeling the relationship between schizophrenia, bipolar disorder, and mixed (or "schizoaffective") psychoses. *Schizophrenia Bulletin*, 35, 482.

El-Mallakh, R. S. (1996). Lithium: Actions and mechanisms. Washington, DC: American Psychiatric Association.

Foster, A., Sheehan, L., & Johns, L. (2011). Promoting adherence in patients with bipolar disorder. *Current Psychiatry*, 10, 45.

Jaffee, W. B., et al. (2009). Depression precipitated by alcohol use in patients with co-occurring bipolar and substance use disorders. *Journal of Clinical Psychiatry*, 70, 171.

Jamison, K. R. (1997). An unquiet mind. Westminster, MD: Vintage.

Janowsky, D. S., Leff, M., & Epstein, R. S. (1970). Playing the manic game. *Archives of General Psychiatry*, 22, 252.

Keltner, N. L., & Folks, D. G. (2005). Psychotropic drugs (4th ed.). St. Louis: Mosby.

Kessler, R. C., et al. (1997). Lifetime co-occurrence of DSM-III-R alcohol abuse and dependence with other psychiatric disorders in the National Comorbidity Survey. *Archives of General Psychiatry*, 54, 313.

Kessler, R. C., et al. (2005a). Prevalence, severity, and comorbidity of 12-month DSM-IV disorders in the National Comorbidity Survey Replication. *Archives of General Psychiatry*, 62, 617.

Kessler, R. C., et al. (2005b). Lifetime and age-of-onset distributions of DSM-IV disorders in the National Comorbidity Survey Replication. *Archives of General Psychiatry*, 62, 593.

Kessler, R. C., et al. (2012). Twelve-month and lifetime prevalence and lifetime morbid risk of anxiety and mood disorders in the United States. *International Journal of Methods in Psychiatric Research*, 21, 169.

Klassen, L. J., Katzman, M. A., & Chokka, P. (2010). Adult ADHD and its comorbidities, with a focus on bipolar disorder. *Journal of Affective Disorders*, 124, 1.

Kosten, T. R., & Kosten, T. A. (2004). New medication strategies for comorbid substance use and bipolar affective disorder. *Biological Psychiatry*, 56, 771.

List of people believed to have been affected by bipolar disorder. (n.d.). <http://en.wikipedia.org/wiki/List_of_people_believed_to_have_been_affected_by_bipolar_disorder> Accessed 29.01.14.

Manji, H. K., & Lenox, R. H. (2000). The nature of bipolar disorder. *Journal of Clinical Psychiatry*, 61(Suppl. 13), 4257.

Marsee, K., & Gross, A. F. (2013). Bipolar disorder or something else? *Current Psychiatry*, 12, 43.

Moon, A. M. (2005). Late-onset bipolar patients not as ill as counterparts. *Clinical Psychiatry News*, 33, 48.

Moore, G. J., et al. (2000). Lithium-induced increase in human brain grey matter. *Lancet*, 356, 1241.

Nejtek, V. A., et al. (2008). Do atypical antipsychotics effectively treat co-occurring bipolar disorder and stimulant dependence? A randomized, double-blind trial. *Journal of Clinical Psychiatry*, 69, 1257.

Nery, F. G., & Soares, J. C. (2011). Comorbid bipolar disorder and substance abuse: Evidence-based options. *Current Psychiatry, 10,* 57.

Orum, M. (1996). Fairytales in reality. Sydney, Australia: Seraline.

Paris, J. (2009). The bipolar spectrum: A critical perspective. *Harvard Review of Psychiatry, 17,* 206.

Shattell, M., & Keltner, N. L. (2004). The case for atypical antipsychotics in bipolar disorder. *Perspectives in Psychiatric Care, 40,* 36.

Sherman, C. (2005). Schizophrenia-bipolar I theory gains traction. *Clinical Psychiatry News, 33,* 27.

Strakowski, S. M., & DelBello, S. P. (2000). The co-occurrence of bipolar and substance use disorders. *Clinical Psychology Review, 20,* 191.

Substance Abuse and Mental Health Services Administration. (2009). Results from the 2008 national survey on drug use and health: National findings. http://www.samhsa.gov/data/nsduh/2k8nsduh/2k8Results.htm, Accessed 13.11.13.

Suppes, T., Denehy, E. B., & Gibbons, E. W. (2000). The longitudinal course of bipolar disorder. *Journal of Clinical Psychiatry, 61*(Suppl. 9), 23.

Wessa, M., et al. (2009). Microstructural white matter changes in euthymic bipolar patients: A whole-brain diffusion tensor imaging study. *Bipolar Disorders, 11,* 504.

Wilf, T. J. (2012). When to treat subthreshold hypomanic episodes. *Current Psychiatry, 11,* 55.

Young, R. C., et al. (1978). A rating scale for mania: Reliability, validity, and sensitivity. *British Journal of Psychiatry, 133,* 429.

Zoler, M. L. (2005a). High impairment found in subthreshold bipolarity. *Clinical Psychiatry News, 33,* 1.

Zoler, M. L. (2005b). Pregnancy often triggers bipolar relapse, studies show. *Clinical Psychiatry News, 33,* 42.

Anxiety-Related, Obsessive-Compulsive, Trauma and Stressor-Related, Somatic, and Dissociative Disorders

*Debbie Steele**

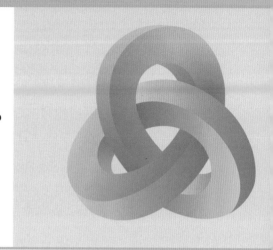

evolve WEBSITE

http://evolve.elsevier.com/Keltner

LEARNING OBJECTIVES

- Explain the relationships between stressors and the neurochemical, emotional, and physiologic responses to anxiety.
- Recognize the special terms related to anxiety-related disorders, obsessive-compulsive disorders, trauma and stressor-related disorders, somatic disorders, and dissociative disorders.
- Describe *DSM-5* criteria for these disorders.

- Describe objective and subjective symptoms of these disorders.
- Develop nursing care plans for individuals with these disorders.
- Evaluate the effectiveness of nursing interventions for individuals with these disorders.
- Recognize issues related to the care of individuals and their families with these disorders.

The disorders discussed in this chapter are classified in *DSM-5* as anxiety-related disorders, obsessive-compulsive and related disorders, trauma and stressor-related disorders, somatic symptom and related disorders, and dissociative disorders. All of these disorders are rooted in stress, anxiety, or fear; it is important to understand their dynamics and how they affect individuals and manifest as mental disorders. When the dynamics of these disorders are understood, appropriate nursing interventions can be instituted.

STRESS

Stress models provide nurses with a framework for understanding how stress affects individuals and their responses. Stress models developed by Selye (1956) and Lazarus (1966, 2006) provide essential concepts that are important for nurses to know as they care for vulnerable patients, especially patients who have experienced trauma. The ability to adapt to stressors leads to conflict resolution, whereas the inability to adapt effectively might result in physical or mental disorders or even death (Figure 27-1).

Selye Stress Adaptation Model

Selye (1956) defined stress as wear and tear on the body. He developed his framework to explain the physiologic response to stress. Selye viewed stressors as any positive or negative occurrence or as any emotion requiring a response. Interaction with the environment and others inevitably produces stress, depending on individual perception and definition of the stressor. However, Selye discovered that many individuals demonstrate the same symptoms, regardless of the stressor. These changes became known as *stress adaptation syndrome*, and they occur in three stages: (1) alarm, (2) resistance, and (3) exhaustion. The three stages are summarized in Table 27-1.

Alarm

Any type of stressor for individuals activates the preparation for "fight or flight." Individuals experience an increase in alertness so as to focus on the immediate task or threat and to mobilize resources and defenses to concentrate on the particular stressor. The levels of anxiety experienced are mild (+1) to moderate (+2). Learning and problem solving can occur. When the stressor continues and is not adaptively or effectively resolved, individuals experience the next stage.

---

*This chapter was previously written by Carol Bostrom.

Resistance

In the resistance stage, individuals strive to adapt to stress. For adaptation to occur, the use of coping and defense mechanisms is increased. Problem solving and learning are difficult but can be accomplished with assistance. The levels of anxiety experienced are moderate (+2) to severe (+3). When stressors become overwhelming or prolonged, individuals experience the next stage.

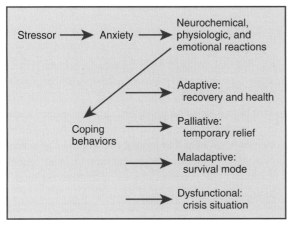

FIG 27-1 Process of anxiety.

Exhaustion

Exhaustion results from stress that lasts too long, is overwhelming, or results from the individual's total inability to cope. The levels of anxiety experienced are severe (+3) to panic (+4). Defenses are exaggerated and dysfunctional, and the personality becomes disorganized, thinking becomes illogical, and decision making becomes ineffective. Delusions and hallucinations can occur, with sensory misperception and a greatly reduced orientation to reality. Individuals might become violent, suicidal, or completely immobilized, without even showing the anxiety. Death might occur when exhaustion continues without intervention.

Lazarus Interactional Model

In contrast to Selye's emphasis on the physiologic effects of stress, Lazarus (1966, 2006) focused on the psychological aspects. According to Lazarus, psychological stress is "a relationship between the person and the environment that is appraised by the person as taxing or exceeding his or her resources and endangering his or her well-being" (Lazarus & Folkman, 1984). Lazarus believed that the basis of coping is not a result of anxiety per se but of the personal, cognitive appraisal of threat. "Anxiety is the response to threat" (Lazarus, 1966). The significance of the threat or what it means to the individual is of primary importance. For one

TABLE 27-1	STRESS ADAPTATION SYNDROME	
STAGE	**PHYSICAL CHANGES**	**PSYCHOSOCIAL CHANGES**
Stage I: Alarm Stage Mobilization of the body's defensive forces and activation of the potential for "fight or flight" (+1 to +2 anxiety)	Release of norepinephrine and epinephrine, causing vasoconstriction, increased blood pressure, and increased rate and force of cardiac contraction Increased hormone levels Enlargement of adrenal cortex Marked loss of body weight Shrinkage of the thymus, spleen, and lymph nodes Irritation of gastric mucosa	Increased level of alertness Increased level of anxiety Task-oriented, defense-oriented, inefficient, or maladaptive behavior might occur
Stage II: Stage of Resistance Optimal adaptation to stress within the person's capabilities (+2 to +3 anxiety)	Hormone levels readjust Reduction in activity and size of adrenal cortex Lymph nodes return to normal size Weight returns to normal	Increased and intensified use of coping mechanisms Tendency to rely on defense-oriented behavior Psychosomatic symptoms develop
Stage III: Stage of Exhaustion Loss of ability to resist stress because of depletion of body resources; fight, flight, or immobilization occurs (+3 to +4 anxiety)	Decreased immune response, with suppression of T cells and atrophy of thymus Depletion of adrenal glands and hormone production Weight loss Enlargement of lymph nodes and dysfunction of lymphatic system If exposure to stressor continues, cardiac failure, renal failure, or death might occur	Defense-oriented behaviors become exaggerated Disorganization of thinking Disorganization of personality Sensory stimuli might be misperceived with appearance of illusion Reality contact might be reduced with appearance of delusions or hallucinations If exposure to stressor continues, stupor or violence might occur

Modified from Kneisl, C.R., & Ames, S.W. (1986). *Adult health nursing: a biopsychosocial approach*. Menlo Park, CA: Addison-Wesley. ©1986. Reprinted by permission of Pearson Education, Inc., Upper Saddle River, NJ.

person, a particular event might be viewed as a challenge; for another, the same event might be viewed as a severe threat or problem.

Three types of cognitive appraisal have been identified. *Primary appraisal* refers to the judgment that individuals make about a particular event. What does it mean personally? What are its effects? *Secondary appraisal* is the individual's evaluation of the way to respond to an event. Possible strategies or solutions as well as resources and supports are examined. *Reappraisal* is further appraisal that is made after new or additional information has been received.

Personal and environmental factors influence appraisal—commitments, beliefs, values, feelings, emotions, and views of what is important. A seemingly appropriate solution might not be useful because it conflicts with individual values and beliefs. For example, a passive wife might be unable to be assertive and confrontational with her husband because she was taught and believes that women should be quiet and submissive.

Stressful events often create demands with which individuals cannot cope effectively. Occasionally, personal resources or social supports are inadequate. Preferred methods of coping might be ineffective in resolving the problem and could result in more problems. Ineffective coping and the creation of additional problems result in additional stress and can lead to physical or mental illness or both.

To assist patients with developing adaptive or effective coping methods, nurses must help patients identify and evaluate palliative, maladaptive, and dysfunctional behaviors as well as assist patients in becoming aware of the consequences of their behavior. Palliative mechanisms decrease the emotions without solving the problems. Maladaptive mechanisms do not manage the emotions sufficiently and do not solve the problems. Dysfunctional mechanisms create new or additional problems (Figure 27-2).

Patients' appraisal of stressors or problems includes their perception of the stressors, the resources or supports they have to help them cope, and the way in which their beliefs and values influence that coping. For example, an individual who is independent and who has sufficient income and savings and a supportive family and believes that divorce is acceptable is likely to cope differently with a partner's affair than an individual who is dependent, unemployed, and without close family and believes that divorce is not an option. In considering a patient's perception of stressors, the nurse can facilitate cognitive restructuring or problem solving by helping patients choose adaptive and appropriate coping behaviors. Together, the patient and the nurse can evaluate the effectiveness of strategies used. When patients exhibit behaviors found in Selye's stage of exhaustion or are using primarily dysfunctional coping, the nurse can assess patients' inability to take constructive action; the nurse might be required to make decisions on behalf of patients. After patients gain some control over their situation, they can benefit from classes on stress management, problem solving, relaxation training, and biofeedback.

ANXIETY

Anxiety has been described as follows:
- Subjective experience that can be detected only by objective behaviors that result from it
- Emotional pain
- Apprehension, fearfulness, or a sense of powerlessness resulting from a threat that is less visible or definable than fear that has a visible object or trigger

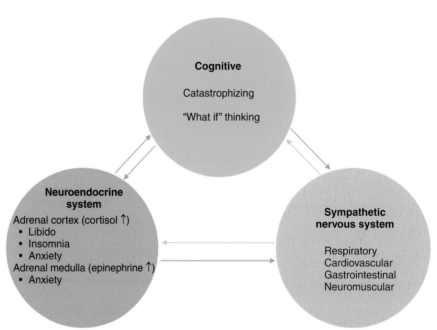

FIG 27-2 Interacting systems of panic attacks. (From Keltner, N.L., Perry, B.A., & Williams, A.R. [2003]. Panic disorder: a tightening vortex of misery. *Perspectives in Psychiatric Care, 39,* 41.)

- Warning sign of a perceived danger or threat
- Emotional response that triggers behaviors (automatic relief behaviors) aimed at eliminating the anxiety
- Alerting an individual to prepare for self-defense
- Occurring in degrees
- Contagious; communicated from one person to another
- Part of a process, not an isolated phenomenon

More recent research on anxiety has identified its biologic basis. Anxiety is the result of neurochemical reactions centered on the hypothalamic-pituitary-adrenal axis, the hypothalamic-pituitary-gonadal axis, and the limbic system reward pathway. The information in this section is meant to convey the significance of the effects of stressful events on the body. For readers particularly interested in psychobiology, the material presented here can be related to the information in Chapter 4.

Major neurochemical changes identified as affected by stressful episodes include the following (Aguilera, 1998; Charney, 2004; Eisner, 2004; Hoffart & Keene, 1998; Koob, 2008; Taylor et al., 2001):

- Increased regional epinephrine and norepinephrine turnover in the locus ceruleus, limbic regions, and cerebral cortex
- Increased corticotropin-releasing hormone and dehydroepiandrosterone
- Increased adrenocorticotropic hormone and corticosterone levels
- Increased dopamine release in the prefrontal cortex and decreased release in the nucleus accumbens
- Increased endogenous opiate release
- Increased glucocorticoid (cortisol) levels
- Increased thyrotropin-releasing hormone
- Increased thyroid-stimulating hormone
- Increased peripheral sympathetic nervous system activity
- Altered function of the serotonin receptors
- Decreased benzodiazepine receptor binding
- Decreased testosterone levels
- Increased estrogen levels

Anxiety-related responses are critical for surviving and tolerating dangerous situations. Increased noradrenergic and dopaminergic system activity (leading to central nervous system hyperarousal and hypervigilance) facilitates rapid behavioral reactions. Tolerating fear and pain associated with serious injuries is enhanced by increased release of endogenous opiates (allowing emotional blunting and physical analgesia) (Martenson et al., 2009). Increased cortisol levels, resulting in metabolic activation, facilitate increased physical activity (Charney, 2004). However, the effectiveness of these responses fades if the individual is continuously exposed to the stressor (Clements & Turpin, 2000). This decrease in effectiveness is related to the alterations in the catecholamine and thyroid systems and the depressed immune system. These effects and a deficiency in serotonin might increase the risk of suicide (Jiwanlal & Weitzel, 2001).

If the threshold set-point for anxiety is changed and the allostatic load (a burden with long-term physiologic and psychological effects) occurs, the individual becomes increasingly sensitive to subsequent stressors, which more easily reactivate the anxiety-related response. The locus ceruleus–norepinephrine system plays a role in chronic anxiety, intrusive memories, and fear (Charney, 2004; Hoffart & Keene, 1998). This tendency is discussed in relation to posttraumatic stress disorder (PTSD) and acute stress disorder (ASD) as explained in this chapter. A stress cycle can begin to occur in which physical and psychological symptoms cause additional stress, negative thinking, and fears. These reactions lead to reactivation of the stress response, resulting in increasingly severe symptoms, increasingly frequent symptoms, or both. Eventually, other symptoms, such as irritability, muscle tension, headaches, back pain, insomnia, gastrointestinal disturbances, hypertension, palpitations, insulin resistance, decreased immune function, increased abdominal fat, and cardiovascular disease, might develop (Charney, 2004; Eisner, 2004; Hoffart & Keene, 1998; Soderstrom et al., 2000). In contrast, if the original stress is resolved, the body can return to normal (a relaxation response) through activation of the parasympathetic nervous system and the decreased activity in the hypothalamus and pituitary gland.

ANXIETY-RELATED DISORDERS

Anxiety-related disorders involve a subset of disorders that are discussed here: (1) anxiety disorders, (2) obsessive-compulsive and related disorders, (3) trauma and stressor-related disorders, (4) dissociative disorders, and (5) somatic symptom and related disorders (see *DSM-5* Diagnoses for Anxiety-Related Disorders box). Anxiety disorders are disorders that share features of excessive anxiety and fear and related behavioral disturbances. Anxiety disorders include (1) generalized anxiety disorder (GAD), (2) social anxiety disorder (social phobia), (3) specific phobias, (4) panic disorder, and (5) agoraphobia (Table 27-2).

GENERALIZED ANXIETY DISORDER

An individual with GAD experiences *excessive or unreasonable worry or apprehension*. The intensity of the worry is out of proportion to the actual likelihood of the anticipated event. The anxiety or worry is chronic, excessive, or unreasonable and may concern everyday events, such as job responsibilities, health, and finances. These individuals have great difficulty in controlling the anxiety, and worrying becomes a habitual way of coping to prevent a negative occurrence or something bad from happening. Decreased concentration and memory problems often exist. Physical symptoms of anxiety, such as difficulty sleeping, fatigue, and muscle tension, are also part of the disorder. The anxiety causes significant distress and impairment in interpersonal, social, or occupational functioning (see *DSM-5* Criteria for Generalized Anxiety Disorder box).

Etiology and Course

Research studies suggest a high genetic correlation between GAD and major depression. Neuroimaging studies

DSM-5 DIAGNOSES FOR ANXIETY-RELATED DISORDERS

Anxiety Disorders
Generalized anxiety disorder (GAD)
Panic disorder
Agoraphobia
Specific phobias
Social anxiety disorder (social phobia)

Obsessive-Compulsive and Related Disorders
Obsessive-compulsive disorder (OCD)
Body dysmorphic disorder
Hoarding disorder
Trichotillomania (hair-pulling disorder)
Excoriation (skin-picking disorder)

Trauma and Stressor-Related Disorders
Posttraumatic stress disorder (PTSD)
Acute stress disorder (ASD)
Adjustment disorder

Somatic Symptom and Related Disorders
Somatic symptom disorder
Illness anxiety disorder
Conversion disorder
Factitious disorder

Dissociative Disorders
Dissociative identity disorder (DID)
Dissociative amnesia
Depersonalization/derealization disorder

From the American Psychiatric Association. (2013). *Diagnostic and statistical manual of mental disorders* (5th ed.). Arlington, VA: APA.

NORM'S NOTES

Anxiety is the most common mental disorder. There are all types of stressors that just get to us, day in and day out. Some people refer to this phenomenon as life. On top of that, some of us just don't handle life as well as others. Among your classmates, you have already identified some people who handle things better than others. Why? There are lots of reasons, and this chapter will help you understand them better. It will also look at some types of anxiety that probably go well beyond anything you have experienced. Just as the chapter on depression can hit a little close to home, so can this chapter.

TABLE 27-2 12-MONTH PREVALENCE RATE OF MENTAL DISORDERS IN THE UNITED STATES*

DISORDERS	APPROXIMATE PERCENTAGE >17 YEARS OLD (%)* (unless noted for children)	GENDER OVERREP-RESENTATION
Anxiety disorders	18.1 overall	
Agoraphobia	1.7	Female
Panic disorder	2.4	Female
Panic attacks	11.2	Female
Social anxiety	7	Female
Specific phobia	7-9	Female
Separation anxiety	1.2	Equal
Generalized anxiety disorder	2	Female
Posttraumatic stress disorder	3.4	Female
Obsessive-compulsive disorder	1.2	Equal
Major depression	8.6	Female
Bipolar disorder I and II	1.8	BD I: ~Equal BD II: Female
Autism spectrum disorders	1 in children	Male
Disruptive, impulse control, and conduct disorders	8.9 overall	
Conduct disorders*	4 in children	Male
Attention-deficit/hyperactivity disorder*	5 in children; 2.5 in adults	Male
Substance use disorders	8.9 overall	
Alcohol use disorder	8.5 in adults; 2.5 in 12- to 17-year-olds	Male
Drug use disorders	1.4	Male
Schizophrenia	1.1	~Equal

*No one source has all of this information. This information has been derived from the following sources: Kessler, R.C., et al. (2012). Twelve-month and lifetime prevalence and lifetime morbid risk of anxiety and mood disorders in the United States. *International Journal of Methods of Psychiatric Research, 21,* 169; Substance Abuse and Mental Health Services Administration (2009). *Results from the 2008 national survey on drug use and health: national findings.* <http://www.samhsa.gov/data/nsduh/2k8nsduh/2k8Results.htm> Accessed November 13, 2013; American Psychiatric Association (2013). *Diagnostic and statistical manual of mental disorders* (5th ed.). Arlington, VA: APA.

have found increased activity in the amygdala or brain fear circuitry and the prefrontal cortex. Cognitive impairment may also be associated with a risk for developing GAD (Stein, 2009). In patients with GAD, there might be neurochemical dysregulation in gamma-aminobutyric acid (GABA)–benzodiazepine, norepinephrine, serotonin, neuropeptide, and glutamate systems (Antai-Ontong, 2003). Further research is needed to clarify the neurobiologic mechanisms involved in GAD.

Psychosocial and environmental factors also play a role in the development of GAD. The median age of onset for GAD is 30 years, and women are more likely to develop the disorder than men. Many affected individuals report they have felt anxious and nervous all their lives (American Psychiatric Association, 2013).

DSM-5 CRITERIA
for Generalized Anxiety Disorder

1. Excessive worry and anxiety
2. Difficulty in controlling the worry
3. Anxiety and worry are evident in three or more of the following:
   - Restlessness
   - Fatigue
   - Irritability
   - Decreased ability to concentrate
   - Muscle tension
   - Disturbed sleep
4. Excessive anxiety and worry (apprehensive expectation), occurring more days than not for at least 6 months, about a number of events or activities (such as work or school performance).
5. The individual finds it difficult to control the worry.
6. The anxiety and worry are associated with three or more of the following six symptoms with at least some symptoms having been present for more days than not for the past 6 months (note: only one item is required in children):
   - Restlessness or feeling keyed up or on edge
   - Being easily fatigued
   - Difficulty concentrating or mind going blank

- Irritability
- Muscle tension
- Sleep disturbance (difficulty falling or staying asleep, or restless, unsatisfying sleep)

7. The anxiety, worry, or physical symptoms cause clinically significant distress or impairment in social, occupational, or other important areas of functioning.
8. The disturbance is not attributable to the physiologic effects of a substance (e.g., a drug of abuse, a medication) or another medical condition (e.g., hyperthyroidism).
9. The disturbance is not better explained by another mental disorder (e.g., anxiety or worry about having panic attacks in panic disorder, negative evaluation in social anxiety disorder [social phobia], contamination or other obsessions in obsessive-compulsive disorder, separation from attachment figures in separation anxiety disorder, reminders of traumatic events in posttraumatic stress disorder, gaining weight in anorexia nervosa, physical complaints in somatic symptom disorder, perceived appearance flaws in body dysmorphic disorder, having a serious illness in illness anxiety disorder, or the content of delusional beliefs in schizophrenia or delusional disorder).

From the American Psychiatric Association. (2013). *Diagnostic and statistical manual of mental disorders* (5th ed.). Arlington, VA: APA.

PUTTING IT ALL TOGETHER

PSYCHOTHERAPEUTIC MANAGEMENT

Nurse-Patient Relationship

The first step in the nurse-patient relationship is for the nurse to assist patients in reducing their level of anxiety and its associated symptoms. Anxiety must be reduced before problem solving can occur. The nurse's ultimate goal is to assist patients with developing adaptive coping responses.

Initially, patients need support and reassurance from the nurse. The nurse promotes trust through acceptance of patients' positive and negative feelings and acknowledgment of their discomfort. Conveying empathy tells patients that the nurse is concerned and understanding and does not minimize the level of distress. For example, the nurse might say, "This must be uncomfortable and painful for you." To help patients manage and reduce their level of anxiety, the nurse should use the interventions found in the Key Nursing Interventions for Reducing Anxiety box.

After the anxiety level has been reduced to a more manageable and comfortable level, the nurse should begin to assist patients in examining their coping behaviors. Through the use of problem-solving methods, adaptive coping skills can increase. The nurse helps the individual to replace ineffective, maladaptive worrying with effective coping methods for dealing with anxiety (see the Key Nursing Interventions for Problem Solving box).

The process of helping individuals learn to use adaptive coping behaviors requires patience and the awareness that individuals learn and change at their own pace. The nurse must also be aware of his or her own verbal and nonverbal

KEY NURSING INTERVENTIONS
for Reducing Anxiety

1. Provide a calm and quiet environment. *Rationale:* To identify and reduce stimulation, which includes exposure to situations and interactions with other patients that might provoke anxiety.
2. Ask patients to identify what and how they feel. *Rationale:* To help patients increase their recognition of what is happening to them.
3. Encourage patients to describe and discuss their feelings with you. *Rationale:* To help patients increase their awareness of the connection between feelings and behaviors.
4. Help patients identify possible causes of their feelings. *Rationale:* To assist patients in connecting their feelings with earlier experiences.
5. Listen carefully for patients' expressions of helplessness and hopelessness. *Rationale:* To assess for self-harm; patients might be suicidal because they want to escape their pain and do not think that they will ever feel better. A comorbid major depression may also be present.
6. Ask patients whether they feel suicidal or have a plan to hurt themselves. *Rationale:* To assess for self-harm, same as above, and to initiate suicide precautions, if necessary.
7. Plan and involve patients in activities such as going for walks or playing recreational games. *Rationale:* To help patients release nervous energy and to discourage preoccupation with the self.

behavior when working with these patients because anxiety is contagious. The nurse should manage his or her own stress and anxiety so that the work between the nurse and the patient is not compromised. The nurse educates the patient about the

1. Discuss with patients their present and previous coping mechanisms. *Rationale:* To reinforce effective adaptive behaviors.
2. Discuss with patients the meaning of problems and conflicts. *Rationale:* To help patients appraise stressors, explore their personal values, and define the scope and seriousness of their problems.
3. Use supportive confrontation and teaching. *Rationale:* To increase patients' insight into the negative effects of their maladaptive and dysfunctional coping behaviors.
4. Assist patients with exploring alternative solutions and behaviors. *Rationale:* To increase adaptive coping mechanisms.
5. Encourage patients to test new adaptive coping behaviors through role playing or implementation. *Rationale:* To provide an opportunity for patients to practice new behaviors.
6. Teach patients relaxation exercises. *Rationale:* To reduce the level of anxiety. These techniques help patients manage or control anxiety on their own.
7. Promote the use of hobbies and recreational activities. *Rationale:* To help patients deal with routine feelings of stress and anxiety.

illness, including the effects of anxiety on the patient's life and on family members.

Psychopharmacology

Antidepressants, such as selective serotonin reuptake inhibitors (SSRIs) and selective serotonin-norepinephrine reuptake inhibitors (SNRIs), are most effective for treating GAD and the presence of comorbid disorders such as depression. Because GAD is a chronic disorder, antidepressants are better than benzodiazepines owing to the possibility of dependency and tolerance with long-term use of benzodiazepines. Benzodiazepines sometimes are used on a short-term basis when a quick-acting medication is needed until the antidepressant takes effect. The benzodiazepine is slowly tapered if necessary and discontinued.

Tricyclic antidepressants are seldom used because of more serious side effects than with SSRIs. Buspirone, a nonaddicting nonbenzodiazepine, is useful for cognitive symptoms of worry, irritability, and apprehension (Davidson, 2009).

Milieu Management

Patients with GAD can benefit from a variety of activities. Cognitive therapy is effective for patients with GAD (Davidson, 2009). Recreational activities help reduce tension and anxiety. The use of relaxation exercises and tapes, meditation, and biofeedback helps decrease tension and promote relaxation and comfort.

Groups that focus on stress management, problem solving, self-esteem, assertiveness, and goal setting are helpful for coping with stress. Depending on the issues and concerns of each patient, various groups can be helpful.

PANIC DISORDER

Patients with panic disorder experience recurrent panic attacks and are worried about having more attacks. A panic attack is an abrupt surge of intense fear or discomfort that peaks within 10 minutes. In addition to somatic symptoms, patients who experience panic attacks fear that they are losing control over themselves, "going crazy," having a heart attack, or dying from a life-threatening illness.

According to *DSM-5*, panic attacks are (1) unexpected, occurring out of the blue, such as when an individual is emerging from sleep, or (2) are situationally bound, meaning that they occur in anticipation of or on exposure to a trigger situation. These patients avoid places where a panic attack has occurred or could occur. The frequency of panic attacks varies widely, from weekly to yearly. Women are more prone to have panic attacks than men (2:1).

Etiology

Psychological and biologic factors contribute to the development of panic disorders (Keltner et al., 2003). Some

CASE STUDY

Sandra Johnson, a 41-year-old white woman, is admitted to the emergency department of a general hospital. Her symptoms are shortness of breath, hyperventilation, palpitations, chest pain, choking sensation, and fear of dying. She stated that these symptoms occurred unexpectedly while she was cooking dinner. She thought she was having a heart attack.

These attacks had happened three times before. The first attack occurred 2 months ago, after which she went to her family physician, who performed an electrocardiogram and a stress test and conducted a complete physical examination. All results were negative for any physiologic cause of the symptoms. After the second attack, Mrs. Johnson stated that she took 2 weeks off from work because she was worried about having another attack. She had been employed for 5 years as a secretary for a small insurance agency. Just before she was about to return

to work, she experienced another attack. After this third attack, she decided not to return to work and to quit her job. She was unable to leave the house to go grocery shopping, drive the children to activities, or go out socially with her friends. Her husband, who is 42 years old, stated that he and their three daughters, aged 15, 12, and 9 years, were very concerned about her and had been helping her with daily tasks.

After her husband leaves, Mrs. Johnson begins to cry and states that she is letting her family down. They have tried to help her, and she cannot do anything at home; she cannot work or even leave the house because she is so afraid of being unable to control the possibility of another attack. She does not understand what is happening to her and wants medication to help her feel better.

◎ CARE PLAN

Name: Sandra Johnson   *Admission Date: _____*
DSM-5 Diagnosis: Panic disorder

Assessment	**Areas of strength:** Patient is managing her role as mother, homemaker, and secretary; was socially active with her friends; is in relatively good health.
	Problems: Fear of dying related to fear of heart attack; unable to leave home; fear of losing her husband; feelings of inadequacy.
Diagnoses	Anxiety: panic related to life stress, as evidenced by somatic symptoms and fear of dying.
	Self-esteem disturbance related to feelings of helplessness, as evidenced by inability to function.
	Fear related to avoidance, as evidenced by difficulty leaving her home.
Outcomes	**Short-term goals**
Date met: _____	Patient will discuss her fears, sense of inadequacy and helplessness, and anger.
Date met: _____	Patient will identify relationship between anxiety and physiologic responses.
Date met: _____	Patient will develop strategies for reducing anxiety, such as relaxation techniques.
Date met: _____	Patient will use problem-solving techniques for life stresses.
	Long-term goals
Date met: _____	Patient will meet with husband and social worker to discuss marital issues.
Date met: _____	Patient will schedule appointment with outpatient therapist for cognitive behavior therapy, systematic desensitization, or self-exposure training.
Date met: _____	Patient will identify schedule for attending a support group.
Planning and Interventions	**Nurse-patient relationship:** Empathy and supportive-suppressive techniques to keep anxiety at a minimum; encourage ventilation of feelings and issues; help patient to identify relationships among stress, anxiety, and physiologic responses; assist with adaptive coping strategies.
	Psychopharmacology: Fluoxetine (Prozac) 20 mg q morning.
	Milieu management: Decrease stimuli and provide quiet, calm atmosphere; monitor anxiety level to prevent escalation; encourage recreational and diversional activities; use quiet room, if necessary; later, encourage problem-solving, assertiveness, communication, problem-centered, self-esteem, and stress-management groups.
Evaluation	Patient reports being less anxious for the past 2 days. Met with husband and social worker.
Referrals	Outpatient appointments for cognitive therapy and self-exposure training.

individuals have an increased sensitivity to anxiety and fear and are more susceptible to the effects of trauma, particularly stressful life events. The center of the fear mechanism is the amygdala, which affects the hippocampus, thalamus, hypothalamus, locus ceruleus, and other sites, setting into motion a chain of events triggering panic (Ninan & Dunlop, 2005).

According to Gorman et al. (2000) and Keltner et al. (2003), three systems work singly or in combination to trigger panic: the sympathetic nervous system, the neuroendocrine system, and cognitive processes (Figure 27-2). An individual's catastrophic or "what-if" thinking can trigger physiologic (somatic symptoms as in the "fight or flight" response), behavioral (avoidant), and affective (fear) responses. Sensitivity to and vigilance about physiologic symptoms can influence cognitive and neuroendocrine responses. Dysregulation of adrenergic receptors, which results in norepinephrine, serotonin, and GABA receptor impairment, causes decreased regulation of the sympathetic nervous system.

▐ PUTTING IT ALL TOGETHER

PSYCHOTHERAPEUTIC MANAGEMENT

Nurse-Patient Relationship

The therapeutic relationship between the nurse and the patient with panic disorder is centered on the same issues and interventions discussed for patients with GAD. Interventions specific for patients experiencing a panic attack are described in the Key Nursing Interventions for Panic Attack box. The rationale for the interventions is to help patients manage the panic attack safely, with as little discomfort as possible. With the nurse's assistance, patients' anxiety can be reduced to a more manageable level.

The nurse educates patients about panic disorder to reassure them that they are not losing their minds or dying during an attack. Patients experience relief when given information about the disorder, symptoms that might be experienced, medications that can relieve symptoms, and effective treatment options (Marcks et al., 2009). The nurse should help

KEY NURSING INTERVENTIONS

for Panic Attack

1. Stay with the patient who is having a panic attack, and acknowledge the patient's discomfort.
2. Maintain a calm style and demeanor.
3. Speak in short, simple sentences, and give one direction at a time in a calm tone of voice.
4. If the patient is hyperventilating, provide a brown paper bag and focus on breathing with the patient.
5. Allow patients to pace or cry, which enables the release of tension and energy.
6. Communicate to patients that you are in control and will not let anything happen to them.
7. Move or direct patients to a quieter, less stimulating environment. Do not touch these patients; touching can increase feelings of panic.
8. Ask patients to express their perceptions or fears about what is happening to them. *Rationale:* To help patients reduce anxiety to a more manageable and comfortable level.
9. Normalize patients' fears related to their physical symptoms.
10. Remind patients that the panic attack episode will be over in less than 10 minutes.

patients realize that attacks are time-limited and that symptoms will abate. Cognitive restructuring helps patients reinterpret and reappraise their beliefs regarding the danger of an event or bodily sensations.

Psychopharmacology

SSRIs and SNRIs are most commonly used for the long-term treatment of panic symptoms. Benzodiazepines, such as alprazolam (Xanax) and lorazepam (Ativan), are used for an immediate effect to decrease somatic symptoms until the antidepressant has started working.

Patients with panic disorder might resist drug therapy because it might mean a loss of control at a time when they are struggling to maintain control over themselves and their symptoms. Some patients fear medications and their side effects. A clear explanation of the disorder and its biologic components can often convince patients that medication is helpful and that taking it is not a sign of weakness.

The nurse must differentiate symptoms of increased anxiety levels from medication side effects. Anxiety symptoms increase when pertinent issues are addressed or stressors are present. When symptoms of anxiety remain constant or decrease immediately before the next dose of medication, the symptoms are probably related to the medication. Strategies for anxiety reduction (e.g., relaxation exercises) might help patients manage anxiety.

Milieu Management

As a patient's anxiety decreases from the panic level, gross motor activities, such as walking, basketball, volleyball,

or the use of a stationary bicycle, are appropriate to help decrease tension and anxiety. Other milieu interventions are located in the previous section on GAD. Cognitive behavior therapy (CBT) plus medication is a first-line treatment for patients; CBT alone has also been found to be effective (Marcks et al., 2009). CBT works on thoughts and substitutes rational interpretations for the misinterpretation of bodily responses and helps reappraise beliefs about the danger of an event. Changes in cognition then lead to decreased avoidant behavior. CBT helps patients control symptoms and improves overall wellbeing (Miller, 2005c). Computer-assisted CBT is a proven evidence-based treatment used in the United Kingdom that it is hoped will be implemented in the United States (Stuhlmiller & Tolchard, 2009).

AGORAPHOBIA

Agoraphobia is characterized by marked fear or anxiety triggered by real or anticipated exposure to certain situations, such as (1) public transportation, (2) being in open spaces (parking lots, marketplaces, bridges), (3) being in enclosed places (shops, cinemas), (4) being in a crowd, and (5) being outside of the home alone. Individuals with agoraphobia avoid these situations because they are afraid they will be unable to escape or help will be unavailable to alleviate panic-like symptoms. Agoraphobic situations are endured with intense fear or anxiety and are out of proportion to the actual danger posed by the situation. The course of agoraphobia is typically chronic and persistent.

SPECIFIC PHOBIAS

Phobias are characterized by marked fear or anxiety in the presence of a specific object or situation (i.e. flying, heights, animals, injections, blood). The feared object or situation provokes immediate fear, which is avoided or endured with intense anxiety. The fear or anxiety is out of proportion to the actual danger posed by the object or situation. The amount of anxiety experienced varies with proximity to the feared object or situation. Specific phobias typically develop after a traumatic event (getting stuck in an elevator) or observing others going through a traumatic event (watching someone drown). Specific phobias are commonly experienced disorders (American Psychiatric Association, 2013).

SOCIAL ANXIETY DISORDER (SOCIAL PHOBIA)

Social phobia is characterized by marked fear or anxiety of being scrutinized in social situations (i.e., meeting new people, eating at a restaurant, giving a speech). There is a fear of being humiliated or embarrassed by a negative evaluation. The individual is afraid that she will be judged as weak, crazy, stupid, boring, intimidating, or unlikable. During social situations, individuals may fear physical evidence of anxiety, such as trembling, sweating, or stumbling over their words. Just thinking about an upcoming social event can produce anticipatory anxiety and dread (American Psychiatric Association, 2013).

Etiology

Research has led to theories stating that specific individual, environmental, family, and genetic factors underlie phobic disorders. Types of phobias develop based on the influence of environment and genetic predisposition. Magnetic resonance imaging scans have shown that when individuals with social phobia read negative statements about themselves, there is increased blood flow to the prefrontal cortex and amygdala, areas of the brain responsible for emotions (Miller, 2009a).

PUTTING IT ALL TOGETHER

PSYCHOTHERAPEUTIC MANAGEMENT

Nurse-Patient Relationship

Patients with phobic disorders are usually treated on an outpatient basis. If the phobia incapacitates a patient to a severe extent, the patient might be hospitalized. For example, hospitalization would be indicated if a person who has a phobia about germs is malnourished or dehydrated because of not eating or drinking. Following are some nursing interventions useful for individuals experiencing phobic disorders:

1. Accept patients and their fears with a noncritical attitude.
2. Provide and involve patients in activities that do not increase anxiety but increase involvement, rather than promote avoidance.
3. Help patients with physical safety and comfort needs.
4. Help patients recognize that their behavior is a method of avoiding anxiety.

Psychopharmacology

CBT is the most successful treatment for phobic patients. Systematic desensitization and exposure therapy by trained counselors has been found to be effective for specific phobias. *Clonidine* and *propranolol* may be taken as needed before social engagements to ease the symptoms associated with social phobia. In addition, SSRIs are used to reduce anxiety and depression if present.

Milieu Management

Assertiveness training and goal-setting groups are beneficial. Social skills groups and other milieu activities help enhance the patient's social interaction and decrease avoidance.

OBSESSIVE-COMPULSIVE AND RELATED DISORDERS

According to *DSM-5*, obsessive-compulsive and related disorders include obsessive-compulsive disorder (OCD), body dysmorphic disorder, hoarding, trichotillomania (hair pulling), and excoriation (skin picking).

Obsessive-Compulsive Disorder

OCD is characterized by the presence of obsessions or compulsions or both. Obsessions are recurrent and persistent thoughts, ideas, impulses, or images that are experienced as intrusive and unwanted (i.e., of contamination, of violent scenes). The performance of compulsions is the individual's attempt to neutralize obsessions with another thought or action. Compulsions or rituals are repetitive behaviors or mental acts the individual feels driven to perform, such as washing hands, checking, counting, and repeating words. The aim is to reduce the anxiety triggered by the obsessions. However, compulsions are typically not connected in a realistic way to the feared thoughts.

Current views concerning the origin of OCD point to genetic transmission. OCD might run in families. Biologic findings in OCD have identified increased brain activity in the frontal lobe and basal ganglia (Glod & Cawley, 1997). Serotonin dysregulation is involved in the development of OCD, which might account for the effectiveness of clomipramine (Anafranil) and SSRIs (Weigartz & Rasminsky, 2005).

An important feature of OCD is that the obsessions or compulsions can be so severe that they significantly interfere with the patient's normal routine and so time-consuming that they interfere with occupational and social functioning. The obsessions and compulsions also interfere with interpersonal relationships because patients are preoccupied with their rituals and magical thinking.

Clinical Example

Josie is married with two small children. Before going to bed, she checks to make sure that the front door is locked. She lays down in bed and begins to think that she might have unlocked the door, rather than lock the door. She can't go to sleep because of her concern, so she gets up to check the door. She lays back down in her bed and begins to wonder if she might have unlocked the door, rather than lock it....

In this society, value is placed on performing well in school and at work. Being responsible and perfectionistic is often rewarded by the boss or by family members. Anyone might be seen as being compulsive at times. However, people generally do not allow their compulsiveness to rule their lives; they are able to maintain a balance between work and play, between role expectations and performance. There is a difference between having characteristics or traits and having an illness. Occasional brooding, rumination, or steadfastness to a task is not usually considered ridiculous or excessively bothersome—these thoughts and feelings do not rule most people's lives.

CRITICAL THINKING QUESTION

1. A patient with OCD washes her hands after each time she touches anything. Her skin is cracked and bleeding. She states to the nurse, "I can't get my hands free of germs." How is this different from the nurse who washes his or her hands before and after each patient contact on a medical-surgical unit?

Body Dysmorphic Disorder

Body dysmorphic disorder is characterized by a preoccupation with perceived flaws in one's physical appearance that are not noticeable to others. The perceived flaws lead the individual to feel ugly, unattractive, abnormal, or deformed. Preoccupations focus on outward appearance, such as acne, scars, wrinkles, paleness, nose, hair, teeth, weight, breasts, or lips. The individuals perform repeated behaviors (mirror checking, excessive surgery) in response to their concerns. The preoccupations are intrusive, unwanted, time-consuming, and difficult to resist or control (American Psychiatric Association, 2013).

Hoarding Disorder

Hoarding disorder is characterized by persistent difficulties parting with possessions, regardless of their actual value. The difficulty is due to the distress associated with discarding, selling, recycling, or throwing them away. This behavior results in the accumulation of possessions that congest and clutter living areas. For example, family members may be unable to cook in the kitchen, sleep in their beds, or sit in the living room because of a pile up of household items. The main motivation for hoarding is related to the perceived value of the items or strong sentimental attachment to them (American Psychiatric Association, 2013).

Trichotillomania (Hair Pulling)

Trichotillomania is characterized by recurrent pulling out of one's hair, resulting in hair loss in various regions of the body (scalp, eyebrows, eyelids, axillary, facial, pubic). Repeated attempts to stop are unsuccessful leading to significant distress, such as feeling a loss of control, embarrassment, and shame. These individuals may attempt to conceal the hair loss by using makeup, scarves, or wigs (American Psychiatric Association, 2013).

Excoriation (Skin Picking)

Excoriation is characterized by recurrent picking at one's own skin, resulting in skin lesions. The most common sites are the face, arms, and hands. Target areas may be healthy skin, pimples, calluses, scabs, or lesions. Individuals pick with their fingernails, tweezers, or pins. Skin picking is preceded by feelings of anxiety or boredom and results in a sense of relief, pleasure, or gratification. Individuals try to conceal tissue damage with makeup or avoid going out in public (American Psychiatric Association, 2013).

PUTTING IT ALL TOGETHER

PSYCHOTHERAPEUTIC MANAGEMENT

Nurse-Patient Relationship

Basic nursing interventions for hospitalized patients with obsessive-compulsive disorders are listed in the Key Nursing Interventions for Obsessive-Compulsive Disorder box. Therapeutic work involves the nurse helping to increase patients' abilities to verbalize feelings, solve problems, and make decisions concerning stressors and problems. The nurse focuses on teaching and helping patients develop adaptive coping behaviors to deal with anxiety. Patients need to learn to substitute positive, anxiety-reducing behaviors for obsessions and rituals. Positive behaviors can include physical exercise, such as walking or using a stationary bicycle. Positive coping behaviors are slowly introduced into the patient's schedule, allowing time for rituals as well as normal activities. The nurse supports patients and positively reinforces nonritualistic behavior. Hobbies and social activities are introduced slowly as patients become more able to handle them.

KEY NURSING INTERVENTIONS

for Obsessive-Compulsive Disorder

1. Ensure that basic needs of food, rest, and grooming are met. Patients are too busy to attend to these tasks. Reminders and specific directions are usually necessary.
2. Provide patients with time to perform rituals. Patients need to keep anxiety in check. Later, work to decrease the rituals by setting limits, but never take away a ritual, or panic might ensue.
3. Explain expectations, routines, and changes. *Rationale:* To prevent an increase or escalation of anxiety.
4. Be empathic toward patients and be aware of their need to perform rituals. *Rationale:* To convey acceptance and understanding.
5. Assist patients with connecting behaviors and feelings. *Rationale:* To promote the ability to identify and understand feelings.
6. Structure simple activities, games, or tasks for patients. *Rationale:* To help patients focus on alternatives to their thoughts and actions.
7. Reinforce and recognize positive nonritualistic behaviors. *Rationale:* To increase patients' self-esteem and self-worth.

Psychopharmacology

SSRIs, such as fluoxetine (Prozac), sertraline (Zoloft), fluvoxamine (Luvox), and paroxetine (Paxil), are effective in treating OCD. Patients tolerate SSRIs better than the antidepressant clomipramine because of a better side effect profile, even though clomipramine is approved for OCD. Patients with OCD usually are started with a higher treatment dosage of SSRIs than patients with depression. Response usually occurs at 10 to 12 weeks instead of 2 to 4 weeks (Miller, 2009b).

Milieu Management

Various milieu activities and groups are beneficial to patients. Of particular importance are relaxation exercises and stress management, recreational or social skills, CBT, problem solving, and communication or assertiveness training groups. Care is always based on the individual needs of patients.

CBT, particularly exposure and response prevention (Miller, 2009b), is effective for patients with OCD and is usually undertaken on an outpatient basis. A technique of cognitive therapy called "thought stopping" can also be used. When an intrusive thought occurs, the patient says "stop" and snaps a rubber band on the wrist or substitutes an adaptive behavior, such as deep breathing, for the ritual. Deep brain stimulation is beginning to show early positive results for patients with severe OCD who have not responded to other treatments (Shah et al., 2008).

TRAUMA AND STRESSOR-RELATED DISORDERS

Trauma and stressor-related disorders include disorders that develop after exposure to a clearly identifiable traumatic event that threatens the self, others, resources, or sense of control or hope. These include PTSD, ASD, and adjustment disorder. Psychological distress is variable after exposure to a traumatic event. The event overwhelms the individual's usual coping strategies. Traumatic stressors that might precipitate the development of these disorders include war, terrorist attack, being a hostage or prisoner of war, torture, disasters, fatalities in fires or accidents, catastrophic illness, rape, and childhood sexual abuse. Among American adults, 7% to 8% are estimated to have PTSD in their lifetime (Antai-Ontong, 2003; Nisenoff, 2008). Examples of more recent events that have the potential for inducing trauma and stressor-related disorders are Hurricanes Katrina and Sandy and the Afghanistan and Iraqi wars.

Anyone experiencing such traumatic events would be distressed and feel intense fear, horror, and a sense of helplessness. To some extent, the type and degree of the initial and later reactions to trauma depend on the individual's prior experiences and psychological factors (Heim & Nemeroff, 2009). See Chapter 33 for additional information about the trauma-related disorders.

Posttraumatic Stress Disorder and Acute Stress Disorder

PTSD and ASD are characterized by intense emotional reactions (fear, helplessness, horror) after exposure to a traumatic event (threatened death, serious injury, sexual violence). Witnessing an event as it occurs to others or learning that a traumatic event occurred to a close family member is considered exposure and can lead to PTSD or ASD. ASD is characteristically similar to PTSD except for onset and duration. The diagnosis of ASD is made when an individual has dissociative symptoms *during or immediately after* the distressing event

(3 days to 1 month), including amnesia, depersonalization, derealization, decreased awareness of surroundings, numbing, detachment, or lack of emotional response. The diagnosis of PTSD is made based on the same characteristic symptoms that occur *1 month or more after* the trauma. It is common for PTSD to be unrecognized for years—sometimes 10 to 20 years. This delay in recognition is a result, in part, of the major characteristic of both ASD and PTSD—numbing of responsiveness, or reduced involvement with the external world. Denial, repression, and suppression are common in both disorders.

Avoidance is an important feature of PTSD and ASD. There is a persistent attempt to avoid situations, activities, and sometimes even people who might evoke memories of the trauma. These efforts include trying to avoid thoughts and feelings related to the event. A constricted or blunted affect, or a limitation in the range of feelings, might occur, such as being unable to show affection. Patients might feel detached or estranged from family and friends. An inability to trust and to love might lead to withdrawal. Patients often lose interest in activities, even activities unrelated to the traumatic event.

Another major characteristic of ASD and PTSD is reexperiencing the traumatic event in some way, which might be in the form of intrusive, unwanted memories; upsetting dreams or nightmares; illusions; or suddenly feeling as if the event were recurring (flashbacks). The triggers for episodes being reexperienced might have obvious connections to the trauma or might not resemble the original situation at all. In either case, patients try to avoid all activities and people in an effort to prevent experiencing the flashback.

Clinical Example

Joan was found wandering around the hospital in which her son was a patient 3 days after a tornado had destroyed her home and seriously injured her son. She was not injured but complained of nightmares and irritability. She said she could not bear to see her son because he "just wanted to talk about what happened—things I can't remember." Joan has not been to work since the tornado. She was taken to the crisis unit and diagnosed with and treated for ASD.

Other criteria of PTSD and ASD include increased arousal, anxiety, restlessness, irritability, disturbances in sleep, and impairment in memory or concentration. Especially with PTSD, there might be occasional outbursts of anger or rage and survivor guilt (guilt about surviving or the actions taken to survive) (Kaplan et al., 2001). For example, combat soldiers might believe that they survived because of a cowardly act; rape victims might feel guilty for not resisting their attacker.

Individuals experiencing posttraumatic symptoms might also develop depression, suicidal ideations and attempts, and substance abuse. Individuals with PTSD are at increased risk to attempt suicide (Wilcox et al., 2009). These symptoms complicate treatment, especially if PTSD and ASD are ignored and only the other diagnoses are treated.

Preexisting psychiatric disorders, including personality disorders, can increase the risk of developing ASD and PTSD after a traumatic event (Axelrod et al., 2005). A history of previous traumas, including torture, childhood abuse, rape, and abuse by a partner, leads to an increased risk for PTSD after later traumas. Conversely, events later in life might trigger previously unrecognized PTSD.

There might be difficulties such as arrests, unemployment, homelessness, abusiveness, divorce, and paranoia toward authority figures or others whom patients perceive as directly or indirectly responsible for not helping with the original traumatic situation (Amaya-Jackson et al., 1999; Beckham et al., 2000). Mistrust, isolation, abandonment fears, workaholism, focusing on the needs of others, feelings of inadequacy, anger toward God, unresolved grief, and fear of losing control of emotions are common (Bille,1993).

The family members, friends, and coworkers of individuals with PTSD or ASD also might develop problems as "secondary victims." In some cases, these individuals have experienced the same trauma (e.g., accident, fire, disaster) and develop symptoms themselves. The family might or might not be able to help their family member with PTSD. The whole family or certain members might need family therapy.

Neurochemical Basis of Acute Stress and Posttraumatic Stress Disorders

Brain structures, neurotransmitters, and the autonomic nervous system are involved in how trauma is processed. During the exposure to trauma, increased heart rate, elevated cortisol levels, and adrenergic overactivity can lead to the development of PTSD. The amygdala, the center for emotional processing and fear response, sends a message to the prefrontal cortex for processing. The hippocampus plays a role in stress responses, memory, and fear conditioning. High glucocorticoid levels and prolonged exposure to stress damage the hippocampi. This damage leads to failure to shut down stress responses and contributes to impaired extinction of conditioned fear (Heim & Nemeroff, 2009). Normally, associations leading to the conditioned response would be erased, or new associations would mask the response-producing associations over time. Conditioned fear responses, after being dormant for years, can be reactivated by trauma-associated stimuli.

Sensitization is the increased magnitude of response to one stimulus, but especially to repeated traumatic stimuli. This behavioral sensitivity produces increased arousal (*hyperarousal*) and stress sensitivity that can endure for a long time (Beckham et al., 2000; Charney, 2004). *Cross-sensitization* can occur so that there is overreaction to other, even minor, stimuli that resemble the original traumatic stimulus (Beckham et al., 2000; Charney, 2004; Friedman, 1997; Solomon & Heide, 2005; van der Kolk, 1997).

Avoidance and numbing, in response to fear conditioning and behavioral sensitization, are likely to be related to increased endogenous opiate release (Charney, 2004; Friedman, 1997), producing emotional blunting, physical analgesia, and depersonalization. Autonomic hyperarousal, also in response to fear conditioning and behavioral sensitization, is related to increased noradrenergic and dopaminergic system activity and to decreased serotonergic activity, causing fear, anxiety, and "fight or flight" readiness. Reexperiencing the trauma, in response to fear conditioning and failure of extinction, is related to activation of the amygdala, locus ceruleus, hypothalamus, thalamus, and hippocampus (limbic system and hypothalamic-pituitary-adrenal axis), which enhances encoding of traumatic memories and sensory and cognitive memory retrieval (Heim & Nemeroff, 2009). Prolonged stress eventually results in down-regulation of corticotropin-releasing hormone, dehydroepiandrosterone, neuropeptide Y, and adrenergic receptors; decreased adrenocorticotropin-releasing hormone release; and increased levels of testosterone and estrogen. The fear-anxiety response can become blunted, and desensitization is induced (Charney, 2004; Solomon & Heide, 2005; van der Kolk, 1997).

? CRITICAL THINKING QUESTION

2. Ron Jenkins' workplace was severely damaged by an explosion. He was found staring at the cars in the parking lot and repeating that he had to find his car and wife. He was unable to give his address or say where his wife would be at that time of day. He refused to be treated for cuts and bruises until he could find his wife. What interventions would you use at the scene?

Adjustment Disorder

Adjustment disorder is characterized by marked emotional distress resulting from an identifiable stressful life event (marital breakup, persistent painful illness, job loss, natural disaster). The symptoms develop within 3 months after the stressor, and the reaction is not severe enough to fit the criteria for PTSD. The symptoms or reactions to the stressful circumstance are considered out of proportion to the severity or intensity of the stressor. The acute reaction interferes with functioning but lasts no longer than 6 months *after* the stressor and its consequences have ended. Chronic symptoms might persist more than 6 months if the consequences of the stressor are more enduring, such as a chronic illness or difficulties resulting from a divorce. The major treatment goals are to recognize the relationship between the stressful situation and current problems and to review and integrate the feelings and memories of the original situation.

PUTTING IT ALL TOGETHER

PSYCHOTHERAPEUTIC MANAGEMENT

An effective approach with PTSD and ASD is to prevent or minimize the symptoms. Principles of critical incident stress management (CISM) are often applied to disaster situations in which the development of posttraumatic symptoms in some victims is likely. This model provides a wide range of services for primary and secondary victims, including seven core integrated elements: (1) precrisis preparation (including individuals and organizations who will assist in CISM); (2) large-scale demobilization procedures for use after mass disasters; (3) individual acute crisis counseling; (4) brief small group discussions called *defusings*, designed to assist in acute symptom reduction; (5) longer small group discussions called *critical incident stress debriefings*, designed to assist in achieving a sense of psychological closure postcrisis or facilitate the referral process; (6) family crisis intervention techniques; and (7) follow-up procedures or referral, or both, for psychological assessment or treatment (Everly et al., 2000). The National Organization of Victims Assistance (NOVA) and the American Red Cross have developed similar models.

The element of CISM related to crisis counseling begins with a discussion of the goals, rules, and roles of the leaders (who are often both mental health workers and trained peers of the victims). This is followed by a cognitive-oriented discussion of the facts of the incident, beginning with thoughts that group members had when they arrived at the scene. The discussion moves to an emotional phase, which allows for the expression of the full range of feelings. The final stage focuses on discussion and education about any symptoms of ASD or PTSD that are being experienced, teaching coping strategies to use with any further stress reactions, and ways to prepare for return to work. Ideally, the goal for group debriefing is psychological closure related to the critical event and a return to a precrisis (or an even more functional) level of adaptation. After the group debriefing, the leaders also debrief each other about what they heard and felt while listening to the traumatic experiences being discussed and about the effectiveness of the group debriefing (Everly et al., 2000). With large-scale disasters, such as at the World Trade Center, closure is much more difficult because of the extended length of time that is required for location and identification of victims and for the final cleanup of the debris.

Nurse-Patient Relationship

The first priority in the nurse's relationship with patients experiencing PTSD or ASD is the development of trust. Because these patients have a tendency to be withdrawn, to feel alienated, and to be suspicious of others, developing trust might be difficult. Seeking help or accepting it when offered is also sometimes difficult for patients. When a patient is aware of the current influence of the trauma, there is often a tendency for him or her to believe that "No one can understand what I've been through unless they have been through it too." The nurse needs to be nonjudgmental, honest, empathic, and supportive. The nurse can convey the message, "I haven't been through what you have, but the more you tell me, the better I will understand what you have been through and are experiencing." It is important to acknowledge any unfairness or injustices that were part of the trauma. Safety and security are other priorities because of the risk for suicide and aggression. Sleep disturbances must also be addressed because of insomnia and nightmares.

These patients also need to hear that they are not crazy but are having typical reactions to a serious trauma. Teaching about the dynamics of PTSD or ASD is often appropriate.

Depending on the nature of the trauma, the nurse must be prepared to hear stories of atrocities and help patients process the losses and changes that have occurred in their lives as a result of the trauma. Nurses might need help for themselves to avoid vicarious victimization (secondary PTSD), compassion fatigue, or burnout when working with trauma victims in settings such as emergency departments, burn units, accidents, or disaster scenes (Badger, 2001; Boscarino et al., 2004).

It might take time for patients to recognize the relationship between their current problems and the original traumatic event. When patients are not initially aware of the connection between the original trauma and current feelings and problems, the nurse should gently clarify these connections as they emerge.

Patients need to evaluate their past behaviors according to the original context of the situation, not by current values and standards (Figley, 2000). For example, a rape victim who did not resist her knife-wielding attacker needs to judge her behavior in the context of the life-or-death situation, not by someone's comment that she "must have asked for it." Another example is the Afghanistan veteran who must evaluate his experience of killing a woman who was holding an assault weapon within the context of war, not by society's current view of war as immoral. Developing a new perspective on the original trauma, which involves clarifying facts, feelings, and values, is not always easy for patients.

Patients need significant help in safely verbalizing feelings, particularly anger, that have often been ignored or repressed; this is especially true if there have been destructive outbursts or if patients are trying desperately to remain in control. Writing in a journal is often helpful. Expressive therapy (art, music, and poetry) can facilitate externalizing painful emotions that are difficult to verbalize (Clark, 1997; Hines-Martin & Ising, 1993).

As patients struggle through the sometimes lengthy process of reexperiencing, reintegrating, and processing memories of and feelings about traumatic experiences, they need empathy and reassurance that they will be safe and need to be taught stress management techniques so they are not overwhelmed with anxiety. It is also important to take time-outs to focus on emergent problems and potential solutions. These problems, such as finances, housing, and divorce, and their associated feelings can be as stressful as the original event. Patients need to be involved in problem solving, decision making, and taking specific actions toward overcoming these stresses. Patients' adaptive coping skills and use of relaxation strategies need to be encouraged, whereas dysfunctional activities, especially avoidance of responsibility for one's actions and the abuse of alcohol and drugs, need to be discouraged.

Involving the family as needed helps patients to reestablish relationships that provide support and assistance. Couple or family education and counseling might be recommended, if appropriate. The box, "Key Nursing Interventions for Posttraumatic Stress Disorder and Acute Stress Disorder," lists additional nursing interventions to use for PTSD and ASD. *Evidence-based therapies* to treat the symptoms of PTSD are trauma-focused CBT, prolonged exposure therapy, and eye movement desensitization and reprocessing (Bisson, 2008;

KEY NURSING INTERVENTIONS

for Posttraumatic Stress Disorder and Acute Stress Disorder

1. Be nonjudgmental and honest; offer empathy and support; acknowledge any unfairness or injustices related to the trauma. *Rationale:* Building trust might be difficult for patients.
2. Assure patients that their feelings and behaviors are typical reactions to serious trauma. *Rationale:* Patients often believe that they are going crazy.
3. Help patients recognize the connections between the trauma experience and their current feelings, behaviors, and problems. *Rationale:* Patients often are unaware of these connections.
4. Help patients evaluate past behaviors in the context of the trauma, not in the context of current values and standards. *Rationale:* Patients often have guilt about past behaviors and are judgmental of themselves.
5. Encourage safe verbalization of feelings, especially anger. *Rationale:* Feelings are or have been repressed or suppressed.
6. Encourage adaptive coping strategies, such as exercise, relaxation techniques, and sleep-promoting strategies. *Rationale:* Patients might have been using maladaptive or dysfunctional coping to avoid dealing with feelings and issues.
7. Encourage patients to establish or reestablish relationships. *Rationale:* Relationships (needed for assistance and support) might have been affected by patients' suspiciousness or fear of asking for help.

Heim & Nemeroff, 2009; Parslow et al., 2008; Rauch et al., 2009; Ray, 2008).

Psychopharmacology

The choice of medications depends on the primary symptoms the patient is experiencing and the presence of other comorbid disorders. SSRIs are the first-line treatment for PTSD. Paroxetine, sertraline, and fluoxetine have been approved for PTSD (Nisenoff, 2008; Parslow et al., 2008). Tricyclic antidepressants and monoamine oxidase inhibitors are second-line treatments. Trazodone helps with insomnia and reduces nightmares in some patients.

Benzodiazepines are effective in reducing anxiety, but there are few studies examining their use for PTSD. There is a risk of dependence, especially for patients who are already abusing alcohol or drugs.

Clonidine and propranolol might produce responses similar to those of benzodiazepines. Both medications can help diminish the peripheral autonomic response associated with fear, anxiety, and nightmares.

Atypical antipsychotics (olanzapine, risperidone, and quetiapine) can be used for severe PTSD or when the patient has a comorbid diagnosis of psychosis or bipolar disorder. These medications might be used for hyperarousal, flashbacks, and nightmares.

Milieu Management

Patients experiencing PTSD or ASD can benefit from many inpatient or outpatient milieu activities. Social activities can help rebuild social skills that have been damaged by suspiciousness and withdrawal. Recreational and exercise programs can help reduce tension and promote relaxation. Moderate-intensity aerobic exercise has been found to decrease symptoms of PTSD in adolescents (Diaz & Motta, 2008). Groups that focus on self-esteem, decision making, assertiveness, anger management, stress management, and relaxation techniques might be useful. Victims of a variety of traumas might benefit from group meetings that focus on the similarities in their reactions and feelings, such as mistrust, helplessness, fear, guilt, numbing, detachment, nightmares, and flashbacks.

Community Resources

Group CBT, group psychotherapy, and self-help groups with others who have experienced the same or a similar trauma are useful. A community might have a Department of Veterans Affairs Hospital or veterans' outreach center for war veterans and their spouses as well as groups for victims of rape, incest, or torture and their family members. A community might hold meetings for victims after a community disaster or national tragedy. There also might be a victim's assistance program for crime victims. Substance abuse programs or groups might be needed.

CASE STUDY

Craig was 19 years old when he spent a year in Afghanistan as the gunman on a tank. His tank was hit several times during his tour of duty, and one of his buddies was seriously injured. In addition, he witnessed several of his colleagues dying as a result of stepping on improvised explosive devices and many others dying or sustaining injury as a result of getting shot. After returning to the United States, he reentered college and tried to resume a normal life in his hometown. Within 2 years he met and married a young woman who was just out of high school. Their marriage lasted less than a year. During this time, Craig flunked out of school and spent much of his time playing video games. He was fired from his part-time job for absenteeism and being late for work. He was able to find another job at a local restaurant as a cook. However, occasionally he would become angry and had a habit of hitting the wall with his fist to relieve his pent-up anger. He was fired after several warnings, again related to absenteeism and showing up late. All the while, he never talked about his experiences in Afghanistan with anyone. Out of work, divorced, and using illegal drugs, his family convinced him to get evaluated at the Veteran's Administration Hospital. During a series of physician visits, he reported having bouts of depression with suicidal ideation, difficulty focusing and concentrating, flashbacks, nightmares, avoidance behavior especially during veteran holidays, avoidance of war movies, and angry outbursts. After 9 months of evaluation, Craig was diagnosed with PTSD, major depression, traumatic brain injury, and attention-deficit disorder. He is currently receiving 65% disability pay and outpatient treatment.

⊚ **CARE PLAN**

Name: Craig Brown   **Admission Date:** _____

DSM-5 Diagnosis: Posttraumatic stress disorder

Assessment	**Areas of strength:** Patient is intelligent, has supportive family, and has Department of Veterans Affairs resources.
	Problems: Suicidal ideation, flashbacks, nightmares, outbursts of anger, isolated, difficulty concentrating and focusing.
Diagnoses	Potential for self-directed and other-directed violence related to suicidal ideation and anger outbursts, as evidenced by suicidal statements.
	Sleep pattern disturbance related to nightmares, as evidenced by interrupted sleep, increasing irritability.
	Posttrauma response related to war experiences, as evidenced by reexperiencing of traumatic events in flashbacks and nightmares.
Outcomes	**Short-term goals**
Date met: _____	Patient will agree to talk to staff if he feels suicidal or aggressive toward others.
Date met: _____	Patient will verbalize feelings of anger and sadness appropriately.
Date met: _____	Patient will describe his experiences in Afghanistan.
	Long-term goals
Date met: _____	Patient will attend outpatient appointments at the veterans' outreach center and attend co-occurring disorders group.
Planning and Interventions	**Nurse-patient relationship:** Assess and monitor suicidal ideations. Assist patient with identification and verbalization of feelings, especially anger. Assist patient in describing Afghanistan experiences.
	Psychopharmacology: Paroxetine (Paxil CR) 20 mg q morning; amphetamine and dextroamphetamine (Adderall XR) 20 mg q morning.
	Milieu management: Co-occurring groups focusing on addiction and anger management, relaxation techniques, social skills, and self-esteem.
Evaluation	Patient verbalizes that he is no longer suicidal. Patient is beginning to verbalize his anger and sadness about Afghanistan and the loss of his buddies.

SOMATIC SYMPTOM AND RELATED DISORDERS

Somatic symptom and related disorders include the following: (1) somatic symptom disorder, (2) illness anxiety disorder, (3) conversion disorder, and (4) factitious disorder. The major characteristic of somatic symptom and related disorders is that patients have physical symptoms for which there is *no known organic cause or physiologic mechanism.* All of these disorders share a common feature: distressing somatic symptoms associated with abnormal thoughts, feelings, and behaviors in response to these symptoms. Individuals with somatic symptoms are usually encountered in primary acute and other medical (nonpsychiatric) settings (American Psychiatric Association, 2013).

The question must be asked: What does the process of somatization achieve for individuals? What does it achieve for the 5-year-old who is afraid of leaving his mother to go to kindergarten for the first time? He tells his mother that he is sick and has a stomachache or headache in hopes of avoiding his fears. Mom comforts him and lets him stay home for the day. This is known as primary gain and secondary gain. *Primary gain* refers to the individual's desire to relieve anxiety to feel better and more secure. *Secondary gain* refers to the attention or support the individual derives from others because of illness. This phenomenon immeasurably complicates the treatment of somatic patients.

Somatic Symptom Disorder

Individuals with somatic symptom disorder (previously known as hypochondriasis) have multiple, recurrent, significant somatic symptoms with no evidence of a medical explanation. They tend to have very high levels of worry about their illness, appraising their bodily symptoms as unduly threatening and harmful. The presumption exists that the physical symptoms are connected to psychological factors or conflicts. These patients are not in control of their symptoms, which are unconscious and involuntary. Patients express conflicts through bodily symptoms (primarily pain) and complaints using the defense of somatization. They do not deal with their anxiety or feelings emotionally but displace the anxiety into bodily symptoms. These patients repeatedly see general practitioners seeking medical diagnosis and treatment even though they have been told that there is no known physiologic or organic evidence to explain their symptoms or disability. Medical interventions rarely alleviate the individual's concern. The overconcern of bodily symptoms assumes a central role in the individual's life, impairing social and occupational functioning (American Psychiatric Association, 2013).

Illness Anxiety Disorder

Individuals with illness anxiety disorder are excessively preoccupied with having or acquiring a serious undiagnosed illness (American Psychiatric Association, 2013). If somatic symptoms are present, they are typically mild in intensity. Similar to somatic symptom disorder, a medical evaluation fails to identify a serious medical condition. The individual feels substantial anxiety over various types of bodily discomfort (i.e., dizziness, tinnitus, belching) because they believe that it means they have a serious undiagnosed disease. These individuals become alarmed when hearing about someone else becoming ill or reading a health-related news story. Regardless of medical reassurances, the anxiety is not alleviated and may even be heightened. Preoccupation with an undiagnosed illness results in the individual researching the suspected disease excessively and making it the prominent topic in social interactions among family and friends.

Conversion Disorder (Functional Neurologic Symptom Disorder)

The major feature of conversion disorder is a deficit or alteration in voluntary motor or sensory function that mimics a neurologic or medical condition (American Psychiatric Association, 2013). Conversion disorder is typically associated with psychological or physical stress or trauma. Individuals have spontaneous attacks of severe physical disability despite a lack of medical evidence. Motor symptoms that most commonly occur include paralysis, tremors, gait abnormalities, and abnormal limb posturing. Frequent sensory symptoms include altered or absent skin sensation, blindness, or inability to hear. Psychogenic or nonepileptic seizures characterized by impaired consciousness and generalized limb shaking may occur. Other symptoms may include dysphonia or aphonia (reduced or absent speech volume), dysarthria (altered articulation), globus (lump in the throat), and diplopia. Dissociative symptoms such as depersonalization, derealization, and amnesia may occur during attacks. Symptoms may be transient or persistent. Individuals also might have an attitude of *la belle indifference*, meaning they express little concern or anxiety about the distressing symptoms. This lack of concern might be interpreted as though individuals with conversion disorder minimize their illness.

Clinical Example

Roberta, age 45, is told by her neurologist that all of her test results are negative and that he cannot find a physiologic reason for her difficulty walking, lump in her throat, dizziness, slurred speech, and foreign accent. He tells her there is nothing else he can do and refers her to psychological services. When she goes to visit a nurse therapist, she arrives in a wheelchair, accompanied by her husband. She is able to ambulate from the wheelchair to the office sofa with help. While talking with the nurse therapist, she asks if she can lay down because of feeling dizzy. When the therapist asks her what she thinks is wrong with her, Roberta replies that she doesn't really know. She also reports that she has recently changed physicians and is still hoping to find out what is wrong with her. After a series of visits with the nurse therapist, Roberta is able to connect her physical symptoms to her anxiety about dying. She had a traumatic experience at age 20 when her fiancé died about a month after a car accident. His death was not anticipated because she was not aware that his injuries were life-threatening. The nurse therapist used cognitive-behavioral therapy, encouraging such techniques as deep breathing, music therapy, and cognitive restructuring.

Factitious Disorder

Factitious disorder is characterized by the falsification of medical or psychological signs and symptoms *in oneself or others*. These individuals impose harm on themselves or others by misrepresenting, exaggerating, fabricating, inducing, simulating, or causing signs or symptoms of illness or injury in the absence of obvious external rewards. Behavioral examples of factitious disorder that can lead to excessive medical intervention include adding blood to urine, ingesting warfarin or injecting insulin, and injecting fecal material to produce an abscess or to induce sepsis (American Psychiatric Association, 2013).

PUTTING IT ALL TOGETHER

PSYCHOTHERAPEUTIC MANAGEMENT

Nurse-Patient Relationship

The focus of the nurse-patient relationship is to improve patients' overall levels of functioning by helping them develop adaptive coping behaviors. Patients with somatoform disorders are often unable to identify and express their feelings, needs, and conflicts. Teaching them ways to verbalize feelings appropriately helps eliminate or diminish the need for physical symptoms.

Patients require time to understand their need for physical symptoms. Awareness and insight develop slowly as patients begin to verbalize their needs. Some patients take longer to develop this awareness and insight. The nurse must convey empathy and reassurance and teach patients about the connection between emotions and physical symptoms.

The physician or psychiatrist orders tests, a physical examination, and a laboratory workup to assess patients thoroughly for the presence of any physiologic or organic disease or etiology (if this has not been done before). The absence of any relevant medical findings strongly suggests that a somatoform disorder is present, especially if stress and conflicts are present in the patient's life.

The box, "Key Nursing Interventions for Somatic Disorders," lists nursing interventions used for patients with somatoform disorders.

Psychopharmacology

Because patients with somatoform disorders might be using too much medication and taking a variety of drugs, medication for pain should be used temporarily and sparingly. SSRIs are helpful for treating anxiety and depression because of the high incidence of comorbidity of these disorders. SSRIs also decrease sensitivity to bodily sensations (Abramowitz & Braddock, 2006).

Milieu Management

Relaxation exercises, meditation, and CBT are used to treat somatoform disorders. Physical therapy might be indicated to prevent muscle atrophy for an individual with conversion disorder (Miller, 2005a). Assertiveness, decision-making, goal-setting, stress management, and social skills groups often benefit these patients. Family therapy is helpful when family conflict is present.

Because patients with somatoform disorders are usually overusers of medical care, some hospitals and clinics provide

KEY NURSING INTERVENTIONS

for Somatic Disorders

1. Use a matter-of-fact, caring approach when communicating with patients. *Rationale:* To decrease secondary gains.
2. Ask patients how they are feeling, and ask them to describe their feelings. *Rationale:* To increase verbalization about feelings (especially negative ones), needs, and anxiety rather than about somatization.
3. Assist patients with developing more appropriate ways to verbalize feelings and needs. *Rationale:* To increase adaptive coping through assertiveness.
4. Use positive reinforcement, and set limits by withdrawing attention from patients when they focus on physical complaints or make unreasonable demands. *Rationale:* To decrease complaining behavior.
5. Be consistent with patients, and have all requests directed to the primary nurse providing care. *Rationale:* To decrease attention-seeking or manipulative behaviors.
6. Use diversion by including patients in milieu activities and recreational games. *Rationale:* To decrease rumination about physical complaints.
7. Do not push awareness of or insight into conflicts or problems. *Rationale:* To prevent an increase in anxiety and the need for physical symptoms.

group interventions as part of the medical care. These groups focus on underlying psychosocial needs, not on physical needs. When successful, this type of treatment approach can result in decreasing hospital costs, while providing more appropriate patient care.

DISSOCIATIVE DISORDERS

Dissociative disorders are characterized by a disruption in consciousness, memory, identity, emotion, perception, body representation, motor control, and behavior (American Psychiatric Association, 2013). The major features of dissociative disorders are depersonalization, derealization, amnesia, numbing, and flashbacks. These disorders are frequently exhibited in the aftermath of trauma and include (1) dissociative amnesia; (2) depersonalization/derealization disorder; and (3) dissociative identity disorder (DID). Dissociative disorders are closely related to trauma and stressor-related disorders. Both PTSD and ASD contain dissociative symptoms (i.e., amnesia, flashbacks, depersonalization).

Dissociation, which is the removal from conscious awareness of painful feelings, memories, thoughts, or aspects of identity, is an unconscious defense mechanism that protects an individual from the emotional pain of experiences or

CASE STUDY

William Robinson, a 62-year-old white man, started attending the community outpatient day program on June 15 at 9 A.M. He walked into the nurse's office limping and supported by his wife, Harriet. He stated to the nurse that he was experiencing horrible pain in his left leg and foot. Anger and irritability were evident in his voice. During the assessment, Mr. Robinson explained that the pain started suddenly about 7 months ago. Since that time, he has seen numerous physicians to obtain treatment and relief from his pain. The last physician told him that his pain was caused by stress and referred him to a therapist trained to manage stress-related disorders. The patient stated that he hoped this therapist would know what to do because none of the other health care professionals did.

Mrs. Robinson brought her husband's medications to the day program. The nurse found that a number of analgesics had been prescribed, along with sleeping medication. Mr. Robinson said that he took what he wanted, when he wanted, and that it was better than not taking anything at all.

Mrs. Robinson told the nurse that Mr. Robinson needed a lot of help with everything. She had been so physically tired that she had called their only daughter, Sheila, for assistance. Sheila lives 400 miles away, and they had not seen her for 3 years. Their daughter was so concerned about her parents that she had come to help for 2 weeks last month.

As the conversation continued, Mrs. Robinson told the nurse that her husband had been in good health except for an occasional cold until about 7 months ago, when he suddenly started to complain about awful pain in his leg and foot. He had never in all his years working for a cabinetmaker experienced anything like this before. Mrs. Robinson did not know why all this pain was occurring now, especially because her husband had retired 9 months earlier. He had been forced to retire early because the company he worked for had not been doing well and all employees aged 60 and older were ordered to retire. She stated that her husband had never said too much about it, and she thought that now they would have time to travel and go on fishing trips, which her husband had always enjoyed. They had gone on many fishing trips as a family while their daughter was growing up and had enjoyed them immensely. Periodically, her husband went fishing with some friends. Since the onset of her husband's pain, however, they had not done anything socially, together or with friends.

From the time he started the day program, Mr. Robinson refused to do anything but sit in a lounge chair in the community room. He needed much assistance from staff members to walk to the dining room and to the restroom. At times, his food was brought to him in the community room because he refused to walk to the dining room.

Interactions with the nurse centered on his pain and on requests for pain medication. He described his pain in detail and would talk of little else. He requested a wheelchair while at the day program so that he could maneuver around the facilities with greater ease. Mr. Robinson was receiving an analgesic for pain, and an antidepressant as ordered by his physician.

CARE PLAN

Name: William Robinson Admission Date: _____

DSM-5 Diagnosis: Somatic symptom disorder

Assessment	**Areas of strength:** Patient enjoyed fishing and traveling; had been in good health. Patient's wife is very supportive. Patient had worked for many years.
	Problems: Experiencing pain in his left leg and foot; social functioning has declined; focus with staff is about his pain; secondary gains maintain his sick role.
Diagnoses	Ineffective coping related to anger, as evidenced by complaints of physical pain.
	Chronic pain, related to low self-esteem, as evidenced by inability to verbalize feelings.
	Severe anxiety, related to dependency, as evidenced by inability to care for self.
Outcomes	**Short-term goals**
Date met: _____	Patient will verbalize feelings and needs.
Date met: _____	Patient will verbalize underlying anger resulting from early retirement.
Date met: _____	Patient will verbalize awareness about connecting emotions with physical symptoms.
Date met: _____	Patient will develop adaptive coping behaviors.
	Long-term goals
Date met: _____	Patient will assume responsibility for self-care and independent functioning.
Date met: _____	Patient will schedule appointments for joint counseling with his wife.
Date met: _____	Patient will identify plans to volunteer in his community.
Date met: _____	Patient will plan leisure activities.
Planning and Interventions	**Nurse-patient relationship:** Convey interest and support; focus on assisting the patient to verbalize feelings and needs related to anxiety, self-esteem, and anger; give positive feedback when the patient focuses on issues other than pain; set limits on need for attention and medication; teach relaxation exercises.
	Psychopharmacology: Decrease the use of analgesics. Paroxetine (Paxil CR) 20 mg q morning.
	Milieu management: Encourage participation in assertiveness and communication, problem-solving, discharge planning, and social skills groups; diversional occupational therapy; and recreational activities.
Evaluation	Patient's focus on pain is decreasing, and he is able to assume self-care activities with little assistance.
Referrals	Appointments for outpatient group therapy and counseling with his wife.

conflicts that have been repressed. This splitting off (removal) helps these individuals to endure and survive intense emotional events or physical pain. Traumatic events such as war, rape, or childhood sexual abuse are closely linked with dissociative episodes.

Dissociative Amnesia

Dissociative amnesia is characterized by the inability to recall important personal information, usually of a traumatic nature (not normal forgetting). The amnesia may be localized, selective, or generalized. Localized amnesia occurs when the individual cannot remember what occurred during a specific period of time (e.g., not being able to remember what happened for hours after a bad car accident). The ability to recall only a specific aspect of an event is called *selective amnesia*. Generalized amnesia, a complete loss of memory related to one's life history, is rare but seen primarily among combat veterans and sexual assault victims (American Psychiatric Association, 2013). Individuals with generalized amnesia are sometimes found by the police wandering aimlessly and are confused and disoriented. They might be taken to a hospital and be frightened and perplexed.

Depersonalization/Derealization Disorder

Depersonalization/derealization disorder is characterized by persistent or recurrent episodes of depersonalization or derealization or both in response to overwhelming stress. The essential feature of depersonalization is a feeling of unreality or detachment from oneself. Individuals feel as if they are watching themselves from outside their bodies, an "out of body experience" (American Psychiatric Association, 2013; Weber, 2007). In addition, individuals may be detached from their emotions, feeling numb. Bodily sensations are altered (e.g., feeling robotic or lacking control of speech and movement).

Derealization is characterized by a feeling of detachment or unfamiliarity with one's surroundings. Individuals experience perceptual distortions such as blurriness, altered distance of objects, heightened acuity, or muted sounds. For example, buildings might appear to be leaning, or everything might seem gray and dull. Some individuals report feeling as if they are in a fog, dream, or bubble.

Dissociative Identity Disorder

DID is characterized by (1) the existence of two or more distinct identities or personality states and (2) recurrent episodes of amnesia (American Psychiatric Association, 2013). Alternative personalities (alters) typically manifest as if another person has taken control, such that the individual begins speaking or acting in a distinctly different way. For example, an alter may seem to be a child, a teenager, or the opposite gender. Alters have distinctive attitudes, emotions, and behaviors. Each personality is different from the others and from the original personality. Each alter has its own name, behavior traits, memories, emotional characteristics, and social relations. The primary identity might carry the person's name and be depressed, dependent, and guilty, whereas alternative personalities might be hostile, controlling, and self-destructive. The person may be aware of alters to varying degrees or completely unaware. Patients can experience memory problems, depersonalization, time loss, voices conversing with each other, and somatic symptoms (Gillig, 2009).

Similar to the other dissociative disorders, DID is a defense against extreme anxiety that is aroused in highly painful and emotionally traumatic situations and is seen most frequently in childhood sexual abuse. The splitting off of these painful events allows the person to survive the trauma but leaves an impaired personality with disconnected parts. The alternative personalities have feelings and behaviors associated with the trauma. Dissociated states represent fragments of the person's sense of identity with different identity states remembering distinct information (Weber, 2007). These states help the person to survive the emotional memories. A shy, quiet woman might have alternative personalities that are promiscuous, flamboyant, childlike, and aggressive. A woman might awaken one morning and find the living room of her apartment littered with toys or strewn with empty alcohol bottles and leftover food. She does not remember what happened because she has amnesia for the span of time when another personality took over, or came out. Dissociative fugue is common, where the individual reports she suddenly found herself at the beach, at work, or in a nightclub with no memory of how she got there.

These patients are admitted to inpatient psychiatric units when they are suicidal or experience hallucinations. Individuals with DID often have comorbid disorders such as major depression, bipolar disorder, PTSD, psychotic disorders, substance use disorders, borderline personality disorder, and somatic disorders. The array of symptoms that these individuals experience is overwhelming. The safe structure of a hospital setting provides emotional safety and security for the patient when working with difficult or overwhelming issues.

DID may be described in some cultures as a possession experience. Possession-form identities typically manifest as a "spirit" that has taken control of the individual. For example, the "ghost" of a girl who died years before possesses the individual and speaks and acts as though she were still alive. In some cases, the individual may be "taken over" by a demon or deity, demanding that a relative be punished for a past act. These identities present recurrently, are unwanted and involuntary, and cause significant distress. (Note: Most possession states around the world are normal spiritual practices and do not meet criteria for DID.)

PUTTING IT ALL TOGETHER

PSYCHOTHERAPEUTIC MANAGEMENT

Nurse-Patient Relationship

The nurse's relationship with individuals experiencing dissociation and amnesia includes interventions to establish trust and support. Patients have physiologic and neurologic workups to rule out organic causations. The nurse assists with gathering data regarding feelings, conflicts, or situations that patients experienced before the dissociative or amnesia state. Patients also might have sessions under hypnosis to gather data about forgotten material. The nurse should slowly help patients deal with anxiety and conflicts in their lives and improve coping skills.

Patients with depersonalization/derealization disorder are not usually found in an inpatient setting unless they have become suicidal, extremely anxious, or depressed. Nurses might work with these patients in outpatient settings.

The treatment goal of DID, ultimately through long-term therapy, is to integrate the personalities or memories, if possible, so that they can survive or coexist in the original personality. The use of hypnosis to retrieve memories is controversial. Some authors think that the use of hypnosis is harmful because it could produce additional alters and false memories (Miller, 2005b).

The nurse caring for these patients provides empathy to establish trust because the relationships of these patients with authority figures might have been inconsistent, rigid, and unpredictable. A contract should be initiated for patients' safety to reduce potential self-harm and violence. An alter might become homicidal because of revelations concerning abuse. Self-mutilation and suicidal behaviors also might be present when overwhelming anxiety or depression occurs. With the presence of a child alter, the nurse needs to remember that the patient is an adult and not a child. Compassionate care must be balanced with education about the disorder (Shusta-Hochberg, 2004). Management of feelings in a supportive environment increases trust and provides a predictable, positive learning environment.

Psychopharmacology

Medication does not eliminate the dissociative disorder itself. If symptoms of anxiety and depression are present, medications might help. For patients with DID, response to medication might be partial, and an alter's response to medication might be different and inconsistent.

Milieu Management

The nurse assumes an important role in the care of patients who are hospitalized in an inpatient psychiatric unit because of suicidal or recurrent attempts to harm themselves. Provisions for a safe environment and a trusting relationship are basic for helping these patients, who usually have not had trusting relationships with anyone. Assisting with group sessions; providing emotional security, empathy, acceptance, and support; and helping patients cope with daily living all are involved in nursing care.

For patients with DID, ongoing process-oriented groups, which might be available in some settings, can become nontherapeutic when patients reveal too much or regress, overwhelming the other group members. Task-oriented groups tend to be more beneficial than process-oriented groups. Long-term individual therapy should be initiated if it is not already occurring. Occupational therapy and art therapy provide patients with a means of non-verbal expression to reveal material that cannot be verbally accessed. Attendance at milieu meetings decreases isolation from the community.

For patients with dissociative disorders, relaxation, stress management, meditation, and exercise are beneficial. Important therapeutic interventions include education about the disorder, symptom management, adaptive coping strategies, and CBT (Gillig, 2009; Turkus & Kahler, 2006). Dialetical behavior therapy can help patients manage their emotional reactions surrounding issues of physical or sexual abuse.

Before discharge, a safety plan and no-harm contract might be necessary as well as initiating or continuing a support system for the patient. Self-help groups provide outpatients with the opportunity to practice social skills and problem solving to develop a sense of empowerment and control.

? CRITICAL THINKING QUESTION

3. A patient with DID is admitted to the inpatient unit because of a suicide attempt. One of the personalities wants to kill the patient, meaning that the patient is suicidal. The patient refuses to sign a no-harm contract. What issues would you expect to help the patient with, including safety precautions?

HIGHLIGHTING THE EVIDENCE

Evidence

Sexual abuse is a strong risk factor in the development of DID. However, not all children who are abused develop psychopathology. New research indicates that the development of DID is best predicted by disorganized attachment and the absence of familial and social support in combination with abuse. Healthy early attachment and solid social support systems contribute to the victim's resiliency and ability to remain psychologically healthy.

Summary

Providing support for children at risk can result in psychological resiliency. Providing social support structures such as mentorship for children in schools is a way to provide role models and support outside the family. Interventions for at-risk expectant mothers and new parents with enduring problems such as substance abuse can promote secure attachment with their child. The child then may have greater resiliency when faced with trauma.

Modified from Korol, S. (2008). Familial and social support as protective factors against the development of dissociative identity disorder. *Journal of Trauma & Dissociation, 9,* 249.

▌ S T U D Y   N O T E S

1. Understanding the process of anxiety is key to understanding and intervening therapeutically with patients who have anxiety-related disorders.
2. The patient's anxiety must be reduced to a mild or moderate level before the nurse can work with the patient on problem solving and adaptive coping.
3. In the category of anxiety-related disorders, patients feel or directly express symptoms of anxiety.
4. With PTSD, ASD, and adjustment disorder, the goals are to integrate traumatic memories and feelings about the original trauma and to move from victim to survivor status.
5. With somatic related disorders, anxiety is expressed through physical symptoms.
6. In DID, traumatic experiences are split off (removed) from conscious awareness, which helps patients survive extreme emotional or physical pain.
7. Key nursing interventions include helping patients to manage feelings, anxiety, conflicts, and life stressors in an adaptive manner so that they can become independent, functioning adults.

REFERENCES

Abramowitz, J. S., & Braddock, A. E. (2006). Hypochondriasis: Conceptualization, treatment, and relationship to obsessive-compulsive disorder. *Psychiatric Clinics of North America, 29,* 503.

Aguilera, D. C. (1998). *Crisis intervention: Theory and methodology* (8th ed.). St. Louis: Mosby.

Amaya-Jackson, L., et al. (1999). Functional impairment and utilization of services associated with posttraumatic stress in the community. *Journal of Traumatic Stress, 12,* 709.

American Psychiatric Association. (2013). *Diagnostic and statistical manual of mental disorders.* (5th ed.). Arlington, VA: APA.

Antai-Ontong, D. (2003). Current treatment of generalized anxiety disorder. *Journal of Psychosocial Nursing and Mental Health Services, 41,* 20.

Axelrod, S. R., Morgan, C. A., & Southwick, S. M. (2005). Symptoms of posttraumatic stress disorder and borderline personality disorder in veterans of Operation Desert Storm. *American Journal of Psychiatry, 162,* 270.

Badger, J. M. (2001). Understanding secondary traumatic stress. *American Journal of Nursing, 101,* 26.

Beckham, J. C., Moore, S. D., & Reynolds, V. (2000). Interpersonal hostility and violence in Vietnam combat veterans with chronic posttraumatic stress disorder. *Aggression and Violent Behavior, 5,* 451.

Bille, D. A. (1993). Road to recovery, posttraumatic stress disorder: The hidden victim. *Journal of Psychosocial Nursing and Mental Health Services, 31,* 19.

Bisson, J. I. (2008). Using evidence to inform clinical practice shortly after traumatic events. *Journal of Traumatic Stress, 21,* 507.

Boscarino, J. A., Figley, C. R., & Adams, R. E. (2004). Compassion fatigue following the September 11 terrorist attacks: A study of secondary trauma among New York City social workers. *International Journal of Emergency Mental Health, 6,* 57.

Charney, D. S. (2004). Psychobiological mechanisms of resilience and vulnerability: Implications for successful adaptation to extreme stress. *American Journal of Psychiatry, 161,* 195.

Clark, C. (1997). Posttraumatic stress disorder. *American Journal of Nursing, 97,* 27.

Clements, K., & Turpin, G. (2000). Life event exposure, physiological reactivity, and psychological strain. *Journal of Behavioral Medicine, 23,* 73.

Davidson, J. R. (2009). First-line pharmacotherapy approaches for generalized anxiety disorder. *Journal of Clinical Psychiatry, 70*(Suppl. 2), 25.

Diaz, A. B., & Motta, R. (2008). The effects of aerobic exercise on posttraumatic stress disorder symptom severity in adolescents. *International Journal of Emergency Mental Health, 10,* 49.

Eisner, R. (2004). Stresses stress in his research: A profile of Bruce McEwen, Ph.D. *NARSAD Research Newsletter, 16,* 1.

Everly, G. S., Flannery, R. B., & Mitchell, J. T. (2000). Critical incident stress management (CISM): A review of the literature. *Aggression and Violent Behavior, 5,* 23.

Figley, C. R. (2000). Families coping with trauma, clinical update: Posttraumatic stress disorder. *American Association for Marriage and Family Therapy, 2,* 1.

Friedman, M. J. (1997). Posttraumatic stress disorder. *Journal of Clinical Psychiatry, 58,* 33.

Gillig, P. M. (2009). Dissociative identity disorder: A controversial diagnosis. *Psychiatry, 6,* 24.

Glod, C., & Cawley, D. (1997). Psychobiology perspectives: The neurobiology of obsessive-compulsive disorders. *Journal of the American Psychiatric Nurses Association, 3,* 120.

Gorman, J. M., et al. (2000). Neuroanatomical hypothesis of panic disorder, revised. *American Journal of Psychiatry, 157,* 493.

Heim, C., & Nemeroff, C. B. (2009). Neurobiology of posttraumatic stress disorder. *CNS Spectrums, 14,* 13.

Hines-Martin, V. P., & Ising, M. (1993). Use of art therapy with post-traumatic stress disordered veteran clients. *Journal of Psychosocial Nursing and Mental Health Services, 31,* 29.

Hoffart, M. B., & Keene, E. P. (1998). The benefits of visualization. *American Journal of Nursing, 98,* 44.

Jiwanlal, S. S., & Weitzel, C. (2001). The suicide myth. *RN, 64,* 33.

Kaplan, Z., Iancu, I., & Bodner, E. (2001). A review of psychological debriefing after extreme stress. *Psychiatric Services, 52,* 824.

Keltner, N. L., Perry, B. A., & Williams, A. R. (2003). Panic disorder: A tightening vortex of misery. *Perspectives in Psychiatric Care, 39,* 41.

Kessler, R. C., et al. (2012). Twelve-month and lifetime prevalence and lifetime morbid risk of anxiety and mood disorders in the United States. *International Journal of Methods in Psychiatric Research, 21,* 169.

Kneisl, C. R., & Ames, S. W. (1986). *Adult health nursing: A biopsychosocial approach.* Menlo Park, CA: Addison-Wesley.

Koob, G. F. (2008). A role for brain stress systems in addiction. *Neuron, 59,* 11.

Korol, S. (2008). Familial and social support as protective factors against the development of dissociative identity disorder. *Journal of Trauma & Dissociation, 9,* 249.

Lazarus, R. S. (1966). *Psychological stress and the coping process.* St. Louis: McGraw-Hill.

Lazarus, R. S. (2006). Emotions and interpersonal relationships: Toward a person-centered conceptualization of emotions and coping. *Journal of Personality, 74,* 9.

Lazarus, R. S., & Folkman, S. (1984). *Stress, appraisal, and coping.* New York: Springer.

Marcks, B. A., Weisberg, R. B., & Keller, M. B. (2009). Psychiatric treatment received by primary care patients with panic disorder with and without agoraphobia. *Psychiatric Services, 60,* 823.

Martenson, M. E., Cetas, J. S., & Heinrecher, M. (2009). A possible neural basis for stress-induced hyperalgesia. *Pain, 142,* 236.

Miller, M. C. (2005a). Conversion disorder. *Harvard Mental Health Letter, 22,* 1.

Miller, M. C. (2005b). Falling apart: Dissociation and its disorders. *Harvard Mental Health Letter, 21,* 1.

Miller, M. C. (2005c). Questions and answers. *Harvard Mental Health Letter, 21,* 8.

Miller, M. C. (2009a). MRI scans reveal altered brain response to criticism in patients with social phobia. *Harvard Mental Health Letter, 25,* 7.

Miller, M. C. (2009b). Treating obsessive-compulsive disorder. *Harvard Mental Health Letter, 25,* 9.

Ninan, P., & Dunlop, B. (2005). Neurobiology and etiology of panic disorder. *Journal of Clinical Psychiatry, 66*(Suppl), 4.

Nisenoff, C. D. (2008). Psychotherapeutic and adjunctive pharmacologic approaches to treating posttraumatic stress disorder. *Psychiatry, 5,* 42.

Parslow, R., et al. (2008). Combined pharmacotherapy and psychological therapies for post traumatic stress disorder. *Cochrane Database of Systematic Reviews, 3,* CD007316.

Rauch, S., et al. (2009). Prolonged exposure effective for PTSD with a variety of traumas. *Journal of Traumatic Stress, 22,* 60.

Ray, S. L. (2008). Evolution of posttraumatic stress disorder and future directions. *Archives of Psychiatric Nursing, 22,* 217.

Selye, H. (1956). *The stress of life.* St. Louis: McGraw-Hill.

Shah, D. B., et al. (2008). Functional neurosurgery in the treatment of severe obsessive compulsive disorder and major depression: Overview of disease circuits and therapeutic targeting for the clinician. *Psychiatry, 5,* 25.

Shusta-Hochberg, S. R. (2004). Therapeutic hazards of treating child alters as real children in dissociative identity disorder. *Journal of Trauma & Dissociation, 5,* 13.

Soderstrom, M., et al. (2000). The relationship of hardiness, coping strategies, and perceived stress to symptoms of illness. *Journal of Behavioral Medicine, 23,* 311.

Solomon, E. P., & Heide, K. M. (2005). The biology of trauma: Implications for treatment. *Journal of Interpersonal Violence, 20,* 51.

Stein, M. B. (2009). Neurobiology of generalized anxiety disorder. *Journal of Clinical Psychiatry, 70*(Suppl. 2), 15.

Stuhlmiller, C., & Tolchard, B. (2009). Computer-assisted CBT for depression and anxiety. *Journal of Psychosocial Nursing and Mental Health Services, 47*, 32.

Substance Abuse and Mental Health Services Administration. (2009). *Results from the 2008 national survey on drug use and health: National findings.* http://www.samhsa.gov/data/nsduh/2k8nsduh/2k8Results.htm, Accessed November 13, 2013.

Taylor, S. E., et al. (2001). Biobehavioral responses to stress in females: Tend-and-befriend, not fight-or-flight. *Psychological Review, 107*, 411.

Turkus, J. A., & Kahler, J. A. (2006). Therapeutic interventions in the treatment of dissociative disorders. *Psychiatric Clinics of North America, 29*, 245.

van der Kolk, B. A. (1997). The psychobiology of post traumatic stress disorder. *Journal of Clinical Psychiatry, 58*, 16.

Weber, S. (2007). Dissociative symptom disorders in advanced nursing practice: Background, treatment, and instrumentation to assess symptoms. *Issues in Mental Health Nursing, 28*, 997.

Weigartz, P. S., & Rasminsky, S. (2005). Treating OCD in patients with psychiatric morbidity: How to keep anxiety, depression, and other disorders from thwarting interventions. *Current Psychiatry, 4*, 57.

Wilcox, H. C., Storr, C. L., & Breslau, N. (2009). Posttraumatic stress disorder and suicide attempts in a community sample of urban American young adults. *Archives of General Psychiatry, 66*, 305.

Cognitive Disorders

Gary Milligan

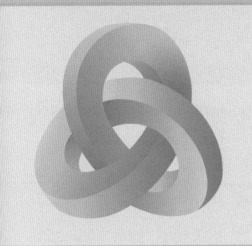

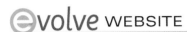

http://evolve.elsevier.com/Keltner

LEARNING OBJECTIVES

- Describe the biologic and functional changes associated with the most prevalent types of dementia.
- Describe the etiologic aspects and behaviors associated with delirium.
- Recognize the *DSM-5* criteria and terminology for neurocognitive disorders.

- Differentiate dementia from delirium.
- Discuss appropriate pharmacologic interventions for patients with dementia.
- Develop a care plan for a patient with dementia.
- Develop effective caregiver interventions.
- Discuss family issues related to cognitive disorders.

Cognitive disorders comprise a variety of assaults on the human brain. Cognition revolves around learning and memory. Loss of these fundamental abilities is a common thread in all cognitive disorders. In some disorders, these losses may be temporary. However, for most disorders, loss of memory is an indicator of future brain function. This chapter describes the most common cognitive disorders the psychiatric nurse may encounter.

Some common changes in cognition include disorientation, decreased concentration, loss of abstract thinking, and language disturbances. Delusions, hallucinations, and misidentification may frighten patients. These individuals may be unable to perform routine activities because of memory loss even though their motor skills are intact.

Cognitive disorders are divided into potentially reversible and irreversible types. These disorders can span a few hours to many years and may or may not be imminently life-threatening. To cloud the diagnostic picture, patients may have more than one cognitive disorder or a coexisting psychiatric illness. In addition, depression and anxiety are common in these patients.

Patients who exhibit a marked change of mental status often have a cognitive disorder. *DSM-5* (American Psychiatric Association, 2013) provides diagnostic criteria for all these disorders. Table 28-1 compares dementia and delirium (Wilson & Helton, 2011). Key terms are included,

and the student should consult the glossary in this text as well. Table 28-2 provides 12-month prevalence rates of mental disorders in the United States. Pertinent *DSM-5* diagnoses are listed as well.

NORM'S NOTES
This chapter is so important. There are more and more of us older people, and we are the ones who tend to develop the cognitive disorders discussed in this chapter. Think about it. When you can no longer reason clearly and rationally, the "real" you has been taken. As a kid, I used to wonder if I would rather lose an arm or a leg. Well, kids think about silly stuff. But I know now that I do not want to lose my cognitive functions. Fortunately, our government (run by a bunch of older people) spends a lot of money studying how these conditions can be stopped or reversed. I just want the researchers to hurry.

In dementia research, dozens of diagnostic tools are used, ranging from pen-and-pencil examinations to sophisticated neuroimaging studies. Genetic studies have isolated chromosomes and genes that are related to certain diseases. Since 1993, five different medications to treat Alzheimer's disease have reached the market.

TABLE 28-1 COMPARISON OF DEMENTIA AND DELIRIUM

CHARACTERISTICS	DELIRIUM	DEMENTIA
Onset	Occurs quickly, is obvious	Slow, unnoticeable at first
Course	Acute: rapid development, usually hours to days, but can last for months	Chronic: slow development over months and years, with a progressive deterioration spanning 3-10 years until death
Causes	Usually the result of other physical problems (e.g., illness, postsurgical complications, toxins)	Usually the primary disorder, but may be related to other illnesses (e.g., AIDS)
Memory	Short-term memory is impaired when assessed during an interim lucid or clear moment	Short-term memory is lost initially; long-term memory fails slowly
Level of consciousness	Fluctuating level of consciousness; alert at times; sleep is erratic; no pattern	No change; sleep patterns are usually consistent; day-night reversal is common
Thought content	Matches level of consciousness	Normal at first; later may be difficult to assess because of confusion or expressive or receptive aphasia and poverty of content
Thought process	Logical alternating with illogical, depending on the level of consciousness	Logical at first, then loss of abstraction (e.g., understanding a joke); concrete thinking occurs as disease progresses
Speech	May have slurred speech	Normal speech
Perceptual differences	Hallucinations—*visual:* seeing animals or unusual colors; picking at the air; *tactile:* feeling bugs on or under skin	Misidentification: calling one relative another's name—for example, calling a daughter "mama"; hallucinations may occur in the later stage, usually not at first; Delusions: grandiose, paranoid; pathologic jealousy
Mood	Anxiety and fear	Wide range of feelings
Affect	Appears bewildered, frightened	Appearance matches feeling

TABLE 28-2 12-MONTH PREVALENCE RATE OF MENTAL DISORDERS IN THE UNITED STATES*

DISORDERS	APPROXIMATE PERCENTAGE > 17 YEARS OLD (%)* (unless noted for children)	GENDER OVERREPRESENTATION
Anxiety disorders	18.1 overall	
Agoraphobia	1.7	Female
Panic disorder	2.4	Female
Panic attacks	11.2	Female
Social anxiety	7	Female
Specific phobia	7-9	Female
Separation anxiety	1.2	Equal
Generalized anxiety disorder	2	Female
Posttraumatic stress disorder	3.4	Female
Obsessive-compulsive disorder	1.2	Equal
Major depression	8.6	Female
Bipolar disorder I and II	1.8	BD I: ~Equal BD II: Female
Autism spectrum disorders	1 in children	Male
Disruptive, impulse control, and conduct disorders	8.9 overall	
Conduct disorders*	4 in children	Male
Attention-deficit/hyperactivity disorder*	5 in children; 2.5 in adults	Male
Substance use disorders	8.9 overall	
Alcohol use disorder	8.5 in adults; 2.5 in 12- to 17-year-olds	Male
Drug use disorders	1.4	Male
Schizophrenia	1.1	~Equal
Alzheimer's disease (≥65 years old)	13 of people ≥65 years	Female

*No one source has all of this information. This information has been derived from the following sources: Kessler, R.C., et al. (2012). Twelve-month and lifetime prevalence and lifetime morbid risk of anxiety and mood disorders in the United States. *International Journal of Methods of Psychiatric Research, 21,* 169; Substance Abuse and Mental Health Services Administration (2009). *Results from the 2008 national survey on drug use and health: national findings.* <http://www.samhsa.gov/data/nsduh/2k8nsduh/2k8Results.htm> Accessed November 13, 2013; American Psychiatric Association (2013). *Diagnostic and statistical manual of mental disorders* (5th ed.). Arlington, VA: APA; Alzheimer's Association (2013). *2013 Alzheimer's disease facts and figures.* <http://www.alz.org/alzheimers_disease_facts_and_figures.asp>.

OVERVIEW OF NONDEMENTIA COGNITIVE DISORDERS

Mild Cognitive Impairment

Mild cognitive impairment (MCI) is a regression in cognition that is not a result of normal aging. Before the publication of *DSM-5*, diagnostic criteria for mild nondementia cognitive disorders were not identified. The diagnostic criteria listed in *DSM-5* for mild nondementia cognitive disorders focus on modest declines in mental cognition that do not prevent independence in everyday activities. More complex activities, such as balancing a checkbook, require increased levels of assistance (American Psychiatric Association, 2013).

When other pathologic causes of MCI have been eliminated, the clinician must gather further information regarding specific cognitive changes in the individual. Individuals who have symptoms of MCI and possess a positive genetic predisposition are more likely to progress to Alzheimer's disease (Albert et al., 2011). In 2009, Lu and associates, on behalf of the Alzheimer's Disease Cooperative Study Group, found that patients with depression as a group were more likely to develop Alzheimer's disease than individuals who were not depressed.

Lyseng-Williamson and McKeage (2013) found that the use of donepezil slows the progression of symptoms of Alzheimer's disease, delaying the need for more intensive levels of care. Although no specific treatments are available, a patient with MCI should develop a variety of healthy habits, such as the following:

- Improve sleep habits or address underlying sleep disturbances.
- Treat any underlying psychiatric disorders such as depression.
- Eat well, reduce alcohol use, and get treatment for physical illnesses.
- Increase socialization and do cognitively stimulating activities.
- Challenge the brain with mental exercises.
- Compare and contrast different things (e.g., the movie version vs. the book).

Other ways to stimulate cognition include playing board games, putting together puzzles, and solving word games. Petersen (2011) stated the use of mnemonics, word association games, and cognition building computer training can be used to stimulate cognition.

Delirium

The word *delirium* literally means "out of one's furrow," which refers to the dramatic behavioral changes that the person may experience. Some have called delirium "brain failure" because it may represent a variety of causes such as heart failure does in cardiac health (Fong et al., 2009). The hallmark sign of delirium is its acute onset, which is key because the disorder rapidly develops in most cases. Other signs include a fluctuating level of consciousness, slurred speech, nonsensical thoughts, and day-night sleep reversal. A delirious patient may have visual hallucinations (e.g., seeing multicolored rats) or tactile hallucinations (e.g., feeling bugs under the skin). The patient may pick at the air as if trying to do some routine task, such as opening a prescription bottle. The patient may be able to follow a conversation for a short period, followed by an acute bout of confusion. Emotions are on edge, and the patient may startle easily. Assessment and treatment of any underlying physical problem or illness should be addressed immediately. The nurse must assess and initiate interventions on patients who are confused, disoriented, and often resistant to ensure the patient's safety and provide the best nursing care for the patient (Phillips, 2013).

Delirium is the most common complication among hospitalized older adults (Phillips, 2013). "ICU psychosis" is another name for hospital-based delirium. Acute changes in the patient's mental status may be a sign that a serious underlying medical illness exists. Delirium is associated with many physical illnesses, especially pneumonia, myocardial infarction, and urinary tract infection. Toxic response to medications occurs with prescribed and over-the-counter (OTC) medications. For example, drugs with anticholinergic properties can cause delirium, such as diphenhydramine (Benadryl), some tricyclic antidepressants, and benztropine (Cogentin). Other drugs, including lithium and divalproex, may become toxic at lower serum levels than the laboratory reference range indicates. Polypharmacy (four or more medications), allergies, hydration, electrolyte imbalance, and bowel and bladder function all are associated with the development of delirium (Phillips, 2013). During the initial medication assessment, the nurse should ask the patient or family member about prescription *and* OTC medications. The nurse should ask specifically about cough syrup; dietary supplements; and medications for allergies, pain, and sedation.

Because delirium is a medical emergency, treatment should start immediately. The severity of delirium can be minimized with timely recognition by clinicians (Phillips, 2013). Once stabilized, the patient may or may not have further episodes.

Clinical Example: Patient with Mild Cognitive Impairment

Mrs. Peacock, a 72-year-old white woman, retired from working as the head librarian in the public library. During her career, she coordinated many regional conferences. Now her daughter has to remind her to take her medication. She recognizes that she is having memory problems, but she is still able to live independently. No problems have been reported by her peers with whom she volunteers in the Friendship Bookstore where donated books are sold.

Clinical Example: Patient with Delirium

Mrs. Edwards, a 64-year-old woman, was found crawling around her bedroom. She thought her husband was plotting to kill her. She found his pistol, took it, and was waiting to shoot him when her daughter found her. At that time, she was taking diphenhydramine in three OTC preparations: a cough syrup, an allergy capsule, and a sleeping aid pill. Discontinuation of these medications resulted in a return to the patient's premorbid level of cognitive function. She did not require any further psychiatric care.

Dementia is a leading risk factor for delirium, and a patient can have both. However, delirium takes treatment priority because it is imminently life-threatening. A diagnosis of a dementing illness can be made only after the delirium has cleared.

Pseudodementia

The term *pseudodementia* is fading from the clinical cognitive literature. For decades, this term had been used to describe patients who had either cognitive deficits or depression but not enough symptoms to make a dementia diagnosis. The diagnostic challenge was to determine if the patient had a true memory disorder or social withdrawal and apathy associated with depression.

The reason for the reduction in use of the previously often used word *pseudodementia* is perhaps related to the increasing knowledge about MCI and the fact that it is now known that depression may be prodromal to dementia. If a patient is depressed, treatment may include medications and various therapeutic modalities such as psychotherapy, occupational therapy, and exercise therapy. Electroconvulsive treatment may be suggested if depression is severe.

DEMENTIA

The word *dementia*, from Latin, literally means "out of one's mind." Dementia is a type of illness with a progressively deteriorating course that ultimately affects cognition, perception, language, behavior, and motor abilities. There are many types of dementing disorders, but the common denominator for these disorders is the progressiveness of dementia. Researchers are focusing on early identification of dementia to initiate early treatment. Caselli and Reiman (2013) have been concentrating on genetic factors that can lead to early detection and subsequent treatment.

> **? CRITICAL THINKING QUESTIONS**
>
> 1. Why is it important to recognize the difference between dementia and delirium?
> 2. Explain why attending a senior center may be therapeutic for a patient with a dementia.

A dementia may be potentially reversible or irreversible. Most dementing illnesses are irreversible, and dementias that can be reversed may not be completely reversible. Normal-pressure hydrocephalus and vitamin B_{12} deficiency are two dementias that are potentially reversible. Alcoholic dementia cannot be reversed. Wernicke's encephalopathy and Korsakoff's psychosis, two neurologic problems often found in patients with chronic alcoholism, are dementia-type neurologic problems that can often be reversed by treating the underlying thiamine (Vitamin B_1) deficiency and malnutrition frequently seen in these patients (Thomson et al., 2012). Some or all of the confusion and retrograde amnesia associated with Wernicke-Korsakoff syndrome may improve. Because these symptoms are similar to symptoms of cognitive dementia, improvement looks like the dementia is being reversed. Before making

a diagnosis of dementia in a patient, all physical illnesses, such as metabolic disturbances and neoplasms, must be ruled out (American Psychiatric Association, 2013).

POTENTIALLY REVERSIBLE DEMENTIAS

Normal-Pressure Hydrocephalus

Patients with normal-pressure hydrocephalus usually present with a classic triad of symptoms: (1) unsteady gait or apraxia, (2) urinary urgency or incontinence, and (3) dementia. A diagnosis is not made in up to 80% of patients because of the difficulty of distinguishing this disorder from other neurologic disorders (Kiefer & Unterberg, 2012). The cause of normal-pressure hydrocephalus is impaired return of cerebrospinal fluid through the subarachnoid space to the venous system. The cerebrospinal fluid has normal pressure or is slightly elevated when monitored.

Problems with gait usually precede the other symptoms. If gait problems are severe, the patient may develop apraxia; this condition is best described as looking as if the patient were walking over a sticky floor.

If detected early, normal-pressure hydrocephalus may be reversed. However, the patient, family, and clinicians often ignore the initial symptoms. Treatment requires neurosurgery. A ventricular shunt is placed in one of the lateral ventricles in the brain, which leads to the peritoneum (ventriculoperitoneal shunt). A small pump is implanted just under the scalp behind the ear. More recent reports indicate that 70% to 90% of patients undergoing surgical intervention show clinical improvement as measured at 1- to 7-year intervals. This improvement is seen in all three aspects of the triad: urinary symptoms, gait, and dementia (Kiefer & Unterberg, 2012).

Public awareness about normal-pressure hydrocephalus has been heightened since a television advertising campaign appeared in the last few years. A commercial featured a man walking as if he had normal-pressure hydrocephalus followed by his dramatic improvement after surgery. When there is improvement, it is usually not as striking as the commercial. After this normal-pressure hydrocephalus advertising campaign, patients' family members started asking if surgery may be done on their loved ones even before the cognitive evaluation began.

Clinical Example: Patient with Normal-Pressure Hydrocephalus

Mrs. Burkhalter, a 66-year-old woman, was admitted for evaluation. Her husband said that she had been diagnosed with Alzheimer's disease by her internist. After a neurologic evaluation, normal-pressure hydrocephalus was the more likely diagnosis. Mrs. Burkhalter's symptoms started with gait instability, noted especially when she had difficulty starting to walk. She complained of urinary urgency and sometimes had incontinence. However, it was unknown if it were true urinary incontinence or her difficulty making it to the bathroom in time. Finally, her memory started failing, and she had some emotional changes. After ventriculoperitoneal shunt surgery, her gait and urinary problems improved, but her memory showed little change.

Vitamin B$_{12}$ Deficiency

Although vitamin B$_{12}$ deficiency is common in older adults, the dementing disorder related to this deficiency is not. If anything interferes with the absorption of vitamin B$_{12}$ in the stomach, inadequate absorption may occur. Pernicious anemia is the most prevalent cause of this deficiency.

Dementia related to vitamin B$_{12}$ deficiency is rare. When the deficiency proceeds to this level, demyelinization of the cerebrum has occurred. Peripheral neuropathy is the most common physical presentation. Delirium, depression, and psychosis may be present. Vitamin B$_{12}$ replacement should be started immediately and continued throughout the patient's lifetime. Intramuscular administration of vitamin B$_{12}$ is the treatment of choice because malabsorption is the usual cause of the deficiency. However, according to Stabler (2013), high-dose oral therapy (2-mg tablets) yielded similar improvements in hematocrit and mean corpuscular volume as 1-mg injections when measured after 4 months of treatment.

Clinical Example: Patient with Severe Vitamin B$_{12}$ Deficiency

Mrs. Washington, an 84-year-old woman, was admitted for cognitive evaluation after the adult protective agency found her living in squalor. She was malnourished and dehydrated with a low vitamin B$_{12}$ level. The patient had forgotten to eat. She was also unstable because of weakness in her upper and lower extremities. Vitamin B$_{12}$ replacement therapy was started and continued in the nursing home after discharge.

IRREVERSIBLE DEMENTIAS

At the present time, no cure is available for any of the dementing disorders discussed in this section, but medications have been developed with U.S. Food and Drug Administration (FDA) indications for Alzheimer's disease. One medication that previously had been approved only for Alzheimer's disease has received FDA approval for dementia related to Parkinson's disease.

The course of irreversible dementias may be slowed and even plateau, but ultimately cognition declines. Through education and support, the nurse can play a pivotal role in assisting both the patient and the family with this devastating diagnosis. Additionally, the nurse can inform patients and family members about available local and national resources.

Each illness is different in origin and clinical manifestation, but they share some common behaviors. Effective interventions and important issues faced by patients and their families are described in this chapter.

Alzheimer's disease is the most prevalent dementia; 50% to 80% of all patients with dementia have Alzheimer's disease. Individuals with vascular dementia account for approximately 20% to 30% of cases of dementia. The remaining types of dementia include frontotemporal dementias (e.g., Pick's disease), dementia related to Parkinson's disease, dementia with Lewy bodies (DLB), AIDS, Huntington's disease, and Creutzfeldt-Jakob disease (CJD) (Alzheimer's Association, 2013).

DSM-5 CRITERIA

for Major and Mild Neurocognitive Disorders

Major Neurocognitive Disorder*
A. Evidence of significant cognitive decline from a previous level of performance in one or more cognitive domains (complex attention, executive function, learning and memory, language, perceptual-motor, or social cognition) based on:
  1. Concern of the individual, a knowledgeable informant, or the clinician that there has been a significant decline in cognitive function; and
  2. A substantial impairment in cognitive performance, preferably documented by standardized neuropsychological testing or, in its absence, another quantified clinical assessment.
B. The cognitive deficits interfere with independence in everyday activities (i.e., at a minimum, requiring assistance with complex instrumental activities of daily living such as paying bills or managing medications).
C. The cognitive deficits do not occur exclusively in the context of a delirium.
D. The cognitive deficits are not better explained by another mental disorder (e.g., major depressive disorder, schizophrenia).
Specify whether due to:
- Alzheimer's disease
- Frontotemporal lobar degeneration
- Lewy body disease
- Vascular disease
- Traumatic brain injury
- Substance/medication use
- HIV infection
- Prion disease
- Parkinson's disease
- Huntington's disease
- Another medical condition
- Multiple etiologies
- Unspecified

* From American Psychiatric Association (2013). *Diagnostic and statistical manual of mental disorders* (5th ed.) (pp. 602-603). Arlington, Virginia: APA.

Alzheimer's Disease

Alzheimer's disease is the most prevalent form of dementia, affecting 5.2 million patients in the United States. It is estimated that by 2025, more than 7 million people older than 65 years will have Alzheimer's disease (Alzheimer's Association, 2013). Alois Alzheimer, a German neurologist, first described a patient with this disease in 1907. He identified the plaques and tangles that are now considered pathognomonic (hallmark signs) for Alzheimer's disease. However, the disease did not attract much attention for many years. For example, *Introduction to Psychiatry*, a psychiatric nursing text published in 1948, included only three sentences about Alzheimer's disease. None of the other aforementioned dementias were mentioned (Biddle & van Sickel, 1948).

A resurgence in interest in this disease has occurred in the last 20 years. Now that Alzheimer's disease has been studied extensively, it is known that the course from onset to death may be longer than 10 years. Alzheimer's disease showed a 68% increase in deaths from 2000 to 2010, and it is the fifth leading cause of death in the United States of people older than 64 years (Alzheimer's Association, 2013). Alzheimer's disease as well as the other types of dementia is diagnosed after all other disorders have been ruled out. MCI, delirium, and other psychiatric illnesses are considered before a dementia diagnosis is made. As previously stated, a patient may have more than one illness, which makes assessment and treatment more difficult.

Age is the most significant risk factor for Alzheimer's disease followed by the presence of the apolipoprotein E4 Apo ε4 allele on chromosome 19. Other risk factors include a family history of the disease, history of heart-related conditions (e.g., hypertension, high cholesterol, stroke, heart disease), and a history of head injury (Alzheimer's Association, 2013).

Stages of Alzheimer's Disease

There are two different ways to stage Alzheimer's disease. The first divides the stages into three parts: mild, moderate, and severe. Each stage has typical characteristics, but symptoms may occur outside their expected stage. Table 28-3 provides information about the three stages of Alzheimer's disease. The stages are based on the scores obtained on the mini-mental state examination. This test was developed in 1975 by Folstein et al. at Johns Hopkins as a teaching tool to assess cognitive status. The second stage-based way to look at the cognitive decline associated with Alzheimer's disease is the Global Deterioration Scale, also known as the Reisberg Scale (Reisberg et al., 1982).

Some find the more specific stages helpful in recognizing the level of the disease process. Nurses and caregivers can plan appropriate interventions when they make accurate assessment of the patient's capabilities. The following summary (Bellenir, 2008) was based on the original article entitled "The Global Deterioration Scale (GDS)."

Stage 1: No cognitive decline
Experiences no problems in daily living
Stage 2: Very mild cognitive decline
Forgets names and locations of objects
May have trouble finding words
Stage 3: Mild cognitive decline
Has difficulty traveling to new locations
Has difficulty handling problems at work
Stage 4: Moderate cognitive decline
Has difficulty with complex tasks (finances, shopping, planning for guests)
Stage 5: Moderately severe cognitive decline
Needs help to choose clothing
Needs prompting to bathe
Stage 6: Severe cognitive decline
Needs help putting on clothing
Requires assistance bathing; may have a fear of bathing
Has decreased ability to use the toilet or is incontinent
Stage 7: Very severe cognitive decline
Vocabulary becomes limited, eventually declining to single words
Loses ability to walk and sit
Becomes unable to smile

> **? CRITICAL THINKING QUESTION**
>
> 3. How do you explain the difference between dementia and Alzheimer's disease?

Causes of Alzheimer's Disease

Alzheimer's Disease Most Likely Has Multiple Etiologies. Many concepts have been introduced and researched, which suggests myriad problems. Alzheimer, with his primitive means, was able to identify the main characteristics still cited today: the

TABLE 28-3	STAGES OF ALZHEIMER'S DISEASE	
STAGE	**DURATION (YR)**	**CHANGES**
Mild (MMSE score = 20-30)	2-3	Decreased short-term memory Word- and name-finding difficulties Decision-making, concentration, reasoning, and judgment problems Difficulty performing usual activities Denial Getting lost Repetitive questioning
Moderate (MMSE score = 10-19)	3-4	Apraxia, agnosia, aphasia with poor comprehension, disorientation, blunting of affect, misidentification, sleep disturbance, delusions, needs assistance with activities of daily living Redirectable, extreme emotional lability, self-absorption, supervision with meals, wandering, urinary incontinence, requires supervision
Severe (MMSE score = 0-9)	5-10	Gait disturbance, unable to feed self, double incontinence, bowel impaction, bed bound, difficulty swallowing, fetal position; requires 24-hour supervision, close observation, or both

MMSE, Mini-mental state examination.
Modified from Folstein, M.F., Folstein, S.E., & McHugh, P.R. (1975). "Mini-mental state." A practical method for grading the cognitive state of patients for the clinician. *Journal of Psychiatric Research, 12,* 189.

presence of β-amyloid plaques and the neurofibrillary tangles in the brain (Tarawneh et al., 2011). After more than a century, researchers still do not know if the plaques and tangles cause Alzheimer's disease or are a result of it. However, Tarawneh et al. examined cerebrospinal fluid to determine if it contains protein markers that indicate Alzheimer's disease pathology is present in adults without clinical symptoms of the illness.

Neuronal Loss. Diagnostic imaging identifies the cerebral cortex, hippocampus, amygdala, and forebrain as the four areas that have neuronal loss in a brain with Alzheimer's disease (Teipel et al., 2013). The nucleus basalis of Meynert in the basal forebrain is the major site of cholinergic cell bodies. The loss of the cholinergic neurons that produce the neurotransmitter acetylcholine has been strongly implicated in Alzheimer's disease—so much so that the first class of medications developed specifically for this disease targeted this deficiency. The cholinergic system forms the basis of memory acquisition, but that is not all. Many other cognitive aspects are affected as well, such as processing new information and making complex decisions. The ability to understand abstract thought may slowly fade away.

The hippocampal volume loss seen on magnetic resonance imaging is an established biomarker used to predict Alzheimer's disease (Teipel et al., 2013). Before this hippocampal change occurs, the entorhinal cortex (entorhinal means "toward the nose") starts reducing in size. This area of the brain acts as a "gateway" to the hippocampi by regulating input. If there is a problem in this area, the hippocampi can no longer receive the kinds of information needed to lay down new memories. Screening for entorhinal cortex atrophy is not commonly done. However, hippocampal atrophy may be seen on magnetic resonance imaging of the brain.

Neurofibrillary Tangles. The microtubules within neurons are responsible for cellular nutrient transport. They function in pairs that are held apart by tau protein. This tau protein provides structural support inside the microtubules and keeps them working properly. In a brain with Alzheimer's disease, extra tau protein gathers causing the microtubules to collapse. The tau protein fibrils (segments), now separated from the microtubules, start twisting. These twists, known as *neurofibrillary tangles*, cause the nutrient-starved neuron to die. The dead nerve cell withers and shrinks (National Institute on Aging, 2011).

β-Amyloid Plaques. When the Alzheimer's disease process starts, an inevitable cascade of events follows. A protein known as *amyloid precursor protein* (APP) is partly inside and partly outside the neuron, "like a toothpick stuck in an orange" (National Institute on Aging, 2011). As the APP moves outside the cell through the semipermeable membrane, the protein is "sniped" or "cleaved" by enzymes known collectively as *secretases*. Some of the resulting APP pieces are shorter, and these are doomed to join others. Ultimately these APP pieces clump to form β-amyloid peptide. Several of the β-amyloid peptides (up to a dozen) form oligomers. These oligomers interfere with the neuronal receptors and the synapses, ultimately causing the cell to die (National Institute on Aging, 2011).

Oxidative stress contributes to neuronal death. Although this process occurs as part of the aging process, a patient with Alzheimer's disease experiences more oxidative stress. A chain reaction of free radicals starts when an atom loses one of its electrons. An odd number of electrons creates an unstable atom. The electron-deficient atom seeks out another electron to stabilize itself (Borda, 2006). The repeated pattern of the "robbed atom becoming the robber" ultimately leads to cell destruction.

Brain Atrophy. Neuronal loss from plaques, tangles, and oxidative stress may contribute to the reduction of the actual size of the brain, leading to another hallmark sign of Alzheimer's disease—the atrophied brain. A normal adult brain weighs approximately 3 lb. The brain of a person with advanced Alzheimer's disease may weigh less than half that amount. This atrophy begins in the temporal and parietal regions and progresses throughout the entire brain (National Institute on Aging, 2011).

Smaller gyri and corresponding larger sulci undergo atrophic changes (Figures 28-1 through 28-4). Atrophy also occurs in the subcortical areas, which is most apparent in the lateral ventricles. The more the brain shrinks, the larger the ventricles become.

Genetics. A genetic predisposition exists for the development of Alzheimer's disease; this is especially true for late-onset Alzheimer's disease, with a 60% to 80% risk factor (Casey, 2012). The genetic components of Alzheimer's disease are described subsequently.

Alzheimer's Disease—Early Onset. Familial Alzheimer's disease has an autosomal dominant inheritance pattern. These patients are diagnosed in their fifties (or earlier) and have a faster course than patients who develop Alzheimer's disease at an older age. The following mutations of chromosomes 1, 14, and 21 have been identified for individuals with early-onset familial Alzheimer's disease:

- Chromosome 1—presenilin 2 gene
- Chromosome 14—presenilin 1 gene
- Chromosome 21—makes abnormal APP

If only one parent has only one of these abnormal chromosomes, offspring have a 50% chance of developing familial Alzheimer's disease (National Institute on Aging, 2011).

Alzheimer's Disease—Late Onset. Additionally, the allele Apo ε4 on chromosome 19 has been linked to the development of β-amyloid plaque seen in Alzheimer's disease. The more β-amyloid plaque deposited in the brain, the greater the impairment is thought to be. If one or both parents provide the Apo ε4 gene, not only is the recipient more likely to develop Alzheimer's disease, but also the recipient is likely to develop the disease at an earlier age than an individual without the allele. In contrast, a person who does not inherit the gene for Apo ε4 may also develop the disease (National Institute on Aging, 2012).

Hormones. Barron and Pike (2012) believed sex hormones provide a degree of protection against the development of Alzheimer's disease, and the decrease in estrogen during menopause is a risk factor for women developing Alzheimer's disease. The most controversial finding of the Women's Health Initiative Memory Study (WHIMS) was that the risk of Alzheimer's disease increased with women using estrogen alone or in combination with progesterone. Henderson (2006) described "the critical window hypothesis" that may be key

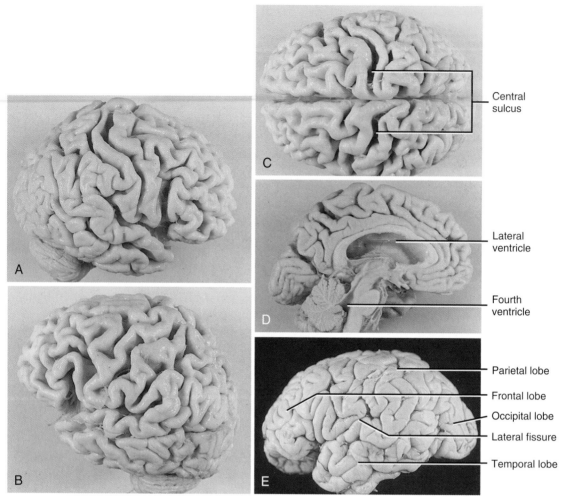

FIG 28-1 A, Right side of the brain of a patient with Alzheimer's disease. Narrow gyri and larger sulci are shown. **B,** Left side of the same brain demonstrates even narrower gyri and larger sulci. **C,** Superior view. The central sulcus is very wide. **D,** Midsagittal view of the left hemisphere. The greatly enlarged lateral and fourth ventricles are demonstrated. **E,** Normal brain. (**A-D,** Photographs by Berto Tarin, Western University of Health Science; **E,** courtesy of Dr. Richard E. Powers, University of Alabama at Birmingham Brain Resource Program.)

regarding hormone replacement therapy. Is it the age when estrogen is started, or does it have to do with when estrogen is started in relation to menopause? As indicated by Maki and Henderson (2012), the question remains largely unanswered but does create controversy regarding the results of WHIMS. Should younger postmenopausal women be treated with estrogen replacement therapy to minimize the risk of dementia, or should the results of WHIMS be generalized to this population?

The debate continues about aluminum and mercury causing Alzheimer's disease. Aluminum is one of the most abundant chemicals in the environment. Also, it is in personal products such as deodorant (aluminum oxide), OTC antacid medications (aluminum hydroxide), and aluminum cookware. It is difficult to control for all of the variables. There is a repeated association of aluminum and Alzheimer's disease but no definitive cause. One view proposed by Rountree (2012) is that the brain initiates an antiinflammatory response to the presence of heavy metals such as aluminum, which possibly results in damage to surrounding

tissue. Mercury composes about 50% of dental amalgams. Mercury vapor is released very slowly in minute amounts over time. The American Dental Association acknowledges the mercury in dental amalgams as safe for dental restoration. The FDA deemed amalgam safe to use for adults and children older than 6 years. It was determined that the mercury contained in amalgam fillings does not constitute a substantial risk to the public. The FDA cited no clinical studies that indicate a relationship between amalgam fillings and health problems for the approved age group (U.S. Food and Drug Administration, 2009).

Nontraditional Findings

The traditional roots of Alzheimer's disease development have been discussed, but the cause of Alzheimer's disease is not without controversy. The *Nun Study*, a longitudinal research study that explored topics related to normal aging and Alzheimer's disease, generated new questions. More than 20 years ago, 678 nuns from the Order of the School Sisters of Notre Dame agreed to undergo physical and mental annual

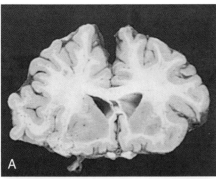

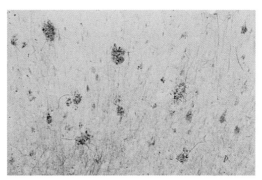

FIG 28-4 The darker objects are plaques, one of two microscopic findings in Alzheimer's disease (the other is the tangles; see Figure 28-3). Plaques can be found in about 50% of individuals older than 70 years; it is the quantity of plaques in relation to the person's age that is significant. (Courtesy of Dr. Richard E. Powers, University of Alabama at Birmingham Brain Resource Program.)

FIG 28-2 **A,** Normal brain. The sulci and gyri are not atrophied. **B,** Brain shows the effects of Alzheimer's disease. Widened sulci and narrowed gyri are demonstrated. In addition, the lateral ventricles are increased in size because of the decrease in brain mass associated with Alzheimer's disease. (Courtesy of Dr. Richard E. Powers, University of Alabama at Birmingham Brain Resource Program.)

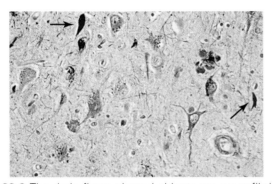

FIG 28-3 The dark, flame-shaped objects are neurofibrillary tangles, or dead neurons *(arrows)*. Tangles are twisted fibrils inside the neuron that disrupt cellular processes and eventually kill the cell. (Courtesy of Dr. Richard E. Powers, University of Alabama at Birmingham Brain Resource Program.)

assessments. In addition, each nun volunteered to have her brain autopsied. The sisters of this order had been teachers while they lived. Their contributions would be a great source of future knowledge about Alzheimer's disease (Snowdon, 2001). Hundreds of professional articles have been published using this unique data set.

The Nun Study had some unexpected findings. One sister who lived to be more than 100 years old showed no signs of cognitive decline, although her brain autopsy showed an abundance of both plaque and tangle formations. Another nun, who died in her seventies, had profound dementia yet

had few tangles and plaques. The Nun Study researchers explored reasons for these unusual findings and concluded that the degree of resistance or cognitive reserve has some effect on the clinical manifestations of Alzheimer's disease (Snowdon, 2003).

Complex use of language and advanced education were two background issues that were isolated in the nuns who had the highest cognitive ability. Also, nuns with a more positive lifetime attitude were found to be in the highest cognitive group (Snowdon, 2001).

Classic Behaviors

Memory loss is most noticeable initially. Impairment of short-term memory usually occurs first. The patient and family may think that this loss is minor because the long-term memory remains intact at first. Long-term memory loss generally follows. Sometimes the patient has a developmental regression. When a female patient confuses her son for her deceased husband, she is most likely remembering the era when her spouse was her son's age. As the regression continues, the patient may think that her children are school-age. Finally, the cries for "Mama" reflect complete memory deterioration and come at the final stages of this disease.

Word-finding difficulty is the easiest problem for the nurse to assess because the nurse likely would be unable to discern short-term memory losses at first. Only people with the patient would know what was served for breakfast. The patient often describes an object rather than names it—"the thing you tell time with" for a watch or "hitting the ball over the fence" for a home run. Describing, rather than identifying, is a common form of aphasia. The two types of aphasia, expressive and receptive, refer to these communication barriers. Expressive aphasia means difficulty expressing oneself, as problems with word finding exemplifies. Receptive aphasia means that the patient has difficulty understanding what is being said. It is common to have both types of aphasias, which complicates communicating with the patient.

Difficulty concentrating may be subtle at first. Trouble understanding a conversation, comprehending the plot in a book, or following a television program are frequent problems. As the disease progresses, the patient usually no longer finds interest in previous pleasurable activities. The lack of mental stimulation further contributes to cognitive decline. Box 28-1 outlines what is referred to as the "four *As* of Alzheimer's disease."

One unusual problem associated with Alzheimer's disease is *misinterpreting the environment.* Patients often have visual hallucinations of dead relatives. One patient was found to be routinely preparing meals for visiting family members, all of whom were deceased. *Voices* or *sounds* typically go along with the visual hallucinations—for example, the perceived deceased relative is *speaking* to the patient. Olfactory, tactile, and gustatory hallucinations are the least common types of hallucinations.

Delusions are common. These are misconceptions that have no basis in reality and are often accusatory. Delusions held by patients with Alzheimer's disease are very different from ones held by patients with psychoses related to chronic mental illnesses (e.g., schizophrenia). Delusions from patients with schizophrenia are typically bizarre and often frightening. Patients with Alzheimer's disease have delusions that are based on reality and are not usually fantastical. Common delusions of patients with Alzheimer's disease may include the following:

- Thinking that a deceased relative is alive (perhaps the most common)
- Pathologic jealousy about the spouse having an extramarital affair
- Stealing something odd, such as the mortgage papers out of a safe while leaving money.

The nurse would need to find out if any of these ideas are factual. The patient's 85-year-old wife may be going out on the town, and the patient's mother may still be alive.

Illusions are almost universal and represent a worsening of the disease. An illusion is a misinterpretation of something that really does exist. Thinking one's image in a mirror is an intruder or trying to give ice cream to a doll means that the patient really *sees* something other than a self-reflection or an inanimate object.

Somatic preoccupations blended with either or both aphasias produce complaints that may not make sense. Patients may say "my stomach hurts" regardless of the question. Frequent somatic complaints often result in diagnostic testing without clear-cut results.

Misidentification is an example of calling a family member or a friend by another person's name. Family members are often devastated when the patient cannot remember their names. The nurse can educate the family about misidentification and dispel any idea that it may be a humorous attempt by the patient.

Sundowning is a period of restless agitated behavior that typically occurs after 4:30 P.M. This type of behavior can be exhibited in 20% of patients with a diagnosis of dementia (Sparks, 2011). The term *sundowning* describes when this behavior classically occurs; however, some patients have problems at other times of the day. No definitive cause has been found for sundowning.

Loss of the ability to care for oneself is difficult for all parties. Over time, the patient forgets how to take care of all

---

BOX 28-1 FOUR *A*s OF ALZHEIMER'S DISEASE* AND ADAPTIVE ACTIONS

Agnosia

Impaired ability to recognize or identify familiar objects and people in the absence of a visual or hearing impairment.

- Assess and adapt for visual impairment.
- Do not expect the patient to remember you; introduce yourself.
- Cover mirrors or pictures if they cause distress.
- Name objects and demonstrate their use.
- Keep area free of ingestible hazards (toiletries, chemical cleaning supplies, checkers, buttons, unmonitored medicine).

Aphasia

Language disturbances are exhibited in both expressing and understanding spoken words. Expressive aphasia is the inability to express thoughts in words; receptive aphasia is the inability to understand what is said.

- Assess and adapt for hearing loss.
- Observe and use gestures, tone, and facial expressions.
- Provide help with word finding.
- Restate your understanding of behaviors and word fragments.
- Acknowledge feelings expressed verbally and nonverbally.
- Use simple words and phrases; be concise and organized.
- Allow time for response.
- Listen carefully and encourage with nonverbal praise.
- Use pictures, symbols, and signs.

Amnesia

Inability to learn new information or to recall previously learned information.

- Do not expect the patient to remember you; introduce yourself.
- Do not test the patient's memory unnecessarily.
- Operate in the here and now.
- Provide orientation cues.
- Remember, *you* must adapt when the patient cannot change.
- Compensate for patient's lost judgment or reasoning.

Apraxia

Inability to carry out motor activities despite intact motor function.

- Assess and adapt for motor weakness and swallowing difficulties.
- Simplify tasks; give step-by-step instructions and time for response.
- Initiate motion for patient with gentle guidance or touch.

*May also be present in other cognitive disorders.

---

personal care needs. Incontinence of bowel and bladder and wandering can become unmanageable behaviors. When the behavioral and functional decline reaches this point, the patient usually requires 24-hour care. Incontinence and wandering often mean that the patient can no longer be cared for in the home.

Vascular Dementia

The second most prevalent dementia is vascular dementia. The diagnosis of vascular dementia is made when the brain has multiple vascular lesions in the cortex and subcortical areas. Memory loss is the most common presenting complaint. In contrast to patients with Alzheimer's disease, patients with vascular dementia usually maintain the ability to speak without word-finding difficulty. Symptoms of vascular dementia typically have an abrupt onset and are related to the area of the brain where the lesions are located (Huether & McCance, 2012). In contrast, patients with Alzheimer's disease have a more global pattern of deterioration. The time the patient remains at a particular cognitive level may be days, months, or years, depending on the vascular changes. If the cognitive levels were plotted periodically on a graph, the decline would assume a stepwise pattern of deterioration. It is impossible to predict the course of the disease because the presence of underlying pathology, such as extreme hypotension, persistent hypertension, or inflammation of blood vessels, influences the illness (National Institute of Neurological Disorders and Stroke, 2013c).

The major risk factors for vascular dementia are hypertension, diabetes mellitus, previous stroke, cardiac arrhythmias, coronary artery disease, tobacco use, and alcohol or substance abuse. Treatments focus on the patient's medical problems and health care issues. No medications have been developed and approved by the FDA for vascular dementia. Treatment is often geared toward interventions designed to minimize the risk factors and subsequently reduce damage to the brain (National Institute of Neurological Disorders and Stroke, 2013c).

Because improving physical health is one treatment for vascular dementia, the Alzheimer's Association advocates lifestyle changes that improve overall cardiovascular health. Such changes include improved dietary habits; regular exercise; and control of blood pressure, blood glucose, and cholesterol levels (Alzheimer's Association, 2013).

? CRITICAL THINKING QUESTION

4. Which risk factors for vascular dementia may be modified by the patient or caregiver?

Frontotemporal Lobe Dementia

Frontotemporal lobe dementia is a type of dementia caused by atrophy of the frontal and anterior temporal lobes of the brain. This atrophy may be symmetric or asymmetric. Pick's disease is a subtype of frontotemporal lobe dementia; it features Pick cells and Pick bodies in the brain. Pick cells are swollen and ballooned neurons. This disease is usually diagnosed when patients are in their fifties or early sixties (National Institute of Neurological Disorders and Stroke, 2013b).

The area of the brain affected is responsible for executive functioning. These behaviors include judgment, decision making, impulse control, and abiding by social norms. Dramatic behavioral changes are usually the first signs that something is wrong. Disinhibition is the most shocking, which explains these common behaviors: disrobing in public, intrusiveness, and hypersexuality. Difficulties with abstraction, reasoning, lack of initiative, and poor planning may occur. Problems with memory, calculations, and visuospatial abilities (common signs seen in Alzheimer's disease) are not usual early findings because the parietal region of the brain is preserved. The outcome for individuals with frontotemporal lobe dementia is poor because the disease may progress rapidly, requiring either institutional or 24-hour care (National Institute of Neurological Disorders and Stroke, 2013).

Dementia Related to Parkinson's Disease

Parkinson's disease is a complex neurologic disorder that affects the extrapyramidal system. All diseases that affect this system have associated aberrant movements. Parkinson's disease is usually diagnosed when patients are in their fifties or sixties, although patients in their thirties, such as the actor Michael J. Fox, have developed the disease.

Barone et al. (2011) indicated that 10% of patients with a diagnosis of Parkinson's disease develop dementia every year. Neurocognitive impairment is insidious. Language skills are usually maintained. In addition to memory problems, patients with Parkinson's disease with dementia have problems with visuospatial skills, attention, and executive functioning. Hallucinations and delusions may occur. Patients who experience visual hallucinations are more likely to develop dementia; one study performed over a 30-month period indicated that 75% of patients experiencing visual hallucinations developed dementia (Barone et al., 2011).

Clinical Example: Patient with Parkinson's Disease

Mr. McGreevy, a 72-year-old man, has had Parkinson's disease for 7 years. He has a blunted affect, excessive drooling, and shuffling gait. He was hospitalized last year for aspiration pneumonia. Managing his parkinsonian signs was made difficult by frequent visual hallucinations caused by the dopamine component in the levodopa-carbidopa that he took. He had a prescription for an atypical antipsychotic drug to reduce the hallucinations. (He and his wife had been told about the FDA black box warning that described the greater risk for stroke and its *off-label* use.)

The delicate balance of prescribing a dopaminergic drug for Parkinson's disease (dopamine deficiency in the nigrostriatal tract) and a dopamine-blocking antipsychotic medication (excessive dopamine in the mesolimbic tract) may be the most difficult prescribing challenge in psychiatry. The medications are seemingly at cross purposes. One is to boost dopamine, and the other is to reduce its effects. With too much dopamine, the patient may hallucinate; with too little, the patient may become stiff. Do not be surprised if a patient prefers flexibility, even if it means hallucinations occur. These patients usually can discern that hallucinations are part of their illness and learn to live with them.

Dementia with Lewy Bodies

DLB is a form of dementia that has both cognitive impairment and extrapyramidal signs. Lewy bodies are intracellular bodies found in neurons. Originally, Lewy bodies were found only in the substantia nigra and were thought to be associated only with Parkinson's disease. With the availability of better tissue staining methods, Lewy bodies have been found in the cortex as well. A patient can have Lewy bodies in both places, which makes diagnosis a challenge. Postural instability gait was found to be associated with dementia. Diagnostic questions arise such as the following: Is DLB a stand-alone diagnosis? Is DLB a variant of Alzheimer's disease or Parkinson's disease? DLB and Parkinson's dementia have similarities and now are seen on a continuum. Although DLB was not a separate diagnosis in *DSM-IV-TR*, "major or mild neurocognitive disorder with Lewy bodies" has been added to *DSM-5*.

Common symptoms of DLB are depression, sleep disturbance, delusions, and hallucinations (Huether & McCance, 2012). These patients may not be disturbed by the hallucinations, which confound their caregivers.

DLB is second only to Alzheimer's disease as a dementing disorder, and it is often difficult for clinicians to distinguish DLB from Alzheimer's disease. A patient with DLB is likely to present with psychomotor rigidity, bradykinesia, tremors at rest, and olfactory and rapid eye movement sleep dysfunction (Fujishiro et al., 2013). The nonmotor symptoms are often helpful in making a diagnosis of DLB.

Clinical Example: Patient with Diffuse Lewy Body Dementia

Mr. Wade, a 68-year-old man, started having recurrent visual hallucinations. He had fallen twice as a result of gait disturbance. He slept well at night despite sleeping off and on throughout the day. According to the family, some days he seemed like his old self, and at other times he became agitated easily. He had been given an intramuscular injection of haloperidol during the night, and he became progressively more agitated. Based on Mr. Wade's symptoms, diffuse Lewy body dementia was diagnosed.

Fluctuation in behavior and mood is pathognomonic for this disease. Families have a difficult time coping with these changes. One day the patient may be lucid, and the next day he may be confused. Because of this waxing and waning, family members sometimes think that the patient is playing tricks. Or family members may not believe that the patient has a dementing illness because he may be clear and not hallucinating at times. The nurse can help the family understand that all of these changes are part of the disease. Another key aspect of DLB is sensitivity to antipsychotic medication. If an atypical antipsychotic medication is used, the patient and family must be told of the FDA-imposed black box warnings. Medication is discussed in more detail in the pharmacology section of this chapter.

Creutzfeldt-Jakob Disease

Until mad cow disease (bovine spongiform encephalopathy) became headline news, little information appeared in the media about CJD. Now, variant CJD has been identified, which is the human form of mad cow disease. Patients contract this variant after ingesting meat infected with bovine spongiform encephalopathy. Subacute spongiform encephalopathy is the key feature of both mad cow disease and CJD.

On microscopic examination, these brain cells appear like sponges. The cells are stripped of their intracellular material. The infecting agent is the prion, a protein particle, which is unlike either a bacterium or a virus. CJD is one of at least 12 prion-related diseases, all of which are transmissible from one person to another. A genetic component also exists, but this accounts for 10% or less of patients with CJD. When a genetic component is suspected, the causative agent is a mutation of the tau protein. There is no diagnostic test that identifies CJD, but the typical age of onset is around 60 (National Institute of Neurological Disorders and Stroke, 2013a). CJD is potentially transferable between people when blood and bodily fluids are present. However, the illness is not contagious by casual contact with the patient. No airborne pathogen is involved either.

Dementia is inevitable and occurs early in the disease. Personality changes, seizures, and myoclonic movements may also occur. Impairment of vision and blindness are not unusual. The course is rapid; on average, 90% of patients die within 12 months (National Institute of Neurological Disorders and Stroke, 2013a). The nurse should focus on anticipatory grief for the family and the patient if he or she is cognitively able. The nurse should also expect that family members will be concerned that they may inherit CJD and will be understandably anxious.

Neuronal tissue is extremely contagious. Anyone who may be involved with the brain and cerebrospinal fluids must observe very strict precautions. If an autopsy is done, the physician and staff doing the autopsy should be told about the patient's illness. The funeral home personnel also need to be told that the deceased individual had this illness.

Clinical Example: Patient with Creutzfeldt-Jakob Disease

Mrs. Mercer, a 65-year-old woman, became openly hostile to her husband while they were dining out. She had never had outbursts like this. Her vision was steadily declining, and in 6 months she was blind. She also developed myoclonic jerks that were not controlled with medication. Based on the change in personality, visual impairment, and movement disorder, CJD was diagnosed. Mrs. Mercer died 9 months later. Postmortem examination confirmed the diagnosis.

AIDS Dementia Complex

A dementia related to the late stages of AIDS occurs in 10% to 20% of patients. This percentage has been reduced to 5% to 10% with better medicine. Cortical atrophy is the most common brain imaging finding. Other common symptoms found with AIDS dementia complex include memory lapses, decreased concentration, and difficulty with reading comprehension (Theroux et al., 2013).There is no specific treatment for dementia related to AIDS. Because AIDS can occur at any age, behavioral and cognitive changes in a younger patient should alert the nurse that the patient may be developing a dementia.

Clinical Example: Patient with AIDS Dementia Complex

Mrs. Halston, a 36-year-old woman, has unknowingly had AIDS for 8 years. Her family reported that she had been raped 10 years ago. The rapist was HIV-positive. Now, Mrs. Halston is agitated, does not eat, and does not sleep well. In the last 6 months, Mrs. Halston's memory began to fail. Because of the early onset of this cognitive disorder, she had a diagnostic HIV test, which was positive. She died 10 months after receiving a diagnosis of AIDS dementia complex.

Dementia Associated with Alcoholism

Excessive alcohol intake over many years can result in dementia. However, before the dementia, two neurologic abnormalities occur. The first is Wernicke's encephalopathy, and the second is Korsakoff's syndrome. Both are attributable to a thiamine deficiency. The alcoholic patient usually has poor eating habits, which is one avenue that leads to this deficiency. The other is the alcohol itself, which causes malabsorption problems in the stomach. Wernicke's encephalopathy occurs first and is considered an acute situation. The typical triad of symptoms is confusion, ataxia, and abnormal extraocular movements (e.g., nystagmus). Thiamine replacement is crucial. The most effective route of administration is either intramuscular or intravenous because the patient most likely has a malabsorption problem.

Korsakoff's syndrome, also known as Korsakoff's psychosis, is a more chronic neurologic problem. Sometimes these two disorders are linked as Wernicke-Korsakoff syndrome. The major symptom of Korsakoff's syndrome is antegrade amnesia. The patient cannot remember anything since he developed these problems. The patient continues to make comments and responds to questions, but if he cannot remember, he makes up something (without being aware of doing so). This attempt to fill in the gaps is called *confabulation*. The patient may talk about some very interesting topics, and the nurse may find out later that none of it really happened. He may also repeat certain comments. In addition to memory loss, the patient may experience fatigue, weakness, apathy, insomnia, and difficulty with concentration (Guerrini & Mundt-Leach, 2013).

Thiamine replacement and abstinence from alcohol are urgently indicated. Any chance for improvement hinges on both. If the patient continues to drink alcohol, he is likely to develop dementia. With abstinence from alcohol, improvement of cognitive function is possible; however, long-term alcohol use leading to Korsakoff's syndrome and subsequent institutionalization is costly not only for the patient but also for society in general (Guerrini & Mundt-Leach, 2013).

If the patient is too cognitively impaired, he will become unable to process new information. The patient will be unable to benefit from participating in a support group such as Alcoholics Anonymous (AA).

Clinical Example: Patient with Dementia Related to Alcoholism

Mr. Kelly, a 75-year-old man, was admitted to a general hospital for chest pain. He was transferred 3 days later to a geriatric psychiatry unit with altered mental status. Mr. Kelly was unable to speak rationally; he made gestures in the air as if he were having visual hallucinations. His spouse said that he did not have a drinking problem, but he did drink wine each evening. After 3 days of abstinence, Mr. Kelly was experiencing delirium related to alcohol withdrawal and was placed on an alcohol withdrawal protocol.

The patient returned to the hospital 2 years later with short-term memory loss. He said that he was in Hawaii when asked where he had been before admission. His wife confirmed that Mr. Kelly had not gone to Hawaii. He was confabulating. He had developed Korsakoff's syndrome. If he continues to drink alcohol, it is likely that he will go on to have alcoholic dementia.

Dementia Related to Huntington's Disease

Huntington's disease is a particularly devastating dementing illness because it is transmitted through an autosomal dominant gene that either parent may provide. It takes only one autosomal dominant gene to produce the illness. The patient may not know he or she has (or will develop) Huntington's disease before having children. Each offspring of a patient with Huntington's disease has a 50% chance of inheriting one of the paired chromosomes, known to be chromosome 4. Huntington's disease does not skip generations. It is transmitted through the generations *if and only if* the person has the affected chromosome 4.

This illness is not usually diagnosed until patients are in their thirties or forties. At the present time, more than 15,000 people in the United States have Huntington's disease, and another 150,000 have a 50% or greater chance of developing the disease (National Institute of Neurological Disorders and Stroke, 2013b). By the time patients are diagnosed with Huntington's disease, they may already have had children and grandchildren. Each offspring has a 50% chance of inheriting the disease. This does not mean that half of the children will inherit the disease and the other half will not. Regarding the affected chromosome, no children may have inherited it, some may have inherited it, or all may have inherited it.

Personality changes are usually the first signs to appear. A mild-tempered person may develop mood swings or start drinking alcohol. Usually, movement disorders occur after personality changes. These movements, known as choreiform movements, begin with facial twitches or involuntary limb movement and progress to myoclonus (jerking movements) of all extremities. These involuntary movements cause a lack of coordination that may make walking and balance difficult (National Institute of Neurological Disorders and Stroke, 2013b).

The Huntington's disease gene has an excessive repeating pattern of the DNA bases cytosine, adenine, and guanine (abbreviated C, A, and G) in the DNA structure. The Huntington's disease gene (the particular allele on chromosome 4) has an excessive repeating pattern of these bases in this order: C-A-G. All normal people have this particular sequence (C-A-G), but people with Huntington's disease have many more. With 26 or fewer repetitions, the gene is not affected; with 26 to 40 repetitions, there's questionable effect; and with more than 40 repetitions, the person will definitely develop Huntington's disease (Huntington Outreach Project for Education at Stanford, 2011).

Dementia may develop before or after the choreiform movements begin. Short-term memory is affected first, followed by long-term memory loss. The course is unpredictable.

The severity of the illness may rest on the number of C-A-G repetitions, particularly if the number is between 26 and 40. A person with 40 repetitions or more most definitely will develop the disease, but persons with this middle range may develop it or may develop a milder form.

There is a rare form of Huntington's disease that affects children and adolescents. These patients typically inherit the disease from their fathers and have more than 60 repetitions of the genetic code C-A-G (National Institute of Neurological Disorders and Stroke, 2013b).

Genetic testing involves a simple laboratory blood sample. Testing must follow rigorous guidelines. Multiple issues are involved; only some of them are listed here. Should individuals at risk be tested before having children, should they decide not to have children, or should they proceed and take the chance that a child will not have Huntington's disease? Testing a fetus is possible, but it is not recommended. If the patient decides to be tested, the testing should follow a strict confidentiality protocol, with extremely limited access to both the testing and the results. This protocol protects the patient from personal struggle with this decision, particularly if the test result is positive. Insurance companies and health maintenance organizations could consider a positive test result for Huntington's disease a preexisting condition, even if the disease has not manifested. Of course, the Patient Protection and Affordable Care Act may rectify this situation. This disease places a great deal of stress on the caregivers (National Institute of Neurological Disorders and Stroke, 2013b). Counseling is always important with these patients and their families.

As the disease progresses, the patient may need more calories to compensate for all of the energy expended with the continual movements. There is no reliable treatment for Huntington's disease; medications are used to address symptoms. The nurse has many variables to take into account when caring for a patient with Huntington's disease. Although a patient with Huntington's disease requires extra nursing care, it is a rare opportunity to work with a patient with this disease.

Clinical Example: Patient with Dementia Related to Huntington's Disease

Mrs. Thompson, a 57-year-old woman with Huntington's disease, was admitted to the psychiatric unit for unmanageable behavior. She had severe myoclonus to the extent that she almost fell out of her wheelchair. She could no longer feed herself and was incontinent of bowel and bladder. She no longer recognized family members, and she did not know that she was in the hospital. Dementia related to Huntington's disease was diagnosed based on Mrs. Thompson's previous diagnosis of Huntington's disease and her obvious memory loss.

? CRITICAL THINKING QUESTION

5. Why is genetic counseling essential with a patient who has Huntington's disease?

Other Dementias

The most prevalent dementias have been described. Dozens of other illnesses may include dementia. For example, progressive supranuclear palsy, thyroid disease, Wilson's disease, neurosyphilis, herpes simplex encephalitis, partial complex status epilepticus, and limbic encephalitis are examples of other types of dementia. Although individual patients have a different presentation of symptoms, all dementias involve cognitive, behavioral, and self-care issues (Casey, 2012).

 CRITICAL THINKING QUESTION

6. Is it important to know the type of dementia that a patient has?

PUTTING IT ALL TOGETHER

PSYCHOTHERAPEUTIC MANAGEMENT

Nurse-Patient Relationship

Nursing care of patients with dementia is challenging. Nothing is more important than getting to know the unique personal qualities of these patients. The golden rule is simply this: Promote maximum functioning and have patience.

 CRITICAL THINKING QUESTION

7. What can the caregiver of a patient with dementia do to reduce stress?

Communication Strategies

The importance of the nurse-patient relationship cannot be overstated. It is important for the nurse to realize and to help subordinates realize that many cognitively impaired individuals live in the moment. They may be incapable of retrieving the past (memory failure) and unable to contemplate the future. The present is what they have. The nurse must be pleasant, be kind, smile, and use good eye contact. The following tips have been used successfully:

- If an interaction is going poorly, stop, walk away (provided that it is safe to do so), and return in a few minutes with a fresh start.
- Effective communication starts with nonverbal behavior, so use a kind voice and make eye contact.
- Be positive and stay with pleasant subjects.
- Do not use sarcasm, jokes, and metaphors because the patient's loss of abstract thinking makes understanding these language subtleties almost impossible.
- Recognize that patients may be unable to tell the difference between a real argument and an impassioned discussion about a new movie. Observing staff members in such a debate can be frightening and confusing to these patients.
- Use short sentences, not complex ones.
- Give directions slowly, one step at a time.
- Do not finish sentences for patients; give them time to finish their thoughts.
- Approach patients from the front in case they have visual or hearing impairment.
- Lots of chatter can be confusing because patients struggle to track one conversation when several are going on around them.

Scheduling Strategies

The way the day of a cognitively impaired patient is structured is crucial in the plan of care. The nurse should do the following:

- Develop a schedule that provides structure to the day because patients adapt better when they have a predictable routine.
- Focus on patient-centered activities.
- Develop singular activities because multiple activities overwhelm the patient. For example, turn off the television while the patient is putting together a puzzle.
- Provide a group experience with one subject approached at a time. Too much stimulation increases anxiety and may lead to agitation.

Nutritional Strategies

Many patients with cognitive impairment do not want to eat, will not eat, and sometimes cannot eat (without great difficulty). Patience and developing a strategy to meet nutritional needs are important. The nurse should consider the following:

- Ensure that patients are eating properly by tailoring dietary needs to the patient. Serve smaller meals several times per day. If too much food is on the plate, the patient may be overwhelmed.
- Finger foods work well for people who will not stay at the table.
- Find out about a patient's favorite foods and provide them as much as possible even if this means spaghetti for breakfast.
- Beverage supplements can provide nutrition when regular food intake decreases.
- If the patient has swallowing difficulties, a consultation with a speech pathologist is in order. This health care professional can determine if the patient needs a change in beverage consistency or if the patient needs foods that all have the same texture.

Toileting Strategies

Toileting is a big issue. This often is *the* issue that causes families to seek placement outside the home. The nurse should do the following:

- Ensure the patient does not have an illness that may be affecting toileting.
- Seek to keep the patient comfortable.
- Provide meticulous attention to personal hygiene and toileting needs.
- Take the patient to the bathroom every 2 hours to promote continence (incontinence contributes to the formation of decubitus ulcers, as does immobility).

Wandering Strategies

Wandering is the second major reason why families choose to place their loved ones in a long-term care facility. Wandering is defined as engaging in ambulatory movement; it may be aimless in that an individual may pace back and forth or seem to be goal-oriented when an individual is trying to leave to go to their home (Halek & Bartholomeyczik, 2012).

Visuospatial perceptions may be disturbed. Individuals may have day-night reversal and be up rambling during the night. Sometimes the person will try to bathe and dress for church or work before the usual time.

To provide a safe place, some long-term care facilities have developed wandering paths. The best paths are continuous, without dead ends. Areas with windows, interesting art on the walls, and an unobstructed hallway provide a safe place to wander as well. By making the exit doors to the facility less obvious and painting them with attractive scenes, escapes may be reduced. Some facilities have painted elaborate scenes on the door, for example, a window with an attractive view or a china hutch complete with dishes and teapot. (Do not paint the floor directly in front of the door black. This appears as a big hole in front of the door and will keep people away from the door. This is potentially very dangerous because some patients with Alzheimer's disease may try to leap over it. Using a STOP sign on the door is a better idea.)

Music is comforting to many and may have a calming effect. The music should be the type the patient prefers and not the type the caregiver does.

Photographs or videos of patients should be available and updated and easy to find. Many law enforcement agencies have partnered with the Alzheimer's Association "Safe Return" program. These patients wear a "Safe Return" armband that identifies them and provides other personal information. Some families may use a bracelet, necklace, or watch with pertinent emergency information from MedicAlert (call 1-800-ID ALERT).

If the patient is still able to use a cellular telephone, a contact entry with the name "ICE," which stands for "in case of emergency," can be made and emergency telephone numbers can be entered. Also, some cellular telephones have an "ICE" key prominently featured as a speed dial number. Some cellular telephones have a global positioning system (GPS) built in that is marketed as a child or adolescent monitoring service. However, it can be used for any age. It sends out a notification when the person has left a predetermined zone, for example, 100 yards. Although originally developed for athletic use, GPS wristbands are another monitoring alternative. The state of New Jersey has a pilot program that provides these wristbands for free for citizens with Alzheimer's disease.

Another option is a lanyard if the patient will keep it on. In this situation, a flash drive can be attached to it. Emergency names, addresses, telephone numbers, allergies, medication lists, names and numbers of physicians, insurance information, and other personal information can be easily stored. The caregiver can keep a duplicate flash drive. The caregiver's flash drive can keep photo and video files of the patient. Because the flash drive can plug into any computer with a Universal Serial Bus (USB) port, instant information can be available to hospitals and the police.

Psychopharmacology

Geriatric patients with cognitive disorders often face the double burden of dealing with a psychiatric diagnosis superimposed on a chronic medical condition. Because of this comorbidity, these individuals are often prescribed many medications. Part of the nurse's role is to ensure that prescribed medications are helping and not harming the patient and to monitor for drug adherence. Because most drugs used in geriatric psychiatry do not have FDA indications specifically for patients with cognitive disorders, nurses must be particularly vigilant in assessing drug effects. However, medications for Alzheimer's disease are the exception. These medications have survived the intense scrutiny of FDA approval and are available for use.

When another psychiatric medication is prescribed for use with patients with dementia, it is called "off-label" usage. This means that the prescriber is using the medication for a symptom or illness that is other than the FDA-approved indication. Off-label drugs are most often used to manage behavior, psychosis, depression, and anxiety associated with Alzheimer's disease and the other dementias. Often, the side effect profile drives the decision on medication choice. For example, some antidepressant medications are activating, and some are more sedating.

Many medications may cause or contribute to delirium. Perhaps the most common source of drug-mediated cognitive impairment is agents that have anticholinergic properties. For example, diphenhydramine (Benadryl) is sold alone and in combination with many OTC medications (e.g., sinus preparations, cough syrups, sleeping agents). For instance, two tablets or gelcaps of Tylenol PM contain 50 mg of diphenhydramine and can significantly add to the cholinergic deficiency.

There is no FDA-approved medication for MCI, although studies using donepezil have shown it to decrease the progression to Alzheimer's disease in subjects for 2 years. The effects do not extend past this 2-year period (Petersen, 2011).

Drugs for Alzheimer's Disease

As previously mentioned, only five medications have FDA approval for Alzheimer's disease, and no drugs have been approved for any of the other dementias. An acetylcholine deficiency is the neurotransmitter problem most often implicated in Alzheimer's disease. The first drug approved for Alzheimer's disease targeting acetylcholine deficiency was released about 20 years ago. Tacrine (Cognex) was the first in a class of medications called cholinesterase or acetylcholinesterase (AChE) inhibitors. Donepezil (Aricept), rivastigmine (Exelon), and galantamine (Razadyne; formerly known as Reminyl [name changed in 2005]) followed. All four have FDA indications for mild to moderate Alzheimer's disease. These medications in effect boost the level of acetylcholine by preventing its metabolic breakdown. Although these drugs increase the amount of available synaptic acetylcholine, the disease itself continues to progress. In other words, if two patients with equal neurodegeneration were followed clinically for 1 year, one receiving an AChE inhibitor (e.g., donepezil) and one not receiving any medication at all, they would have approximately equal brain pathology. The patient taking donepezil may function better during the year, but the underlying disease process would continue in both patients. There is much research to be done before treatment of Alzheimer's disease is adequate.

Memantine (Namenda) is an agent approved for moderate to severe Alzheimer's disease; it is the only approved medication for Alzheimer's disease that is *not* an AChE inhibitor. Memantine works by blocking abnormal signaling by glutamate at the *N*-methyl-D-aspartate receptor; it does not interfere with normal receptor activation and transmission of neuronal activity. This action moderates the symptoms of Alzheimer's disease (Lyseng-Williamson & McKeage, 2013). Glutamate is the most abundant excitatory neurotransmitter in the brain and is involved with learning and memory; however, overstimulation of these pathways leads to cell death (neuronal excitotoxicity). As opposed to the AChE inhibitors, in which the disease progression continues, memantine is thought to slow the onset of neurodegeneration. Memantine can be used alone or with an AChE inhibitor.

Note to Students: *In this chapter, we do not make a distinction between AChE and butyrylcholinesterase. We refer to all cholinesterase inhibitors as AChE inhibitors. See Chapter 18 for more detailed information.*

All five of the Alzheimer's disease medications may be effective, although to caregivers improvements can be subtle. Prescribers usually start with an AChE inhibitor. Tacrine is rarely used now because of the potential for severe hepatic toxic side effects. Donepezil, rivastigmine, or galantamine is usually started first. Each of these has FDA approval for mild to moderate Alzheimer's disease. In addition, donepezil has an indication for severe Alzheimer's disease. Convenience in giving medications is always important, but it is particularly so with these patients (Table 28-4). Similar to most people, caregivers prefer simple medication regimens. Donepezil and extended-release galantamine provide once-daily dosing. Rivastigmine and galantamine are given twice daily with meals. Tacrine is given four times daily. Gastrointestinal adverse effects are common, and dosing at mealtime helps lessen these.

Patient and family education about these medications poses a perplexing situation. Most medications are prescribed to produce improvements, but these medications usually level out the decline. While the disease continues to progress, AChE inhibitors increase the amount of acetylcholine in the areas of the brain most affected, which masks the deterioration of the disease. *Staying the same* (and not regressing) for a patient with Alzheimer's disease can be theoretically seen as an improvement. However, the illness continues to take its toll on the cholinergic system. The AChE inhibitors have been artificially boosting the acetylcholine in the brain. Stopping the medications can cause a precipitous drop in the patient's cognitive status.

Memantine, by working on glutamate, affects a different neurotransmitter system. Typically, it works on behavioral and functional aspects of the disease rather than cognition.

Families may want to stop these medications for a variety of reasons. Some cannot accept the idea that the patient is not getting better. Some do not want to delay the inevitable. Others have seen the patient go through months and even years of unmanageable behavior. They question the value of this type of medication.

Expense is another consideration for many families. These drugs are expensive. Some pharmaceutical companies have initiated cost-saving programs, including medication samples, vouchers for free medications, and patient-assistance programs.

? CRITICAL THINKING QUESTIONS

8. How do you explain that patients taking an AChE inhibitor (e.g., donepezil, rivastigmine, or galantamine) may stay the same over a period of 6 months?
9. Should patients take AChE inhibitors for the rest of their lives?

Milieu Management

Much is involved in making the patient comfortable. At home or in a specialized care facility, the room temperature and lighting should be at the patient's preference and not that of family or staff. Nursing staff should seek to reduce noxious sounds that may offend or frighten patients. Television should not be allowed unless there is purposeful viewing. For patients in a specialized care facility, it is important to match roommates' personalities when possible.

TABLE 28-4 ANTIDEMENTIA DRUGS

DRUG	TYPICAL DAILY DOSAGE	HALF-LIFE (HR)	PROTEIN BINDING (%)	CYTOCHROME P-450 ENZYMES	MECHANISM OF ACTION
Donepezil (Aricept)	5-10 mg at bedtime	~70	~95	2D6, 3A4	Cholinesterase inhibitor
Rivastigmine (Exelon)	6-12 mg in two divided doses	~2	~40	Not metabolized	Cholinesterase inhibitor
Galantamine (Razadyne)	8-16 mg twice a day	~6	Insignificant	2D6	Cholinesterase inhibitor
Memantine (Namenda)	20 mg in two divided doses	~60-80	~45	Not extensively metabolized	NMDA antagonist

NMDA, N-methyl-D-aspartate.

Memory Aids

A person does not have to have a cognitive disorder to benefit from memory aids. Many patients keep track of appointments on a calendar that has big blocks for each date. Notes are good reminders, but the patient must know to look for them. Directions may be written in large print to instruct patients about how to operate new appliances, such as a new microwave. One patient bought a new television system that required three separate remote controls to operate all the features of the television, cable television box, and DVD player. The daughter made a color photocopy of these remote controls and took it home. When the patient had difficulty turning on his television, finding the right channel, or operating the DVD player, he would call his daughter to talk him through it.

In another example, a patient's son took digital photographs of each of his mother's pills. He then made a daily grid for her with pictures of the real pills placed according to the time of day that she needed to take them.

Medication administration accuracy and patients' adherence to their medication regimens make a critical combination. A deficit on either side can cause major problems.

Pillboxes for the day, week, or month help patients keep their medications sorted out. Some pillboxes have an alarm in them to remind patients when to take their medications. Sometimes all a patient needs is a telephone reminder to take the medication. Here are some examples of medication errors that could have been prevented:

1. A patient did not know which medication to take, so he took all his blue pills on one day and all his white pills on another.
2. Another patient took both lorazepam prescribed by one physician and Ativan prescribed by another. She did not know that they were chemical equivalents.

If there is any doubt about a patient's ability to take medication, the nurse should ask the patient to demonstrate which medication to take and when.

CASE STUDY

Roberta Evans, an 81-year-old white woman with type 2 diabetes, lived in a retirement community apartment before admission to a geropsychiatric unit. This retired high school science teacher had been living independently since her husband died 5 years ago. Her only child, a son, had moved to Texas about a year ago.

Mrs. Evans drove her car to a local discount store 3 weeks before her admission. Two women approached her in the parking lot and told her that they knew a way to invest her money that would double it overnight. Mrs. Evans went to the bank with them, withdrew $1000, and gave it to them. The women were con artists and disappeared with the money. When her son learned about the scam, instead of calling the retirement community director to report what had happened, he called a friend who lived locally and had him disable his mother's car battery. When Mrs. Evans' car would not start, she started walking out on the busy streets. She never considered that her car could be repaired. Mrs. Evans wandered away from the retirement community 2 weeks later and was found several blocks away. She did not know where she was going and could not remember how to get back to her apartment. A police officer brought her back to the apartment director, who called her son. He flew in from Texas the next morning.

When he visited his mother in her apartment, he saw plates with dried half-eaten food all over the kitchen and living room. He found a plastic bag with her diabetes supplies and prescription in it. Dirty clothes were strewn about the apartment. Her bathtub faucet did not work. He did not know how long it had been since she had bathed, and his mother could not tell him. She agreed to be evaluated for this change in cognitive status, although she thought nothing was wrong. She was admitted to the geriatric psychiatric unit in a university hospital in her town. The multidisciplinary treatment team met the day after Mrs. Evans was admitted to plan her care. Her son did not know what her most recent baseline behavior was because he had only spoken with her over the telephone. He said he could not detect any changes in their telephone conversations. The patient was able to take care of her activities of daily living independently when she had prompts, especially for hygiene and grooming. Mrs. Evans attended all the unit activities and enjoyed being with her peers. However, she needed to be reminded to go to each session. She told the music therapist that she was glad that he had started the music group that day. She did not remember participating in music therapy the week before. Mrs. Evans ate well and slept through the night.

She participated in all the diagnostic testing and did not complain. A magnetic resonance imaging scan of her brain showed some atrophy. Electroencephalography showed mild background slowing. A single-photon emission computed tomography scan of her brain demonstrated lower perfusion in the frontoparietal lobes. Neuropsychological testing showed that the patient had difficulty with short-term memory and visuospatial difficulties. On admission, she scored 23 out of 30 on the mini-mental state examination. She said, "I don't keep up with these things anymore since I've retired." These findings were consistent with a diagnosis of Alzheimer's disease. She was started on an AChE inhibitor.

Before discharge, the geriatric psychiatrist, nurse, and social worker met with the patient and her son to make treatment recommendations. The results of the diagnostic testing were discussed. The patient had asked the team members while she was being evaluated to tell her what was wrong. "I'm not crazy, you know!" she insisted.

The son agreed that it was in his mother's best interest that she be told her diagnosis. The physician told her that she had Alzheimer's disease. She said at first, "I don't believe it." Later, she admitted that she had "memory problems, but I do not have Alzheimer's disease." She reluctantly agreed to move to the assisted-living facility in the same retirement community. "I know I need some help with my cooking."

The patient did well in the assisted-living facility. She liked the various activities; in addition, her roommate was a woman who had taught in the same high school in which she had taught. Mrs. Evans responded favorably to the AChE inhibitor. She was able to live in the assisted-living facility for 3 more years before she had to move to the nursing home.

◎ CARE PLAN

Name: Roberta Evans
DSM-5 Diagnosis: Alzheimer's disease — a patient who wanders

Admission Date: _____

Assessment	**Areas of strength:** Patient is willing to be evaluated, has good relationships with fellow residents and staff at the retirement community, and has a strong faith.
	Problems: Short-term memory loss, confusion, poor judgment, wandering.
Diagnoses	Acute confusion (got lost)
	Memory impairment (forgot that she had been diagnosed with type 2 diabetes mellitus)
	Impaired judgment (was conned out of $1000)
	Social isolation—relationship with her son; although their relationship is a good one, he lives at a distance
	Self-care deficits—poor personal hygiene and apartment filth
	Wandering

Outcomes

Short-term goals

Date met: _____ Patient will have a comprehensive geriatric psychiatric evaluation.
Date met: _____ Patient will be medically stable, especially related to new-onset type 2 diabetes mellitus.
Date met: _____ Patient will participate in group activities.
Date met: _____ Patient and son will meet with multidisciplinary treatment team to discuss diagnosis, patient's progress, and plans for discharge.

Long-term goals

Date met: _____ Patient will be safe and free of injury (both physical and emotional).
Date met: _____ Patient will be discharged to appropriate level of care.
Date met: _____ Patient will maintain her independence as long as possible, even though she now needs assistance.
Date met: _____ Patient will be introduced to a variety of social activities in which she can participate at her new residence.
Date met: _____ Patient will have medical and psychiatric follow-up scheduled before discharge.
Date met: _____ Patient will have her dignity preserved and her self-esteem enhanced.

Planning and Interventions

Nurse-patient relationship:

Explain the process of evaluation and treatment by the nursing staff and the rest of the multidisciplinary treatment team.
Educate the patient about her recent-onset diabetes mellitus, even though she will not be doing the monitoring herself.
Educate and support the patient regarding this hospitalization, especially the patient's concern that others will think that she is "crazy" (her term).

Psychopharmacology:

Educate the patient and her son about AChE inhibitors and the specific one she is taking.
Educate the patient and her son about the oral hypoglycemic agent that she is taking for type 2 diabetes mellitus.
Monitor for any adverse reactions.

Milieu management:

Assess and provide the level of care for her activities of daily living associated with bathing, hygiene, and grooming.
Facilitate interaction between patients who are at her cognitive and functional level in preparation for discharge to a facility where she will have the opportunity to make new acquaintances.

Evaluation

Patient will meet her short-term and long-term goals. She will be prepared to move to the assisted-living facility in her retirement community.
Patient's son has agreed to visit his mother every 3 months and to call her at least once a week. To comply with the Health Insurance Portability and Accountability Act regulations, the patient has signed a release of information so that her son can call the assisted-living facility director with any concerns that he may have.

Referrals

The referral was made to the assisted-living facility in her retirement community about her transfer from her apartment.
The police department was notified about the scam artists because this had not been done at the time.

STUDY NOTES

1. The normal aging process does not include the development of any cognitive disorder.

2. On first glance, delirium and dementia share some commonalities. However, in contrast to dementia, delirium can be imminently life-threatening, and treatment for delirium must be started immediately.

3. Most types of dementia feature a progressive cognitive deterioration over time. Only a few types are potentially reversible. Normal-pressure hydrocephalus, vitamin B_{12} deficiency, and alcohol-related dementia may be reversed in early stages. Alzheimer's disease, DLB, and vascular dementia—the three types of dementia that account for most of these illnesses—are characterized by chronic deterioration.

4. Alzheimer's disease is not a new disease. Alois Alzheimer, a German neurologist, first described a patient with these signs in 1907. Frederic Lewy, also a neurologist and a contemporary of Alzheimer, first described Lewy bodies.

5. Although not a perfect predictor of Alzheimer's disease, a person with mild cognitive impairment is more likely to develop Alzheimer's disease than a person who has no cognitive impairment.

6. Vascular dementia is caused by little strokes. The progression is unpredictable because it depends on the occurrence of another vascular event. The deterioration takes a stepwise progression, meaning that the patient may stay on a plateau for days to years before another ischemic event occurs. Risk factors include hypertension, diabetes mellitus, smoking, and obesity. The reduction of these risk factors may also reduce the likelihood of a subsequent ischemic event.

7. A pathognomonic (hallmark) sign of diffuse Lewy body dementia is the hypersensitivity that the patient demonstrates with antipsychotic medication.

8. A patient with Parkinson's disease may also have a dementia or depression or both.

9. Patients with dementia who exhibit disruptive behavior may be delirious, confused, or uncomfortable. Many cannot make their needs known.

10. Nursing care must be patient-focused. Dignity must be preserved, and safety must be maintained. The nurse promotes as much independence for the patient as possible.

11. Genetics plays a part in some types of dementia (e.g., Huntington's disease is an autosomal dominant transmitted disease). Several chromosomes that are related to Alzheimer's disease have been identified. The most prominent ones are chromosomes 1, 14, and 21, which have been linked to familial Alzheimer's disease, and the Apo ε4 allele on chromosome 19, which has been linked to β-amyloid plaque.

12. Caregiver burden is a significant stressor felt by many caregivers of patients with dementia. The caregivers are at risk for developing or exacerbating physical illnesses (e.g., diabetes mellitus, hypertension) as well as psychiatric disorders (e.g., depression, anxiety).

REFERENCES

Albert, M. S., et al. (2011). The diagnosis of mild cognitive impairment due to Alzheimer's disease: Recommendations from the National Institute on Aging-Alzheimer's Association workgroups on diagnostic guidelines for Alzheimer's disease. *Alzheimer's & Dementia, 7*, 270.

Alzheimer's Association. (2013). *2013 Alzheimer's disease facts and figures.* http://www.alz.org/alzheimers_disease_facts_and_figures.asp, Accessed 17.02.14.

American Psychiatric Association. (2013). *Diagnostic and statistical manual of mental disorders* (5th ed.). Arlington, Virginia: APA.

Barone, P., et al. (2011). Cognitive impairment in nondemented Parkinson's disease. *Movement Disorders, 26*, 2483.

Barron, A. B., & Pike, C. J. (2012). Sex hormones, aging, and Alzheimer's disease. *Frontiers in Bioscience (Elite edition), 4*, 976.

Bellenir, K. (Ed.), (2008). *Alzheimer disease sourcebook* (4th ed.). Detroit: Omnigraphics.

Biddle, W., & van Sickel, M. (1948). *Introduction to psychiatry* (2nd ed.). Philadelphia: Saunders.

Borda, C. (2006). *Alzheimer's disease and memory drugs.* New York: Chelsea House Publishers.

Caselli, R. J., & Reiman, E. M. (2013). Characterizing the preclinical stages of Alzheimer's disease and the prospect of presymptomatic intervention. *Journal of Alzheimer's Disease, 33*(Suppl. 1), S405.

Casey, G. (2012). Alzheimer's and other dementias. *Kai Tiaki Nursing New Zealand, 18*, 20.

Folstein, M., Folstein, S., & McHugh, P. (1975). "Mini-mental state." A practical method for grading the cognitive status of patients for the clinician. *Journal of Psychiatric Research, 12*, 189.

Fong, T. G., et al. (2009). Delirium accelerates cognitive decline in Alzheimer disease. *Neurology, 72*, 1570.

Fujishiro, H., et al. (2013). Dementia with Lewy bodies: Early diagnostic challenges. *Psychogeriatrics, 13*, 128.

Guerrini, I., & Mundt-Leach, R. (2013). Preventing long-term brain damage in alcohol-dependent patients. *Nursing Standard, 27*, 43.

Halek, M., & Bartholomeyczik, S. (2012). Description of the behaviour of wandering in people with dementia living in nursing homes—A review of the literature. *Scandinavian Journal of Caring Sciences, 26*, 404.

Henderson, V. (2006). Estrogen-containing hormone therapy and Alzheimer's disease risk: Understanding discrepant inferences from observational and experimental research. *Neuroscience, 138*, 1031.

Huether, S. E., & McCance, K. L. (2012). *Understanding pathophysiology* (5th ed.). St. Louis: Mosby.

Huntington Outreach Project for Education at Stanford. (2011). *The basics of Huntington's disease.* https://www.stanford.edu/group/hopes/cgi-bin/wordpress/2011/06/the-basics-of-huntingtons-disease-text-and-audio/, Accessed 17.02.14.

Kessler, R. C., et al. (2012). Twelve-month and lifetime prevalence and lifetime morbid risk of anxiety and mood disorders in the United States. *International Journal of Methods of Psychiatric Research, 21*, 169.

Kiefer, M., & Unterberg, A. (2012). The differential diagnosis and treatment of normal-pressure hydrocephalus. *Deutsches Ärzteblatt International, 109*, 15.

Lu, P., et al. (2009). Donepezil delays progression to AD in MCI subjects with depressive symptoms. *Neurology, 72*, 2115.

Lyseng-Williamson, K. A., & McKeage, K. (2013). Once-daily memantine. *Drugs & Aging, 30*, 51.

Maki, P. M., & Henderson, V. W. (2012). Hormone therapy, dementia, and cognition: The Women's Health Initiative 10 years on. *Climacteric, 15*, 256.

National Institute of Neurological Disorders and Stroke. (2013a). *Creutzfeldt-Jakob disease information page.* http://www.ninds. nih.gov/disorders/cjd/cjd.htm, Accessed 17.02.14.

National Institute of Neurological Disorders and Stroke. (2013b). *Huntington's disease: Hope through research.* http://www. ninds.nih.gov/disorders/huntington/detail_huntington. htm#160593137, Accessed 17.02.14.

National Institute of Neurological Disorders and Stroke. (2013c). *Dementia: Hope through research.* http://www.ninds.nih.gov/ disorders/dementias/detail_dementia.htm#2531319213.

National Institute on Aging. (2011). *Alzheimer's disease: Unraveling the mystery.* Bethesda, MD: National Institutes of Health, U.S. Department of Health and Human Services.

National Institute on Aging. (2012). *Alzheimer's disease genetics: Fact sheet.* Bethesda, MD: National Institutes of Health, U.S. Department of Health and Human Services.

Petersen, R. C. (2011). Clinical practice. Mild cognitive impairment. *New England Journal of Medicine, 364*, 2227.

Phillips, L. A. (2013). Delirium in geriatric patients: Identification and prevention. *Medsurg Nursing, 22*, 9.

Reisberg, B., et al. (1982). The Global Deterioration Scale for assessment of primary degenerative dementia. *American Journal of Psychiatry, 139*, 1136.

Rountree, R. (2012). Neurodegenerative disease: Part 1—Common pathways to brain injury in Alzheimer's and Parkinson's disease. *Alternative and Complementary Therapies, 18*, 4.

Snowdon, D. (2001). *Aging with grace: What the Nun Study teaches us about leading longer, healthier, and more meaningful lives.* New York: Bantam Books.

Snowdon, D. (2003). Healthy aging and dementia: Findings from the Nun Study. *Annals of Internal Medicine, 139*(5 Pt. 2), 450.

Sparks, M. (2011). Preventing and managing sundowning. *Long-Term Living for the Continuing Care Professional, 60*, 58.

Stabler, S. P. (2013). Clinical practice. Vitamin B12 deficiency. *New England Journal of Medicine, 368*, 149.

Substance Abuse and Mental Health Services Administration. (2009). *Results from the 2008 national survey on drug use and health: National findings.* http://www.samhsa.gov/data/ nsduh/2k8nsduh/2k8Results.htm, Accessed 13.11.13.

Tarawneh, R., et al. (2011). Visinin-like protein-1: Diagnostic and prognostic biomarker in Alzheimer disease. *Annals of Neurology, 70*, 274.

Teipel, S. J., et al. (2013). Relevance of magnetic resonance imaging for early detection and diagnosis of Alzheimer disease. *Medical Clinics of North America, 97*, 399.

Theroux, N., et al. (2013). Neurological complications associated with HIV and AIDS: Clinical implications for nursing. *Journal of Neuroscience Nursing, 45*, 5.

Thomson, A. D., Guerrini, I., & Marshall, E. J. (2012). The evolution and treatment of Korsakoff's syndrome: Out of sight, out of mind? *Neuropsychology Review, 22*, 81.

U.S. Food and Drug Administration. (2009). *About dental amalgam fillings.* http://www.fda.gov/MedicalDevices/ ProductsandMedicalProcedures/DentalProducts/ DentalAmalgam/ucm171094.htm, Accessed 17.02.14.

Wilson, J., & Helton, B. (2011). PSYCHed: Continuing education and consultation dementia module. In N. Keltner, C. Bostrom, & T. McGuinness (Eds.), *Psychiatric nursing.* (6th ed.). St. Louis: Mosby.

Personality Disorders

Karmie M. Johnson

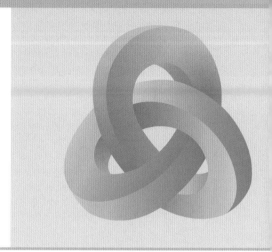

LEARNING OBJECTIVES

- Recognize characteristics of each personality disorder.
- Describe behaviors of individuals with personality disorders.

- Describe nursing interventions for patients with personality disorders.
- Recognize issues related to the care of patients with personality disorders.

This chapter focuses on patients with personality disorders either hospitalized in the inpatient psychiatric setting or treated in outpatient programs. Except for patients with a borderline personality disorder (BPD), these patients usually are not hospitalized because of their personality disorders but because of other diagnosed mental disorders. Although a patient may present because of another diagnosis, it is important to note that treatment options and their efficacy are greatly impacted by the personality disorder. Interventions focus primarily on the nurse-patient relationship unique to each personality disorder; however, this chapter does not repeat the general nurse-patient interventions described in Chapter 9. Milieu issues and psychopharmacologic factors are not addressed for each disorder because unique milieu and pharmacologic interventions are not appropriate for all disorders. Medication might be given if a patient has a comorbid diagnosis or if a symptom is severe enough to interfere with functioning, such as severe anxiety or depression.

PERSONALITY

All individuals have personality traits and characteristics that make them unique and interesting human beings. Traits are exhibited in the way individuals think about themselves and others and in the way they behave. Although experience varies across environmental, cultural, and social lines, there are expected and persistent facets of behavior and cognition that

every human possesses to one extent or another. Because these traits are evident across the diversity of humanity, they can be used to dimensionalize personality (Adelstein et al., 2011). The five-factor model categorizes these as *emotional stability, extroversion, agreeableness, conscientiousness,* and *openness* (Table 29-1) (Blais, 2008).

Emotional stability can best be conceptualized by contrasting it with its polar opposite—negative affectivity or neuroticism. Neuroticism is associated with negative emotion and pessimism. People with high negative affectability might be described as "worriers." An individual who displays an excessive amount of neuroticism has a high probability of having a mental illness, such as anxiety or depression, at some point in his or her life. Extroversion reflects the degree of positive emotion and optimism a person possesses. Extroverted people tend to favor interacting with others and being the life of the party. They are usually responsive to positive reinforcement and enjoy praise for their efforts. The opposite of extroversion is introversion. Introverted individuals prefer a solitary existence with little social interaction and are less influenced by certain types of positive encouragement. Agreeableness is an interpersonal trait. Individuals who are high in agreeableness are cooperative and easygoing, sometimes to a fault. People with low agreeableness are the opposite; they are often oppositional, easy to anger, and prone to contentious relationships. Individuals with little agreeableness fall in the domain of antagonism. Conscientiousness reflects the level of self-control and focus an individual has. High conscientiousness manifests itself in an

TABLE 29-1	RELATIONSHIP OF *DSM-5* PERSONALITY DISORDERS TO THE FIVE-FACTOR MODEL DOMAINS				
DSM PD	**NEUROTICISM**	**EXTROVERSION**	**OPENNESS**	**AGREEABLENESS**	**CONSCIENTIOUSNESS**
Paranoid	+			−	
Schizoid		−			
Schizotypal	+		+	−	
Antisocial				−	−
Borderline	+			−	
Histrionic		+			
Narcissistic			+	−	
Avoidant	+	−			
Dependent	+			+	
Obsessive		−			+

PD, Personality disorder.

Modified from Blais, M.A., et al. (2008). Personality and personality disorders. In T.A. Stern, et al. (Eds.), *Massachusetts General Hospital Clinical Psychiatry* (pp. 527–540). Philadelphia: Mosby.

organized, goal-oriented approach to life. These people work to achieve their long-term goal and are considered responsible and dependable. Individuals with low conscientiousness are impulsive and disorganized and prefer immediate gratification. People with these traits fit in the domain of disinhibition. Openness is associated with curiosity and imagination. Individuals with high openness are interested and engaged in a variety of intellectual and cultural pursuits. People with low openness can be just as intelligent as their counterparts on the opposite end of the spectrum, but they are more pragmatic and utilitarian with their learning experiences (Blais et al., 2008). Too much of anything is often a bad thing: individuals with difficulties regulating their amount of openness can exhibit psychoticism.

Personality traits are usually *egosyntonic*; they are consistent and acceptable to the ego or one's sense of self. Individuals with personality disorders have traits and habits that are rigidly fixed on one end of the five-factor model spectrum. These personality features become inflexible and dysfunctional. Individuals with personality disorders exhibit lifelong, inflexible, and dysfunctional patterns of relating and behaving. These dysfunctional patterns and behaviors usually cause distress to others. However, because personality traits are egosyntonic, individuals with personality disorders might not find their behaviors distressing to themselves; they become distressed because of other people's reactions or behaviors toward them. These reactions affect these individuals by causing immense emotional pain and discomfort. Difficulty in managing complicated symptoms and significant impairment in functioning have resulted in increased contact with the mental health system and use of services. Patients do not seek treatment to change their personality but want help for depression, anxiety, somatic symptoms, alcohol and chemical dependency, and difficulties in work and personal relationships. If a patient does present to a provider with a personality complaint, it is usually not of their own accord: "I don't think there's anything wrong with me, but my wife thinks I'm too hard on our kids. What's so bad about having high standards!"

NORM'S NOTES
In my opinion, these disorders are the toughest to treat. For instance, someone with a narcissistic personality disorder can be charming and delightful company, but at their center they are always scheming and looking out for number one. They tend to be subversive and undermine authority whenever they can. Note that personality disorders were placed on axis II in *DSM-IV-TR*. The other category of disorders placed under axis II was mental retardation. Why were personality disorders placed there? I will answer with another question, "How deep does the yellow go in a banana?" Our personalities go to our core. Although *DSM-5* brings some needed changes, I think the *DSM-IV-TR* axis system reflected the uniqueness of personality disorders better by differentiating these conditions as innately tied in with who we fundamentally are.

Personality disorders were listed on axis II per *DSM-IV-TR*. Axis II was used to designate developmental disorders, personality traits, or habitual use of particular defense mechanisms. For example, compulsive traits are not the same as obsessive-compulsive personality disorder, which is not the same as obsessive-compulsive disorder. Many high-functioning people have compulsive traits, whereas only a few have compulsive personality disorders. Patients benefit from the fact that some nurses might have compulsive traits—for example, rechecking labels, dressings, and drainage tubes. *DSM-5* removed the multiaxial system because there was no fundamental difference between axis I and axis II disorders, and some clinicians thought the distinction was burdensome and time-consuming. *DSM-5* retained the categorical approach used in *DSM-IV-TR* and introduced an alternative model in Section III that uses a dimensional-categorical methodology (American Psychiatric Association, 2013).

DSM-IV-TR criteria for a personality disorder include experiences and behaviors that are very different from those that are usually expected in an individual's culture. The individual must have disturbances in two of the following areas: cognition, affect, interpersonal functioning, and impulse control. The categorical approach to diagnosing personality disorders presents general criteria for a personality disorder and criteria specific to each personality disorder (American Psychiatric Association, 2000); see the *DSM-5 Criteria for General Personality Disorder* box.

DSM-5 CRITERIA

for *General Personality Disorder*

A. An enduring pattern of inner experience and behavior that deviates markedly from the expectations of the individual's culture. This pattern is manifested in two (or more) of the following areas:
   1. Cognition (i.e., ways of perceiving and interpreting self, other people, and events).
   2. Affectivity (i.e., range, intensity, lability, and appropriateness of emotional response).
   3. Interpersonal functioning.
   4. Impulse control.
B. The enduring pattern is inflexible and pervasive across a broad range of personal and social situations.
C. The enduring pattern leads to clinically significant distress or impairment in social, occupational, or other important areas of functioning.
D. The pattern is stable and of long duration, and its onset can be traced back at least to adolescence or early adulthood.
E. The enduring pattern is not better explained as a manifestation or consequence of another mental disorder.
F. The enduring pattern is not attributable to the physiological effects of a substance (e.g., a drug of abuse, a medication) or another medical condition (e.g., head trauma).

Cluster A: Personality Disorders
Criteria for Paranoid Personality Disorder (p. 649)

A. A pervasive distrust and suspiciousness of others such that their motives are interpreted as malevolent, beginning by early adulthood and present in a variety of contexts, as indicated by four (or more) of the following:
   1. Suspects, without sufficient basis, that others are exploiting, harming, or deceiving him or her.
   2. Is preoccupied with unjustified doubts about the loyalty or trustworthiness of friends or associates.
   3. Is reluctant to confide in others because of unwarranted fear that the information will be used maliciously against him or her.
   4. Reads hidden demeaning or threatening meanings into benign remarks or events.
   5. Persistently bears grudges (i.e., is unforgiving of insults, injuries, or slights).
   6. Perceives attacks on his or her character or reputation that are not apparent to others and is quick to react angrily or to counterattack.
   7. Has recurrent suspicions, without justification, regarding fidelity of spouse or sexual partner.
B. Does not occur exclusively during the course of schizophrenia, a bipolar disorder or depressive disorder with psychotic features, or another psychotic disorder and is not attributable to the physiological effects of another medical condition.
Note: If criteria are met prior to the onset of schizophrenia, add "premorbid," i.e., "paranoid personality disorder (premorbid)."

Criteria for Schizoid Personality Disorder (p. 653)

A. A pervasive pattern of detachment from social relationships and a restricted range of expression of emotions in interpersonal settings, beginning by early adulthood and present in a variety of contexts, as indicated by four (or more) of the following:
   1. Neither desires nor enjoys close relationships, including being part of a family.
   2. Almost always chooses solitary activities.
   3. Has little, if any, interest in having sexual experiences with another person.
   4. Takes pleasure in few, if any, activities.
   5. Lacks close friends or confidants other than first-degree relatives.
   6. Appears indifferent to praise or criticism of others.
   7. Shows emotional coldness, detachment, or flattened affectivity.
B. Does not occur exclusively during the course of schizophrenia, a bipolar disorder or depressive disorder with psychotic features, another psychotic disorder, or autism spectrum disorder and is not attributable to the physiological effects of another medical condition.
Note: If criteria are met prior to the onset of schizophrenia, add "premorbid," i.e., "schizoid personality disorder (premorbid)."

Criteria for Schizotypal Personality Disorder (p. 655)

A. A pervasive pattern of social and interpersonal deficits marked by acute discomfort with, and reduced capacity for, close relationships as well as by cognitive or perceptual distortions and eccentricities of behavior, beginning by early adulthood and present in a variety of contexts, as indicated by five (or more) of the following:
   1. Ideas of reference (excluding delusions of reference).
   2. Odd beliefs or magical thinking that influences behavior and is inconsistent with subcultural norms (e.g., superstitiousness, belief in clairvoyance, telepathy, or "sixth sense"; in children and adolescents, bizarre fantasies or preoccupations).
   3. Unusual perceptual experiences, including bodily illusions.
   4. Odd thinking and speech (e.g., vague, circumstantial, metaphorical, overelaborate, or stereotyped).
   5. Suspiciousness or paranoid ideation.
   6. Inappropriate or constricted affect.
   7. Behavior or appearance that is odd, eccentric, or peculiar.
   8. Lack of close relationships or confidants other than first-degree relatives.
   9. Excessive social anxiety that does not diminish with familiarity and tends to be associated with paranoid fears rather than negative judgments about self.
B. Does not occur exclusively during the course of schizophrenia, a bipolar disorder or depressive disorder with psychotic features, another psychotic disorder, or autism spectrum disorder.

DSM-5 CRITERIA—CONT'D

Note: If criteria are met prior to the onset of schizophrenia, add "premorbid," e.g., "schizotypal personality disorder (premorbid)."

Cluster B: Personality Disorders (p. 659)
Criteria for Antisocial Personality Disorder

A. A pervasive pattern of disregard for and violation of the rights of others, occurring since age 15 years, as indicated by three (or more) of the following:
   1. Failure to conform to social norms with respect to lawful behaviors, as indicated by repeatedly performing acts that are grounds for arrest.
   2. Deceitfulness, as indicated by repeated lying, use of aliases, or conning others for personal profit or pleasure.
   3. Impulsivity or failure to plan ahead.
   4. Irritability and aggressiveness, as indicated by repeated physical fights or assaults.
   5. Reckless disregard for safety of self or others.
   6. Consistent irresponsibility, as indicated by repeated failure to sustain consistent work behavior or honor financial obligations.
   7. Lack of remorse, as indicated by being indifferent to or rationalizing having hurt, mistreated, or stolen from another.
B. The individual is at least age 18 years.
C. There is evidence of conduct disorder with onset before age 15 years.
D. The occurrence of antisocial behavior is not exclusively during the course of schizophrenia or bipolar disorder.

Criteria for Borderline Personality Disorder (p. 663)

A pervasive pattern of instability of interpersonal relationships, self-image, and affects, and marked impulsivity, beginning by early adulthood and present in a variety of contexts, as indicated by five (or more) of the following:
   1. Frantic efforts to avoid real or imagined abandonment. (Note: Do not include suicidal or self-mutilating behavior covered in Criterion 5.)
   2. A pattern of unstable and intense interpersonal relationships characterized by alternating between extremes of idealization and devaluation.
   3. Identity disturbances: markedly and persistently unstable self-image or sense of self.
   4. Impulsivity in at least two areas that are potentially self-damaging (e.g., spending, sex, substance abuse, reckless driving, binge eating). (Note: Do not include suicidal or self-mutilating behavior covered in Criterion 5.)
   5. Recurrent suicidal behavior, gestures, or threats, or self-mutilating behavior.
   6. Affective instability due to a marked reactivity of mood (e.g., intense episodic dysphoria, irritability, or anxiety usually lasting a few hours and only rarely more than a few days).
   7. Chronic feelings of emptiness.
   8. Inappropriate, intense anger or difficulty controlling anger (e.g., frequent displays of temper, constant anger, recurrent physical fights).
   9. Transient, stress-related paranoid ideations or severe dissociative symptoms.

Criteria for Narcissistic Personality Disorder (p. 669)

A. Pervasive pattern of grandiosity (in fantasy or behavior), need for admiration, and lack of empathy, beginning by early adulthood and present in a variety of contexts, as indicated by five (or more) of the following:
   1. Has a grandiose sense of self-importance (e.g., exaggerates achievements and talents, expects to be recognized as superior without commensurate achievements).
   2. Is preoccupied with fantasies of unlimited success, power, brilliance, beauty, or ideal love.
   3. Believes that he or she is "special" and unique and can only be understood by, or should associate with, other special or high-status people (or institutions).
   4. Requires excessive admiration.
   5. Has a sense of entitlement (i.e., unreasonable expectations of especially favorable treatment or automatic compliance with his or her expectations).
   6. Is interpersonally exploitative (i.e., takes advantage of others to achieve his or her own ends).
   7. Lacks empathy: is unwilling to recognize or identify with the feelings and needs of others.
   8. Is often envious of others or believes that others are envious of him or her.
   9. Shows arrogant, haughty behaviors or attitudes.

Criteria for Histrionic Personality Disorder (p. 667)

A pervasive pattern of excessive emotionality and attention seeking, beginning by early adulthood and present in a variety of contexts, as indicated by five (or more) of the following:
   1. Is uncomfortable in situations in which he or she is not the center of attention.
   2. Interaction with others is often characterized by inappropriate sexually seductive or provocative behavior.
   3. Displays rapidly shifting and shallow expression of emotions.
   4. Consistently uses physical appearance to draw attention to self.
   5. Has a style of speech that is excessively impressionistic and lacking in detail.
   6. Shows self-dramatization, theatricality, and exaggerated expression of emotion.
   7. Is suggestible (i.e., easily influenced by others or circumstances).
   8. Considers relationships to be more intimate than they actually are.

Cluster C: Personality Disorders (p. 675)
Criteria for Dependent Personality Disorder

A pervasive and excessive need to be taken care of that leads to submissive and clinging behavior and fears of separation, beginning by early adulthood and present in a variety of contexts, as indicated by five (or more) of the following:
   1. Has difficulty making everyday decisions without an excessive amount of advice and reassurance from others.
   2. Needs others to assume responsibility for most major areas of his or her life.
   3. Has difficulty expressing disagreement with others because of fear of loss of support or approval. (Note: Do not include realistic fears of retribution.)

(Continued)

DSM-5 CRITERIA—CONT'D

4. Has difficulty initiating projects or doing things on his or her own (because of a lack of self-confidence in judgment or abilities rather than a lack of motivation or energy).
5. Goes to excessive lengths to obtain nurturance and support from others, to the point of volunteering to do things that are unpleasant.
6. Feels uncomfortable or helpless when alone because of exaggerated fears of being unable to care for himself or herself.
7. Urgently seeks another relationship as a source of care and support when a close relationship ends.
8. Is unrealistically preoccupied with fear of being left to take care of himself or herself.

Criteria for Avoidant Personality Disorder (p. 672)
A pervasive pattern of social inhibition, feelings of inadequacy, and hypersensitivity to negative evaluation, beginning by early adulthood and present in a variety of contexts, as indicated by four (or more) of the following:
1. Avoids occupational activities that involve significant interpersonal contact because of fears of criticism, disapproval, or rejection.
2. Is unwilling to get involved with people unless certain of being liked.
3. Shows restraint within intimate relationships because of fear of being shamed or ridiculed.
4. Is preoccupied with being criticized or rejected in social situations.
5. Is inhibited in new interpersonal situations because of feelings of inadequacy.
6. Views self as socially inept, personally unappealing, or inferior to others.

7. Is unusually reluctant to take personal risks or to engage in any new activities because they may prove embarrassing.

Criteria for Obsessive-Compulsive Personality Disorder (p. 678)
A pervasive pattern of preoccupation with orderliness, perfectionism, and mental and interpersonal control, at the expense of flexibility, openness, and efficiency, beginning by early adulthood and present in a variety of contexts, as indicated by four (or more) of the following:
1. Is preoccupied with details, rules, lists, organization, or schedules to the extent that the major point of the activity is lost.
2. Shows perfectionism that interferes with task completion (e.g., is unable to complete a project because his or her own overly strict standards are not met).
3. Is excessively devoted to work and productivity to the exclusion of leisure activities and friendships (not accounted for by obvious economic necessity).
4. Is overconscientious, scrupulous, and inflexible about matters of morality, ethics, or values (not accounted for by cultural or religious identification).
5. Is unable to discard worn-out or worthless objects even when they have no sentimental value.
6. Is reluctant to delegate tasks or to work with others unless they submit to exactly his or her way of doing things.
7. Adopts a miserly spending style toward both self and others; money is viewed as something to be hoarded for future catastrophes.
8. Shows rigidity and stubbornness.

From American Psychiatric Association. (2013). *Diagnostic and statistical manual of disorders* (5th ed.). Arlington, Virginia: APA.

The *DSM-5* alternative model for personality disorders characterizes impairments across two main criteria: personality functioning and pathologic personality traits. Personality functioning comprises self-functioning and interpersonal functioning. Within these two elements of personality, self-functioning involves identity and self-direction, whereas interpersonal functioning includes empathy and intimacy. Pathologic personality traits are organized into five broad domains of negative affectivity, detachment, antagonism, disinhibition, and psychoticism. Within these five domains, there are 25 specific trait facets (American Psychiatric Association, 2013).

Regardless of the model used, personality disorders display an enduring pattern of dysfunction that can be traced back to adolescence or early adulthood. The personality impairments should be relatively pervasive and stable and not considered normal as they relate to development and sociocultural environment. For these reasons, most personality disorders, although in evidence, are usually not diagnosed before age 18.

ETIOLOGY: CONTEMPORARY VIEWS

Historically, the causes of personality disorders were thought to be only psychological in origin based on problems experienced in childhood, growth and development disturbances, reactions to childhood experiences, family, and environmental factors. Current biologic research and neuroimaging studies have produced data that add to our understanding of the psychopathology of some personality disorders. Childhood trauma and disordered attachment have been found to affect the prefrontal cortex; the secretion of cortisol; and the functioning of neurotransmitters, particularly serotonin (Saradjian et al., 2010). Adverse childhood experiences also affect the functioning of the amygdala, altering perceptions of risk (Plodowski et al., 2009).

Some personality disorders have been studied more than others, resulting in information for borderline, antisocial, and schizotypal disorders and little or no data for other disorders. Biologic factors alone are not totally responsible for the occurrence of these disorders. The social environment, coupled with psychological vulnerability, strongly influences the individual. Along with biologic factors, the effects of societal changes, a stressful environment, and negative childhood experiences are important in the genesis of personality disorders.

PERSONALITY DISORDER CLUSTERS

According to the *DSM*, the personality disorders are grouped into three clusters based on descriptive features.

Cluster A includes the schizoid, schizotypal, and paranoid disorders, characterized by odd or eccentric behaviors. Cluster B includes the narcissistic, histrionic, antisocial, and borderline disorders, characterized by dramatic, emotional, or erratic behaviors. Cluster C includes the dependent, avoidant, and obsessive-compulsive disorders, characterized by anxious or fearful behaviors. The box below lists these three clusters.

DSM-5 PERSONALITY DISORDERS

Cluster A—Odd, Eccentric Behaviors
Paranoid personality disorder
Schizoid personality disorder
Schizotypal personality disorder

Cluster B—Dramatic, Emotional, Erratic Behaviors
Antisocial personality disorder
Borderline personality disorder
Histrionic personality disorder
Narcissistic personality disorder

Cluster C—Anxious, Fearful Behaviors
Avoidant personality disorder
Dependent personality disorder
Obsessive-compulsive disorder

Prevalence estimates are 5.7% for cluster A disorders, 1.5% for cluster B disorders, and 6% for cluster C disorders. Data from the 2001-2002 National Epidemiologic Survey on Alcohol and Related Conditions suggest 15% of Americans have at least one personality disorder (American Psychiatric Association, 2013).

CLUSTER A: ODD-ECCENTRIC

PARANOID PERSONALITY DISORDER

Suspiciousness and mistrust of people characterize a person with a paranoid personality disorder. These individuals interpret the actions of others as personal threats, which results in an increase in anxiety and the need for defensiveness. They are hypersensitive to other people's motives and feel vulnerable because they think others treat them unfairly. Individuals with paranoid personality disorder are unable to laugh at themselves and are often humorless, rigid, and guarded. Speech is logical and goal-directed, although the basis of an argument is false because of their suspiciousness. Other symptoms include prejudice and sometimes ideas of reference. These individuals have a blunted affect, so they might appear to be cold, although they are capable of close relationships with a select few. However, they might be suspicious and jealous of people close to them. For example, an individual with paranoid personality disorder might unjustifiably believe that his spouse is having an affair.

In contrast to patients with paranoid schizophrenia, people with paranoid personality disorder do not have fixed delusions or hallucinations. Transient psychotic symptoms might be precipitated by extreme stress. People with paranoid personality disorder are hospitalized when their behavior is out of control in response to a threat perceived as overwhelming or immediate. Because they are quick to respond with anger or rage if they feel threatened, these individuals might be brought to the hospital because of their potential loss of control and potential for violence. Treatment may be court ordered for these individuals.

Unique Causes

Evidence has suggested that paranoid personality disorder tends to occur in biologic relatives of identified patients with schizophrenia and is diagnosed more often in men than in women (American Psychiatric Association, 2000).

Clinical Example

James Sneed is admitted to the hospital accompanied by a female friend. Mr. Sneed states, "My neighbor is taking my land. He built a fence on my property instead of his. He's always trying to pull one over on me." The female friend states that James had barricaded himself in his house, was surrounded by his collection of shotguns, and was threatening to "blow away" his neighbor. James then becomes angry with her, accusing "You would side with him! In fact, I think you bringing me here isn't to help me at all but to get me out of the picture so you two can take everything I've worked for all my life."

SCHIZOID PERSONALITY DISORDER

People with schizoid personalities do not want to be involved in interpersonal or social relationships and keep people at an emotional distance. These individuals rarely have close friends and appear uncomfortable interacting with others; they might be thought of as hermits or loners because of their shyness and introversion; they respond with short answers to questions and do not initiate spontaneous conversation; they can function at work successfully if they can work in isolation, where little verbal interaction is required; and although they are reality-oriented, solitary activities are more gratifying compared with social situations. In the description of these individuals, you may think of another diagnosis: autism spectrum disorder. Research is still ongoing with both diagnoses, but the shared deficits in interpersonal and social interaction may be an indicator that schizoid personality disorder is a variant of high functioning autism.

If a person with schizoid personality disorder is hospitalized, usually because of another axis I diagnosis, the nurse-patient relationship should focus initially on building trust, followed by the identification and appropriate verbal expression of feelings. At first, the patient might be able to participate only on the fringe of unit activities because he or she has no need or desire to be with people. Slowly involving the patient in milieu and group activities, if possible, might help increase social skills.

SCHIZOTYPAL PERSONALITY DISORDER

Individuals with schizotypal personality disorder appear similar to patients with mild schizophrenia but do not meet enough of the criteria for a diagnosis of psychosis or schizophrenia. These patients have problems in thinking, perceiving, and communicating. Their outward appearance might be eccentric, and their thinking and behavior might be odd; they are sensitive to the behaviors of others, especially rejection and anger, and feel that they are different and do not fit in. Paranoid ideation, ideas of reference, and odd beliefs are some of the most prevalent and unchangeable criteria for this disorder (McGlashan et al., 2005).

When a person with schizotypal personality disorder is hospitalized, interventions offering support, kindness, and gentle suggestions help the patient become involved in activities with others. It is essential for the nurse to help the patient improve interpersonal relationships, social skills, and appropriate behaviors. Social situations are uncomfortable and cause discomfort and anxiety because of the reactions of others to the patient's appearance and behavior. These patients can benefit from socializing experiences if the interactions are carefully orchestrated. Vocational counseling and assistance with job placement increase the patient's opportunity for success.

Unique Causes

Schizotypal personality disorder is viewed as part of the schizophrenia spectrum. Individuals who have a family member with schizophrenia are at increased risk for developing schizotypal personality disorder. Neurobiologic findings indicate a preservation of frontal lobe volume in individuals with schizotypal personality disorder, which may protect them from psychosis and severe decline in functioning despite their cognitive-perceptual and interpersonal disturbances (New et al., 2008a).

PUTTING IT ALL TOGETHER

PSYCHOTHERAPEUTIC MANAGEMENT

Nurse-Patient Relationship

The most important psychotherapeutic task centers on dealing with trust issues. A professional demeanor coupled with honesty and nonintrusiveness assists in developing trust. Clear, simple explanations and requests reduce the patient's feelings of being threatened or controlled. These patients do not tolerate group therapies that expect or involve confrontation or much emotional involvement.

CLUSTER B: DRAMATIC-ERRATIC

ANTISOCIAL PERSONALITY DISORDER

The main feature of antisocial personality disorder is a pattern of disregard for the rights of others, which is usually demonstrated by repeated violations of the law. Before the age of 15 years, these behaviors are diagnosed as conduct disorder. Affected individuals engage in unlawful behavior, as evidenced by driving while intoxicated and engaging in spouse or child abuse. They abuse alcohol and other substances and can be promiscuous and feel no guilt about hurting others. Lying, cheating, and stealing are common. Their criminal behavior places them within the judicial and prison systems more than it does the mental health system. However, not all criminals have antisocial personality disorder.

The diagnosis of antisocial personality disorder is based on a history of disordered life functioning rather than on mental status. These individuals might experience distress and anxiety because of others' hostility toward them, but they see the problem as being in others and not in themselves. They use others to their advantage and do not assume responsibility for their behaviors. People with antisocial personality disorder might appear to be charming and intellectual; they are smooth talkers and deny and rationalize their behavior. Expected anxiety over their predicament is absent. Guilt, sorrow for offenses, or loyalty is nonexistent, as if they do not have a conscience.

> **? CRITICAL THINKING QUESTION**
>
> 1. A patient with antisocial personality disorder is verbally threatening to the staff when limits are set on his manipulative behaviors. How would the nurse manage the patient's threatening behavior?

Unique Causes

Both genetics and the environment are known to influence the development of antisocial personality disorder. Parents establish an environment in which the parent-child relationship is unstable, resulting in delinquency in their children. Genetic studies of twin or adoptive siblings and family history data have provided significant evidence that suggests a genetic predisposition to this disorder. In other words, children inherit traits that could lead to the development of antisocial personality disorder. Various genes have been identified in antisocial personality disorders. For example, the gene *C-521 T*, which is involved in the creation of the dopamine 4 receptor, has been implicated in novelty-seeking behavior and impulsivity, two personality traits that are dysfunctional in an individual with antisocial personality disorder (Basoglu et al., 2011).

A genetic abnormality of the monoamine oxidase (MAO) A gene has also been linked to antisocial behavior. Dysfunction of this gene produces less MAO to break down dopamine and serotonin, resulting in elevated levels of these neurotransmitters and subsequent aggressive behavior (Merriman & Cameron, 2007). There are also correlations between MAO activity and adverse childhood experiences such as abuse. Even with the genetic predisposition of low MAO A activity, Caspi et al. (2002) found that between children who were maltreated and children who were not, the seriously abused children were most likely to express antisocial behaviors.

Another common biologic finding seen in individuals with antisocial personality disorder is a weak response to stress in the autonomic nervous system, as evidenced by a low heart rate and a lack of increase in level of anxiety. These individuals are insensitive to the emotional connotations of language, which might explain their inability to learn from punishment. Brain scans of individuals with antisocial personality disorder indicate dysfunction in the prefrontal cortex, frontal temporal, and amygdala-hippocampal regions of the brain. Frontal regions of the brain function inefficiently. Dysfunctional processing of harmful stimuli and decreased amygdala activity in response to negative words exist (Goodman et al., 2007). Additionally, a growing body of evidence suggests an association between altered hypothalamic-pituitary-adrenal axis reactivity resulting in a diminished cortisol response and the development of antisocial behavior in children (Von Polier et al., 2013).

PUTTING IT ALL TOGETHER
PSYCHOTHERAPEUTIC MANAGEMENT
Nurse-Patient Relationship

Long-term treatment is necessary for any type of lasting changes to occur. With short-term hospitalization, the nurse can initiate the therapeutic process by setting firm limits. These patients try to manipulate staff and bend rules for their own desires and needs. The nurse must be steadfast and consistent in confronting behaviors and enforcing rules and policies. Consequences of behavior, both on the unit and for the patient's life, are also a point of focus. Helping the patient be aware of consequences is a concrete way to assist the patient in realizing what the results of behaviors are or will be. The patient must learn to be responsible for his behaviors. Pointing out the effects that the patient's behaviors have on others is also part of the therapeutic process. The patient must begin to understand others' reactions to his behaviors and why people react the way they do. The nurse avoids moralizing and assists the patient in identifying and verbalizing feelings that might reflect anxiety and depression. Membership in a group can help the patient feel accepted as a person, even if the patient's behaviors are unacceptable. Groups of other individuals with this same diagnosis can be effective in confronting inappropriate and manipulative behavior because these individuals are experts in spotting smooth talking, rationalizing, and lying. Such groups can be effective in helping antisocial patients. The keys to working with an antisocial patient are consistency by the nursing staff and fostering responsibility in the patient.

BORDERLINE PERSONALITY DISORDER

Features of borderline personality disorder (BPD) include emotional dysregulation, anger, impulsivity, unstable relationships, identity or self-image disturbance, abandonment fears, self-mutilation, and suicidality. Of all personality disorders, BPD is the one most commonly treated, triggering high mental health care utilization (Gunderson, 2009; New et al., 2008b). However, because the full range of symptoms and behaviors is not typically demonstrated during one short-term inpatient hospitalization, it is often difficult to appreciate fully the complexity of these individuals' symptoms, which can fluctuate and increase in intensity. Also, somatic symptoms result in numerous physician office visits, telephone calls, and prescriptions (Sansone & Sansone, 2008). These patients usually require hospitalization when they are in a crisis or exhibit self-injurious or suicidal behaviors.

Problems with identity, self-image, relationships, thinking, mood, and impulsive behaviors greatly impair functioning. Identity problems are apparent in the individual, who is uncertain about his or her self-image, career goals, personal values, and sexual orientation. Interpersonal relationships are chaotic, and problems exist in choosing unhealthy relationships and short-term intimate relationships. Sexual impulsiveness is seen in casual sexual relationships and multiple sexual partners (Sansone & Wiederman, 2009). The individual alternates between overidealization and devaluation of individuals. For example, an individual with BPD "falls in love" with the perfect person and, shortly thereafter, can find no redeeming qualities in the formerly idealized person. A person with BPD cannot appreciate the mixed bag of qualities that most people have. These individuals have great difficulty in being alone and seek intense but brief relationships.

Projective identification is used to protect the self. Patients displace their angry feelings onto others to justify their own feelings. Blaming others, although dysfunctional and inappropriate, helps the patient deal with feelings. Mood disturbances are exhibited in symptoms of depression, intense anger, and labile mood. Intense emotional pain contributes to mood shifts, which range from euphoria to crying to acting-out behaviors, such as temper tantrums, physical fights, self-mutilation, and suicidal behaviors. Impulsiveness is exhibited in the use of substances and in a tendency toward anorexia-bulimia. Other common impulsive activities include overspending, promiscuity, compulsive overeating, and unhealthy risk taking and decision making. Some behaviors, such as self-injury, are frantic efforts to avoid abandonment and attempts to cope with affective dysregulation and impulsive aggression (McGlashan et al., 2005).

Research findings indicate that 20% to 45% of individuals with BPD have no history of childhood sexual abuse and that 80% of victims of abuse do not have personality disorders (New et al., 2008b). Previously, it was thought that 75% were victims of childhood sexual abuse (American Psychiatric Association, 2000). Research indicates that other forms of childhood adversity, such as bullying, violence in schools, and emotional abuse, have a higher association with personality disorders, particularly BPD, than sexual abuse (Hengartner et al., 2013). The complexity of behaviors associated with BPD can include severe symptoms of posttraumatic stress disorder and dissociative disorder related to a history of abuse and adversity. See Chapters 27 and 36 for related discussions.

The dissociation used by a child abuse victim might result in *splitting*, which is found in a patient with BPD. The defense mechanism of splitting is defined as the inability to view both the self and others as having both good and bad qualities. Patients with BPD use all-or-nothing thinking to view themselves and others as either all good or all bad. One minute you can be on a pedestal and the "the greatest thing ever," and as soon as you disappoint, you are "evil" and "the worst." Splitting also extends to patients' views of themselves. When they see themselves in the worst light, patients are prone to self-injurious or impulsive behaviors. Splitting helps the individual avoid the pain and feelings associated with past abuse and adversity and current situations involving threats of rejection or abandonment.

On admission to an inpatient psychiatric unit, a patient with BPD might exhibit a need for attention and affection by contradictory behaviors of manipulation, dependency, or acting out. Frustration on the part of the staff might be seen as rejection. This perception by the patient can lead to increased anger and withdrawal because of fear of abandonment. Shifts between depression, anxiety, euphoria, and anger are seen in the patient's labile mood. Under stress, the patient regresses to immature behaviors and is unable to cope with conflict. The patient vacillates between clinging and disengaged behaviors, as demonstrated by wanting the staff to solve all problems or by the patient viewing the inpatient treatment as unnecessary and meaningless. When progress seems to be occurring, a patient with BPD might suddenly exhibit opposite behaviors, and it might seem as if the staff will need to start over.

Patients with BPD use self-mutilation or self-injurious behavior for the purpose of self-punishment reflecting a self-perception of "badness" as a result of their cognitive distortion of splitting. Self-injurious behavior provides relief from psychic pain and intolerable feelings with a resulting focus on physical pain and a release of neurohormones (Gunderson, 2009). Self-injury can be seen in cutting, burning, and severe skin scratching resulting in the patient feeling better (Muehlenkamp, 2005). Patients who mutilate themselves are at a serious risk for suicide. Their feelings of hopelessness, despair, and depression contribute to their suicidality, and their self-mutilation should never be interpreted as manipulation or as attention-seeking behavior. Patients with BPD are at risk for suicide because of their depression, aggression, impulsivity, underestimation of the lethality of their behavior, and longer and more frequent occurrence of suicidal thoughts. These patients are often unaware of the likelihood of death and misperceive the lethality of their attempts. The lethality of individuals who self-mutilate and attempt suicide is as serious as that of individuals who do not self-mutilate and attempt suicide (Stanley et al., 2001). Self-mutilation and suicide attempts should never be minimized or ignored. Comorbid diagnoses of posttraumatic stress disorder and major depression increase the risk for suicide.

Unique Causes

The development of BPD is multifactorial. Heredity, genetics, environmental factors, childhood experiences, hyperresponsiveness to stress, and neurologic and biochemical dysfunction contribute to the complexity of BPD (Goodman et al., 2007; Gunderson, 2009; New et al., 2008a, 2008b). Biologic studies have indicated neurotransmitter dysregulation of the serotonin system, as seen in affective disturbances and impulsive behaviors. Defects in serotonin function might be associated with specific genetic risk factors, but the precise molecular nature of this abnormality is unclear (Leichsenring et al., 2011). Environmental factors include a chaotic home environment, such as emotional discord in the family; neglect of the child's feelings and needs; and verbal, emotional, physical, and sexual abuse.

Stress-related events might trigger the individual's genetically based vulnerable temperament and create misery and frustration. The individual can be reminded of earlier stress or trauma, which results in the development of some of the symptoms of this disorder (Goodman et al., 2007). Early trauma and stress affect the hippocampus. Reduced hippocampal volume in adults has been studied with brain imaging in adults who were abused as children. Additionally, the lack of integration of the right and left hemispheres results in abused children using their right hemispheres for frightening memories and left hemispheres when thinking of neutral memories. This might account for the use of splitting by the patient (Gabbard, 2005).

Neuroimaging studies indicate a weakening of the prefrontal cortex, which helps to inhibit or control behaviors and hyperactivity in the amygdala. These neuroimaging findings been identified as a hyperarousal-dyscontrol syndrome (Goodman et al., 2007).

Another area of research is dysregulation of neuropeptides, such as opioids, oxytocin, and vasopressin (Stanley & Siever, 2010). Endogenous opioids are implicated in the regulation of emotion and stress. Oxytocin is involved in affiliation and trust and may be deficient in patients with BPD. Vasopressin is correlated with aggression and irritability. Because the behaviors regulated by these neuropeptides are associated with BPD, investigation may yield improved treatment.

> **? CRITICAL THINKING QUESTION**
>
> 2. A 22-year-old woman is admitted to the unit with BPD and self-injurious behaviors. What are the nurse's priorities in caring for this patient?

PUTTING IT ALL TOGETHER

PSYCHOTHERAPEUTIC MANAGEMENT

Nurse-Patient Relationship

The use of empathy by the nurse while maintaining clear boundaries is important in establishing a relationship with a patient with a diagnosis of BPD. The nurse is not a friend but a health care professional. The nurse acknowledges the reality of the patient's pain; offers support; and empowers and works with the patient to understand, control, and change dysfunctional behaviors. The patient is ultimately in control of her own behaviors, even when the behaviors seem out of control (Smith et al., 2001). With the nurse's assistance, the patient can identify and verbalize feelings, control negative behaviors, and slowly begin to replace the negative behaviors with more appropriate actions.

The patient is usually in a crisis situation when hospitalized because of suicidal behavior, self-mutilation, acute personality disorganization, or inability to function. The nurse conducts a suicide assessment and provides a safe environment to decrease self-harm and contain impulses and then works with the patient to find less destructive ways to handle anger, rage, and psychic pain. Alternatives might include ventilation and discussion of feelings, punching pillows, and the use of foam bats. For self-harm behaviors to diminish, the nurse helps the patient identify feelings and verbally

express them nonaggressively, which enables the patient to understand that his actions are habitual responses to handling emotions. Recognizing behavioral and emotional cues can help the patient decrease impulsive and self-harming behaviors. The nurse then discusses with the patient safe, alternative methods to handle feelings. The use of a behavioral contract to decrease self-injurious behaviors in inpatient and outpatient settings provides the patient with clear expectations of behavior. Patients need to recognize that they can choose to harm themselves or choose alternative methods to manage feelings and reduce anxiety (Aviram et al., 2004).

Patients can be helped with understanding themselves and their feelings by having them write in a notebook or journal on a daily basis. In sharing the journal with the nurse, the patient gains an understanding of self and a sense of autonomy and responsibility. This technique can be useful for many patients with BPD.

Patients with BPD who are victims of abuse need to talk about their trauma in a safe environment. The nurse should acknowledge their pain and convey empathy and the appropriateness of their feelings. When patients understand that current behaviors are linked to past trauma, they can learn to recognize and work toward changing dysfunctional actions toward self and others. See Chapter 33 for more detailed interventions.

Patients with BPD are often manipulative. Consistency, limit setting, and supportive confrontation are necessary interventions to provide clear expectations regarding patient behaviors. These patients are adept at sidestepping rules, avoiding consequences, and pitting staff members against each other, all for the sake of getting what they want. Enforcing unit rules, providing clear structure, and placing the responsibility for appropriate behaviors on the patient, although vigorously resisted, benefits a patient with BPD. Helping the patient develop realistic short-term goals must be part of the treatment plan if the patient's responsibility for self is to increase.

The psychiatric nurse is in a perfect position to help a patient with BPD with the daily give-and-take issues of life that create the many problems for such patients. The nurse should work with the patient on appropriate verbal expression of feelings and assertiveness, even though the nurse's ability to be empathic, nonjudgmental, and therapeutic is sometimes severely tested by the patient's behaviors. Individuals with BPD may have a pattern of undermining themselves when a goal is soon to be achieved (American Psychiatric Association, 2013). After a therapy session that went well, a patient with BPD may decompensate and regress back to previous self-harming or impulsive behaviors. The nurse might feel frustrated and ineffective as a caregiver because of the patient's anger and defenses. Offering superficial solutions to problems, pointing out rules, and interacting superficially might be less frustrating and safer. However, understanding and working with the patient therapeutically can result in a positive experience for the nurse and be of lasting import to the patient.

CASE STUDY

Sherry Morgan, a 27-year-old woman, is brought to the psychiatric inpatient unit from the emergency department. Both wrists were bandaged after suturing. She vacillates between being angry and crying. Sherry states, "I know I am bad. I should not have done it. I do not want to die, but I am tired of the hassles. You wouldn't understand." During the admission interview, the nurse finds that Sherry has had three previous admissions to this inpatient unit during the past 8 years. Sherry states that she refuses to return to work because her boss accuses her of bothering the other employees instead of doing her own work. She states that her boss is falsely accusing her of using alcohol and drugs and does not accept her reasons for being absent from work. On the morning of admission, she called her outpatient therapist, whom she had not seen in a year and a half; he agreed to see her at 3 P.M. When she called the therapist back at noon and found that he was at lunch, she used her scissors to cut her wrists. "I used to think he understood me, but now I know he doesn't care." Her parents are on vacation out of state, and her only close friend is busy with a sick child. She had taken some of her mother's Valium, but it did not calm her down. She has averaged only 3 to 4 hours of sleep each night for the past 5 days and has been unable to eat regular meals. Her attempts to clean her parents' house were not completed. She could not even finish watering her mother's plants. A male acquaintance of 2 weeks was no longer calling her, so she was frequenting several bars and inviting men home. She never heard from these men again, even though she thought that their relationships were sexually satisfying.

Sherry completed 2 years of college and is dressed attractively. She enjoys reading romance novels and has brought five of her favorite books.

CARE PLAN

Name: Sherry Morgan   **Admission Date:** _____
DSM-5 Diagnosis: Axis I—major depression; borderline personality disorder

Assessment	**Areas of strength:** Patient is well groomed, neat, and clean; is intelligent; enjoys reading.
	Problems: Self-mutilating behavior, absence of support system, loss of job, decreased sleeping and eating, irresponsible and impulsive sexual behavior.
Diagnoses	Risk for self-directed violence related to absence of support system and history of cutting wrists
	Defensive coping related to low self-esteem, as evidenced by angry and labile emotions
Outcomes	**Short-term goals**
Date met: _____	Patient will eliminate self-mutilating behavior and appropriately verbalize feelings of anger and sadness.
Date met: _____	Patient will use alternative methods of coping with emotions.
	Long-term goals
Date met: _____	Patient will schedule outpatient appointment and meeting with boss regarding job problems.
Planning and Interventions	**Nurse-patient relationship:** Monitor and set limits on acting-out behaviors. Assist patient with identification and verbalization of feelings. Teach healthy coping behaviors. Discuss fears about accepting responsibility for self and decision making. Discuss behaviors interfering with job performance.
	Psychopharmacology: Fluoxetine (Prozac) 20 mg q morning; trazodone 150 mg q at bedtime.
	Milieu management: Groups focusing on self-esteem, stress and anger management, assertiveness training, social skills, problem-solving skills, and discharge planning.
Evaluation	Patient has not engaged in self-mutilating behavior. Patient is appropriately verbalizing feelings of anger and sadness. Patient has identified and is using two methods of coping with feelings. Patient has a crisis plan when overwhelmed by emotions.
Referrals	Appointment weekly after discharge with therapist at outpatient mental health clinic.

Psychopharmacology

Psychopharmacology is used for specific symptoms for patients with BPD. The symptoms are divided into three domains: (1) cognitive-perceptual symptoms, (2) affective or emotional dysregulation, and (3) impulsive-behavioral dyscontrol (Lively, 2000; Soloff, 2000). Medications are only part of the treatment plan and do not solve all the patient's problems. Cognitive-perceptual symptoms might include transitory hallucinations, suspiciousness, paranoid thinking, and delusions. Transient psychotic states resulting from overwhelming stress are treated with low-dose typical and atypical antipsychotics for 3 to 12 weeks to decrease symptoms.

Affective or emotional dysregulation might include depression, labile mood, anger, anxiety, hostility, and mistrust. Selective serotonin reuptake inhibitors are used to reduce anger, anxiety, chronic emptiness, and temper outbursts (New et al., 2008a). Clonazepam might be useful for anxiety management, if needed (Soloff, 2000). Lithium, valproic acid, and carbamazepine can be used for rapid mood swings. Impulsive-behavioral dyscontrol symptoms might include suicidal threats and attempts; assaultiveness; impulse aggression; and binge behaviors involving alcohol, drugs, or sex. Selective serotonin reuptake inhibitors are used to decrease impulsive behaviors.

Milieu Management

Interventions mentioned in the discussion of the nurse-patient relationship regarding firm limits, consistency, and clear structure are basic to the milieu for patients with BPD. The patient's manipulation of other patients must be confronted because patients with BPD can mobilize others against the staff. Consistent communication among staff members is essential to minimize the patient's attempts to divide them.

Dialectical behavior therapy has been proven to benefit these patients (DuBose & Linehan, 2005; Paris, 2008). Therapeutic activities that are important for these patients in both inpatient and outpatient settings include assertiveness training, problem solving, stress management, and anger management.

Referral to self-help groups for alcohol and drug problems, eating disorders, and victimization is also important. Vocational counseling and training are important to foster autonomous and independent functioning. Residential treatment might need to be considered, particularly for patients with chronic self-destructive behavior.

CRITICAL THINKING QUESTION

3. Staff members on the unit are frustrated and angry with a patient with a diagnosis of BPD who is attempting to pit members on the various shifts against each other. They are even beginning to be angry with each other for the inconsistencies occurring with this patient's care. What strategies should the head nurse employ to help the staff and ultimately the treatment of the patient?

Balanced Therapy: How to Avoid Conflict and Help Patients with Borderline Personality Disorder

Description

Dialectical behavior therapy (DBT) is an evidence-based, comprehensive treatment modality that helps patients with BPD who have problems regulating emotions and who are suicidal. The outpatient model for DBT requires patients to meet weekly in individual psychotherapy and skills training groups. Patients consult with their therapist between sessions by telephone to decrease suicide crisis behaviors, increase behavioral skills, and decrease feelings of conflict and alienation or distance from the therapist.

DBT consists of four stages. In stage 1, patients move from severe behavioral dyscontrol to behavioral control to decrease suicidal and other life-threatening behaviors. Stage 2 consists of moving from desperation to emotional experiencing. In stage 3, patients address problems in living and moving toward happiness/unhappiness. In stage 4, patients move from incompleteness to a capacity for joy and freedom.

Results

In seven randomized control trials, DBT was shown to be useful to patients with BPD. In the initial trial by DuBose and Linehan (2005), subjects were assessed every 4 months while in treatment for 1 year and for 1 year afterward. DBT was effective in reducing suicide attempts and self-injury; decreasing premature dropout from therapy; reducing emergency department admission and length of psychiatric hospitalization; and reducing drug use, depression, hopelessness, and anger.

Implications

Nurses trained in DBT can offer patients with BPD effective, evidence-based, comprehensive, and compassionate treatment.

Modified from DuBose, A.P., & Linehan, M.M. (2005). Balanced therapy: how to avoid conflict and help "borderline" patients. *Current Psychiatry, 4,* 12.

NARCISSISTIC PERSONALITY DISORDER

A key component of narcissistic personality disorder is grandiosity (Pincus & Lukowitsky, 2010). A patient with narcissistic personality disorder displays grandiosity about his importance and achievements. This grandiosity differs from the delusions of grandeur found in schizophrenia or bipolar disorders. The grandiosity of narcissistic personality disorder is based in reality but is distorted, embellished, or convoluted to meet the patient's needs of self-importance. For example, a man with narcissistic personality disorder might say that he was a star football player in high school and that he could have played for the Indianapolis Colts; he does not tell the nurse that he barely made the second-string football team in high school.

The grandiosity of a patient with narcissistic personality disorder is displayed through interpersonal exploitation, lack of empathy, arrogance, intense envy, and entitlement. These individuals may also superficially seem supportive to others but secretly harbor contempt for the person being helped

and manipulate the interaction to reflect their own specialness, goodness, or superior capabilities (Pincus & Lukowitsky, 2010).

The other key component is narcissistic vulnerability. Individuals with narcissistic personality disorder are intensely troubled when faced with disappointments and threats to their extreme positive self-image. Because no one is perfect, these patients must use maladaptive strategies to manage the constant obstacles and challenges to the unfulfilled or unattainable perfection they see in themselves. A person with vulnerable narcissism might appear nonchalant or indifferent to criticism while hiding feelings of anger, rage, or emptiness. Constant reinforcement from others is needed to boost self-esteem. Relationships with others seem shallow but might be meaningful if the patient's self-esteem is positively enhanced. The patient can empathize with others but is very self-centered. These individuals use others selfishly to meet their own needs and to assuage their loneliness and feelings of inadequacy.

Clinical Example

A patient has been admitted to the unit and insists on a private room with a telephone and television because he needs to keep up with the reports on the financial news network. He says he's "not like these other people up here" and that he can't let their problems keep him from his important work. When you are unable to meet his demands, he smugly states, "You wouldn't understand all the big decisions I have to make for others. You're just a nurse."

Unique Causes

Studies of biologic and genetic factors in narcissistic personality disorder have not been conducted. Some theorists believe that the self-centered person is arrested in emotional development because the parents failed to mirror that which was appropriate or inappropriate back to the child (Miller, 2004). Consequently, the child developed without any feedback about his or her behaviors.

PUTTING IT ALL TOGETHER

PSYCHOTHERAPEUTIC MANAGEMENT

Nurse-Patient Relationship

If a patient with narcissistic personality disorder is hospitalized, the nurse must deal with decreasing the constant recitation of self-importance and grandiosity. The nurse must mirror what the patient sounds like, especially if contradictions exist, and help the patient focus on the identification and verbal expression of feelings. Supportive confrontation is used to point out discrepancies between what the patient says and what actually exists to increase responsibility for self. Limit setting and consistency in approach are used to decrease manipulation and entitlement behaviors. Realistic short-term goals focused on the here and now are important to decrease the patient's use of fantasy and rationalization and to increase responsibility for self. The patient needs to be taught that everyone has worth, even if he or she makes mistakes and has imperfections. Group therapy provides the opportunity for the patient to see how his behavior affects others and, perhaps for the first time, gives the patient a chance to become involved with the problems of others. Caution must be exercised not to give the patient free rein to talk about himself (Miller, 2004).

HISTRIONIC PERSONALITY DISORDER

A person with histrionic personality disorder dramatizes events and draws attention to self. The person is extroverted and thrives on being the center of attention. Behavior is silly, colorful, frivolous, and seductive. Speech is vague, descriptive, superficial, and overembellished but lacking in detail, insight, and depth. The person seems to be in a hurry and restless. Temper tantrums and outbursts of anger as well as overreactions to minor events are seen. Patients with a diagnosis of histrionic personality disorder might use somatic complaints to avoid responsibility and support dependency. Dissociation is a common defense to avoid feelings. This patient cannot deal with his or her true feelings. The patient views relationships with others as special or possessing greater intimacy than is real. Individuals the patient recently met are thought of as being dear friends.

Unique Causes

The causes of histrionic personality disorder are unknown but are probably a result of many factors.

PUTTING IT ALL TOGETHER

PSYCHOTHERAPEUTIC MANAGEMENT

Nurse-Patient Relationship

Positive reinforcement in the form of attention, recognition, or praise is given for unselfish or other-centered behaviors. Because the patient needs much reassurance and feels helpless, the nurse must provide support to facilitate independent problem solving and daily functioning. Because the patient is unaware of and does not deal with feelings, the nurse must help clarify the patient's true feelings and help the patient learn appropriate ways to express them. Working with this type of patient can be frustrating for the nurse because the patient needs time to internalize the meaning of what the nurse is trying to accomplish.

CLUSTER C: ANXIOUS-FEARFUL

DEPENDENT PERSONALITY DISORDER

The main characteristic of dependent personality disorder is a "pervasive and excessive need to be taken care of that leads to submissive and clinging behaviors and fears of separation" (American Psychiatric Association, 2013). Dependent individuals want others to make daily decisions for them, such as the type of clothes to wear and the type of job to seek. They need direction and reassurance. These individuals feel inferior and cling to others excessively because they are afraid that they will be left alone. Avoiding responsibility and expressing helplessness, the person maintains the need to rely on others. These persons perceive themselves as being unable to function without the help of others.

Dependent individuals also expect that if they perform good deeds for others, they will be rewarded by someone doing something for them. An intimate relationship with a spouse who is abusive, unfaithful, or an alcoholic is tolerated so as not to disturb the sense of attachment. Passivity and concealing of sexual feelings and anger are a means of avoiding conflict.

Clinical Example
A patient has been telling the nurse about her alcoholic abusive husband. She has been married to him for 16 years. She expresses sadness and frustration about her marriage but states, "How could I leave him? Who will take care of me? I could never live alone. He's not perfect, but at least he cares about me." The patient continues to ask the nurse what she should do.

Unique Causes

Biochemical and genetic factors have not been correlated with dependent personality disorder. Psychosocial theories consider culture to be the basis of the development of this disorder. Parents or society might believe that the child should not exhibit certain autonomous behaviors, and the child might believe that disapproval and loss of attachment are consequences of these behaviors. Research from different countries has shown that dependent adults are at increased risk for physical illness, suggesting a dependency-dysfunction link that crosses culture and has a basis in other factors (Bornstein, 2012).

PUTTING IT ALL TOGETHER

PSYCHOTHERAPEUTIC MANAGEMENT

Nurse-Patient Relationship

The nurse slowly works on decision making with the patient to increase responsibility for self in daily living. The patient needs assistance with managing anxiety because it will increase as the patient assumes more responsibility for self. Assertiveness is an important area of the nurse's teaching, which enables the patient to state clearly his or her feelings, needs, and desires. Verbalization of feelings and ways to cope with them are essential.

AVOIDANT PERSONALITY DISORDER

Patients with the avoidant personality disorder are timid, socially uncomfortable, and withdrawn. They feel inadequate and are hypersensitive to criticism. Although they are fearful and shy, patients with avoidant personality disorder desire relationships; however, they need to be certain of being liked before making social contacts (McGlashan et al., 2005). To keep their anxiety at a minimal level, these individuals avoid situations in which they might be disappointed or rejected. When interacting with someone, this person sounds uncertain and lacks self-confidence and is afraid to ask questions or speak up in public, withdraws from social support, and conveys helplessness.

Unique Causes

Few biologic, genetic, and psychological studies have been conducted on avoidant personality disorder. It is known that amygdala hyperactivity causes anxiety and fearfulness in humans (Goodman et al., 2007). Shyness is common in childhood, but increased shyness and avoidant behavior during adolescence might lead to this disorder. Avoidant personality disorder appears to be specifically associated with social phobia and may be considered the extreme end of this spectrum (Borge et al., 2010).

PUTTING IT ALL TOGETHER

PSYCHOTHERAPEUTIC MANAGEMENT

Nurse-Patient Relationship

The nurse helps the patient gradually confront his or her fears. Discussing the patient's feelings and fears before and after doing something that he is afraid to do is an essential part of the relationship. The nurse supports and directs the patient in accomplishing small goals. Helping the patient to be assertive and develop social skills is necessary. The nurse includes the patient in interactions with others and progresses to small groups as the patient is able to tolerate them. Because of the patient's anxiety, relaxation techniques are taught to enable the patient to be successful in interactions. The nurse gives positive feedback to the patient for any real success and for any attempts to engage in interactions with others to promote self-esteem.

OBSESSIVE-COMPULSIVE PERSONALITY DISORDER

Individuals with obsessive-compulsive personality disorder are perfectionistic and inflexible. These individuals are overly strict and often set standards for themselves that are too high; their work is never good enough. They are preoccupied with rules, trivial details, and procedures. When others are asked to describe them, the phrase "control freak" might be used. These individuals find it difficult to express warmth or tender emotions. There is little give-and-take in their interactions with others, and they are rigid, controlling, and cold. The person is serious about all of his activities, so having fun or experiencing pleasure is difficult. Because the person is afraid of making mistakes, he can be indecisive or put off decisions until all the facts have been obtained. The person's affect is constricted, and he might speak in a monotone. Because personality traits are egosyntonic, their perfectionism does not disturb these individuals; they see nothing wrong with a rigorous, orderly approach. In contrast, obsessive-compulsive disorder is part of the anxiety spectrum and is *egodystonic*; the need to check obsessions compulsively does cause these patients tremendous distress because they recognize the abnormality of their thoughts and behaviors.

Unique Causes

Early parent-child relationships around issues of autonomy, control, and authority might predispose a person to this disorder. Many of the features of obsessive-compulsive personality disorder resemble a "type A" personality and may be present in people at risk for myocardial infarction. There is an association between obsessive-compulsive personality disorder and eating disorders, and their etiologies may be similar (American Psychiatric Association, 2013).

PUTTING IT ALL TOGETHER

PSYCHOTHERAPEUTIC MANAGEMENT

Nurse-Patient Relationship

The nurse needs to support the patient in exploring his feelings and in attempting new experiences and situations. The nurse helps the patient with decision making and encourages follow-through behavior. Sometimes a need exists to confront the patient's procrastination and intellectualization. The nurse teaches the patient the importance of leisure activities and exploring interests in this area. Because the patient lacks awareness of the way he affects others, the patient needs to look at and understand others' view of him. Teaching the patient that he is human and that it is all right to make mistakes helps decrease irrational beliefs about the need to be perfect.

STUDY NOTES

1. Personality traits are enduring approaches to the world expressed in the way a person thinks, feels, and behaves.
2. When personality traits become rigid and dysfunctional and cause distress in self and others, a personality disorder might be diagnosed. Personal discomfort arises primarily from others' reactions to or behaviors toward the person.
3. The odd-eccentric cluster of personality disorders includes the following:

a. Paranoid, characterized by suspiciousness and mistrust
b. Schizoid, characterized by aloneness and a hermit-like lifestyle
c. Schizotypal, characterized by symptoms similar to but less severe than symptoms of schizophrenia

4. The dramatic-erratic cluster of personality disorders includes the following:

a. Antisocial, characterized by disregard of others' rights without guilt

b. Borderline, characterized by problems with self-identity, interpersonal relationships, emotional dysregulation, and self-injurious behaviors

c. Narcissistic, characterized by overevaluation of self, arrogance, and indifference to the criticism of others

d. Histrionic, characterized by dramatic behaviors, attention seeking, and superficiality

5. The anxious-fearful cluster of personality disorders includes the following:

a. Dependent, characterized by submissiveness, helplessness, fear of responsibility, and reliance on others for decision making

b. Avoidant, characterized by timidity, socially withdrawn behavior, and hypersensitivity to criticism

c. Obsessive-compulsive, characterized by indecisiveness, perfectionism, inflexibility, and difficulty expressing feelings

6. Nursing interventions for individuals with personality disorders help the patient recognize specific behaviors distressing to self, others, or both; manage feelings; and develop coping behaviors that are less dysfunctional.

REFERENCES

Adelstein, J. S., et al. (2011). Personality is reflected in the brain's intrinsic functional architecture. *PLoS One, 6*, 11.

American Psychiatric Association. (2000). Diagnostic and statistical manual of mental disorders, text revision (4th ed.). Arlington, Virginia: APA.

American Psychiatric Association. (2013). Diagnostic and statistical manual of mental disorders (5th ed.). Arlington, Virginia: APA.

Aviram, R. B., et al. (2004). Adapting supportive psychotherapy for individuals with borderline personality disorder who self-injure or attempt suicide. *Journal of Psychiatric Practice, 10*, 145.

Basoglu, C., et al. (2011). Synaptosomal-associated protein 25 gene polymorphisms and antisocial personality disorder: Association with temperament and psychopathy. *Canadian Journal of Psychiatry, 56*, 341–347.

Blais, M. A., et al. (2008). Personality and personality disorders. In T. A. Stern, et al. (Eds.), Massachusetts General Hospital clinical psychiatry (pp. 527–540). Philadelphia: Mosby.

Borge, F. M., et al. (2010). Pre-treatment predictors and in-treatment factors associated with change in avoidant and dependent personality disorder traits among patients with social phobia. *Clinical Psychology & Psychotherapy, 17*, 87–99.

Bornstein, R. F. (2012). Illuminating a neglected clinical issue: Societal costs of interpersonal dependency and dependent personality disorder. *Journal of Clinical Psychology, 68*, 766–781.

Caspi, A., et al. (2002). Role of genotype in the cycle of violence in maltreated children. *Science, 297*, 81.

DuBose, A. P., & Linehan, M. M. (2005). Balanced therapy: How to avoid conflict and help "borderline" patients. *Current Psychiatry, 4*, 12.

Gabbard, G. O. (2005). Mind, brain, and personality disorders. *American Journal of Psychiatry, 162*, 648.

Goodman, M., et al. (2007). Neuroimaging in personality disorders: Current concepts, findings, and implications. *Psychiatric Annals, 37*, 2.

Gunderson, J. G. (2009). Borderline personality disorder: Ontogeny of a diagnosis. *American Journal of Psychiatry, 166*, 5.

Hengartner, M. P., et al. (2013). Childhood adversity in association with personality disorder dimensions: New findings in an old debate. *European Psychiatry, 28*, 476–482.

Leichsenring, F., et al. (2011). Borderline personality disorder. *The Lancet, 377*, 74–84.

Livesly, W. J. (2000). A practical approach to the treatment of patients with borderline personality disorder. *Psychiatric Clinics of North America, 23*, 211.

McGlashan, T. H., et al. (2005). Two-year prevalence and stability of individual DSM-IV criteria for schizotypal, borderline, avoidant, and obsessive-compulsive personality disorders: Toward a hybrid model of axis II disorders. *American Journal of Psychiatry, 162*, 883.

Merriman, T., & Cameron, V. (2007). Risk-taking: Behind the warrior gene story. *The New Zealand Medical Journal, 120*, 1250.

Miller, M. C. (2004). Narcissism and self-esteem. *Harvard Mental Health Letter, 20*, 1.

Muehlenkamp, J. J. (2005). Self-injurious behavior as a separate clinical syndrome. *American Journal of Orthopsychiatry, 75*, 324.

New, A. S., et al. (2008a). Recent advances in the biological study of personality disorders. *Psychiatric Clinics of North America, 31*, 3.

New, A. S., Triebwasser, J., & Charney, D. S. (2008b). The case for shifting borderline personality disorder to axis I. *Biological Psychiatry, 64*, 653.

Paris, J. (2008). Clinical trials of treatment for personality disorders. *Psychiatric Clinics of North America, 31*, 3.

Pincus, L., & Lukowitsky, M. (2010). Pathological narcissism and narcissistic personality disorder. *Annual Review of Clinical Psychology, 6*, 421–446.

Plodowski, A., Gregory, S. L., & Blackwood, N. J. (2009). Persistent violent offending among adult men. In S. Hodgins, E. Viding, & A. Plodowski (Eds.), The neurological basis of violence: Science and rehabilitation. Oxford: Oxford University Press.

Sansone, R. A., & Sansone, L. A. (2008). Borderline personality disorder: Are proliferative symptoms characteristic? *Psychiatry, 5*, 18.

Sansone, R. A., & Wiederman, M. W. (2009). Borderline personality symptomatology, casual sexual relationships, and promiscuity. *Psychiatry, 6*, 36.

Saradjian, J., Murphy, N., & McVey, D. (2010). Fundamental treatment strategies for optimising interventions with people with personality disorder. In N. Murphy, & D. McVey (Eds.), Treating personality disorder. Creating robust services for people with complex mental health needs. London: Routledge, Taylor & Francis Group.

Smith, G. W., Ruiz-Sancho, A. R., & Gunderson, J. G. (2001). An intensive outpatient program for patients with borderline personality disorder. *Psychiatric Services (Washington, D.C.), 52*, 532.

Soloff, P. H. (2000). Psychopharmacology of borderline personality disorder. *Psychiatric Clinics of North America, 23*, 169.

Stanley, B., & Siever, L. (2010). The interpersonal dimension of borderline personality disorder: Toward a neuropeptide model. *American Journal of Psychiatry, 167*, 24.

Stanley, B., et al. (2001). Are suicide attempters who self-mutilate a unique population? *American Journal of Psychiatry, 158*, 427.

Von Polier, G. G., et al. (2013). Reduced cortisol in boys with early-onset conduct disorder and callous-unemotional traits. *BioMed Research International, 2013*, 349530.

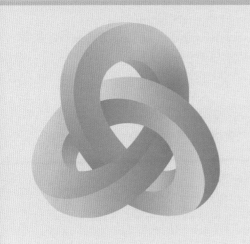

Sexual Disorders

Karmie M. Johnson

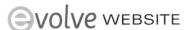 WEBSITE

http://evolve.elsevier.com/Keltner

LEARNING OBJECTIVES

- Recognize the importance of the nurse's role in assessing patients' sexual concerns and problems.
- Describe the categories of sexual dysfunctions, paraphilic disorders, and gender dysphoria.

- Identify the issues related to the care of patients with sexual disorders.
- Demonstrate an understanding of the need for referring patients with sexual disorders for further assessment and treatment.

This chapter presents an overview of sexual disorders and sexual dysfunctions. Normal sexuality and sexual preference issues, such as homosexuality, are not included.

Individuals engage in a wide range of sexual activities, resulting in a wide range of sexual responses. Sexual activity might focus on objects or people; it is unacceptable legally when it involves a nonconsenting individual or a child. Other laws regarding illegal sexual activity vary from area to area and can include laws that prohibit the sexual use of objects in a way that might interfere with healthy relationships. Sexual activity is unacceptable morally when it violates the norms, standards, and values of the culture. Sexual activity should be evaluated according to its effects on the individual and others, such as the level of functioning, self-esteem, and relationships with others.

Considering coercion versus consent between sexual partners is important. An individual's rights and needs should never be violated. Power and control issues affect the definition of consent and the degree of coercion. For example, some clinicians believe that a sexual relationship between a powerful political figure and a young office worker, although apparently consensual, is actually coercive at its core.

DSM-5 CRITERIA AND TERMINOLOGY

DSM-5 (American Psychiatric Association, 2013a) categorizes sexual disorders according to sexual dysfunctions, the

paraphilias, and gender dysphoria. Sexual dysfunctions are typically characterized by a significant disturbance in a person's ability to respond sexually or to experience sexual pleasure. Paraphilic disorders are characterized by intense sexual urges focused on abnormal sexual activities or preferences. Gender dysphoria is characterized by persistent distress with one's biologic sex versus one's desired or expressed gender. As with all disorders, sexual disorders must cause clinically significant distress or an impairment of social function before a diagnosis can be made.

NORM'S NOTES

We will now discuss a topic that evokes a kind of morbid curiosity. Sexual disorders come in many varieties, from the inability to participate in healthy sexual activity to behaviors that are illegal, immoral, and sometimes weird. You probably will not run into these individuals during your clinical rotation, but I think you will find this short chapter interesting.

DSM-5 DIAGNOSES RELATED TO SEXUAL DISORDERS

Sexual dysfunctions
Paraphilic disorders
Gender dysphoria

SEXUAL DYSFUNCTIONS

As part of the admission interview, the nurse assesses each patient for potential or actual problems with sexual functioning. Box 30-1 lists initial questions that the nurse might use to assess the patient's feelings and concerns about sexuality. Potential or actual problems can occur as a result of emotional factors, physiologic factors, or both. Medications and chemicals also can alter sexual desire and functioning. A thorough assessment or evaluation is necessary for appropriate referral and treatment. Treatment is individualized according to the cause or combination of causes. For example, an individual who becomes impotent because of a medical illness or a medication side effect might also have diminished self-esteem and self-confidence that compounds the problem. Treatment would focus on both the physiologic aspects and the emotional needs of the individual.

In the past, the four phases of human sexual activity were called the sexual response cycle and identified as the desire phase, the excitement phase, the orgasm phase, and the resolution phase. Research now suggests that sexual response is not always a linear, uniform process and that the distinction between certain phases (e.g., desire and arousal) may not be as appropriate as previously delineated. For example, *DSM-IV-TR* differentiated female sexual desire disorders and arousal disorders. In *DSM-5*, these two disorders are combined into female sexual interest/arousal disorder (American Psychiatric Association, 2013b). Sexual dysfunctions are also divided into subtypes related to time. *Lifelong* problems have been present since the patient's first sexual experience, whereas *acquired* disorders have developed after a period of normal sexual functioning. *Generalized* difficulties are not limited by certain types of stimulation, situations, or partners, whereas *situational* disorders occur only with certain types of stimuli, circumstances, or partners (American Psychiatric Association, 2013b).

Other factors may also influence the onset and duration of sexual dysfunction, such as a partner's own separate problems, relationship issues, cultural or religious attitudes and inhibitions, and medical causes. The patient may also have personal factors such as poor body image, history of abuse, mental health issues, or other stressors. The duration of symptoms within the disorder must be at least 6 months to be considered dysfunctional and a disorder.

BOX 30-1 INITIAL NURSING ASSESSMENT OF SEXUAL CONCERNS

Describe any difficulties that you have experienced with sexual performance or satisfaction.

What are your feelings and concerns about sexuality?

How satisfied are you with your sexual relationship?

What type of changes would you like to make in your sexual relationship?

What type of negative sexual experiences have you had?

Specific Sexual Dysfunction Disorders

Male Hypoactive Sexual Desire Disorder

Men with hypoactive sexual desire disorder have little or no interest in sexual fantasies or activities and have hypoactive sexual desires.

Erectile Disorder

Men with erectile disorder have erectile dysfunction and either cannot obtain or cannot maintain an erection sufficient for sexual activity.

Ejaculation Disorders

The two disorders related to ejaculation are delayed and premature (early). Men with delayed ejaculation experience a marked delay or absence of orgasm. In premature ejaculation, a man reaches orgasm within 1 minute of vaginal penetration and before he wishes it, frustrating both himself and his partner.

Female Sexual Interest/Arousal Disorder

Women with sexual interest/arousal disorder have little or no interest in sexual fantasies or activities. The reduction or absence of sexual interest makes sexual arousal difficult so that sensations and pleasure from sexual activity are also affected.

Female Orgasmic Disorder

Women with orgasmic disorder experience a marked delay or absence of orgasm. Women also may experience a reduction in the intensity of orgasmic sensations.

Genito-Pelvic Pain/Penetration Disorder

Women with genito-pelvic pain/penetration disorder experience pain or anticipate pain with vaginal penetration.

Treatment

The first step in treating sexual dysfunction disorders is to determine if there is an underlying medical cause, such as illness, side effects from medication, or lifestyle choices such as diet and exercise. Sexual dysfunction may be a symptom of another psychiatric condition such as depression and will abate once the primary condition is corrected. After a preexisting illness or condition has been ruled out, there are many pharmacologic and medical-surgical interventions that have proved useful. Psychologically based treatments that improve communication between partners and decrease stress and performance pressure as well as other behavioral techniques can also be effective.

❓ CRITICAL THINKING QUESTION

1. A patient with insulin-dependent diabetes states, "After I leave the hospital, I'm going to use only half of the prescribed insulin because I heard insulin might affect my sexual performance." What are your interventions with this patient?

PARAPHILIC DISORDERS

A paraphilia is an intense and persistent sexual interest in anything other than a physically normal and mature consenting adult (Box 30-2). The paraphilia may be directed toward an abnormal activity or target. Abnormal activities can be divided further into *courtship* disorders that are distortions of acceptable human courtship behaviors and *algolagnic* disorders, which involve pain and suffering. Anomalous target preferences can be directed at humans or objects. For a paraphilia to be considered a disorder, there must be negative consequences, such as distress, impairment to functioning, or harm to self or others (American Psychiatric Association, 2013a).

BOX 30-2 SEXUAL DISORDERS

Paraphilic Disorders

The following paraphilic activities last over a period of 6 months and cause distress or impairment in social, occupational, or other important areas of functioning.

Exhibitionistic Disorder
- Recurrent, intense sexually arousing fantasies, urges, or behaviors involving exposing one's genitals to unsuspecting strangers.

Fetishistic Disorder
- Recurrent, intense sexually arousing fantasies, urges, or behaviors using nonliving objects.

Frotteuristic Disorder
- Recurrent, intense sexually arousing fantasies, urges, or behaviors involving touching and rubbing against a nonconsenting person.

Pedophilic Disorder
- Recurrent, intense sexually arousing fantasies, urges, or behaviors that involve sexual activity with a child or children generally 13 years old or younger.
- The person is at least 16 years old and at least 5 years older than the child or children involved.

Sexual Masochism Disorder
- Recurrent, intense sexually arousing fantasies, urges, or behaviors involving the act of being humiliated, beaten, restrained, or otherwise made to suffer.

Sexual Sadism Disorder
- Recurrent, intense sexually arousing fantasies, urges, or behaviors involving acts in which the psychological or physical suffering of the victim is sexually exciting to the person.

Transvestic Disorder
- Recurrent, intense sexual arousing fantasies, urges, or behaviors involving cross-dressing or dressing as the opposite sex.

Voyeuristic Disorder
- Act of observing an unsuspecting person who is naked, in the process of disrobing, or engaging in sexual activity.

Modified from McManus, M., et al. (2013). Paraphilias: definition, diagnosis and treatment. *F1000Prime Reports, 5,* 36.

Individuals with paraphilia might seek inpatient treatment because of another psychiatric diagnosis that does not reflect a sexual disorder. The nurse on an inpatient unit might encounter individuals admitted with major depression and suicidal ideation who might be trying to avoid criminal prosecution or to be given a lesser sentence by seeking psychiatric treatment. Others might be admitted to inpatient or outpatient care because of axis I disorders and not their paraphilia. Mood disorders, anxiety disorders, and substance disorders might be the reason for seeking treatment. The nurse intervenes with therapeutic techniques relevant to the axis I diagnosis, rather than specifically addressing the paraphilia.

Individuals with paraphilias often do not consider their sexual activities or interests a disorder and do not seek psychiatric treatment for them. However, when examining the scope of the disorder, it is found that individuals with a paraphilia have difficulty forming socially acceptable relationships and at best lead lonely, dissatisfied lives or at worst engage in destructive criminal activities.

Treatment for pedophilia, exhibitionism, and voyeurism generally occurs on an outpatient basis. Information about pedophilia comes from individuals who have been arrested and incarcerated and from their victims. Outpatient treatment programs and programs for incarcerated individuals also provide information about assessment and treatment, with most research being carried out on convicted sex offenders (Hall, 2007).

Paraphiliacs might be men or women, and paraphilic activity might be limited to a period of stress rather than following a chronic or repetitive pattern. Generally, paraphiliacs with a chronic pattern of behavior have a large number of victims. Paraphilias usually begin in adolescence. There is evidence that mood disorders; anxiety and impulse disorders; substance-related disorders; and personality disorders, especially the antisocial and cluster C personality disorders, are frequently comorbid diagnoses. Research studies involving neuropsychological testing, endocrine functioning, brain imaging, and personality characteristics have been conducted. The results are mixed and sometimes contradictory.

Pedophilic Disorders

Pedophilia involves recurrent intense sexual urges and sexually arousing fantasies involving sexual activity with children. The individual acts on the urges or is distressed by them (American Psychiatric Association, 2013a). By definition, the victim of pedophilia must be younger than 13 years old, and the pedophile must be 16 years old or older and at least 5 years older than the victim. Pedophilic behavior can be expressed for opposite-sex children, same-sex children, or both.

Typical pedophilic behaviors are fondling, inappropriate touching, masturbating in a child's presence, and penetration of the mouth, anus, or vagina. Pedophiles also engage in other paraphilias, such as exhibitionism and voyeurism (Hall, 2007). These individuals may justify their actions by thinking that they are educating the child or that the child liked the attention or pleasure. To compensate for feelings of powerlessness, the pedophile might need to feel power over the victim through control and domination. Some sex offenders are nonaggressive; others use aggression in the form of trickery or bribery. The threat of violence might be used to encourage the victim's silence. The pedophile might seek an occupation that provides easy access to children. Typical occupations are teaching school, working in a day care center, babysitting, coaching, or scout leadership. In June 2012, Jerry Sandusky, an assistant football coach at Pennsylvania State University, was convicted on 45 counts of sexual abuse of 10 adolescent boys beginning in the mid-1990s. Sandusky used his position as a coach and founder of a charity to impress the disadvantaged youths and engage them in illegal and abusive sexual activity.

The psychological features or motivations underlying pedophilic behavior are varied. Antisocial personality disorder and a history of sexual abuse as a child may be considered risk factors for pedophilic disorder. Brain imaging has demonstrated that neurobiologic abnormalities exist in the frontotemporal regions and amygdala and other limbic structures of some perpetrators (Cohen & Galynker, 2009).

The accessibility and anonymity of the Internet have facilitated an increase in child pornography. Child pornography is any visual depiction of sexually explicit conduct involving someone younger than 18 years old. Children are extremely vulnerable and should be protected from sexual abuse and exploitation, which is why there are distinct legal ramifications for child pornography as opposed to adult pornography. Although viewing child pornography by itself is not a risk factor for contact pedophilic disorder, multiple studies have shown a correlation toward sexual aggression and relapse of offending. In other words, not every individual who views child pornography becomes a sex offender, but almost every child molester has viewed child pornography (Burgess et al., 2012).

A study by John Jay College on Catholic clergy who abuse children indicated that most victims were boys 11 through 17 years old (Cartor et al., 2008). The victimization usually occurred in hotel rooms, parish residences, or vacation homes. The offenders were more likely to view sexual involvement as being two-sided and included sexual touching, mutual masturbation, and oral sex. Victims were likely to experience guilt and self-blame for participation in the sexual activity. This was one of the first studies done on a nonforensic population.

The typical perpetrator of child sexual abuse is likely to be a trusted person in the child's immediate network of family or friends. Most child molesters are men who have been engaged in a long-term adult heterosexual relationship with a female relative of the victim (Jenny et al., 1994). A distinction should also be made between a victim's gender and a perpetrator's sexual orientation. Even if the perpetrator abuses a child of the same gender, the perpetrator's identified sexual orientation toward adults may be heterosexual. Patients with pedophilic disorders bear a slight difference from child sexual abusers in that their sexual fixation on children persists over time and is not limited to a crime of opportunity or exploitation.

The goal of treatment is to stop offenses against children rather than to change the paraphilia toward children (Hall, 2007). Treatment includes a combination of various cognitive behavioral methods, antiandrogen medication to decrease sexual desires, and selective serotonin reuptake inhibitors. Specialized groups include victim empathy training, psychoeducation about the illness and medication, coping and social skills training, and relapse prevention.

Incest

Incest is pedophilia with child and adolescent relatives and involves relationships by blood, marriage (stepparents), or live-in partners. Incest is traumatic to children because they are victimized by someone they depend on and trust and are unable to escape their victimization.

The characteristics of the perpetrator of incest are as varied as the characteristics of the pedophile. Families in which incest occurs might be generally disorganized and exhibit disturbed relationships. Although sex is always involved between the perpetrator and the victim, the perpetrator turns to the child for gratification, intimacy, emotional fulfillment, power, and control. The perpetrator's distorted thinking includes denial of any wrongdoing as well as thinking that he or she is teaching the child about sexuality and giving the child pleasure. In contrast to pedophiles, perpetrators of incest do not typically select occupations for access to potential victims because their victims are easily accessible. Treatment is offered to victims and spouses. Some family studies have indicated that victims and spouses do not hate the abuser and do not want others to condemn them (Scheela, 1999).

Exhibitionistic Disorder

The primary characteristic of exhibitionism is sexual pleasure derived from exposing one's genitals to an unsuspecting stranger. The stereotypical offender is a young man in a raincoat who flashes women while walking down the street. No other sexual activity is attempted. The exhibitionist is stimulated by the effect of shocking or frightening the victim.

Fetishistic Disorder

The primary characteristic of fetishism is sexual pleasure derived from inanimate objects. Common fetish objects are bras, underpants, stockings, and shoes. Less common fetish objects include urine-soaked and feces-smeared items. The individual with fetishism often masturbates while holding or rubbing these items. An individual with fetishism may also have a sexual partner wear the fetish object to increase arousal.

Frotteuristic Disorder

The primary characteristic of frotteurism is sexual pleasure derived from touching or rubbing one's genitals against a nonconsenting individual's thighs or buttocks. An individual with frotteurism might also attempt to fondle the person's breasts or genitals. Frotteurism usually occurs in a crowded place in which escape into the crowd is possible.

Sexual Masochism Disorder

The primary characteristic of sexual masochism is that sexual pleasure is derived from physical or mental abuse or humiliation. These urges and behaviors involve being humiliated, beaten, or otherwise made to suffer. Some sexually masochistic individuals enjoy being urinated or defecated on and might pay prostitutes to do so. Hypoxyphilia or erotic asphyxiation is the act of enhancing sexual arousal by strangulation or some other oxygen-depleting activity. Apparently, sexual response is heightened by these activities. People have died in their search for enhanced orgasms.

Sexual Sadism Disorder

The primary characteristic of sexual sadism is sexual pleasure derived from inflicting psychological or physical suffering on another. Partners can be consenting or masochistic. Sadistic behaviors include spanking, whipping, pinching, beating, burning, and restraining. Some sadistic individuals derive great pleasure from torturing or even killing their victims. Sexual sadism affects mostly men and can progress to sadistic rape.

Transvestic Disorder

The primary characteristic of transvestic disorder is sexual arousal derived from cross-dressing or dressing as the opposite sex. This behavior is almost exclusively seen in heterosexual men who continue to identify with the male gender and do not meet criteria for gender dysphoria. The female partner may be unaware of the activity or may help in the selection of clothing (Blanchard, 2010).

Voyeurism

The primary characteristic of voyeurism is sexual arousal derived from observing unsuspecting people who are naked or undressing or who are engaged in sexual activity. The voyeur is commonly referred to as a *peeping Tom*. The voyeur often masturbates during peeping or after returning home.

GENDER DYSPHORIA

Gender dysphoria in adults involves feelings of incongruence between one's assigned or biologic sex and one's gender identity. When conceptualizing this disorder, it is important to understand the distinctions in terminology. *Sex* refers to the biologic indicators of male and female such as sex chromosomes, sex hormones, and genitalia. *Gender* refers to a lived role in public of either a man or a woman. *Gender assignment* denotes the initial assignment as male or female, occurring usually at birth and corresponding to sex. *Gender identity* refers to how an individual identifies himself or herself as male or female and is a facet of social identity.

Gender dysphoria replaces the older term *gender identity disorder* to focus on the distress caused by the incongruence between sex and gender. In adults, this disorder can include the desire to live as the other gender or can involve feelings and reactions of the other gender (see the *DSM-5* Criteria for Gender Dysphoria box). Another characteristic is a preoccupation with getting rid of primary and secondary sexual characteristics. These individuals believe that they were born as the wrong gender, experience unhappiness with their own biologic gender, and might desire hormones and surgery to become the opposite gender.

Sexual reassignment surgery is not undertaken immediately on request. Individuals requesting sexual reassignment surgery must be thoroughly assessed for the presence of other psychiatric disorders that may be the primary dysfunction for which gender incongruence is a symptom. An individual who desires sexual reassignment generally receives psychotherapy for 6 to 12 months. Counseling should help the individual clarify issues surrounding his or her problems and desires. Emotional, medical, surgical, financial, and legal issues are explored, along with the risks involved. Sexual reassignment surgery is not the answer for everyone with gender dissatisfaction (Fee et al., 2003). Some gender dysphoria programs require a written second opinion from another physician or psychologist before proceeding with surgical reassignment. Hormonal treatment and living and relationship changes are slowly made over months while the individual is in therapy. During this time, the individual's attitudes toward sexual reassignment might change, and sexual reassignment surgery might not be chosen. People who do choose sexual reassignment surgery can be helped to live more comfortable and productive lives.

DSM-5 CRITERIA

Gender Dysphoria

Diagnostic Criteria
Gender Dysphoria in Children:

A. A marked incongruence between one's experienced/expressed gender and assigned gender, of at least 6 months' duration, as manifested by at least six of the following (one of which must be Criterion A1):

1. A strong desire to be of the other gender or an insistence that one is the other gender (or some alternative gender different from one's assigned gender).
2. In boys (assigned gender), a strong preference for cross-dressing or simulating female attire; or in girls (assigned gender), a strong preference for wearing only typical masculine clothing and a strong resistance to the wearing of typical feminine clothing.
3. A strong preference for cross-gender roles in make-believe play or fantasy play.
4. A strong preference for the toys, games, or activities stereotypically used or engaged in by the other gender.
5. A strong preference for playmates of the other gender.
6. In boys (assigned gender), a strong rejection of typically masculine toys, games and activities and a strong avoidance of rough-and-tumble play; or in girls (assigned gender), a strong rejection of typically feminine toys, games and activities.

(Continued)

7. A strong dislike of one's sexual anatomy.
8. A strong desire for the primary and/or secondary sex characteristics that match one's experienced gender.
B. The condition is associated with clinically significant distress or impairment in social, school or other important areas of functioning.

Gender Dysphoria in Adolescents and Adults:
A. A marked incongruence between one's experienced/expressed gender and assigned gender, of at least 6 months' duration, as manifested by at least two of the following:
1. A marked incongruence between one's experienced/expressed gender and primary and/or secondary sex characteristics.
2. A strong desire to be rid of one's primary and/or secondary sex characteristics because of a marked incongruence with one's experienced/expressed gender (or in adolescents, a desire to prevent the development of the anticipated secondary sex characteristics).
3. A strong desire for the primary and/or secondary sex characteristics of the other gender.
4. A strong desire to be of the other gender (or some alternative gender different from one's assigned gender).

5. A strong desire to be treated as the other gender (or some alternative gender different from one's assigned gender).
6. A strong conviction that one has the typical feelings and reactions of the other gender (or some alternative gender different from one's assigned gender).
B. The condition is associated with clinically significant distress or impairment in social, occupational, or other important areas of functioning.
Specify if:
With a disorder of sex development (e.g., a congenital adrenogenital disorder such as 255.2 [E25.0] congenital adrenal hyperplasia or 259.50 [E34.50] androgen insensitivity syndrome). Coding note: Code the disorder of sex development as well as gender dysphoria.
Specify if:
Posttransition: The individual has transitioned to full-time living in the desired gender (with or without legalization of gender change) and has undergone (or is preparing to have) at least one cross-sex medical procedure or treatment regimen—namely, regular cross-sex hormone treatment or gender reassignment surgery confirming the desired gender (e.g., penectomy, vaginoplasty in the natal male; mastectomy or phalloplasty in a natal female).

From American Psychiatric Association (2013). *Diagnostic and statistical manual of mental disorders* (5th ed.) (pp. 452-453). Arlington, VA: APA.

PUTTING IT ALL TOGETHER

PSYCHOTHERAPEUTIC MANAGEMENT

Nurse-Patient Relationship

The nurse must have an accepting, empathic, and nonjudgmental attitude if patients are to be comfortable enough to disclose problems with sexuality. This trust comes about only after the nurse has reconciled and accepted his own feelings related to sexuality. Patients might interpret the nurse's discomfort with sexual issues and sexuality as disapproval of them and of their sexual issues and concerns. A private area in which to discuss fears or concerns about sexuality and victimization helps patients disclose and discuss their feelings. The nurse discusses options for dealing with sexual issues and problems. Clarification and education might be needed about sexual functioning, effective communication, and healthy relationships. The nurse might also need to intervene with self-esteem issues, anxiety, and guilt.

Helping patients who are perpetrators deal with physical and emotional dimensions is necessary. Physical dimensions might include anorexia, insomnia, and weight loss. Emotional dimensions might include guilt, helplessness, shame, and relief about getting caught. Setting limits on how much information the patient discloses in a group setting, especially if other group members might be victims of sexual assault, must be discussed.

The nurse is involved in the planning of patients' care regarding the specific issues and problems that are addressed during an inpatient stay versus issues and problems addressed in outpatient treatment. The nurse also collaborates with social workers and chaplains, if patients so choose, about feelings and religious views. The nurse is legally obligated to report suspected and actual sexual abuse of children to police or appropriate agencies. All states have mandatory child abuse reporting statutes. The nurse discusses possible referrals with patients and family members and refers patients to sex therapists, if necessary. Referrals to outpatient treatment programs or therapy groups for specific disorders might be necessary. Individual, group, and family treatment for incest and support groups for perpetrators and victims might be appropriate.

> **? CRITICAL THINKING QUESTION**
>
> 2. What approaches would the nurse use while working with patients with sexual problems?

Psychopharmacology

Patients with other diagnoses are prescribed psychotherapeutic medication for the specific disorders. The nurse assesses all medications for side effects that affect sexual performance or dysfunction.

Men with sexual arousal disorders might choose to be prescribed vardenafil (Levitra), tadalafil (Cialis), or sildenafil (Viagra). Men with paraphilias can be treated with agents to decrease testosterone levels, reducing their sex drive. Antiandrogen medications have been proven to suppress pedophilic urges by diminishing sexual desire and fantasy. They can be taken orally or by intramuscular injection for slow release over several months. Medroxyprogesterone (Provera) and leuprolide acetate (Lupron) inhibit the release of luteinizing hormone by the pituitary gland, which decreases the production of testosterone by the testes (Miller, 2004). Luteinizing hormone–releasing hormone agonists inhibit the production of testosterone or produce a pharmacologic castration and reduce sex drive (Briken, 2002). This medication might become another option in the treatment of paraphilias. In addition to antiandrogens, selective serotonin reuptake inhibitors are used for paraphilias and related disorders. It is unclear if the medication helps by reducing depression and compulsive behavior or sexual functioning (Cohen & Galynker, 2009).

Milieu Management

Patients with sexual disorders and dysfunctions benefit from groups dealing with self-esteem, assertiveness, anger management, social and relationship skills, sex education, and stress management. Referrals might be indicated as mentioned previously. Self-help groups such as Sex Addicts Anonymous can benefit some individuals. A multidimensional treatment plan employing a combination of education and cognitive behavioral and family intervention should be used to reduce recidivism for sexual offenders. It is hoped that longitudinal research studies will eventually help determine treatment plans that are effective in reducing recidivism rates.

CASE STUDY

Bill Wood, 62 years old, has been admitted to the inpatient unit. His wife died 2 years earlier; he has one daughter and three grandchildren. Bill is presently employed but has few friends or hobbies. He visits his daughter and grandchildren approximately once a month. He does not date and does not have any female companions. For the past year, he has noticed an increase in sexual fantasies concerning children. He did not act on the fantasies until a week ago when he was babysitting for his youngest grandchild, 8-year-old Stephanie. He admits to fondling Stephanie's breasts but denies other sexual contact with her. Bill states to the nurse, "I never thought I could be capable of such a horrible thing. I deserve to die. I even thought of killing myself."

◎ CARE PLAN

Name: Bill Wood   *Admission Date: _____*
DSM-5 Diagnosis: Major depression and pedophilia

Assessment	**Areas of strength:** Patient is employed, visits daughter and grandchildren, has remorse for contact with child; first offense.
	Problems: Death of wife, few friends, disturbing sexual fantasies, suicidal ideation.
Diagnoses	Risk for self-directed violence related to guilt and suicidal ideation
	Sexual dysfunction related to lack of significant other, as evidenced by fondling child
	Social isolation related to lack of social support, as evidenced by loneliness
Outcomes	**Short-term goals**
Date met: _____	Patient will state that he no longer has thoughts of suicide.
Date met: _____	Patient will discuss sexual concerns and needs and methods to satisfy these needs.
	Long-term goals
Date met: _____	Patient will contact support groups and senior citizen organizations.
Date met: _____	Patient will attend outpatient appointment for further assessment and treatment of sexual disorder.
Planning and Interventions	**Nurse-patient relationship:** Instruct patient to approach staff when suicidal thoughts occur. Discuss feelings of guilt, remorse, anger, loneliness, and low self-esteem. Discuss the patient's beliefs and values about sexuality with him. Discuss and help the patient to identify sexual concerns, needs, and methods to satisfy needs.
	Psychopharmacology: Fluoxetine (Prozac) 20 mg q morning.
	Milieu management: Groups focusing on self-esteem, stress and anger management, assertiveness training, social skills, and discharge planning.
Evaluation	Patient reports that he is no longer suicidal.
Referrals	Patient will attend senior citizen activities at his church with a friend. Appointment is scheduled at a sexual disorders clinic.

▌STUDY NOTES

1. Sexual dysfunctions might occur as the result of psychological, physiologic, and pharmacologic factors.
2. Paraphilic disorders involve sexual activity with objects, children, and consenting or nonconsenting adults that are socially prohibited, unacceptable, or biologically undesirable.
3. Efforts to achieve sexual pleasure do not give individuals the right to violate the rights of others through coercion and control.
4. Currently, cognitive behavioral techniques and the use of antiandrogen medications are effective treatments for paraphilic disorders.
5. Gender dysphoria in adults involves persistent discomfort with one's biologic gender.
6. The nurse's role in the treatment of sexual disorders is primarily one of referral.

REFERENCES

American Psychiatric Association. (2013a). *Diagnostic and statistical manual of mental disorders* (5th ed.). Arlington, Virginia: APA.

American Psychiatric Association. 2013b. *Highlights of changes from DSM-IV-TR to DSM-5.* Arlington, Virginia: APA.

Blanchard, R. (2010). The DSM diagnostic criteria for transvestic fetishism. *Archives of Sexual Behavior, 39*, 363.

Briken, P. (2002). Pharmacotherapy of paraphilias with luteinizing hormone-releasing hormone agonists. *Archives of General Psychiatry, 59*, 469.

Burgess, A. W., Carretta, C. M., & Burgess, A. G. (2012). Patterns of federal Internet offenders: A pilot study. *Journal of Forensic Nursing, 8*, 112.

Cartor, P., Cimbolic, P., & Tallon, J. (2008). Differentiating pedophilia from ephebophilia in cleric offenders. *Sexual Addiction & Compulsivity, 15*, 311.

Cohen, L. J., & Galynker, I. (2009). Psychopathology and personality traits of pedophiles: Issues for diagnosis and treatment. *The Psychiatric Times, 26*, 6.

Fee, E., Brown, T. M., & Laylor, J. (2003). One size does not fit all in the transgender community. *American Journal of Public Health, 93*, 899.

Hall, R. C. W. (2007). A profile of pedophilia: Definition, characteristics of offenders, recidivism, treatment outcomes, and forensic issues. *Mayo Clinic Proceedings, 82*, 4.

Jenny, C., Roesler, T., & Poyer, K. (1994). Are children at risk for sexual abuse by homosexuals? *Pediatrics, 94*, 41.

McManus, M., et al. (2013). Paraphilias: Definition, diagnosis and treatment. *F 1000 Prime Reports, 5*, 36.

Miller, M. C. (2004). Pedophilia. *The Harvard Mental Health Letter, 20*, 1.

Scheela, R. A. (1999). A nurse's experiences, working with sex offenders. *Journal of Psychosocial Nursing and Mental Health Services, 37*, 25.

Substance-Related Disorders

Gordon I.G. Pugh, Susanne Fogger

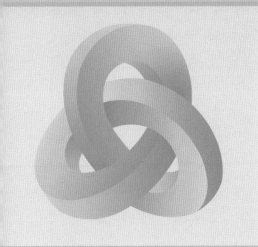

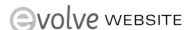

evolve WEBSITE

http://evolve.elsevier.com/Keltner

LEARNING OBJECTIVES

- Recognize the personal and societal toll of misuse of alcohol and other substances.
- Recognize *DSM-5* criteria and terminology for substance use disorders.
- Recognize and describe objective and subjective symptoms of substance use disorders.
- Describe physiologic, emotional, and interpersonal theoretical explanations for the development of substance use disorders.

- Develop a nursing care plan for patients with substance use disorders.
- Understand the contributions of nonmedical interventions in recovery from substance use disorders.
- Understand the impact of substance use disorders on the family.
- Identify evidenced-based websites for additional information and teaching material on substance use disorders.

A single death is a tragedy; a million deaths is a statistic.
Joseph Stalin

An estimated 22,600,000 (8.9 per cent of) Americans aged 12 or older were current illicit drug users.
Substance Abuse and Mental Health Services Administration, 2011

INTRODUCTION

A University of Wisconsin-Milwaukee student "lost his life after celebrating New Year's eve, ... drowned in the Milwaukee River and ... found nearly three months later. Tests showed his blood alcohol level to be 0.22."
Alcohol-Related Student Deaths-Spring 2013
<http://compelledtoact.com/Tragic_listing/Main_list-ing_Spring_2013.htm>

Drug use statistics vary from time to time and from culture to culture. Because of the enormity of these numbers, most people find it difficult to grasp the extent of societal and individual suffering produced by substance use and misuse. Because it is beyond the scope of this text to cover all

addictions in detail, this chapter is an overview of drugs of addiction. The stories about real patients in this chapter represent the many individuals who make up the startling statistics. The effects of drug and alcohol use ripple through our society, touching everyone to some degree and at a staggering cost to the U.S. economy of $559 billion (National Institute on Drug Abuse, 2012).

Humans have used mood-altering substances since at least the beginning of recorded history. Whether using Far Eastern opium, South American cocaine, North American peyote, French wine, prescribed drugs, or a morning cup of Starbuck's coffee, humans consistently find ways to alter their mood. Use of mind-altering substances can lead to many complications and problems. However, mind-altering drugs often provide therapeutic benefit (e.g., pain relief, decreased anxiety), clouding the distinction between therapeutic and abusive use. Table 31-1 outlines the extent of drug use in a given month.

Substance Use as a Brain Disorder

All addicting substances affect the dopamine pathway because dopamine is the common neurotransmitter that is associated with the reinforcing effect of the substance. The substance

TABLE 31-1 NUMBER OF USERS WITHIN THE PREVIOUS 30 DAYS (2009)

SUBSTANCE	CURRENT USERS
Heroin	200,000
Methamphetamine	502,000
Ecstasy	760,000*
Inhalants	600,000
Hallucinogens	1,300,000*
Cocaine/crack	1,600,000
Legal drugs abuse	6,200,000
Marijuana	16,700,000
Cigarette smoking	69,700,000
Alcohol	130,600,000

*The number of users for the hallucinogens also includes the users for ecstasy.
From Substance Abuse and Mental Health Services Administration (2010). *Results from the 2009 national survey on drug use and health: national findings.* <http://www.oas.samhs.gov/NSduh.htm> Accessed September 13, 2013.

TABLE 31-2 12-MONTH PREVALENCE RATE OF MENTAL DISORDERS IN THE UNITED STATES*

DISORDERS	APPROXIMATE PERCENTAGE >17 YEARS OLD (%)* (unless noted for children)	GENDER OVERREPRE-SENTATION
Anxiety disorders	18.1 overall	
Agoraphobia	1.7	Female
Panic disorder	2.4	Female
Panic attacks	11.2	Female
Social anxiety	7	Female
Specific phobia	7-9	Female
Separation anxiety	1.2	Equal
Generalized anxiety disorder	2	Female
Posttraumatic stress disorder	3.4	Female
Obsessive-compulsive disorder	1.2	Equal
Major depression	8.6	Female
Bipolar disorder I and II	1.8	BD I: ~Equal
		BD II: Female
Autism spectrum disorders	1 in children	Male
Disruptive, impulse control, and conduct disorders	8.9 overall	
Conduct disorders*	4 in children	Male
Attention-deficit/hyperactivity disorder*	5 in children; 2.5 in adults	Male
Substance use disorders	8.9 overall	
Alcohol use disorder	8.5 in adults; 2.5 in 12- to 17-year-olds	Male
Drug use disorders	1.4	Male
Schizophrenia	1.1	~Equal

*No one source has all of this information. This information has been derived from the following sources: Kessler, R.C., et al. (2012). Twelve-month and lifetime prevalence and lifetime morbid risk of anxiety and mood disorders in the United States. *International Journal of Methods of Psychiatric Research, 21,* 169; Substance Abuse and Mental Health Services Administration (2009). *Results from the 2008 national survey on drug use and health: national findings.* <http://www.samhsa.gov/data/nsduh/2k8nsduh/2k8Results.htm> Accessed November 13, 2013; American Psychiatric Association (2013). *Diagnostic and statistical manual of mental disorders* (5th ed.). Arlington, Virginia: APA.

directly or indirectly increases dopamine intracellularly in the limbic regions, including the nucleus accumbens. Drug exposure causes dopamine levels to spike much higher and for a longer time than with any natural reward such as food or sex. With repeated use, the brain no longer responds to natural rewards. Exposure to the substance is thought to alter neurons permanently; although an individual may become free of a substance for years, he remains vulnerable to the effects of the substance on reexposure. Substance use disorders must be considered a chronic disease because of this ongoing risk. An old Alcoholics Anonymous (AA) saying that illustrates this concept is to consider the brain like a cucumber—once it has been exposed (to substances) and changed to a pickle, it can never be anything but a pickle—once a pickle, always a pickle.

Adolescents are especially at risk for substance use because the frontal lobe, which regulates decision making and executive function, is not fully developed. Risk taking and impulsive behavior is an aspect of adolescent development that increases the potential for drug use. When substance exposure occurs later in life, it is less likely the individual will have the brain "hijacked" by substances. The adult brain may not experience the same degree of neuroadaptive changes with exposure to substances because the adult brain has a more completed myelination of the frontal lobe region (Cavacuiti, 2011).

As a nurse, you will see patients suffering from the consequences of substance use as part of your work (Table 31-2). You

NORM'S NOTES

Substance use disorders are a big problem in the United States, and the problem does not seem to be getting any better. Whenever you hear or read about someone shot dead in a car somewhere, or three young men gunned down in a low-rent motel, or a mother abandoning her children, it is probably related to drugs. Yes, this is a big problem in our country.

probably know people personally who have substance-related disorders and who have experienced problems associated with substance use; you might suspect that other people you know have substance-related disorders as well. Your ability to recognize the possibility and to suggest appropriate referrals or interventions might save a home, a family, a friendship, or a life. Friends and acquaintances might turn to you as a nurse first when they realize that their substance use has become a problem. We hope that you take the time to study this information carefully and diligently. The road to recovery begins with the initial assessment.

Clinical Example- Back From the Brink of Self Destruction

Robert had an average childhood and made good grades in school. He grew up in a home with both parents and with other siblings. In other words, Robert had a good start in life. His parents were active in the community. In high school, he was particularly talented in sports and was popular among his peers. Robert was, and is, an immensely likable fellow. He began drinking beer when he was 15 years old with his baseball teammates. After graduation from high school with honors, he went to college on a baseball scholarship. In college, he was known to smoke some marijuana, but "never let it get in the way" of his sports or his studies. He was good at hiding his drug use. It would never have occurred to him that he "had a problem," not even later when his self-destruction was blatantly apparent to everyone else in his life. However, Robert has since learned that he suffers from addiction and has learned how to manage his condition.

At first, he stayed out a little too late one night before a big game, and he had a bad game or two because of his slightly decreased performance. Eventually, he was introduced to cocaine, discovered intravenous use (mainlining), lost his promising sports career, was divorced by his wife, stole from people, lied to his family, tried to kill himself, and spent time in prison. While he was incarcerated, he realized how self-destructive his drug use had become, and he vowed to do whatever it would take to become and remain drug-free. He reasoned that he had been willing to do a great many things in his search for dope, so he ought to be willing to exert the same amount of energy in his search to break free from its grip on his life. Robert had been hospitalized for detoxification in the past but "wasn't ready," he says. When he attended a small treatment group at the county jail, he was ready to listen and learn. At that time, he was in his late twenties.

As of this writing, Robert is in his late forties. After he cleared up his legal troubles, he earned his bachelor's degree, found a good career in which he advanced, no longer has legal problems, plays ball in a local community league, is married to a wonderfully supportive spouse, and—most importantly—remains drug-free more than 20 years later. His life is full of love, hope, and happiness. Today, no one would believe the path of self-destruction that he was following at one time. Robert's life did not get back together overnight, however. Undoing most of the damage that his drug use caused took several years. Some of the damage he caused can never be repaired, but he is far better off now than he was before he recognized the extent of the problems caused by his drug use.

Assessment Strategies for Chemical Dependency

As a component of every assessment, the nurse should inquire about the amount and type of alcohol and other drugs (AOD) used by the patient or family. The nurse should always ask about the amount of prescription medication the patient actually takes (not simply the amount prescribed because many people abuse prescription medications as well). The nurse should also question the patient about medical problems associated with AOD use by the patient or family members. Because many substance abusers tend to minimize their level of AOD use (and the consequences of their use), many facilities routinely use blood or urine drug screens to obtain objective information. The importance of this objective data lies in its prevention of AOD minimization. Probably 40% to 60% of AOD users underreport use during their initial interview. Many addicted patients do not readily reveal in an initial interview more than what the nurse can already discover by other means. For example, someone referred to treatment because alcohol use has led to problems with the legal system often does not admit to cocaine or marijuana use until objective testing reveals it. Some patients even deny use of the substance detected. Signs and symptoms raising the index of suspicion of a substance-related disorder might include the following:

- Absenteeism, especially after days off
- Frequent accidents or injuries
- Drowsiness
- Slurred speech
- Inattention to appearance
- Increasing isolation
- Frequent secretive disappearances
- Tremors
- Flushed face
- Watery or reddened eyes
- Appearing spaced out
- Odor of alcohol on the breath or strong mouthwash or breath mint smell
- High number of physical complaints
- Disappearing prescriptions (raiding the medicine cabinet)

The primary defense mechanism of an individual addicted to substances is frequently denial. A person with substance-related disorder does not recognize the destructive nature of AOD use, although it may be obvious to others. Denial prevents the individual from linking his or her problems with AOD use. This inability to see self-destructive behavior and attitudes, to discontinue use despite knowledge of worsening mental and physical condition, or to link life problems with AOD use defines substance use disorders. Figure 31-1 identifies the drug most often used when beginning the use of illicit drugs. Figure 31-2 illustrates the high percentage of AOD users who do not believe they need treatment.

Urinalysis often provides the most objective measure of recent drug use (Table 31-3). Blood and saliva levels can also detect recent use and trigger treatment protocols. Hair toxicology effectively determines long-term patterns of use but costs more than other methods of detection. Hair toxicology

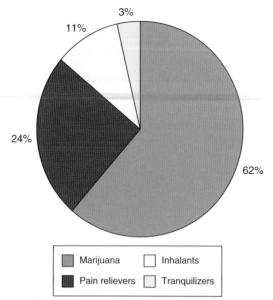

FIG 31-1 Specific drug used when initiating illicit drug use.

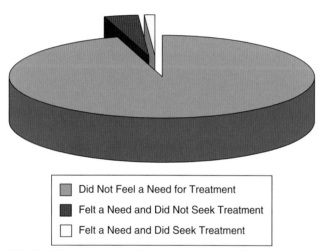

FIG 31-2 Perceived need for treatment and effort to receive treatment.

TABLE 31-3	PERIOD OF TIME AFTER INGESTION THAT DRUGS CAN BE DETECTED IN THE URINE
DRUG	**URINE**
Opioids	1-3 days
Barbiturates	1-7 days
Benzodiazepines	24-36 hr up to 30 days for long-acting agents
Amphetamines	2-3 days
Cocaine	2-3 days occasional use; up to 8 days with heavy use
Marijuana	3-30 days
PCP	7-14 days

PCP, Phencyclidine.
Modified from Standridge, J., Adams, S., & Zotos, A. (2010). Urine drug screening: a valuable office procedure. *American Family Physician, 81,* 635-640.

kits available on the retail market enable parents to test the hair of children if they suspect drug use.

Interview Approaches

Because underreporting can lead to misdiagnosis, it is important for the nurse to approach the patient in a manner that encourages forthrightness. The nurse should be *matter-of-fact* and *nonjudgmental* while eliciting information that might carry with it some feelings of shame. Most nurses are not prepared for the defensiveness that a person with substance-related problems displays, but *genuine concern* for the patient can help overcome this barrier. Because drugs and alcohol have personally affected many nurses, it is important for them to be aware of their own feelings and to avoid projecting any negative attitudes onto the patient.

Gathering accurate information during the interview is a high priority. As a nurse, you might find it difficult to elicit accurate clinical information. Phrases such as "problem with drinking" or "difficulties with drug use" might be more palatable compared with the labels *alcoholic* or *addict*, but these, too, might not elicit the accurate information sought by the nurse. It also might be helpful initially to focus more on legally or culturally accepted substances such as caffeine and nicotine. The patient's consumption should be evaluated in more detail if the initial assessment data identify the patient as being at higher risk for substance-related problems. Using the phrases *problems because of drinking* and *using more than intended* is more accurate and diagnostic, less threatening, and more likely to link patients' AOD use with the problems in their lives. The last-mentioned factor is important both in effective care planning and in providing the patient with positive internal motivation.

Various assessment guides are available to the nurse, including both subjective interview and objective assessment instruments. Early diagnosis of substance-related disorders is often missed because of misdiagnosing or underdiagnosing related to misunderstandings about AOD disorders, inadequate training, or both. Selected instruments are discussed later in this chapter.

Substance use is widespread in North America and demands the attention of psychiatric nurses, both as a singular phenomenon and as a variable in other psychiatric disorders. The degree of individuals with substance use disorders may be underestimated as "in 2012, the use of illicit drugs was more likely among adults age 18 or older with mental illness than it was among adults without mental illness (13.2%)." (Substance Abuse and Mental Health Services Administration, 2013). Patients with both mental illness and substance use disorders are considered to have co-occurring disorders. In the United States, a large percentage of smokers with nicotine dependence have mental disorders. A 2012 Surgeon General's report highlighted health care concerns: "Prevention efforts must focus on both adolescents and young adults because among adults who become daily smokers, nearly all first use of cigarettes occurs by 18 years of age (88%), with 99% of first use by 26 years of age" (U.S. Surgeon General, 2012). Helping young people to avoid use is the mainstay of preventive efforts.

To assess the health condition of a person with problematic substance use effectively, the nurse must understand tools and methods for screening, including how to perform a brief intervention to recognize the patient's readiness for change. Motivational interviewing can help many individuals participate in their health care decisions, with the nurse providing support, encouragement, and education.

Transtheoretical Model

The transtheoretical model developed by Prochaska and DiClemente (1983) is helpful in working with individuals who have substance use issues because it assists the nurse to identify the individual's readiness to change behaviors that may be harmful or in some way interfering with their life plans. Using the model as a guide, the nurse can determine the individual's current stage of change and plan for future opportunities to support or assist the individual's move toward a healthier lifestyle. The nurse assists the individual to examine relevant factors, such as objective data to understand the consequences of their choices. Should behavioral changes be desirable, the nurse helps the individual frame his or her goals and follows up during each visit. Translating laboratory work, individual physical strengths, and other data can be helpful supporting evidence concerning milestones toward change. The stages of change are precontemplation, contemplation, preparation, action, maintenance, and relapse.

Precontemplation: The person is not thinking about change in the foreseeable future. He may not recognize behavior is problematic. He is not interested in changing behavior.

Contemplation: The person recognizes behavior as problematic. Pros and cons of change are starting to be considered.

Preparation: The person intends to take action and may take small steps toward change.

Action: The person makes specific overt modifications to behavior or acquires new healthy behaviors.

Maintenance: The person is able to sustain action and works to prevent relapse to old behaviors.

Relapse: The person recycles from action or maintenance to an earlier stage.

Behavioral changes may not be linear and are considered fluid and in flux. An individual may progress or digress at any time. Each issue should be considered separately because it is the behavioral change of that one issue that is in flux, not the individual. The individual may attend Weight Watchers meetings weekly (action) yet does not want to eliminate alcohol from her diet (precontemplation). To be successful in her weight loss goal, she may have to move to action by decreasing her intake of alcohol.

DSM-5 CRITERIA

for Alcohol Use Disorder

Diagnostic Criteria

A. A problematic pattern of alcohol use leading to clinically significant impairment or distress, as manifested by at least two of the following, occurring within a 12-month period:
1. Alcohol is often taken in larger amounts or over a longer period than was intended.
2. There is a persistent desire or unsuccessful efforts to cut down or control alcohol use.
3. A great deal of time is spent in activities necessary to obtain alcohol, use alcohol, or recover from its effects.
4. Craving, or a strong desire or urge to use alcohol.
5. Recurrent alcohol use resulting in a failure to fulfill major role obligations at work, school, or home.
6. Continued alcohol use despite having persistent or recurrent social or interpersonal problems caused or exacerbated by the effects of alcohol.
7. Important social, occupational, or recreational activities are given up or reduced because of alcohol use.
8. Recurrent alcohol use in situations in which it is physically hazardous.
9. Alcohol use is continued despite knowledge of having a persistent or recurrent physical or psychological problem that is likely to have been caused or exacerbated by alcohol.
10. Tolerance, as defined by either of the following:
    a. A need for markedly increased amounts of alcohol to achieve intoxication or desired effect.
    b. A markedly diminished effect with continued use of the same amount of alcohol.
11. Withdrawal, as manifested by either of the following:
    a. The characteristic withdrawal syndrome for alcohol (refer to Criteria A and B of the criteria set for alcohol withdrawal, pp. 499-500 of *DSM-5*).
    b. Alcohol (or a closely related substance, such as a benzodiazepine) is taken to relieve or avoid withdrawal symptoms.

Specify if:

In early remission: After full criteria for alcohol use disorder were previously met, none of the criteria for alcohol use disorder have been met for at least 3 months but for less than 12 months (with the exception that criterion A4, "Craving, or a strong desire or urge to use alcohol," may be met).

In sustained remission: After full criteria for alcohol use disorder were previously met, none of the criteria for alcohol use disorder have been met at any time during a period of 12 months or longer (with the exception that criterion A4, "Craving, or a strong desire or urge to use alcohol," may be met).

Specify if:

In a controlled environment: This additional specifier is used if the individual is in an environment where access to alcohol is restricted.

From American Psychiatric Association (2013). *Diagnostic and statistical manual of mental disorders* (5th ed.). Arlington, Virginia: APA.

DSM-5 CRITERIA

DSM-5 (American Psychiatric Association, 2013a) contains a common language for the psychiatric health care community and specifies criteria for classifications of substance use disorders, substance intoxication, and substance withdrawal. In addition, substance use severity can be defined as mild, moderate, or severe. Criteria include using longer and more than intended; desiring to cut back but failing when attempted; spending a great deal of time seeking, using, and recovering from use; experiencing cravings for the substance; failing to fulfill role obligations; using despite potential for worsening social or interpersonal problems; giving up important obligations to use; using when it is physically hazardous; and using despite known physical or psychological problems that worsen with use. Additional criteria include tolerance—the need to use more of the substance to obtain the desired effect and not experiencing the same effect if using the same amount as previously. Withdrawal is defined as experiencing withdrawal symptoms when cutting back or stopping use. The individual may use more of the substance or a similar drug to avoid the withdrawal symptoms.

Researchers have defined the use of substances as a problem when the effects of such use interfere with and disrupt family, work, or social relationships. If these areas of a person's life are being adversely affected, the person is viewed as having a problem and as being in need of treatment. Drugs that can be misused fall into several classes: alcohol, barbiturates and other central nervous system (CNS) depressants, opioids, stimulants, nicotine, and hallucinogens (Table 31-4).

ALCOHOL

Alcohol misuse is the primary drug problem in North America and is addressed separately because of the enormity of the problem it poses. The cost to the United States in terms of health problems, lost work hours, family disruption and disintegration, and criminal activity has been estimated at more than $223 billion annually (Gordis, 2000; Rehm et al., 2009). More than 52.1% of Americans older than 12 years of age drink alcohol, 23% engage in binge drinking, and approximately 6.5% drink heavily (defined as five or more drinks per sitting five or more times per month) (Substance Abuse and Mental Health Services Administration, 2013). Most binge and heavy drinkers (~75%) were employed. An estimated 6.8% of the adult population in the United States exhibits symptoms of alcohol use disorder. Alcoholism ranks as one of the leading causes of death and disability in the United States (Kessler et al., 2005). Alcoholics have a premature death rate two to four times higher than nonalcoholic individuals that may be related to increased cardiovascular and cancer risks.

Etiology

Psychodynamic Theories

Many older psychological theories have attempted to explain substance dependence. Alcohol-dependent individuals have often been viewed as individuals who easily succumb to the escape that alcohol provides. More recent theories have described people likely to become dependent on alcohol as more fearful and with greater feelings of inferiority compared with social drinkers. Over time, the search for an "alcoholic personality" has given way to a multivariate model that incorporates the biopsychosocial components of addiction. Current researchers believe that many of the stereotypical characteristics found in alcohol-dependent individuals (e.g., dependency, low self-esteem, passivity, introversion) are the result of and not the cause of substance dependence. Psychodynamically oriented treatment tends to emphasize behavioral management techniques and rejects the disease model of substance use disorders.

Biologic Theories

Heredity as an etiology has been studied for many years and continues to provide insight into understanding the genesis of alcoholism. Genetic predisposition is considered to be the most significant piece of information in identifying alcoholism (Spanagel, 2009), with children of alcoholics 4 to 10 times more likely to become alcoholics themselves (Mayfield et al., 2008). Genetic material can protect against substance use. Individuals who inherit alterations in alcohol dehydrogenase are protected against alcoholism; however, individuals with a genetic alteration in gamma aminobutyric acid (GABA) type A are predisposed to alcoholism (Cavacuiti, 2011). Although studies have indicated different degrees of effect, hereditary explanations at least provide a satisfactory basis for understanding a person's vulnerability to alcohol dependency. However, predisposition suggests neither fatalism nor determinism. For example, even patients who are genetically predisposed to certain types of cancer can take steps to minimize their risk. Recognizing their familial predisposition to alcoholism or addiction, individuals can avoid the use of alcohol and drugs.

Pharmacokinetics of Alcohol

Absorption

Alcohol is a lipid that is highly water-soluble. Alcohol is absorbed partially from the stomach (20%) but mostly from the small intestine (80%). If a person with an empty stomach ingests alcohol, 50% is in the bloodstream within 15 minutes, and peak levels are reached in 40 to 60 minutes (Colyar, 2003). The form of alcohol consumed affects the rate of absorption. Alcohol in beer and wine is absorbed more slowly compared with alcohol in liquor. This characteristic might be a result, in part, of dilution; beer contains 4% ethanol; wine, 12% ethanol; and whiskey, 40% to 50% ethanol. However, dilution of the alcohol in its beverage medium cannot completely account for slower absorption. Food also slows alcohol absorption.

Distribution

Ethanol is distributed equally in all body tissue according to water content. Larger individuals (who have greater amounts

TABLE 31-4   DRUG INFORMATION

CLASS	EXAMPLES OR OTHER NAMES	WITHDRAWAL SYNDROME	WITHDRAWAL TREATMENT	PSYCHIATRIC SYMPTOMS DURING CHRONIC USE	OVERDOSE FATAL?*	UNASSISTED WITHDRAWAL FATAL?*	OVERDOSE SYMPTOMS
CNS depressants	Barbiturates; other depressants	Tremors, sweats, autonomic irritability, seizures, anxiety, irritability, hallucinations, death*	Tapering doses of long-acting benzodiazepine, barbiturates	Mood disorder, depression, psychosis, dementia	Yes*	Yes*	Shallow respirations, clammy skin, dilated pupils, weak and rapid pulse, coma, death
Opioids	Demerol, heroin, morphine, opium, codeine, OxyContin	Lacrimation, runny nose, diaphoresis, chills, muscle aches, n/v, diarrhea, leg spasm, goose bumps	Taper of methadone or buprenorphine, clonidine, supportive medications	Psychosis, mood disorder	Yes	No	Respiratory depression, pulmonary edema, pinpoint pupils, seizures, coma, death
Cannabinoids	Marijuana, hash	Craving, irritability		Psychosis, paranoia	No	No	Hallucinations, paranoia, insomnia, hyperactive
Cocaine	Crack, coke, snow	Anhedonia, craving, irritability, fatigue, mood disorder, anxiety	Dopamine agonists, catecholamine precursors	Psychosis	Yes	No	Delirium, psychosis, violence, tachycardia, hypertension, coma, hyperreflexia, myocardial infarction
Methamphetamine	Oral: speed, meth; smokable: ice, crystal, crank	Dsyphoria, fatigue, insomnia	Supportive	Psychosis, mood disorder, anxiety disorder	Yes	No	Delirium, psychosis, violence, tachycardia, hypertension, coma, hyperreflexia
Inhalants	Gasoline, Freon, paint, and others	Mouth ulcers, gastrointestinal problems, anorexia, confusion, headache	Supportive	Psychosis, panic, memory loss	Yes	No	Seizures, coma
Hallucinogens	LSD, psilocybin, PCP	None specific	Supportive	Psychosis, panic	No	No	Seizures, panic, depression

*These are generalizations that are typically true.
CNS, Central nervous system; *LSD,* lysergic acid diethylamide; *n/v,* nausea and vomiting; *PCP,* phencyclidine.

of body water) can ingest more alcohol than smaller people, who have less body water. Because muscle contains more water than fat tissue, men tend to have lower blood alcohol levels than women, even when weight is controlled. Alcohol affects the cerebrum and cerebellum before it affects the spinal cord and the vital centers because the cerebrum and cerebellum contain more water.

Metabolism

Although the rate of absorption largely determines how quickly a person becomes intoxicated, a person's metabolic rate largely determines how long alcohol affects the body. A healthy body can metabolize 15 mL of alcohol per hour, or roughly the alcohol content in a 1-oz. shot of whiskey, 12-oz. can of beer, or 4-oz. glass of wine. Individuals who drink alcohol constantly over a number of years have increased hepatic drug-metabolizing enzymes that hasten alcohol metabolism (metabolic tolerance [pharmacokinetic tolerance]). Hot coffee, sweating it out, and other home remedies do not increase alcohol metabolism, and they do not hasten the sobering-up process. Attempts by scientists to develop a pill to prevent or decrease intoxication have been unsuccessful. In late-stage alcoholism, tolerance decreases because the abused liver can no longer metabolize the alcohol adequately.

The chemical name for alcohol is *ethanol* (CH_3CH_2OH). Alcohol is primarily metabolized in the liver, but 10% is excreted unchanged in the breath, sweat, and urine (Colyar, 2003). The oxidation process can be described chemically as follows:

Alcohol is converted to **acetaldehyde** *(a toxic molecule),* which is converted to **acetic acid** *(nontoxic).*

At each step of the metabolic process, an enzyme breaks down the chemical and speeds up the reaction. *Alcohol dehydrogenase* breaks down alcohol (CH_3CH_2OH) to acetaldehyde (CH_3CHO) and H_2. The H_2 molecule causes the liver to bypass normal energy sources (H_2 from fat) and to use the H_2 from alcohol. Fat accumulates because it is not being used as a primary energy source; this leads to fatty liver, hyperlipemia, hepatitis, and, ultimately, cirrhosis. Acetaldehyde is *toxic* to the body; it compromises normal cell function in the liver. If the metabolism of acetaldehyde is impaired, acetaldehyde accumulates in the liver, causing cell death and necrosis. Acetaldehyde also interferes with vitamin activation. *Aldehyde dehydrogenase* breaks down acetaldehyde to acetic acid (CH_3COOH), which is a harmless substance. When enzymatic action on acetaldehyde is blocked by the aldehyde dehydrogenase blocker disulfiram (Antabuse), acetaldehyde accumulates, causing severe sickness.

Research confirms the suspicion that women become intoxicated more easily than men, even when studies are controlled for size differences. Frezza and colleagues (1990) discovered that the gastrointestinal tissue of women and of alcohol-dependent men contains little alcohol dehydrogenase. The alcohol dehydrogenase in the gastrointestinal tissue of men who are not dependent on alcohol oxidizes a significant amount of CH_3CH_2OH in the gut before it enters the bloodstream. The inability of women's bodies to undergo this first-pass metabolism accounts for their enhanced vulnerability to alcohol. For example, a 140 lb male drinks two drinks in one hour and his blood alcohol level is 0.038. A 140 lb female drinks two drinks in one hour and her blood alcohol level is 0.048. In addition, women's alcohol levels are affected by other issues. "Research suggests that menstrual cycle and the use of any medications that affects the liver (because of the hormones) may intensify a woman's response to alcohol. Women have been shown to develop their highest blood alcohol concentrations immediately before menstruation and the lowest on the first day of menstruation" (Office of Alcohol and Drug Education, 2014). Another enzyme system, cytochrome P-450 2E1 enzyme, breaks down some alcohol. This metabolic pathway becomes more important after chronic heavy alcohol consumption because chronic drinking induces the synthesis of this enzyme (Lieber, 2003). An important adverse effect can develop when acetaminophen is taken after chronic drinking. Because cytochrome P-450 2E1 metabolizes acetaminophen and alcohol creates more cytochrome P-450 2E1, more acetaminophen is broken down. The first metabolite of acetaminophen is very toxic and, in some cases, cannot be metabolized further to a nontoxic molecule before liver damage occurs.

Blood Alcohol Levels

Blood alcohol levels accurately indicate the amount of ethanol to which the brain is exposed. Behavioral and physiologic effects are predictable for most drinkers. For example, at a 0.05% blood alcohol level, most individuals are predictably feeling good and experience disinhibition (i.e., they might do and say things they would typically just think or think about doing). The following box outlines the typical responses for a given blood alcohol level.

Tolerance to Alcohol

Tolerance to alcohol is probably related to elevated hepatic enzyme levels (pharmacokinetic tolerance) and to cellular

CLINICAL EFFECTS OF ALCOHOL

BLOOD ALCOHOL LEVEL (%)	PHYSIOLOGIC EFFECT
0.05	Euphoria, decreased inhibitions
0.10-0.15	Labile mood, talkative, impaired judgment
0.15-0.20	Decreased motor skills, slurred speech, double vision
0.25	Altered perceptions
0.30	Altered equilibrium
0.34	Apathy, inertia
0.40	Stupor, coma
0.40-0.50	Severe respiratory depression, death

adaptation (pharmacodynamic tolerance). At the point at which the normal drinker might be noticeably drunk after 10 to 12 drinks, the long-term drinker with pharmacodynamic tolerance might seem unaffected by drinking the same amount. However, tolerance to the respiratory depressing effects of alcohol does not develop appreciably. Blood levels just slightly higher than the levels required to get a buzz have resulted in the deaths of long-term, pharmacodynamically tolerant drinkers.

Physiologic Effects

Alcohol targets several neurotransmitter receptors: glutamate, N-methyl-D-aspartate (NMDA), GABA, 5-hydroxytryptamine 3, and nicotinic acetylcholine receptors. Each of these receptors influences dopamine, the "pleasure" neurotransmitter. Alcohol activates the pleasure pathway of the brain. A secondary effect—what Spanagel (2009) called a "second hit"—occurs when alcohol modulates opioids and endocannabinoids. These plus dopamine are thought to be responsible for the "rewarding" effect of alcohol (Spanagel, 2009).

People generally begin consuming alcohol because it causes a reaction they desire. Disinhibition, impaired judgment, and fuzzy thinking are initial responses to alcohol ingestion. These signs represent cerebral intoxication. In many situations, this mental relaxation is pleasant. Alcohol also depresses psychomotor activity. Alcohol has been described as a social lubricant because it relaxes self-imposed barriers that inhibit sociability. Anxiety and tension are relieved, usually for several hours after a drink is taken. Eventually, at least for an alcoholic, drinking becomes defensive; that is, an alcoholic often drinks to avoid the effects of many years of drinking. For example, when the anxiety-reducing effect wears off, more tension and anxiety are produced, and the drinker must consume more alcohol to regain the anxiety-free state. Many people with severe alcohol use disorder, even after drinking all they can hold, are unable to quell the rebound psychomotor upheaval caused by years of alcohol-related CNS irritation. Many individuals who seek treatment for alcohol dependence have anxiety or depression directly related to their substance use.

Central Nervous System Effects

The adverse effects of alcohol can be categorized as central or peripheral. CNS effects are related to sedation and toxicity. As the vital centers become affected, a slowed, stuporous to unconscious mental state develops. Large amounts of alcohol can cause sleep, coma, deep anesthesia, or death. Other common symptoms of intoxication include slurred speech, short retention span, loud talk, and memory deficits. "Blackout" refers to a period during which the drinker functions socially but afterward the drinker has no memory. Large amounts of alcohol prevent the hippocampus from recording short-term memory, and "blackout" occurs. The individual has no recall of an event despite appearing as if they were functioning normally.

Even when a nutritious diet is maintained, brain damage occurs with drinking. Neuronal death is probably related to changes in NMDA receptor sensitivity over time (as opposed to the reinforcing effect of NMDA modulation mentioned previously), heightening the excitotoxicity potential of glutamate (Harper & Matsumoto, 2005). Brain changes include reduced brain weight, frontocortical gray matter loss, atrophy, reductions in white matter, hippocampal changes, hypothalamic neuronal loss, and cerebellar neuronal loss (Harper & Matsumoto, 2005; Quertemont et al., 2005). Acetaldehyde, the first metabolic product, also contributes to the effects of alcohol (Quertemont et al., 2005).

Increased psychomotor activity as a consequence of alcohol is called *alcohol withdrawal syndrome.* Sedation is the predominant effect of alcohol, but as sedation wears off, psychomotor activity increases. This state is referred to as a *rebound phenomenon.* As the CNS becomes more irritated, a normal drinker feels sick and irritable (a hangover) but lives through it, perhaps vowing never to go through this again. Heavy drinkers and alcoholics have to drink again to sedate the psychomotor system. Eventually, a person has to drink larger amounts to feel normal. A few drinkers reach the point at which they cannot drink enough alcohol, and alcoholic tremors, sweating, palpitations, and agitation occur. Although these symptoms usually occur when alcohol ingestion has stopped or been reduced, CNS irritability of withdrawal may begin when the blood alcohol level decreases; sometimes drinkers still may be legally intoxicated but in withdrawal. Blood pressure and pulse may spike in response to the CNS rebound (Table 31-5).

Alcohol induced psychotic disorder (formerly referred to as alcoholic hallucinosis) may manifest as short-lived delusions or hallucinations. This phenomenon that alcohol-dependent people experience may begin 48 hours or so after drinking has stopped. Most hallucinations are auditory and may be considered rare and should resolve within one week. Frightening voices or sounds are heard, usually within the context of a clear sensorium.

The ultimate level of CNS irritability is delirium tremens (DTs). In DTs, the body not only invents sensory input but also has extreme motor agitation. Hallucinations become visual (e.g., the proverbial pink elephants), and the drinker is tremulous and terrified. Tonic-clonic seizures (grand mal seizures) are associated with a high risk for aspiration or death.

Wernicke-Korsakoff syndrome is a mental disorder characterized by amnesia, clouding of consciousness, may have confabulation (falsification of memory) and memory loss, and peripheral neuropathy. This disorder results from the poor nutrition of the alcoholic (specifically, inadequate amounts of thiamine and niacin in the diet) and from the neurotoxic nature of alcohol. Thiamine is given as an intramuscular injection as a standard protocol for alcohol detoxification to halt the progression.

Peripheral Nervous System Effects

Peripheral nervous system (PNS) effects are varied and cause many problems. For a complete discussion of these various processes, the reader is directed to a medical-surgical textbook. Cirrhosis and peripheral neuritis are the physical health problems most commonly associated with alcohol. As liver function becomes impaired in the alcohol-dependent person, he is less able to tolerate alcohol. The drinker who once boasted of drinking exploits becomes drunk after only a few drinks. Physical consequences of cirrhosis include obstructed blood flow (which leads to portal hypertension, ascites, and possibly esophageal varices), decreased liver cell function, low serum albumin levels, high ammonia and high bilirubin serum levels, and clotting problems. Peripheral neuritis causes numbness and subsequent injury in the legs and changes in gait.

Alcohol is also an irritant; it burns the mouth and throat and prompts the stomach to secrete more hydrochloric acid. Gastric ulcers develop and are worsened by alcohol. Alcoholics can experience ulcers, gastritis, bleeding, and hemorrhage in the stomach. Ulcers can eventually perforate, creating a life-threatening situation. In addition, chronic alcohol use increases the risk of oral and stomach cancers (Cavacuiti, 2011).

The pancreas is affected by alcohol in many ways. Pancreatitis and diabetes are common consequences of alcoholism. A malabsorption syndrome is caused by irritation of the intestinal lining. This condition seems to affect B vitamins generally and to lead to a deficiency of vitamin B_1 (thiamine) in particular. Thiamine deficiency contributes to peripheral neuritis. Alcohol also has a direct effect on muscle tissue, a condition known as *alcoholic myopathy*. Other organs affected by alcohol include the eyes (loss of peripheral and night vision), the heart (hypertension, enlarged left ventricle), and reproductive organs. As a depressant, alcohol can cause impotence. Prolonged drinking shrinks the testicles and decreases testosterone. Sexual potency is compromised further by a failing liver that is unable to detoxify female hormones, increasing the level of estrogen and adding to sexual decline in a male drinker. As many men have experienced, alcohol can increase interest in sex but can lead to decreased sexual performance.

TABLE 31-5 COURSES OF WITHDRAWAL FROM ADDICTIVE DRUGS

DRUGS	LENGTH OF ACUTE DETOXIFICATION	COMMON DETOXIFICATION AGENTS	WITHDRAWAL SIGNS AND SYMPTOMS
CNS Depressants			
Alcohol	3-5 days	Librium, Serax, Valium, Vistaril, alcohol	Anxiety, sweats, tremors, flushed face, irritability, sleeplessness, confusion, seizures, delirium
Valium	Slow drug taper, up to 2 weeks	Librium, Valium	
Phenobarbital	Slow drug taper, 2-4 weeks	Librium, phenobarbital	
Opioids			
Heroin	3-5 days	Methadone, buprenorphine, other tapering opioid, or nonopioid withdrawal regimen	Yawning, dilated pupils, gooseflesh, vomiting, diarrhea, runny nose and eyes, sleeplessness, anxiety, irritability, elevated blood pressure and pulse, craving for narcotics
Morphine	3-5 days		
Demerol	3-5 days		
Methadone	2 weeks		
Stimulants			
Amphetamines	3-5 days	Drug intervention usually not required	General fatigue, apathy, depression, drowsiness, irritability, paranoia, suicidal ideation
Cocaine	3-5 days		
Hallucinogen			
Marijuana	2-3 days (metabolites remain in the body up to 2 weeks)	Drug intervention usually not required	Few signs of withdrawal, craving for marijuana, general anxiety and restlessness

CNS, Central nervous system.
From Mueller LA and Ketcham K (1987): Recovering: how to get and stay sober, New York, Bantam Books.

Clinical Example- AA Saved His Life

Anthony is a 36-year-old man with alcohol use disorder so severe that he has physiologic dependence. He also uses other substances. He has a long history of presentations at the emergency department for suicidal ideations. Alcohol and other drugs are always found in his system. He presents at a local treatment facility, saying, "I just can't keep it up any more. I've been drinking for 23 years and my life is falling apart. Everyone I know hates me. I can't keep a job. No one trusts me. I have to have some help." First, Anthony needed detoxification. He then went through a 28-day treatment program. He attended AA five times each week and had a sponsor, someone in whom he could confide and from whom he could "learn to live life on life's terms." He also attended an aftercare treatment group three times a week to focus on dealing with his shame. After 108 days of sobriety, Anthony began to think that he was cured and no longer needed his sobriety support system. He drank again. Just before he was pulled over for driving under the influence, he managed to throw away the cocaine he had just bought.

The consequences of his past lifestyle have begun to catch up with him 5 months later. He is considered a habitual offender and has been offered 20 years in prison by the district attorney. After getting the alcohol out of his system and reconnecting with AA, Anthony is now prepared to go to prison if necessary, rather than trying to run from his obligations. The AA program teaches responsibility for one's actions and surrender of self-will to one's "higher power." "I did it. I don't want to go to prison, but if that's what God has in mind for me because of my foolish decisions, then so be it. Might be there's somebody out there who needs to hear my story. I can share my experience, strength, and hope, and let them know that God is a way maker." These attitudes of surrender of self-will to one's "higher power" are characteristic of 12-step programs and are considered essential to recovery.

Nursing Issues

Overdose

People die as a result of overdoses of alcohol because it depresses the CNS. Vital centers become anesthetized, compromising breathing and heart rate and leading to a comatose state or death. People consistently underestimate the potency of alcohol, and deaths have occurred simply because individuals have consumed too much. Almost every year, newspapers report deaths of college students by alcohol poisoning (see earlier in the chapter). Although alcohol alone can kill, most overdose-related deaths are the result of combining alcohol with other CNS depressants.

Interactions

Alcohol taken with other CNS depressants causes profound CNS depression and can lead to death. For instance, diazepam, which is not lethal when taken alone, has led to death when combined with alcohol. Alcohol should be avoided when a person is taking barbiturates, antipsychotic drugs, antidepressants, benzodiazepines, and other sedatives.

Use by Older Adults

Older adult alcoholics can be roughly divided into the following two groups:

1. Lifelong users
2. Late-onset users responding to stress

Lifelong users tend to have increased physical, cognitive, and emotional problems associated with their drinking. Late-onset alcoholics include individuals who, as they grow older, tend to cope with the many and persistent losses of later life by drinking. If not effectively treated, these individuals can deteriorate rapidly. However, late-onset alcoholics have a robust response when treated.

Alcohol use in older adults is underreported, frequently unrecognized, and rarely treated. As the population of older adults has grown, so have substance-related problems in older adults. People with impaired liver function do not metabolize alcohol efficiently and can have a low tolerance for alcohol. Decreased liver function is a product of aging, and consequently older individuals cannot drink much alcohol without becoming inebriated, confused, and sedated. The nurse should be particularly watchful for combinations of alcohol with other CNS depressants among patients in this age group.

Withdrawal and Detoxification

Withdrawal from alcohol can be painful, scary, and lethal. As a person abstains from alcohol, he begins to experience CNS irritation caused by alcohol: tremulousness, nervousness, anxiety, anorexia, nausea and vomiting, insomnia and other sleep disturbances, rapid pulse, high blood pressure, profuse perspiration, diarrhea, fever, unsteady gait, difficulty concentrating, exaggerated startle reflex, and a craving for

CASE STUDY

Evan Franklin, a 28-year-old man, was brought to treatment by his wife after his third DUI offense in which he ran off the road and into a neighbor's mailbox. He has had a history of alcohol and drug use since age 14. Although neither of his parents drank, his grandfather died of cirrhosis of the liver and bleeding esophageal varices.

Evan has been in counseling twice before in an effort to salvage his previous marriage. After the breakup of the marriage, he lost his business and became extremely depressed. When Evan drank, he became belligerent and, at one point, threatened his ex-wife and child, forcing her to file for sole custody of their son. During this period, he also began gambling in an effort to make quick money.

Evan says that he is willing to enter treatment at this time so that he does not lose his wife and because he fears the men to whom he owes gambling debts. He knows that he will be safe in the hospital until he can figure out what to do. He does not believe that he has a problem with alcohol, drugs, or gambling and attributes his misfortunes to the ill will of others. He denies suicidal ideation at this time. Blood alcohol level on admission was 0.02%.

His current lifestyle involves hunting and doing things with his wife and two stepchildren, Ann, 4, and Steve, 6. He misses his 2-year-old son, who lives with his ex-wife.

◎ **CARE PLAN**

Name: Evan Franklin   *Admission Date:* _____

DSM-5 Diagnosis: Alcohol use disorder, severe (or alcoholism)

Assessment	**Areas of strength:** Patient has no medical problems and denies suicidal ideation, has been in counseling twice previously, and enjoys hunting and doing things with his family.
	Problems: Has a family history of chemical dependency and long-term use of alcohol and drugs. Denies that alcohol is a problem in his life despite family and occupational problems.
Diagnoses	Ineffective individual coping related to alcohol abuse as evidenced by legal and financial problems
	Ineffective family coping; disabled related to alcohol abuse, as evidenced by potential marriage separation and financial difficulties
Outcomes	**Short-term goals**
Date met: _____	Patient will state that his marital and occupational problems are the result of drinking.
	Long-term goals
Date met: _____	Patient will remain chemical-free on monthly testing, which will be assessed through urine testing by his probation officer.
Planning and Interventions	**Nurse-patient relationship:** Recognize the patient's initial need to use denial; discuss the natural consequences of his drinking and the need for total abstinence; educate regarding the diagnosis of alcoholism, offering hope for long-term recovery; encourage attendance at AA meetings.
	Psychopharmacology: No caffeine or sugar; multivitamin daily.
	Milieu management: Family treatment; encourage activities of daily living.
Evaluation	According to probation officer, E.F. is sober after 1 month.
Referrals	Refer to AA and make appointment with substance treatment counselor.

alcohol or other drugs. As the withdrawal symptoms become increasingly pronounced, a few individuals can experience hallucinations.

The level of supervision needed depends on the severity of alcoholism. Mild dependence can be handled on an outpatient basis. Because of the misery and risk of death associated with unattended withdrawal, more severe alcoholics have medical supervision of some sort. Drugs that have a cross-dependence with alcohol—that is, other CNS depressants—can be used to diminish symptoms of withdrawal.

ILLICIT DRUGS

There are three categories of illicit drug use: depressants, stimulants, and hallucinogens. Each of these categories has distinct subgroups. Not all drugs are described in this section, but rather a representation of each class is provided to illustrate the drug effect.

DEPRESSANTS

BARBITURATES

Barbiturates depress the CNS. Barbiturates were first used medicinally as sedatives in the last half of the nineteenth century. In 1950, researchers confirmed that barbiturates could produce physical dependence. CNS depressants decrease the awareness of and response to sensory stimuli. These medications are effective for seizure disorders, can decrease pain related to severe headaches, and are still prescribed today.

Withdrawal and Detoxification

Symptoms of withdrawal from barbiturates are severe and can cause death. Symptoms usually begin 8 to 12 hours after the last dose. Because barbiturates depress the CNS, a rebound effect can occur when a person stops taking them. Minor withdrawal symptoms include anxiety, muscle twitching, tremor, progressive weakness, dizziness, distorted visual perception, nausea and vomiting, insomnia, and orthostatic hypotension. More serious withdrawal symptoms include convulsions and delirium. Untreated withdrawal symptoms might not decline in intensity for about 1 week (Lehne, 2007). Detoxification requires a cautious and gradual reduction of these drugs.

BENZODIAZEPINES

Benzodiazepines have many legitimate uses and are reviewed in an earlier chapter (Chapter 17). However, one benzodiazepine, flunitrazepam (Rohypnol; also known as *roofies, rophies, roche, roaches,* and *ruffies*), is known primarily for its abuse potential (Taylor & Donoghue, 2001). Because of its sedative and amnesic effects, flunitrazepam as Rohypnol has been used for date rape. Until more recently, it was manufactured as a colorless, odorless, and tasteless substance that could be mixed with liquids. Sexual predators were able to slip it easily into the beverage of an unsuspecting woman and then perpetrate date rape. This drug is not available legally in the United States.

SUMMARY OF HOW ABUSED DRUGS WORK

ABUSED SUBSTANCE	MECHANISM OF ACTION
Barbiturates	Increase effect of GABA
Opioids	Mimic endogenous neurotransmitters by stimulating opioid receptors; increase release of dopamine in the nucleus accumbens
Cocaine	Decreases reuptake of dopamine
Amphetamines	Increase release of norepinephrine; enhance dopamine release; block reuptake of dopamine, and retard dopamine reuptake
Methamphetamine	Blocks breakdown of dopamine, enhances release, and blocks its reuptake
Ecstasy	Increases release of serotonin; increases release of dopamine
Marijuana	Stimulates dopamine pathways in the nucleus accumbens
LSD	Binds tightly to 5-HT$_{2A}$ receptors causing a psychedelic effect

GABA, Gamma-aminobutyric acid; *5-HT$_{2A}$,* 5-hydroxytryptamine 2A; *LSD,* lysergic acid diethylamide.

INHALANTS

Inhalants are absorbed by the transpulmonary route nasally or orally through inhaling the gaseous product. They are commonly used because they are cheap, readily available, and typically legal. Examples include airplane glue, gasoline, rubber cement, polyvinylchloride cement, hair spray, air freshener, spot remover, polish remover, paint remover, white out, keyboard cleaner, and lighter fluid. Most users are male with gasoline as the most common inhalant. Inhalants usually depress the CNS and increase hilarity; they can also cause excitability. Inhalants are particularly dangerous because the amount inhaled cannot be controlled. Deaths from asphyxiation, suffocation, and choking (e.g., on vomit) have been reported. Inhalants cross the blood-brain barrier quickly. Common side effects include mouth ulcers, gastrointestinal problems, anorexia, confusion, headache, and ataxia. Some inhalants are highly lipid-soluble to the extent that they become sequestered in fatty tissues, having a prolonged effect. Brain damage has been reported with inhalant use, including frontal lobe, cerebellar, and hippocampal damage, leading to diminished problem solving, ataxic gait, and memory dysfunction. Inhalants can be breathed in by sniffing fumes from a container, by bagging (inhaling fumes from a paper bag), and by huffing (inhaling fumes from an inhalant-soaked rag stuffed in the mouth). Signs of use include rash around the nose and mouth and residue on the face and clothing.

OPIOIDS (NARCOTICS)

Opioids include opium, morphine, codeine, heroin, hydromorphone (Dilaudid), meperidine (Demerol), methadone (Dolophine), and others. The illicit use of legal prescription medications has increased substantially in the past 10 years. Opioids can be swallowed, smoked, snorted, injected into soft tissue (skin popping), and mainlined (intravenous injection). The use of heroin is anticipated to increase as the prescribing of opioids has become more restrictive. Opioid dependent individuals are projected to switch to the cheaper and easier to access heroin.

Clinical Example- Booze, MJ, and Painkillers

Sam Jones is a 32-year-old maintenance man. He has a history of drinking and using marijuana since junior high. He began showing a strong preference for opioids after a visit to the dentist to have a tooth extracted. Since that visit, Sam has had several other teeth extracted and has been to the emergency department several times for various situations requiring treatment for one type of intense pain or another. Sam has lost several jobs because of suspected stealing. Actually, he was only trying to get people's prescriptions that they weren't using anyway, and he "would never steal from people." Sam recently started injecting drugs and became obviously impaired quickly. When he was found wandering around the apartment complex with slurred speech and confused thinking, his boss fired him. He left angrily and had a motorcycle accident in which he almost lost his life. He was taken to the trauma unit of the medical center where he began to exhibit narcotic withdrawal the following day. Sam's injuries were so severe that he was "sobered" into agreeing to be evaluated for treatment in the substance abuse treatment program of the medical center. Sam has a long way to go to recover successfully, but exposing him to treatment will at least help him learn more about another way of life, even if he is not ready to participate fully in recovery right now.

Physiologic Effects

Opioids relieve pain by increasing the pain threshold and by reducing anxiety and fear. These drugs accomplish this by stimulating opioid receptor sites in the brain. The naturally occurring neurotransmitters, the endorphins, produce various responses, including being able to mediate pain and regulate mood by activating opioid receptors. The opioids are endorphin agonists. Users are attracted by the drug's effect on mood (a feeling of euphoria) and frequently refer to the euphoric mood created by morphine and heroin as being better than sex. Intravenous heroin delivers a rush (lasting < 1 minute) described as similar to a sexual orgasm. In addition to the euphoria, an overall CNS depression occurs. Drowsiness and sleep are common effects.

Heroin has a higher abuse potential compared with morphine and other opioids because it more readily passes the blood-brain barrier. When heroin enters the brain, its chemical structure is changed to that of morphine, so it becomes trapped in the brain, causing a more sustained high. CNS effects of opioids include respiratory depression related to decreased sensitivity to carbon dioxide stimulation by the medullary center for respiration. Respiratory depression is the primary cause of death when death occurs as a result of opioid use. PNS effects include constipation; decreased gastric, biliary, and pancreatic secretions; urinary retention; hypotension; and reduced pupil size. Pinpoint pupils (miosis) are a sign of opioid overdose. Another opioid, meperidine, is typically the drug of choice for physicians and nurses. Readily available in the health care setting, this drug produces less pupil constriction (hard to detect), is effective if taken orally, and causes less constipation than other opioids (Lehne, 2007).

Nursing Issues

Overdose

At therapeutic doses prescribed and administered by professionals, opiates are helpful and safe analgesics. However, adolescents who buy someone else's prescription may be opiate-naïve and die of overdose. Users who purchase street drugs cannot be sure of the amount of opioid they are taking. Street purchases are not standardized, and users occasionally obtain a purer drug form than they anticipated. Inadvertent overdose might be due to the unexpected strength of the opiate. The primary effect of overdose is respiratory depression. A respiratory rate 12 breaths/minute or less is cause for alarm. There is a narrow window between an intoxicating dose and one that is lethal. Concomitant use of other CNS depressants (e.g. alcohol, benzodiazepines) increase, the risk of fatal overdose.

Symptoms of overdose—respiratory rate less than 12 breaths/ minute:

- The person becomes stuporous and then sleeps.
- The skin is wet and warm.
- A coma develops, accompanied by respiratory depression and hypoxia.
- The skin becomes cold and clammy.
- The pupils dilate.
- Death quickly follows.

Provision of an adequate airway and assisted ventilation, if needed, are treatment priorities. A narcotic antagonist is administered to reverse the effects of opioids.

Narcotic Antagonists: Antidote to Opioids

The opioids are the only class of commonly abused drugs that have a specific antidote. Naloxone (Narcan), a narcotic antagonist, is the intervention of choice if opioid overdose is suspected. Naloxone blocks the neuroreceptors affected by opioids; the patient responds in a few minutes to an intravenous injection of naloxone. Respiration improves, and the patient consciously responds. However, because most opioids have a longer lasting effect than naloxone, it is often necessary to repeat the antagonist to maintain adequate respiration. The nurse who administers naloxone must observe the patient carefully to determine whether additional antagonist will be needed. If the dose of the antagonist is proportionately higher than the dose of opioids in the system, it is possible to precipitate narcotic withdrawal or abstinence syndrome. Patients using opiates for chronic pain and opiate-dependent individuals will be in significant pain after reversal of the opiate.

Clinical Example-What They Don't Know May Kill You

A hospice team member told the following story. The patient was a 70-year-old man with prostate cancer and painful bone metastases. A nursing concern is maintaining a balance between the need for pain management and the risk of respiratory suppression. The patient built up tolerance to his pain medication. His family members were afraid that he was becoming an "addict," so they decided to reduce his medication intake without consulting the physician. Cutting in half and administering a time-release pain pill (a synthetic morphine that lost its time-release properties when broken), they quickly noticed that the patient was not very responsive. He was taken to the hospital, and naloxone (Narcan) was administered. Because it blocks the opioid receptor sites, there was no effective pain relief for this patient. The man was in extreme physical pain because his family was afraid of the legitimate medical uses of pain medication. Additionally, lack of knowledge about how time-release medications work led to an erratic and potentially fatal dose being administered.

Use by Older Adults

Some older patients might have chronic medical conditions associated with chronic pain for which long-term narcotic pain medication has been prescribed. Older adults are particularly at risk for decreased pulmonary ventilation associated with opioids.

Withdrawal and Detoxification

Unassisted withdrawal from alcohol or barbiturates can be fatal, but unassisted withdrawal from opioids is rarely fatal, although often painful. The term *kicking the habit* or *going cold turkey* comes from the leg spasms associated with the withdrawal from opioids. Withdrawal symptoms are related to the degree of dependence and the abruptness of the discontinuance. Maximal intensity is reached within 36 to 72 hours and subsides in about 1 week. Withdrawal symptoms include yawning, rhinorrhea, sweating, chills, piloerection (goose bumps), tremor, restlessness, irritability, leg spasm, bone pain, diarrhea, and vomiting.

Clonidine has been used successfully for withdrawal by relieving some of the autonomic symptoms (e.g., vomiting and diarrhea). However, clonidine does not reduce craving or insomnia. A controlled taper with buprenorphine (Buprenex) or methadone can assist with the pain related to withdrawal. Treatment is primarily symptomatic and supportive.

Methadone

Methadone (Dolophine), although an opioid similar to morphine, is used specifically to prevent withdrawal symptoms; it is also used as an analgesic in conditions associated with severe pain, such as cancer. Methadone is used as replacement therapy when the addict is unable to discontinue opiate use successfully. Methadone is given orally and is poorly metabolized in the liver. Methadone has a much longer half-life (15 to 30 hours) than morphine (about 2 hours). Because of its long half-life, once-daily dosing is effective and useful for outpatient care. In addition, the use of methadone for management of chronic pain has increased with the potential for accidental overdose if misused.

Heroin

Heroin was derived from morphine as a cure for morphine addiction, but proved to be more addictive by comparison. It is highly favored by opioid abusers. Heroin is typically injected intravenously (its effect is felt within 7 to 8 seconds) or smoked, snorted, or mixed with other substances such as cocaine (10 to 15 minutes for effect) (Lehne, 2007). Heroin is more potent and lipid soluble than morphine; therefore it crosses the blood-brain barrier faster with more rapid onset.

Clinical Example-Dying From Overdose and Nobody Knew

A 32-year-old mother of two was seen in the emergency department in a medium-sized city. She had a history of psychiatric disorders and substance use. She admitted to ingesting a large number of oxycodone (OxyContin) pills, along with other CNS depressants. She was alert at times but at other times displayed slurred speech and psychomotor retardation. After an initial assessment, it was decided that she should be sent to a free-standing psychiatric facility. Several hours later, she was taken to that facility. On admission late in the day, her speech was unintelligible, and her respirations were noted to be slowed (12/minute) and irregular. A full assessment was deferred. She died as a result of opioid-induced respiratory depression before morning. Because only nurses were involved in the admissions process, those nurses were deemed negligent (settled out of court however).

STIMULANTS

Use of stimulants containing caffeine such as soda, coffee, and tea is widespread. Many people feel sluggish if they do not start their day with a cup of coffee. Other, more powerful stimulants, such as amphetamines and cocaine, are widely abused and cause immeasurable harm to society in the United States. Caffeine intoxication occurs at 300 mg with symptoms of jitters and increased heart rate. For example, a 12 oz. Starbuck's coffee contains about 250 mg of caffeine. Caffeine increases attention and alertness and decreases fatigue; however it can also increase anxiety and, when heavy use stops, may result in withdrawal.

COCAINE

Coca plants grow high in the Andes Mountains, and the Incas chewed coca leaves long before the Spanish explorers arrived. This plant is not cocoa, from which we get chocolate, but *coca*. Cocaine is still legitimately used today in some parts of Andean South America. As a mild tea, cocaine can help bring relief for altitude sickness. Cocaine is a fine, white, odorless powder with a bitter taste that was introduced to Western medicine as an anesthetic in 1858. Sigmund Freud was known to use co-

caine and believed it to be a remedy for morphine addiction; he reported on the effects of cocaine in his book, *Cocaine Papers*. Cocaine was once used in some cola drinks (e.g., Coca-Cola), and advertisements extolled the ability of cola as well as of other brain tonics to refresh. After the Pure Food and Drug Act passed in 1906, cocaine was eliminated from these beverages. Cocaine (cocaine hydrochloride) and crack (freebase cocaine) are now responsible for a major drug problem.

Physiologic Effects

Cocaine's exhilarating effect is related to its ability to block dopamine reuptake, particularly in the nucleus accumbens pleasure center in the brain. Euphoria, increased mental alertness, increased strength, anorexia, and increased sexual stimulation are desired effects of these drugs. Increased motor activity, tachycardia (up to 200 beats/minute), and high blood pressure are PNS effects. CNS effects include deep respirations (from medullary stimulation), euphoria, increased mental alertness, dilated pupils, anorexia, and increased strength. The cocaine user can be loquacious and stimulated sexually (libido is increased; ejaculation is retarded). This latter characteristic undoubtedly adds to the drug's overall appeal. Intense paranoia is common.

Less common reactions are specific hallucinations and delusions. Cocaine users report what they think are bugs crawling beneath their skin (formication) and foul smells. Nasal septum perforation has been associated with snorting cocaine and is the result of extreme vasoconstriction, which impedes blood supply to this area and causes nasal necrosis. Death from cocaine is linked to metabolic and respiratory acidosis and hyperthermia associated with prolonged seizures. Tachyarrhythmias and coronary artery spasm have also led to death.

Routes of Cocaine Use

Cocaine hydrochloride is snorted or injected intravenously but not smoked. Crack (freebase cocaine) is smoked. Cocaine passes the blood-brain barrier quickly, causing an instantaneous high. When administered intravenously (mainlining), cocaine is rapidly metabolized by the liver; the rush, although exhilarating, does not last long. Cocaine exerts both CNS and PNS effects because of its ability to block norepinephrine and dopamine reuptake into presynaptic neurons; it depletes these neurotransmitters. With the discovery of smoking an adulterant-free cocaine crystalline base, freebasing became popular and paved the way for the advent of crack or rock cocaine.

Crack

Crack is a less expensive way of using cocaine compared with snorting or mainlining, primarily because it is sold and marketed in smaller packages. It is produced in a relatively uncomplicated procedure (mixed with baking soda and water, heated, and hardened) and smoked; it is reported to produce an instantaneous high and almost as instantaneous a crash. It is thought that the faster a drug's effect builds and then

Jerry Random (J.R.) is a 25-year-old unemployed carpenter who lives with his aunt. One night, he began tearing the house apart, then locked himself in the bathroom, yelling that he was going to kill himself. His aunt called the police, who brought J.R. to the emergency department of the local hospital. The emergency department examiner noted that J.R. was suicidal and having auditory hallucinations, delusions of persecution, disorganized thinking, anorexia, insomnia, anxiety, and agitation. He had been threatening the police and continued to be extremely agitated, threatening the emergency department personnel. Based on a history provided by his aunt, the diagnosis of cocaine intoxication was made.

J.R.'s aunt stated that she had been concerned about possible drug use for the last couple of years but had never pursued the issue with J.R. He was often belligerent and was fired from his job until he was able to get "cleaned up." She had noticed things missing around the house but never questioned J.R. about this.

The emergency department physician decided to keep J.R. in the emergency department until his thinking cleared and to monitor him for tachycardia, cardiac arrhythmia, and seizure activity. The physician ordered 5 mg of diazepam (Valium) administered intravenously for 2 to 3 minutes every 10 to 15 minutes if needed for seizures and propranolol (Inderal) (0.1 to 0.15 mg/kg administered intravenously at a rate of 0.5 to 0.75 mg every 1 to 2 minutes) should the patient experience cardiac arrhythmias. J.R. was transferred to the psychiatric unit after 4 hours of observation in which there was no seizure activity or cardiac abnormalities.

On arrival at the unit, J.R. was noticeably irritable, agitated, and anxious, and he complained of a headache. His responses to questions indicated continuing difficulty in concentration and some disorganized thinking.

🔅 CRITICAL THINKING QUESTION

1. Some cocaine users turn to heroin as they grow older. Can you think of a reason why this might be so?

Clinical Example- Cocaine and Would Do Anything For It

Gladys, a 32-year-old woman with severe cocaine use disorder, was referred to outpatient treatment through the legal system because of a possession charge. After her second group therapy session, she requests an individual session with her counselor. She reveals to the counselor that 1 month earlier, other "customers" at the local crack house that she has frequented had raped her. Gladys is frightened and embarrassed; her urge to use drugs to escape the emotional pain she feels is strengthened by her traumatic experience at the crack house. Although Gladys says that she has a supportive family, she is further ashamed and terrified because she thinks that she is pregnant. In her helplessness, Gladys experiences some suicidal ideation and talks about aborting the pregnancy. After she is calm, Gladys agrees to consult with her physician. After she does not return to treatment, no one answers the telephone, and there is no response to letters sent, Gladys is lost to contact. Gladys calls her counselor 6 months later to say that she put aside her shame and talked with her pastor, her mother, and her 12-year-old daughter. She reports that all is going well, although the baby was stillborn. She has not used since that time.

diminishes, the more addictive it is—this explains why crack is considered to be the most addictive drug. When the user's money is gone, however, the crash often gives way to cocaine-induced depression. This depression is sometimes so severe because of the neurotransmitter depletion that the user may attempt suicide.

AMPHETAMINES AND RELATED DRUGS

Amphetamines, which were developed in 1887, have medicinal uses, such as short-term treatment of obesity, attention-deficit/hyperactivity disorder (ADHD) in childhood, and narcolepsy. Amphetamines and some variants referred to as *speed, crystal, meth, ice,* or *crank* are widely abused. Related drugs include methylphenidate (Ritalin), a drug used in the treatment of ADHD, and 3,4-methylenedioxymethamphetamine (MDMA or ecstasy). These drugs are often "traded" or sold to high school or college students so that they can achieve improved test performance or remain alert while completing assignments.

Methamphetamine

Methamphetamine use probably reached its peak during World War II and then had a revival of sorts over the past decade. The Combat Meth Act of 2005, which restricted the sale of some ingredients for methamphetamine (meth) production, such as pseudoephedrine and ephedrine, has been particularly effective. These drugs now must be kept behind the pharmacy counter, and there is a limitation on the quantity sold. Instructions for home production are still available on the Internet. One of the main causes of burns significant enough to warrant hospitalization is from explosions experienced by meth cooks.

Methamphetamine (also referred to as *speed, meth, crystal, crank,* or *ice*) produces a longer high than cocaine and is typically less expensive by comparison (Table 31-6). It stays in the body 10 times longer (Herrick, 2005, Medline Plus, 2013). Methamphetamine is frequently used as an adulterant of cocaine; it can be snorted, swallowed, injected, or smoked. It causes an immediate intense feeling of pleasure, followed by a lasting high. When the high wears off, an equally intense crash occurs. Users become paranoid and might hallucinate or experience violent rages. Long-term use of methamphetamine can cause damage to dopaminergic systems and other brain areas (Zickler, 2000).

Ecstasy

Ecstasy (MDMA; also known as *XTC, E, X, rolls,* or *Adam*) was synthesized in the early 1900s and briefly used some time later as an adjunct to psychotherapy. It use seems to be leveling off at about 0.2% of individuals older than 12 years of age, or about 869,000 (average age of first use, 20.3 years)people in the United States (Substance Abuse and Mental Health Services Administration, 2013). The chemical structure of ecstasy is closely related to mescaline and methamphetamine. Ecstasy is a popular club drug, promoted as enhancing closeness to others, affection, and communication abilities (Keltner & Folks, 2005). At higher doses, an amphetamine-like stimulation occurs, including euphoria, heightened sexuality, diminished self-consciousness, and disinhibition. Unpleasant amphetamine-type side effects also occur, such as tachycardia, increased blood pressure, anorexia, dry mouth, and teeth grinding (Taylor & Donoghue, 2001). Ecstasy has made headlines related to its use at all-night dance parties where drugs are used to enhance dancing and other activities. Hyperthermia, dehydration, rhabdomyolysis, renal failure, and deaths have been reported.

Metabolism

Amphetamines are taken orally, well absorbed from the gastrointestinal tract, excreted basically unchanged by the kidney, and continue to have an effect until cleared.

Physiologic Effects

Amphetamines are indirect-acting sympathomimetics that cause the release of norepinephrine from nerve endings. Amphetamines also block norepinephrine reuptake in presynaptic nerve endings. Similar to cocaine, amphetamines also have a profound effect on the pleasure pathway by enhancing dopamine, sometimes referred to as the pleasure neurotransmitter. Amphetamines block dopamine reuptake but also stimulate excess release of dopamine and retard its enzymatic breakdown. This effect on dopamine and the dopamine system probably accounts for the so-called addicting effects of amphetamines. CNS effects range from wakefulness, alertness, heightened concentration, energy, and improved mood to euphoria, insomnia (sometimes desired, sometimes not), and amnesia. The most common side effects of amphetamine use are restlessness, dizziness, agitation, and insomnia. PNS effects are palpitations, tachycardia, and hypertension. Respirations also increase because amphetamines, similar to cocaine, stimulate the medulla. A psychiatric side effect of amphetamine use is amphetamine-induced psychosis. In the emergency department, this psychotic presentation can be almost indistinguishable from paranoid schizophrenia.

Nursing Issues
Overdose

Cocaine and amphetamine overdoses have resulted in numerous deaths, resulting primarily from cardiac arrhythmias and respiratory collapse. Smoking cocaine adds to the problem because large amounts reach the system quickly. Toxic levels of amphetamines cause tachycardia, severe hypertension, cardiac ischemia, cerebral hemorrhage, seizures, and coma. Treatment includes induction of vomiting, acidification of the urine, and forced diuresis.

Withdrawal and Detoxification

Although cocaine and amphetamines are highly addictive, physical withdrawal is mild. However, psychological withdrawal is severe because the drugs are highly pleasurable and

---

◎ CARE PLAN

Name: Jerry Random   **Admission Date:** _____

DSM-5 Diagnosis: Cocaine intoxication

Assessment	**Areas of strength:** Patient is young (25 years old); lives with his aunt who wants him to return once he begins to feel better; previous employer will rehire him if he gets "clean."
	Problems: Suicidal ideation, hallucinations (auditory), delusions that someone wants to kill him, thinking disorganized (has difficulty completing thoughts), anorexia, insomnia, anxious (has exaggerated startle reflex), agitated.
Diagnoses	Risk for self-directed violence related to substance abuse or CNS agitation
	Sensory perceptual alteration related to substance abuse or CNS agitation, as evidenced by suicidal ideation, disorganized thinking, hallucinations, and delusions
	Imbalanced in nutrition; less than body requirements related to anorexic effect of cocaine, as evidenced by weight loss
Outcomes	**Short-term goals**
Date met: _____	Patient will not experience physical injury during hospitalization.
Date met: _____	Patient will not experience symptoms of cocaine withdrawal.
Date met: _____	Patient will sleep 6 to 8 hours per night.
Date met: _____	Patient will admit that cocaine is a problem in his life.
	Long-term goals
Date met: _____	Patient will maintain optimal levels of nutrition and maintain at least 90% of normal weight.
Date met: _____	Patient will attend outpatient Cocaine Anonymous meetings.
Date met: _____	Patient will practice abstinence from psychoactive drugs.
Date met: _____	Patient will verbalize and show some evidence of developing non–drug-using friends.

(Continued)

◎ **CARE PLAN—CONT'D**

Planning and Interventions	**Nurse-patient relationship:** Develop a contract with the patient to report to the nurse if suicidal thoughts occur. Establish trusting relationship with the patient. Provide reality-based conversation. Accept the patient. Set limits on behavior, confront the patient with inconsistencies, and do not allow the patient to manipulate. All staff must be consistent. Allow the patient to verbalize anxiety and fear. Teach the patient the effects of drugs on his body. Encourage independence in self-care, and reinforce examples of self-denial and delayed gratification. **Psychopharmacology:** Lorazepam for cocaine withdrawal for 2 weeks. Haloperidol (Haldol) 5 mg orally q4h as needed (prn) for agitation; benztropine mesylate (Cogentin) 2 mg orally with first dose of haloperidol on days it is given. Acetaminophen (Tylenol) 2 tabs q4h prn for headache. **Milieu management:** Provide patient with a quiet room to decrease stimulation and agitation. Provide safe environment, including frequent observation by staff, monitoring of smoking, and assessing vital signs prn. Monitor environment for dangerous objects such as glass, razors, and belts. Provide foods the patient likes to increase interest in food. Provide group setting for patient to explore the issues of substance abuse with other patients and to help the patient get past the notion that no one understands his problems. Orient to surroundings.
Evaluation	Patient has not experienced significant cocaine withdrawal; appetite returning. Beginning to sleep better (4 to 6 hours). Patient has not attempted self-injury and denies suicidal intent.
Referrals	Outpatient treatment for aftercare, including Cocaine Anonymous meetings and random urine screens for increased accountability.

because of the depletion of monoamines, which is known to be associated with depression. For individuals withdrawing from amphetamines under medical supervision, the withdrawal process is gradual and safe. Cold turkey withdrawal without medical supervision causes agitation, irritability, and severe depression, frequently with suicidal ideation. As a rule of thumb, the low of withdrawal is inversely proportional to the high experienced.

HALLUCINOGENS

Hallucinogens, also referred to as *psychotomimetics* or *psychedelics*, cause hallucinations. Hallucinogens are divided into two basic groups, natural and synthetic. Natural hallucinogenic substances include mescaline (peyote [from cactus]), psilocybin (psilocin [from mushrooms]), and marijuana (*Cannabis sativa*). Synthetic or semisynthetic substances include lysergic acid diethylamide (LSD) and phencyclidine (PCP). In general, hallucinogens can heighten awareness of reality or can cause a terrifying psychosis-like reaction. Users report distortions in body image and a sense of depersonalization.

TABLE 31-6	**COMPARISON OF METHAMPHETAMINE AND COCAINE**
METHAMPHETAMINE	**COCAINE**
Synthetic	Plant derived
Smoking produces high that lasts 8-24 hr	Smoking produces high lasting 20-30 min
Half-life, 12 hr	Half-life, 1 hr
Limited medical use	Can be used as local anesthetic

National Institute on Drug Abuse. http://www.drugabuse.gov/publications/me. Accessed February 23, 2014.

Marijuana

Marijuana (also known as *pot, weed,* and *grass*) has been cultivated for more than 5000 years. Marijuana is the most widely used illegal drug in the United States. It has become legalized in some states, and others regulate its use for medical purposes only. Marijuana and other related drugs (hashish and tetrahydrocannabinol [THC]) come from an Indian hemp plant. Marijuana varies significantly in strength depending on the climate and soil conditions in which it is grown.

Metabolism

The active ingredient in marijuana is THC. THC, which is changed to metabolites in the body and stored in fatty tissues, can remain in the body for 6 weeks after it is smoked and can be detected in blood and urine for 3 days to about 4 weeks, depending on its level of use. The effects of smoked marijuana last 2 to 4 hours. If marijuana is ingested, effects might last 12 hours.

Physiologic Effects

Marijuana produces a sense of well-being, is relaxing, and alters perceptions. Euphoria results and is the cause of drug-seeking behaviors. Increased hunger (known as the *munchies*) is an effect that makes marijuana useful for anorexic individuals (e.g., patients with cancer who are undergoing chemotherapy). Marijuana's antiemetic properties make it useful for treating nausea and vomiting associated with chemotherapy.

Balance and stability are impaired for 8 hours after marijuana use. Short-term memory, decision making, and concentration are also impaired. Dry mouth, sore throat, increased heart rate, dilated pupils, conjunctival irritation (i.e., red eyes), and keener sight and hearing are physical

2. If you believe that marijuana is benign, would you want your neurosurgeon to "take the edge off" by taking a few tokes just before surgery to remove your mother's brain tumor? Explain and justify your answer.

responses to marijuana. Marijuana has also been thought to be amotivational; however, a few individuals react with agitation or aggression.

Other effects associated with the use of marijuana include harmful pulmonary effects (bronchitis), weakening of heart contractions, immunosuppression, and reduction of the serum testosterone level and sperm count. Anxiety, impaired judgment, paranoia, and panic are common reactions to marijuana. Memory is also impaired, owing to THC receptors occupying the hippocampus.

Nursing Issues
Interactions
Marijuana should not be used with alcohol because marijuana masks the nausea and vomiting associated with excessive alcohol consumption. Respiratory depression, coma, and death can occur.

Lysergic Acid Diethylamide
Lysergic acid diethylamide (LSD), which stimulates the nervous system by binding tightly to serotonin receptors (i.e., 5-hydroxytryptamine 2A), is taken orally, and the effects are experienced for up to 12 hours. LSD causes a phenomenon known as *synesthesia*, which is the blending of senses (e.g., smelling a color or tasting a sound). Expectations and environment govern the quality of the LSD trip. LSD causes an increase in blood pressure, tachycardia, trembling, and dilated pupils. CNS effects include a sense of unreality, perceptual alterations and distortions, and impaired judgment.

Clinical Example-Seeing The Real Meaning of Life With LSD
Mary Sky is an 18-year-old high school student who has recently become involved with peers who use various hallucinogenic drugs to help them with their spiritual quests. Mary attended a ceremony last night during which she had LSD for the first time. Initially, she experienced anxiety as the sky became a brilliant blue and particular stars seemed to shine brightly, as if they were directly in front of her. Mary soon began smiling a lot and realized the depth of "this process called life" and how we are all "a part of the stars." This heightened experience continued throughout the evening. By the next day, all that remained was memory of bliss and insights, but Mary's actual state of consciousness had returned to its usual state, with all her previously standing inner conflicts.

RELATED ISSUES
EFFECTS ON FAMILY
All family members are affected in some way by substance abuse. The family can benefit from treatment and often fluctuate between enabling (e.g., making excuses, lying for, doing things for) or blaming the abuser. A point that has been repeatedly verified is that some families are better at coping with a substance-abusing family member than dealing with a recovered family member.

Family members, while not actively using substances, are still affected by the behaviors of the addicted person. Past behaviors, which may have included deception and resulted in disappointment and loss of respect, may require family members to seek assistance for their own recovery. Family therapy can help families develop new methods of coping. Al-Anon can also help families heal while the addict goes to AA or NA.

Clinical Example-Dying From Mother's Milk
The Eureka (California) *Times-Standard* reported that Maggie Jean Wortman was convicted of voluntary manslaughter of her 6-week-old son. She was sentenced to a 6-year prison term. The infant died as a result of a methamphetamine overdose through his mother's breastfeeding. Wortman's own childhood included domestic violence, a family history of alcoholism, sexual abuse, and foster care from the age of 3 years. She was a victim of physical and sexual abuse until she was 11 years old. She began smoking marijuana at age 8 and methamphetamine at age 13. She has carried on the family history of domestic violence, drug use, legal problems, and child endangerment. She now lives with the terrible reality that she contributed to the death of her son. (Greenson, T. [2012]. *The tragic case of Maggie Jean Wortman: a woman who never had a chance gives her son the same fate.* <http://www.times-standard.com/ci_20252302/tragic-case-maggie-jean-wortman-woman-who-never> Accessed July 14, 2013.)

TREATING A CHEMICALLY DEPENDENT PERSON
The most common goal of treatment for a chemically dependent person is abstinence from alcohol or drugs. It is believed that a person who is dependent on one substance can easily become dependent on another. The term *cross-dependence* describes this condition. Professionals working with chemically dependent individuals realize their patients' vulnerability and usually refrain from thinking of anyone as being cured. Professionals treat substance use disorders as a chronic, remitting, ongoing, lifelong process in which the person is in recovery while working to remain substance-free. A chronic disease model includes the concept of *recovery*, which indicates a current and dynamic process but also indicates the ever-present possibility of relapsing to substance use.

DIAGNOSTIC TOOLS FOR CHEMICAL DEPENDENCY

Many tools exist for the evaluation of chemical dependency. Early diagnosis can mean a better treatment prognosis. Misdiagnosis can lead to unsuspected withdrawal, drug interactions, or both. Ultimately, an accurate diagnosis might mean the difference between life and death. It is most important that the nurse look for behavioral and physical clues when making diagnostic evaluations with the treatment team.

Tools for Alcoholism

Several screening questionnaires have been developed to assist the health care professional in diagnosing alcohol use disorders. Among the easiest to use are the Michigan Alcoholism Screening Test (MAST) and the CAGE questionnaire. The problem with most screening tools, particularly for drug users, has been their susceptibility to faking and denial on the part of the patient. Part of this process of discovery is to assist the patient in identifying behaviors they want to change.

Michigan Alcoholism Screening Test

The MAST is a good screening tool that can help an unconvinced patient gain insight into at least the possibility of a problem if questions are answered honestly. This test can also aid the clinician in diagnostic assessment and can be easily modified to identify other drug problems.

CAGE Questionnaire

The CAGE questionnaire is another valid instrument. Even easier to administer and possibly perceived as less accusatory compared with the MAST, the following four questions compose this tool:

1. Have you ever felt you should *Cut* down on your drinking?
2. Have people *Annoyed* you by criticizing your drinking?
3. Have you ever felt bad or *Guilty* about your drinking?
4. Have you ever had an *Eye*-opener in the morning to steady your nerves or get rid of a hangover?

Two positive responses are suggestive of alcoholism, and three or four positive responses are diagnostic (Whitfield et al., 1986).

PSYCHOTHERAPEUTIC MANAGEMENT

Alcoholism is highly treatable. Success of treatment for abuse of other chemical substances varies, but recovery is possible with all chemical dependencies. However, the success of treatment depends first on the patient's motivation (Box 31-1) and then on the clinician's. The importance of understanding the role of each of the three psychotherapeutic management interventions is crucial. In working with these individuals, the nurse must realize that milieu management has the potential to be more important for this group of patients than for other types of patients.

The ideal goal of treatment is total abstinence. However, with some individuals not ready to commit to abstinence, risk

---

> **BOX 31-1 MOTIVATION**
>
> Whether external coercion is a positive influence on treatment outcome is a matter of disagreement. Participants who voluntarily seek treatment are more compliant with their therapists than are those coerced into treatment. Participants who are coerced into treatment might be compliant only while the coercive influence is present and might be compliant only with behaviors specified by the coercive agent. One example would be the person who does not drive after drinking, but insists on continuing alcohol use, which has proven to contribute to problems in others areas of life.

reduction may be the goal. When something as significant as alcohol in an alcoholic's life is removed, something must take its place. This replacement can be in the form of counseling groups facilitated by nurses or other professionals or 12-step programs directed by successfully recovering individuals.

Nurse-Patient Relationship

Because most addicted people are experiencing problems in many areas of their lives when they seek treatment, understanding positive motivators can help in establishing new goals and directions for the patient's life. The patient's ability to function at work, at home, in society, and in many roles has been compromised by alcohol and drugs. Stated another way, almost no one comes to treatment because life is going well. The converse is almost always true: the boss is going to fire the person, the spouse is going to leave, or the judge is sending the person to jail. Treatment for chemically dependent people is usually initiated out of a crisis. To the degree that treatment can help the patient replace ineffective behaviors with new coping skills, the patient has a better chance of getting and staying sober. Coping skills worthy of nursing effort include work skills and habits, parenting, family communication, family role responsibilities, and exploration of leisure activities.

Establishing a trusting therapeutic relationship with the patient requires that the rules for treatment are consistently applied. Genuineness is the most important quality of this relationship. Expressing empathy and providing a safe environment that minimizes anxiety are also important, especially in the early stages of treatment. Engendering feelings of hope for the future is also necessary as the patient begins to establish new life goals. Nurses working with chemically dependent patients must become skilled at confronting denial and managing manipulation.

Because denial is the most predominant defense of an alcoholic, treating it appropriately is important. A group therapy setting seems to provide the best avenue for treatment because groups are especially effective in breaking down the denial process. The group is able to point out the disparity between what is believed to be true and what others know to be true. Assisting the substance user to recognize these discrepancies, by gentle confrontation can help the individual recognize his own cognitive inconsistencies. Group support of individuals who share a common goal diminishes isolation and builds a sense of belonging and trust.

Confrontation

Here are two common examples of confrontation:
1. "You say you have not been drinking (or using drugs), but I can smell alcohol on your breath (or cocaine was detected in your urine sample)."
2. "I hear you saying that you are in treatment because you believe you need help, so help me understand how you see your need, given your absence from treatment all week without a medical excuse."

What seems to be most effective is when the patient's peers provide appropriate confrontation. For example, Lloyd reported to the group that he had not used alcohol in the last 3 months. Lloyd's peer, Christy, had appropriately used the group for support earlier that session to process her own recent relapse episode. Christy was able to confront Lloyd directly about the fact that she had seen him at the same club where she had been the previous weekend.

Personal Responsibility of Recovery

It is important to help the patient learn to foster personal responsibility for recovery. The nurse must cultivate awareness by the patient that he is responsible for change. Although the nurse expresses support and concern for the patient in recovery, the nurse must not shield the patient from the negative consequences of the patient's own addictive behavior.

Milieu Management

All six dimensions of milieu management are important when shaping the milieu of a chemically dependent inpatient. Some dimensions are significant for the patient who receives outpatient care as well. Safety issues such as a drug-free environment are critical. Nurses and others must be vigilant to protect the environment from individuals who might bring drugs into the milieu. Psychiatric units are not necessarily drug-free; multiple avenues exist for illicit contraband. Other safety issues, such as suicide prevention and thwarting inappropriate sexual behavior, are the responsibility of nursing staff. Effective unit structure maximizes what the milieu has to offer the patient. Norms of nonviolent behavior, openness, feedback, and the prohibition of nonprescribed drugs are critical to an effective treatment program. As previously noted, confrontation and coaching are useful techniques for working with chemically dependent individuals.

Limit setting is perhaps the most important and most challenged (i.e., by patients) milieu management technique that the nurse uses. Limit setting can be characterized as providing an environment that protects patients from themselves and from other patients. The nurse needs to recognize the symptoms of a still actively addicted mind (i.e., mood swings and substance-seeking, stubborn, belligerent, violent, and aggressive behavior) and set limits on these behaviors. Urine drug screens are also a dimension of limit setting because these tests reinforce the no-drug policy. If drugs are found, the patient must be confronted and held accountable.

Balance and environmental modification also play significant roles in a well-managed milieu for chemically dependent patients. Balance is especially important—for example, when using the technique of confrontation. Although confrontation is important and therapeutic, in the hands of less skilled staff and some patients it can become little more than a heavy-handed counterpart to the abuse patients might have experienced years ago. The proper technique requires sensitivity to confront without crushing or totally alienating the patient. Skillful confrontation combines knowledge, empathy, and concern with accurate timing.

Psychopharmacology

Treatment for chemical dependency using medication is becoming increasingly important as knowledge about brain biochemistry increases. Many of the current available pharmacologic agents for treatment of substance use disorders are helpful for some and ineffective for others. At the present time, there are no common methods of discovering which medication would work on a particular person as substance use disorders may affect more than one neurotransmitter or area of the brain. However, all of the medications offer added support to the individual's recovery process. Medication for nicotine dependence such as varenicline (Chantrix) assists smokers to become nicotine-free, yet some people who are sensitive to neurochemical changes of the serotonin and nicotine receptors experience mood changes such as suicidal ideation or extreme irritability. As scientists continue to explore brain function, understanding of ideal prescribing practices will improve recovery outcomes. Developing research in genetics may help identify who will respond favorably to medication supporting sobriety (Arias & Sewell, 2012; Johnson et al., 2013).

Drugs to Treat Substance Use Disorders

Naltrexone: Decreases the Pleasure of Drinking. Naltrexone hydrochloride (ReVia) is an opioid receptor antagonist used to treat narcotic dependence and is approved for the treatment of alcohol dependence. This would be the first choice when treating alcoholism. Naltrexone increases abstinence and reduces alcohol craving when used as a part of a comprehensive treatment plan (Sinclair, 2001). Naltrexone interferes with opioid functioning, which probably compromises the pleasurable effects of alcohol. Naltrexone is also available as an intramuscular injection that is given on a monthly basis. The medication does not stop the individual from drinking, but it can lengthen the periods of sobriety. Only about 20% to 30% of patients have been reported to respond to anticraving drugs (Spanagel, 2009). The response may improve as studies examining genetic material help to identify what treatment works best for individual genetic makeup. This personalized method of treatment holds promise for the future.

Acamprosate: Restores Chemical Balance in the Alcoholic Brain. Although the mechanism of action of acamprosate (Campral) is not precisely known, it is thought that continuous consumption of alcohol alters the balance between neuronal inhibition and excitation (Forest Laboratories, 2004). This drug can be used when abstinence has begun but not while an alcohol-dependent person is drinking. It causes neither the aversive effects of disulfiram nor the pleasure-stealing effects of naltrexone. Initial reports have suggested that acamprosate enhances abstaining behaviors. It may be used in conjunction with other medications to support recovery.

Disulfiram: Makes Drinking Painful. Disulfiram is an aversive drug. Disulfiram inhibits the breakdown of CH_3CHO (acetaldehyde) by the enzyme aldehyde dehydrogenase. Because CH_3CHO is toxic, a person who drinks alcohol while taking disulfiram becomes ill (as evidenced by sweating, flushing of the neck and face, tachycardia, hypotension, throbbing headache, nausea and vomiting, palpitations, dyspnea, tremor, weakness, or any combination of these effects). Disulfiram and alcohol can also cause arrhythmias, myocardial infarction, cardiac failure, seizures, coma, and death. The unpleasant response to alcohol is intended to help reinforce the alcoholic's efforts to stop drinking alcohol. Basically, a patient taking disulfiram has to make only one decision a day about drinking: once the pill is taken, the patient dare not drink. A person who is very sensitive to the effects of disulfiram may also have to avoid skin bracers or cologne because alcohol is absorbed through the skin and can trigger a reaction. Anecdotal accounts note that some alcoholics experience an ostensibly spontaneous relapse episode that coincides with their forgetting to take disulfiram for 1 or 2 weeks before their return to alcohol use. Disulfiram is most effective in patients with significant internal motivation for long-term change who have someone willing to oversee daily medication ingestion. Research has found that disulfiram has also been helpful in reducing cocaine use in individuals who have been unsuccessful in stopping use. This potential treatment option is still being explored and is not yet approved by the U.S. Food and Drug Administration.

Off Label Use to Reduce Alcohol Consumption. These medications may be useful to reduce the number of heavy drinking days in people who have heavy drinking but are not ready to stop drinking alcohol altogether. The reduction in consumption may be a much more workable goal than total abstinence as many people are more likely to discuss and commit to "cutting back" rather than to quitting altogether. Reduction of heavy drinking can reduce negative consequences of excessive alcohol use (Aubin & Daeppen 2013).

Topiramate –Anticonvulsant which helps decrease the number of heavy drinking days as well as increases the likelihood the individual will remain abstinent. It can enhance GABA functioning and reduce glutamate. Topiramate can improve sense of well-being and decrease alcohol seeking, and harmful drinking such as binge drinking. It may also decrease craving. Dosage ranges from 50 mg-200 mg per day. This medication may be combined with naltrexone for increased effectiveness.

Ondansetron - An antiemetic medication used with chemotherapy – (5HT3 antagonist). Given in doses of 8 ug/kg/day the results seem to be more favorable to specific individuals such as those with genotype group LL or type B early-onset alcoholic patients. Ondansetron does not interfere with breakdown of alcohol, so it can be taken when the person is still drinking. It may be helpful with early-onset alcoholism. Blockade of 5HT3 receptors is thought to decrease craving and increase abstinence (Myrick et al., 2008).

Sertraline – SSRI which helps to reduce the number of heavy drinking days in type A late-onset alcoholic men. It was not as effective for women who were type A or type B alcoholics.

Medications Used to Treat Alcohol Withdrawal

Long-acting benzodiazepines such as chlordiazepoxide (Librium), diazepam (Valium), and lorazepam (Ativan) are useful for treatment of alcohol withdrawal. The principle behind this treatment is the rapid substitution of the benzodiazepine for the alcohol to suppress withdrawal symptoms. Benzodiazepines bind to the GABA-benzodiazepine receptor sites, explaining their mechanism of action. The next step is a gradual tapering of benzodiazepines over several days. Some clinicians prefer barbiturates for alcohol withdrawal, but respiratory depression and safety concerns dissuade most prescribers.

All patients being treated for alcoholism should be given thiamine. Thiamine specifically prevents the development of Wernicke's encephalopathy.

Medications Used to Treat Opioid Dependence

Drugs used to treat opioid dependence can be divided into agents for opioid overdose and agents for long-term replacement therapy.

Naloxone for Opioid Overdose. Naloxone (see previous discussion) blocks the receptors affected by opioids. In case of an opioid overdose, naloxone can be given to reverse opioid-induced CNS depression. Although improvement occurs rapidly in a patient who has taken an overdose, the effect of naloxone is short-lived because of its short half-life. Symptoms of opioid overdose may reemerge.

Methadone and Buprenorphine for Maintenance Treatment of Opioid Dependence. Methadone is an opioid with a much longer half-life compared with the prototype opioid morphine and can be given in once-daily doses. Methadone relieves the drug hunger associated with opioid abuse. When used for opiate replacement therapy, it is given in high doses and causes receptor blockade and prevents uptake of other opiates.

Buprenorphine is an agonist-antagonist opioid, a partial agonist for the mu receptor and an antagonist for the kappa receptor. This pharmacologic activity seems to reduce the craving for opioids. Two different formulations are available that can prevent illicit opiate use: Subutex, which can be used for opiate replacement therapy or for opiate taper for detoxification, and Suboxone, a combination drug that combines buprenorphine with naloxone. This combination for opiate replacement therapy prevents the individual from achieving the benefit of the injected opiate.

INTERVENTION AND TREATMENT PROGRAMS

Many programs exist for the treatment of chemical dependency. The fact that these various programs exist gives testimony to the complexity and seriousness of chemical dependencies in North America.

The best-known intervention programs are AA and Narcotics Anonymous (NA) (see Box 31-1). These programs use a self-help, support group model made up of fellow users in various stages of recovery. Philosophically, AA and NA view psychosocial problems as stemming from substance abuse and generally reject the idea that an underlying psychopathology is responsible for the abuse. AA (>1 million members in the United States) has established the 12 steps (see Box 31-2), which start with a person admitting personal powerlessness over alcohol and end with the person being available, night or day, to help another alcoholic in need (Bates, 2005). The popular bumper sticker slogan, "Easy does it," reflects a philosophy of taking life one day at a time and avoiding a frenetic lifestyle. AA and NA subscribe to the belief that only total abstinence can free a chemically dependent person from the bondage of alcohol and drugs because they maintain "a drug is a drug is a drug," meaning that if someone is addicted to one substance, that person is by definition addicted (at least potentially) to all substances. Although AA in particular has a program that has helped many people, it does not appeal to everyone. Reasons vary, but some professionals believe that the spiritual nature of AA is a deterrent to some who are seeking help; 8 of the 12 steps have a spiritual perspective. Specifically, the concept of a higher power, the expectation that a person tell his or her story publicly, of making a searching and fearless moral inventory, and then making amends when needed are incongruent with some people's belief systems. AA continues to be an important treatment alternative for thousands of individuals with alcoholism.

BOX 31-2 TWELVE STEPS OF ALCOHOLICS ANONYMOUS

1. Admitted we were powerless over alcohol—that our lives had become unmanageable.
2. Came to believe that a power greater than ourselves could restore us to sanity.
3. Made a decision to turn our will and our lives over to the care of God as we understood Him.
4. Made a searching and fearless moral inventory of ourselves.
5. Admitted to God, to ourselves, and to another human being the exact nature of our wrongs.
6. Were entirely ready to have God remove all these defects of character.
7. Humbly asked Him to remove our shortcomings.
8. Made a list of all persons we had harmed and became willing to make amends to them all.
9. Made direct amends to such people wherever possible, except when to do so would injure them or others.
10. Continued to take personal inventory, and when we were wrong promptly admitted it.
11. Sought through prayer and meditation to improve our conscious contact with God as we understood Him, praying only for knowledge of His will for us and the power to carry that out.
12. Having had a spiritual awakening as the result of these steps, we tried to carry this message to alcoholics, and to practice these principles in all our affairs.

The Twelve Steps are reprinted with permission of Alcoholics Anonymous World Services, Inc. Permission to reprint this material does not mean that AA has reviewed or approved the contents of this publication. AA is a program of recovery from alcoholism only—use of the Twelve Steps in connection with programs and activities that are patterned after AA, but that address other problems, does not imply otherwise.

A STUDENT'S CLINICAL LOG*

I went to the substance abuse program the week of November 2. When the two other students and I arrived, we were amazed to see all the teenagers standing in front of the building. As I waited in line to sign in, I heard several of them talking. They were talking about the party they went to last weekend, how they got "messed up," and how they were planning on doing it again the next weekend. They talked about how they hated the substance abuse program and they thought it was a waste of their time. I was bothered by this conversation. If they had that kind of attitude, they did not need to be there. They were wasting their time and money. I should have expected this type of attitude from them. Most of them were there because they had to be there. Some judge thought it was the solution to their problem. I wonder if they were paying for this program or was somebody else "throwing their money away." I think most of them viewed this as a social gathering. I wish I did not think this way. I want to believe that these kids want to "get better," but based on their actions I do not think some of them are ready. They will have to hit rock bottom before they see the error of their ways.

* After an evening at an intensive outpatient program meeting.

? CRITICAL THINKING QUESTION

3. The founders of AA were clear that the recovery process was a spiritual journey. However, we now live in times in which most people are reluctant to speak of spiritual matters for fear of offending others or of imposing their views on others. Do you think that in our efforts not to "offend" people we have deemphasized an important part of psychiatric nursing?

SPECIAL NOTES

The traditional stereotype of an addict or alcoholic is the "skid row bum." One is shocked and dismayed to find professionals, especially health care professionals, using drugs. However, all individuals are at risk and health care providers ae often at a higher risk because of medication availability. A common form of drug use is addiction to prescription medications, such as pain medications or anxiolytics. People who are addicted to prescriptions have a particularly difficult denial through which to break.

Prescriptions, being legally obtained, are justified as legitimate by the prescription drug addict. The skills acquired by a prescription drug addict in maintaining an increasing supply of their drug of choice are accompanied by significant rationalization and sophisticated denial. Because their drugs are acquired legally, prescription drug addicts have a difficult time seeing their use in the same way as a street addict. Concern about the problem of prescription drug use has increased considerably over the last 20 years (Meadows, 2001; Vastag, 2001). Pain medications have become recreational with adolescents and young adults, who often get prescription drugs from a friend or relative (SAMHSA, 2013).

Addicted Health Care Professionals

Substance use among health care professionals is a particularly difficult problem because it is an ethical violation of the professional's relationship with the patient. However, health care professionals are vulnerable to the effects of substance use (Fogger & McGuinness, 2012). Often the substance use has a slow, insidious onset with "rationalized" use to manage stress. Substance use becomes the individual's coping mechanism for managing life demands with often easier access than other people. Health care professionals who divert (take

---

Clinical Example-Stealing a Patient's Meds

Terry is a 39-year-old, opioid-dependent registered nurse whose presentation in treatment is precipitated by the state nursing board. Nursing was Terry's life, and her identity centered on being a nurse. Reporting that it was common to "share medication" with patients, Terry told of how easy it was at first to document giving the maximum as-needed pain medications in a patient's chart but not always giving them to the actual patient. "I never let one of my patients be in pain, though," Terry reported.

Terry's supervisor did not suspect a problem until medications were unaccounted for. Terry thought that all areas had been covered but was eventually caught, not because of stupidity, but from the kind of impaired judgment that results from drug use.

Terry's nursing license was put on probationary status. Most facilities were unwilling to hire a nurse on probation; the limitations placed by the board were strict. Terry cannot work the night shift and cannot hold the keys to the medication storage; she must also submit to random drug testing. Without a job, Terry cannot begin to fulfill the conditions of the probation.

Terry was hired as a nurse at a health care facility and has 6 months remaining until another hearing date can be set.

---

drugs) from patients are particularly scorned (Bachman, 2001). Many states have adopted nonpunitive monitoring programs that allow nurses an opportunity to work under strict guidelines while actively participating in recovery.

Clinical Example-Working Hard to Get a Nursing License Only to Smoke it Away

Bill was 27 years old when he started nursing. He was a bright young man but had limited financial resources, so making ends meet was a continual struggle. There were periods during nursing school in which he had to sleep in his car. He finished his nursing program and found a position in a large teaching hospital. Before his first month of work was complete, he failed a random drug screen (for marijuana). After 4 years, he still did not have his license back.

Follow-up Care

Follow-up care is essential for preventing relapse. Patients and nurses need to be aware that recovery has begun only when an inpatient or outpatient program is completed. The few months immediately after completion of a treatment program can be dangerous for a chemically dependent person. Relapse is most common during this period. A relapse prevention plan can be developed during treatment that can assist the patient to avoid "triggers" to use. The nurse should confirm that arrangements for aftercare, outpatient counseling, and self-help support group meetings are made before discharge. One saying used in treatment is "H.A.L.T.: Don't get too hungry, angry, lonely, or tired" because any of these states increases the chance of poor decision making, increasing the risk of return to using.

Helpful Websites for Additional Information

American Society of Addiction Medicine. <http://www.asam.org/>

International Nurses Society on Addictions. <http://www.intnsa.org/home/index.asp>

National Institute on Drug Abuse. <http://www.drugabuse.gov>

Substance Abuse and Mental Health Services Administration. <http://www.samhsa.gov/>

? CRITICAL THINKING QUESTION

4. What can you do to assist adolescents to avoid substance use?

STUDY NOTES

1. Chemical dependency is a major physical and mental health problem in North America, and most nurses, whether they want to or not, will take care of patients with chemical dependencies.

2. Drugs of abuse can be categorized into the following basic groups: (1) alcohol, (2) CNS depressants, (3) opioids, (4) stimulants, and (5) hallucinogens.

3. *DSM-5* defines substance use disorders as mild, moderate, and severe, depending on the degree of problems related to use. Alcohol represents the leading drug problem in North America; it exacts a high price economically from society and is responsible for much suffering and death.

4. Alcohol causes disinhibition and impaired judgment and is relaxing when first used. The primary concern with respect to alcohol overdose is severe and often fatal CNS depression. Withdrawal causes tremors, nausea, vomiting, tachycardia, diaphoresis, seizures, anxiety, and depression. Withdrawal can be fatal as well.

5. Prevention of nicotine use in children, adolescents, and young adults is a health priority.

6. Depressants cause euphoria, disinhibition, and drowsiness. The primary effect of overdose is respiratory depression. Withdrawal from CNS depressants can be life-threatening.

7. Opioids (narcotics) come from the juice of the opium poppy or are synthetic substances, with opium being the natural product and morphine, codeine, and the semi-synthetic heroin being easily derived from the poppy juice. Opioids are taken intravenously, orally, intramuscularly, and subcutaneously (skin popping). Overdose can be fatal, with respiratory depression being the most serious side effect. Withdrawal, although unpleasant (influenza-like symptoms), is not life-threatening.

8. Naloxone is an opioid receptor blocker and is given in emergency departments to treat opioid overdose. Naloxone causes an opioid abstinence syndrome.

9. Stimulants include amphetamines and cocaine. Stimulants cause elation, grandiose thinking, talkativeness, and other less pleasant effects. The primary concerns in the event of overdose are agitation, tachycardia, cardiac arrhythmias, and convulsions. Hallucinogens include mescaline, marijuana, LSD, and PCP. Hallucinogens cause illusions, hallucinations, diminished ability to perceive time and distance, anxiety, and paranoid thinking. The primary effects of hallucinogenic overdose are intense trips, psychotic reactions, and panic. Although several treatment approaches are effective, the therapeutic goal for most approaches is abstinence from the substance, although the patient might still be seeking a way to engage in controlled use. If the patient is not ready to quit, the nurse can assist the patient to identify through motivational interviewing what changes the patient is willing to make to decrease the harm risk of the substance.

10. Medications such as buprenorphine, naltrexone, and disulfiram can support recovery and decrease cravings or diminish the effect of the illicit drug should relapse occur.

11. Nursing interventions include group work, education, confrontation, tough love (simply not allowing oneself to be a participant in the patient's self-destruction), providing for physical and nutritional needs, and helping the patient become involved in groups such as AA and NA.

12. Health care professionals have access to medications that can be diverted for their personal use. Most licensing boards monitor recovery by ensuring individuals in recovery remain abstinent through long-term monitoring programs.

REFERENCES

American Psychiatric Association. 2013a. *Diagnostic and statistical manual of mental disorders* (5th ed.). Arlington, Virginia: APA.

Arias, A., & Sewell, R. (2012). Pharmacogenetically driven treatment for alcoholism: Are we there yet? *CNS Drugs, 6,* 461.

Aubin, H., & Daeppen, J. (2013). Emerging pharmacotherapeutics for alcohol dependence: A systemic review focusing on reduction in consumption. *Drug and Alcohol Dependence, 133,* 15.

Bachman, J. (2001). One nurse's story of addiction and recovery. *Colorado Nurse, 101,* 11.

Bates, F. (2005). Study detects some "heretics" among AA program faithful. *Clinical Psychiatry News, 33,* 50.

Cavacuiti, C. (2011). *Principles of addiction medicine: The essentials.* Philadelphia: Lippincott Williams & Williams.

Colyar, M. R. (2003). Testing for drugs of abuse. *Advance for Nurse Practitioners, 9,* 30.

Fogger, S., & McGuinness, T. (2012). Relationship between addictions and bariatric surgery for nurses in recovery. *Perspectives in Psychiatric Care, 48,* 10–15.

Forest Laboratories. (2004). *Campral delayed-release tablets prescribing information.* St. Louis: Forest Laboratories.

Frezza, M., et al. (1990). High blood alcohol levels in women: The role of decreased gastric alcohol dehydrogenase activity and first-pass metabolism. *New England Journal of Medicine, 322,* 95.

Gordis, E. (2000). Alcohol and the brain. Neuroscience and neurobehavior. In C. Armstrong, et al. (Eds.), *Tenth special report to the U.S. Congress on alcohol and health.* Washington, DC: National Institutes of Health.

Greenson, T. (2012). *The tragic case of Maggie Jean Wortman: A woman who never had a chance gives her son the same fate.* http://www.times-standard.com/ci_20252302/tragic-case-maggie-jean-wortman-woman-who-never, Accessed 14.07.13.

Harper, C., & Matsumoto, I. (2005). Ethanol and brain damage. *Current Opinion in Pharmacology, 5,* 73.

Herrick, T. (2005). The meth epidemic. *Clinician News, 9,* 21.

Johnson, B., et al. (2013). Determination of genotype combinations that can predict the outcome of the treatment of alcohol dependence using the 5-HT3 antagonist ondansetron. *American Journal of Psychiatry, 170,* 1020–1031.

Keltner, N. L., & Folks, D. G. (2005). *Psychotropic drugs* (4th ed.). St. Louis: Mosby.

Kessler, R. C., et al. (2005). Prevalence, severity, and comorbidity of 12-month DSM-IV disorders in the national comorbidity survey replication. *Archives of General Psychiatry, 62*, 617.

Kessler, R. C., et al. (2012). Twelve-month and lifetime prevalence and lifetime morbid risk of anxiety and mood disorders in the United States. *International Journal of Methods in Psychiatric Research, 21*, 169.

Lehne, R. A. (2007). *Pharmacology for nursing care* (6th ed.). Philadelphia: Saunders.

Lieber, C. S. (2003). Relationships between nutrition, alcohol use, and liver disease. *Alcohol Research & Health, 27*, 220.

Mayfield, R. D., Harris, R. A., & Schuckit, M. A. (2008). Genetic factors influencing alcohol dependence. *British Journal of Pharmacology, 154*, 275.

Meadows, M. (2001). Prescription drug use and abuse. *FDA Consumer, 34*, 18.

Medline Plus. (2013). *How is methamphetamine different from other stimulants, such as cocaine?* http://www.nida.nih.gov/researchreports/methamph/methamph4.html, Accessed 04.03.13.

Myrick, H., Anton, R. F., Li, X., et al. (2008). Effect of naltrexone and ondansetron on alcohol cue-induced activation of the ventral striatum in alcohol-dependent people. *Archives of General Psychiatry, 65*, 466.

National Institute on Drug Abuse. (2012). *Understanding drug abuse and addiction. DrugFacts.* http://www.nida.nih.gov/PDF/InfoFacts/Understanding08.pdf, Accessed 23.02.14.

National Institute on Drug Abuse. (2013). http://www.drugabuse.gov/publications/me. Accessed 23.02.14.

Office of Alcohol and Drug Education. (2014). *Differences between men and women.* http://oade.nd.edu/educate-yourself-alcohol/al, Accessed 23.02.14.

Prochaska, J., & DiClemente, C. (1983). Stages and processes of self-change of smoking: Toward an integrative model of change. *Journal of Consulting and Clinical Psychology, 51*, 390–395.

Quertemont, E., et al. (2005). Is ethanol a pro-drug? Acetaldehyde contribution to brain ethanol effects. *Alcoholism, Clinical and Experimental Research, 29*, 1514.

Rehm, J., et al. (2009). Global burden of disease and injury and economic cost attributable to alcohol use and alcohol-use disorder. *The Lancet, 373*, 2223.

Sinclair, J. D. (2001). Evidence about the use of naltrexone and for different ways of using it in the treatment of alcoholism. *Alcohol, 36*, 2.

Spanagel, R. (2009). Alcoholism: A systems approach from molecular physiology to addictive behavior. *Physiological Reviews, 89*, 649.

Standridge, J., Adams, S., & Zotos, A. (2010). Urine drug screening: A valuable office procedure. *American Family Physician, 81*, 635–640.

Substance Abuse and Mental Health Services Administration. (2011). *Results from the 2010 national survey on drug use and health: Summary of national findings.* http://oas.samhsa.gov/NSDUH/2k10NSDUH/2k10Results.htm, Accessed 04.03.14.

Substance Abuse and Mental Health Services Administration. (2013). *Results from the 2012 national survey on drug use and health: National findings.* http://www.samhsa.gov/data/nsduh/2k8nsduh/2k8Results.htm, Accessed 25.02.14.

Taylor, B., & Donoghue, J. (2001). Club drugs—Its effects on our youth. *The Alabama Nurse, 28*, 20.

U.S. Surgeon General. (2012). *2012 Surgeon General's report: Preventing tobacco use among youth and young adults.* Washington, DC: U.S. Department of Health and Human Services.

Vastag, B. (2001). Mixed message on prescription drug abuse. *JAMA, 285*, 2183.

Whitfield, C., Davis, J., & Barker, L. (1986). Alcoholism. In L. R. Barker, J. R. Burton, & P. D. Zieve (Eds.), *Principles of ambulatory medicine.* Baltimore: Williams & Wilkins.

Zickler, P. (2000). Brain imaging studies show long-term damage from methamphetamine abuse. *NIDA Notes, 15*, 11.

Eating Disorders

Joan S. Grant

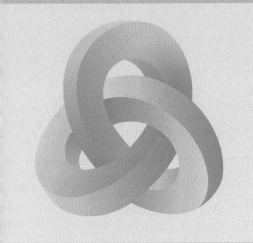

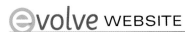 WEBSITE

http://evolve.elsevier.com/Keltner

LEARNING OBJECTIVES

- Recognize criteria and terminology for eating disorders used in *DSM-5*.
- Recognize and describe objective and subjective symptoms of eating disorders.
- Describe current etiologies for eating disorders.
- Describe treatment issues for professionals who deal with patients with eating disorders.

- Recognize the continuum from dieting to an obvious eating disorder.
- Develop nursing care plans for patients with eating disorders.
- Evaluate the effectiveness of nursing interventions for patients with eating disorders.

Hospitalizations have increased by 13% for anorexia nervosa and decreased by 14% for bulimia nervosa. Although hospitalizations for men have increased by 53%, 9 in 10 cases of hospitalizations for eating disorders are still for women (Agency for Healthcare Research and Quality, 2011). These hospitalizations increased most sharply for children younger than 12 years old (119%) and adults 45 to 64 years old (48%). Hospitalizations related to mental health eating disorders also increased by almost 25% for older adults (Agency for Healthcare Research and Quality, 2009). Finally, hospitalizations for less common eating disorders, such as pica (an obsession with eating nonedible substances such as clay) increased by 93% (Agency for Healthcare Research and Quality, 2011). However, the severity of eating disorders declined, with symptoms such as an irregular heartbeat and menstrual disorders decreasing by 39% and 46%, respectively.

Eating disorders are associated with devastating psychological and physical sequelae. Serious secondary conditions include fluid and electrolyte imbalances; cardiac dysrhythmias; nutritional deficiencies or other nutritional, endocrine, or metabolic disorders; menstrual disorders; iron deficiency and anemia; acute renal or liver failure; and convulsions and epilepsy (Agency for Healthcare Research and Quality, 2009; MacDonald, 2009). Other symptoms associated with eating disorders include distractibility, depression, anxiety, anger, sadness, agitation, sleep disturbance, and obsessive-compulsive

patterns of behavior (Ansell et al., 2008; Attia, 2009; Cuzzocrea et al., 2012; Fox, 2009; Fox & Froom, 2009; Hütter et al., 2009).

These disorders affect not only the patient but also family members. Family members commonly report feelings of sadness, fear, guilt, hopelessness, and ambiguity when another member has an eating disorder. They feel lack of control over the situation and manipulated, with feelings of helplessness and impotence (Espindola & Blay, 2009). Nurses and other health care professionals have a role in assisting both patients with eating disorders and their families to address these feelings and to identify potentially useful treatments for eating disorders.

This chapter focuses on patients with anorexia nervosa and bulimia nervosa, the most common eating disorders. The similarities and differences of these two disorders are highlighted as well as the continuum of eating behavior from dieting to anorexia, bulimia, and other eating disorders. Some professionals also consider obesity an eating disorder, but a detailed discussion is beyond the scope of this chapter.

ANOREXIA NERVOSA

DSM-5 Criteria

Viewed with the context of age, sex, developmental trajectory, and physical health, a core feature of anorexia nervosa is a restriction of caloric intake relative to body requirements, which leads to a significantly low body weight. People with anorexia nervosa have an intense fear of gaining weight or of becoming overweight. They also may have persistent behaviors that focus on not gaining weight, despite their low weight (APA, 2013). Although anorectics limit their intake or refuse to eat, they generally do not lose their appetites. They suppress their appetite in an effort to remain thin or get thinner (Kaye et al., 2000). Anorectics think about food and eating much of the time. They have a disturbance in the way they view their weight or shape but these two factors are the most important influence on the anorectic's sense of worth. They might deny that they are dangerously thin or might acknowledge their underweight status but then deny that their condition is problematic (Halmi, 2005, APA 2013).

NORM'S NOTES

When I was a younger psychiatric nurse, it was difficult for me to believe that eating disorders were legitimate mental health concerns. I just could not grasp that someone could not stop purging or could not start eating if they really wanted to. I held that uninformed view until I worked with a few young people who could not stop or not start whatever their particular problem was. I saw how it dominated and, in a few cases, ruined their lives. I can only say this—it is real, and it can be devastating.

Amenorrhea is no longer a diagnostic criterion for anorexia nervosa (American Psychiatric Association, 2013). However, empirical data support that menstrual difficulties or irregularities may occur in this disease. For example, menstruation might cease early in the illness, before significant weight loss has taken place, or menstruation might continue but be irregular and spotty. If menarche has not been reached, menstruation might not begin. One theory for the cause of amenorrhea suggests that lack of nourishment significantly slows pituitary functioning, which is fundamental to the menstrual cycle. Women must maintain a body mass index (BMI) of 18 or greater to support menstruation (Muscari, 2002). A BMI less than 18 can result in amenorrhea, with accompanying reduction of hormone levels and inadequate development of secondary sexual characteristics. In anorectic men, low sex drive and low testosterone levels might be the equivalent of amenorrhea in female patients (Misra et al., 2008; Treasure et al., 2010).

Anorexia is less common than bulimia, affecting up to 3.7% of women during their lifetime (Finelli, 2001). Women account for approximately 90% of reported cases of anorexia nervosa, although anorexia in men appears to be increasing, as noted later in this chapter (Cohane & Pope, 2001). Onset varies from preadolescence to early adulthood, with an increasing incidence at early adolescence (12 to 13 years old) as well as some new-onset cases that may develop from about age 8 onward (MacDonald, 2009) to cases in middle and later adulthood

---

DSM-5 CRITERIA

for Anorexia Nervosa

A. Restrictions of energy intake relative to requirements, leading to a significantly low body weight in the context of age, sex, developmental trajectory, and physical health. Significantly low weight is defined as a weight that is less than minimally normal or, for children and adolescents, less than that minimally expected.

B. Intense fear of gaining weight or becoming fat, or persistent behavior that interferes with weight gain, even though at a significantly low weight.

C. Disturbance in the way in which one's body weight or shape is experienced, undue influence of body weight or shape on self-evaluation, or persistent lack of recognition of the seriousness of the current low body weight.

Coding note: The ICD-9-CM code for anorexia nervosa is 307.1, which is assigned regardless of the subtype. The ICD-10-CM code depends on the subtype (see below).

Specify whether:

(F50.01) Restricting type: During the last 3 months, the individual has not engaged in recurrent episodes of binge eating or purging behavior (i.e., self-induced vomiting or the misuse of laxatives, diuretics, or enemas). This subtype describes presentations in which weight loss is accomplished primarily through dieting, fasting, and/or excessive exercise.

(F50.02) Binge-eating/purging type: During the last 3 months, the individual has engaged in recurrent episodes of binge eating or purging behavior (i.e., self-induced vomiting or the misuse of laxatives, diuretics, or enemas).

Specify if:

In partial remission: After full criteria for anorexia nervosa were previously met. Criterion A (low body weight) has not been met for a sustained period, but either Criterion B (intense fear of gaining weight or becoming fat or behavior that interferes with weight gain) or Criterion C (disturbances in self-perception of weight and shape) is still met.

In full remission: After full criteria for anorexia nervosa were previously met, none of the criteria have been met for a sustained period of time.

Specify current severity:

The minimum level of severity is based, for adults, on current body mass index (BMI) (see below) or, for children and adolescents, on BMI percentile. The ranges below are derived from World Health Organization categories for thinness in adults; for children and adolescents, corresponding BMI percentiles should be used. The level of severity may be increased to reflect clinical symptoms, the degree of functional disability, and the need for supervision.

Mild: BMI ≥ 17 kg/m²
Moderate: BMI 16–16.99 kg/m²
Severe: BMI 15–15.99 kg/m²
Extreme: BMI < 15 kg/m²

From American Psychiatric Association. (2013). *Diagnostic and statistical manual of disorders* (5th ed.). Washington, DC: Author; (pp. 338–339)

(Bulik et al., 2005). These ages correspond with transitional stages in people's lives. Initial morbidity and relapse from adolescent episodes are seen in adulthood. Of anorectic patients, 6% to 20% die as a result of their illness, usually through starvation or suicide; anorexia nervosa is associated with a higher suicide rate than most other psychiatric disorders (Andrist, 2003; Keel et al., 2003; Pompli et al., 2004).

Behavior

The onset of anorexia is often insidious because the typical adolescent victim, who is usually female, appears compliant and does not cause problems for others. Because dieting and fad foods are common in adolescence and young adulthood, often no one notices until the young woman has lost a significant amount of weight. A common premorbid personality profile is that of a perfectionistic and introverted girl with self-esteem and peer relationship problems, but patients might also be accomplished and active in school activities (Bulik et al., 2005; Holland et al., 2013; Karpowicz et al., 2009). Empirical data also suggest that individuals with anorexia nervosa appear to have decision-making deficits, with more risky decision making occurring in eating disorders (Boisseau et al., 2013).

Objective Signs

The most observable behavior of anorexia nervosa is deliberate weight loss in an effort to control weight through changing eating behaviors. Patients with anorexia nervosa are in two groups: the restricters and the vomiters-purgers. The restricters are more often young people in the normal or slightly above normal weight range for height and build before the eating disorder begins. This group views losing weight as more probable if they simply eat less and avoid social situations in which they are expected to eat. Restricters often withdraw to their rooms and avoid family and friends. It is common for them to be competitive, compulsive, and obsessive about their activities. They might participate in rigid exercise programs to help reduce their weight (Kaye et al., 2000). Many restricting anorectics become hyperactive to lose weight and because they are highly anxious and unable to relax. They might take early morning walks because of insomnia and a need to burn off calories.

Clinical Example

Kristin Chambliss, age 15, was in the normal weight range when she joined the school volleyball team with her friends. The first time they donned their uniforms, one of Kristin's friends called her "piano legs." Kristin was horrified and began to diet. In addition, she asked her parents to join the local health club so she could exercise to keep in shape for the team. Her entire day revolved around participation on the team to the extent that she forfeited all other social involvement. She did not arrive home until after 9 P.M. each night because she went to the health club to exercise after a volleyball game or after practice. Kristin lost 21 lb before anyone noticed.

Compared with restricters, vomiters-purgers are more often overweight before the eating disorder begins, and their weight tends to fluctuate (Kaye et al., 2000). These young women who are prone to dangerous methods of weight reduction, such as induction of vomiting or excessive use of laxatives or diuretics. These anorectic patients commonly deny concerns about weight and typically eat normally in social situations. After the meal, they retreat to the nearest bathroom and purge themselves of the consumed food, although the amount is not excessive, as it is with bulimics. Dental problems frequently occur in these patients because the acidic vomitus decays the enamel on their teeth (Orbanic, 2001). This group also might be susceptible to times when they uncontrollably eat large amounts of food if unsuccessful in maintaining the severe dietary restriction they impose on themselves. Purging anorectics are more likely to have histories of behavior problems, substance abuse, and open family conflict than restricting anorectics (Kaye et al., 2000). In an interview analysis of 680 women with anorexia nervosa, Zerwas et al. (2013) indicated that self-induced vomiting and greater trait anxiety predicted a lower likelihood of recovery.

Clinical Example

Tina Easterling was always a chubby child. When she was 23 years old, she lost considerable weight by dieting. Shortly thereafter, she began seriously dating and was married. Tina was thrilled with her new look and worked hard to maintain her weight loss, consistently keeping her weight slightly under the ideal for her height. After 2 years of marriage, Tina became pregnant. The thought of gaining weight during her pregnancy upset Tina greatly, and she vowed to herself never to let herself become chubby again. Before long, Tina's physician noticed that she was not gaining weight at her monthly prenatal checkups and asked what she was eating. When she did a food log for the office nurse, her anorectic behavior was revealed.

A study by Easter et al. (2013) examined eating disorder diagnostic status and related symptoms in early pregnancy of 739 women. During pregnancy, 7.5% of women met diagnostic criteria for an eating disorder compared with a prepregnancy prevalence of 9.2%. About one fourth of women reported high weight and shape concerns during their pregnancy. Binge eating was endorsed by 8.7% of these women. This clinical example depicts the importance of an increased understanding of symptoms of eating disorders during pregnancy and for appropriate screening tools to be incorporated into antenatal care.

Because the intake of nutrients is so low in anorectic patients, their bodies try to adjust by using less energy. Consequently, other physiologic processes are affected. Hypotension, bradycardia, and hypothermia are common. The skin is often dry, and lanugo might appear. Many patients have delayed gastric emptying, causing them to feel full much longer than most people, and they do not have the normal desire to eat as often as others. They believe they can get by on one small meal a day. Slower abdominal peristalsis combined with decreased intake leads to constipation, which fuels the use of laxatives, leading to dehydration and giving the anorectic a false sense of decreased weight. Dehydration can lead to irreversible renal damage. Refeeding syndrome involving severe shifts in fluid and electrolyte levels from extracellular to intracellular spaces in severely emaciated patients can occur, causing cardiovascular, neurologic, and hematologic complications and death (Katzman, 2005). Refeeding must be done slowly and under very close supervision to prevent serious problems (Usdan et al., 2008). Pitting edema occurs in some anorectic patients, most often after attempts to gain weight by eating more food during the refeeding process while in treatment. Noticing the swelling, the patient often becomes anxious about the weight gain, immediately stops eating, and might attempt to counteract the perceived weight gain, further complicating the emaciated condition. In addition, osteopenia or osteoporosis might develop as a consequence of prolonged amenorrhea and malnutrition (Lock & Fitzpatrick, 2009; Muscari, 2002). Bone mass loss might be irreversible if the anorexia goes on long enough. Studies have found ventricular dilation, decreases in thickness of the left ventricular wall, alterations in the size of the cardiac chambers, and decreased myocardial oxygen uptake, which can lead to life-threatening cardiac arrhythmias (Bulik et al., 2005; Katzman, 2005).

Anorectic patients become preoccupied with food and eating (Bulik et al., 2005). This preoccupation involves all aspects of life. Patients are often found reading many materials on food and dieting and attempting to control family meals because they believe that they are the nutrition authorities in their household. Patients might engage in bizarre behavior regarding food and eating, such as hoarding food or preparing elaborate meals for others but not eating the food they prepare. Elaborate rituals before and during eating might become a compulsion, which adds to the patient's problems and might result in the patient being diagnosed with obsessive-compulsive disorder as well as anorexia (Kaye et al., 2004).

Subjective Symptoms

An outstanding feature of anorexia nervosa is the conscious fear that these patients have of losing control over the amount of food eaten, resulting in becoming fat. Patients are concerned about being obese, losing weight, or preventing weight gain. Some patients even say that they would rather be dead than fat. This fear motivates them to begin dieting. The fear might be triggered by an event that seems trivial to others, such as an offhand comment by a friend or relative or one or more traumatic events for the patient. These patients might feel abandoned or inadequate, which can precipitate an overall feeling of helplessness. They try to combat helplessness by controlling what they can control—how much food they eat and their weight. Much of the patient's energy becomes invested in this effort (Troop, 2012; Williamson et al., 2004).

In addition to problems with eating behavior and weight concern, anorectic individuals have other psychological symptoms known to be consequences of semistarvation. These patients exhibit depression, irritability, social withdrawal, lessened sex drive, and obsessional symptoms, which are also seen in research studies of starvation. It is believed that some of an anorectic's bizarre behavior might be the result of starvation (Finelli, 2001; Treasure et al., 2010). These

symptoms often diminish with weight gain, but if they do not, the patient might have a comorbid condition, such as obsessive-compulsive disorder, major depression, substance abuse, or a personality disorder (Ro et al., 2005).

Etiology

Bruch (1973) believed that anorexia was caused by many disturbances. Today, most experts agree that eating disorders have multifactorial causes, with significant variance among individuals (Kaye et al., 2000). Suggested contributing factors include biologic, sociocultural, family, cognitive, behavioral, and psychodynamic factors.

Biologic Factors

Earlier in the twentieth century, physiologic disturbances were postulated as causative in anorexia. Currently, researchers believe that the physiologic abnormalities found in anorectic patients are mostly a result of semistarvation and purging behavior rather than the cause of disordered eating. An exception might be increased serotonin levels. Studies have found that even after long-term weight restoration and recovery, anorectics have increased cerebrospinal fluid levels of 5-hydroxyindoleacetic acid, the major metabolite of serotonin (Kaye et al., 2005). However, the binding potential of the serotonin (5-HT) receptor 1A (5-HT1A) also is increased in individuals with eating disorders (Bailer et al., 2007; Galusca et al., 2008). Some studies met the sample size needed to obtain 80% power, suggesting that the 5-HT1D receptor gene is significantly associated with anorexia nervosa (Bergen et al., 2003; Brown et al., 2007; Kiezebrink et al., 2010), especially for the restricting type (Brown et al., 2007; Kiezebrink et al., 2010). The neuronal circuits that control the ingestion of food are mainly related to catecholaminergic, serotonergic, and peptidergic systems. Disturbances in the serotonin system contribute to vulnerability for restricted eating, behavioral inhibition, and a bias toward anxiety and error prediction, whereas disturbances in the dopamine system contribute to an altered response to reward (Kaye et al., 2009). The use of selective serotonin reuptake inhibitors (SSRIs), which regulate serotonin levels in depressed patients, has not been as effective in treating anorexia as in treating bulimia. Researchers such as Kaye and associates (2005) have suggested that the malnutrition of anorexia might negate the positive effects of SSRI medication in early treatment; if SSRIs are used to treat anorexia, they should not be started until weight restoration has been achieved.

Sociocultural Factors

Feminist theorists have highlighted the role of Western philosophical, political, and cultural history in the development of eating disorders. The increased incidence of eating disorders in the twentieth century has been recognized as corresponding to an increasingly and unrealistically thin beauty ideal for women—almost a culture of thinness (Bachner-Melman et al., 2009; Rand & Wright, 2000). In addition, American culture has advanced the notion that body weight is a matter of personal choice and that shape can be changed at will.

Computer imaging technology has resulted in the enhancement of photos on the Internet in response to the current societal standard of beauty. These images encourage dieting, which is a major predisposing factor to both anorexia nervosa and bulimia nervosa (White, 2000).

Another factor is the relational orientation of women, which creates a vulnerability to the opinions of others, particularly during adolescence (Andrist, 2003). American culture stresses the importance of physical attractiveness in obtaining approval; because of the thin beauty ideal, some girls believe that thinness leads to approval by others. Lack of approval is interpreted as being caused by a less than ideal body size, which causes girls, in particular, to begin dieting.

Family Factors

Several studies of identical and fraternal twins have suggested a genetic component to the etiology of anorexia (Dauncey, 2013; Kaye et al., 2008; Trace et al., 2013). Family environment might also play a role. Emotional restraint, enmeshed relationships, rigid organization in the family, tight control of child behavior by parents, and avoidance of conflict are other factors (Kaye et al., 2000). Odd eating habits and an emphasis on appearance and weight by other family members, especially mothers and sisters, have also been described (Mazzeo et al., 2005). However, the extent to which the observed family problems of anorectics are consequences of the disorder rather than etiologies is still undetermined. Preliminary evidence suggests that family-based treatment may be useful for younger patients with anorexia nervosa (Attia, 2009).

Cognitive and Behavioral Factors

Behavioral theorists have noted that anorectic behavior develops and is maintained as a function of environmental contingencies. Rejecting food and losing weight might be reinforced by positive attention from others (Finelli, 2001). The use of behavioral treatments such as assertiveness training and cognitive restructuring is based on such cognitive factors. A study by Ohlmer et al. (2013) examined the effectiveness of a prevention program for women at risk for anorexia nervosa. In the study, 36 women were selected by high weight and shape concerns, low BMI, or high restrained eating and participated in a 10-week, Internet-based cognitive behavior prevention program for anorexia nervosa. Although investigators suggested examining the usefulness of testing the program in a larger randomized controlled trial, 88% of the women completed the program, satisfaction with the program was high, and anorexia nervosa–specific eating and associated psychopathology improved significantly and differentially in three weight-related subgroups: low weight and normal weight, underweight, and binge eating.

Dahlgren et al. (2013) also conducted a feasibility study of cognitive remediation for adolescents with anorexia nervosa. Each participant received 7 to 12 sessions (average of 10 sessions) delivered twice weekly. The investigators found that the intervention appeared feasible for both inpatient and outpatient females as well as for clinicians delivering the therapy.

Psychodynamic Factors

Modern psychoanalytic theorists have stressed the role of sexuality in anorexia nervosa. In addition, some clinicians have suggested that eating disorders might be related to an early history of sexual abuse. Some research indicates that childhood sexual abuse seems to be related to increased body shame, which is a risk factor for eating disorders and self-mutilation (Wonderlich et al., 2001). Sexual abuse might predispose a person to psychiatric disorders in general, rather than to eating disorders in particular.

Some researchers have suggested that anorexia involves a regression to a prepubertal state, so that the adolescent does not mature physically or emotionally. Regression is reinforced when the anorectic adolescent's dependency needs are met. The conscious fear of becoming fat is thought to be the symbolic expression of becoming bigger, or growing up, supposedly the real unconscious fear of the anorectic. Other psychoanalytic theorists have suggested that the drive for thinness might be an attempt to reduce the control of an overcontrolling maternal figure (Stein & Corte, 2003).

Another theory has described anorexia nervosa as an obsession with weight stemming from a fear of being out of control because of the lack of a well-defined self. Patients use reaction formation to organize their lives with a set of rules and regulations for everything they do. They experience a tremendous amount of anxiety if their rules are broken and attempt to regain control by tightening the rules and punishing themselves for their failure (Stein & Corte, 2003).

Experts agree that the causes of anorexia nervosa are multifactorial. Biologic, sociocultural, family, cognitive, behavioral, and psychodynamic factors all might contribute to the disease. Factors contributing to the maintenance of anorexia might differ from factors leading to its development. Today, most research focuses on factors contributing to the onset of dieting (White, 2000). Greater emphasis on factors contributing to the development and maintenance of eating-disordered behavior might result in a better understanding of this disorder and more effective prevention of the disease. Research on adult-onset eating disorders might also prove fruitful because this phenomenon has been observed more frequently in recent years (Bulik et al., 2005).

❓ CRITICAL THINKING QUESTION

1. Some theorists contend that adolescent eating disorders are an expression of ambivalence toward becoming an adult. Explain how this might have some validity.

BULIMIA NERVOSA

DSM-5 Criteria

Bulimia nervosa is characterized by three behaviors: recurrent episodes of binge eating, continuing inappropriate compensatory behaviors to avoid weight gain, and an evaluation of self that is significantly influenced by body weight and shape. These behaviors must be present an average of at least once per week, for a minimum of 3 months (APA, 2013). Bulimia nervosa usually begins in adolescence or early adult life, primarily in women, although it has been diagnosed more often in men than in the past (Scagliusi et al., 2009). The prevalence of bulimia among adolescents and young women is thought to be approximately 1% to 2% of adolescents and 4% of young adults (Orbanic, 2001). The usual course of the disorder is chronic and intermittent over many years. Most commonly, the binge periods alternate with periods of restrictive eating, complicating the diagnosis and treatment (Orbanic, 2001).

Behavior

The word *bulimia* literally means to have an insatiable appetite. The term is often used to describe massive overeating and is used interchangeably with *binge eating* or *bingeing*. Until recently, bulimia nervosa was considered to be part of anorexia nervosa because almost half of patients with a diagnosis of anorexia were observed to have binge-eating episodes. Bulimia nervosa is now considered a separate disorder, although there is still much overlap between the disorders (Kaye et al., 2000). The true prevalence of bulimia nervosa is unknown because many patients hide their eating-disordered behaviors. In these patients, diagnosis of other more familiar psychiatric disorders, such as major depression, personality disorder, or posttraumatic stress disorder, may be made (Orbanic, 2001). Individuals who seek medical attention (usually for gastrointestinal or menstrual disturbances) could be identified as having bulimia, but the lack of weight loss might blind the treatment provider to the patient's bulimia (Orbanic, 2001).

The onset of the illness is usually between the ages of 15 and 24 years. The disease might develop after anorexia nervosa or after a period of dieting. The dieting predisposes the individual to binge eating, and purging develops as a means of compensating for calories ingested during the binge in an attempt to prevent weight gain. The individual continues restrictive eating during the disorder, which precipitates binge eating and then purging, perpetuating the cycle.

Clinical Example

Mary Franklin, age 28, was a young professional with an active social life. Although she was approximately 15 lb overweight, Mary used her sense of humor to hide any serious concern she had about her appearance. However, Mary worried that her weight might deny her a highly prized job that she wanted. Before applying for the job at a prestigious banking firm, Mary began dieting and ate less food than her friends did at lunch. However, when she arrived home, Mary felt hungry and secretly raided her refrigerator, making several sandwiches before dinner. Despite feeling guilty over her uncontrolled snacking, Mary ate dinner with her roommate. After dinner, feeling uncomfortably full, Mary retreated to the bathroom and vomited until she felt empty. She vowed to try harder to diet the next day, only to have a similar experience.

DSM-5 CRITERIA
for Bulimia Nervosa

A. Recurrent episodes of binge eating. An episode of binge eating is characterized by both of the following:
  1. Eating, in a discrete period of time (e.g., within any 2-hour period), an amount of food that is definitely larger than what most individuals would eat in a similar period of time under similar circumstances.
  2. A sense of lack of control over eating during the episode (e.g., feeling that one cannot stop eating or control what or how much one is eating).
B. Recurrent inappropriate compensatory behavior in order to prevent weight gain, such as self-induced vomiting; misuse of laxatives, diuretics or other medications; fasting; or excessive exercise.
C. The binge eating and inappropriate compensatory behaviors both occur, on average, at least once a week for 3 months.
D. Self-evaluation is unduly influenced by body shape and weight
E. The disturbance does not occur exclusively during episodes of anorexia nervosa.

Specify if:

In partial remission: After full criteria for bulimia nervosa were previously met, some, but not all, of the criteria have been met for a sustained period of time.

In full remission: After full criteria for bulimia nervosa were previously met, none of the criteria have been met for a sustained period of time.

Specify current severity:

The minimum level of severity is based on the frequency of inappropriate compensatory behaviors (see below). The level of severity may be increased to reflect other symptoms and the degree of functional disability.

Mild: An average of 1—3 episodes of inappropriate compensatory behaviors per week.

Moderate: An average of 4—7 episodes of inappropriate compensatory behaviors per week.

Severe: An average of 8—13 episodes of inappropriate compensatory behaviors per week.

Extreme: An average of 14 or more episodes of inappropriate compensatory behaviors per week.

From American Psychiatric Association. (2013). *Diagnostic and statistical manual of disorders* (5th ed.). Washington, DC: Author; (p. 345)

It is important to distinguish overeating from binge eating. To meet *DSM-V* diagnostic criteria for a binge episode, the eating behavior must qualify as an "objective bulimic episode." That is, the person consumes an unusually large amount of food in a relatively short period (e.g., several thousand calories in <2 hours). The amount of food eaten is considered by others to be atypically large for the particular situation. Additionally, there is a feeling of lack of control over eating during the binge (Orbanic, 2001).

Objective Signs

Most bulimic patients are secretive about their behavior. A variety of foods might be eaten during a binge, but the most common is high-calorie, high-carbohydrate "snack" food easily ingested in a short period. Some bulimics visit several different fast food restaurants or grocery stores during a binge so that no one knows how much they are eating at one time. Some patients with bulimia have been caught shoplifting food. Most binges occur during the evening or at night. The amount of calories consumed during a binge varies but is considerably more than the recommended daily allowance (Orbanic, 2001). There is a tendency to eat rapidly during the binge.

Patients report that their bulimic episodes usually end when they begin to induce vomiting, are physically exhausted, suffer from painful abdominal distention, are interrupted by others, or have run out of food. After a binge, patients promise themselves to adhere to a strict diet and vow never to binge again, only to return to this behavior because they find themselves addicted to the high they experience when bingeing. Many bulimics resume their usual schedules as if they had never been interrupted. The frequency of binges varies greatly, depending on the patient. Some patients report having several episodes a day; others report losing control two or three times a week (Orbanic, 2001).

Medical complications in bulimic patients depend on the form and frequency of purging and can include previously described mechanical irritation and dilation of the stomach resulting from binge eating. Fluid and electrolyte abnormalities might result from self-induced vomiting or abuse of laxatives or diuretics; these can include dehydration, hyponatremia, hypochloremia, hypokalemia, and metabolic alkalosis and acidosis. Self-induced vomiting and laxative abuse can cause mechanical irritation and injuries to the gastrointestinal tract. Abuse of laxatives, diuretics, and diet pills can result in addiction. Laxatives can lead to reflex constipation, and both laxatives and diuretics are associated with rebound edema (Orbanic, 2001).

Use of ipecac syrup to induce vomiting is dangerous and can cause fatal cardiomyopathy. Bulimics often have menstrual irregularities or enlarged salivary glands, particularly the parotid glands. Erosion of the dental enamel from chronic vomiting often occurs. Russell's sign, callusing of the knuckles of the fingers used to induce vomiting, is also common. Pancreatitis also has been reported in bulimics (Muscari, 2002).

Subjective Symptoms

Although most bulimic patients have a normal body weight, they are gravely concerned about their body shape and weight. Loss of control over eating causes them great anxiety and shame and, similar to anorectic patients, they express a fear of becoming fat (Orbanic, 2001).

Moods vary considerably among bulimic patients. Some bulimics have reported feeling weak before a binge, followed either by continued anxiety or relief from tension during the binge (Orbanic, 2001). Patients have reported feeling anxious, lonely, or bored or uncontrollably craving food before the binge. The anxiety present before the binge is replaced with guilt after the binge. If the anxiety is not relieved after

the binge, patients feel angry and agitated and might become depressed. Depression appears to be common in bulimic patients. The relationship between bulimia and depression might be one in which one causes the other, or there might be independent factors contributing to both disorders. Researchers have found a high rate of mood disorders, particularly depression, in families in which bulimia occurs (Keel et al., 2003). Substance abuse and anxiety disorders also occur at a higher than normal rate among bulimics. It appears that although pharmacotherapy can be helpful, it should be combined with psychotherapy for the most effective long-term outcome.

Most bulimic patients induce vomiting to reduce the fear of becoming fat. Patients might self-induce vomiting by sticking their fingers, a toothbrush, or an eating utensil down their throats; this is a dangerous practice because patients have swallowed objects used to induce vomiting. Over time, vomiting becomes easier and might require only slight abdominal pressure or no physical manipulation at the end of the binge (Mendell & Logemann, 2001). Some bulimics eat what is known as a *marker* food at the beginning of the binge and then vomit until this food comes back up. This practice is ineffective because food is quickly mixed in the stomach. Although bulimics believe that self-induced vomiting rids them of all binge calories, researchers have determined that only a partial amount of calories consumed can be regurgitated. Abuse of laxatives or diuretics primarily causes fluid loss rather than a reduction in absorbed calories (Orbanic, 2001). Other compensatory behavior might include the neglect of insulin requirements by patients with diabetes mellitus (Poirier-Solomon, 2001).

Etiology

Similar to anorexia, the causes of bulimia nervosa are thought to be multifactorial, with biologic, sociocultural, family, cognitive, behavioral, and psychodynamic contributing factors. Many of the factors thought to precipitate anorexia are also thought to be involved in bulimia. The focus of this discussion is on the proposed causes of bulimia that differ from the causes stated for anorexia.

Biologic Factors

Brain chemistry has been increasingly implicated in studies relating to the cause of eating disorders, with several neuroendocrine and neurotransmitter abnormalities demonstrated in dieters and in individuals demonstrating symptoms of eating disorders. Biologic and genetic factors have also been implicated in the causes of bulimia and anorexia. Most researchers believe that illness symptoms are related to the physiologic state of the victims and lessen when weight is restored. However, serotonin activity appears to be an exception. It has been proposed that, as in depression, there is generally lowered serotonin activity in the brains of bulimics (Kaye et al., 2000). Binge eating is seen by some as a form of self-medication to raise the levels of serotonin. Abnormalities in peripheral 5-HT uptake are observed in individuals with bulimia nervosa in both acute and recovery stages of illness

(Steiger et al., 2011), suggesting that these findings may be trait features rather than the outcome of abnormal eating patterns (Trace et al., 2013). Findings of near infrared spectroscopy reported by Sutoh et al. (2013) indicated that individuals with bulimia nervosa had decreased cognitive abilities and prefrontal hyperactivation patterns associated with self-regulatory functions, which correlated with their symptoms. These findings suggested inefficient prefrontal self-regulatory function of bulimia nervosa, which correlates with bulimia nervosa–associated symptoms. Treatment of bulimia with SSRI antidepressants, particularly fluoxetine (Prozac), appears to be helpful whether or not patients have comorbid depression, so it is unknown whether or not the antidepressant has a direct effect on the bulimia (Goldstein et al., 1999).

Sociocultural Factors

Sociocultural factors are thought to be the same as factors for anorexia nervosa, as noted earlier in this chapter.

Family Factors

As with anorexia nervosa, a heritable component for bulimia has been proposed. Twin studies have found a higher concordance rate for bulimia in identical than in fraternal twins (Trace et al., 2013). In addition, mood disorders and substance abuse disorders are found at a higher rate in the families of bulimics (Kaye et al., 2000), which might be a result of both biologic and environmental factors.

Families of bulimics are seen as having a great deal of conflict, being disorganized, lacking in nurturance, and not being cohesive (Kaye et al., 2000). Observations of family interactions have yielded similar data, lending credence to the idea that the bulimia might be a response to chaos in the family.

Cognitive and Behavioral Factors

Fairburn and colleagues pioneered work on cognitive behavioral theory for the maintenance of bulimia nervosa after its onset. According to this theory, bulimia nervosa is maintained by cycles of low self-esteem, extreme concerns about body shape and weight, strict dieting, binge eating, and compensatory behavior, which interact and affect each other. Bulimia is maintained by the behaviors of dieting, bingeing, and purging, which are both affected by and contribute to distorted and negative cognitions about the self and the body (Williamson et al., 2004). This theory has led to the development of successful cognitive behavior therapy programs for bulimia nervosa that target both eating-disordered behaviors and cognitions (Bakke et al., 2001; O'Dea & Abraham, 2000). The role of binge eating in decreased self-awareness and how restriction can reduce emotional awareness are incorporated into these contemporary cognitive therapy models of eating disorders (Fox, 2009). Cognitive behavior therapy for the treatment of bulimia nervosa was supported in a review of 48 studies using this therapy.

In a review of 106 meta-analyses regarding the efficacy of cognitive behavior therapy, the strongest support was found for bulimia and some other disorders (e.g., anxiety disorders, anger control problems), although future research concerning randomized controlled trials and using other subgroups, such as ethnic minorities and low-income samples, was recommended (Hofmann et al., 2012). McClay et al. (2013) also examined patients' experiences using an online self-help cognitive behavior therapy package (Overcoming Bulimia Online) for bulimia nervosa and eating disorders not otherwise specified (NOS). Eight participants participated in semistructured interviews about the program and indicated that overall the online cognitive behavior therapy self-help was generally a desirable and acceptable treatment option. In reviewing technology use within the treatment of eating disorders over 11 years (2002-2012), Shingleton et al. (2013) found that technology (e.g., televideo, e-mail, CD-ROM, Internet, text messaging) may be successfully integrated within eating disorder treatment and may offer new ways to extend interventions to individuals who otherwise may not have access to specialty care for eating disorders. Other psychotherapies were also efficacious, particularly psychotherapy in the longer term, although psychotherapy alone is unlikely to reduce or change body weight in people with bulimia nervosa or similar eating disorders (Hay et al., 2009).

Psychodynamic Factors

Some psychodynamic theorists have placed particular emphasis on ambivalent feelings of self-esteem in bulimics. The binge eating and purging behavior is thought to express the ambivalence that patients feel toward themselves. On the one hand, patients believe that they are worthy of the nurturing they lack, and because food is a symbolic form of nurturing they binge. On the other hand, patients feel unworthy of nurturing, so they purge. Bingeing and purging can also be seen as patients' attempts to numb themselves from the pain in their lives resulting from abuse, neglect, trauma, and strong feelings (Orbanic, 2001).

PUTTING IT ALL TOGETHER
PSYCHOTHERAPEUTIC MANAGEMENT

Psychotherapeutic management for anorexia and bulimia shares many characteristics and has some differences. In this section, the commonalities and differences are highlighted. The psychotherapeutic management of each disorder varies, depending on the period of treatment being considered and whether the focus is on short-term or long-term treatment. For example, when an anorectic patient is hospitalized because of extreme weight loss and its life-threatening physical effects, the focus must be on weight restoration before any treatment dealing with changing the patient's perceptions about his or her body or any long-term goals can be addressed.

COMPARING ANOREXIA AND BULIMIA

Shared Features
Restriction of intake at times, especially anorectics
Bingeing or overeating at times, especially bulimics
Purging through vomiting, laxatives, or diuretics
Overexercise
Extreme concern about appearance
Perfectionistic traits—dissatisfaction with appearance and performance in aspects of life such as work or school
Belief that self-worth is based solely on appearance
Discomfort in social settings, especially with the opposite gender
Misperception of body size, shape, and level of fat
Low self-esteem

Differentiation of Behaviors

ANOREXIA	BULIMIA
Early onset	Later onset
Very low weight	More normal weight
Hormonal imbalance	Fluid and electrolyte imbalance
Constipation if not using laxatives	Gastrointestinal problems related to bingeing and purging

Management of anorexia is geared toward three primary objectives: (1) increasing weight to at least 90% of the average body weight for the patient's height; (2) helping patients reestablish appropriate eating behavior; and (3) increasing self-esteem, so patients do not need to attain the perfection that they believe thinness provides. The objectives for bulimics are similar but, rather than the need for weight increase, are more likely to focus on stabilizing weight without purging because bulimics are more likely to be of normal weight.

When patients are in the starvation phase of anorexia and malnutrition has become a serious medical problem, treatment occurs in a medical environment in which appropriate supplies and equipment, such as intravenous lines and feeding tubes, are readily available for feeding the patient if he or she will not eat voluntarily. Refeeding and weight restoration in anorexia must be done slowly and carefully, with close monitoring by experts to avoid life-threatening physical complications and possible death. Medical stabilization of the patient is the initial treatment goal. After medical stabilization, psychotherapy is the treatment of choice (Castro et al., 2004). When medical crises are resolved, patients are transferred to a psychiatric unit or are seen in an outpatient program, in which effective psychotherapeutic intervention can occur.

Cognitive behavior therapy has the greatest research support, especially for people with bulimia (National Collaborating Centre for Mental Health, 2004). The results of the highlighted study by Fairburn and colleagues (2009) represent a significant advance in knowledge about the treatment of eating disorders with cognitive behavior therapy because it demonstrates the efficacy of a manual-based treatment for a more heterogeneous sample than in previous studies (Crow & Peterson, 2009). Limited evidence also exists

suggesting that interpersonal psychotherapy might have similar effectiveness (McIntosh et al., 2000). Pharmacotherapy is used as an adjunct to psychotherapy for bulimics, when indicated (Nakash-Eisikovits et al., 2002).

Nurses might encounter anorectic or bulimic patients on an inpatient basis in a medical or psychiatric unit or on an outpatient basis in a physician's office, clinic, or school. Bulimics are less likely to be encountered in inpatient settings unless their purging has led to medical complications, but these individuals should be hospitalized in the following circumstances: (1) to treat a psychiatric or medical crisis, (2) when respite is needed from a chaotic home life so that the bulimic patient can examine his or her living situation more objectively, and (3) if the patient cannot obtain treatment in his or her home community. In any setting, a multidisciplinary treatment approach is crucial. Members of the treatment team should include a physician, nurse, dietitian, and psychotherapist specializing in the treatment of eating disorders. These patients need thorough medical and psychiatric assessment, medical monitoring, nutritional education and counseling, and psychotherapy (Stewart & Williamson, 2004). Assessment should include use of instruments from self-reporting to more structured interview tools as well as differential diagnosis of other psychiatric conditions, including affective disorders, personality disorders, anxiety disorders such as obsessive-compulsive disorders, and substance abuse or dependence (Pike, 2005).

Empirical evidence for the effectiveness of family therapy for adolescent anorexia nervosa is gaining strength (Cook-Darzens et al., 2008). See the accompanying Highlighting the Evidence boxes; the first three studies highlight family therapy, and the remaining two studies contrast the value of cognitive behavior therapy and limitations of therapy with bulimia nervosa.

HIGHLIGHTING THE EVIDENCE

Comparison of Family Therapy and Family Group Psychoeducation in Adolescents with Anorexia Nervosa

Description: This study, completed in the late 1990s at an eating disorders program in Toronto, Canada, compared 4 months of family therapy with a psychiatrist and two social workers with 4 months of family psychoeducation with an occupational therapist, dietitian, and registered nurse. A group of 25 adolescent girls meeting *DSM-IV-TR* criteria for anorexia and admitted to the hospital needing treatment for weight restoration met the criteria for the study and were randomly placed in the family therapy or family psychoeducation group. The study was undertaken to determine which of the two treatment methods was more effective.

Results: In both groups, weight restoration (from 77% to 96% of ideal body weight) was achieved for most patients. Hospital length of stay was also similar for both groups. Both groups acknowledged more family pathology at the end of treatment than at the beginning. There appeared to be no significant difference between the treatment modalities, although family group psychoeducation was less expensive than family therapy.

Implications: Because family group psychoeducation is a less expensive and more easily administered treatment, in part owing to the type of personnel needed to present the program, it might be a more effective treatment in situations in which costs of care are severely constrained.

Modified from Geist, R., et al. (2000). Comparison of family therapy and family group psychoeducation in adolescents with anorexia nervosa. *Canadian Journal of Psychiatry, 45,* 173.

HIGHLIGHTING THE EVIDENCE

Comparison of Acceptance and Commitment Therapy with Treatment-as-Usual for Eating Disorders

Description: This study compared acceptance and commitment therapy (ACT) with treatment-as-usual (TAU) groups at a residential treatment facility for eating disorders. A group of 140 participants with either anorexia nervosa or bulimia nervosa were randomly assigned using three sequential phases (TAU, ACT, TAU), so that half of the participants received ACT plus TAU, whereas the other half received TAU alone. The study was undertaken to determine which of the two treatment methods was more effective.

Results: There appeared to be no significant difference between the treatment modalities, although there were trends toward larger decreases in eating pathology in the ACT group.

Implications: Overall, results suggest that ACT might be a valuable treatment option for individuals with eating disorders and warrants further research.

Modified from Juarascio, A., et al. (2013). Acceptance and commitment therapy as a novel treatment for eating disorders: an initial test of efficacy and mediation. *Behavior Modification, 37,* 459.

HIGHLIGHTING THE EVIDENCE

Early Response to Family-Based Treatment for Adolescent Anorexia Nervosa

Description: This study examined whether early weight gain predicted remission at the end of treatment in a clinic sample of 65 adolescents (mean age, 14.9 years; standard deviation, 2.1) with anorexia nervosa who received a course of family-based treatment (FBT). The treatment was manual-based. The study used two sites (Chicago, n = 45; Columbia, n = 20). Response to treatment was assessed using percent ideal body weight (IBW) with remission defined as having achieved 95% or greater IBW at end of treatment (session 20).

Results: A weight gain of at least 2.88% in IBW by session 4 best predicted remission at the end of treatment (area under the curve = 0.674; $p = 0.024$).

Implications: Results suggest that adolescents with anorexia nervosa receiving family-based therapy who do not show early weight gain are unlikely to experience remission at the end of treatment.

Modified from Doyle, P.M., et al. (2009). Early response to family-based treatment for adolescent anorexia nervosa. *International Journal of Eating Disorders, 43,* 659.

HIGHLIGHTING THE EVIDENCE

Comparison of Two Cognitive Behavioral Treatments for Outpatients with Eating Disorders

Description: This study compared two cognitive behavioral treatments for outpatients with eating disorders. One was a focused form of cognitive behavior therapy that concentrated on eating-related psychopathology, and the other was a more complex form of cognitive behavior therapy that used several treatment sessions to address mood intolerance, clinical perfectionism, low self-esteem, or interpersonal difficulties. A group of 154 patients with bulimia nervosa or an eating disorder NOS and BMI greater than 17.5 were enrolled in a two-site randomized controlled trial involving 20 weeks of treatment and a 60-week follow-up. The control condition was an 8-week waiting list period preceding treatment.

Results: Patients in the waiting list control condition showed little change in their clinical status, whereas patients in the two treatment conditions exhibited substantial differences in symptom severity, which were well maintained during follow-up. At the 60-week follow-up assessment, more than half of the sample had a level of eating disorder features less than 1 standard deviation above the community mean. Treatment outcome did not depend on eating disorder diagnosis. Patients with marked mood intolerance, clinical perfectionism, low self-esteem, or interpersonal difficulties appeared to respond better to the more complex treatment, with the reverse pattern evident among the remaining patients.

Implications: Both transdiagnostic treatments appear to be suitable for most outpatients with an eating disorder, with the more complex treatment reserved for patients with marked additional psychopathology (e.g., marked mood intolerance, clinical perfectionism, low self-esteem, or interpersonal difficulties).

Modified from Fairburn, C.G., et al. (2009). Transdiagnostic cognitive-behavioral therapy for patients with eating disorders: a two-site trial with 60-week follow-up. *American Journal of Psychiatry, 166,* 311.

HIGHLIGHTING THE EVIDENCE

Outcomes of Bulimia Nervosa

Description: In this analysis, 79 studies using 5653 patients suffering from bulimia nervosa were analyzed with regard to recovery, improvement, chronicity, crossover to another eating disorder, mortality, and comorbid psychiatric disorders. Forty-nine studies dealt with prognosis only, and prognostic factors were based on 4639 patients.

Results: Using 27 studies examining recovery, improvement, and chronicity, close to 45% of the patients on average showed full recovery of bulimia nervosa, whereas 27% on average improved considerably and nearly 23% on average had a chronic protracted course. Patients with crossover diagnoses for another eating disorder at the follow-up evaluation amounted to over 20%. The crude mortality rate was 0.32%, and other psychiatric disorders at outcome were very common. For most prognostic factors, there was only conflicting evidence.

Implications: One-quarter of a century of specific research in bulimia nervosa shows that the disorder still has an unsatisfactory outcome in many patients. More refined interventions may contribute to more favorable outcomes in the future.

Modified from Steinhausen, H.C., & Weber, S. (2009). The outcome of bulimia nervosa: findings from one-quarter century of research. *American Journal of Psychiatry, 166,* 1331.

Treatment for comorbid diagnoses with psychotherapy and medication enhances the success of treatment for the eating disorder. Premorbid physical conditions that should be ruled out include thyroid conditions, bowel disease or other gastrointestinal conditions, pancreatitis, cancer, or the effects of medications. If eating behaviors are caused by one of these conditions, therapeutic effectiveness involves different treatments than if the eating behaviors were solely the result of an eating disorder. Patients with diabetes might also develop eating disorders, increasing their risk of serious medical complications of diabetes in the future and the risk of ketoacidosis in the present (Poirier-Solomon, 2001).

Working with anorectic or bulimic patients presents a challenge to the psychotherapeutic team as patients continue their struggle to maintain control. When the treatment team requires weight gain or an end to bingeing and purging, patients perceive themselves as losing control, which triggers unconscious feelings of helplessness and resistance to treatment goals and interventions. Consciously, patients again experience the fear of becoming fat. This fear underlies the need to gain more control, restarting the vicious cycle of disordered eating. Nurses need to confront this fear openly and help patients to find ways to deal with it (Cummings et al., 2001). See the Tips for Professionals and Families from Persons Recovering from Eating Disorders box and the Key Nursing Interventions for Patients with Eating Disorders box.

Nurse-Patient Relationship

Because most anorectic patients have been forced into treatment by concerned family or friends, developing a therapeutic alliance is a challenge. Patients might believe that the nurse's purpose is simply to make them gain weight, so the nurse is perceived as an enemy, not an ally. Bulimic patients differ from anorectic patients in that bulimics are more likely to want help. They are more likely to enter therapy of their own volition, are eager to please, and so behave in a manner that will lead therapists to like them. However, in trying to please, bulimic patients have a tendency to become manipulative and might conceal the full extent of their problem. The desire to be helped is the greatest strength of bulimic patients. See Chapter 9 for general information about communicating with patients and developing rapport and trust with patients.

Psychopharmacology

No psychopharmacologic agent is approved specifically for anorexia nervosa at the present time. Medication management of anxiety, depression, somatic disturbances, or other comorbid conditions is appropriate and might assist in treatment of the patient's anorexia. Small amounts of anxiolytics might help patients with eating if given just before meals when refeeding is occurring. Anxiolytics can also be used to decrease the anxiety that fuels bingeing and purging in a bulimic patient, although antidepressants are a safer, more effective way to achieve that end. Long-term use of anxiolytics

TIPS FOR PROFESSIONALS AND FAMILIES FROM PERSONS RECOVERING FROM EATING DISORDERS

Be wary of rigidly applying *DSM* criteria in the detection of eating disorders.

* Some patients never binge or purge but control weight with exercise and restriction of intake.
* Some patients do not stop menstruating, although there might be changes in their cycles.
* Depression, anxiety, neglect, and domestic violence might predispose patients to eating disorders or be seen concurrently with them. If only these conditions or problems are addressed without treating the eating disorder, efforts are likely to fail.
* Patients' concentration on exactness and perfection might lead them to deny their illness by rationalizing that if they do not exhibit *all* the criteria of the disorder, they do not have the disorder.
* Patients might recognize that their body image is distorted but might be unable to stop their destructive behavior.
* Not all patients with eating disorders have rituals about eating. They might simply avoid being in situations in which they have to eat in front of others.

When educating adolescents about eating disorders, avoid using films or other graphic materials that might teach the teens more ways to beat the system regarding eating and maintaining healthy weight.

Dishonesty (lying to self and others) is a hallmark of patients with eating disorders. Honesty toward self and others is the key to recovery and relapse prevention.

Watch for the onset of eating disorders at times of major life transition with increased pressure on an individual to fit in or adjust. These times include the move to middle school from elementary school, to high school from junior high or middle school, and graduation from high school with the move to college or a job.

Patients with eating disorders believe that calories are everywhere and go to great lengths to avoid them, including not smelling food or licking stamps for fear calories will be absorbed.

Media images of very thin models and celebrities might be viewed by very young girls as an ideal to be achieved, but most patients use media images of thinness to justify their behavior after the start of the eating disorder rather than motivation to begin their disordered eating.

The author acknowledges the sharing of a local chapter of the Anorexia and Associated Disorders Association of Indianapolis support group in 2000, whose members offered their experience and information to help professionals deal with individuals such as themselves.

KEY NURSING INTERVENTIONS
for Patients with Eating Disorders

- Monitor daily caloric intake and electrolyte status while in the hospital; patients should not gain too much weight too quickly.
- Observe patients for signs of purging or other compensation for food consumed.
- Monitor activity level, and encourage appropriate levels of activity for patient.
- Weigh daily while in the hospital, but encourage patient to diminish focus on weight after refeeding.
- Plan for a dietitian to meet with patients and families to (1) provide accurate information on nutrition, (2) discuss a realistic and healthy diet, and (3) assist the nurses in monitoring the nutritional intake of the patient (particularly crucial for patients who are diabetic or pregnant).
- Encourage use of therapies or support groups to attain healthy weight and prevent relapse.
- Promote patient decision making concerning issues other than food.
- Promote positive self-concept and perceptions of body as well as interactions with others.
- Convey warmth and sincerity. Patients must believe that the nurse genuinely understands and cares about their concerns and efforts to overcome their ambivalence about treatment (Sloan, 1999).
- Listen empathically. Although anorectic patients are likely to deny that weight is a problem, they do admit being lonely and tired of compulsively striving to meet unreachable goals. Bulimics are more likely to admit their problems with weight but still feel helpless in addressing them (Muscari, 2002; Sloan, 1999).
- Be honest. Patients enter treatment distrustful of everyone. Honesty is essential to developing a trusting relationship with any patient with an eating disorder.
- Set appropriate behavioral limits. Because of control needs, patients are likely to attempt to manipulate the nurse. A clear contract between the nurse and patient helps establish trust and minimize power struggles.
- Assist patients in identifying their positive qualities. Because self-esteem is low, patients need to see concrete evidence of their positive qualities. Improving patients' self-worth is a primary objective in recovery (Sloan, 1999).
- Collaborate with patients. To elicit cooperation, engage patients in planning to foster trust and a sense of control, which will diminish their need to maintain control through disordered eating (Sloan, 1999).
- Teach patients about their disorders. Providing accurate information about eating disorders should decrease denial and help patients understand the effects of the disease on their bodies and minds (Sloan, 1999).
- Determine the anorectic's ability to be weighed in the early stages of treatment. Often, anorectics need to be weighed with their backs to the scale to help reduce their focus on body weight.
- Initiate a behavior modification program with patient input that rewards weight gain or lack of purging with meaningful privileges or rewards. Although the idea of gaining weight is stressful to patients, it is crucial to recovery. When a safe weight is attained, allow patients more control of their own progress and program as long as they do not backslide. Patients must eventually take control of maintaining a safe weight.
- Model and teach appropriate social skills. Acquiring social skills, particularly expressing emotions assertively, is crucial for patients with eating disorders. Encourage patients to examine their interpersonal relationships and work to decrease their loneliness.
- Help patients identify and express bodily sensations and feelings related to their disorders. Anorectic patients have little bodily awareness other than a distorted perception of their size (Sloan, 1999).
- Identify non–weight-related interests of the patient. Involvement with these interests can reduce anxiety as patients invest their energies in areas not related to eating. Encourage the development of new hobbies and interests that are not food-related.

can lead to medication dependence, adding to the patient's problems. The atypical antipsychotic olanzapine (Zyprexa) has been tried to promote weight gain with some success, but it is unclear whether the weight gain is a result of the medication's tendency to cause weight gain or its effect on disturbed thought content and process, such as that experienced by anorectic patients (Attia & Schroeder, 2005).

Other Treatments

There has been initial investigation using the virtual environment for normalizing eating patterns in eating disorders. In a study comprising 22 patients with eating disorders and 37 individuals with healthy eating patterns, Perpiñá et al. (2013) examined the clinical validation of a virtual reality environment developed to normalize eating patterns. Compared with subjects with healthy eating patterns, subjects with eating disorders paid more attention and had greater emotional involvement and dysphoria when eating a virtual

pizza, suggesting that the virtual environment may be a useful therapy tool for normalizing eating patterns in these patients. Similarly, Marco et al. (2013) did a controlled study of 34 individuals comparing cognitive behavior therapy for eating disorders with and without a component for body image treatment using virtual reality techniques. Patients who received the component for body image treatment improved more than the group without this component.

The safety of deep brain stimulation (DBS) has been explored more recently for treatment of treatment-refractory anorexia nervosa. This disorder has one of the highest mortality rates of any psychiatric disorder. In a review of literature regarding treatment and management of patients with eating disorders who fail to change over prolonged periods of time, Wonderlich et al. (2012) indicated that treatments for these individuals are not based on evidence-based findings, but rather there is a lack of standardized treatment approaches and consistent definitions of chronicity for this population.

These investigators emphasized the need for an integrative and practical clinical protocol for these patients.

In a phase 1 trial, Lipsman et al. (2013) performed subcallosal cingulate DBS in six patients with severe and enduring treatment-refractory anorexia nervosa. Patients were followed for 9 months after DBS activation. DBS was associated with a seizure in one patient, within the context of a serious, illness-related metabolic problem. Other adverse events also occurred (i.e., panic attack, air embolus) intraoperatively, which were managed. Improved mood, anxiety, affective regulation, and anorexia nervosa–related obsessions and compulsions occurred in four patients, with improvements in quality of life in three patients after 6 months of stimulation. The usefulness of this intervention for treatment-refractory anorexia nervosa is pending, subsequent to further research.

Treatment with antidepressants, especially SSRIs, has proved helpful in reducing bingeing, purging, and depression in bulimic patients (Nakash-Eisikovits et al., 2002). These drugs have been shown to have a positive effect on associated mood disturbances and preoccupation with shape and weight. Antidepressants appear to be equally effective in both depressed and nondepressed patients with bulimia nervosa. These results suggest that the mechanism of the drug action might not be the antidepressant, but rather the drug might have direct central effects on neurotransmitter systems, particularly serotonin and norepinephrine. However, although antidepressants have beneficial effects in the short term, this improvement does not appear to be maintained over the long term (Nakash-Eisikovits et al., 2002). Generally, psychotherapy is recommended before a trial of an antidepressant. Antidepressants are considered when the patient has failed to respond adequately to psychotherapy alone or when there is comorbidity with severe clinical depression.

Milieu Management

- Provide an orientation to the setting to prepare the patient for inpatient or outpatient treatment so that fears are reduced.
- Provide a warm, nurturing atmosphere. It is important for patients to feel support to reduce anxiety and increase trust.
- Closely observe patients. Avoidance behaviors should be identified to plan appropriate interventions. Common behaviors include hiding food in a paper napkin to be discarded later, leaving bread crusts on the plate and discarding the rest, discarding food into plants or out the window, spilling food while eating so it cannot be determined how much the patient really ate, and holding food in the mouth to be discarded when the patient brushes his or her teeth. Respond to such behaviors with nonjudgmental confrontation, conveying understanding of weight gain fears.
- Encourage the patient to approach a team member if feeling the need to purge. Expression of feelings reduces anxiety and helps patients discover alternatives to restricting food or vomiting.
- Involve the patient's family in treatment, when appropriate. If the family denies the problem or is not supportive

of treatment, the family might need to be temporarily excluded from the treatment team. If parents, particularly of minors, provide emotional support, treatment efforts have a greater chance of success. Families must understand the disorder and its treatment. Family therapy and family education are crucial components for helping adolescents with eating disorders in both short-term and long-term treatment (Geist et al., 2000; Melrose, 2000).

- Respond with consistency. The behavioral program or treatment regimen implemented must be constantly adhered to by the entire staff to diminish patient manipulation and avoid sabotage of treatment.
- Encourage participation in art, recreation, and other types of therapy. These modalities teach patients alternative ways to express their feelings and provide activities other than focusing on food and dieting.
- Involve a dietitian in the treatment plan who can teach proper nutrition while providing patients with an opportunity to select menus. Increase caloric intake gradually to increase patient cooperation in the weight gain program, maintain patient safety, and avoid the medical risks in adding weight too quickly. Encourage compliance with planned schedules for meals and snacks. Regularization of eating prevents the precipitation of binge eating resulting from dieting or restrictive eating practices. Encourage all patients to follow the advice of dietitians regarding normalization of eating (Stewart & Williamson, 2004).
- Encourage patient attendance at group therapy sessions. Providing an opportunity for patients to participate in a group with peers helps them see that they are not alone in having difficulty expressing feelings and dealing with developmental issues. Nurse-led support groups encourage patients to share issues, feelings, and fears (Muscari, 2002).
- Recommend follow-up psychotherapeutic groups and support groups for patients and their families and individual psychotherapy for patients with a qualified therapist. These sessions are particularly beneficial after significant weight gain and after discharge from a treatment program (Castro et al., 2004). Patients might relapse or die because of lack of appropriate outpatient follow-up or might attempt suicide (Pompli et al., 2004). A comprehensive continuum of care provides the best option for relapse prevention in view of the chronic nature of the disease (Cummings et al., 2001).

Treatment in various settings from outpatient to day treatment and inpatient treatment for the most physically compromised patients has been attempted, but research has not shown any clear difference in results related to the treatment setting (Fairburn, 2005). A stepped care approach might be useful, in which patients first participate in a simple treatment, such as guided self-help or a psychoeducational group with their families, and then, if they do not respond, are referred for cognitive behavior therapy. Group therapies usually address issues such as social skills training, social anxiety, and body image distortion (Halmi, 2009). Patients who do not improve with therapy can be referred for a more intensive form of treatment, such as interpersonal psychotherapy, partial or full hospitalization, and possibly antidepressant medication.

CASE STUDY

Sarah Hodge, a 17-year-old girl, was brought to the hospital by her parents and outpatient therapist, whom she had been seeing weekly for 1 month. Sarah and the therapist had a contract of a 2-lb weight gain every week, but Sarah had continued to lose weight. On admission, she was 5 feet 5 inches tall and weighed 86 lb. Sarah strongly opposed her hospitalization and denied she had a problem.

Sarah is the youngest of three daughters, ages 27, 24, and 17, a late addition to her middle-class family. Sarah's parents admitted that she had been steadily losing weight for the last 6 months. At first, Sarah's parents believed that she was just dieting, but when they began to see her ribs and vertebrae through her nightgown, they became gravely concerned.

Sarah was recently named recipient of a college scholarship. She has been active in school activities and was well-liked by her teachers because of her hard work. Although she appeared to have many friends, Sarah claimed that she had only one real friend, another anorectic.

Sarah said her obsession with weight began approximately 6 months ago, when the family went to visit the oldest daughter, whom Sarah idolized. One afternoon, the three sisters went berry picking, and the oldest daughter told Sarah, "Don't eat all the berries, or you'll grow into a real chub!" Sarah interpreted this to mean that her sister thought she was fat. She became obsessed with food and became a vegetarian. She adopted the role of planning menus and educating the family on proper nutrition. When her mother attempted to intervene, Sarah screamed that she knew what she was doing and was tired of being treated like a baby. If her mother attempted further control over Sarah's eating behavior, Sarah refused to eat at all. The situation at home deteriorated until there was little communication between family members and Sarah. She engaged in irrational rituals and lost 30 lb. When Sarah began to look very thin, they persuaded her to seek help, although she continued to lose weight during outpatient therapy.

Sarah is a likable girl. The other adolescents in the hospital were attracted to her and wanted to be her friend. However, they noticed Sarah's odd eating habits, such as mixing cornflakes in vanilla pudding and pouring cranberry juice over cereals. At first, she resisted eating meals and snacks, but she complied when faced with tube feeding to replace what she refused to eat. Sarah always dressed in baggy overalls and wore oversized sweaters. When other patients asked Sarah if she felt cold, she quietly told them that she did not want them to stare at her fat body, a comment that tended to put off her peers.

During break times, Sarah was found writing morbid poetry, which contained subtle suicidal messages. She preferred to be alone and became irritable and rude when asked to participate in group therapy sessions. Sarah tried to be as compliant as she thought others wanted her to be; however, the lack of control she experienced in the hospital added to her anxiety and discomfort and fueled her denial that she had a problem.

◎ CARE PLAN

Name: Sarah Hodge.   **Admission Date:** _____

DSM-5 Diagnosis: Anorexia nervosa

Assessment	**Areas of strength:** Intelligence; past achievements; likableness; past healthy interpersonal relationships; good personal hygiene; some insight into reasons for hospitalization; family support.
	Problems: Low weight, disturbed body image, low self-esteem, depression, lack of accurate knowledge regarding nutrition, manipulative behavior.
Diagnoses	Imbalanced nutrition; less than body requirements, related to not eating enough nutrients, as evidenced by continued weight loss and inappropriate eating habits
	Disturbance in body image, related to feeling fat when actually underweight, as evidenced by inappropriate dress and comments about how fat she is
	Disturbance in self-esteem, related to fear of becoming fat and repulsive, as evidenced by suicidal messages in poetry and by social withdrawal
	Knowledge deficit in proper nutrition, related to fear of being fat, as evidenced by odd eating habits and refusal to eat certain foods
Outcomes	**Short-term goals**
Date met: _____	Patient will gain 1 lb per week.
Date met: _____	Patient will identify two positive qualities about herself.
Date met: _____	Patient will discuss fears of losing control.
	Long-term goals
Date met: _____	Patient will gain at least 20 lb within 6 months.
Date met: _____	Patient will verbalize knowledge of illness and proper nutrition.
Date met: _____	Patient will identify at least three alternative coping mechanisms to use when feeling out of control.
Date met: _____	Patient will verbalize increased comfort in relating to peers.
Planning and Interventions	**Nurse-patient relationship:** Establish a contract to meet with the patient daily to discuss feelings; express concern for the patient; encourage verbalization of feelings about depression and lack of control; encourage patient to identify positive qualities about herself.

CARE PLAN—CONT'D

	Milieu management: Encourage patient to attend meals and sit with peers; encourage participation in group therapy to discuss feelings with peers; encourage patient to share positive qualities of herself with peers; maintain consistency of unit rules, and ensure that patient is adhering to them.
Evaluation	Patient gained 2 lb in the first 10 days of hospitalization; attended all unit activities; attended individual therapy with nurse therapist, and stated one positive thing about herself.
Referrals	Patient has been given information about an eating disorder support group in her community and a person to contact regarding group attendance after discharge.

EATING DISORDERS IN MEN

The incidence of eating disorders among men is currently 11% of the population with eating disorders (Agency for Healthcare Research and Quality, 2009), with speculation that this figure might increase as men become more comfortable seeking treatment (Ray, 2004). Although 9 out of 10 cases of eating disorders were women, cases in men increased by 53% (Agency for Healthcare Research and Quality, 2011). Identification of men with partial and full syndromes of eating disorders has increased the numbers of men with eating disorders. Although diagnoses, etiologies, and treatment of men and women with eating disorders are similar, there appear to be differences in onset, presentation, and assessment. Men are more likely than women with eating disorders to have a history of obesity before the onset of symptoms of an eating disorder and to have a later onset and higher initial BMI before engaging in disordered eating. Men also tend to feel less guilt than women about episodes of bingeing and purging. Comorbidity with other psychiatric disorders is higher in men than in women with eating disorders (Woodside et al., 2001). Dieting or bingeing is more often related to a desire to build a lean body for participation in sports, such as competing in a lower weight class in wrestling (Ray, 2004).

Although controversial, some research has shown that male patients with eating disorders exhibit a higher frequency of concerns about gender or sexual identity, homosexual orientation, and asexuality (Austin et al., 2009; Ray, 2004). Although some men with eating disorders have a homosexual orientation, this is still a minority of cases. Sexual orientation might represent a risk factor for eating disorders because homosexual men might place particular emphasis on physical attractiveness (Ray, 2004).

Treatment for men with eating disorders is similar to that for women. From a psychotherapeutic management standpoint, the following three areas need particular focus with men:
1. The excessive attention that adolescent boys can place on attaining a masculine physique and its effect on their body image
2. Dietary habits to promote health, fitness, and muscle mass without using disordered eating patterns
3. The expression of feelings and the exploration of any underlying sexual identity concerns

Although most adolescents with eating disorders have difficulty expressing their feelings, boys seem to have more difficulty than girls. A therapeutic relationship can be especially instrumental in the recovery of these young men (Ray, 2004).

> **? CRITICAL THINKING QUESTION**
>
> 2. A 17-year-old boy remarks to you that he feels too fat and is afraid that he will not be able to "make weight" for wrestling. You do not observe that the patient is overweight. How do you begin to assess whether the patient has an eating disorder?

BINGE-EATING DISORDER

DSM-5 lists binge-eating disorder (BED) as a condition that has not met diagnostic criteria for inclusion in *DSM-5* but might warrant further research and study. BED shares many criteria of bulimia nervosa (lack of control over intake, patient distress, and guilt over bingeing) but without the regular compensation for excess intake through purging, laxatives, fasting, or overexercise. As a consequence, individuals with BED tend to be overweight to a moderate or greater degree, and their weight tends to fluctuate more compared with individuals with anorexia or bulimia. As with bulimia, the onset of this disorder tends to be later than in anorexia, generally beginning in late adolescence to early adulthood. These patients are given a diagnosis of eating disorder NOS, with the notation that the patient's symptoms meet the research criteria for BED. Empirical data suggest that familial and genetic factors influence the risk of this disorder (Javaras et al., 2008; Mitchell et al., 2010).

Other examples of NOS disorders include patients who have a regular pattern of vomiting for weight control after normal eating. These individuals might not be underweight or demonstrate binge eating and so are not identified as having an eating disorder. Clinicians should recognize the importance of early detection and treatment before the NOS illness becomes more severe (American Psychiatric Association, 2013).

WEB RESOURCES

The following websites represent a small sampling of available resources for professionals, patients, and families. Nurses should evaluate the appropriateness of web resources as with all other resources before giving them to patients and families. There is a disturbing phenomenon on the Internet known as *pro anorexia* (pro ana) and *pro bulimia* (pro mia) websites, bulletin boards, and chat rooms hosted by individuals with eating disorders and proclaiming anorexia and bulimia as lifestyle choices rather than life-threatening illnesses. These sites offer tips on how to be the "best anorectic" or "best bulimic" and often feature alarming pictures of individuals with the disorders in a macabre competition of thinness. The web addresses of these sites are often passed from patient to patient, making them very difficult to track and control (Andrist, 2003).

National Association of Anorexia and Associated Disorders (ANAD)
http://www.anad.org
This site is sponsored and maintained by ANAD, the oldest national nonprofit organization devoted to helping patients with eating disorders and their families through providing networking, support groups, and advocacy for patients and their families. Current efforts are directed at monitoring and advocating against media references that portray eating disorders as funny and that the organization believes are dangerous and demeaning.

Eating Disorders Referral and Information Center (EDRIC)
http://www.edreferral.com
This site is sponsored and maintained by the International Eating Disorders Referral Organization, a nonprofit organization. The website contains much information and many links to other resources as well as referrals worldwide to caregivers experienced in treating eating disorders.

Academy for Eating Disorders (AED)
http://aedweb.org/web/index.php
The AED is the international source for state-of-the-art information in the field of eating disorders. The organization is a global, multidisciplinary, professional association committed to leadership in eating disorder research, education, treatment, and prevention. AED advocates for the field on behalf of patients, the public, and eating disorder professionals.

Something Fishy Web Site on Eating Disorders
http://www.something-fishy.org/
This site serves as a clearinghouse for eating disorder resources and information. It provides discussion forums for people with eating disorders and another forum for loved ones of individuals with eating disorders and proclaims itself as pro recovery.

STUDY NOTES

1. Anorexia nervosa is characterized by a refusal to maintain body weight at or above a minimally normal weight for age and height, an intense fear of becoming fat, a distorted body image, and amenorrhea or irregular menstrual cycles in women and low testosterone levels in men.

2. Anorectic dieters might begin their illness in a normal weight range but then isolate themselves socially from others, become competitive concerning weight loss, and exercise excessively.

3. Bulimia is characterized by episodes of binge eating, a feeling of lack of control over eating, use of compensatory behavior, and an overconcern with body shape and weight. Depression commonly coexists with bulimia.

4. Anorectic and bulimic patients experience a variety of physiologic problems that can lead to death. Personality and emotional changes are also evident in these patients, which might result from the eating disorder or might be a contributing factor in its genesis.

5. The causes of eating disorders are thought to be multifactorial, including biologic, sociocultural, familial, cognitive, behavioral, and psychodynamic factors.

6. Cognitive behavior therapy has the most research support in the treatment of eating disorders.

7. The incidence of eating disorders in men is increasing, with similarities in presentation and treatment to those in women with eating disorders, although eating disorders in men seem to manifest at a later age than in women.

8. Nursing interventions with patients with eating disorders require caring, supportive relationships; limit setting; a behavior modification program; and a consistent milieu. Family involvement, individual psychotherapy, and group therapy are also essential.

9. Hospitalization with a structured milieu and antidepressant medications might be needed if weight decreases below what is appropriate for the patient's height or if medical complications related to the patient's condition are present.

REFERENCES

Agency for Healthcare Research and Quality. (2009). *Statistical brief #70.* http://www.hcup-us.ahrq.gov/reports/statbriefs/sb70.jsp, Accessed 22.08.13.

Agency for Healthcare Research and Quality. (2011). *Hospitalizations for eating disorders declined, but big increase seen in pica disorder.* http://www.ahrq.gov/news-and-numbers/090811.html, Accessed 22.08.13.

American Psychiatric Association. (2013). *Diagnostic and statistical manual of mental disorders* (5th ed.). Arlington, Virginia: APA.

Andrist, L. (2003). Media images, body dissatisfaction and disordered eating in adolescent women. *The American Journal of Maternal Child Nursing, 28*, 119.

Ansell, E. B., et al. (2008). Structure of diagnostic and statistical manual of mental disorders, fourth edition criteria for obsessive-compulsive personality disorder in patients with binge eating disorder. *Canadian Journal of Psychiatry, 53*, 863.

Attia, E. (2009). Anorexia nervosa: Current status and future directions. *Annual Review of Medicine, 61,* 425.

Attia, E., & Schroeder, L. (2005). Pharmacologic treatment of anorexia nervosa: Where do we go from here? *International Journal of Eating Disorders, 37,* S60.

Austin, S. B., et al. (2009). Sexual orientation disparities in purging and binge eating from early to late adolescence. *The Journal of Adolescent Health, 45,* 238.

Bachner-Melman, R., et al. (2009). Protective self-presentation style: Association with disordered eating and anorexia nervosa mediated by sociocultural attitudes towards appearance. *Eating and Weight Disorders, 14,* 1.

Bailer, U. F., et al. (2007). Exaggerated 5-HT1A but normal 5-HT2A receptor activity in individuals ill with anorexia nervosa. *Biological Psychiatry, 61,* 1090.

Bakke, B., et al. (2001). Administering cognitive-behavioral therapy for bulimia nervosa via telemedicine in rural settings. *International Journal of Eating Disorders, 30,* 454.

Bergen, A. W., et al. (2003). Candidate genes for anorexia nervosa in the 1p33-36 linkage region: Serotonin 1D and delta opioid receptor loci exhibit significant association to anorexia nervosa. *Molecular Psychiatry, 8,* 397.

Boisseau, C. L., et al. (2013). The relationship between decision-making and perfectionism in obsessive-compulsive disorder and eating disorders. *Journal of Behavior Therapy and Experimental Psychiatry, 44,* 316.

Brown, K. M., et al. (2007). Further evidence of association of OPRD1 & HTR1D polymorphisms with susceptibility to anorexia nervosa. *Biological Psychiatry, 61,* 367.

Bruch, H. (1973). *Eating disorders.* New York: Basic Books.

Bulik, C. M., et al. (2005). Anorexia nervosa: Definition, epidemiology, and cycle of risk. *International Journal of Eating Disorders, 37,* S2.

Castro, J., et al. (2004). Predictors of rehospitalization after total weight recovery in adolescents with anorexia nervosa. *International Journal of Eating Disorders, 36,* 22.

Cohane, G. H., & Pope, H. G. (2001). Body image in boys: A review of the literature. *International Journal of Eating Disorders, 29,* 373.

Cook-Darzens, S., Doyen, C., & Mouren, M. C. (2008). Family therapy in the treatment of adolescent anorexia nervosa: Current research evidence and its therapeutic implications. *Eating and Weight Disorders, 13,* 157.

Crow, S., & Peterson, C. B. (2009). Refining treatments for eating disorders. *American Journal of Psychiatry, 166,* 266.

Cummings, M. M., et al. (2001). Developing and implementing a comprehensive program for children and adolescents with eating disorders. *Journal of Child and Adolescent Psychiatric Nursing, 14,* 167.

Cuzzocrea, F., Larcan, R., & Lanzarone, C. (2012). Gender differences, personality and eating behaviors in non-clinical adolescents. *Eating and Weight Disorders, 17,* e282.

Dahlgren, C. L., et al. (2013). Developing and evaluating cognitive remediation therapy (CRT) for adolescents with anorexia nervosa: A feasibility study. *Clinical Child Psychology and Psychiatry,* June 11 [Epub ahead of print].

Dauncey, M. J. (2013). Genomic and epigenomic insights into nutrition and brain disorders. *Nutrients, 15,* 887.

Doyle, P. M., et al. (2009). Early response to family-based treatment for adolescent anorexia nervosa. *International Journal of Eating Disorders, 43,* 659.

Easter, A., et al. (2013). Recognising the symptoms: How common are eating disorders in pregnancy? *European Eating Disorders Review, 21,* 340.

Espindola, C. R., & Blay, S. L. (2009). Anorexia nervosa treatment from the patient perspective: A metasynthesis of qualitative studies. *Annals of Clinical Psychiatry, 21,* 38.

Fairburn, C. G. (2005). Evidence-based treatment of anorexia nervosa. *International Journal of Eating Disorders, 37,* S26.

Fairburn, C. G., et al. (2009). Transdiagnostic cognitive-behavioral therapy for patients with eating disorders: A two-site trial with 60-week follow-up. *American Journal of Psychiatry, 166,* 311.

Finelli, L. (2001). Revisiting the identity issue in anorexia. *Journal of Psychosocial Nursing and Mental Health Services, 39,* 23.

Fox, J. R. (2009). Eating disorders and emotions. *Clinical Psychology & Psychotherapy, 16,* 237.

Fox, J. R., & Froom, K. (2009). Eating disorders: A basic emotion perspective. *Clinical Psychology & Psychotherapy, 16,* 328.

Galusca, B., et al. (2008). Organic background of restrictive type anorexia nervosa suggested by increased serotonin1A receptor binding in right frontotemporal cortex of both lean and recovered patients: [18F]MPPF PET scan study. *Biological Psychiatry, 64,* 1009.

Geist, R., et al. (2000). Comparison of family therapy and family group psychoeducation in adolescents with anorexia nervosa. *Canadian Journal of Psychiatry, 45,* 173.

Goldstein, D. J., et al. (1999). Effectiveness of fluoxetine therapy in bulimia nervosa regardless of comorbid depression. *International Journal of Eating Disorders, 25,* 19.

Halmi, K. (2005). Psychopathology of anorexia nervosa. *International Journal of Eating Disorders, 37,* S20.

Halmi, K. A. (2009). Salient components of a comprehensive service for eating disorders. *World Psychiatry, 8,* 150.

Hay, P. P., et al. (2009). Psychological treatments for bulimia nervosa and binging. *The Cochrane Database of Systematic Reviews,* (4), CD000562.

Hofmann, S. G., et al. (2012). The efficacy of cognitive behavioral therapy: A review of meta-analyses. *Cognitive Therapy and Research, 36,* 427.

Holland, L. A., Bodell, L. P., & Keel, P. K. (2013). Psychological factors predict eating disorder onset and maintenance at 10-year follow-up. *European Eating Disorders Review, 21,* 405.

Hütter, G., Ganepola, S., & Hofmann, W. K. (2009). The hematology of anorexia nervosa. *International Journal of Eating Disorders, 42,* 293.

Javaras, K. N., et al. (2008). Familiality and heritability of binge eating disorder: Results of a case-control family study and a twin study. *International Journal of Eating Disorders, 41,* 174.

Juarascio, A., et al. (2013). Acceptance and commitment therapy as a novel treatment for eating disorders: An initial test of efficacy and mediation. *Behavior Modification, 37,* 459.

Karpowicz, E., Skärsäter, I., & Nevonen, L. (2009). Self-esteem in patients treated for anorexia nervosa. *International Journal of Mental Health Nursing, 18,* 318.

Katzman, D. K. (2005). Medical complications in adolescents with anorexia nervosa: A review of the literature. *International Journal of Eating Disorders, 37,* S52.

Kaye, W. H., Fudge, J. L., & Paulus, M. (2009). New insights into symptoms and neurocircuit function of anorexia nervosa. *Nature Reviews. Neuroscience, 10,* 573.

Kaye, W. H., et al. (2000). Anorexia and bulimia nervosa. *Annual Review of Medicine, 51,* 299.

Kaye, W. H., et al. (2004). Comorbidity of anxiety disorders with anorexia and bulimia nervosa. *American Journal of Psychiatry, 161,* 2215.

Kaye, W. H., et al. (2005). Neurobiology of anorexia nervosa: Clinical implications of alterations of the function of serotonin and other neuronal systems. *International Journal of Eating Disorders, 37,* S15.

Kaye, W. H., et al. (2008). The genetics of anorexia nervosa collaborative study: Methods and sample description. *International Journal of Eating Disorders, 41,* 289.

Keel, P. K., et al. (2003). Predictors of mortality in eating disorders. *Archives of General Psychiatry, 60,* 179.

Kiezebrink, K., et al. (2010). Evidence of complex involvement of serotonergic genes with restrictive and binge purge subtypes of anorexia nervosa. *The World Journal of Biological Psychiatry, 11,* 824.

Lipsman, N., et al. (2013). Subcallosal cingulate deep brain stimulation for treatment-refractory anorexia nervosa: A phase 1 pilot trial. *Lancet, 381,* 1361.

Lock, J. D., & Fitzpatrick, K. K. (2009). Anorexia nervosa. *Clinical Evidence (Online),* 1011.

MacDonald, A. (Ed.). (2009). Treating anorexia nervosa. A multidisciplinary approach is best, but relapses are common. In *The Harvard Mental Health Letter, 26,* 1.

Marco, J. H., Perpiñá, C., & Botella, C. (2013). Effectiveness of cognitive behavioral therapy supported by virtual reality in the treatment of body image in eating disorders: One year follow-up. *Psychiatry Research, 209,* 619.

Mazzeo, S. E., et al. (2005). Parenting concerns of women with histories of eating disorders. *International Journal of Eating Disorders, 37,* S77.

McClay, C. A., et al. (2013). Online cognitive behavioral therapy for bulimic type disorders, delivered in the community by a nonclinician: Qualitative study. *Journal of Medical Internet Research, 15,* e46.

McIntosh, W. V., et al. (2000). Interpersonal psychotherapy for anorexia nervosa. *International Journal of Eating Disorders, 27,* 125.

Melrose, C. (2000). Facilitating a multidisciplinary parent support and education group guided by Allen's developmental health nursing model. *Journal of Psychosocial Nursing and Mental Health Services, 38,* 19.

Mendell, D. A., & Logemann, J. A. (2001). Bulimia and swallowing: Cause for concern. *International Journal of Eating Disorders, 30,* 252.

Misra, M., et al. (2008). Bone metabolism in adolescent boys with anorexia nervosa. *The Journal of Clinical Endocrinology and Metabolism, 93,* 3029.

Mitchell, K. S., et al. (2010). Binge eating disorder: A symptom-level investigation of genetic and environmental influences on liability. *Psychological Medicine, 40,* 1899.

Muscari, M. (2002). Effective management of adolescents with anorexia and bulimia. *Journal of Psychosocial Nursing and Mental Health Services, 40,* 23.

Nakash-Eisikovits, O., Dierberger, A., & Westen, D. (2002). A multidisciplinary meta-analysis of pharmacotherapy for bulimia nervosa: Summarizing the range of outcomes in controlled clinical trials. *Harvard Review of Psychiatry, 10,* 193.

National Collaborating Centre for Mental Health. (2004). *Eating disorders: Core interventions in the treatment and management of anorexia nervosa, bulimia nervosa, and related eating disorders.* London: British Psychological Society and Royal College of Psychiatrists.

O'Dea, J. A., & Abraham, S. (2000). Improving the body image, eating attitudes and behaviors of young male and female adolescents: A new educational approach that focuses on self-esteem. *International Journal of Eating Disorders, 28,* 43.

Ohlmer, R., Jacobi, C., & Taylor, C. B. (2013). Preventing symptom progression in women at risk for AN: Results of a pilot study. *European Eating Disorders Review, 21,* 323.

Orbanic, S. (2001). Understanding bulimia. *American Journal of Nursing, 101,* 35.

Perpiñá, C., et al. (2013). Clinical validation of a virtual environment for normalizing eating patterns in eating disorders. *Comprehensive Psychiatry, 54,* 680.

Pike, K. (2005). Assessment of anorexia nervosa. *International Journal of Eating Disorders, 37,* S22.

Poirier-Solomon, L. (2001). Eating disorders and diabetes. *Diabetes Forecast, 11,* 43.

Pompli, M., et al. (2004). Suicide in anorexia nervosa: A meta-analysis. *International Journal of Eating Disorders, 36,* 99.

Rand, C. S. W., & Wright, B. A. (2000). Continuity and change in the evaluation of ideal and acceptable body sizes across a wide age span. *International Journal of Eating Disorders, 28,* 90.

Ray, S. L. (2004). Eating disorders in adolescent males. *Professional School Counseling, 8,* 98.

Ro, O., et al. (2005). Two-year prospective study of personality disorders in adults with long-standing eating disorders. *International Journal of Eating Disorders, 37,* 112.

Scagliusi, F. B., et al. (2009). Nutritional knowledge, eating attitudes and chronic dietary restraint among men with eating disorders. *Appetite, 53,* 446.

Shingleton, R. M., Richards, L. K., & Thompson-Brenner, H. (2013). Using technology within the treatment of eating disorders: A clinical practice review. *Psychotherapy (Chicago, Ill.), 50,* 576.

Sloan, G. (1999). Anorexia nervosa: A cognitive behavioural approach. *Nursing Standard, 13,* 43.

Steiger, H., Bruce, K. R., & Groleau, P. (2011). Neural circuits, neurotransmitters, and behavior: Serotonin and temperament in bulimic syndromes. *Current Topics in Behavioral Neurosciences, 6,* 125.

Stein, K. F., & Corte, C. (2003). Reconceptualizing causative factors and intervention strategies in the eating disorders: A shift from body image to self-concept impairments. *Archives of Psychiatric Nursing, 17,* 57.

Steinhausen, H. C., & Weber, S. (2009). The outcome of bulimia nervosa: Findings from one-quarter century of research. *American Journal of Psychiatry, 166,* 1331.

Stewart, T. M., & Williamson, D. A. (2004). Multidisciplinary treatment of eating disorders—Part 2. *Behavior Modification, 28,* 831.

Sutoh, C., et al. (2013). Changes in self-regulation-related prefrontal activities in eating disorders: A near infrared spectroscopy study. *PLoS One, 8,* e59324.

Trace, S. E., et al. (2013). The genetics of eating disorders. *Annual Review of Clinical Psychology, 9,* 589.

Treasure, J., Claudino, A. M., & Zucker, N. (2010). Eating disorders. *Lancet, 375,* 583.

Troop, N. A. (2012). Helplessness, mastery and the development of eating disorders: Exploring the links between vulnerability and precipitating factors. *Eating and Weight Disorders, 17,* e274.

Usdan, L. S., Khaodhiar, L., & Apovian, C. M. (2008). The endocrinopathies of anorexia nervosa. *Endocrine Practice, 14*, 1055.

White, J. H. (2000). The prevention of eating disorders: A review of the research on risk factors with implications for practice. *Journal of Child and Adolescent Psychiatric Nursing, 13*, 76.

Williamson, D. A., et al. (2004). Cognitive-behavioral theories of eating disorders. *Behavior Modification, 28*, 711.

Wonderlich, S. A., et al. (2001). Eating disturbance and sexual trauma in childhood and adulthood. *International Journal of Eating Disorders, 30*, 401.

Wonderlich, S., et al. (2012). Minimizing and treating chronicity in the eating disorders: A clinical overview. *International Journal of Eating Disorders, 45*, 467.

Woodside, D. B., et al. (2001). Comparisons of men with full or partial eating disorders, men without eating disorders, and women with eating disorders in the community. *American Journal of Psychiatry, 158*, 570.

Zerwas, S., et al. (2013). Factors associated with recovery from anorexia nervosa. *Journal of Psychiatric Research, 47*, 972.

CHAPTER

33

Survivors of Violence and Trauma

Lee H. Schwecke

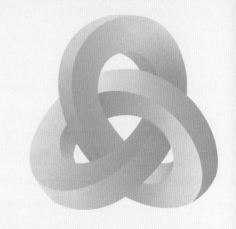

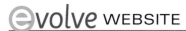 WEBSITE

http://evolve.elsevier.com/Keltner

LEARNING OBJECTIVES

- Recognize the seriousness of violence and trauma in the United States.
- Describe the emotional reactions of adult victims of crime, workplace violence, terrorism, torture, ritual abuse, mind control, human trafficking, rape and sexual assault, childhood sexual abuse, and partner and elder abuse.
- Recognize the dynamics involved in interpersonal violence crimes.

- Analyze the way in which the cycle of violence inhibits individuals from leaving abusive relationships.
- Identify the needs of victims of violence and trauma.
- Describe strategies for facilitating the transition from victim to survivor of violence or trauma.
- Develop a nursing care plan for survivors of violence and trauma.

The victimization of any individual by another creates serious mental health, social, community, and legal problems. Violence in all forms is prevalent in U.S. society. Nurses, regardless of their areas of practice, will come into contact with the victims—as inpatients, outpatients, home care patients, emergency care patients, parents of patients, friends, and relatives. Although victims are typically seen initially for physical injuries, their psychological needs require attention if long-term mental health problems are to be prevented.

Forensic nursing (including sexual assault nurse examiners [SANEs]) is a vital aspect of the holistic care of victims and perpetrators of violent crimes and their families (Peternelj-Taylor, 2001). This care includes obtaining clinical histories, documenting evidence including photographs of injuries, and carrying out quality nursing interventions in a holistic care framework, which includes consideration of all

the medicolegal aspects of the patient's problems (Hammer, 2000; Jackson, 2011). The rights of the alleged perpetrators of crime, suspects, and victims must be protected so that the legal cases are not jeopardized.

This chapter focuses on victims of violence and trauma, beginning with an overview of general reactions to any crime, workplace violence, terrorism, torture, ritual abuse, and human trafficking, followed by a more in-depth look at rape survivors, adult survivors of childhood sexual abuse, individuals abused by their partners, and abused older adults. Although a few perpetrators of rape, sexual abuse, and partner abuse are female, the more common pattern of this victimization is men against women. The short-term and long-term reactions of victims described in this chapter are generally true for both male and female victims; however, men sometimes have a more difficult time admitting to and dealing with their emotional victimization than women. The added impact on men of sexual violation by other men, both as children and as adults, is a result in part of fears about homosexuality (Masho & Anderson, 2009; Shea, 2008).

NORM'S NOTES

If ever there was a timely topic, this is it. I read notes weekly, and a high number of adult patients were abused as children—sexually or physically or both. Sometimes the behavior of some child pornographers is so barbaric that newscasters refuse to describe them on the air. The victims, when they survive such abuse, are potentially scarred for life. How in the world do they ever learn to trust again? Whatever your views on capital punishment, I have no mercy in my heart for these people (mostly men). The Bible says, "But whoso shall offend one of these little ones ...., it were better for him that a millstone were hanged about his neck, and that he were drowned in the depth of the sea." AMEN! Lee Schwecke has had a lot of experience with survivors of violence and trauma and has a lot to share in this chapter.

Beyond the scope of this chapter are the issues of crime and violence by and against children and adolescents, dating violence, gangs, school shootings, bullying, hate crimes against certain populations, robbery, property damage, fighting (with or without weapons), cyber sex, cyber bullying, and drug-related crimes.

VIOLATION BY CRIME

Effects of Crimes

Each year over 11 million people in the U.S. experience at least one violent victimization with 1.6 million being seen in emergency departments for physical injuries caused by these assaults (Simon Kresnow & Bossarte, 2008). Not all crimes involve physical violence, injury, and threat to life; however, all crimes involve emotional violation and trauma. The victim's identity is affected, even with the loss or destruction of possessions and property, because these are a representation of an individual's identity and have personal significance. Crime undermines foundations formed in the first two stages of human development, regardless of the victim's age when the crime occurred (see Chapter 9). There is a loss of *trust*, not only in the criminal but also to some degree in all other individuals. Victims also lose self-esteem and a sense of ability to control their own lives and themselves (*autonomy* issues) as well as having *identity* issues (Rowell, 2005).

Emotional reactions to crime vary greatly according to the individual, his or her resources and past history, the situation, and the meaning of the crime to that person. However, common reactions are denial, fear, anxiety, anger, powerlessness, and depression. A sense of failure and guilt is common; victims wonder what they did to cause the crime and how they might have prevented or stopped it. Victims usually feel ashamed and unworthy as well as contaminated or dirty, whether or not they were physically touched by the perpetrator. Fantasies

of revenge or a wish for legal retribution are typical. The relationships of victims to family and friends can be disturbed in part because of the loss of trust but also because of the response of others. Caring individuals often imply that the victim was responsible for the crime with questions such as the following: "Why were you there alone at night?" "Why were you carrying so much cash?" "Why didn't you install that burglar alarm?" The victim might feel alienated and isolated. Hospital personnel, the police, and the legal system might also unwittingly convey what could be called a "blame the victim" attitude in their manner of questioning and in focusing only on the facts, without any emotional support or empathy. Long-term effects of crime may result in prolonged stress, posttraumatic stress disorder (PTSD), depression, substance abuse, suicidality, and unhealthy weight control (Amar & Clements, 2009).

Workplace violence is a particular crime that more recently has received increased employer and media attention, and it is included here because in two surveys in nonpsychiatric and psychiatric settings, 13% to 21% of nurses reported incidences of physical violence, and 34% to 55% reported emotional or verbal violence in the past year (Lanza et al., 2009). Workplace violence includes betrayal of employee trust, verbal abuse, sexual harassment, stalking, assault and battery, rape, and murder perpetrated by patients or their visitors, other employees, former or current partners of employees, and intruders from the outside looking for specific items such as money or drugs (Institute for Safe Medication Practices, 2004; Twibell & Townsend, 2011). One study by the National Institute of Occupational Safety and Health in 2006 found that nearly 5% of 7.1 million private industry business establishments had an incident of workplace violence within 12 months (Amar & Clements, 2009). According to a study published in *Nursing Management*, 80% of nurse leaders have experienced some form of workplace violence at work. Of these nurse leaders, 73% reported that "workplace violence is experienced occasionally," 19% reported that it was experienced "frequently," and 1.7% said "always" (Hader, 2008).

Verbal abuse (horizontal/vertical) by other employees includes intimidation, condescending language or tone, reluctance or refusal to answer questions, withholding information, scapegoating, negative or threatening language, angry outbursts, rude gestures, property damage, threats to or actual reporting of the nurse to a manager, ostracism, offensive notes or e-mail, criticism, humiliation, screaming, sabotage, and threats with weapons (American Psychiatric Nurses Association, 2008; Broome & Williams-Evans, 2011; Center for American Nurses, 2008; Hader, 2008; Institute for Safe Medication Practices, 2004; Leiper, 2005; Walrafen et al., 2012). Verbal abuse, especially when the abusers are nurses, physicians, nurse managers, or supervisors, has been linked to high turnover of nursing staff (American Psychiatric Nurses Association, 2008; Broome & Williams-Evans, 2011; Center for American Nurses, 2008) and, indirectly, to the nursing shortage.

Sexual harassment is defined as "an unwelcomed sexual advance or conduct on the job that creates an intimidating, hostile, or offensive working environment … [ranging from] repeated offensive or belittling jokes to pornography or outright sexual assault" (Farella, 2001, p. 14). According to a 1988 survey of the federal workforce, 42% of all women and 15% of all men have experienced some form of harassment (Farella, 2001).

Stalking is a crime that can occur anywhere but often occurs in the workplace. Stalking is obsessional pursuit, harassment, and intimidation by a person who has or believes that he or she has a significant personal relationship with the object of his or her unwanted attention. Stalkers might send letters, packages, or e-mails; make harassing phone calls; or follow and appear repeatedly at the victim's home or workplace. Sometimes they kill pets, vandalize or destroy property, and physically or sexually assault or even murder their victims (Hughes et al., 2007; Muscari, 2005). Surveys indicate that 2% to 7% of all men and 8% to 16% of all women have been stalked at least once in their lifetimes (Amar, 2007; Hughes et al., 2007). Men account for 87% of stalkers, and women are victims in 60% of cases. However, some cases involve female-male, male-male, or female-female stalking (Muscari, 2005).

The media tends to focus on the stalking of celebrities and public officials by strangers. The stalkers in these cases tend to be psychotic or have delusions about their victims and a supposed love relationship. However, most cases of stalking occur as the victim is trying to end a casual, dating, or marital relationship. This pattern is more likely than celebrity stalking to involve physical violence (80%) and sexual assault (30%) and to be carried out by nondelusional individuals (Mawson, 2005).

The Occupational Safety and Health Administration encourages voluntary compliance by employers with their workplace violence guidelines, published in 1998. Briefly, these and other guidelines suggest the following: (1) systematic education of all employees about verbal abuse, sexual harassment, and other forms of violence, along with ways to prevent and deal with them, including conflict resolution and negotiation skill training; (2) development of corporate policies and procedures related to workplace violence and reporting procedures; (3) definition of roles for supervisors, employee health staff, and security personnel; and (4) provision for treatment and counseling for employee victims (American Psychiatric Nurses Association, 2008; Broome & Williams-Evans, 2011; Walrafen et al., 2012). Counseling is most often provided by Employee Assistance Programs (Paul & Blum, 2005).

Recovery from Violence and Trauma

Many models have been formulated about the process of recovery from traumas such as crimes and disasters. Most researchers agree that the duration and severity of the trauma, the victim's resources, and the nature of help available during and immediately after the crime or trauma, influence recovery. Typically, three stages of recovery are defined: (1) initial disorganization (impact), (2) a struggle to adapt (recoil), and (3) reconstruction (reorganization). The brief summary here is derived from the views of Foa (2005), Lacy and Benedek

(2003), and Tynhurst (1951). The stages are not clearly separated, and the readjustment process is not smooth. Vacillation among the stages might occur, and recovery might take months or years, especially if revictimization or secondary victimization (from involvement with the criminal justice system) continues after the crime (Baliko & Tuck, 2008).

Impact

The initial reaction to a single-event trauma usually lasts a few minutes to a few days. Common responses are shock, denial, disbelief, and confusion. There might be paralyzing fear, hysteria, horror, anger, rage, shame, guilt, a sense of helplessness and vulnerability, physiologic responses, and disturbed sleeping and eating. These reactions might occur for a longer time when the trauma is ongoing, such as harassment or stalking. Some victims react less visibly or in a delayed manner; they look calm, organized, and rational, and they take all the necessary actions initially needed. Later, the other reactions might occur. Occasionally, the victim's reaction might include dissociative symptoms (amnesia, depersonalization, numbing, detachment), intrusive memories (nightmares, flashbacks), and severe anxiety. These symptoms might indicate that the victim is experiencing acute stress disorder (see Chapter 27).

Recoil

In the recoil stage, victims begin the struggle to adapt. The immediate danger might be over, but a great deal of emotional stress remains. In the beginning of this phase, there are periods in which victims look and act normal and are able to carry out daily routines at home and at work. Activity helps suppress fears, anger, and sadness. Later in this phase, there is a desire to talk about all the details of and feelings about the trauma ("What happened?"). Victims often need support and become temporarily dependent. Fantasies of revenge for the crime are natural during this stage. In the weeks and months after trauma, victims gradually become aware of the full impact that the event has had on their lives.

Reorganization

Reorganization might take months or years to accomplish. Although the trauma is not forgotten, the anxiety, fear, and anger diminish, and victims reconstruct their lives. The beginning of this phase includes reviewing and organizing what happened and why ("Why me?"); attributing blame to self, others, or both; justifying one's own actions at the time and later ("Why did I act the way I did then and since then?"); and regaining a sense of control and self-protection. Grief over losses resolves slowly. Lingering nightmares, frustrations, and disillusionment might occur; however, these subside as victims become reengaged in life and activities. If reorganization is not effective, victims might experience degrees of symptoms that, in some cases, are clinically diagnosable (e.g., PTSD) and need appropriate treatment (Alim et al., 2008; Lacy & Benedek, 2003; Naifeh et al., 2008; Roberts et al., 2009) (see Chapter 36).

Even with satisfactory recovery, victims sense that they and their lives are, and always will be, different as a result of the crime ("What if it happens again?"). Moving from victim to survivor or victor status is the goal for individuals experiencing trauma (Rowell, 2005), which can be accomplished by integrating the memories of the trauma and moving on in life with restored functioning, a reasonable sense of safety and security, healthy relationships, improved self-esteem, and a sense of purpose in life (Alim et al., 2008).

PUTTING IT ALL TOGETHER

PSYCHOTHERAPEUTIC MANAGEMENT

Nurse-Patient Relationship

Although trust, empathy, emotional support, and a willingness to listen are important in all stages of recovery, specialized care is needed in each stage. During the *impact stage*, the focus is on the survivor's need for physical safety and emotional security. Reassurance, protection from further harm, and sometimes medical care are needed. Survivors might need clear, simple directions on what to do, where to go, and what to avoid. It is crucial that nurses avoid accusations (blaming), intimidation, unnecessary intrusions, and invasion of privacy. In most instances, crisis intervention occurs face to face at the scene of the trauma or in the emergency department. For survivors who are superficially calm and in control, the crisis intervention might be needed a few hours or days later, when the impact of the trauma reality hits. Phone numbers for crisis telephone or walk-in services can be given to survivors before they leave the police interview at the scene or the emergency department.

During the *recoil stage*, survivors need validation of their worth and rights as victims. Referrals can be made to a victim's assistance program and for legal, insurance, or financial assistance if needed. If family and friends are not fully available during the episodes of emotional turmoil in the recoil phase, short-term counseling might be beneficial. During the struggle to adjust, support groups with other survivors can be useful. Whether the group is of short duration (6 to 8 weeks) or ongoing, and whether the group is professionally led or self-led, there is value in receiving information, encouragement, and companionship from others "who have been there."

During the *reorganization stage*, most survivors are able to recover and grow with minimal assistance. Long-term counseling is sometimes needed to overcome anxiety, phobias, depression, suicidal ideation, or other posttraumatic symptoms. It is uncommon for survivors to need hospitalization beyond initial medical care. Exceptions are survivors who are unable to function or meet their basic needs and individuals who become suicidal.

Psychopharmacology

Survivors of crime do not generally need medications. Antianxiety agents (benzodiazepines) are prescribed occasionally for short-term use to decrease anxiety, and trazodone (Desyrel) is prescribed to facilitate sleep.

Milieu Management

Many communities have temporary or ongoing groups for survivors of divorce, death of a loved one, sudden infant death syndrome, rape, incest, and physical and emotional abuse as well as for people affected by suicide or homicide, mass murders, torture, and abduction of children.

TERRORISM

Nature of the Problem

September 11, 2001, is the day that awakened the United States to the realities of terrorism and its unpredictability and devastation. Before this day, terrorism was a news story about terrible acts in foreign countries. Terrorism can be perpetrated under the justification of military, political, social, cultural, or religious reasons. Acts of terrorism can involve plane crashes, bombings, military warfare, biologic and chemical agents, trained or programmed assassins, and suicide/homicide bombers. Terrorism rarely affects only a single individual; victimization can involve thousands who have been injured or killed in a single event. The victims of terrorism include people who were injured or killed; police, fire, and rescue personnel; businesses and their employees; friends and families of all the victims; and potentially anyone who witnessed the tragedy (directly or through the media).

Effects

Terrorism can have more devastating results than natural disasters or major accidents because terrorism is not only perpetrated by humans, but it is also not accidental. The purpose of terrorism is to terrorize, kill, or injure targeted groups and to generate fear that it will happen again (Foa, 2005). The trauma of terrorism is more pervasive, long-lasting, and severe than other violent crimes. Survivors typically experience some degree of grief and mourning and acute or posttraumatic stress symptoms, which are expected reactions to an abnormal and horrifying event (Zawahir & Scudder, 2012). Box 33-1 lists typical reactions to terrorism. The event might also retrigger memories of previous traumatic experiences or lead to new or exacerbation of preexisting disorders (Ai et al., 2005).

Recovery

Most individuals recover with the support of loved ones, coworkers, and friends; memorial or religious services and community meetings; sleep, stress management techniques, relaxation techniques, and physical activities; and a return to normal activities (Foa, 2005; Miller, 2005). Critical incident stress management strategies can also facilitate recovery and prevent other untoward consequences.

A major goal of recovery is to regain some sense of trust, safety, and security, while acknowledging that future terrorist attacks are possible. In general, recovery parallels the stages of recovery described earlier (*impact*, *recoil*, and *reorganization*)

BOX 33-1	SPECIFIC RESPONSES RESULTING FROM TERRORISM, TORTURE, SERIAL RITUAL ABUSE, MIND CONTROL, AND HUMAN TRAFFICKING

Shock, disbelief, fear, anxiety, powerlessness
Insecurity, guilt, shame, spiritual distress
Unresponsiveness, dissociation, numbness
Decreased concentration, confusion
Panic, terror, sense of violation, anger, rage
Aggression, fantasies of revenge, impulsiveness
Helplessness, hopelessness, despair
Suicidal or homicidal ideation, self-mutilation
Mistrust, suspiciousness, paranoia, alienation
Estrangement, withdrawal, isolation
Fatigue, insomnia, nightmares, flashbacks
Memory disturbances, amnesia
Hyperarousal, stress sensitivity, startle response
Denial, repression, suppression, intellectualization
Body kinesthetic memories, psychosomatic symptoms
Extreme passivity, loss of self-esteem
Depression, prolonged grieving, substance abuse, PTSD
Sexual dysfunction, eating disorders, anxiety disorders
Labile emotions, personality changes
PTSD, Posttraumatic stress disorder.

Modified from Anorexia Nervosa and Associated Disorders (2002). *Anorexia Nervosa and Associated Disorders (Indianapolis Chapter of ANAD): Personal interviews.* Indianapolis: ANAD; Cole, H. (2009). Human trafficking: implications for the role of the advanced practice forensic nurse. *Journal of the American Psychiatric Nurses Association, 14,* 6; Lacy, T.J., & Benedek, D.M. (2003). Terrorism and weapons of mass destruction: managing the behavioral reaction in primary care. *Southern Medical Journal, 96,* 394; Miller, M.C. (2002). Disaster and trauma. *The Harvard Mental Health Letter, 18,* 1; Sarson, J., & MacDonald, L. (2009, May 8). *Behavioural harms: enforced and survival tactics in ritual abuse-torture.* Presented at the Thirty-first SALIS Conference.; Trossman, M. (2009). Supporting the mental health and psychosocial wellbeing of former child soldiers. *Journal of the American Academy of Child and Adolescent Psychiatry, 48,* 6; Turkus, J.A. (2000). The treatment challenge. *Many Voices, 12,* 6; Valente, S. (2000). Controversies and challenges of ritual abuse. *Journal of Psychosocial Nursing and Mental Health Services, 38,* 8; Van der Kolk, B., McFarlane, A.C., & Weissaeth, L. (1996). *Traumatic stress: the effects of overwhelming experience on mind, body, and society.* New York: Guilford Press.

but might be lengthier and more complicated, depending on the severity and duration of the trauma. On a larger scale, most cities and hospitals are reviewing their disaster plans for the capability to respond to terrorist attacks, biologic and chemical warfare, large-scale bombings, and other disasters. For many cities, an effort has been made to improve citywide, coordinated plans among police, fire, and rescue agencies; hospitals and mental health facilities; and local, state, and federal emergency management administrations. Psychiatric nurses and mental health personnel are included in the planning.

TORTURE, RITUAL ABUSE, MIND CONTROL, AND HUMAN TRAFFICKING

Nature of the Problem

Public and professional attention to the effects of torture, serial ritual abuse (SRA), mind control (MC), and human trafficking on mental health has waned in recent years, although the crimes have not, according to the victims. These crimes might be perpetrated by individuals, relatives, gangs, cults (satanic or nonsatanic), hate groups, organized crime, work/sex trade traffickers, or military-political organizations (e.g., Al Qaeda, the Taliban regime, Abu Ghraib Prison) (Lacter, 2011; Schwartz, 2011). Gangs are responsible for an increased number of homicides, other physical violence, and intimidation according to the U.S. Federal Bureau of Investigation (Ragavan & Guttman, 2004). The actions of members of drug cartels in Mexico are another example of the destruction that can occur in a country. The effect of this criminal activity is more severe because it involves multiple, calculated, and organized crimes against each victim or group of victims. This type of crime is used to create fear, humiliation, and submission in individuals, communities, and societies and is usually done for power or profit or both.

Statistics on the prevalence of torture, SRA, and MC are not readily available because of the problems in acknowledging, reporting, and proving occurrences. The threat of further harm to the self, family, or pets tends to keep victims silent. Especially in SRA and MC, perpetrators might use triggers to maintain victims' silence or to control their actions, such as special words, hand signals, or greeting cards (Anorexia Nervosa and Associated Disorders, 2002; Lacter, 2011).

Drug and MC experiments began before the 1970s (e.g., lysergic acid diethylamide experiments and covert military-political operation [MK-ULTRA] programming that trained or programmed assassins for U.S. security forces) (Katchen, 2005; Lacter, 2011; Schwartz, 2011; Shurter, 2012). MK-ULTRA operations (noted in movies, such as *Conspiracy Theory*, and the *Bourne Identity* series) are becoming more widely known because the Freedom of Information Act has resulted in the declassification of military and political documents.

"Human trafficking (HT) is the equivalent of modern-day slavery" (Cole, 2009). It involves the transportation and harboring of individuals for the very profitable purpose of slavery, sex, forced labor, or organ harvesting (profits as estimated to be $32 billion a year at least) (Cole, 2009; de Chesnay, 2013; Newby & McGuinness, 2012). Women and children, especially those in poverty, are particularly vulnerable. Estimates for international trafficking are 4 to 40 million (Hoerrner & Hoerrner, 2013). Each recent Super Bowl event has been described as "the single largest human trafficking incident in the U.S." (e.g., Miami in 2010, Dallas in 2011, and Indianapolis in 2012) (Goldberg, 2013; Sabella, 2013). Germany has the largest market for trafficking of women and children, and the United States has the second largest (Newby & McGuinness, 2012).

Tactics

According to survivors, torture involves physical, psychological, pharmacologic, MC, or sexual manipulation, or any combination of these aimed at damaging the victim's identity, personality, emotional stability, spirit, and physical integrity. Human trafficking tactics may include recruitment based on offers of money (to the victims or their families who sell the individual), a promise of a "better life," deceptions, threats, coercion, force, or kidnapping (Cole, 2009). Torture, SRA, and MC can begin with abduction and detention and end with execution or can be ongoing over time. Tactics can include using hot irons, electric shock, submersion, suffocation, large doses of drugs/alcohol, beatings, physical restraint, confinement in cramped or buried containers, watching or forced participation in others' torture/killings, gang rape, sexual and physical mutilation, being tied or hung in the air, being photographed during the abuse, starvation, and sensory and sleep deprivation. There might also be prolonged interrogation, brainwashing, indoctrination, personality destruction/creation of multiple personalities, programming, threats to or lies about the safety of loved ones and pets, overstimulation, mock executions, cannibalism, electronic harassment (microchip implants, as in the movie *Manchurian Candidate*), and threats with weapons (Anorexia Nervosa and Associated Disorders, 2002; Crane, 2013; Lacter, 2011; McCollough-Zander & Larson, 2004; Rutz, 2007; Schwartz, 2011; Sarson & MacDonald, 2004, 2009; Tolces, 2005).

Effects

Common outcomes of torture, SRA, MC, and human trafficking are injuries to the head (including traumatic brain injury), teeth, and genitals; infections, sexually transmitted diseases, malnutrition, poor hygiene, reproductive problems, bone fractures/dislocations, scars, burns, pain, chronic headaches, and forced pregnancies/abortions (Hoerrner, 2013; Lapp & Overman, 2013; Newby & McGuinness, 2012; Rutz, 2007). There may be disruptions in the functioning of the prefrontal cortex as a result of the prolonged stress (Liston, 2009). The emotional and other effects are more severe and longer lasting than effects caused by other crimes and include a sense of violation, dehumanization, humiliation, horrification, compulsive spending, guilt about harming others or animals, identity and personality changes, and damaged social and family relationships. In addition, victims may reveal a fear of leaving home/work, of authority, and of revealing personal information (Rutz, 2007). Trauma-specific fears (e.g., small dark spaces or nudity); hypersexuality; and obsessions with rituals, magic, or devils are common. Victims might have been forced or programmed to commit crimes against others. They might talk about topics that do not make sense to professionals, such as the Greek alphabet, sex trade, "Dr. Black," "Dr. White," white slavery, witchcraft, drinking blood, satanic rituals and holidays, and the *Satanic Bible* (written by Anton LaVey) (Anorexia Nervosa and Associated Disorders, 2002; Rutz, 2007; Shurter, 2012). Other specific responses resulting from torture, SRA, MC, and human trafficking are listed in Box 33-1.

There is much controversy about assigning psychiatric diagnoses (e.g., PTSD, adjustment disorder, major depression, dysthymia, anxiety disorder, dissociative identity disorder, or other dissociative disorders) to victims who are having *typical* reactions to *horrific* crimes (de Chesnay et al., 2013; Lapp & Overton, 2013). The major concern is that diagnosis is another form of victimization, stigmatization, and discounting of the validity of reports of these crimes. Blaming the victim draws attention away from the individual, social, cultural, and political variables creating and fostering torture, SRA, MC, and human trafficking and from research on strategies for prevention. Some professionals even view PTSD as insufficient for acknowledging the catastrophic effects experienced by victims and their families. The Salvation Army and the U.S. Department of Health and Human Services have developed guides for identifying and assessing victims of human trafficking. Another resource is *The Crime of Human Trafficking* (Anonymous, not dated).

Recovery

Because torture, SRA, MC, and human trafficking tend to be ongoing, the *impact* stage of recovery persists but might wax and wane over the years. In the *recoil* stage, adaptation is difficult because of the severity of the emotional stress remaining after these crimes end. Although supportive, cognitive behavioral, psychodynamic, and pharmacologic approaches (Anonymous, 2012; Lacy & Benedek, 2003; McCollough-Zander & Larson, 2004) are useful in helping these survivors *reorganize* their lives, this stage is likely to be prolonged, with more relapses during other life crises. Admission to a specialized program or psychiatric unit might be needed during intense therapy periods, when the risk of self-mutilation, suicide, or increased substance abuse is present. Major goals for recovery (Alim et al., 2008; Cole, 2009; Howe, 2003; Lacy & Benedek, 2003; McCollough-Zander & Larson, 2004; Sarson & Macdonald, 2009) include the following:

1. Decreasing and eventually eliminating self-destructive behaviors (self-mutilation, suicide attempts, substance abuse, and manipulation)
2. Developing emotion management skills and acknowledging the thoughts, feelings, and behaviors as "normal reactions to abnormal situations"
3. Expressing and dealing appropriately and safely with the intense emotions, especially anxiety, guilt, anger, rage, and desire for revenge
4. Becoming aware of suppressed or repressed thoughts and feelings, positive emotions, and body memories and reactions
5. Allowing oneself to grieve for the various losses experienced
6. Processing and integrating the memories of the experiences, often from the least to the most bizarre experiences (as in the recovery from PTSD and the integration of multiple personalities)
7. Developing or reestablishing healthy relationships with family, friends, and the community

8. Developing boundaries, a sense of privacy, self-integrity, and empathy
9. Using complementary or alternative medicine and spiritual practices that are helpful
10. Developing occupational and community living skills that lead to economic and social independence
11. Becoming aware of new perspectives in life and reasons to live despite the past
12. Regaining a sense of hope, personal power, and control over oneself and one's life

PUTTING IT ALL TOGETHER

PSYCHOTHERAPEUTIC MANAGEMENT

Nurse-Patient Relationship

Conveying acceptance, caring, and support; ensuring confidentiality; and believing what is being described are crucial if survivors are going to trust someone enough to discuss their experiences (Cole, 2009; McCollough-Zander & Larson, 2004; Sarson & MacDonald, 2009). Survivors must have time and space to process the issues at their own pace and within their own cultural framework; this is known as culturally appropriate and trauma-informed care (Lapp & Overman, 2013). Strategies used with patients experiencing PTSD are particularly useful for survivors of torture, SRA, MC, and human trafficking. Depending on the origin of the torture, SRA, MC, or human trafficking (individuals, relatives, gangs, hate groups, cults, organized crime, traffickers, military-political organizations), it might be crucial to understand the survivor's family, religious, cultural, or political background (Crane, 2013; Sabella, 2013). Referrals for treatment or correction of physical injuries and other outcomes might be appropriate, such as to dentists, plastic surgeons, gynecologists, neurologists, endocrinologists, or gastroenterologists (Rutz, 2007). Survivors may also need support and protection while they are involved with the criminal justice system when their perpetrators are being investigated and prosecuted. Foreign survivors may require the use of translators and may face immigration charges and deportation (Cole, 2009; Trossman, 2008).

Psychopharmacology

Using medication for treating survivors of torture, SRA, and MC is highly controversial, especially because drugs were often a part of the abuse as it occurred. Sometimes medications used in treating PTSD, anxiety disorders, depression (especially selective serotonin reuptake inhibitors), sleep disturbances, and psychosis are effective (Lacy & Benedek, 2003; McCollough-Zander & Larson, 2004).

Milieu Management

Specialized treatment centers, such as the St. Paul Healing Center at the Center for Victims of Torture in Minnesota (612-436-4800) and The Center: Post-Traumatic Disorders Program (800-369-2273) in Washington, D.C., use a multidisciplinary approach in providing treatment and rehabilitation for survivors and their families. Some of the 30 or more centers and programs use bicultural counselors to facilitate counseling with immigrants and former gang members. Self-help and therapy groups might be useful for survivors with similar experiences and needs, such as political refugees; rape, childhood sexual abuse, and partner abuse survivors; and former cult and gang members. Nurses and survivors of human trafficking can access information and resources from the national hotline (888-373-7888) of the U.S. Department of Health and Human Services or The Trafficking in Persons and Worker Exploitation Task Force (888-428-7581). Grants through the Partnership for Freedom: Innovation Awards to Stop Human Trafficking was launched in 2013 ((http://www.acf.hhs.gov/programs/orr/resource/atip-website-resources; 2013).

For further information about torture, SRA, MC, and human trafficking, the following autobiographers have written their own personal stories:

Family torture: David Pelzer, Richard Pelzer, deJoly LaBrier
Fundamentalist/religious/polygamous cults: Jenna Hill, Brent Jeffs, Carolyn Jessop, Flora Jessop, Elissa Wall
Military-political/satanic SRA and MC: Carol Rutz, David Shurter, Kathleen Sullivan

RAPE AND SEXUAL ASSAULT

Nature of the Problem

Statistics indicate that rape is an underreported crime in the United States; probably only 20% to 33% of rapes are reported (Amar & Clements, 2009; Annan, 2011; Jordan, 2004). Valid statistics are unavailable for sexual assault and rape because of this lack of reporting. It is estimated that 20% of women in the general population and up to 40% of women in rural areas have had an attempted or completed rape in their lifetime (Annan, 2011; Campbell & Wasco, 2005). In one survey, 14.8% of women and 2.1% of men reported having been raped in the past year (Courey et al., 2008). In the U.S. military, 1 in 500 men and 1 in 5 women on active duty were found to have "some form of 'military sexual trauma'" (Burgess et al., 2013). Older adults are vulnerable at home and in extended care facilities, especially if they have medical conditions, a physical or mental disability, or dementia (any of which might result in their reports being discounted by caregivers, family, and officials) (Burgess et al., 2005). In the general population, rape of men by men is increasing (an estimated 1 in 10 rape victims is a man) (Amar & Clements, 2009) but is rarely reported. Of reported sexual assaults and rapes, probably 90% involve a male perpetrator and a female victim (Brown, 2001). The increasing availability of adult and child pornography through electronic media may have a role in the increasing rate of rape, sexual assault, and child sexual exploitation (Alexy et al., 2009; Burgess et al., 2008; Courey et al., 2008).

One major problem in reporting rape is that laws and attitudes vary in different states and communities. In general, rape is considered forcible penetration of the victim's body by the perpetrator's penis, fingers, or an object without consent (Martin et al., 2000). Any other form of forced sexual contact (from touch to mutilation) is considered sexual assault. Despite sexual contact, it is generally acknowledged that rape is not sexually motivated but involves a desire for power and control, a wish to humiliate the victim, and the playing out of a (sexual) fantasy (Brown, 2001). Some police and prosecutors still do not pursue rape as a charge if the two individuals know each other (Jordan, 2004), despite the fact that in 90% of reported rapes, the victim knows the offender at least casually (Brown, 2001). A longitudinal study of adolescents found that 46% experienced sexual aggression and 65% of those adolescents experienced a repeated incident of sexual aggression (Young & Furman, 2008). Date or acquaintance rape might be complicated by the use of amnesiacs (date rape drugs), other drugs, and alcohol, which interfere with remembering the rape (Osterman et al., 2001). Some states lack marital rape statutes, or prosecutors are reluctant to charge husbands with raping their wives. Many people in our society ignore rape or convey the message that anyone who is raped asked for it (blaming the victim) (Annan, 2011).

Effects

Similar to all crime victims, the rape victim experiences a severe violation and all the possible emotions of the *impact* stage. In addition to internal and external bodily injuries, there might be a threat to life with weapons, to return and rape again, or to kill the victim if the rape is reported, or the perpetrator might kill the victim during or after the rape (Brown, 2001). Victims usually live but wish they had died. The traumatic memories of the rape usually include tastes, smells, sounds, and sights as well as tactile sensations and physical pain (Brown, 2001). These memories and the powerlessness, loss of control, fear, shame, guilt, humiliation, rage, and feelings of being contaminated or dirty might be overwhelming. A typical reaction of the victim is the wish to regain a sense of control and retreat to a safe place, take a thorough shower, and destroy any damaged belongings. However, these actions would destroy most of the evidence that is required if the victim decides to report the rape and prosecute. Avoiding medical attention also places victims at risk for AIDS, hepatitis B infection, sexually transmitted diseases, pregnancy, and improper healing of any physical injuries (Campbell & Wasco, 2005; Marchetti, 2012). Beyond the injuries, there may be long-term effects of headaches, gastrointestinal disturbances, obesity, hypertension, human papillomavirus infections, chronic pain, depression, anxiety, substance abuse, dissociative disorders, personality disorders, eating disorders, bipolar disorders, and PTSD (Burgess et al., 2013; Courey et al., 2008).

Recovery

Despite an outward appearance of calm composure and a denial at times of the need for help (as in silent or delayed reactions), the rape survivor needs assistance, information, and support. It might not be until the survivor begins the up-and-down struggle of the *recoil* stage that the losses, anger, and needs are recognized. In an emergency department, collecting

---

BOX 33-2   NEEDS AND RIGHTS OF RAPE SURVIVORS

1. Crisis intervention—information, counseling, and referrals
2. Help with basic needs—housing, transportation, child care, safety
3. Medical information and care—information about pregnancy prevention, testing for sexually transmitted diseases, follow-up care, and counseling
4. Advocacy for whatever choices are made about reporting or prosecuting
5. Protection of rights—to privacy, confidentiality, gentleness, sensitivity, and explanations of procedures and tests (trauma-informed care)
6. Protection of rights—to refuse collection of evidence, to determine who will and will not be present during examinations, to get copies of all medical and legal reports, and to apply for reimbursement through victim's compensation
7. Fairness, information, and protection of legal rights during investigations, hearings, and trial, including not being asked about prior sexual experiences with anyone other than the suspect or defendant
8. Reasonable protection against further harm—escorts to court, restraining order, additional patrols, relocation if necessary

---

evidence, taking away clothes, and other procedures might be a priority for staff, but for the survivor it is perceived as further intrusion and violation (Courey et al., 2008). To staff, survivors might seem resistant and uncooperative, whereas survivors are trying to protect themselves and regain a sense of control (Brown, 2001). Box 33-2 lists some of the needs and rights of rape survivors.

Many communities have developed specialized services for rape survivors (e.g., Centers for Hope) within clinics or emergency departments. SANEs have skills in collecting forensic evidence while providing empathy, support, and information (Campbell & Wasco, 2005; Jackson, 2011). Nurses also can encourage the beginning of the recovery process by avoiding a "blame the victim" attitude and by challenging any myths stated by the survivors, such as, "I should have fought him off" or "I shouldn't have been drinking" (Annan, 2011; Girardin, 2001; Willis, 2009).

Specialized rape services have information packets prepared for rape survivors and staff in hospitals, counseling centers, and other crisis areas. Survivors can be encouraged to keep the information sheets and phone numbers of resources for later use. A victim who appears temporarily composed and calm and denies the need for help should be especially encouraged to take materials home. A SANE might also call a sexual assault advocate, an advocate from a victim's assistance program, or a rape crisis counselor to initiate contact with the survivor and make periodic follow-up contact days, weeks, and months later when emotional, physical, or legal issues and concerns might arise (Campbell & Wasco, 2005; Jackson, 2011). Women in rural areas and women who are on active military duty may not have the same access to these services (Annan, 2011; Burgess et al., 2013).

In the *recoil* stage, most survivors begin to react to the significant effect that rape has had on their lives; they might alternately deny and admit to experiencing turmoil. Fear and mistrust are major issues and might be directed toward individuals resembling the perpetrator or toward everyone around them, especially if others convey any hint of blaming the victim. Survivors might be afraid to leave the one place they designate as safe. They might be able to go out with family and friends, but they more often avoid strangers; places similar to the rape scene; and intimacy, especially sexual relationships. If the rapes occurred in their residence, survivors might move or at least make safety-related changes to prevent recurrence, or they might ask for someone to stay with them at night for a while. Being alone and unprotected is usually frightening, especially when nightmares and traumatic memories occur. Survivors need help in reaffirming that they are worthwhile individuals, with dignity and rights, who did not cause and did not deserve the rape. They need to know that their anger is natural, especially about the violation of person and privacy, the humiliation, and the sense of powerlessness. Survivors often question whether they might have fought off the attacker. Survival is most important; if the victim survived the rape, he or she did exactly what was necessary to stay alive.

Rape Trauma Symptoms

One way to monitor and evaluate the responses of the rape survivor to the trauma and recovery process through the recoil and reorganization stages is to assess periodically for improvements in the following rape trauma symptoms (DiVasto, 1985):

- Sleep disturbances, nightmares
- Loss of appetite, somatic symptoms
- Fears, anxiety, phobias, suspicion
- Decrease in activities and motivation
- Disruptions in relationships with partner, family, friends
- Self-blame, guilt, shame
- Lowered self-esteem, feelings of worthlessness

Survivors vacillate in the recoil stage between repression or suppression and dealing with the trauma. Progress in the reorganization stage is not smooth; backslides occur at times, especially if new situations trigger memories of the rape. Survivors might avoid future routine gynecologic and rectal examinations to avoid reexperiencing the trauma (Osterman et al., 2001). The use of restraints during an inpatient stay might also reactivate the trauma symptoms (Chandler, 2008). The goals of recovery from rape and sexual assault are the same as the goals for all survivors of crime. In addition, rape survivors might need to develop or regain healthy sexual functioning and relationships (Osterman et al., 2001). Victims need to transfer traumatic memories to narrative or past memories by processing the sensory memories and decreasing their strength and influence, enabling them to move from victim to survivor status (Brown, 2001).

PUTTING IT ALL TOGETHER

PSYCHOTHERAPEUTIC MANAGEMENT

Nurse-Patient Relationship

The rape or sexual assault survivor needs continual empathy, support, and an opportunity to process the events and manage the intense feelings as well as to regain a sense of psychological and physical safety (Osterman et al., 2001). Although it is more time-consuming and energy-consuming, the best approach in collecting evidence and providing nursing care is to move slowly and supportively at the individual survivor's pace and to give rationales for and descriptions of procedures and referrals (using trauma-informed care strategies). Nurses can be particularly helpful to rape survivors. Male and especially female survivors tend to feel safer with a woman and might refuse to talk to a man, especially alone. The presence of a SANE or sexual assault advocate during examinations and interrogations can be reassuring. Survivors might or might not choose to have a friend or family member stay with them for additional support or help them get home. A sense of shame or guilt might interfere with reaching out for support (Osterman et al., 2001).

Crisis intervention is the most appropriate approach during the impact stage. Short-term counseling and a rape support group can be beneficial during the recoil stage. Long-term counseling might be needed during the reorganization stage, especially if the survivor decides to prosecute the perpetrator. On the one hand, a lengthy legal process can seriously delay recovery because of having to relive the events and emotions, and the survivor is treated as a criminal during cross-examinations in many trial situations. On the other hand, conviction and imprisonment of the perpetrator can help survivors feel vindicated, compensated, and safer in their environments.

If the symptoms of rape trauma do not gradually diminish and if reorganization of lifestyle does not seem to occur, the survivor needs to be assessed for and helped with any new problems, such as PTSD, anxiety, excessive anger and guilt, depression, acting out, isolation, suicidal thoughts, self-destructive behaviors, eating and sexual disorders, substance abuse, phobias, negative or destructive relationships with others, and reactivation of childhood sexual abuse memories (Campbell & Wasco, 2005; Faravelli et al., 2004). With any of these behaviors, longer term counseling might be necessary, and hospitalization for safety becomes essential.

Psychopharmacology

Although rarely prescribed to rape survivors, benzodiazepines to reduce anxiety and provide for sleep might be used on a temporary basis. Alternatively, an antidepressant taken at bedtime (especially trazodone) might be ordered if symptoms of depression exist with a sleep disturbance. If nightmares or traumatic memories are severe, a low dose of an atypical antipsychotic such as risperidone (Risperdal), quetiapine (Seroquel), or the alpha-1-adrenergic antagonist prazosin (Minipress) might be indicated (Zawahir & Scudder, 2012).

Milieu Management

Referral can be made to a rape support group or center, which encourages expressing anger safely, overcoming guilt and shame, building self-esteem and trust, and assisting in regaining control of the survivor's life and a sense of safety. Support groups are sometimes available for relatives, especially partners, of rape survivors to help them deal with the trauma; stereotyping and myths; and changes occurring in the survivors, themselves, and their relationship with the survivors. Also available are the Rape, Abuse and Incest National Network (RAINN) National Sexual Assault Hotline (800-656-Hope) and the National Sexual Assault On-line Hotline (http://rainn.org) (Anonymous, 2008).

Clinical Example- A Case of Rape

A 24-year-old woman called a rape crisis line complaining of anxiety at work, not sleeping, fear of being out at night, overwhelming anger, and feeling dirty and ashamed. For several weeks she thought that a coworker was watching her. Last Friday, as she was leaving work late, the coworker pushed her into her car and raped her. She did not report the rape and hid in her apartment all weekend. She forced herself to go to work on Monday. The man acted friendly toward her, as if nothing had happened.

ADULT SURVIVORS OF CHILDHOOD SEXUAL ABUSE

Nature of the Problem

Approximately 1 million cases of child abuse (including childhood sexual abuse) are reported each year. However, child abuse is grossly underreported (Rick & Douglas, 2007). It is likely that the Internet is compounding the problem. One study found that approximately 14% of 10- to 17-year-olds who were online received a sexual solicitation (Burgess et al., 2008). The childhood sexual abuse crimes of child pornography, childhood sexual abuse (by nonrelatives), and incest (by relatives) are especially destructive for two major reasons: (1) the crimes usually are not one-time occurrences, and (2) the perpetrators may be known and trusted. These crimes are common, but more are getting attention (e.g., victims of Jerry Sandusky at Penn State, Catholic priests, and child actors in California). Studies have indicated that 15% to 30% of all girls and 4% to 16% of all boys have experienced childhood sexual abuse (Cook, 2005; Valente, 2005). The incidence of sexual abuse of boys might be much higher. One estimate is that 25% to 35% of all childhood sexual abuse victims are boys (Masho & Anderson, 2009). It is sometimes harder for men to reveal the abuse because of the fear of being seen as unable to protect themselves, weak, or gay (Cook, 2005; Masho & Anderson, 2009; Shea, 2008; Valente, 2005).The number of children who have been sexually abused and never reported it, even when they became adults, is unknown.

Sexual abuse and incest include voyeurism and exhibitionism, which can lead to intercourse and mutilation and always involve a younger victim who is not capable of giving consent to the older, more powerful individual. For 75% of the adult female survivors in one study, the abuse began before age 7 years, and 62% had multiple perpetrators (Jonzon & Lindblad, 2005; Valente, 2005). Male perpetrators are commonly fathers, uncles, stepfathers, older brothers, cousins, grandfathers, neighbors, scout leaders, camp counselors, coaches, and religious leaders. Less frequently, the perpetrators are women—mothers, older sisters, other relatives, day care workers, teachers, coaches, neighbors, and babysitters. Perpetrators tend to choose either male or female victims, so there can be male-to-male, male-to-female, female-to-male, and female-to-female abuse. However, in one study, 92% of the women were victimized by male perpetrators, and 38% of the men were victimized by female perpetrators (Lie & Barclay, 2005). Victims are from every social, cultural, ethnic, and economic group (Cook, 2005).

Although sexual abuse can be violent, it often is not. Coercion is possible because of the victim's dependent, trusting, or loving relationship with the perpetrator. The victim is urged to maintain the secret with various threats, such as the following: the victim will be taken away from the family; the perpetrator will be put in a mental hospital or jail; the parents will divorce; the other parent will get sick; there will be no abuse of siblings if the victim is compliant; love will be withdrawn; no one would believe the victim anyway; or there will be physical abuse if the victim does not comply. Even when no physical violence takes place, victims usually fear that it will occur if they resist the perpetrator. Factors such as family conflicts or disorganization, witnessing violence, parental loss, parental mental illness, economic instability, secrecy and communication difficulties, substance abuse, and other forms of abuse (emotional, verbal, physical) and neglect seem to correlate with sexual abuse (Davis & Petretic-Jackson, 2000; Gladstone et al., 2004; Goodwin, 2005).

Even if the young victims want to disclose the abuse, it is difficult for them because they lack the words and concepts to describe the event. An emotional reaction of fear and confusion usually occurs, and some physical pain but not a moral, ethical, or legal concept of right or wrong. Most victims who, as children, tried to tell a parent or other adult were met with disbelief, denial, or pressure to retract their accusations. It is difficult for a parent to believe that the partner they love or a respected member of the community is capable of sexual abuse. Police, prosecutors, judges, mental health professionals, and the general public might discount a child's report as unreliable, a fantasy, distorted, or faked at the urging of a parent, especially if there is a custody dispute in progress (Davis & Petretic-Jackson, 2000). There are also potential "benefits" from the sexual relationship; the child is made to feel special, with extra attention from and time with the perpetrator that other children do not have. A certain power comes from pleasing the adult and receiving a degree of (distorted) affection (Davis & Petretic-Jackson, 2000). At times, the child might even have the physical experience of sensual pleasure (Valente, 2005). However, the emotional pleasure and concept of adult sexual love are absent. (It should be noted that all children make bids for attention and affection. Even if they are cute, coy, or flirtatious, these bids should not be viewed as seduction. Perpetrators of sexual abuse choose to misinterpret the child's behavior to meet their own needs and should still be held responsible for the crime.)

Effects of Childhood Sexual Abuse

On the Child

For the victim, the prolonged stress of the abuse might lead to changes in his or her neurobiology, neurotransmitters, hypothalamic-pituitary-adrenal axis, and noradrenergic systems (Waite et al., 2010; Zawahir & Scudder, 2012). "Stress hormones affect myelination, neural morphology, neurogenesis, and synaptogenesis" (Rick & Douglas, 2007). Specific areas of the brain likely to be affected by childhood trauma include the amygdala, cerebellar vermis, cerebral cortex, corpus callosum, and hippocampus (Rick & Douglas, 2007). Other results are disturbed growth and development (beginning with trust and autonomy issues), ambivalence about the experience (both the benefits and the pain), and denial of what is happening to protect the whole family or the community. The young child is fulfilling the roles of child and lover to the perpetrator and roles of child and protector to the rest of the family or community (protecting them from the horrible secret). As a result, the child begins a long-term process of taking care of others to the exclusion of personal needs. Basically, the child wishes for love, not sex, but eventually feels guilty, exploited, betrayed, angry, dirty, helpless, and responsible. Denial, repression, suppression, rationalization, and dissociation are mechanisms used by young victims to cope with this no-win situation. Sleep and eating disturbances, enuresis, anxiety, depression, aggression, an active fantasy life, masturbation, sexualized play, sexual aggression, poor impulse control, cruelty to animals, spiritual distress, somatization, alienation, fear, shame, self-blame, self-destructive behaviors, running away, and truancy are common (Cook, 2005; Davis & Petretic-Jackson, 2000; Valente, 2005; Waite et al., 2010). The more severe the abuse, the more likely that repression will begin near puberty. If the sexual abuse continues throughout adolescence, repression is less likely. Repression normally lasts until victims are in their twenties or thirties and are having trouble with intimate relationships or parenting or both.

Clinical Example- A Child Tortured

Children who were examined following ritual abuse in a day care center reported being locked in a cage, put in a coffin, held underwater, injected with needles, tied and hung from hooks, sexually assaulted, and threatened with guns and knives. The children were told that if they told anyone about the abuse, their parents, siblings, or pets would be killed.

On the Adolescent

As adolescents, sexual abuse victims show mostly overt methods of dysfunctional coping, such as impulsive acting out, violence toward or abuse of others, cruelty to animals, self-destructive behaviors, sleeping and eating disorders, suicide attempts, running away, truancy, delinquency, substance abuse, spiritual distress, sexual acting out, prostitution, early pregnancy, and early marriage (Cook, 2005; Davis & Petretic-Jackson, 2000; Valente, 2005). For victims who cope through self-mutilation, these behaviors tend to begin between the ages of 12 and 14 years (Cerdorian, 2005).

Adolescents might have fantasies of revenge and wish for the perpetrator's death. The anger toward the perpetrator and other adults (for not protecting them) approaches rage but is not directly expressed. Victims might not even be aware of the reason for their rage, shame, guilt, confusion, sense of alienation, and isolation and might not realize that their acting-out behaviors are related to the abuse. Regression, depression, depersonalization, dissociation, manipulation, low self-esteem, impaired social skills, spiritual distress, thought and memory disturbances, self-neglect, aimlessness, and withdrawal are common. Sexual abuse survivors are also more likely than the general population to be raped and battered by partners in adolescence and later in life (Annan, 2011; Davis & Petretic-Jackson, 2000; Gladstone et al., 2004; Valente, 2005).

On the Adult

For many victims of childhood sexual abuse, the process of surviving childhood and adolescence and becoming an adult is similar to delayed PTSD responses: repression of memories (even nonsexual ones), followed by a breakthrough of unwanted, intrusive memories. The memories might begin as nightmares, kinesthetic sensations (e.g., flinching or vaginal pain when touched by a partner in the same way as the perpetrator), or flashbacks. The memories might return gradually, in pieces, or in a sudden, overwhelming flood. Victims cannot be rushed to remember the abuse before they are ready to cope with it.

On the surface, adult victims might look relatively uninjured because of denial, dissociation, amnesia, emotional deadening, or repression. They enter counseling for manifestations of the abuse rather than for the incest or sexual abuse itself. The list of typical reactions in Box 33-3 can be used as a checklist to identify the issues to be addressed in counseling. Victims who see this list typically express amazement (that so much has resulted from the sexual abuse) and relief (that there is finally an explanation for all their "craziness"). Up to this point, victims might tend to deny or minimize the relationship of the sexual abuse to any of their current problems. It becomes evident to victims that the event has disturbed their entire growth and development process and their self-esteem and has set them up for other abusive relationships (Waite et al., 2010). Only 33% of victims ever receive counseling specifically focusing on the childhood sexual abuse (Gladstone et al., 2004). Until counseling finally focuses on the anger and underlying cause of their reactions, victims tend to seek treatment repeatedly, without relief.

The inability to handle the memories of abuse and the painful emotions, especially anger, often induces thoughts of suicide to escape the pain and depression, to die with the secret, to avoid conflict with the family or perpetrator, to stop

BOX 33-3 ADULT MANIFESTATIONS OF CHILDHOOD SEXUAL ABUSE

Memory disturbances
  Amnesia about abuse
  Memory gaps about childhood
  Inability to think straight
Keeping unnecessary secrets
Relationship issues
  Trouble connecting with others
  Running away from others
  Fear of men or fear of women
  Trouble trusting others and their motives
  Fear of intimacy, inability to maintain intimacy
  Fear of abandonment and rejection
  Trouble giving and receiving affection
  Feeling alienated from others
  Fear of being used, abused
  Trouble saying no, taking care of others
  Trouble with parenting
  Entering abusive relationships
  Poor choices of partners
Body symptoms
  Vague and transient pains
  Memories of physical pain
  Chronic pain or migraine headaches
  Gagging, nausea, vomiting
  Unpleasant sensation when touched
  Negative, distorted body image
  Self-conscious about body
  Overly conscious of appearance
Anger issues
  Fear of expressing anger
  Holding anger in
  Crying instead of being angry
  Fantasies of revenge
  Feeling violent, full of rage
  Fear of violence
  Homicidal thoughts
Anxiety issues
  Easily startled, inability to relax
  Fear of being attacked, exposed
  Hypervigilance
  Feeling like a frightened child
  Fear of the dark
  Panic attacks, phobias, agoraphobia
Addiction issues
  Alcohol or drug abuse or dependence
  Compulsive spending
Intrusive thoughts and memories

Intense nightmares, unwanted thoughts
  Flashbacks—feeling, seeing, smelling, tasting,
    hearing
Detachment issues
  Feeling numb, unreal
  Disconnected from feelings from body
  Feeling as if there are "personalities" inside
  "Out-of-body" experiences
Control issues
  Fear of authority, rules
  Need to be in control, feeling out of control
  Pretending to be out of control (or helpless)
  Fear of being vulnerable
  Ambivalent about being taken care of
  Letting others be in control or trying to control others
  Allowing children to be abused
Identity issues
  Confusion about identity or roles
  Negative self-image
  Need to be perfect or perfectly bad
  Underachievement or overachievement
  Need to be totally competent
Sexual issues
  Concealing sexual feelings, feeling nonsexual
  Discomfort with sexual touching
  Lack of orgasms, sexual dysfunction
  Confusion about sexuality, sexual identity
  Feeling "dirty," contaminated
  Trading sex for favors
  Promiscuity, prostitution
  Wondering if one is gay
Self-punishment
  Suicidal thoughts, attempts
  Wanting to die or to be dead
  Self-mutilation
  Compulsive eating or dieting
  Bingeing, purging
Other feelings
  Low self-esteem, guilt, shame
  Fear of feelings
  Feeling stuck
  Feeling like a failure
  Chronic dissatisfaction
  Frozen emotions
  Lack of a sense of humor
  Feeling inadequate
  Feeling walled in or "crazy"

feeling "crazy," and to end the nightmares and flashbacks that are so frightening. Self-harm or mutilation, without even feeling the pain, is a common way of dealing with the emotional pain, loss, rage, and abandonment. Dissociation during the mutilation is common. Victims describe the following various patterns of their mutilation (Anorexia Nervosa and Associated Disorders, 2002; Cerdorian, 2005; Isaacs, 2011; Starr, 2004; Williams & Bydalek, 2009):

1. When feeling overwhelmed, they inflict harm as a cry for help when they believe that no one is listening or cares.

2. When emotions build up, they go numb or dissociate and have to inflict pain to make sure that they can still feel.

3. When they are feeling unreal (depersonalization), they draw blood to make sure that they are alive.

4. They cause physical pain so that they do not have to focus on the emotional pain.

5. They punish themselves when they are feeling self-loathing, guilt, shame, or fear.

6. They use the mutilation as a way of avoiding suicide.

7. They use the mutilation to relieve the anger or rage toward self and others.

8. They might use the mutilation as an attempt to manipulate others.

9. The mutilation might become chronic and addictive, especially if it produces a high (related to endogenous opiates/endorphins).

Some evidence has suggested that suicide attempts might share similar, as well as unique, dynamics as self-mutilation and might become a chronic pattern or addiction (Mynatt, 2000). According to U.S. studies, 4% to 38% of adolescents use self-harming behaviors for stress relief whether or not they have experienced childhood sexual abuse (Williams & Bydalek, 2009).

Alcohol and drugs are often used to avoid or numb the pain and memories and to bring fleeting pleasure that is otherwise elusive (Davis & Petretic-Jackson, 2000; Gladstone et al., 2004). Food might also provide brief pleasure or fill emptiness inside (bingeing) but leads to feeling bloated and guilty and a need to purge. Although sex is not usually enjoyable, it can bring relief from loneliness, temporary attention, affection, and approval. Sexual encounters also might trigger traumatic flashbacks, anxiety, fear, shame, disgust, or a sense of helplessness. Healthy adult relationships and sexual intimacy are difficult because of problems in trusting anyone and the history of linking abuse and love. Victims have boundary issues, trouble setting limits with others, and difficulty with asking for what they really need (Davis & Petretic-Jackson, 2000). Victims also tend to be caretakers, rescuers, and codependents.

Reactions of victims to the trauma (see Box 33-3) are often labeled as clinical symptoms. In addition, other problems resulting from the effects of trauma on the brain may include temporal lobe epilepsy or changes on electroencephalography, autism, and attention-deficit/hyperactivity disorder (Rick & Douglas, 2007; Isaacs, 2011; Waite et al., 2010) as well as migraines, irritable bowel syndrome, fibromyalgia (Cassels & Vega, 2007), and chronic fatigue syndrome (Heim et al., 2009). When an axis I diagnosis is given to patients, it is commonly depression (atypical type), PTSD, substance abuse disorder, eating disorder, anxiety disorder, somatoform disorder, dissociative disorder (including dissociative identity disorder), bipolar disorder, schizophrenia, or impulse-control disorder. Personality disorder diagnoses are commonly borderline, narcissistic, histrionic, avoidant, dependent, atypical, or mixed disorders (Davis & Petretic-Jackson, 2000; Rick & Douglas, 2007).

Receiving a diagnosis is a major problem not only because of the stigma and blaming the victim but also because the diagnosis often becomes the focus of treatment rather than the underlying issues; this is especially true when the symptoms of childhood sexual abuse are labeled as a diagnosis of borderline personality disorder instead of PTSD (Schwecke, 2009). Lack of appropriate treatment carries a major risk not only for adult survivors but also for their children, especially if the survivors are still in a stage of repression. Evidence has suggested that victims who go untreated or are improperly treated occasionally set up dysfunctional, disorganized families, in which there is incestuous abuse of the children. With their own denial, repression, amnesia, or other mechanisms, survivors have trouble relating to their partners and are unable to see the partners' involvement with their children. Perpetrators (and occasionally victims) might sexually abuse their younger siblings, children, grandchildren, nieces, nephews, and others. Examples of incest have surfaced within three and four generations of a family. Breaking this cycle is crucial.

Clinical Example- A Man Rapes His Own Daughter

Jan Lester, 30 years old, was admitted to a psychiatric unit as a result of suicidal ideations and 12 superficial cuts on her wrists. She began having nightmares 9 months ago about being awakened at night as a child with someone on top of her. During the nightmares, she would wake up crying with strange body sensations, gagging, pressure on her chest, and vaginal pain. As the nightmares and memories became more complete and vivid, she realized her father had frequently had sex with her while her mother was asleep. As her father's fiftieth birthday approached, she felt as if she could not tolerate going to his party. She wanted to be dead but was unable to force herself to cut her wrists more deeply. She wanted help.

Recovery

In some ways, recovery from childhood sexual abuse or incest is similar to recovery from all crimes and from PTSD, but it tends to be more complex, difficult, and lengthy by comparison, especially if emotional abuse by the family is ongoing or if the survivor still lives with the abuser. The memories and emotions are strong, painful, and confusing. The intense anger and ambivalence toward the perpetrator (because the victim is still seeking approval and love from the perpetrator) are hard for both the survivor and the nurse to handle. Survivors need to know in the beginning that the symptoms and emotional pain will probably worsen before they improve as the experiences are reviewed. Survivors need to learn emotion management and regulation to tolerate the distress and use safety measures before using imaginal exposure techniques (Dunbar, 2004; Goodwin, 2005; Spinhoven et al., 2009). (See the discussion of dialectical behavioral therapy in Chapter 7).

Although outpatient counseling often takes 2 years or longer, survivors tend to engage in treatment sporadically. It is common for survivors initially to disclose, discuss, vent, and feel cured. Then as new crises or relationship problems emerge, survivors return to counseling to deal with each issue and its possible connection to the original trauma. Getting a patient to commit to continuous, long-term counseling is sometimes difficult, but the nurse can emphasize the desirability and value of at least sporadic counseling.

The overall goals of recovery are safety and security; rebuilding trust; improved self-esteem and self-acceptance; forgiveness of self; adaptive coping with life and its stresses; assertiveness skills; the capacity for intimate relationships and genuine sexual pleasure; improvements in affect; reduced anxiety, anger, shame, guilt, fear, and dissociation; and the prevention of suicide, self-mutilation, and sexual abuse of future generations (Davis & Petretic-Jackson, 2000; Waite et al., 2010).

PUTTING IT ALL TOGETHER

PSYCHOTHERAPEUTIC MANAGEMENT

Nurse-Patient Relationship

Much depends on the ability of the nurse to develop a trusting relationship with the survivor quickly. Empathy, active support, compassion, warmth, and being nonjudgmental are crucial. Survivors need to be calmly and matter-of-factly asked about childhood sexual abuse because they are not likely to reveal it spontaneously. The old and perhaps current coercions to keep the secret remain strong in the minds of survivors; they need to feel safe about confidentiality and the nurse's acceptance before disclosure can occur. How much detail is revealed and how soon depend in part on the nurse's ability to be receptive to the experiences without being critical of the perpetrator, of other adults in the family, or of the survivor's loyalty to them. The survivor needs to be reassured that all the emotions (positive, negative, and ambivalent) are valid and that exploring them is the beginning of the process of working through recovery (Davis & Petretic-Jackson, 2000). It is usually helpful for survivors to be reminded periodically that they were not responsible for and did not deserve the sexual abuse, that they are not to be blamed, that they were not in control of the situation, and that the way they coped in the past was the best they could do at the time. Cognitive behavioral approaches and education about the dynamics of sexual abuse and reassurances about recovery can be useful in correcting faulty perceptions about the abuse, decreasing self-blame and guilt, and instilling hope for the future despite the inability to change the past. (See Key Nursing Interventions for Survivors of Childhood Abuse box.)

Mentally and emotionally reexperiencing traumatic memories and emotions is disturbing; only periodic, small doses might be tolerable. In contrast, excessive rumination on events can be counterproductive (Schwecke, 2009). It is helpful to remind survivors that they went through the abuse alone but do not have to remember it alone. If traumatic flashbacks or dissociation occurs, it is important to bring the survivors back to the present by reminding them where they are now and that the nurse is with them. The nurse and survivors can monitor their safety and tolerance of the process to prevent becoming overwhelmed, retreating, attempting suicide, or self-mutilating. Anger release strategies, such as using a foam bat (batacca) while talking to a chair that represents the perpetrator or nonprotective adult and other productive anger management techniques, often help the survivor express thoughts and feelings that could not be expressed in childhood. Play therapy, therapeutic stories, and art therapy can be especially useful in helping children and adults process their abuse (Bennett, 1997; Hinds, 1997; Isaacs, 2011; Prugh, 2011; Rick & Douglas, 2007). Writing memories and painful feelings in an ongoing journal and writing "letters" that will not be sent to the perpetrator and nonprotectors can be useful (Cerdorian, 2005; Kreidler & Einsporn, 2012; Miller, 2011).

Confrontation of the family or perpetrator by the survivor is not a desired outcome or safe option. Confrontation might be done symbolically or verbally with the nurse and in the "letters," rather than directly with the perpetrator

KEY NURSING INTERVENTIONS

For Survivors of Childhood Abuse

- Contract for safety and control of impulses to harm self or others.
- Set limits on self-destructive or self-harm patterns.
- Establish a trusting and supportive environment.
- Accept all feelings and reactions as normal responses.
- Ask permission before touching survivors.
- Reinforce that recovery is possible, even if it is difficult.
- Educate about the dynamics of abuse and recovery processes.
- Assist survivors in understanding current behaviors as reflections of survival strategies used in childhood.
- Facilitate reevaluation of the sexual abuse and its effects but without pressuring or excessive rumination.
- Encourage coping choices that are in survivors' best interests.
- Discuss safeguarding other children if the perpetrator still poses a risk.
- Support choices about future disclosures, confrontation, or reporting.
- Be aware that family members and others might feel split loyalty and engage in dysfunctional roles and interaction patterns.

- Decrease feelings of isolation, shame, and stigma.
- Encourage self-acceptance.
- Facilitate acknowledgment, forgiveness, and love for the child within.
- Teach and encourage stress management and anger reduction.
- Facilitate the transfer of responsibility and anger to the perpetrator, but set limits on acting out fantasies of revenge.
- Foster separation and individuation from the family and its patterns.
- Help to find meaning in the experience and mourning of all the losses (grieving is a very painful experience).
- Facilitate the change from victim to survivor status (reexperiencing and integrating the positive, negative, and ambivalent feelings and memories).
- Facilitate reexperiencing and reworking of maturational tasks that were missed or experienced prematurely.
- Educate about life skills, communication skills, coping skills, assertiveness, decision making, conflict resolution, boundary setting, friendship, intimacy, sexuality, and parenting.
- Refer to outpatient counseling and appropriate support groups.

and other family members. If survivors choose to confront directly, much preparation is needed before this can happen. Survivors need to consider, plan for, and rehearse their reactions to all the typical responses of family members, such as denial, rationalization, and blaming the victim. Confessions and apologies are unlikely. Survivors can be helped to debate the benefits and risks of confrontation as well as the degree and type of contact they want to have with the family, even if they do not confront them or if the survivors need to protect their own children. An important consideration for the nurse and survivor to discuss is the mandatory reporting of child abuse if younger children are currently victims of abuse by the same perpetrators. This type of reporting is understandably difficult for both the nurse and the survivor but needs to be carefully and directly addressed.

When survivors are in outpatient counseling, it is important to consider priorities in each counseling session. Current crises and problems need to be addressed (instead of the sexual abuse) as they arise. For example, gynecologic and physical examinations might be distressing and trigger flashbacks (Roberts, 2000). This aspect is also critical for self-destructive behaviors that are increased because of counseling, such as suicidal ideation, self-mutilation, and substance abuse. Hospitalization might be necessary if the crisis is severe. Staff should avoid use of restraints that could cause retraumatization (Chandler, 2008). Although survivors view recovery as frightening and painful, they also experience relief that they are making progress.

Psychopharmacology

Medications are not always needed or desirable for adult survivors of childhood sexual abuse, especially if substance abuse is a problem or potential problem. For the small number of survivors with serious psychopathology, medications should be given according to the DSM-5 diagnosis, such as depression. An antidepressant such as trazodone might be used if the depressive symptoms are interfering with sleep. Benzodiazepines or clonidine might be given on a short-term basis to help control the emotional or autonomic arousal that occurs during the reexperiencing of traumatic memories. Occasionally, low doses of risperidone, aripiprazole (Abilify), prazosin, quetiapine, or topiramate (Topamax) are given for persistent and severely disturbing nightmares, flashbacks, disinhibition, negative affectivity, and agitation (Ripol, 2012; Zawahir & Scudder, 2012).

Milieu Management

On an outpatient basis and during any brief hospitalizations, trauma-informed care and cognitive behavioral and affect management groups can be a useful adjunct to nursing care (Kreidler & Einsporn, 2012). If available, a short-term or ongoing sexual abuse or incest recovery group is beneficial. Some self-help groups include Incest Survivors Anonymous, Survivors of Sexual Abuse, and Daughters and Sons United. Parents United (for the nonperpetrator parent) can be suggested, if appropriate. The perpetrator might also be referred

to counseling. Family therapy is sometimes appropriate but needs to be well planned.

Other groups that might be recommended, depending on the symptoms and needs of the survivor, are Co-dependency Anonymous, Adult Children of Alcoholics, and Alcoholics or Narcotics Anonymous. Survivors might also be directed to classes or short-term groups that address issues such as decision making, problem solving, communication or relationship skills, conflict resolution, anger management, parenting skills, and human sexuality.

> **? CRITICAL THINKING QUESTION**
>
> 1. You are working with a patient who was sexually abused as a child by her father. The father insists on visiting his daughter and telling you about her history of emotional problems and lying about the family. What is your approach in working with the father?

PARTNER AND ELDER ABUSE

Nature of the Problem

A woman is beaten every 9 seconds in the United States; approximately 2 million are injured in a year (Solnit, 2013). Estimates are that more than 7% to 21% of men and women have suffered physical assault by a partner in the past year. In a national survey, young adults reported violence in the past year toward an intimate: 35% for women (often in self-defense) and 37% in men (Carretta, 2008; Gratz et al., 2009). The number is even higher when psychological abuse and other violations of rights are considered (Figure 33-1) (Daniels, 2005; Dutton & Nicholls, 2005). It is difficult to collect statistics on female-to-female, female-to-male, and male-to-male abuse because of the lack of reporting (Brown, 2008; Dutton & Nicholls, 2005). Women are abused, raped, tortured, or beaten by their husband, boyfriend or girlfriend, male or female lover, former partner, or estranged partner (Carretta, 2008; Daniels, 2005), and most of this abuse goes unreported, even when injuries are severe enough to require treatment. Prior partner abuse increases the risk of it occurring during pregnancy (Tilley & Brackley, 2004). In primary care practice, it has been estimated that 34% to 46% of female patients are victims of partner abuse (Lie and Barclay, 2006).

Dating violence among adolescents is estimated to be 10% to 35%. Among children 11 to 14 years old, up to 20% are affected as they begin emotional and sexual dating relationships (Anonymous, 2008). Contributing factors for these children include witnessing parental violence, prior victimization or abuse, early puberty, typical stresses and issues of early adolescence, early use of drugs and alcohol, and exposure to media and Internet violence (Close, 2005; Gratz et al., 2009; Miller, 2004).

Finally, among older adults, sexual, physical, and psychological abuses exist as well as forced suicide or homicide of widows for economic reasons (Carretta, 2008). Elder abuse also includes violation of personal rights, abandonment, and material and financial exploitation (Baker, 2007). It

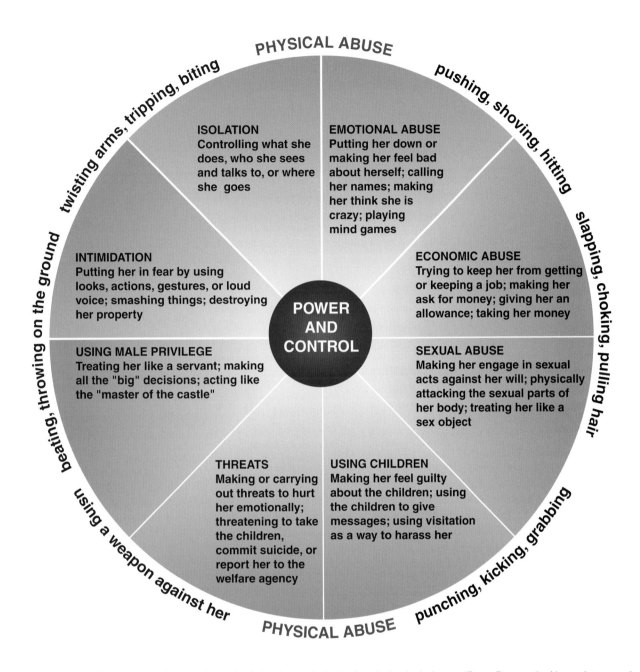

FIG 33-1 The desire for power and control results in both psychological and physical abuse. (From Domestic Abuse Intervention Project [1987]. *Power and control.* Duluth, MN: Domestic Abuse Intervention Project.

is estimated that 3.2% of adults 65 years old and older are abused while they still live in a private home, but only one in five cases are likely reported (Baker, 2007).

Victims of partner abuse tend to conceal their victimization. They are acutely aware that disclosure of their plight will be met with denial or be minimized by the partner, friends, and relatives and by increased abuse by the partner (Merrell, 2001). As abused women become more independent (both emotionally and financially), the incidence of violence by their partners increases as well. The fact that 30% to 50% of all women killed in the United States are killed by a partner as they tried to leave or after they left supports women's fears

(Carretta, 2008; Jordan, 2004; Logan & Walker, 2004). About 50% of victims murdered by partners were seen in the emergency department for injuries at other times before they died (Gerard, 2000). Men are also killed by their partners (4% of all male homicides) (Carretta, 2008; Daniels, 2005). Homicide sometimes occurs in self-defense during the abuse or after a history of beatings.

Studies have shown that partner abuse crosses all social, racial, cultural, and economic classes, including both homosexual and heterosexual relationships, but it is more often reported by individuals on welfare. This tendency is because the victims are more likely to be in contact with reporting agencies, such as public health nurses, welfare offices, public clinics, and emergency departments. Individuals with higher incomes are likely to obtain private services that do not report the abuse (Poirier, 2000). Nurses in any setting need to screen patients for any past or current abuse. Questions about domestic violence need to be asked routinely because victims are reluctant to disclose such information (Howard et al., 2010; Trevillion et al., 2012).

The relationship of alcohol and drug abuse to violent behavior has been the subject of many studies on partner abuse. Some abusers are abstainers, but more are substance abusers (Murphy et al., 2005). Rather than hold the batterers accountable for their violent behavior, the victim's view is that abusers use alcohol and drugs as an excuse for their violence and drink when they are about to become violent. Victims have also reported a correlation between increased intake of alcohol and the severity of violence (Murphy et al., 2005). Women often describe their abusers as "Dr. Jekyll and Mr. Hyde," with changing personalities—gentle, loving, and kind at times; rude, uncaring, and violent at other times. This change is explained in part by the cycle of violence described later.

In some relationships, violence is mutual (Dutton & Nicholls, 2005; Whitaker, 2007) and is the result of efforts to resolve negative communications and escalating conflicts. These couples are often motivated to change and can be taught more effective skills for handling conflict and anger. This mutual violence pattern differs from, but can become, the more common pattern of using violence to exploit and control a partner, often arising out of anger, fear of abandonment, and jealousy (McClellan & Killeen, 2000). This second pattern almost always involves a man abusing a woman, and the man has little motivation to change. Separate interventions and therapy with the man, such as motivational interviewing, might interrupt the cycle of violence (Alexander & Morris, 2008). Other studies have reported that men and women use violence almost equally in the nonmutual abuse pattern, and individuals with personality disorders have higher rates of violence with their partners (Dutton & Nicholls, 2005).

The nature of modern society is a factor to be considered in partner abuse. The portrayal of physical and sexual violence in the media (e.g., the Internet, television, music videos, and films) continues to increase in frequency and severity. Women are still portrayed by the media as second-class citizens at times. However, women younger than 30 are more aggressive in their intimate relationships than women older than 30 (Dutton & Nicholls, 2005). In addition, it is well documented that witnesses of family violence and victims of child abuse and neglect tend to become perpetrators of other violence or the abusers and partners of abusers (Hill & Nathan, 2008; Kelly et al., 2010; Stith et al., 2004; Woods & Wineman, 2004).

In cases of elder abuse and neglect, 90% of the perpetrators are family members, especially adult children and spouses. Other relatives, grandchildren, friends, neighbors, and home service providers may be abusive or neglectful (Baker, 2007).

Elder abuse, sexual abuse, and neglect also occur in long-term care facilities by staff and other residents (Ramsey-Klawsnik et al., 2007). Elder abuse shows power and control dynamics similar to partner abuse (see Figure 33-1) (Spangler & Brandl, 2007).

Effects

Most experts acknowledge the development of learned helplessness, hopelessness, isolation, and resignation in response to ongoing emotional and physical abuse. Abused women report that they fear and hate the abuse but have a tendency to believe their partner's view that they deserve the abuse. Box 33-4 lists common reasons why women endure long-term abuse. Another accepted view of why women endure abuse is the cycle of violence (Box 33-5). During the honeymoon stage, the good side of the man is evident, and the woman is reminded of their love and the happy potential of the relationship (Farella,

---

BOX 33-4 WHY WOMEN STAY AS LONG AS THEY DO

Situational Factors
- Economic dependence; lack of job skills
- Fear of greater physical danger to themselves and their children if they attempt to leave or have partner arrested
- Fear of emotional damage to children because of being without a father
- Fear of losing custody of children
- Lack of alternative housing
- Social isolation; lack of support from family or friends
- Lack of information regarding alternatives
- Fear of involvement in court processes
- Fear of retaliation from partner or partner's family

Emotional Factors
- Poor self-image; fear of being alone
- Being in a state of denial and living a secret
- Personal embarrassment and protecting the image of husband and family
- Insecurity over potential independence and lack of emotional support
- Guilt about failure of marriage or relationship
- Fear that partner is unable to survive alone
- Belief that partner is sick and needs her help
- Belief that partner will change
- Ambivalence and fear about making formidable life changes and having increased responsibility

Cultural Factors
- Knowing that batterers are not held accountable for their violent actions
- Believing that the abuse is her fault
- Being raised to be passive and submissive
- Developing survival skills instead of escape skills
- Recognizing that the legal system is a male-dominated system

Plus: She Still Loves Him

Modified from Julian Center Shelter, Indianapolis, IN, and Task Force on Families in Crisis, Nashville, TN.

BOX 33-5   CYCLE OF VIOLENCE

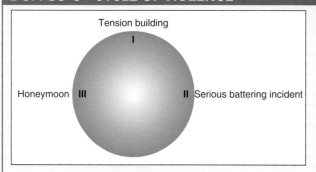

Man

I. Tension Building
He has excessively high expectations of her.
He blames her for anything that goes wrong.
He does not try to control his behaviors.
He is aware of his inappropriate behaviors but does not admit it.
Verbal and minor physical abuse increase.
Afraid that she will leave, he gets more possessive to keep her captive.
He gets frantic and more controlling.
He misinterprets her withdrawal as rejection.

II. Serious Battering Incident
The trigger event is an internal or external event or substance.
The battering usually occurs in private.
He will threaten more harm if she tries to get help (police, medical).
He tries to justify his behaviors but does not understand what happens.
He minimizes the severity of the abuse.
His stress is relieved.

III. Honeymoon
He is loving, charming, begging for forgiveness, making promises.

He truly believes that he will never abuse again.
He feels that he taught her a lesson and she will not act up again.
He preys on her guilt to keep her trapped.

Woman

I. Tension Building
She is nurturing, compliant, tries to please him.
She denies the seriousness of their problems.
She feels she can control his behaviors.
She tries to alter his behavior to stay safe.
She tries to prevent his anger.
She blames external factors—alcohol, work.
She takes minor abuse but does not feel she deserves it.
She gets scared and tries to hide (withdrawal).
She might call for help as the tension becomes unbearable.

II. Serious Battering Incident
In cases of long-term battering, she might provoke it just to get it over with.
She might call for help if she is afraid of being killed.
Her initial reaction is shock, disbelief, and denial.
Fearing more abuse if police come, she might plead for them not to arrest him.
She is anxious, ashamed, humiliated, sleepless, fatigued, depressed.
She does not seek help for injuries for a day or more and lies about the cause of injuries.

III. Honeymoon
She sees his loving behaviors as the real person and tries to make up.
She wants to believe that the abuse will never happen again.
She feels that if she stays, he will get help; the thought of leaving makes her feel guilty.
She believes in the permanency of the relationship and gets trapped.

Modified from Gerard, M. (2000). Domestic violence: how to screen and intervene, *RN, 63,* 52; McFarlane, J., et al. (2004). Increasing the safety-promoting behaviors of abused women. *American Journal of Nursing, 104,* 40; Walker, L. (1979). *The battered woman.* New York: Harper & Row.

2000; Gerard, 2000; Walker, 1979). Women report thinking that they can help their partners overcome their problems and violent behaviors. There is still a shortage of safe places to go as well as a shortage of services to help victims become independent. Many states have ineffective or outdated laws that indirectly perpetuate abuse rather than foster arrest of the abuser for assault and battery. Arrest is a way that batterers get the message that their violence is a crime and not their right (Jordan, 2004; Williams, 2005).

Battered woman syndrome has been suggested as a subclassification of PTSD because repetitive abuse is a serious threat to the victim's health and life. Victims often report nightmares, flashbacks, recurrent fears of more violence, emotional detachment, numbness, startle response, sleep problems, guilt, impaired concentration, and hypervigilance. However, there are other symptoms, such as depression,

hostility, low self-esteem, self-blame, relative passivity, impaired decision making, psychosomatic complaints, fatalism, social isolation, and an unwillingness to seek help (Anorexia Nervosa and Associated Disorders, 2002; Carretta, 2008; Logan & Walker, 2004). Similar to patients with PTSD, battered women show typical reactions to a chronic trauma, not symptoms of psychopathology. Labeling and blaming the victims shifts responsibility away from the perpetrators.

According to victims, it is unlikely that abused women will leave their partners until they realize that the cycle is not going to stop and they have the emotional support to leave and a safe place to go. Fearing that the next beating might be fatal, finding that their partners are physically or sexually abusing their children, and realizing that their children are learning to be abusive are incentives for leaving permanently (Anorexia Nervosa and Associated Disorders, 2002; Miller, 2004).

Recovery

Immediately preceding or at the beginning of a serious battering incident, victims are frightened, amenable to crisis intervention, and more likely to call the police or a crisis service agency for help. Getting victims and their children to a shelter or other safe place, if they will go, is desirable when immediate danger of injury is present. If injuries have occurred, victims should be encouraged to go to an emergency department. In any case, crisis workers, shelter workers, or nurses can begin the important process of assessment and providing information that can make a dent in the cycle of abuse. Even if the survivors are not yet ready to leave their partners, they can be given an easily concealed card with telephone numbers of police, prosecutors, crisis services, victims' assistance, shelters, and support groups and perhaps a short message about the inevitability of the cycle of violence and the fact that no one deserves to be abused. If contact is only by phone or if they are worried that the abusers will find the card, they can be asked to write down the phone numbers on the back of a picture in their wallets or be told to call 911. (In some cities, such as Indianapolis, dialing 211 provides a direct connection to the Domestic Violence Network.) Survivors can also be given ideas for developing a safety or escape plan (Daniels, 2005), such as packing a bag with medicines and clothes for them and their children, house and car keys, money and change for a pay telephone (if they do not have a cell phone), and important phone numbers and papers (e.g., bank account numbers, birth certificates, social security numbers, medical insurance cards, no contact/protective orders). They should also be informed of the protections afforded by legal statutes, protective orders, and more recent antistalking laws. In elder abuse and neglect situations, all states have mandatory reporting laws and procedures, and the survivors need to know this. These affect confidentiality and may pose more safety issues. Adult protective and advocacy services and the judicial system are essential resources (Spangler & Brandl, 2007). Long-term goals for survivors of partner abuse are to develop self-confidence; self-respect; independence; healthy support systems; and a sense of freedom, safety, and empowerment.

PUTTING IT ALL TOGETHER

PSYCHOTHERAPEUTIC MANAGEMENT

Nurse-Patient Relationship

Because most abused women seek help for their injuries and somatic symptoms at least once, nurses can be instrumental in offering information and assistance. Nurses in emergency departments, clinics, physicians' offices, psychiatric facilities, and community health agencies need to be educated on domestic violence and know how to recognize a survivor, make an assessment, offer support, and make a referral to available services (Carretta, 2008; Trevillion et al., 2012). Some common cues to abuse are listed in Box 33-6. In older adults, there also may be malnutrition, frailty, immune suppression, pressure ulcers, and early mortality (Baker, 2007). Inadequate

---

BOX 33-6 COMMON CUES TO PARTNER ABUSE

- Repeated, vague symptoms or illnesses that are not confirmed by tests, such as backache, abdominal pain, indigestion, headaches, hyperventilation, anxiety, insomnia, fatigue, anorexia, heart palpitations
- Unexplained injuries or injuries with unlikely explanations and embarrassment about them
- Hidden injuries such as in areas concealed by clothes or visible on physical or x-ray examination only—for example, head and neck injuries, internal injuries, genital injuries, scars, burns, joint pain or dislocations, numbness, hearing problems, or bald spots
- Injuries with recognizable marks such as from a belt, iron, raised ring, teeth, fingertips, cigarette, gun, or knife
- Multiple fractures or bruises in various stages of healing
- Jumpiness or flinching in the presence of the abuser
- Substance abuse and suicidal thoughts or attempts
- Attempts to conceal fear of the abuser
- Continual efforts to keep the abuser from getting angry
- Denial of any problems in the relationship
- Lack of relationships with family or friends
- Isolation or confinement to home
- Guilt, depression, anxiety, low self-esteem, sense of failure, concealed anger
- Continual justification of own actions and whereabouts of the abuser
- Continual justification of the abuser's actions in public; excusing or rationalizing the behaviors
- Believing in family unity at all costs and in traditional stereotypes
- Believing in managing alone, even when help is offered
- An oversolicitous abuser who does not want to leave the victim alone with hospital or agency staff or even with family and friends

Modified from Carretta, C.M. (2008). Domestic violence: a worldwide exploitation. *Journal of Psychosocial Nursing and Mental Health Services, 46,* 3; Constantine, R.E., & Bricker, P.L. (1997). Social support, stress, and depression among battered women in the judicial setting. *Journal of the American Psychiatric Nurses Association, 3,* 8; Merrell, J. (2001). Social support for victims of domestic violence. *Journal of Psychosocial Nursing and Mental Health Services, 39,* 30; Miller, M.C. (2004). Countering domestic violence. *The Harvard Mental Health Letter, 20,* 1.

---

provision of safety, clothes, shelter, food, water, hygiene, medications, glasses, hearing aids, dentures, and comfort are also common (Strasser & Fulmer, 2007). The assessment process is often difficult because survivors fear disclosure, are embarrassed about the situation, and desire to be treated quickly and leave, and sometimes the abusers are present. It is important to interview the victim privately and with sensitivity, empathy, and compassion. Box 33-7 lists other responses that survivors consider helpful.

The most crucial information to document in an initial contact includes the following:

1. Identity and current location of the abuser
2. Location and safety of any children
3. Length and frequency of abuse

BOX 33-7	HELPFUL RESPONSES TO PARTNER OR ELDER ABUSE

- Be nonjudgmental, objective, and nonthreatening.
- Ask directly if abuse is occurring.
- Identify the abuser's behavior as abusive.
- Acknowledge the seriousness of the abuse.
- Assist the victim in assessing internal strengths.
- Encourage the use of personal resources.
- Give the victim a list of resources—shelters, financial aid, police, and legal assistance.
- Allow victim to choose own options.
- Offer names of relevant support groups.
- Help victim to develop a safety or escape plan.
- Tell the abuser to stop the abuse and get help.
- Do not disbelieve or blame the victim.
- Do not get angry with the victim.
- Do not refuse to help if the victim is not ready to leave the abuser.
- Do not align with the abuser against the victim.
- Do not push the victim to leave the abuser before ready.

BOX 33-8	IF YOU HAVE LEFT AN ABUSIVE MAN …

1. Your problems are not over.
2. Your abuser will try to locate you through family and friends. He will play on their sympathy or intimidate them.
3. He will repeatedly apologize, make promises about changing, and give gifts.
4. Next, he will threaten or intimidate you, your children, family, and friends.
5. He might threaten to kill himself because of you.
6. He will often threaten to take your children away.
7. In another step, he will enter counseling and/or will express religious fervor.
8. He might try to find a counselor or religious leader to try to convince you to return to him.
9. Next, he might harass and stalk (begging, crying, phone calls, written or verbal threats, legal actions, or following you from location to location).

Regardless of his tactics, use legal, community, and personal resources to protect yourself and your children.

Modified from the Salvation Army Domestic Violence Program, Indianapolis, IN.

4. Types of abuse (physical, psychological, sexual, financial) and use of weapons
5. Types and locations of injuries (photographs and body maps are preferred)
6. Availability of weapons at the place of residence
7. Use and abuse of substances and medications by victim and abuser
8. Active and passive suicidal ideation (with or without a plan or a wish to be dead)
9. Types of service desired (police, legal, shelter, crisis counseling, knowledgeable clergy, social service agencies, transportation)
10. Referrals made

Even if the initial contact is brief, it is important to convey to survivors that they are not alone in their abuse and there are people who are willing and able to help when they are ready. Survivors also need to be told more than once that they do not deserve the abuse. The nurse must convey to survivors that they are important and have dignity and worth. These individuals need acknowledgment of their mental and physical exhaustion; fears; and ambivalence about the abuser, leaving, and their wish to help the abuser as well as themselves. It is difficult for nurses and all professionals to accept that survivors cannot be pushed, rushed, or coerced into leaving the abuser before they are ready. Survivors might want to try couples/family counseling and personal counseling (when the abuser refuses counseling) more than once before giving up hope of saving the relationship and of helping the ones they love. It is important to recognize and to acknowledge that it is common for survivors to leave and return several times; it is a process, not a single event (Leone et al., 2007; Spangler & Brandl, 2007). Survivors need not feel guilty or ashamed for trying to improve the relationship. The guilt of leaving will be lessened if they believe they have tried everything and are finally able to acknowledge that nothing will change because the abusers are the only ones who can control the violence and stop the abuse.

When an abused woman does leave her partner, the problems are not over. Box 33-8 lists some of the common reactions the abuser might have and ways in which he might behave. Psychological and physical abuse might continue after separation (Logan & Walker, 2004). Survivors frequently need long-term counseling and social services to recover and become independent, especially if the abuser is unwilling to participate in couples' counseling or an abusers' program (often a court-ordered program of group education and counseling lasting ≥26 weeks). Nursing interventions for survivors (individually or in groups, using cognitive behavioral and trauma-informed care techniques) generally focus on the following:

1. Monitoring safety from partner abuse and preventing suicide
2. Reiterating information about abuse, the cycle of violence, and the abuser's accountability
3. Building self-esteem, confidence, independence, and sense of hope
4. Sharing of feelings, especially anger, frustration, fear, and anxiety
5. Decreasing shame, guilt, embarrassment, manipulation, isolation, and codependency
6. Confirming personal and legal rights
7. Teaching techniques for stress management, communication, conflict resolution, and assertiveness
8. Teaching parenting techniques
9. Building a new, improved support system
10. Setting goals and specific plans for the immediate future
11. Resolving grief

Referrals might also be needed for job counseling or training, legal assistance, financial aid, child care, and permanent housing. At any stage during working with survivors, brief hospitalization might be needed because of injuries, suicide attempts, self-mutilation, or substance abuse and for treatment of serious problems such as depression, anxiety, or panic attacks. Assessment and treatment for ongoing headaches, gastrointestinal complaints, back and pelvic pain, hyperventilation or chest pains, and insomnia are also needed (Amar & Clements, 2009).

> **? CRITICAL THINKING QUESTION**
>
> 2. Your coworker is sharing with you that she is thinking about leaving her husband because of his drinking and long-term emotional abuse of her. She expresses a fear that he might try to kill her and a fear of raising her two children alone. What information would you offer her?

Psychopharmacology

Medications normally are not needed but are commonly given to survivors. Often misprescribed medications are antidepressants, benzodiazepines, and hypnotics. These medications might be used appropriately if the survivor's symptoms of depression, anxiety, sleeplessness, or nightmares or flashbacks are severe. Continual assessment is needed to determine when medications are no longer needed to prevent abuse and addiction.

Milieu Management

Groups in inpatient or outpatient settings that might be relevant for survivors are groups focusing on self-esteem, problem solving, assertiveness, relationship issues, stress management, and codependency. Substance abuse groups should be recommended if necessary. In the community, a group for abused women is desirable. One form of intervention is a telephone support program that focuses on safety-promoting behaviors. Six calls over 8 weeks have encouraged increased use of these behaviors, which were more likely to be practiced 18 months later (McFarlane et al., 2004). The National Domestic Violence Hotline is also available (800-799-SAFE) and online (www.ndvh.org).

> **? CRITICAL THINKING QUESTION**
>
> 3. As an emergency department nurse, you are treating a 19-year-old male victim who was tortured and raped by a local gang. The victim refuses to give any details or to identify members of the gang. Describe what information you would give him about being a victim and the benefits of follow-up counseling.

CASE STUDY

Rachael Benton, a 26-year-old survivor of incest by her father, is married to Richard. She has an 8-year-old child, Matthew; Richard has three boys, Robert, James, and Daniel, ages 11, 8, and 7, who live with them. Angela, age 5, was born after Rachael and Richard were married. Matthew was removed from the home after being abused by Robert, his oldest stepbrother. Rachael sought help by attending a battered women's group.

Rachael's situation was difficult to resolve. Because of heavy drinking, Richard was missing work and changing jobs. His income declined and was sporadic, but expenses did not decline. Without insurance, Rachael's repeated treatment of menstrual irregularities, back pain, chronic and severe headaches, and diarrhea were not paid for. She avoided treatment for bruises, a superficial knife wound, head cuts, and contusions. Richard repeatedly punched her stomach during a pregnancy, causing a miscarriage.

When Richard raped her, Rachael realized that there was no hope for change and that she had to leave. As Rachael became more assertive and independent, Richard demanded that she stay home, bought a shotgun to convince her to stay, and took the starter off the car. He rode to work with coworkers. Rachael had not adopted Richard's boys, so she could not take them with her. She was afraid that his verbal abuse of them would turn to physical violence when she left. Richard knew about all the places she thought of going.

It took 4 months to develop, coordinate, and implement arrangements so that Rachael and Angela were safe in leaving Richard. Neighbors, friends, and teachers were warned of the potential abuse of the boys and given the phone number for anonymously reporting child abuse. Rachael's mother rented her a small trailer in a rural town and obtained forms for Aid to Families with Dependent Children. Rachael secretly and gradually packed clothes and important documents in the trunk of a group member's car.

One night Richard got drunk, beat Rachael, and tried to rape her again. She fought him off and waited until he passed out. The group member with the packed car drove her to the new trailer. As expected, Richard got his shotgun and went to every friend of Rachael's, but none knew where she was. He drove to Rachael's mother's home, and she called the sheriff when his car pulled into the driveway. Richard was escorted out of the county and warned not to return. Within a week, Daniel's teacher filed a child abuse report about bruises found on him. Within 2 weeks, the boys were removed from the home and returned to their biologic mother.

Rachael has received proper medical treatment and feels healthier. She is now divorced, attending a job training program, and maintaining her secret location. She feels safe but is still in counseling once a month to complete her emotional recovery. She attends a support group for battered women once a week.

◎ CARE PLAN

Name: *Rachael Benton*   ***Admission Date:*** _____

DSM-5 Diagnosis: Child Sexual Abuse

Assessment	**Areas of strength:** Patient is bright, articulate, and capable of problem solving; mother and one friend are willing to help; patient is developing trust in group and beginning to process her feelings and rights.
	Problems: Lack of safe housing and employment; inability to remove husband's children from the house and fear he will abuse them; fear of increased abuse of her, even death, if she tries to leave; severe headaches.
Diagnoses	Decisional conflict related to dysfunctional marriage, as evidenced by attendance in a battered women's support group
	Posttrauma syndrome related to previous sexual abuse and physical, emotional, and economic abuse, as evidenced by physical wounds, fear, and emotional trauma
	Fear (of leaving husband) related to potential abuse of sons, as evidenced by reluctance to leave without stepsons
Outcomes	**Short-term goals**
Date met: _____	Patient will remove bullets from gun; design an escape plan.
Date met: _____	Patient will verbalize ability to survive on her own; confirm housing in rural county.
	Long-term goals
Date met: _____	Patient will enroll in job training program.
Date met: _____	Patient will obtain legal assistance for divorce.
Date met: _____	Patient will seek medical treatment for chronic problems.
Planning and Interventions	**Nurse-patient relationship:** Listen nonjudgmentally and empathically; accept strange behaviors related to secrecy and self-protection; avoid disparaging spouse and pressuring to leave; locate resources for training, finances, counseling, and medical care in rural county.
	Psychopharmacology: Trazodone (Desyrel) 50 mg at bedtime to alleviate moderate depression and improve sleep; ibuprofen as needed for severe headaches.
	Milieu management: Encourage continuing in local support group; locate support group in rural county; continue assessment of safety of patient and children.
Evaluation	Patient has moved to rural county and joined support group; is receiving counseling and medical care. Husband's children were removed and placed with their biologic mother.
Referrals	Has an appointment with a job training program in rural county.

▮ STUDY NOTES

1. Not all crimes involve physical violence and injury; however, all crimes involve emotional violation and injury. Victims lose a sense of the ability to control their own lives as well as losing trust in others.

2. Progression through the stages of recovery from a crime might take years. Crisis intervention and group meetings with other survivors can facilitate recovery.

3. In assisting survivors, sensitivity to their needs is crucial to build trust and to avoid blaming the victim.

4. Information about counseling resources and support groups can be given to the survivors of any crime or trauma for later use, even if there is an initial denial of the need for help.

5. The reexperiencing and working through of any trauma or crime memories is a painful, lengthy, and sometimes sporadic process that requires intense support and empathy.

6. Adult survivors of childhood sexual abuse might repress memories for years as a result of the emotional turmoil and sense of being betrayed by the abuser and others.

7. Adult survivors of childhood sexual abuse typically enter counseling for a variety of overt problems, unaware of how these are related to childhood trauma.

8. The concept of learned helplessness; the cycle of violence; and other situational, emotional, and cultural factors help explain why survivors often remain with their abusive partners.

9. Abuse victims are most amenable to crisis intervention and referrals for needed services immediately preceding or at the beginning of a serious battering incident.

10. Patience, support, and information are critical aspects of nursing interventions with all survivors.

REFERENCES

Ai, A. L., et al. (2005). Hope, meaning, and growth following the September 11, 2001, terrorist attacks. *Journal of Interpersonal Violence, 20,* 523.

Alexander, P. C., & Morris, E. (2008). Stages of change in batterers and their response to treatment. *Violence and Victims, 23,* 4.

Alexy, E. M., Burgess, A. W., & Prentky, R. A. (2009). Pornography use as a risk marker for an aggressive pattern of behavior among sexually reactive children and adolescents. *Journal of the American Psychiatric Nurses Association, 14,* 6.

Alim, T. N., et al. (2008). Trauma, resilience, and recovery in high-risk African-American population. *American Journal of Psychiatry, 165,* 12.

Amar, A. F. (2007). Behaviors that college women label as stalking or harassment. *Journal of the American Psychiatric Nurses Association, 13,* 4.

Amar, A. F., & Clements, P. T. (2009). The intersection of violence, crime, and mental health. *Journal of the American Psychiatric Nurses Association, 14,* 6.

American Psychiatric Nurses Association. (2008). *APNA 2008 position statement: Workplace violence executive summary.* Falls Church, VA: APNA.

Annan, S. L. (2011). "It's not just a job. This is where we live. This is our backyard": The experiences of expert legal and advocate providers with sexually assaulted women in rural areas. *Journal of the American Psychiatric Nurses Association, 17,* 2.

Anonymous. (2008). RAINN hotline for sexual assault victims goes digital. *Journal of Psychosocial Nursing and Mental Health Services, 46,* 10. http://www.healio.com/psychiatry/journals/jpn/%7B4c27c25e-02db-4ddc-89ef-716256a2593a%7D/news?fulltext=1

Anonymous. (2012). Obama commits to fight human trafficking. *Journal of Psychosocial Nursing and Mental Health Services, 50,* 12.

Anorexia Nervosa and Associated Disorders. (2002). *Anorexia Nervosa and Associated Disorders (Indianapolis Chapter of ANAD): Personal interviews.* Indianapolis: ANAD.

Baker, M. W. (2007). Elder mistreatment: Risk, vulnerability, and early mortality. *Journal of the American Psychiatric Nurses Association, 12,* 6.

Baliko, B., & Tuck, I. (2008). Perception of survivors of loss by homicide: Opportunities for nursing practice. *Journal of Psychosocial Nursing and Mental Health Services, 46,* 5.

Bennett, L. (1997). Projective methods in caring for sexually abused young people. *Journal of Psychosocial Nursing and Mental Health Services, 35,* 18.

Broome, B. S., & Williams-Evans, S. (2011). Bullying in a caring profession: Reasons, results, recommendations. *Journal of Psychosocial Nursing and Mental Health Services, 49,* 10.

Brown, K. (2001, August 29). Rape and sexual assault: The nursing role. *Nursing Spectrum (DC/Baltimore Metro Ed.),* 29.

Brown, C. (2008). Gender-role implications on same-sex intimate partner abuse. *Journal of Family Violence, 23,* 457.

Burgess, A. W., Slattery, D. M., & Herlihy, P. A. (2013). Military sexual trauma: A silent syndrome. *Journal of Psychosocial Nursing and Mental Health Services, 51,* 2.

Burgess, A. W., et al. (2005). Sexual abuse of older adults. *American Journal of Nursing, 105,* 66.

Burgess, A. W., et al. (2008). Cyber child sexual exploitation. *Journal of Psychosocial Nursing and Mental Health Services, 46,* 9.

Campbell, R., & Wasco, S. M. (2005). Understanding rape and sexual assault. *Journal of Interpersonal Violence, 20,* 127.

Carretta, C. M. (2008). Domestic violence: A worldwide exploration. *Journal of Psychosocial Nursing and Mental Health Services, 46,* 3.

Cassels, C., & Vega, C. (2007, September 7). *Childhood abuse linked to migraine with major depression.* http://cme.medscape.com/view article/562572, Accessed 14.09.07.

Center for American Nurses. (2008, February 27). *The Center for American Nurses calls for an end to lateral violence and bullying in nursing work environments.* http://www.thefreelibrary.com/The center for American nurses calls for an end to lateral violence…-a0179457552, Accessed 10.03.14.

Cerdorian, K. (2005). The needs of adolescent girls who self-harm. *Journal of Psychosocial Nursing and Mental Health Services, 43,* 40.

Chandler, G. (2008). From traditional inpatient to trauma-informed treatment: Transferring control from staff to patient. *Journal of the American Psychiatric Nurses Association, 14,* 5.

Close, S. M. (2005). Dating violence in middle school and high school youth. *Journal of Child and Adolescent Psychiatric Nursing, 18,* 2.

Cole, H. (2009). Human trafficking: Implications for the role of the advanced practice forensic nurse. *Journal of the American Psychiatric Nurses Association, 14,* 6.

Cook, L. J. (2005). The ultimate deception: Childhood sexual abuse in the church. *Journal of Psychosocial Nursing and Mental Health Services, 43,* 19.

Courey, Y. J., et al. (2008). Hildegard Peplau's theory and the health care encounters of survivors of sexual violence. *Journal of the American Psychiatric Nurses Association, 14,* 2.

Crane, P. (2013). A human trafficking toolkit for nursing intervention. In M. de Chesnay (Ed.), *Sex trafficking: A clinical guide for nurses.* New York: Springer Publishing Company.

Daniels, K. (2005). Violence and depression: A deadly comorbidity. *Journal of Psychosocial Nursing and Mental Health Services, 43,* 45.

Davis, J. L., & Petretic-Jackson, P. A. (2000). The impact of child sexual abuse on adult interpersonal functions: A review and synthesis of the empirical literature. *Aggression and Violent Behavior, 5,* 291.

de Chesnay, M. (2013). Sex trafficking as a new pandemic. In M. de Chesnay (Ed.), *Sex trafficking: A clinical guide for nurses.* New York: Springer Publishing Company.

de Chesnay, M., et al. (2013). First-person accounts of illnesses and injuries sustained while trafficked. In M. de Chesnay (Ed.), *Sex trafficking: A clinical guide for nurses.* New York: Springer Publishing Company.

DiVasto, P. (1985). Measuring the aftermath of rape. *Journal of Psychosocial Nursing and Mental Health Services, 23,* 33.

Dunbar, B. (2004). Anger management: A holistic approach. *Journal of the American Psychiatric Nurses Association, 10,* 16.

Dutton, D. G., & Nicholls, T. L. (2005). The gender paradigm in domestic violence research and theory: Part I—the conflict of theory and data. *Aggression and Violent Behavior, 10,* 680.

Faravelli, C., et al. (2004). Psychopathology after rape. *American Journal of Psychiatry, 161,* 1483.

Farella, C. (2000, November). Love shouldn't hurt: Understanding domestic violence. *Nursing Spectrum (D.C./Baltimore Metro Ed.).*

Farella, C. (2001, September 14). Hot and bothering: Sexual harassment in the workplace is no joke. *Nursing Spectrum (D.C./Baltimore Metro Ed.),* 14.

Foa, E. B. (2005). The psychological aftermath of Hurricane Katrina. *Medscape Psychiatry & Mental Health, 8,* 1.

Gerard, M. (2000). Domestic violence: How to screen and intervene. *RN, 63,* 52.

Girardin, B. (2001). Is this forensic specialty for you? *RN, 64,* 37.

Gladstone, G. L., et al. (2004). Implications of childhood trauma for depressed women. *American Journal of Psychiatry, 161,* 1417.

Goldberg, E. (2013, February 3). Superbowl is single largest human trafficking incident in U.S: Attorney General. *The Huffington Post.* http://www.huffingtonpost.com/2013/02/03/super-bowl-sex-trafficking_n_2607871.html, Accessed 05.02.13.

Goodwin, J. M. (2005). Redefining borderline syndromes as posttraumatic and rediscovering emotional containment as a first stage in treatment. *Journal of Interpersonal Violence, 20,* 20.

Gratz, K. L., et al. (2009). Exploring the relationship between childhood maltreatment and intimate partner abuse: Gender differences in the mediating role of emotion dysregulation. *Violence and Victims, 24,* 1.

Hader, R. (2008). Workplace violence: Survey 2008. *Nursing Management, 39,* 13.

Hammer, R. (2000). Caring in forensic nursing: Expanding the holistic model. *Journal of Psychosocial Nursing and Mental Health Services, 38*(18), 200.

Heim, C., et al. (2009). Childhood trauma and risk for chronic fatigue syndrome. *Archives of General Psychiatry, 66,* 1.

Hill, J., & Nathan, R. (2008). Childhood antecedents of serious violence in adult male offenders. *Aggressive Behavior, 34,* 329.

Hinds, J. (1997). Once upon a time: Therapeutic stories as a psychiatric nursing intervention. *Journal of Psychosocial Nursing and Mental Health Services, 35,* 46.

Hoerrner, M. (2013). Working with law enforcement. In M. de Chesnay (Ed.), *Sex trafficking: A clinical guide for nurses.* New York: Springer Publishing Company.

Hoerrner, M., & Hoerrner, K. (2013). Human trafficking. In M. de Chesnay (Ed.), *Sex trafficking: A clinical guide for nurses.* New York: Springer Publishing Company.

Howard, L. M., et al. (2010). Domestic violence and severe psychiatric disorders: Prevalence and interventions. *Psychological Medicine, 40,* 881.

Howe, E. G. (2003). Treating torture victims and enhancing human rights. *Psychiatry, 66,* 65.

Hughes, F. A., Thom, K., & Dixon, R. (2007). Nature and prevalence of stalking among New Zealand mental health clinicians. *Journal of Psychosocial Nursing and Mental Health Services, 45,* 4.

Institute for Safe Medication Practices. (2004). For most nurses, intimidation is commonplace. *RN, 67,* 17.

Isaacs, M. M. (2011). Therapist's page. *Many Voices, 23,* 6.

Jackson, J. (2011). The evolving role of the forensic nurse. *American Nurse Today, 6,* 11.

Jonzon, E., & Lindblad, F. (2005). Adult female victims of sexual abuse. *Journal of Interpersonal Violence, 20,* 651.

Jordan, C. E. (2004). Intimate partner violence and the justice system. *Journal of Interpersonal Violence, 19,* 1412.

Katchen, M. H. (2005). Ritual abuse vs. religious abuse: The development of an artificial distinction. *MKzine, 3,* 9, 2005.

Kelly, P. J., et al. (2010). Profile of women in a county jail. *Journal of Psychosocial Nursing and Mental Health Services, 48,* 4.

Kreidler, M., & Einsporn, R. (2012). A comparative study of therapy duration for survivors of childhood sexual abuse. *Journal of Psychosocial Nursing and Mental Health Services, 50,* 4.

Lacter, E. P. (2011). Torture-based mind control: Psychological mechanisms and psychotherapeutic approaches to overcoming mind control. In O. B. Epstein (Ed.), *Ritual abuse and mind control: the manipulation of attachment needs.* London: Karnac Books.

Lacy, T. J., & Benedek, D. M. (2003). Terrorism and weapons of mass destruction: Managing the behavioral reaction in primary care. *Southern Medical Journal, 96,* 394.

Lanza, M. L., Zeiss, R. A., & Rierdan, J. (2009). Multiple perspectives on assault: The 360-degree interview. *Journal of the American Psychiatric Nurses Association, 14,* 6.

Lapp, C. A., & Overman, N. (2013). Mental health perspectives on care of human trafficking victims within our borders. In M. de Chesnay (Ed.), *Sex trafficking: A clinical guide for nurses.* New York: Springer Publishing Company.

Leiper, J. (2005). Nurse against nurse: How to stop horizontal violence. *Nursing, 35,* 44.

Leone, J. M., Johnson, M. P., & Cohan, C. L. (2007). Victim help seeking differences between intimate terrorism and situational couple violence. *Family Relations, 56,* 427.

Lie, D., & Barclay, L. (2005). *Consequence of childhood sexual abuse similar for both sexes.* www.medscape.com, Accessed 11.07.05.

Lie, D., & Barclay, L. (2006). *Patients might prefer that physicians ask about family conflict.* www.medscape.com, Accessed 03.06.06.

Liston, C. (2009, June). Some brain effects of stress may be reversible. *The Harvard Mental Health Letter.*

Logan, T. K., & Walker, R. (2004). Separation as a risk factor for victims of intimate partner violence: Beyond lethality and injury. *Journal of Interpersonal Violence, 19,* 1478.

Marchetti, C. A. (2012). Regret and police reporting among individuals who have experienced sexual assault. *Journal of the American Psychiatric Nurses Association, 18,* 1.

Martin, L., et al. (2000). Psychological and physical health effects of sexual assaults and nonsexual traumas among male and female United States Army soldiers. *Behavioral Medicine, 26,* 23.

Masho, S. W., & Anderson, L. (2009). Sexual assault in men: A population-based study of Virginia. *Violence and Victims, 24,* 98.

Mawson, A. R. (2005). Intentional injury and the behavioral syndrome. *Aggression and Violent Behavior, 10,* 375.

McClellan, A. C., & Killeen, M. R. (2000). Attachment theory and violence toward women by male intimate partners. *Journal of Nursing Scholarship, 4,* 353.

McCollough-Zander, K., & Larson, S. (2004). "The fear is still in me": Caring for survivors of torture. *American Journal of Nursing, 104,* 54.

McFarlane, J., et al. (2004). Increasing the safety-promoting behaviors of abused women. *American Journal of Nursing, 104,* 40.

Merrell, J. (2001). Social support for victims of domestic violence. *Journal of Psychosocial Nursing and Mental Health Services, 39,* 30.

Miller, M. C. (2004). Countering domestic violence. *The Harvard Mental Health Letter, 20,* 1.

Miller, M. C. (2005). The biology of child maltreatment. *The Harvard Mental Health Letter, 21,* 1.

Miller, L. (2011, July). Expressive writing for mental health. *The Harvard Mental Health Letter.*

Murphy, C. M., et al. (2005). Alcohol consumption and intimate partner violence by alcoholic men: Comparing violent and nonviolent conflicts. *Psychology of Addictive Behaviors, 19,* 35.

Muscari, M. E. (2005). What should I do when a client is being stalked? *Medscape Nurses.* www.medscape.com, Accessed 11.07.05.

Mynatt, S. (2000). Repeated suicide attempts. *Journal of Psychosocial Nursing and Mental Health Services, 38*, 24.

Naifeh, J. A., et al. (2008). Clinical profile differences between PTSD-diagnosed military veterans and crime victims. *Journal of Trauma & Dissociation, 9*, 3.

Newby, A., & McGuinness, T. M. (2012). Human trafficking: What psychiatric nurses should know to help children and adolescents. *Journal of Psychosocial Nursing and Mental Health Services, 50*, 4.

Osterman, J. E., Barbiaz, J., & Johnson, P. (2001). Emergency interventions for rape victims. *Psychiatric Services (Washington, D.C.), 52*, 733.

Paul, J., & Blum, D. (2005). Workplace disaster preparedness and response: The employee assistance program continuum of services. *International Journal of Emergency Mental Health, 7*, 169.

Peternelj-Taylor, C. (2001). Forensic psychiatric nursing: A work in progress. *Journal of Psychosocial Nursing and Mental Health Services, 39*, 8.

Poirier, N. (2000). Psychosocial characteristics discriminating between battered women and other women psychiatric inpatients. *Journal of the American Psychiatric Nurses Association, 6*, 144.

Prugh, P. (2011). Art, art therapy and the inpatient experience. *Many Voices, 23*, 5.

Ragavan, C., & Guttman, M. (2004, December 13). Terror on the streets. *US News and World Report*, 21.

Ramsey-Klawsnik, H., et al. (2007). Sexual abuse of vulnerable adults in care facilities: Clinical findings and a research initiative. *Journal of the American Psychiatric Nurses Association, 12*, 6.

Rick, S., & Douglas, D. H. (2007). Neurobiological effects of childhood abuse. *Journal of Psychosocial Nursing and Mental Health Services, 45*, 47.

Ripol, L. H. (2012, January 29). *Clinical psychopharmacology*. Medscape.com, Accessed 08.02.12.

Roberts, S. J. (2000). Primary health care of survivors of childhood sexual abuse: How can psychiatric nurses be helpful? *Journal of the American Psychiatric Nurses Association, 6*, 191.

Roberts, N. P., et al. (2009). Systematic review and meta-analysis of multiple-session early interventions following traumatic events. *American Journal of Psychiatry, 166*, 3.

Rowell, P. A. (2005). The victor(y) over interpersonal trauma. *Journal of the American Psychiatric Nurses Association, 11*, 103.

Rutz, C. (2007, August 11). *The world will know: Preliminary results of the 2007 International Survey for Adult Survivors of Extreme Abuse*. Presented at the Tenth Annual Ritual Abuse, Secretive Organizations and Mind Control Conference, Windsor Locks, CT.

Sabella, D. (2013). Health issues and interactions with adult survivors. In M. de Chesnay (Ed.), *Sex trafficking: A clinical guide for nurses*. New York: Springer Publishing Company.

Sarson, J., & MacDonald, L. (2004). Human trafficking and ritual abuse-torture. *Persons Against Non-State Torture (NST)*. http://nonstatetorture.org/, Accessed 05.08.04.

Sarson, J., & MacDonald, L. (2009, May 8). *Behavioural harms: Enforced and survival tactics in ritual abuse-torture*, Presented at the Thirty-first SALIS Conference. Halifax, Nova Scotia, Canada.

Schwartz, J. (2011). Introduction. In O. B. Epstein, J. Schwartz, & R. W. Schwartz (Eds.), *Ritual abuse and mind control: The manipulation of attachment needs*. London: Karnac Books.

Schwecke, L. H. (2009). Childhood sexual abuse, PTSD, and borderline personality disorder. *Journal of Psychosocial Nursing and Mental Health Services, 47*, 7.

Shea, D. J. (2008). Effects of sexual abuse by Catholic priests on adults victimized as children. *Sexual Addiction and Compulsivity, 15*, 250.

Shurter, D. (2012). *Rabbit hole: A satanic ritual abuse survivor's story*. Council Bluffs, IA: Consider It Creative.

Simon, T. R., Kresnow, M., & Bossarte, R.M. (2008). Self reports of violent victimization of U.S. adults. *Violence and Victims, 23*, 6.

Solnit, R. (2013, January 24). Violence against women. *The Huffington Post*. www.huffingtonpost.com/rebecca-solnit/violence against women b 254194, Accessed 26.01.13.

Spangler, D., & Brandl, B. (2007). Abuse in later life: Power and control dynamics and a victim centered response. *Journal of the American Psychiatric Nurses Association, 12*, 6.

Spinhoven, P., et al. (2009). Childhood sexual abuse differentially predicts outcome of cognitive-behavioral therapy for deliberate self-harm. *The Journal of Nervous and Mental Disease, 197*, 455.

Starr, D. L. (2004). Clients who self-mutilate. *Journal of Psychosocial Nursing and Mental Health Services, 42*, 33.

Stith, S. M., et al. (2004). Intimate partner physical abuse perpetration and victimization risk factors: A meta-analytic review. *Aggression and Violent Behavior, 10*, 65.

Strasser, S. M., & Fulmer, T. (2007). The clinical presentation of elder neglect: What we know and what we can do. *Journal of the American Psychiatric Nurses Association, 12*, 6.

Tilley, D. S., & Brackley, M. (2004). Violent lives of women: Critical points for intervention-phase I, focus groups. *Perspectives in Psychiatric Care, 40*, 157.

Tolces, R. (2005). Electronic harassment. *MKzine, 3*, 5.

Trevillion, K., et al. (2012). The response of mental services to domestic violence: A qualitative study of service users' and professionals' experiences. *Journal of the American Psychiatric Nurses Association, 18*, 6.

Trossman, S. (2008). Issues up close: The costly business of human trafficking. *American Nurse Today, 12*, 26.

Twibell, R., & Townsend, T. (2011). Trust in the workplace: Build it, break it, mend it. *American Nurse Today, 6*, 11.

Tynhurst, J. S. (1951). Individual reactions to community disaster. *American Journal of Psychiatry, 107*, 764.

Valente, S. M. (2005). Sexual abuse of boys. *Journal of Child and Adolescent Psychiatric Nursing, 18*, 10.

Waite, R., Gerrity, P., & Arango, R. (2010). Assessment for and response to adverse childhood experiences. *Journal of Psychosocial Nursing and Mental Health Services, 48*, 12.

Walker, L. (1979). *The battered woman*. New York: Harper & Row.

Walrafen, N., Brewer, M. K., & Mulvenon, C. (2012). Sadly caught up in the moment: An exploration of horizontal violence. *Nursing Economic$, 30*, 1.

Whitaker, D. J. (2007). Domestic violence: Not always one sided. *The Harvard Mental Health Letter, 24*, 3.

Williams, K. R. (2005). Arrest and intimate partner violence: Toward a more complete application of deterrence theory. *Aggression and Violent Behavior, 10*, 660.

Williams, K. A., & Bydalek, K. (2009). Self-mutilation: The cutting truth. *American Nurse Today, 4*, 8.

Willis, D. G. (2009). Male-on-male rape of an adult man: A case review and implications for interventions. *Journal of the American Psychiatric Nurses Association, 14*, 6.

Woods, S. J., & Wineman, N. M. (2004). Trauma, posttraumatic stress disorder symptom clusters, and physical health symptoms in post-abused women. *Archives of Psychiatric Nursing, 18*, 26.

Young, B. J., & Furman, W. (2008). Interpersonal factors in the risk for sexual victimization and its recurrence during adolescence. *Journal of Youth and Adolescence, 37*, 297.

Zawahir, N., & Scudder, L. E. (2012, January 26). *PTSD: Principles of diagnosis and treatment.* Medscape.org, Accessed 06.02.12.

Children and Adolescents

Teena M. McGuinness

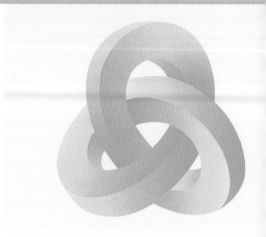

LEARNING OBJECTIVES

- Describe the major categories of child and adolescent psychiatric disorders.
- Describe the frequency of serious psychiatric disorders in children and adolescents.
- Identify genetic and environmental factors associated with development of psychiatric disorders.

- Describe the symptoms of selected child and adolescent psychiatric disorders.
- Identify principles of nursing intervention with child and adolescent psychiatric patients.

Billy is a 9-year-old boy who admitted to setting fires. He states that he set fires in the mail box, trash can, and the alley. He has increased anger and has been aggressive towards his younger sister and brother. He destroyed his bedroom. He is currently in the third grade and has been refusing to go to school. He has no history of significant medical problems or physical/sexual abuse. He struggles to sleep through the night and has a history of difficulty with concentration. He denies suicidal ideation. Both his father and an uncle have been diagnosed with bipolar disorder. Billy's diagnosis is attention deficit hyperactivity disorder.

Vulnerability to psychiatric disorders is a complex interaction between genetic, biologic, and environmental factors. Sometimes, against all odds, an individual transcends early adversities (e.g., parental addiction, poverty, and placement in foster care) and emerges as a stable, competent person. The concept of resilience accounts for why all vulnerable children do not develop mental disorders (Geschwind et al., 2010). Both individual and family factors work together to create resilience, including an easygoing temperament, the ability to form supportive relationships with other adults, family resources, and emotional intelligence (the capacity to delay gratification and understand other people's signals) (Miller et al., 2013; Rutter, 2006).

There is no recipe for resilience, and it is important for nurses to understand child and adolescent mental health and the context in which it develops. Adverse childhood experiences shape later mental health. Childhood adversities such as parental mental illness, addiction, and criminality and physical and sexual abuse are known to be strongly associated with later psychiatric disorders (Green et al., 2010). An example of how the effects of trauma persist into adulthood is illustrated in the accompanying box.

A 30-year-old patient named Alan came to the mental health clinic requesting help with depression and nightmares. On further assessment, an additional diagnosis of posttraumatic stress disorder was revealed. Careful history taking about Alan's childhood revealed that he had endured years of physical and sexual abuse at the hands of older male cousins. The nightmares had persisted throughout his adolescence and his young adulthood. The psychiatric nurse practitioner recommended sertraline (Zoloft) for his depressive symptoms and prazosin for nightmares.

Multiple hardships cause the most risk; about 45% of all childhood-onset psychiatric disorders are associated with the presence of multiple childhood adversities (Green et al., 2010). The onset of other mental disorders later in life is also associated with childhood adversities. The presence of

BOX 34-1   THE DUTCH FAMINE OF 1944

A perfect storm of negative events created what history has called the Dutch Famine of 1944. Scarce food, an unusually hard winter making canals impassable, and German soldiers destroying everything as they retreated in what was proving to be the death rattles of World War II. By the end of the famine in early 1945, adults in Amsterdam were living on a ration of 580 calories per day. Downstream effects of the chronic food shortage include depression for youngsters surviving the "hongerwinter" and schizophrenia for those riding out the famine in their mother's womb.

From Lumey, L.H., & Van Poppel, F.W. (1994). The Dutch famine of 1944-45: mortality and morbidity in past and present generations. *Social History of Medicine, 7,* 229.

multiple childhood hardships is also associated with more adult physical health problems and earlier death (Brown et al., 2009). Conversely, a childhood free of trauma and abuse is associated with greater overall physical and mental health (McGuinness, 2010).

Mental health starts in the womb. Maternal malnutrition is associated with the development of schizophrenia (Box 34-1), mood disorders, and addiction later in life (Franzek et al., 2008). In the United States, prenatal substance exposure is the most common cause of nongenetic mental retardation; alcohol causes the most physical, cognitive, and behavioral difficulties (O'Connor & Paley, 2009; Salisbury et al., 2009). Secondary disabilities of fetal alcohol exposure include school failure and psychiatric illnesses such as mood and anxiety disorders (Paintner et al., 2012). However, it is possible for a range of psychiatric illnesses to develop even if there was no prenatal exposure to substances.

The major diagnostic categories that can occur in childhood and adolescence are discussed in this chapter. These include depression, bipolar disorder (BPD), anxiety disorders, attention-deficit/hyperactivity disorder (ADHD), and autism spectrum disorders (ASDs). In addition to these disorders, the phenomenon of bullying is discussed.

NORM'S NOTES
Child and adolescent psychiatric nursing is a specialty within psychiatric nursing. Whole books are devoted to describing these mental health issues and prescribing their treatment. In this chapter, we try to provide a snapshot of this specialty. The clinical examples should give you a good idea of the problems these patients face and the pain and disappointment their families often endure.

COMMON PSYCHIATRIC DISORDERS

Depression

Conventional wisdom once held that young people did not experience mood disorders. However, several studies have indicated that both unipolar and bipolar depression do occur in children (Costello et al., 2003; Merikangas et al., 2010).

Approximately 12.5% of youth have experienced some form of depression by age 18, with approximately two thirds experiencing severe impairment (Merikangas et al., 2010). After puberty, girls surge ahead of boys in depression rates by a factor of two (Hyde et al., 2008). Girls are more likely to rely on close emotional communication and responsiveness as a source of self-definition; extreme concern about social evaluations by others also contributes to higher rates of depressive symptoms in girls (McGuinness et al., 2012). Higher rates of depression and anxiety also occur in women.

Similar to adults, youth with major depression may experience feelings of helplessness, hopelessness, low energy, and social withdrawal (Zalsman et al., 2006). Children often express depression via somatic complaints and feeling unloved; they are less likely to experience psychosis than adults. Suicidal ideation is possible and is the third leading cause of death among adolescents (Cash & Bridge, 2009; Thapar et al., 2012). Rates of suicide by youth continue to increase, and Internet bullying has been associated with increased risk of suicide (Cash & Bridge, 2009).

Clinical Example: Young and pregnant
"I've been depressed since I lost my baby, and my mom thought I should see someone." Tonya is a 14-year-old African-American girl who presents with complaints of depression. Her mother accompanies her to see the nurse. Tonya states that she has been doing poorly in school. Her grades were "A's" and "B's," but now she is receiving "D's" and "F's." She finds it difficult to concentrate and focus on her work. Her mother reports periods of extreme anger, which is not characteristic of Tonya. The mother thinks Tonya is a "good girl," but she has been having problems with her boyfriend. According to the mother, problems started about 8 months ago when Tonya started dating a 16-year-old boy. Tonya became pregnant and gave birth at 5 months gestation. The baby lived only for a few hours. Tonya became depressed and attempted to get pregnant again by the same boyfriend. The boyfriend had already moved on to another girl. He would call Tonya, often with the new girlfriend on the line, and together they would taunt Tonya and call her names. Nonetheless, Tonya became pregnant a second time by the same boy. Tonya lost this baby as well. Tonya became even more depressed and angry when her sister (also unmarried) became pregnant and talked about her baby. The mother brought Tonya to the hospital to "get on an antidepressant." Tonya was given a diagnosis of major depression with provisional rule-out of postpartum depression diagnosis. She was prescribed escitalopram (Lexapro) 20 mg/day with scheduled follow-up appointments with the nurse.

? CRITICAL THINKING QUESTION

1. If your child had a mental health problem that required hospitalization, what questions would you ask of the staff? What would you look for in the environment? What kind of behaviors by the staff would you consider to be red flags?

Bipolar Disorder

BPD in children differs from the adult type in that irritability is a more prominent symptom, and there are high rates of co-occurring attention problems and anxiety (Carbray & McGuinness, 2009). As children mature, approaching the later teen years, bipolar symptoms begin to conform more to symptoms experienced by adults.

In contrast to adults, who often exhibit grandiosity, hypersexuality, and intrusive behavior, pediatric bipolar symptoms may be quite understated. Mood instability, temper tantrums, impulsivity, and subtle depressive symptoms are more likely to be displayed (Carbray & McGuinness, 2009).

Clinical Example: Wanting to die

Willie is an 8-year-old white boy who was admitted to the hospital because he says that he "wants to be dead." He has trouble getting along with peers at school. He is a second grader and has been involved in fights at school. He was brought to the hospital by the Sheriff's department for fighting. Willie has no history of physical or sexual abuse. He currently lives with his biologic mother and a 12-year-old half-sister. He has no contact with his biologic father, who has a history of BPD and schizophrenia. Testing reveals an IQ of 72, which is 2 points above a mental retardation diagnosis. After a thorough workup, Willie is given a diagnosis of ADHD and BPD.

The clinical example featuring Willie depicts what is often observed clinically: BPD and ADHD look alike and overlap in presentation. Willie was given a diagnosis of both ADHD and BPD. There are also symptoms that suggest depression (he wants to be dead) and anxiety. Because of this array of symptoms, numerous medications might be prescribed. In Willie's case, he was prescribed a drug for impulse control (clonidine), a drug for ADHD (methylphenidate [Concerta]), a drug for mood instability (oxcarbazepine [Trileptal]), and a drug for aggression and unrealistic thinking (risperidone [Risperdal]). Although this medication regimen is well meaning and may be exactly the combination that is needed, it can also cause Willie other problems. For example, in a child with BPD, drugs to elevate a depressed mood or to control hyperactivity might have paradoxical responses and result in extreme irritability or mania (McClellan et al., 2007). In other words, antidepressants can cause the expression of BPD (McNamara et al., 2012). It has also been shown, at least anecdotally, that when a child does not respond to stimulants and antidepressants and when combined with a family history of bipolar illness, as in Willie's case, the clinician should suspect BPD as the primary cause.

? CRITICAL THINKING QUESTION

2. Many people are very concerned about the increased numbers of children and adolescents with ASDs and ADHD. These concerns/debates are as current as the morning paper. What explanations seem to make most sense to you?

Anxiety Disorders

Anxiety disorders in children occur at a rate of about 10% by age 16; girls outpace boys with respect to all anxiety disorders (Costello et al., 2003). Childhood-onset anxiety disorders foreshadow adult anxiety disorders (Rockhill et al., 2010) and are thought to be caused by genetic and environmental factors. Pediatric obsessive-compulsive disorder (OCD) involves recurring thoughts (obsessions) and repetitive ritualistic behaviors (compulsions) in an effort to decrease anxiety (Mancebo et al., 2008). Perfectionism, intolerance for uncertainty, and overestimation of threats are cognitive beliefs that perpetuate OCD (Jacob & Storch, 2013). Pediatric OCD is often associated with disruptive behavioral disorders such as conduct disorder and oppositional defiant disorder (characterized by argumentativeness, testing limits, and aggressive behaviors) (Mancebo et al., 2008).

Symptoms of posttraumatic stress disorder (PTSD) in children are similar to many of the symptoms as adults and include nightmares, intrusive memories, and hypervigilance (Wu et al., 2010). PTSD can be caused by a single traumatic event, such as an automobile accident, or long-term sexual and physical abuse. The greater the magnitude of the stressor, the more likely the child will develop PTSD (Fairbank & Fairbank, 2009). For example, a child who has experienced a major natural disaster such as Hurricane Katrina, in which the child's life was in danger and home and family members were lost, has a great risk for developing PTSD.

Other anxiety disorders, such as separation anxiety, social anxiety disorder, and panic disorder, all may appear in childhood. Panic attacks are more likely to occur in later adolescence and continue into adulthood if not treated. Harsh parenting, stressful life events, and a genetic predisposition to anxiety disorders increase vulnerability to anxiety disorders (Hirshfeld-Becker et al., 2008).

Clinical Example: "I can't breathe!"

"I'm having a lot of anxiety, and I feel really uncomfortable in class sometimes." Brady is a 17-year-old white boy who has panic attacks and anxiety. He reports being this way most of his life. In the past, his anxiety has been manageable and did not impair his ability to function at school. He is now a senior and has done well enough to remain on the honor roll. Until recently, Brady had panic attacks about once per month. Recently the attacks have increased to one to two times per week. Brady reports that he worries about everything. He cannot sit still. His legs never stop moving, and he changes positions nonstop. Occasionally, when meeting with the psychiatrist at the outpatient clinic, he cannot even remain in his seat. He is up and down, pacing back and forth. Having to stay in his seat in class "drives him crazy," and he reports defying his teacher even though he does not want to hurt her feelings. He states that sometimes getting up and moving seems like a matter of life and death to him. Anxiety symptoms include sweating, a racing heart, and feeling that he will faint. Sometimes he "can't breathe" and senses tingling in his body. On a scale of 1 to 10, Brady rates his anxiety at that time as a 10. He is diagnosed with anxiety disorder with agoraphobia. The physician prescribes sertraline (Zoloft) 25 mg/day for 2 weeks with an increase to 50 mg/day thereafter. The physician also recommends cognitive behavior therapy with a trained practitioner.

Attention-Deficit/Hyperactivity Disorder

ADHD is the most common childhood psychiatric disorder; it affects about 2 million children in the United States (Costello et al., 2003). ADHD is a complex brain disorder that involves subtle abnormalities in central nervous system functioning (Kieling et al., 2008). ADHD is probably a group of conditions rather than a distinct entity and is often seen with co-occurring behavior disorders (Spencer, 2006). A vexing issue with ADHD is that symptoms are highly inconsistent. For some children, inattention is the most notable characteristic; for others, hyperactivity, inattention, and defiant behaviors all may be exhibited. All children at times behave hyperactively, are inattentive, or act defiantly. However, for a diagnosis of ADHD to be made, the behavior must last at least 6 months; appear before age 7; and create noteworthy troubles for the child academically, socially, or at home. The best treatment plan includes management and understanding from parents and teachers. In many cases, there is a lack of educational or behavioral assessment, and medication management becomes the first and only intervention.

Clinical Example: ADHD

Burt is a 7-year-old white boy with a diagnosis of ADHD. He is in the first grade and presents to the psychiatric nurse practitioner for follow-up care. He was initially referred to the clinic by his school. He was fidgety, could not sit still for long, talked uncontrollably in class, and performed academically well below what his standardized test scores predicted. He was prescribed methylphenidate (Concerta) 18 mg via 2 tablets in the morning.

During the visit, the father states, "He's doing a little better, but there's not a whole lot of change in him. He seems to be doing a bit better in school." He currently receives tutoring related to his very poor grades in school. He lives with both biologic parents and has two older brothers. One of the brothers has ADHD as does Burt's father and a maternal aunt. His mother has multiple sclerosis. Burt's father reports that his son has trouble sleeping and cannot seem to settle down at night. Burt is cleanly dressed, and the nurse reports that his speech, mood, affect, and thought production are within normal limits. Methylphenidate is increased to 54 mg/day each morning, and clonidine 0.1 mg/day is added for insomnia. No other referrals are offered, and his father is instructed to bring Burt back in 4 weeks for a follow-up visit.

Autism Spectrum Disorders

In 2013, there were significant changes made in the definition of autism in *DSM-5* (American Psychiatric Association, 2013). Most notable was the exclusion of pervasive developmental disorders (including Asperger's disorder), which were subsumed into the category of ASD. There are updated criteria that must be met for the *DSM-5*, as follows: (a) persistent deficiencies in social communication and interaction across settings; (b) restricted and repetitive behaviors, interests, or activities; (c) symptoms must be present early in childhood (but may be delayed to a later age when social demands exceed the limits of the child); and (d) symptoms limit and impair functioning daily. *DSM-IV-TR* required only one symptom of fixed interests and repetitive behaviors for diagnosis, whereas *DSM-5* requires at least two (American Psychiatric Association, 2000; Simons Foundation Autism Research Initiative, 2012).

Additionally, *DSM-IV-TR* required that symptoms must have occurred before age 3 years. Individuals who are higher functioning sometimes do not display impairments until social or educational demands increase at an older age; the new *DSM-5* guidelines do not specify an age, allowing for this consideration. Conversely, with behavioral interventions or improved environment, some symptoms of autism may improve. *DSM-5* allows a diagnosis to be made by history, even though an individual no longer exhibits behavioral criteria. The ASD diagnosis is still retained.

A wide array of behaviors remains within the ASD category. Specific behaviors are often responses to stimuli based on age and developmental level. A young nonverbal child with a diagnosis of autistic disorder might flap his hands in response to stress. However, a teenager may behave disruptively, lashing out with verbal attacks (McGuinness & Johnson, 2013).

ASDs have three major commonalities:

1. *Arrested social skills* are manifested by withdrawal and low interest in others. Demonstrations of reciprocity may be rare because of a lack of understanding about social cues.
2. *Speech and language delays* are common; some children have no speech ability at all. Pitch and intonation are noticeably different with repetition of words or phrases; facial expressions may also be limited.
3. *Narrow interests and repetitive behaviors* are exhibited by a preoccupation with numbers or mechanical objects. Flapping, spinning, and twisting provide specific stimulation that may aid in blocking other sources of stimuli for a person with ASD (McGuinness & Johnson, 2013).

Sensory problems are exhibited as sensitivity to odors, noise, or light as well as problems with certain textures in food or clothing (Iarocci & McDonald, 2006). A clothing tag or a button on clothing may cause great distress to a child with ASD.

Mental retardation can co-occur with ASD; however, estimates vary widely. Chakrabarti and Fombonne (2001) found that 26% of children had some degree of mental retardation, but children with ASDs as a whole were "less impaired than what has been classically described" (p. 3098).

An estimate of the prevalence of ASDs was 116 per 10,000 (Baird et al., 2006), reflecting an alarming 20-fold increase since the early 1980s (Kurita, 2006). Whether this increase is due to better assessment methods, changing diagnostic criteria, or other factors is a subject for debate (Bishop et al., 2008). The theory that immunizations with the measles-mumps-rubella (MMR) vaccine fueled the increase in ASDs has not been supported (Grigorenko, 2009). ASDs are syndromes with genetic and nongenetic causes (Muhle et al., 2004). "Autism is perhaps the most highly heritable behavioral disorder" (Ronald et al., 2006, p. 952). Multiple genes and their variants are thought to be the cause of ASDs.

Clinical Example

Trey is a 7-year-old boy with severe autism. He was diagnosed at about 2 years of age. Before the diagnosis, Trey's mother told her husband, parents, and in-laws that something was wrong with Trey, but they did not hear or, more likely, did not want to hear. Trey's mother first noticed that his head would drop when he was in his high chair. Slowly, others in the family began to notice what would later be diagnosed as atonic seizures. Trey's lack of social development became more and more obvious. By the age of $2\frac{1}{2}$, there was no longer room for anyone to doubt that a problem existed. His seizures became more frequent, sometimes up to 50 per day. Occasionally, Trey would have a grand mal seizure. The parents searched desperately for a physician who could stop the seizures. Several precious years went by before this was accomplished. After trying numerous anticonvulsants, a pediatric neurologist in a town 100 miles away found the right combination, and the seizures ended. Now, at age 7, Trey is in special education and looks forward to school each day. He struggles to communicate because of his inability to articulate. His voice is high-pitched and unintelligible to all but his parents. He demonstrates what the family has learned are typical autistic behaviors (e.g., flapping, obsession with trucks, and screaming when he is frustrated). Although Trey has been prescribed many medications, he now takes only one medication, risperidone, an atypical antipsychotic.

? CRITICAL THINKING QUESTION

3. As noted, the idea that childhood immunizations (MMR) may have caused autism has not been supported by research findings. However, many parents believe these immunizations were the culprit and refuse inoculations for their other children. What does the scientific evidence say on this issue? How would you discuss the importance of immunizations to parents who fear immunizations might be dangerous?

BULLYING

Who hasn't heard of bullying? Most of us have seen it happen or known someone who has been bullied. The study of bullying began after three boys who had been targeted by bullies committed suicide in Norway in 1983. Olweus (1993) was commissioned by the Norwegian government to study the trend of bullying, and during his research, he found that 20% of Norwegian children had been bullied. Since he completed his work, many other studies have been completed, leading to a better understanding of the prevalence, etiology, and potential remediation of bullying behavior. However, bullying has increased in magnitude, and, with the ever-present Internet, bullying can be done any time of the day or night.

Olweus (2001) defined bullying as the repeated negative actions of one or more students toward a victim. Bullying usually entails a systematic abuse of power involving repetition, harm, and unequal power (Nansel & Overpeck, 2003). Playful teasing, one-time aggression, and joking are not bullying; the crucial elements of bullying are that it is both intentionally cruel and unprovoked. Surprisingly, bullies can have friends and followers, and bullying can become a social activity.

Although there has been a great deal of research interest in bullying behavior in recent years, findings from the research have yet to filter into daily lives of school personnel or nurses. Youth who are being bullied often visit the school nurse's office because of somatic symptoms, and the bullying goes unrecognized unless the nurse understands its devastating impact. Complaints of bullying made to school authorities are low, and the true number of incidents is likely underreported.

The incidence of bullying varies from country to country. In a U.S. study, 53% of children reported having been targets of agents of verbal bullying (Liu & Graves, 2011), whereas a South African study of a parochial high school reported that 90% had either been victims of or had witnessed bullying during their high school years (Dussich & Maekoya, 2007). Another study in the U.S. found that among school-age children 21% had been physically bullied, 51% socially bullied, and 14% electronically bullied (Wang, 2009).

Both the targets and the perpetrators endure significantly higher rates of emotional problems, but the effects varied. Perpetrators had higher rates of alcohol abuse. Making friends was more difficult for the victims but was easier for the bullies themselves. In reality, some individuals admired the bullies. All involved in bullying behavior paid a price; smoking and poorer academic achievement were associated with bullying—for the victims, the perpetrators, and the individuals who cheered the bullies on (Nansel et al., 2001).

Verbal bullying is the most frequent type of bullying, with name calling and derogatory remarks being most common (Stassen Berger, 2007). Racial and gender slurs are often components of the verbal assaults. *Slander* (defined as malicious, untrue statements) and *name calling* are the most common bullying methods (Dussich & Maekoya, 2007). *Relational bullying* involves shunning and ignoring the victim (Dussich & Maekoya, 2007). The goal is to disrupt shared relationships between peers and is more common among girls than boys (Raskauskas & Stoltz, 2004). Because of its indirect nature, relational bullying may go unrecognized by parents and teachers. The victim experiences isolation and humiliation.

Physical bullying can range from slight shoving to burns and broken bones (Dussich & Maekoya, 2007). An obvious physical attack at school usually is addressed by a principal, but physical bullying also occurs after school in other locales. The U.S. Secret Service investigated 37 acts of targeted school violence (including Columbine in 1999) and found that three quarters of the attackers (29) had been physically bullied, attacked, or injured by others (usually just before the shooting incidents) (Vossekuil et al., 2002). Some cases involved chronic, severe bullying in which the threats directly contributed to the decision to target the school and demand revenge. In witness statements from one incident, "schoolmates alleged that nearly every child in the school at some point had thrown the attacker against a locker, tripped him in the hall, held his head under water in the pool or thrown things at him" (Vossekuil et al., 2002, p. 21).

Cyberbullying is the newest type of bullying and receives the most media attention. The Cyberbulling Research Center (http://cyberbullying.us) shows that approximately 19.4% of students are cyberbullied in the United States (Hinduja & Patchin, 2010). These messages may take the form of private text messages or e-mails being forwarded; pictures being posted without permission (especially unbecoming or embarrassing photos); and rumors being spread via e-mails, text messages, or social networking websites. Facebook and other social networking websites have exponentially grown; tens of millions of Internet users visit these websites daily. The media has taken notice of cyberbullying more recently because of several suicides that have occurred as the result of electronic bullying activity. Previously contained in the hallways of schools, bullying has become omnipresent and promises to become an even greater threat to the emotional well-being of youth (Stanbrook, 2014).

Although bullying can never be totally prevented, nurses can take action by understanding that bullying can be a daily occurrence (McGuinness, 2007). Additionally, nurses can take a stand against bullying. Although some schools say they have a "zero tolerance policy for bullying," the policy may refer only to physical aggression and not to more subtle relational and cyberbullying. Nurses can and should educate teachers, administrators, and parents about the realities (frequency and types) of bullying because it can happen in any school setting, does untold damage, and ultimately may result in suicide and murder.

Clinical Example: Bullied to death

"Bullied student kills herself leaping from I-65 overpass"

Jemison, Alabama

The father of a Jemison teen who took her life by jumping from an interstate overpass in Chilton County said the family is devastated by the loss and the belief that bullying may have led to her suicide.

"I'm just so sad, you wouldn't believe," Jim Moore said. "We knew she had been picked on some, but we thought it had been dealt with."

Alex Moore, a sophomore at Jemison High School, leaped onto Interstate 65 from a bridge near her home just before 7 a.m. Wednesday. She was pronounced dead on the scene, said Chilton County Coroner Randall M. Yeargen.

She had walked to the overpass after her parents went to work. A Christian, Alex left a note saying she was going to see Jesus.

Moore said his 15-year-old daughter was sometimes teased about her appearance, mainly her weight.

By Carol Robinson, news staff writer, *Birmingham News*, Friday, May 14, 2010, p. 1C

PSYCHOTHERAPEUTIC MANAGEMENT

This chapter has provided glimpses into some of the mental health issues confronted by children and adolescents and their families. The nurse, as with other patients, has three tools: the relationship with the patient and family (Me) medications, and the environment (Milieu). A general overview of these tools is provided.

Nurse-Patient Relationship for Patients and Families—Me

When nurses work with children who receive psychiatric care and their families, an important goal is mental health literacy. Ignorance abounds when it comes to children with psychiatric disorders; often parents also feel stigmatized by the experience of seeking help for their child's mental illness. To add insult to injury, psychiatric care for children is terribly difficult to obtain. Consider that Safe Haven Laws (where mothers can surrender their newborns to child welfare authorities with no questions asked) have been used frequently in recent years to obtain psychiatric care for children with mental illness (Warner, 2009). These children are not just overly energetic youth who tested parental limits. Most are severely mentally ill children who had made homicide or suicide threats. Faced with no access to care (after spending months on waiting lists for a medication appointment or a spot in residential treatment), parents made the difficult decision to terminate their own parental rights. The gradual closing of child/adolescent psychiatric services and general unavailability of care over the last 15 years led to child welfare authorities becoming custodians of many youth with serious psychiatric disorders. Many inpatient and residential mental health services have been closed in the past 20 years. Steep decreases in the reimbursement for residential treatment for children have led to these closures. Where residential facilities remain, they serve the most seriously mentally ill youth with public funds supporting the treatment costs (McGuinness, 2009). The trend toward psychotropic medications for youth as the primary treatment strategy has caused a shift toward medication-based outpatient treatment as a cost-containment strategy. In some locales, there is a 9-month wait for a medication evaluation.

Psychopharmacology—Meds

Psychopharmacology is not the only intervention for mental disorders of childhood, but it remains a major avenue with which to approach most of these patients. Few drug trials have focused on neuropsychiatric disorders in children, and the trials that do exist provide evidence for only a fraction of available drugs used for treatment of these conditions (Murthy et al., 2013). As of 2012, the only drug approved by the U.S. Food and Drug Administration (FDA) for treatment of depression for children younger than 12 years old is fluoxetine (Prozac). Between 2007 and 2011, four drugs were approved for treatment of schizophrenia in adolescents, but no treatment has been approved for children younger than 12.

This chapter is not meant to substitute for a text dedicated to child and adolescent psychiatric nursing, so the student is referred to such a specialty book for very specific information. The medication discussion that follows is meant to provide

---

BOX 34-2   A CONSERVATIVE APPROACH TO DRUG PRESCRIPTION

An important first step in working with children and adolescents when contemplating psychopharmacologic interventions is "prescription hygiene." Prescription hygiene is the removal of selected medications to clarify their effect, interactions, and adverse effects. In other words, one has to attempt to determine what medication is doing what to limit speculations about the treatment approach. If prescription hygiene is performed, adverse effects of medications can be minimized, and a stepwise approach to psychopharmacologic intervention can be realized. This conservative approach to medication dosing is particularly important because it facilitates management of side effects and adverse effects.

BOX 34-3   INVOLVING THE FAMILY

An important component of psychopharmacologic treatment is engagement of the family. Family members take care of the child or adolescent typically, and perhaps no one is more invested in the patient's treatment than the family. Family members can be powerful allies in attempting to overcome the mental disorder but can also be powerful roadblocks to success. Roadblocks can be erected directly or in more indirect, passive-aggressive ways. Family members can be very instrumental in recording symptoms and in tracking symptom frequency, intensity, number, and duration.

---

general information for students who may work with child and adolescent psychiatric patients during their psychiatric nursing clinical rotation. Box 34-2 presents a basic philosophy of care. When dealing with this age group, it is important to be conservative in one's approach to medications. Box 34-3 reinforces the need to work with families.

Drugs for Depression

Numerous drugs are explicitly manufactured for the treatment of depression (see Chapter 15). Some but not all of these are available for use in children and adolescents. Some of these categories of drugs are discussed briefly.

Tricyclic Antidepressants. Tricyclic antidepressants (TCAs) are older agents, are cheap, and have a variety of concerns associated with their use. As in adults, TCAs in children have a narrow therapeutic index rendering them sensitive to changes in serum levels. Historically, deaths of children have been associated with the use of some TCAs, with desipramine being particularly singled out. TCAs used in the treatment of children include imipramine, clomipramine, and desipramine. These drugs produce many side effects, including dry mouth, fatigue, dizziness, sweating, weight gain, urinary retention, tremor, tachycardia, and agitation. *Because all TCAs affect cardiac conduction, baseline cardiograms should be taken and repeated on a scheduled basis thereafter.* In addition, TCAs are susceptible to drug-drug interactions and the aforementioned changes in serum level. Their narrow therapeutic index is responsible for the bothersome to life-threatening adverse effects spawned from drug-caused high serum levels.

Selective Serotonin Reuptake Inhibitors. Selective serotonin reuptake inhibitors (SSRIs) are frequently used in children and adolescents. These agents increase intrasynaptic serotonin over time, and this presumably has an antidepressant effect. It is obvious now that this increase also has other effects. Numerous aggressive, violent, self-destructive, and death-causing behaviors have been linked to these serotonin-enhancing drugs, so a black box warning has been demanded by the FDA warning of SSRI-induced suicidal thoughts and behavior.

SSRIs include fluoxetine, sertraline (Zoloft), paroxetine (Paxil), fluvoxamine (Luvox), citalopram (Celexa), and escitalopram (Lexapro). Fluvoxamine, fluoxetine, and sertraline have been approved to treat OCD in children, and fluoxetine has been approved to treat depression in children older than 8 years of age. As with many medications for many different conditions, drugs are often prescribed for children and adolescents without FDA approval.

SSRIs cause many side effects. The most troublesome are the aforementioned behavioral effects: the risk of suicidal thoughts and suicidal behavior. Beyond these effects, some young people have become very agitated. As noted in Chapter 15, a website, www.ssristories.com, features summaries of violent behaviors purportedly driven by SSRIs or SSRI discontinuance. No one knows whether or not these behaviors were really SSRI driven. However, it can be said that a perception exists that SSRIs can induce morally indifferent thinking. See Chapter 15 for more information on SSRIs and other antidepressants.

Drugs for Bipolar Disorder

Many drugs are available for treating BPD in children and adolescents. Although not dedicated to their use in children and adolescents, Chapter 16 provides a review of the basic drugs used to treat this disorder.

The medication management goals with BPD are straightforward: initially intervene to stabilize both mood and sleep, and then seek to manage comorbid symptoms such as hyperactivity or anxiety (McClellan et al., 2007). As of 2013, only four agents have been approved by the FDA: (1) risperidone, for ages 10 to 17; (2) lithium, for ages 12 and older; (3) aripiprazole, for ages 11 to 17; and (4) olanzapine, for ages 13 to 17 (U.S. Food and Drug Administration, 2013). Dosages are weight based; a 10-year-old child who weighs 125 lb requires more medication to achieve a therapeutic effect than a 17-year-old child who weighs 95 lb. In actual practice, many agents used for mood stabilization are used off label (McClellan et al., 2007). First-line medication choices typically include either an atypical antipsychotic or a mood stabilizer, depending on which mood symptoms are most disrupting the child's life. After mood symptoms are well controlled, residual symptoms, such as inattention, anxiety, or depressive symptoms, can be addressed using symptom-specific medications.

As shown in the clinical example of Willie, BPD is not always "clean"—there are often other comorbidities. In Willie's case, he also required medication for impulse control, ADHD, and aggression.

Drugs for Anxiety Disorders

As with adult patients, antidepressants typically are good choices for anxiety in children and adolescents, albeit with all the concerns and cautions already mentioned. Specifically, some TCAs and some SSRIs are particularly beneficial in treating OCD and separation anxiety. The nonbenzodiazepine buspirone (BuSpar) and the long-acting (and less addicting) benzodiazepine clonazepam (Klonopin) have been found to reduce anxiety in some young patients.

Drugs for Attention-Deficit/Hyperactivity Disorder

Throughout this chapter, several instances of ADHD have been mentioned. The medications to treat ADHD include several stimulants: methylphenidate (Ritalin), long-acting methylphenidate (Concerta), dextroamphetamine with the amino acid lysine attached (lisdexamfetamine [Vyvanse]), plain dextroamphetamine (Dexedrine), an amphetamine mixture (Adderall), and other stimulant formulations such as pemoline (Cylert). It is still not understood exactly how these drugs improve attention and decrease hyperactivity. However, it is known that they affect dopaminergic and noradrenergic systems. Presumably by activating these neurotransmitters (the parts of the prefrontal brain where attention and concentration are centered), these areas are empowered to function as was intended—to attend, concentrate, control impulsive thoughts, and maintain emotional equilibrium. These drugs work better in some children and adolescents than they do in others.

A host of other agents are used at times to treat symptoms associated with ADHD. An increasingly common approach is to treat ADHD with an alpha-2 agonist such as clonidine (Catapres) or guanfacine (Tenex). These drugs work by "tricking" the presynaptic neuron into "thinking" that there are adequate amounts of brain norepinephrine. Over time, this "trickery" results in a lower level of norepinephrine synthesis and release. For many patients with ADHD, alpha-2 agonists are effective, and, as seen in the case of Willie earlier in the chapter, clonidine is prescribed to help control impulsive behavior.

Drugs for Autism Spectrum Disorders

Numerous drugs have been used to treat patients with ASDs. For example, many of the drugs previously mentioned can and have been used to treat symptoms of autism, including antidepressants, antimanic drugs, antianxiety drugs, alpha-2 agonists, and stimulants. However, mainstays of pharmacotherapy in the treatment of autism that have not been mentioned are the atypical antipsychotics. These drugs block both dopamine and serotonin receptors, and it is theoretically this dual action that allows both a superior therapeutic effect and a manageable side effect profile. Included in this category are aripiprazole (Abilify), risperidone (Risperdal), olanzapine (Zyprexa), quetiapine (Seroquel), and ziprasidone (Geodon). Beyond their treatment of psychotic thinking, atypical antipsychotics are used for their ability to modulate aggressive behaviors, tantrums, tics, and various self-injurious behaviors. The dosage of these agents is quite low. In the example mentioned earlier, Trey is prescribed only 0.5 mg twice per day of risperidone (the most commonly prescribed of these drugs). Neurologic side effects are typically benign. Traditional antipsychotics can be used occasionally for aggressive behavior; however, caution because of their side effect potential is always warranted. Chapter 14 provides a thorough review of antipsychotic drugs.

Environmental Issues—Milieu

There are many environmental issues confronting psychiatric nurses, patients, and families. Some issues are more relevant for an autistic child than for a depressed adolescent. Following are some general guidelines first covered in Chapter 1 and again in Chapter 20: safety, structure, norms, limit setting, and balance.

Safety

There is no other nursing responsibility more important than safety. Think about it for just a moment and you will agree. A family entrusts their child into your care and expects that you will, above all, "do no harm." Safety concerns include physical safety such as protecting the patient from aggressive peers, harmful objects (e.g., sharps, glass items, plastic bags), and incompetent medication administration. Safety also means protecting the patient from psychological harm (e.g., ridicule, verbal abuse, or harassment). Finally, and this subject is so terrible it is difficult to broach, patients must be protected from staff. Background checks are essential for people working with vulnerable children and adolescents.

Structure

Structure can mean the layout of the physical environment or the organization of the treatment plan. For an inpatient setting, how the unit is designed can add a therapeutic element to the patient's care. Furnishings, color selection, areas for privacy, areas for visiting, visibility of nursing staff, and visibility of patients by nurses should be carefully considered when developing the environment for children and adolescent patients. Structure and safety issues overlap. An environment where patients can get away and not be noticed is poorly designed. A well-organized treatment approach is important too. Without being overly rigid, nurses and other staff members should do what they indicate they will do when they indicate they will do it. Even when patients resist, it is therapeutic to provide the structure of doing what is supposed to be done.

Norms

Norms are expectations of behavior. For example, norms of nonviolence, cleanliness, participation in chores, and participation in therapeutic activities are minimal expectations on an inpatient unit. Although some patients might resist, it is therapeutic to establish norms and enforce them. For patients who are coming from chaotic home environments, the ability to count on adults to be consistent can be enormously beneficial.

Limit Setting

Limit setting means putting "limits" on certain kinds of behaviors. In particular, acting-out behavior, self-destructive conduct, aggressiveness toward others, and inappropriate sexual actions are behaviors that are off limits on an inpatient unit. Other behaviors that might need to be limited are use of phones and texting, choice of visitors or "friends," and seclusive behaviors. Often limit setting takes the form of rules of behavior. It is important that rules be clearly communicated. No one at any age wants to be held accountable for violating an unknown rule. Some nominal levels of behavior should be expected, and nurses should not get bogged down in attempting to outline every possible deed that is unacceptable. Some adolescent patients can be particularly adept at splitting hairs. In such cases, it is probably better not to "argue" and still enforce the commonly accepted rule.

Balance

Balance involves "balancing" between dependence and independence. Part of maturing is the ability to make decisions for oneself. Some individuals never achieve full independence, but just being aware that appropriate independence is a therapeutic goal is important. A 2-year-old child often brushes away a parent's hand and says "I do it." It is innate to want to do things by yourself for yourself. The nurse must also balance a specific patient's needs (rights) with the needs and rights of another patient. Perhaps an example we can all identify with can better illustrate this point. You have the right to listen to any kind of music you want to listen to. However, do you have the right to play it so loudly that I cannot hear the music I have the right to listen to? As simple as this illustration is, it conveys another aspect of balance that the nurse attempts to achieve.

CONCLUSION

Having a child with a significant mental disorder changes the family—sometimes forever. The impact that the child has on the family is not neutral: some families grow stronger, whereas others disintegrate. A simple pleasure such as going out for dinner may not be able to transpire, or if it does, only with great planning and trepidation. Johnny might explode or have a tantrum. One couple reported these challenges during a coast-to-coast flight with their 5-year-old autistic son. They had overestimated their ability to control his behavior. Shortly after takeoff, the boy had a "meltdown." He was screaming, jumping, and flapping, and the parents had nothing at their disposal to calm him. The boy's behavior ruined the flight for many people. Some passengers were sympathetic, but others accused the couple of poor parenting. One person suggested she might sue because a dress was stained. The couple never attempted another flight with their son.

▌ STUDY NOTES

1. Psychiatric disorders in children and adolescents are caused by an interaction of genetic, biologic, and environmental factors.
2. Resilience is the ability to encounter negative factors successfully and emerge mentally healthy.
3. Common psychiatric disorders of children and adolescents include depression, BPD, anxiety disorder, ADHD, and ASDs.
4. ADHD is the most common pediatric behavioral disorder. Central nervous system stimulants are the drugs most frequently used to treat children with ADHD.
5. Symptoms of ASDs include arrested social skills; impaired verbal and nonverbal communication; and restricted, repetitive, and stereotypical behavior, interests, and activities.
6. Psychotherapeutic management, in which the nurse manages the nurse-patient relationship, psychopharmacologic intervention, and the environment, remains the best strategy to treat the child or adolescent holistically.

REFERENCES

American Psychiatric Association. (2000). *Diagnostic and statistical manual of mental disorders, test revision* (4th ed.). Washington, D.C.: APA.

American Psychiatric Association. (2013). *Diagnostic and statistical manual of mental disorders, test revision* (5th ed.). Arlington, VA: APA.

Baird, G., et al. (2006). Prevalence of disorders of the autism spectrum in a population cohort of children in South Thames: The Special Needs and Autism Project (SNAP). *Lancet, 368,* 210–215.

Bishop, D. V., et al. (2008). Autism and diagnostic substitution: Evidence from a study of adults with a history of developmental language disorder. *Developmental Medicine and Child Neurology, 50,* 341.

Brown, D. W., et al. (2009). Adverse childhood experiences and the risk of premature mortality. *American Journal of Preventive Medicine, 37,* 389.

Carbray, M. J., & McGuinness, T. (2009). Pediatric bipolar disorder. *Journal of Psychosocial Nursing and Mental Health Services, 47,* 22.

Cash, S. J., & Bridge, J. A. (2009). Epidemiology of youth suicide and suicidal behavior. *Current Opinion in Pediatrics, 21,* 613.

Chakrabarti, S., & Fombonne, E. (2001). Pervasive developmental disorders in preschool children. *JAMA, 285,* 3093–3099.

Costello, E. J., et al. (2003). Prevalence and development of psychiatric disorders in childhood and adolescence. *Archives of General Psychiatry, 60,* 837.

Dussich, J. P., & Maekoya, C. (2007). Physical child harm and bullying-related behaviors: A comparative study in Japan, South Africa, and the United States. *International Journal of Offender Therapy and Comparative Criminology, 51,* 495–509.

Fairbank, J. A., & Fairbank, D. W. (2009). Epidemiology of child traumatic stress. *Current Psychiatry Reports*, *11*, 289.

Franzek, E. J., Sprangers, N., & Janssens, A. C. (2008). Prenatal exposure to the 1944-45 Dutch "hunger winter" and addiction later in life. *Addiction*, *103*, 433.

Geschwind, N., et al. (2010). Meeting risk with resilience: High daily life reward experience preserves mental health. *Acta Psychiatrica Scandinavica*, *122*, 129–138.

Green, J. G., et al. (2010). Childhood adversities and adult psychiatric disorders in the national comorbidity survey replication I: Associations with first onset of DSM-IV disorders. *Archives of General Psychiatry*, *67*, 113.

Grigorenko, E. L. (2009). Pathogenesis of autism: A patchwork of genetic causes. *Future Neurology*, *4*, 591.

Hinduja, S., & Patchin, J. W. (2010). Bullying, cyberbullying, and suicide. *Archives of Suicide Research*, *14*, 206.

Hirshfeld-Becker, D. R., et al. (2008). High risk studies and developmental antecedents of anxiety disorders. *American Journal of Medical Genetics Part C, Seminars in Medical Genetics*, *148C*, 99.

Hyde, J., Mezulis, A., & Abramson, L. (2008). The ABCs of depression: Integrating affective, biological, and cognitive models to explain the emergence of the gender difference in depression. *Psychological Review*, *115*, 291–313.

Iarocci, G., & McDonald, J. (2006). Sensory integration and the perceptual experience of persons with autism. *Journal of Autism and Developmental Disorders*, *36*, 77–90.

Jacob, M., & Storch, E. (2013). Pediatric obsessive-compulsive disorder: A review for nursing professionals. *Journal of Child and Adolescent Psychiatric Nursing*, *26*, 138.

Kieling, C., et al. (2008). Neurobiology of attention deficit hyperactivity disorder. *Child and Adolescent Psychiatric Clinics of North America*, *17*, 285.

Kurita, H. (2006). Disorders of the autism spectrum. *Lancet*, *368*, 179–181.

Liu, J., & Graves, W. (2011). Childhood bullying: A review of constructs, concepts, and nursing implications. *Public Health Nursing*, *28*(6), 556–668.

Lumey, L. H., & Van Poppel, F. W. (1994). The Dutch famine of 1944-45: Mortality and morbidity in past and present generations. *Social History of Medicine*, *7*, 229.

Mancebo, M. C., et al. (2008). Juvenile-onset OCD: Clinical features in children, adolescents and adults. *Acta Psychiatrica Scandinavica*, *118*, 149.

McClellan, J., et al. (2007). Practice parameter for the treatment of children and adolescents with bipolar disorder. *Journal of the American Academy of Child and Adolescent Psychiatry*, *46*, 107–125.

McGuinness, T. M. (2007). Dispelling the myths of bullying. *Journal of Psychosocial Nursing and Mental Health Services*, *45*, 19–22.

McGuinness, T. M. (2009). Youth in the mental health void: Wraparound is one solution. *Journal of Psychosocial Nursing and Mental Health Services*, *47*, 23.

McGuinness, T. (2010). Childhood adversities and adult health. *Journal of Psychosocial Nursing and Mental Health Services*, *48*, 15–16.

McGuinness, T. M., Dyer, J., & Wade, E. (2012). Gender differences in adolescent depression. *Journal of Psychosocial Nursing and Mental Health Services*, *50*, 17–20.

McGuinness, T. M., & Johnson, K. (2013). DSM-5 changes in the diagnosis of autism spectrum disorder. *Journal of Psychosocial Nursing and Mental Health Services*, *51*, 17.

McNamara, R., et al. (2012). Interventions for youth at high risk for bipolar disorder and schizophrenia. *Child and Adolescent Psychiatric Clinics of North America*, *4*, 739.

Merikangas, K. R., et al. (2010). Prevalence and treatment of mental disorders among US children in the 2001-2004 NHANES. *Pediatrics*, *125*, 75.

Miller-Lewis, L., et al. (2013). Resource factors for mental health resilience in early childhood: An analysis with multiple methodologies. *Child and Adolescent Psychiatry and Mental Health*, *22*, 6–22.

Muhle, R., Trentacoste, S. V., & Rapin, I. (2004). The genetics of autism. *Pediatrics*, *113*, e472.

Murthy, S., Mandl, K., & Bourgeois, F. (2013). Analysis of pediatric clinical drug trials for neuropsychiatric conditions. *Pediatrics*, *131*, 1125–1131.

Nansel, T. R., & Overpeck, M. D. (2003). Operationally defining "bullying." *Archives of Pediatrics & Adolescent Medicine*, *157*, 1135–1136.

Nansel, T. R., et al. (2001). Bullying behaviors among US youth: Prevalence and association with psychosocial adjustment. *JAMA*, *285*, 2094–2100.

O'Connor, M. J., & Paley, B. (2009). Psychiatric conditions associated with prenatal alcohol exposure. *Developmental Disabilities Research Reviews*, *15*, 225.

Olweus, D. (1993). *Bullying at school: What we know and what we can do*. Oxford, UK: Blackwell.

Olweus, D. (2001). Peer harassment: A critical analysis and some important issues. In J. Juvonen & S. Graham (Eds.), *Peer harassment in school: the plight of the vulnerable and the victimized* (pp. 3–20). New York: Guilford.

Paintner, A., Williams, A., & Burd, L. (2012). Fetal alcohol spectrum disorders—Implications for child neurology, part 1: Prenatal exposure and dosimetry. *Journal of Child Neurology*, *27*, 258.

Raskauskas, J., & Stoltz, A. D. (2004). Identifying and intervening in relational aggression. *The Journal of School Nursing*, *20*, 209–215.

Rockhill, C., et al. (2010). Anxiety disorders in children and adolescents. *Current Problems in Pediatric and Adolescent Health Care*, *40*, 66.

Ronald, A., Happe, F., & Plomin, R. (2006). Genetic research into autism. *Science*, *311*, 952.

Rutter, M. (2006). Implications of resilience concepts for scientific understanding. *The Annals of the New York Academy of Sciences*, *1094*, 1.

Salisbury, A. L., Ponder, K. L., & Padbury, J. F. (2009). Fetal effects of psychoactive drugs. *Clinics in Perinatology*, *36*, 595.

Simons Foundation Autism Research Initiative. (2012). *Proposed DSM-5 criteria for autism spectrum disorders*. https://sfari.org/news-and-opinion/news/2012/proposed-dsm-5-criteria-for-autism-spectrum-disorders, Accessed 05.03.14.

Spencer, T. J. (2006). ADHD and comorbidity in childhood. *Journal of Clinical Psychiatry*, *67*(Suppl. 8), 27.

Stanbrook, M.B. (2014). *Stopping cyberbullying requires a combined societal effort*. www.cmaj.ca/site/misc/about.xhtml, Accessed 07.04.14.

Stassen Berger, K. (2007). Update on bullying at school: Science forgotten? *Developmental Review*, *27*, 90–126.

Thapar, A., et al. (2012). Depression in adolescence. *Lancet*, *379*, 1056.

U.S. Food and Drug Administration. (2013). *New pediatric labeling information database*. http://www.accessdata.fda.gov/scripts/sda/sdNavigation.cfm?filter=&sortColumn=14d&sd=labelingdatabase&displayAll=true, Accessed 05.03.14.

Vossekuil, B., et al. (2002). *The final report and findings of the Safe School Initiative: Implications for the prevention of school attacks in the United States*. United States Secret Service and United States Department of Education. http://www.secretservice.gov/ntac/ssi_final_report.pdf, Accessed 05.03.14.

Wang, J. (2009). School bullying among adolescents in the United States: Physical, verbal, relational, and cyber. *Journal of Adolescent Health*, 45(4), 368–375.

Warner, J. (2009, February 19). Children in the mental health void. *The New York Times*.

http://warner.blogs.nytimes.com/2009/02/19/is-there-no-place-on-earth/?scp=1andsq=children%20in%20the%20voidandst=cse, Accessed 11.05.10.

Wu, P., et al. (2010). Trauma, posttraumatic stress symptoms, and alcohol-use initiation in children. *Journal of Studies on Alcohol and Drugs*, 71, 326.

Zalsman, G., Brent, D. A., & Weersing, V. R. (2006). Depressive disorders in childhood and adolescence: An overview: Epidemiology, clinical manifestation and risk factors. *Child and Adolescent Psychiatric Clinics of North America*, 15, 827.

35

Older Adults

Aida J. Sapp

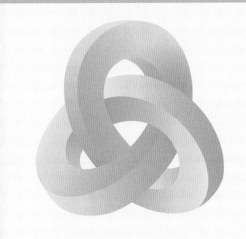

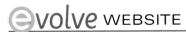

WEBSITE

http://evolve.elsevier.com/Keltner

LEARNING OBJECTIVES

- Describe the barriers to mental health care that exist for older adults.
- Describe the various treatment options and care settings available to older adults.
- Identify the unique variations in symptoms of mental disorders evidenced by older adults.

- Identify major substance use issues in older adults.
- Recognize pharmacokinetic and pharmacodynamic changes in older adults that affect pharmacotherapy.
- Perform a psychological assessment on an older adult.
- State therapeutic goals for older adults.

INTRODUCTION

The number of adults aged 65 and older is projected to soar to 72.1 million by 2030 – up from 40.3 million in 2010 according to the Institute of Medicine (2012). An estimated 25% of adults, approximately 8.6 million Americans older than age 65, experience a mental disorder (Substance Abuse and Mental Health Services Administration, 2008), and the National Institute of Mental Health projects that 15 million older adults will need mental health services by 2030 (Administration on Aging, 2005; National Institute of Mental Health, 2012). This number includes individuals who experience mental disorders for the first time in late life as well as individuals whose early-onset psychiatric disorders persist as chronic or recurrent conditions. Mental disorders in older adults might have a clear biochemical basis or might be a reaction to stressors that commonly occur in late adulthood.

Rapid growth in the older population (≥65 years old; 40.3 million in 2010) is fueling interest in issues surrounding mental health and aging. In 2010, 13.1% of the U.S. population was older than age 65. By 2030, the number of Americans older than age 65 will be twice as large as in 2000, growing from 35 million to 72 million and representing nearly 20% of the total U.S. population (Administration

on Aging, 2011a). This segment represents aging members of the baby boom generation, a group that already has relatively high rates of anxiety, depression, schizophrenia, and substance abuse (Administration on Aging, 2005). Life expectancy is also lengthening. By 2050, the number of Americans older than age 85, known as the old-old, will increase fourfold or more, placing a significantly greater number of people at risk for mental disorders (National Institute on Aging, 2009). Box 35-1 provides an overview of the prevalence rates of selected psychiatric diagnoses in older adults. The personal and economic consequences of mental disorders in this rapidly expanding cohort require heightened attention to the special mental health needs of older adults.

Modern American culture, which tends to celebrate youth, has placed little emphasis on understanding old age. This bias has contributed to insufficient knowledge about

❓ CRITICAL THINKING QUESTION

1. Think of the last patient older than age 65 for whom you cared during a medical-surgical clinical rotation. What factors could have placed the patient at risk for depression? If you noted any signs of depression, what actions were in the plan of care?

mental health disorders in the older population and public policies that adversely affect access to care. Research results have increased the ability of health care providers to differentiate illness from normal aging and to identify differences between the clinical presentation and course of mental disorders in older adults and other age groups. Government agencies have joined together to investigate factors that influence older adults. A better understanding of the complex interplay of physical health, social factors, and emotional well-being in older adults is leading to mental health strategies tailored for the special needs of this group.

Nurses involved in the care of older adults should be familiar with prevention, detection, and treatment strategies for mental

NORM'S NOTES
The geriatric population, people older than 65, is growing rapidly. There are more and more older people and more of their mental health problems for the health care system to deal with. Sometimes, older people in need of mental health care had the same problems during their younger years and have simply grown older. However, others are growing older in a society in which work defines the person, and they no longer are working. Coupled with the mobility of our society, many older people find themselves without purpose (i.e., no job to do) and alone. I get depressed just thinking about it.

disorders throughout the continuum of care. This chapter presents an overview of mental health issues in older adults that differ from those of other age groups. Stressors, policy issues, barriers to mental health care, and common mental disorders occurring in older adults are discussed along with assessment and psychotherapeutic management. Cognitive disorders, which account for some of the most frequently occurring mental disorders in older adults, are discussed in Chapter 28.

Barriers

Patient Barriers

Attitudes of older adults themselves serve as a barrier to seeking mental health care. Patients and families who subscribe to stereotypes about normal aging might delay seeking care if they believe that conditions such as depression or memory loss are a normal part of aging. Additionally, older individuals might be reluctant to seek psychiatric care because admitting to mental health problems is seen as a weakness and is more stigmatizing than it might be for a younger person. Seeking psychiatric care might also represent a loss of control and elicit fear of institutionalization. When outside help is required, people who grew up in an era that emphasized self-reliance are more likely to rely on family, friends, and other informal supports than on mental health professionals, who are often viewed with skepticism.

Provider Barriers

Older adults are more likely to receive care from primary care physicians than from geriatric specialty providers. Despite the rapid growth in the population 65 years old and older and recognition of their unique needs, geriatric specialists are scarce. Nurses and other health care providers who are not attuned to the complexities of geriatric care might miss opportunities to identify mental health disorders or predisposing factors.

Accurate assessment and diagnosis require familiarity with diagnostic tools, such as the Geriatric Depression Scale (available on Evolve website). Individuals working with older adults must recognize that mental disorders might be expressed through somatic complaints and that symptoms of comorbid physical problems might compound the difficulty of diagnosing a mental disorder. Ageism, the negative stereotyping and devaluation of people solely because of their age, is also a significant barrier. Ageism includes the stereotypical view that mental health problems are part of the aging process. To serve older adults effectively, professionals must be attentive to their biases and stereotypes and increase their geriatric-specific knowledge.

System-Economic Barriers

Funding issues, along with a lack of collaboration and coordination among primary care, mental health, and aging services providers, thwart the provision and receipt of adequate mental health care for older adults (Administration on Aging, 2005). The cost of mental health care has been a major disincentive to providers and older adults who might otherwise seek psychiatric assistance. Historically, insurers, including federally funded Medicare and Medicaid, have placed severe limits on reimbursement for mental health care. Only in the last few years has legislative effort addressed parity in mental health coverage with the Domenici-Wellstone amendment.

Analysis of Medicare claims over 1 year uncovered that participants with a diagnosis of depression incurred about $22,960 in total health care costs, whereas participants without depression incurred costs of about $11,956. Participants with possible depression, based on depression screening or reported antidepressant use, incurred costs of $14,365. Specialty mental health care costs, when compared with every other health care cost category, accounted for less than 1% of total health care costs for the participants in the study (Unützer et al., 2009).

 CRITICAL THINKING QUESTION

2. Many older adults have no insurance coverage to offset the high cost of prescription medications. How might this affect adherence?

CONTINUUM OF CARE

Because of the prevalence and profound negative consequences of mental disorders in late life, nurses who encounter older adults in any setting should consider their physical, social, and emotional needs. Whenever possible, factors that place older adults at risk for mental disorders or problems stemming from mental illness should be identified, and plans should be developed to meet the needs.

Prevention

A balance of physical, social, spiritual, and emotional functioning contributes to mental health. Many of the changes that accompany advancing age affect this balance, increasing vulnerability of older adults to mental disorders. A primary stressful event (e.g., broken hip [physical]) might lead to secondary stressors (e.g., emotional isolation). Acute and chronic health problems might lead to dependence, relocation, isolation, and financial hardship. A closer examination of these consequences might prove enlightening.

Dependence: Loss of independence, even temporarily, is terribly threatening to an older person because having to rely on others might signal a continued dependency.

Relocation: Moving from familiar surroundings to a new environment is also threatening. To many older individuals, familiar surroundings represent a connection to all that is important in life, and the related changes could be overwhelming for some individuals.

Isolation: Most older individuals have fewer meaningful connections than they had earlier in life. Death, a mobile society, and estrangements are only a few reasons for this reality. Health care–related isolation can be particularly devastating for some older adults.

Financial hardship: Although many older individuals are financially secure, a significant number find unexpected medical expenses to be difficult or impossible to meet on

---

BOX 35-2   LOSSES THAT OCCUR MORE FREQUENTLY AMONG OLDER ADULTS

Loss of health
Loss of loved ones
Loss of hearing and vision
Loss of status
Loss of work
Loss of income
Loss of friends
Loss of cognitive skills
Loss of home and community
Loss of mobility (physical abilities; driving privileges)

---

a fixed income. Most older adults have little, if any, ability to increase their income to meet additional unplanned expenses.

Adaptive Mechanisms: Meaning, Control, Support

Losses common in later years of life are listed in Box 35-2 and often precede the onset of mental disorders in older adults. Despite numerous inevitable changes, most older adults adjust well and express a high degree of satisfaction with life (U.S. Department of Health and Human Services, 1999b). Exposure and adaptation to stressors vary with each older adult's economic and social resources, physical status, ethnicity, gender, and life experiences (Administration on Aging, 2005). Successful adaptation is enhanced by the ability to give *meaning* to experiences. Part of this process is comparing problems with what is experienced and expected by others who are the same age (Federal Interagency Forum on Aging Related Statistics, 2008). This observation might account for 72% of older Americans reporting their health as good to excellent, despite multiple coexisting medical conditions and impairments. As one sage older adult noted, at some point, simply being alive can be seen as a sign of good health. This coping skill is especially helpful when the stressor, such as a chronic health problem, is not easily modified.

Another adaptive mechanism that assists older adults to cope with stressful events is the use of mastery—the sense of ability to exercise *control* over circumstances. Adequate planning for the social and financial implications of retirement significantly affects adjustment to this major life change. Nurses can reinforce mastery by encouraging the older person's participation in care decisions.

Support systems (family, friends, spiritual communities, and private and government organizations) are valuable sources of emotional support and aid and are important predictors of physical and mental health and delay institutionalization (Federal Interagency Forum on Aging, 2008). Measures that contribute to physical health and promote social functioning are important components of preventing mental disorders in older adults. Improved health care and programs developed to target needs of older adults have resulted in declines in the rates of disability and poverty, which are key indicators of well-being in older adults, as reported by the Administration on Aging, 2011.

Caregiver Training and Transportation

Specific legislation has led to funding programs to meet the special needs of an aging population. One example is the National Aging Network and Transportation Assistance program, which was established to address transportation needs (Administration on Aging, 2005) and then reauthorized in 2009 to improve the availability and accessibility of transportation services for older Americans (National Association of Area Agencies on Aging, 2011). Lack of transportation has been cited as a factor in isolation and is a barrier to accessing health care. Nurses play a key role in illness prevention by providing information about mental health and available resources at sites where older adults are likely to visit.

LOCAL AREA AGENCY ON AGING

The government section of the telephone book contains the telephone number for a local Area Agency on Aging (AAA). This organization also can be found on the web (www.n4a. org). This organization is a valuable resource for older adults and their caregivers, who often have difficulty initiating a search for or negotiating access to care.

? CRITICAL THINKING QUESTION

3. If you have had the opportunity to meet the caregiver of an older adult with a mental disorder, were both the patient and the caregiver participants involved in decision making? Did the caregiver treat the patient in the way that you would want to be treated in that situation? Describe both the positive and the negative aspects of nurse-patient-caregiver interactions.

Detection

Measures that promote early detection of mental disorders in older adults include increasing public awareness of mental health issues, encouraging collaboration among service providers, and providing education for health professionals. Public education that emphasizes symptoms of mental disorders and treatment options does much to dispel the myths and stigma surrounding mental illness and empowers older adults to seek treatment. Some programs have been established to enhance community involvement. Public service workers such as grocery clerks, postal employees, and public utility workers are recruited and trained to identify and report vulnerable older adults to significant others. Nurses in all settings can contribute to early detection by assessing and reporting stressors and symptoms. Healthy IDEAS, an initiative aimed at identifying depression and empowering activities for older adults, is an evidence-based program that integrates depression awareness and management into existing case management services provided to older adults. The focus of

this program is to ensure availability of the help older adults need to manage symptoms of depression and live full lives (Care for Elders, 2012).

Treatment Sites

Federal legislation has strongly influenced the care of older adults who have mental disorders. The Community Mental Health Act of 1963 initiated deinstitutionalization, resulting in a large number of individuals with serious mental illness (SMI) being discharged from state and county mental hospitals to less restrictive settings. Many discharged older adults were placed in nursing homes, where inappropriate and inadequate care, including excessive use of physical and chemical restraints, led to the passage of the Nursing Home Reform Act, known as the Omnibus Reconciliation Act of 1987 (OBRA). This legislation set stringent limits on the use of physical restraints and established guidelines for psychotropic drug use that regulate drug selection, dosing, and duration of treatment. In addition, to prevent nursing home placement for individuals who need psychiatric care in hospital or community programs, OBRA requires preadmission screening for all individuals with suspected mental disorders. Nursing home residents whose only need for nursing care stemmed from mental disorders were to be discharged. Nonetheless, many institutionalized older people with SMI continue to live in nursing homes. Most of these residents do not receive adequate psychiatric treatment because of a lack of mental health training for nursing home staff and inadequate Medicare and Medicaid funding to cover behavioral health care (Administration on Aging, 2005; Shea et al., 2000).

Most older adults with SMI live in the community. At the present time, only a small percentage of community mental health centers have staff or services that target the needs of older adults, and primary care physicians are ill prepared and typically too rushed to treat mental disorders adequately. When care is provided, it is common for older adults to receive inappropriate psychotropic medication (U.S. Department of Health and Human Services, 1999b). The services needed to help community-based older adults with SMI include the following:

1. Mental health outreach programs
2. Adult day services
3. Respite care and caregiver programs
4. Support groups
5. Self-help groups

PSYCHOPATHOLOGY IN OLDER ADULTS

Unit V of this text provides an in-depth review of diagnostic classifications. This section is meant to supplement that information by detailing unique information on the presentation, course, and treatment of mental disorders in older adults. It is important for nurses in all practice areas to note that treating older adults with mental disorders benefits overall health by improving functional ability and collaboration with health care instructions.

DEPRESSION

Depression, along with the experience of anxiety disorders, are the most prevalent mental health problems among older adults (U.S. Department of Health and Human Services, 1999b) and by 2020 is expected to be the second most common cause of disability and death in established market economies such as the United States (Care for Elders, 2012). Behavioral risk factor surveillance data from the U.S. Centers for Disease Control and Prevention indicated that among adults age 50 or older, 7.7% reported current depression, and 15.7% reported a lifetime diagnosis of depression (U.S. Centers for Disease Control and Prevention and National Association of Chronic Disease Directors, 2008). An estimated 15% to 30% of U.S. adults 65 years old and older experience depressive symptoms on any given day, and severe depressive symptoms in this group appear more commonly among women than men; however, by age 85, symptoms occur equally in both groups—22.5% in men and 23% in women (Care for Elders, 2012). And according to the National Alliance on Mental Illness (NAMI), depression affects more than 6.5 million of the 35 million Americans aged 65 years or older. For most, depression has occurred during much of life. For others, depression has a first onset in later life—even persons in their 80s and 90s. Depression in older persons is closely associated with dependency and disability and causes great suffering for the individual and the family (NAMI, 2014). As in other age groups, depression in older adults might result from psychosocial stress, biochemical changes, comorbid medical conditions, pharmaceutical agents, or a combination of factors. The effects of depression extend beyond well-known and emotionally distressing symptoms such as sadness, worthlessness, hopelessness, helplessness, fear, shame, and guilt. Less obvious effects include diminished social, cognitive, and physical functioning as well as increased mortality.

Incidence

Table 35-1 details the prevalence of late-life depression and the increased risk for women over men. Clinically relevant depressive symptoms are present in 11% of men and 17% of women age 65 and older. The percentage is 19% for all adults age 85 and older (Federal Interagency Forum on Aging, 2008). Of clinical relevance is that depression occurs concurrently with other serious illnesses of older adults, such as heart disease, cerebrovascular accident, diabetes, cancer, and Parkinson's disease. Approximately 8% to 15% of community-dwelling older adults and 30% of institutionalized adults are clinically depressed (Tabloski, 2006).

Presentation

Depression in older adults frequently does not align neatly with current *DSM-V* criteria, and many depressive symptoms can be attributed to physical causes in individuals with comorbid medical illnesses such as chronic pain, prior depression, or traumatic brain injury (Maurer, 2012). Older adults are more likely to present with memory disturbance or somatic complaints than with the feelings associated with

TABLE 35-1	PERCENTAGE OF NONINSTITUTIONALIZED PERSONS, AGE 65 AND OLDER, WITH SEVERE DEPRESSIVE SYMPTOMS (1998)		
AGE (YEARS)	TOTAL (%)	MEN (%)	WOMEN (%)
65-69	15.4	12.1	18
70-74	14.3	10.3	17.2
75-79	14.6	10.4	17.4
80-84	20.5	17.1	22.4
≥85	22.8	22.5	23

From Federal Interagency Forum on Aging-Related Statistics (2000). *Older Americans 2000: key indicators of well-being, appendix A: detailed tables.* Washington, D.C.: Federal Interagency Forum on Aging-Related Statistics. Also available at http://www.agingstats.gov/agingstatsdotnet/Main_Site/Data/2008_Documents/Health_Status.aspx

depression for which younger patients seek care. Older adults also might lack the range of vocabulary that younger individuals commonly possess to describe emotions. Rather than expressions of sadness, diminished self-esteem, irritability, or apathy, for example, older adults are more likely to complain of having the blues or feeling worthless. Also, cultural competence demands that professionals recognize differences in expression common to ethnic and cultural subgroups within the older population. For example, You and colleagues (2009) found that among community-dwelling Korean older adults, individuals living alone were significantly more depressed than individuals living with family.

For nurses working with older adults, a deeper understanding of how loneliness may contribute to the development of depression, a diminished quality of life, or cognitive decline is important. In a sample of Swedish older adults and their caregivers, a report of loneliness was the most important factor in predicting quality of life (Ekwall et al., 2006). Another group of researchers recommended that loneliness be targeted for cognitive intervention because it was the strongest predictor for depression in the participants in their study (Cohen-Mansfield & Parpura-Gill, 2007). Advocating for routine assessments of depression and assessments of loneliness in older adults could lead to the development of interventions that would serve as a primary prevention for depression (Theeke, 2009). Another complicating factor in the occurrence of depression in elders is that only a minority receives treatment (Holvast et al., 2012; Jokela et al., 2013). Therefore, continuing studies of barriers and opportunities for recognition and access to services is imperative.

In addition to diagnostic barriers already discussed, the connection between medical conditions and depression complicates diagnosis. The clinician should consider cerebrovascular disease in a first episode of depression occurring in a person older than 60 years of age (Sherman, 2005).

It is difficult to determine whether or not common physical indicators of depression in older adults, including weight loss, fatigue, insomnia, constipation, and multiple vague aches and pains, are the result of a mood disorder or symptoms of a medical problem. The *DSM-V* diagnosis of "mood disorder due to a general medical condition" can be given when mood symptoms are a direct physiologic consequence of medical conditions (American Psychiatric Association, 2013).

Although depression is caused by a medical illness in some cases, depression causes physiologic changes that enhance susceptibility to disease in other cases (Casey, 2012). Depression adversely affects endocrine, neurologic, and immune processes by increasing sympathetic tone, decreasing vagal tone, and causing immunosuppression (Penninx et al., 1999). People with depression are more likely to smoke, drink alcohol excessively, be physically inactive, and have poorer eating habits than people who are not depressed. These changes and health habits might be factors in depression as a predictor of coronary artery disease and diabetes and the increased risk of death after myocardial infarctions (Creed, 1999; Kayton, 2001).

Depression or Dementia?

Because of the shared cognitive symptoms of depression and dementia, misdiagnosis of dementia occurs frequently. Depression that mimics dementia is termed *pseudodementia*. Shared symptoms include poor memory, disorientation, poor judgment, and agitation or psychomotor retardation. In addition to psychological tests, nursing observations can be critical to correcting a misdiagnosis. Nurses should assess for higher functioning than would be expected in dementia and can look for a downcast mood, which can help distinguish depression from the blander affect of true dementia. Differentiating these disorders is important for treatment because depression is highly treatable. Psychotic depression might also be confused with cognitive or other psychiatric disorders. When depression occurs for the first time after age 60, delusions are more common than with early-onset depression. Delusions of persecution or of having an incurable illness and nihilistic delusions are more frequent than delusions associated with guilt (Blazer & Koenig, 1996). However, hallucinations are an uncommon feature of psychotic depression. Many older adults with psychotic depression might ruminate, express suspiciousness, and voice multiple physical complaints. Psychotic depression is often resistant to traditional antidepressant medications and psychotherapy. As a result, electroconvulsive therapy (ECT) is frequently used in treatment.

Electroconvulsive Therapy

ECT is often the treatment of choice for severe depression in older adults, especially individuals who are poor candidates for drug therapy or who have failed to respond to other treatments. ECT offers a rapid response that is necessary when patients are suicidal or in danger of medical crisis. The safety and efficacy of ECT have been demonstrated for all age groups, including the old-old (Tew et al., 1999). The decision-making process of older adults electing to receive ECT is highly individualized and relates to family support, trust, past experience, a feeling of desperation, and the stigma of mental illness (Amazon et al., 2008). Chapter 25 provides a thorough review of ECT process.

Suicide

Older Americans are disproportionately more likely to die by suicide, the most serious consequence of missed or undertreated depression. Suicide is preventable and needs to be addressed in older adults. Although adults 65 years old and older compose only 12% of the U.S. population, older adults accounted for 16% of reported suicide deaths in 2004 (U.S. Centers for Disease Control and Prevention National Center for Injury Prevention and Control, 2005). Considering the occurrence of suicide in the general population to be at a rate of about 11 per 100,000, the older adult rate is higher at 14.3 per 100,000 people age 65 and older in 2004. Table 35-2 shows that the incidence of suicide increases with age and that white men older than age 65 have the highest rate of all (Hoyert et al., 1999). Estimates support that non-Hispanic white men age 85 and older were most likely to die by suicide. They had a rate of 49.8 suicide deaths per 100,000 persons in that age group (U.S. Centers for Disease Control and Prevention National Center for Injury Prevention and Control, 2005). Suicidal gestures and impulsiveness, common among young adults, are rare in older adults. In older adults, attempts are usually not a cry for help; rather, they are a serious suicide warning (Kjolseth & Ekeberg, 2012). To underscore this point, older people tend to select highly lethal methods for suicide. For example, firearms are the most common method of suicide by both men and women 65 years old and older, accounting for 78% of male suicides and 34.8% of female suicides (Jancin, 2005; National Institute of Mental Health, 2007a).

The rate of suicide might be even higher than reported because statistics do not include what is known as *chronic suicide*. This term characterizes death caused by slower, less obvious means than the abrupt acts usually associated with suicide. Refusing to eat, inconsistent medication usage, excessive alcohol intake, and physical risk taking might result

TABLE 35-2	RATE OF SUICIDE AMONG OLDER ADULTS*	
POPULATION GROUP	**SUICIDE RATE (%)**
55-64 years old	13.5
65-74 years old	14.4
75-84 years old	19.3
≥85 years old	20.8
White men >85 years old	65
Average rate across the life span	10.6

*Rates per 100,000 population based on 1997 data.
Modified from Hoyert, D.L., Kochanek, K.D., & Murphey, S.L. (1999). *Deaths: final data for 1997. National vital statistical report.* U.S. Department of Health and Human Services Publication No. 99-1120. Hyattsville, MD: National Center for Health Statistics.

in deaths that are not recorded as suicides (Butler & Lewis, 1995). The "silent suicide" of older adults who have experienced a loss of health status and independence is of particular interest in nursing research (Fitzpatrick, 2005). Depression is a strong predictor of patients' decisions to support euthanasia or forego life-sustaining treatment (Blank et al., 2001). Suicide does not always arise from depression. For some individuals who face life-threatening illness, suicide is the ultimate means of exercising control over a situation. There are differences between ethnic groups in the methods employed in deliberate self-harm. Social and cultural backgrounds play a part in structuring cognitive patterns and problem-solving mechanisms that may influence the expression of any of the risk factors identified in Box 35-3. In addition, defining the barriers individuals experience in seeking help from support networks and health care professionals is imperative (Chan et al., 2007).

Perceived burdensomeness (Joiner, 2005) is also noted in the literature related to suicide risk in older adults. The perception that one is a burden on others, even if those people do not feel burdened, is present. In one study, the role of perceived burdensomeness was a mediator of the relationship between depressive symptoms and suicide ideation in older adults (Jahn et al., 2011).

In a research study regarding suicide risk and precipitating circumstances among male veterans, the veterans were found to be at higher risk for suicide compared with their nonveteran counterparts. Suicide was influenced by health problems in the older veteran decedents. Nearly all elderly veterans used firearms for suicide, punctuating the importance of assessing for access and intervening appropriately in this population (Kaplan et al., 2012).

Suicide prevention begins with the detection of risk (see Box 35-3). It is important for nurses to listen to the themes of conversation and observe for signs that might signal suicidal risk or thoughts (Plawecki & Amrhein, 2010; Monteso et al., 2012). Particular attention should be given to older individuals who are beginning to recover from depression because as energy returns, the risk of suicide increases. Intent might be signaled by a new preoccupation with religious issues, giving away possessions, changing a will, or other new behaviors. People might feel ashamed to voice ideas of self-harm plainly, so if negative statements or behaviors are detected, it is essential to ask directly about any intentions. The notion that these discussions can exacerbate suicidal thought is a myth.

Clinical Example: Despondency related to loss

Mr. Nelson is an 86-year-old African-American man who has outlived two wives. Mr. Nelson has remained sexually active into his eighties, but within the last 2 years he has had difficulty attaining an erection. Mr. Nelson relates that a younger woman (mid-fifties) recently asked about spending the night. She did, and Mr. Nelson was unable to perform sexually. He said, "I'm just no good anymore." Mr. Nelson said he was embarrassed by his sexual dysfunction. He states that he has had thoughts of suicide but would not act on them. He promises the nurse that he will call if he has an urge to harm himself.

Clinical Example: I'd be better off dead

Mr. Timchuk is a 77-year-old Pacific Islander with chronic obstructive pulmonary disease. He has great difficulty doing any physical activity. Mr. Timchuk is very despondent over his condition, and there is little hope that he will improve. Although he has not verbalized a desire to "end it all," he states that he "would be better off dead." The nurse understands that he is at great risk for self-harm.

MANIC EPISODES

Manic symptoms in older adults might be associated with bipolar disorder, medical and neurologic conditions, substance abuse, or medication. In older adults, bipolar disorder accounts for about 5% to 20% of mood disorders, most often as a recurrence of an existing disorder (Cassano et al., 2000). Late-onset bipolar disorder is defined as bipolar disorder in which symptoms first occur after age 40. Differences between early-onset and late-onset bipolar disorder suggest that they might be different types of manic-depressive illness (Schurhoff et al., 2000). For example, affective disorders are less common in first-degree relatives of patients with late onset compared with patients with early onset (Cassano et al., 2000; Schurhoff et al., 2000). Late-onset bipolar disorder is generally less severe, with fewer and milder manic symptoms compared with early-onset bipolar disorder (Moon, 2005). Features might include grandiosity or irritability, disorientation, and euphoria. A substantial proportion of new-onset manic symptoms in older adults is associated with cerebral disorders or injuries and might run a bipolar course, with intervening periods of euthymia (Snowdon, 2000). Because of self-reported cognitive complaints in elderly patients with bipolar disorder, an evaluation of cognitive functioning in such patients is an important part of treatment (Schouws et al., 2012). Nursing interventions must address the negative impact of agitation and distractibility on self-care and self-protection in older adults.

BOX 35-3	**PREDICTORS OF SUICIDE RISK IN OLDER ADULTS**

Age >65 years
Male sex
White
Chronic or uncontrolled pain
Bereavement
Unmarried (single, widowed, divorced)
Social isolation
Retirement
Financial difficulty
Hopelessness or helplessness
Alcohol or drug abuse
History of previous attempt
Major depressive disorder, particularly psychotic depression
 or depression caused by a general medical condition

Clinical Example: Evicted

The local police department's community service officer brought Ms. Ellington, a 72-year-old white woman, to the hospital. She was found sitting outside a homeless shelter surrounded by boxes of personal belongings, drinking orange juice that had a strong odor of alcohol. She wore tight animal print leggings, a transparent blouse, and thigh-high white boots. A decorated wide-brimmed hat covered her sparse, flame-red hair. On admission, Ms. Ellington was cursing loudly and threw her dentures at the first staff person who approached. Although she was well known to the staff, Ms. Ellington claimed that she was a Hollywood star who had been kicked out of her own mansion by friends, robbed of identification, and shipped to this city where she would be unknown. According to police, she had been evicted from several shelters for disruptive behavior. An empty bottle of lithium and an unfilled prescription for more lithium were found in her purse.

PSYCHOTIC DISORDERS

Psychotic disorders, characterized by delusions, hallucinations, disordered thoughts, bizarre behavior, or other evidence of impaired reality testing, are among the most severe psychiatric disorders. Symptoms often contribute to the institutionalization of older adults. Active psychosis is as disabling as quadriplegia on the disability component of the disability-adjusted life-years measure. Nurses should be familiar with the numerous physical conditions and medications associated with psychosis in older adults (Box 35-4). A comprehensive assessment, including the nature and content of delusions and hallucinations, can facilitate identification of reversible causes and contribute to the accurate diagnosis necessary for determining the most effective course of treatment.

Schizophrenia

Although generally regarded as an illness with onset in late adolescence or early adulthood, symptoms first occur after age 40 in approximately 23.5% of all patients with schizophrenia, with a high female-to-male ratio (Howard et al., 2000). The most important characteristics for assessing a schizophrenic episode in an older person are hallucinations, delusions, and a history of a psychotic disorder (Alexopoulous et al., 2004).

Patients with late-onset psychosis are more likely than their counterparts with earlier onset to present with bizarre, persecutory delusions; visual, tactile, and olfactory hallucinations; and accusatory or abusive auditory hallucinations (Howard et al., 2000; McClure et al., 1999). Disorganization and negative symptoms (withdrawal, apathy, and anhedonia) are less prominent than in early-onset psychosis. Most individuals in whom schizophrenia is diagnosed late in life have abnormal premorbid personality traits but are more likely to have better employment and marital histories compared with persons with early-onset schizophrenia. For many individuals, late-onset schizophrenia marks the beginning of a chronic disorder with periods of remission and symptom recurrence. The insidious deterioration of personality and social adjustment characteristic of early-onset schizophrenia

BOX 35-4 DISORDERS ASSOCIATED WITH PSYCHOSIS IN OLDER ADULTS

Disorders
Parkinson's disease
Alzheimer's disease
Pick's disease
Diffuse Lewy body disease
Vascular dementia
Seizure disorders
Hydrocephalus
Demyelinating diseases
Neoplasms (undetected cancer)
Encephalopathies
Neurosyphilis
Spinocerebellar degeneration

Endocrinopathies
Hyperthyroidism, hypothyroidism
Hyperparathyroidism, hypoparathyroidism
Addison's disease
Cushing's disease
Hypoglycemia

Vitamin Deficiencies
Thiamine
Niacin
Vitamin B_{12}
Folate

Other Conditions
Iatrogenic (secondary to drugs)
Lupus
Alcohol intake or withdrawal
Temporal arteritis
Hyponatremia
Delirium

Differential Diagnosis
Psychotic disorder caused by a general medical condition
Delirium
Dementia with delusions and hallucinations
Mood disorder with psychotic features
Delusional disorder
Psychosis secondary to substance abuse or dependence
Brief reactive psychosis
Psychosis not otherwise specified or schizophreniform disorder
Schizophrenia

From Benros, M.E., et al. (2009). Psychiatric disorder as a first manifestation of cancer: a 10-year population-based study. *International Journal of Cancer, 124,* 2917; Jeste, D.V., Harris, M.J., & Paulsen, J.S. (1996). Psychosis. In J. Sadavoy, et al. (Eds.), *Comprehensive review of geriatric psychiatry—II* (2nd ed.) (pp. 593-614). Washington, DC: American Psychiatric Press; McClure, F.S., Gladsjo, J.A., & Jeste, D.V. (1999). Late-onset psychosis: clinical, research, and ethical considerations. *The American Journal of Psychiatry, 156,* 935.

also occurs; however, cognitive declines are no faster in older noninstitutionalized patients with schizophrenia than in normal comparison subjects (Eyler Zorrilla et al., 2000). In all age groups, antipsychotic medications are an effective treatment for many of the positive symptoms, especially when coupled with a structured environment (milieu), including social skills training and supportive nurse-patient interactions.

Research documenting the long-term course of schizophrenia is extremely limited; however, many patients with chronic schizophrenia reach late life despite the high mortality associated with chronic early-onset schizophrenia. Mortality is associated with a high risk of suicide and medical problems, often related to comorbid substance abuse—especially nicotine dependence. The increase of movement disorders and metabolic syndrome (weight gain, obesity, hyperglycemia, and hypertriglyceridemia) in older patients treated with traditional antipsychotics complicates medical management, increases the degree of disability associated with the disorder, and contributes to the high cost of services for older adult patients with schizophrenia. However, though remission in elderly patients with schizophrenia has been little studied, aging does not adversely affect remission in the elderly (Barak & Swartz, 2012). Therefore, management of elders with schizophrenia should be targeted toward remission.

Older patients with schizophrenia, especially individuals who returned to the community after long-term institutionalization, might have significant deficits in daily living skills and lack the social networks important to successful adaptation. Similar to what has been reported in younger patients, psychological and social needs appear to be underserviced in the elderly who experience schizophrenia. Having more unmet needs was associated with a lower perceived quality of life (Meesters et al., 2013). These individuals have a higher need for daily living services. Caregivers should emphasize problem-solving skills and interventions that promote socializing and access to social interactions.

Clinical Example: Just can't get along

Ms. Yu is a 68-year-old Asian-American woman brought to the hospital by her sister, with whom she lives. She accuses her sister of forcing her into the hospital so that the sister can steal her money and car. The sister can recall no recent major stressor or signs of physical illness. She states that Ms. Yu has no history of psychiatric symptoms but has always been a "loner." Despite obtaining a college degree, she had a stormy employment history because she was "unable to get along" with coworkers. She also was unable to sustain a long-term relationship with any man she dated. Ms. Yu's appearance is evidence of her inattention to dress and grooming. Although cooperative with the examination, her mood is dysphoric, and she has a flat affect. She admits to auditory hallucinations, particularly voices of people she knows, often conversing with each other. The voices tell her that they will steal from her, and they sometimes tell her to hurt herself. A complete evaluation resulted in a diagnosis of schizophrenia. The geropsychiatrist ordered olanzapine (Zyprexa) 2.5 mg at bedtime.

Paranoid Thinking

Paranoid symptoms are common in older adults. Delusions are generally chronic and well systematized and, unless associated with dementia or delirium, are not associated with memory loss, disorientation, or diminished cognitive function (Koenig et al., 1996). The content often involves persecution, jealousy (e.g., infidelity), or unusual situations that might conceivably occur in real life. It is important to investigate actual facts before labeling beliefs as delusional because patients might relate bizarre tales that have a basis in reality. Because physicality is compromised with age, paranoid thinking often emerges as a defense mechanism against a potentially hostile environment. Walking to the corner store in some neighborhoods might be perilous for older individuals because they are less able than younger people to fend off aggressors. A retreat into an environment that the fearful older adult can control results in increasing isolation. Although the threat might be based on reality, the resulting isolation and decrease in external stimuli, along with suspicious behaviors, can lead to paranoid thinking.

Clinical Example: A cruel hoax

Mrs. Justice is an 81-year-old African-American woman who was referred to the community mental health center by her primary care physician for treatment of psychosis. The neatly attired and spry woman tearfully relates that "haunts" have been breaking into her house at night, stealing money and other possessions. She sees the ghostly apparitions at least once a month, and when they appear, they speak to her, most often saying, "You stay out of the way, old woman, or we'll get you!" Before initiating pharmacologic intervention, a nurse practitioner conducted a home visit and found Mrs. Justice's home in disarray. Broken windows, gaps where kitchen appliances had been removed, and other findings led the nurse to request a police investigation. On the first night of their home surveillance, police arrested two young men dressed in white sheets who were hiding behind high shrubbery in front of the house. Interventions that were social rather than pharmacologic were instituted. This actual case is an example of how cultural awareness and careful investigation prevented subsequent inappropriate diagnosis and treatment.

ANXIETY DISORDERS

Anxiety disorders along with depression are the most prevalent of the mental disorders in older adults. Little research has specifically addressed anxiety symptoms and syndromes in older adults, perhaps because epidemiologic data have revealed lower rates of anxiety disorders in community-dwelling older adults compared with younger groups (Lenze et al., 2000; U.S. Department of Health and Human Services, 1999b). As with other mental disorders, most anxiety disorders do not begin in later life but are a recurrence or worsening of a preexisting condition (Lang & Stein, 2001). Cognitive, behavioral, somatic, and physiologic symptoms are similar to those of other age groups (Box 35-5).

Many older adults have symptoms of anxiety that fail to meet diagnostic criteria for an anxiety disorder. Among older adults with depression, 23% to 38% also experience anxiety, sometimes at a level that meets *DSM* criteria for generalized anxiety disorder, panic disorder, or a phobia (Lenze et al., 2000). Two anxiety disorders defined in *DSM* might

BOX 35-5   SIGNS AND SYMPTOMS OF ANXIETY

Gastrointestinal or Genitourinary Symptoms
Abdominal pain
Anorexia
"Butterflies"
Diarrhea
Dry mouth
Nausea
Urinary frequency
Vomiting

Cardiovascular Symptoms
Chest discomfort
Diaphoresis
Dyspnea
Flushing
Hyperventilation
Pallor
Palpitations
Tachycardia

Musculoskeletal Symptoms
Backache
Fatigue
Muscle tension
Tremulousness

Neurologic Signs
Dizziness or faintness
Paresthesia

Psychological Manifestations
Apprehensive
Compulsive
Fearful
Feelings of dread
Irritable
Intolerant
Panicky
Phobic
Preoccupied
Tense or worried

Modified from Keltner, N., & Folks, D. (2005). *Psychotropic drugs* (4th ed.). St. Louis: Mosby.

be overrepresented in older adults. "Anxiety due to a general medical condition" is a commonly used diagnosis resulting from the frequency of anxiety related to cardiovascular, endocrine, respiratory, and neurologic disorders in this age group. "Substance-induced anxiety disorder" might be present in 10% of community-dwelling older adults and 40% of nursing home residents, a consequence of substance abuse and dependence as well as toxicity from prescription drugs (Folks & Fuller, 1997). Although anxiety is a normal emotion that alerts a person to impending danger or an unpleasant event, it can be considered maladaptive when it interferes with functioning. A trusting nurse-patient relationship in which consistent, reliable care is provided can be crucial in managing patients' anxiety (Flood & Buckwalter, 2009a).

SUBSTANCE USE

Substance use and dependence place older adults at tremendous risk of negative physical, psychological, and social consequences but often go undetected. Late-life alcohol and drug use and dependence are problems that have received little attention until recent years; a great deal is yet to be learned about geriatric-specific prevention, detection, and treatment options. In 2006, 41 million adults age 50 and older drank alcohol in the past month (Blank, 2009). This number is expected to increase rapidly as a result of aging baby boomers, who have a greater history of alcohol abuse than the current older cohort. In addition, the data from 2006 show that adults aged 50 and older who entered treatment for the first time had a median duration of alcohol use of 38 years (Substance Abuse and Mental Health Services Administration, 2006).

Similar expansion is expected with illicit drug use, currently a problem for approximately 2.2 million adults aged 50 and older who reported using illicit drugs in the past month when surveyed (Substance Abuse and Mental Health Services Administration, 2006). Marijuana use alone (54%), prescription drugs used nonmedically (28%), and use of a different illicit drug such as cocaine or heroin were also noted. Concern exists with the potential of a monumental increase in the need for treatment services by the aging baby boom generation, although many are not seeking treatment; 83% (of 3.2 million adults ≥50 years old who needed treatment based on standard criteria) *felt no need* for treatment and did not seek help.

An even larger problem is the frequent misuse of prescription and over-the-counter (OTC) drugs, sometimes to the point that it can be characterized as drug abuse. It is important for nurses to understand factors that contribute to substance abuse and recognize presenting symptoms and potential consequences. Unless nurses and other health care providers recognize the serious problems that alcohol and prescription drugs pose for older adults and take measures to intervene, quality of life is diminished, independence is compromised, and physical deterioration is accelerated.

Alcohol Abuse and Dependence

Alcohol abuse and dependence might occur for the first time in late life or might represent an unresolved problem from earlier life. More men than women approach late life with problem drinking; although men represent most older adults who abuse alcohol, late-onset alcohol abuse is more common in women than in men (Blow, 2000; Ludwick et al., 2000). Numerous risk factors have been identified for late-onset problematic drinking. The presence of chronic medical disorders and sleep disturbances might lead some older adults to self-medicate with alcohol to control pain or induce sleep. Some isolated older adults or older adults with excessive free time use drinking to combat boredom or loneliness. Individuals who have lost a spouse are particularly at risk (Byrne et al., 1999). In addition, a recent comparison study amplifies the presence of alcohol use disorders in elderly suicide attempters (Morin et al., 2013). For some individuals, alcohol is seen as a means of decreasing or escaping the emotional distress of psychiatric disorders. When an alcohol use disorder is associated with another mental disorder, the term *co-occurring disorders* is used. The treated prevalence of substance use disorders and co-occurring disorders decreases with age, declining to approximately 10% in adults older than age 65. Questions remain regarding the possibility of underdiagnosis of substance use disorders in older adults (Kerfoot et al., 2011).

Problematic alcohol use in older adults is often minimized or undetected by health care providers. Recognition may be difficult because of challenges in recognizing alcohol abuse secondary to the aging process itself. Disorientation, forgetfulness, hoarding, inadequate diet, and neglect of personal appearance all may be attributed to the aging process but are also symptomatic of alcohol misuse (Flood & Buckwalter, 2009b). Older adults often underreport alcohol consumption as a result of impaired recall, guilt, or shame. Social stigma is especially strong in older women, who are more likely than men to drink secretly at home and make efforts to conceal their drinking behavior (Ludwick et al., 2000). Along with assessment of the quantity of alcohol consumed, physiologic changes that occur with aging, medications, and certain conditions (e.g., cognitive disorders) that intensify the effects of alcohol must be considered. Older adults show greater central nervous system sensitivity to alcohol than younger drinkers, so adverse effects on cognition and coordination are more pronounced by comparison. Because of age-related changes, the same amount of alcohol produces a blood alcohol level about 20% higher in a 65-year-old than in a 30-year-old (Ganzini & Atkinson, 1996). Even if older adults do not increase their level of alcohol consumption over consumption of earlier years, their bodies react as if they were drinking more.

Screening tools such as the CAGE questionnaire and the Geriatric Michigan Alcohol Screening Test (G-MAST) can assist identification of at-risk drinkers and should be included in health assessments of older adults. It is important to ask questions about alcohol consumption and its effects on life.

Nurses should also be attuned to the possibility of alcohol as a contributing factor in many problems seen in older medical and psychiatric patients. Box 35-6 lists some presenting features of older adult problem drinkers. Problem drinkers generally have more health-related complaints than their peers, and older women are particularly susceptible to the toxic effects of alcohol (Ludwick et al., 2000). Withdrawal symptoms might be the first indication of alcohol dependence. Alcohol withdrawal includes a broad spectrum of symptoms, and although the severity of withdrawal symptoms is not appreciably different across age groups, physiologic changes and comorbid physical conditions place older adults at an increased risk (Wetterling et al., 2001). Nurses have a significant role in the management of alcohol withdrawal (Box 35-7).

Various interventions are available to support continued abstinence after withdrawal. For some late-onset drinkers, education and abstinence advice are effective (Blow, 2000). For other drinkers, including long-term alcohol abusers, formal structured programs are necessary. Greatest success

---

BOX 35-6 POTENTIAL ALCOHOL-RELATED PROBLEMS IN OLDER ADULTS

Fluctuations in activities of daily living and instrumental activities of daily living
Self-neglect
Trauma (e.g., falls, burns, accidents)
Weight loss
Dehydration
Gastrointestinal complaints (e.g., pain, bleeding, chronic diarrhea)
Incontinence
Increased medical complaints
Neuropathy
Jaundice
Ascites
Unexpected drug effects
Confusion or delirium
Dementia (Wernicke-Korsakoff syndrome)
Depression
Sleep disturbance
Family discord
Legal trouble (especially driving under the influence)

BOX 35-7 NURSING CARE OF ALCOHOL WITHDRAWAL SYNDROME IN OLDER ADULTS

Assess withdrawal symptoms.
Assess vital signs.
Educate about withdrawal process.
Assist with activities of daily living.
Reduce environmental stimuli.
Supplement diet to meet nutritional needs.
Reorient patient.
Provide relaxation exercises.

---

is achieved when the program is geared specifically for older adults. Programs for older adults emphasize peer bonding and shared reminiscing in addition to cognitive behavioral training that addresses themes such as self-efficacy, self-esteem, and relapse prevention strategies. Whenever possible, it is of paramount importance to address the factors that initially led to problem drinking.

Outcomes of Alcoholics Anonymous (AA) for special populations to include the elderly are an area of discussion. Existing studies and the need for future ones among these groups focus on outcomes of AA participation and spirituality in addiction recovery (Timko, 2008).

Drug Misuse and Abuse

Problems may result from the overuse and misuse of prescription and OTC medications. Older adults use 25% to 30% of all prescription drugs and an even larger share of OTC agents (Substance Abuse and Mental Health Services Administration, 2001). Many prescriptions for this age group are for psychoactive, mood-changing drugs that have the potential for misuse, abuse, or dependency. Box 35-8 provides guidelines for the use

BOX 35-8 GUIDELINES FOR PSYCHOTROPIC DRUG USE IN OLDER ADULTS

Initial Dose (Start Low-Go Slow)
- Usually one third to one half of dose used for younger adults is effective.
- Start with a small dose and gradually increase until therapeutic effect or adverse side effects occur.

Daily Dosage
- Use the smallest dose that produces relief.
- Simplify dosing schedule.

Individualization
- Monitor blood levels when possible.
- Consider effects of other drugs and conditions.
- Partial symptom relief might be the most judicious and realistic goal.

Discontinuation
- Gradually taper off psychotropic drugs.
- If patients can manage without drug therapy, they should be allowed to do so.

of psychotropic drugs in older adults. Benzodiazepines, used for the treatment of anxiety and insomnia, are of particular concern because they are frequently prescribed at inappropriately high doses and for excessive periods. This practice might lead to tolerance, physiologic dependence, and psychological dependence. Older women are more likely to receive and abuse psychoactive drugs than men (Blow, 2000; U.S. Department of Health and Human Services, 1999a).

Variable usage of prescribed drugs is a significant problem, exacerbated by poor vision and hearing, physical deficits, confusion, mental disorders, and inadequate instructions. Drug costs and packaging should also be considered as factors that impede optimal usage. Further complicating the situation, older adults might add several OTC agents, combine medications with alcohol, or take medication prescribed for others without notifying their prescriber. Many older adults see multiple providers, each of whom might prescribe drugs without reliable information about medications that the others have prescribed. Confusion caused by generic and trade names can result in older adults taking the same medication under two names at the same time. Polypharmacy is common, so the nurse should be aware of potential complications and encourage patients to show the nurse all medications for cataloging. Drug regimens should be simplified and carefully explained, verbally and in writing.

? CRITICAL THINKING QUESTION

4. Do nurses at the facility where you have clinical rotations routinely include the same questions for alcohol and other drugs in their assessments of older adults as they do for younger adults? Do you feel comfortable asking your patients questions about alcohol or drugs?

ASSESSMENT OF OLDER ADULTS WITH MENTAL DISORDERS

Mental disorders are not isolated phenomena in older adults. Comprehensive psychosocial and physical assessments are required to determine factors that influence the older adult's level of function. Family members or other caregivers, who often play a pivotal role in the function of older adults, should be included in the assessment process whenever possible. The goals of the initial assessment and subsequent reassessments are to collect accurate information, identify problems and assets, plan interventions, predict outcomes, and measure changes over time. Because of the amount and depth of information needed, the nurse often works collaboratively with the health care team to complete the assessment in collaboration with the patient and caregivers and develops goals and methods for care.

Nurses who are sensitive to the unique psychosocial and physical needs of older adults and adapt the assessment to accommodate these needs increase the chances of obtaining data that accurately represent the patient. Interviews might produce anxiety because older adults are often reluctant to discuss problems with a stranger, especially a younger one. Older adult patients might be irritated by direct questions and view them as intrusive. Open-ended questions, which provide an opportunity for the patient to vent feelings and describe concerns and problems, often foster a healthy understanding of the patient's perspective of life and functioning. Strategies such as giving older people a measure of control, increasing self-esteem, using nonjudgmental wording, and providing positive reinforcement facilitate truthful information. Other strategies to enhance communication with older adults are listed in Box 35-9.

PSYCHOSOCIAL ASSESSMENT

A wealth of clinical data can be obtained by listening to the stories that many older adults love to tell. Listening not only conveys a sense of appreciation for the individual's contributions across the life span but also provides the patient a nonthreatening means of communicating pertinent information. The nurse should listen carefully during these conversations for persistent themes, such as guilt, stress, grief, fear, or despair (Cully et al., 2001). By accepting expressed fears and concerns, the nurse assures the patient that these expressions will not result in rejection. Information about past experiences and coping strategies along with personal strengths and weaknesses might also be revealed. Formal assessment tools previously described might also be used to assess mental status, depression, and problem alcohol or other drug consumption. Box 35-10 lists information to obtain during the initial assessment.

Caregivers should be included in the assessment process. Not only can they provide information to clarify or expand on that given by the patient, but also their perspective of problems is important for inclusion in a plan of care. Family members might be embarrassed to contradict information

BOX 35-9 ENHANCING COMMUNICATION WITH OLDER ADULTS

CONSIDERATIONS	NURSING IMPLICATIONS
Slowed information processing	Do not rush; allow adequate time for questions to be answered.
	Use common words and short sentences.
	Avoid unnecessary interruptions.
Establishment of rapport	Offer a handshake; if appropriate culturally, physically acceptable (not painful). Ask permission first.
	Make eye contact.
	Position at equal or lower level than patient while remaining in view.
	Address by title and last name unless asked to use another name.
	Use a calm, clear voice.
Hearing deficits	Articulate words clearly.
	Face patient when speaking.
	Adjust volume of speech to patient's need; do not shout.
	Ensure use of hearing aid or amplifier.
	Use complementary nonverbal strategies (e.g., facial expressions, gestures).
Visual deficits	Provide adequate nonglare lighting.
	Ensure use of corrective lens.
Competing stimuli	Minimize background noise.
	Avoid times when patient is excessively tired, is in pain, is hungry, or has toileting needs.
	Provide privacy.
Education level	Match vocabulary to patient's level of use.
Decreased physical tolerance	Avoid overtiring.

BOX 35-10 INITIAL ASSESSMENT INFORMATION

Demographics (age, marital status)
Spiritual and cultural values
Personal and family history
History of legal difficulties
Economic status and sources of income
Education and work history
Lifestyle and perception of current life situation
Current living arrangements
Interests, pleasures, and activities
Friendship and social interactions
Sexual functioning
Medical information and history
Prescription and over-the-counter drugs
Alcohol, tobacco, and other chemical use
Cognitive, behavioral, and emotional status
Goals and plans for the future

given by the patient in a joint interview. Because assessing family interaction is important, time should be spent interviewing the patient and family members both separately and together. Nurses should use time with caregivers to assess their ability and willingness to provide care and support for the patient. Many caregivers, often spouses or children, fail to take care of their own needs and lack information about support services and respite care. In addition, special attention must be given to male caregivers based upon levels of stress, gender roles, age, income, and social support in interaction with physical and emotional health (Neri et al., 2012).

PHYSICAL ASSESSMENT

Throughout this chapter, the connection between physical conditions and mental disorders has been stressed. A complete physical examination is an essential component in the assessment of any older adult presenting with symptoms of mental disorders. The examination techniques for each subsystem do not differ substantially from the examination of younger adults. Adaptations for decreased mobility and obvious impairments must be made. Careful attention to every subsystem is required because, in older adults, examination might reveal abnormalities in a system not suggested by the presenting symptoms. For example, subtle hearing loss can result in bizarre or incorrect responses, leading to erroneous assumptions about psychopathologic conditions. The nurse should use all senses during the examination, attending to the patient's visual presentation, odors, voice tone, and content. Blood tests, electroencephalography, and neuroimaging studies might be ordered to identify conditions that contribute to symptoms of mental disorders.

Special attention should be given to defining how physical problems interfere with the patient's functional ability. Older adults assign a great value to independence, and loss of independence can contribute to lower self-esteem and declines in mental health. The loss of key abilities might result in shame and frustration. Older adults who are dependent on others might resent the idea that others have to provide care and might believe that they have become a burden. The resulting anger can be directed internally and result in depression or withdrawal, or it might be directed at caregivers. Assessment of activities of daily living (ADLs) and instrumental activities

BOX 35-11 FUNCTIONAL ASSESSMENT

ACTIVITIES OF DAILY LIVING	INSTRUMENTAL ACTIVITIES OF DAILY LIVING
Bathing	Preparing meals
Dressing	Shopping
Eating	Managing money
Transferring	Using the telephone
Walking	Toileting
Doing housework	Taking medication

BOX 35-12 SAMPLE QUESTION: INSTRUMENTAL ACTIVITIES OF DAILY LIVING SCALE

A. Ability to use telephone
  1. Operates telephone on own initiative—looks up and dials numbers, and so forth.
  2. Dials a few well-known numbers.
  3. Answers telephone but does not dial.
  4. Does not use telephone at all.
  There are eight variables on this scale. The higher the score, the greater the disability. Other variables include shopping, food preparation, housekeeping, laundry, mode of transportation, responsibility for own medications, and ability to handle finances.

From Lawton, M.P., et al. (1992). A research and service-oriented multilevel assessment instrument. *Journal of Gerontology, 37,* 91.

of daily living (IADLs) provides a measure of the older adult's functional ability and guides the selection of interventions and services to meet identified needs. Box 35-11 identifies some of the variables for both ADLs and IADLs; Box 35-12 provides a sample question from the IADLs scale. Patients and sometimes their families are often unable or unwilling to describe functional difficulties because of the threat to established patterns of lifestyle and interactions. According to the Administration on Aging (2008), more than 27% of community-resident Medicare beneficiaries older than age 65 in 2006 had difficulty carrying out ADLs, and 12.5% reported difficulties with IADLs. By contrast, 91% of institutionalized Medicare beneficiaries had difficulties with one or more ADLs, and 73.4% experienced difficulty with three or more ADLs. Observing task performance and carefully listening both to the patient and to collateral sources (e.g., family or caregiver) as they describe daily activities might provide a more accurate picture of functional ability than direct questioning.

The physical examination should be used as an opportunity to assess for signs of abuse or neglect. Each state has laws that specify reporting requirements for intentional abuse, neglect, and exploitation of older adults. Laws also cover endangerment resulting from mental disorders. Chapter 3 discusses some legal issues that might stem from abuse or neglect.

PSYCHOTHERAPEUTIC MANAGEMENT

Nurse-Patient Relationship

Attitude

Ageist attitudes, intergenerational differences, communication deficits, and the multiple problems of older adults can pose significant obstacles to developing a therapeutic nurse-patient relationship. Nurses who are aware of their own feelings and reactions are able to focus on patients and their significant others in a therapeutic manner. By empathizing with the patient and caregivers and focusing on the patient's needs, the nurse can assist patients and their families to manage the activities and demands of daily living and improve the overall quality of both physical and mental health.

CASE STUDY

Ms. Othelia Thatcher, a 78-year-old white woman with a 10-year history of severe depression, has been hospitalized twice in the last 2 years. She received a series of electroconvulsive therapy (ECT) treatments during each stay, with the last treatment given 11 months ago. Ms. Thatcher's cousin, a woman about 60 years old, brought the patient to the hospital emergency department this morning. The cousin described a gradual worsening of depressive symptoms over the past few months and says that Ms. Thatcher seems to need ECT approximately once a year. About 6 or 7 months after a course of ECT has been completed, the patient "goes bad again."

Ms. Thatcher complains of erratic sleep patterns and decreased appetite. She will not eat unless her cousin spoon-feeds her. The cousin reports that after a series of ECT, the patient is "easier to live with," plays with children, takes care of herself, helps with household tasks, and will "eat anything not nailed down."

The cousin estimates that the patient's depression began in the 1990s when "her only son, to whom she was very devoted," abandoned Ms. Thatcher to the welfare of the state and sold all her furniture. This occurred after the patient's extended hospitalization for treatment of pneumonia and a urinary tract infection. Since that time, Ms. Thatcher had reportedly lived in five different boarding homes before her cousin took her to the hospital 3 years ago.

The cousin states that Ms. Thatcher has never verbalized suicidal or homicidal thoughts, but she has a basically "paranoid view of life." The cousin cannot recall Ms. Thatcher ever having hallucinations.

Communication

Communicating a sense of unconditional acceptance of the patient might be the most important intervention that the nurse can provide. Spending time with the patient beyond that required for tasks such as medication administration and ADLs communicates an appreciation for the patient as a person of worth. Providing opportunities for the patient to participate in care decisions and to control the sequence of events, such as allowing the patient to choose when to bathe, enhances self-esteem, self-worth, and decision-making skills. The nurse must be aware of problems and unspoken needs and incorporate them into the plan of care.

Realistic Goals

Establishing short-term and long-term goals is important for nurses and patients. Discussions should be held with patients to stress the importance of goal setting. ADLs often can be a challenge, and developing a schedule of the day's activities with goals can help patients make decisions and cope with demands. Simple decisions might be difficult for older adults with mental disorders. Reducing the options available before allowing the patient choices can diminish frustration. For example, when it is time to dress, the nurse might restrict the choices of attire to two rather than offering an entire closet of options. The caregiver must be gentle and supportive because additional time might be needed to achieve goals. Caregivers who base care decisions on the goal of restoring the patient to maximal independent function are likely to resist the urge to save time and energy by taking over tasks. Nurses should provide information on self-care and disease management at a pace that facilitates understanding. Patience, positive reinforcement, and consistency by the nurse benefit the patient.

Psychopharmacology

Polypharmacy, physiologic changes, and comorbid physical disorders combine to increase the risk of unexpected drug effects in older adults. The negative impact of typical side effects is also exacerbated. Age-related changes that affect drug absorption, distribution, metabolism, and elimination are listed in Table 35-3 (Gareri et al., 2000). Knowledge of *pharmacokinetics* is important, particularly when elderly patients take multiple drugs. For example, antacids might delay absorption; proximal loop and potassium-sparing diuretics affect lithium excretion. Knowledge of drugs' characteristics and their site and mechanism of action is important to understanding the sensitivity that older adults exhibit. For example, antipsychotic medications that act by blocking dopamine receptors have an increased likelihood of causing extrapyramidal side effects (EPSEs) in older adults who already have diminished dopamine concentrations. Nurses must observe and report expected therapeutic and adverse medication reactions and plan interventions to minimize the negative consequences of drug therapy.

Antidepressants

Target symptoms of depression, side effect profiles, dosing schedules, and cost are factors in antidepressant drug selection. Selective serotonin reuptake inhibitors (SSRIs), which are generally favored for older adults, are effective, have a favorable side effect profile, and are not lethal in overdose. SSRIs are also used to treat primary anxiety disorders common in older adults (Compton & Nemeroff, 2001). Tricyclic antidepressants (TCAs) can be used in older adults, but their anticholinergic, antiadrenergic, and antihistaminic properties cause side effects that are particularly problematic for older adult patients. TCAs are not recommended for patients with known cardiac problems because of their association with changes in cardiac conduction, arrhythmias, and orthostatic hypotension. TCAs are not frequently prescribed.

Antidepressant agents such as bupropion (Wellbutrin) and trazodone (Desyrel) have a better side effect profile than TCAs and are widely used. Bupropion causes little sedation, hypotension, anticholinergic response, or cardiotoxicity. Trazodone does not have anticholinergic effects, but it is

TABLE 35-3 AGE-RELATED CHANGES: EFFECTS ON PHARMACOKINETICS

PHYSIOLOGIC CHANGE	EFFECTS	SPECIAL CONSIDERATIONS
↑ Gastric pH ↓ Absorptive surface ↓ Splanchnic blood flow ↓ Gastrointestinal motility ↓ Gastric emptying	Absorption	Delayed absorption of oral medication Acid drugs more rapidly absorbed than base drugs
↑ Body fat ↓ Lean body mass ↓ Total body water ↓ Serum albumin ↓ Cardiac output	Distribution	Extended half-life of lipid-soluble drugs, which accumulate in adipose tissue (e.g., barbiturates, phenothiazines, benzodiazepines, phenytoin, TCAs) ↓ Total plasma albumin = ↓ binding sites for protein-bound drugs, resulting in increased amount of free or active drug
↓ Hepatic blood flow ↓ Hepatic mass ↓ Hepatic enzyme activity	Metabolism	Multiple drugs competing for same enzyme—might ↓ liver metabolism High degree of genetic variability in available hepatic enzymes
↓ Renal blood flow ↓ Glomerular filtration rate ↓ Tubular secretion ↓ Number of nephrons ↓ Creatinine production ↓ Creatinine clearance	Elimination	Creatinine clearance—can be reduced despite normal serum creatinine levels because of ↓ lean body weight and ↓ creatinine production Reduction in renal clearance—might reduce dose requirements

TCAs, Tricyclic antidepressants.
From Gareri, P., et al. (2000). Conventional and new antidepressant drugs in the elderly. *Progress in Neurobiology, 61,* 354; Keltner, N., & Folks, D. (2005). *Psychotropic drugs* (4th ed.). St. Louis: Mosby.

CARE PLAN

Name: Ms. Othelia Thatcher   **Admission Date:** _____

DSM-5 Diagnosis: Major depression

Assessment	**Areas of strength:** Patient is willing to be treated; is cooperative, has a good support system (cousin very concerned and wants patient back in home).
	Problems: Withdrawn, decreased interest in interactions and activities, decreased self-esteem, decreased energy, hopelessness, poor judgment.
Diagnoses	Ineffective coping, disturbed sleep pattern, dysfunctional grief (son's behavior, loss of contact, and loss of home, & belongings, imbalanced nutrition; less than body requirements, impaired social interaction, self-care deficits
Outcomes	**Short-term goals**
Date met: _____	Patient can maintain safety.
Date met: _____	Patient can express feelings verbally.
Date met: _____	Patient will have increased energy for self-care.
	Long-term goals
Date met: _____	Patient will initiate and respond to social interactions.
Date met: _____	Patient will be able to talk about anger and disappointment related to son.
Date met: _____	Patient will have an increase in self-concept.
Date met: _____	Patient will maintain independence although living in cousin's home.
Planning and Interventions	**Nurse-patient relationship:** Convey concern and acceptance without sympathy, encourage expression of feelings, encourage interactions with others as tolerated, help patient explore anger with son.
	Psychopharmacology: fluoxetine (Prozac) 20 mg every morning; risperidone (Risperdal) 0.5 mg q12h; docusate sodium 100 mg twice a day (prophylactic).
	Milieu management: Provide adequate nutrition and hydration. Monitor patient for safety issues. Keep patient around others (not alone in her room) as much as is reasonable. Keep naps short to facilitate sleep at night.
Evaluation	Patient expressed feelings of anger at being abandoned by son. Activity level increased. Able to perform ADLs independently. Minimal confusion after ECT. Medication maintained. Patient will be discharged to return to cousin's home.
Referrals	Schedule visit with home health nurse for follow-up care. Schedule appointment with outpatient program coordinator within 7 days.

sedating. The sedation distinction between antidepressants is important because depression is sometimes exhibited by agitation or sleep disturbance, and affected patients might benefit from the sedating properties of an antidepressant. When depression is exhibited by lethargy and excessive sleep, a more activating antidepressant is in order (e.g., bupropion, SSRIs). Patients should be carefully monitored for orthostatic changes, especially individuals who are also taking diuretics or vasodilators. Monoamine oxidase inhibitors (MAOIs) are rarely used in older adults because these medications have potentially serious side effects and require dietary restrictions (Compton & Nemeroff, 2001). Similar to TCAs, MAOIs are lethal in overdose.

For most antidepressants, full therapeutic response takes at least 2 to 4 weeks. Many patients fail to respond to the first antidepressant prescribed. When failure to respond occurs, the nurse can reassure patients that this is common and that other drugs can be effective. Education about the importance of adherence and the need to continue antidepressant therapy even when depressive symptoms resolve is important. In most cases, antidepressants are continued for at least 6 months after symptom resolution to prevent relapse. Patients who are at high risk of relapse are maintained on antidepressants for longer periods (Whooley & Simon, 2000).

Antipsychotics

Antipsychotic drugs are used in the treatment of schizophrenia, acute psychosis, aggressive behavior, and agitation. Atypical antipsychotics are regarded as the drugs of choice for treatment of older adults because of favorable side effect profiles and efficacy of these drugs. The term *atypical* was introduced to describe the low propensity of these agents to cause EPSEs and tardive dyskinesia, a significant advantage for older adults who are at risk for developing disabling and stigmatizing movement disorders because of neurodegenerative processes. Over a 1-year period taking conventional antipsychotics, older adults develop tardive dyskinesia at a cumulative incidence rate of 28% compared with only 5% in younger patients (Jeste, 2004). With atypical drugs, such as risperidone, this rate decreases significantly to 2.7% (Jeste, 2004). Compared with traditional antipsychotics, atypical antipsychotics also show greater efficacy for both the positive and the negative symptoms of schizophrenia and have fewer adverse cardiac effects and reduced sedative effects. Table 35-4 presents guidelines for treating schizophrenia in older adult patients.

If a traditional antipsychotic is used, it tends to be haloperidol. Antipsychotic drug dosages for older adults tend to be 50% or less than the dosages given to younger

TABLE 35-4 EXPERT GUIDELINES FOR TREATING SCHIZOPHRENIA IN OLDER PATIENTS

FIRST-LINE ANTIPSYCHOTIC	SECOND-LINE ANTIPSYCHOTICS
risperidone (Risperdal) 1.25-3.5 mg/day (median dose 2 mg/day*)	quetiapine (Seroquel) 100-300 mg/day
	olanzapine (Zyprexa) 7.5-15 mg/day (median dose 10 mg/day*)
	aripiprazole (Abilify) 15-30 mg/day

*Median doses from Suzuki et al. (2011).
From Alexopoulous, G., et al. (2004). The expert consensus guidelines: using antipsychotic agents in older patients. *The Journal of Clinical Psychiatry, 65*(Suppl. 2), 1.

patients. Nurses must monitor patients carefully for side effects. Assessment tools, such as the Abnormal Involuntary Movement Scale, can be used to identify EPSEs and tardive dyskinesia.

Antianxiety Agents

Anxiety is a common late-life problem, and management often involves SSRIs, benzodiazepines, and buspirone (BuSpar). A disproportionate share of prescriptions for benzodiazepines is written for older adults, despite the fact that this age group is particularly vulnerable to common side effects, such as drowsiness, cognitive suppression, and ataxia. An increased risk of falls, disinhibition characterized by violence or agitation, and retrograde amnesia are additional related concerns. Federal guidelines and improved practice guidelines for management of anxiety in older adults have encouraged the use of benzodiazepines such as lorazepam (Ativan) and oxazepam (Serax), which are metabolized by phase II mechanisms (i.e., nonoxidative). Benzodiazepines are recommended only for short-term management of anxiety. Because withdrawal syndrome (including withdrawal seizure) can occur when benzodiazepines are removed after 30 or more days of use, they should be withdrawn slowly over several weeks or longer. Benzodiazepines are safe drugs when taken alone but can cause severe sedation and respiratory suppression when combined with alcohol or other sedatives. Buspirone, a nonbenzodiazepine antianxiety agent, effectively manages anxiety without concerns for physical or psychological dependence. Buspirone is not sedating and has no additive effect with alcohol. Its chief disadvantage is that its full therapeutic effects are delayed for 3 to 6 weeks.

Additionally, many older adults with depression experience comorbid anxiety. Careful assessment is critical to provide appropriate interventions. Treating these symptoms with anxiolytic medications alone has been associated with suboptimal outcomes. Choosing antidepressant drugs with known anxiolytic effects is preferable (Lindsey, 2009).

Mood Stabilizers

Mood-stabilizing drugs used for treating bipolar disorders and mixed depressive episodes include lithium, valproates such as divalproex (Depakote), and atypical antipsychotics. Lithium has long been the drug of choice for manic symptoms in patients of all ages; however, in recent years, the most commonly prescribed class of mood stabilizer appears to be the valproates. As a group of drugs, atypical antipsychotics are prescribed about as often as valproates and even more often in patients with late onset at age 60 or older (Sajatovic et al., 2005). Recently, in a small open-label study of elderly patients with bipolar mania, benefit was derived from asenapine in both total improvement of outcome score measurements and reaching remission of symptoms (Baruch et al., 2013).

With lithium, the serum levels are closely monitored in all patients and in older adults; both a therapeutic response (serum levels 0.4 to 0.8 mEq/L) and a toxic response occur at lower levels. Older adults are also at a higher risk for toxic reactions related to altered fluid and electrolyte balance and coadministered medications, especially diuretics. Because therapeutic effects of mood stabilizers take weeks to manifest, short-acting benzodiazepines are often considered as adjuncts to manage dangerous behaviors in the interval (Snowdon, 2000).

In a qualitative-quantitative study of medication therapy in older adults with bipolar disorder, da Cruz et al. (2011) found that a low level of adherence to pharmacologic treatment and a deficit in knowledge in relation to the medication were identified. This deficit in knowledge especially applied to dose and frequency of administration. Among the difficulties inherent to pharmacotherapy, the obligation, the desire to quit, the limitation in the self-administration, collateral effects, and feeling doubt about the need for the medication all were related. Investment is needed in educational activities and in the promotion of adherence that addresses the difficulties experienced by elders with bipolar disorder to ensure safety.

Milieu Management

Nurses responsible for older adults with mental disorders in inpatient or day care settings have a therapeutic responsibility to facilitate optimal function. Attention to all elements of the milieu can increase psychological functioning and prevent the deterioration resulting from withdrawal and disuse of skills that has been well documented in institutionalized older adults.

Normalizing the Environment

Effective milieu management changes the quality of life in institutional environments by working with residents to normalize the environment as much as possible. The traditional associations of home involve control over people who come and go as well as control of personal spaces, furnishings, and accessories. Furniture, at a height that facilitates independent mobility, can be placed in conversational groupings. Common rooms are best equipped with large-print books, games with large print and pieces, and stimulating pictures.

Individual rooms can be deinstitutionalized by encouraging residents to use their own bedspreads, family pictures, favorite calendars, and other personal items. This same strategy, even in acute care settings, has the added benefit of providing orientation cues. Staff members often wear street clothes rather than traditional uniforms to encourage social interaction with residents and eliminate artificial barriers. It is important to remember privacy needs and respect personal space. Environmental adaptations that promote safety and independence for older adults are listed in Table 35-5.

NURSING INTERVENTIONS FOR ASSISTING OLDER ADULTS WITH DEPRESSION

Assess and meet physical needs.
Promote healthy behavior.
Maximize independence.
Promote sense of control.
Provide consistency.
Reinforce self-esteem.
Acknowledge individual's feelings.
Appreciate individual's uniqueness in context of entire life span and culture.
Reinforce genuine hope.
Identify available supports.
Consider family and caregivers (Ramsay et al., 2012).

Controlling Aggression

Controlling aggression is a major component of maintaining individual and environmental safety. Violent or agitated behavior might be the result of poor frustration tolerance, ineffective coping strategies, impulsivity, or real or imagined threats to personal space. Nurses must look at the environment and develop strategies to minimize precipitating factors. Careful attention should be paid to the potential for background stimuli such as constant music or television to cause distress. Physical and chemical restraints to control behavior have numerous negative consequences, and alternative interventions should be attempted before use. Managing environmental stimuli, providing productive outlets for energy, and practicing redirection and diversion are important for reducing outbursts.

Tailoring Activities

Therapeutic approaches should be based on the concept that all individuals have a need for human contact, social participation, and meaningful activity to maintain function. Individual and group interactions and activities should be planned to foster the greatest degree of independence and develop interpersonal and communication skills. Various activities can be tailored to match individual levels of physical and psychological function. Pet therapy helps fulfill patients' needs to give and receive affection through supervised sessions of holding, stroking, and playing with specially screened animals. Pet therapy is efficient in improving depressive symptoms and cognitive function in residents of long-term care facilities with mental illness (Moretti et al., 2011). Exercise therapy, tailored to all needs, including the needs of patients with limited physical ability, provides outlets for the excess energy of anxiety and provides stimulation and socialization opportunities. Music is also an effective way to make contact with patients. Songbooks, hymnals, and various forms of music via technology offer an array of choices familiar to older adults, who often enjoy sing-alongs or simply listening to familiar and comfortable tunes. Listening to music can help older people reduce their depression level (Chan et al., 2011). Nurturing and tending to plants can enhance physical function, relieve tension, and provide a sense of responsibility and accomplishment. These therapeutic activities and others are important opportunities to provide patients with positive experiences and help them attain realistic goals.

Valuing the Person through Reminiscence

Reminiscence is the process of recalling past experiences, which allows the listener insight into the patient's history and perspective. Patients can benefit from multiple dimensions of

---

TABLE 35-5   ENVIRONMENTAL ADAPTATIONS

CONSIDERATIONS	INTERVENTIONS
Decreased ability to distinguish colors	Use high-contrast colors in vivid hues
Mobility impairments	Ensure nonslip floor surfaces
	Provide adequate, nonglare lighting
	Ensure well-fitting footwear
	Provide chairs and toilets at comfortable height with armrests or handrails
	Avoid placing rolling tables where patients might attempt to use them for stability
	Provide shower stools, nonskid tub guards, and grab bars
	Provide ambulation rails
	Remove obstacles, clutter, and spills promptly
Inability to read	Mark spaces with pictures or universal symbols
Decreased thermoregulation	Ensure comfortable temperature
	Observe for signs of hypothermia or hyperthermia
	Provide sweaters, blankets
	Ensure safe water temperature

reminiscence, including clarifying their sense of self, connecting with others, providing instruction, restructuring recalled events, recalling previously used problem-solving strategies, and bringing closure and calmness in death preparation (Cully et al., 2001). Reminiscence groups can provide validation for each member and help participants establish new relationships, while enhancing valuable communication and socialization skills. Older women participating in 6 weeks of reminiscence group sessions experienced an increase in self-transcendence compared with a control group (Stinson & Kirk, 2006). In a more recent study, screening of all older women admitted to assisted living facilities for depression on admission and offering education to nurses working with older adults to educate them on the benefits of this cognitive behavioral approach, a structured protocol of reminiscence, for dealing with depression in older women were supported. Structured reminiscence group interventions can be especially beneficial because medications do not always decrease depression (Stinson et al., 2010).

STUDY NOTES

1. Despite the increase in the population of individuals 65 years old and older, this group experiences major barriers to obtaining quality mental health care because of issues such as ageism, their own attitudes, lack of transportation, and cost of care.

2. Depression is a common mental disorder among older adults, but it is often overlooked, misdiagnosed, and inadequately treated.

3. Symptoms of other illnesses might mask depression because older adults might be preoccupied with physical rather than emotional symptoms.

4. Age-related life events, losses, changes, and physical decline are associated with the onset of depression.

5. The nurse-patient relationship focuses on helping patients achieve their highest level of functioning. Caregivers, when available, should be included in planning strategies to manage the activities and demands of daily living.

6. Adequate nutrition, socialization, and achievement of small realistic goals in ADLs help reduce anxiety and maintain or restore psychological functioning.

7. Use of medications in older adults involves risks associated with polypharmacy, variable usage, and altered pharmacokinetics.

8. Recommended agents for treating depression in older adults include SSRIs, bupropion, and trazodone.

9. When treating psychotic disorders, atypical antipsychotics are usually prescribed. If an older traditional agent is to be used, haloperidol is the most often used agent because of fewer antiadrenergic and anticholinergic effects.

10. Benzodiazepines using phase II metabolism, lorazepam and oxazepam, SSRIs, and nonbenzodiazepine anxiety agents are prescribed most often for older adults.

11. ECT can be an effective treatment for older adults with depression.

12. Milieu management in the care of older adults includes special attention to normalization, controlling aggression, specifically tailoring activities, and valuing the person through reminiscence.

REFERENCES

Administration on Aging. (2005). *Factsheets*. http://www.aoa.gov/factsheets, Accessed 15.03.10.

Administration on Aging. (2008). *A profile of older Americans: 2008. Disability and activity limitations*. http://www.aoa.gov/AoAroot/Aging_Statistics/Profile/2008/16.aspx, Accessed 12.11.09.

Administration on Aging. (2011a.). *Factsheets*. http://acl.gov/NewsRoom/Publications/Index.aspx#AoAfs, Accessed 18.03.13.

Alexopoulous, G., et al. (2004). The expert consensus guidelines: Using antipsychotic agents in older patients. *The Journal of Clinical Psychiatry*, *65*(Suppl. 2), 1.

Amazon, J., et al. (2008). The decision making process of older adults who elect to receive ECT. *Journal of Psychosocial Nursing and Mental Health Services*, *46*, 45.

American Psychiatric Association. (2013). *Diagnostic and statistical manual of mental disorders* (5th ed.). Arlington, Virginia: APA.

Barak, Y., & Swartz, M. (2012). Remission amongst elderly schizophrenia patients. *European Psychiatry*, *27*, 62–64.

Baruch, Y., Tadger, S., Polpski, I., & Barak, Y. (2013). Asenapine for elderly bipolar manic patients. *Journal of Affective Disorders*, *145*, 130–132.

Benros, M. E., et al. (2009). Psychiatric disorder as a first manifestation of cancer: A 10-year population-based study. *International Journal of Cancer*, *124*, 2917.

Blank, K. (2009). Older adults and substance use: New data highlight concerns. *SAMSHA News*. http://www.samhsa.gov/samhsaNewsletter/Volume_17_Number_1/OlderAdults.aspx, Accessed March 18, 2013.

Blank, K., et al. (2001). Life-sustaining treatment and assisted death choices in depressed older patients. *Journal of the American Geriatrics Society*, *49*, 153.

Blazer, D. G., & Koenig, H. G. (1996). Mood disorders. In E. Busse, & D. Blazer (Eds.), *Textbook of geriatric psychiatry*. (2nd ed.) (pp. 235–264). Washington, DC: American Psychiatric Press.

Blow, F. (2000). Treatment of older women with alcohol problems: Meeting the challenge for a special population. *Alcoholism: Clinical and Experimental Research*, *24*, 1257.

Butler, R. N., & Lewis, M. L. (1995). Late-life depression: When and how to intervene. *Geriatrics*, *50*, 44.

Byrne, G., Raphael, B., & Arnold, E. (1999). Alcohol consumption and psychological distress in recently widowed older men. *The Australian and New Zealand Journal of Psychiatry*, *33*, 740.

Care for Elders. (2012). *Healthy IDEAS. Addressing depression in older adults*. http://careforelders.org/files/DDF/mental_health_brief_2.pdf, Accessed 06.04.14.

Casey, D. A. (2012). Depression in the elderly: A review and update. *Asia-Pacific Psychiatry*, *4*, 160–167.

Cassano, G., et al. (2000). Current issues in the identification and management of bipolar spectrum disorders in "special populations". *Journal of Affective Disorders*, *59*, S69.

Chan, J., Draper, B., & Banerjee, S. (2007). Deliberate self-harm in older adults: A review of the literature from 1995 to 2004. *International Journal of Geriatric Psychiatry, 22,* 720.

Chan, F. M., et al. (2011). Effects of music on depression in older people: A randomized controlled trial. *Journal of Clinical Nursing, 21,* 776.

Cohen-Mansfield, J., & Parpura-Gill, A. (2007). Loneliness in older persons: A theoretical model and empirical findings. *International Psychogeriatrics, 19,* 279.

Compton, M., & Nemeroff, C. (2001). The evaluation and treatment of depression in primary care. *Clinical Cornerstone, 3,* 10.

Creed, F. (1999). The importance of depression following myocardial infarction. *Heart, 82,* 406.

Cully, J., LaVoie, D., & Gfeller, J. (2001). Reminiscence, personality, and psychological functioning in older adults. *Gerontologist, 41,* 89.

da Cruz, L. P., et al. (2011). Medication therapy: Adherence, knowledge and difficulties of elderly people from bipolar disorder. *Revista Latino-Americana de Enfermagem, 19,* 944.

Ekwall, A. K., Sivberg, B., & Hallberg, I. R. (2006). Loneliness as a predictor of quality of life among older caregivers. *Journal of Advanced Nursing, 49,* 23.

Eyler Zorrilla, L. T., et al. (2000). Cross-sectional study of older outpatients with schizophrenia and healthy comparison subjects: No differences in age-related cognitive declines. *The American Journal of Psychiatry, 157,* 1324.

Federal Interagency Forum on Aging-Related Statistics. (2000). *Older Americans 2000: Key indicators of well-being, appendix A: Detailed tables.* Washington, D.C.: Federal Interagency Forum on Aging-Related Statistics.

Federal Interagency Forum on Aging-Related Statistics. (2008). *Older Americans 2008: Key indicators of well-being.* Washington, D.C.: Federal Interagency Forum on Aging-Related Statistics.

Fitzpatrick, J. J. (2005). Signs of silent suicide among depressed hospitalized geriatric patients. *Journal of the American Psychiatric Nurses Association, 11,* 290.

Flood, M., & Buckwalter, K. C. (2009a). Recommendations for mental health care of older adults: Part 1—An overview of depression and anxiety. *Journal of Gerontological Nursing, 35,* 26.

Flood, M., & Buckwalter, K. C. (2009b). Recommendations for mental health care of older adults: Part 2—An overview of dementia, delirium, and substance abuse. *Journal of Gerontological Nursing, 35,* 35.

Folks, D., & Fuller, W. (1997). Anxiety disorders and insomnia in geriatric patients. *The Psychiatric Clinics of North America, 20,* 137.

Ganzini, L., & Atkinson, R. (1996). Substance abuse. In J. Sadavoy, et al. (Eds.), *Comprehensive review of geriatric psychiatry— II.* (pp. 659–692). (2nd ed.). Washington, D.C.: American Psychiatric Press.

Gareri, P., et al. (2000). Conventional and new antidepressant drugs in the elderly. *Progress in Neurobiology, 61,* 354.

Holvast, F., et al. (2012). Determinants of receiving mental health care for depression in older adults. *Journal of Affective Disorders, 143,* 69–74.

Howard, R., et al. (2000). Late-onset schizophrenia and very-late-onset schizophrenia-like psychosis: An international consensus. *The American Journal of Psychiatry, 157,* 172.

Hoyert, D. L., Kochanek, K. D., & Murphey, S. L. (1999). *Deaths: Final data for 1997. National vital statistical report.* U.S. Department of Health and Human Services Publication No. 99-1120, Hyattsville, MD: National Center for Health Statistics.

Institute of Medicine. (2012). *The mental health and substance use workforce for older adults; In whose hands?* . http://www.iom.edu/Reports/2012/The-Mental-Health-and-Substance-Use-Workforce-for-Older-Adults.aspx, Accessed 06.04.2014.

Jahn, D. R., et al. (2011). The mediating effect of perceived burdensomeness on the relation between depressive symptoms and suicide ideation in a community sample of older adults. *Aging & Mental Health, 15,* 214.

Jancin, B. (2005). New suicide data highlight toxicity of depression. *Clinical Psychiatry News, 33,* 6.

Jeste, D. V. (2004). Tardive dyskinesia rates with atypical antipsychotics in older adults. *The Journal of Clinical Psychiatry, 65*(Suppl. 9), 21.

Jeste, D. V., Harris, M. J., & Paulsen, J. S. (1996). Psychosis. In J. Sadavoy, et al. (Eds.), *Comprehensive review of geriatric psychiatry—II* (pp. 593–614) (2nd ed.) Washington, DC: American Psychiatric Press.

Joiner, T. E., Jr. (2005). *Why people die by suicide.* Cambridge, MA: Harvard University Press.

Jokela, M., Batty, G. D., & Kivimaki, M. (2013). Ageing and the prevalence and treatment of mental health problems. *Psychological Medicine, 43,* 2037–2045.

Kaplan, M. S., et al. (2012). Suicide risk and precipitating circumstances among young, middle-aged, and older male veterans. *American Journal of Public Health, 102,* S131.

Kayton, W. (2001). The impact of major depression in patients with chronic medical illness. In *Proceedings of the 154th annual meeting of the American Psychiatric Association, New Orleans.*

Keltner, N., & Folks, D. (2005). *Psychotropic drugs* (4th ed.). St. Louis: Mosby.

Kerfoot, K. E., Petrakis, I. S., & Rosenheck, R. A. (2011). Dual diagnosis in an aging population: Prevalence of psychiatric disorders, comorbid substance abuse, and mental health service utilization in the Department of Veteran Affairs. *Journal of Dual Diagnosis, 7,* 4.

Kjolseth, I., & Ekeberg, O. (2012). When elderly people give warning of suicide. *International Psychogeriatrics, 24*(9), 1393–1401.

Koenig, H., et al. (1996). Schizophrenia and paranoid disorders. In E. Busse & D. Blazer (Eds.), *Textbook of geriatric psychiatry* (pp. 265–278) (2nd ed.) Washington, D.C.: American Psychiatric Press.

Lang, A., & Stein, M. (2001). Anxiety disorders. How to recognize and treat the medical symptoms of emotional illness. *Geriatrics, 56,* 24.

Lawton, M. P., et al. (1992). A research and service-oriented multilevel assessment instrument. *Journal of Gerontology, 37,* 91.

Lenze, E., et al. (2000). Co-morbid anxiety disorders in depressed elderly patients. *The American Journal of Psychiatry, 157,* 722.

Lindsey, P. L. (2009). Psychotropic medication use among older adults: What all nurses need to know. *Journal of Gerontological Nursing, 35,* 29.

Ludwick, R., et al. (2000). Alcohol use in elderly women: Nursing considerations in community settings. *Journal of Gerontological Nursing, 26,* 44.

Maurer, D. M. (2012). Screening for depression. *American Family Physician, 85,* 139.

McClure, F. S., Gladsjo, J. A., & Jeste, D. V. (1999). Late-onset psychosis: Clinical, research, and ethical considerations. *The American Journal of Psychiatry, 156,* 935.

Meesters, P. D., et al. (2013). The care needs of elderly patients with schizophrenia spectrum disorders. *The American Journal of Geriatric Psychiatry, 21,* 129–137.

Monteso, P., et al. (2012). Depression in the elderly: Study in a rural city in southern Catalonia. *Journal of Psychiatric and Mental Health Nursing, 19*, 426–429.

Moon, M. A. (2005). Late-onset bipolar patients not as ill as counterparts. *Clinical Psychiatry News, 33*, 48.

Moretti, F., et al. (2011). Pet therapy in elderly patients with mental illness. *Psychogeriatrics, 11*, 125.

Morin, J., et al. (2013). Alcohol use disorder in elderly suicide attempters: A comparison study. *The American Journal of Geriatric Psychiatry, 21*, 196–203.

National Alliance on Mental Illness. (2014). *Depression in older persons fact sheet.* http://www.nami.org, Accessed on April 6, 2014.

National Association of Area Agencies on Aging. (2011). *Policy priorities.* http://www.n4a.org/files/advocacy/campaigns/policy-priority-11.pdf, Accessed 05.03.13.

National Institute of Mental Health. (2007a.). *Older adults: Depression and suicide facts (fact sheet).* http://www.nia.nih.gov/about/health-disparities-strategic-plan-fiscal-years-2009-2013, Accessed 18.03.13.

National Institute of Mental Health. (2012). *Rethinking mental illness: The view from 2022.* http://www.nimh.nih.gov/about/presentations/rethinking-mental-illness.pdf, Accessed 18.03.13.

National Institute on Aging. (2009). *Health disparities strategic plan: Fiscal years 2009–2013.* http://www.nia.nih.gov/about/health-disparities-strategic-plan-fiscal-years2009-2013, Accessed 06.04.14.

Neri, A. L., et al. (2012). Relationships between gender, age, family conditions, physical and mental health, and social isolation of elderly caregivers. *International Psychogeriatrics, 24*(3), 472–483.

Penninx, B., et al. (1999). Minor and major depression and the risk of death in older persons. *Archives of General Psychiatry, 56*, 889.

Plawecki, L. H., & Amrhein, D. W. (2010). Someone to talk to: The nurse and the depressed or suicidal older patient. *Journal of Gerontological Nursing, 36*, 15.

Ramsay, C. E., et al. (2012). An exploration of perceptions of possible depression prevention services for caregivers of elderly or chronically ill adults in rural Georgia. *Community Mental Health Journal, 48*, 167–178.

Sajatovic, M., et al. (2005). New-onset bipolar disorder in later life. *The American Journal of Geriatric Psychiatry, 13*, 282.

Schouws, S.N.T.M., Comijs, H. C., Stek, M. L., & Beekman, A. T. F. (2012). Self-reported cognitive complaints in elderly bipolar patients. *The American Journal of Geriatric Psychiatry, 20*, 700–706.

Schurhoff, F., et al. (2000). Early and late onset bipolar disorders: Two different forms of manic-depressive illness? *Journal of Affective Disorders, 58*, 215.

Shea, D., Russo, P., & Smyer, M. (2000). Use of mental health services by persons with a mental illness in nursing facilities: Initial impacts of OBRA, 87. *Journal of Aging and Health, 12*, 560.

Sherman, C. (2005). Modify depression treatment for older patients. *Clinical Psychiatry News, 33*, 54.

Snowdon, J. (2000). The relevance of guidelines for treatment of mania in old age. *International Journal of Geriatric Psychiatry, 15*, 779.

Stinson, C. K., & Kirk, E. (2006). Structured reminiscence: An intervention to decrease depression and increase self-transcendence in older women. *Journal of Clinical Nursing, 15*, 208.

Stinson, C. K., et al. (2010). Use of a structured reminiscence protocol to decrease depression in older women. *Journal of Psychosocial Nursing and Mental Health Services, 17*, 665.

Substance Abuse and Mental Health Services Administration. (2001). *The national clearinghouse for alcohol and drug information: Use and abuse of psychoactive prescription drugs and over the counter medications.* Rockville, MD: SAMHSA.

Substance Abuse and Mental Health Services Administration. (2006). *Results from the 2005 national survey on drug use and health: National findings.* Publication No. SMA 06-4194, Rockville, MD: Office of Applied Studies NSDUH Series H-30, D1-1 1-15.

Substance Abuse and Mental Health Services Administration. (2008). Mental health and mental disorders. In *Healthy people 2010—Conference edition.* Rockville, MD: SAMHSA. http://www.samhsa.gov/samhsanewsletter/Volume_18_Number_1/OlderAdults.aspx, Accessed 18.03.13.

Suzuki, T., et al. (2011). Management of schizophrenia in late life with antipsychotic medications: A qualitative review. *Drugs and Aging, 28*, 961.

Tabloski, P. (2006). *Psychological and cognitive function.* In *Gerontological nursing* (pp. 188–241). *Upper Saddle River, NJ*: Pearson Prentice Hall.

Tew, J. D., Jr., et al. (1999). Acute efficacy of ECT in the treatment of major depression in the old-old. *The American Journal of Psychiatry, 156*, 1865.

Theeke, L. A. (2009). Predictors of loneliness in U.S. adults over age sixty-five. *Archives of Psychiatric Nursing, 23*, 387.

Timko, C. (2008). Outcomes of AA for special populations. In M. Galanter & L. A. Kaskutas (Eds.), *Research on alcoholics anonymous and spirituality in addiction recovery* (pp. 373–392). New York: Springer Science+Business Media.

U.S. Centers for Disease Control and Prevention and National Association of Chronic Disease Directors. (2008). *The state of mental health and aging in America issue brief 1: What do the data tell us?* . http://www.cdc.gov/aging/pdf/mental_health.pdf, Accessed 05.03.13.

U.S. Centers for Disease Control and Prevention National Center for Injury Prevention and Control. (2005). *Web-based injury statistics query and reporting system (WISQARS).* http://www.cdc.gov/ncipc/wisqars, Accessed 30.03.13.

U.S. Department of Health and Human Services. (1999a.). *Mental health: A report of the Surgeon General.* Rockville, MD: U.S. Department of Health and Human Services, Substance Abuse and Mental Health Services Administration, Center for Mental Health Services, National Institutes of Health, National Institute of Mental Health. http://profiles.nlm.nih.gov/ps/access/NNBBHS.pdf, Accessed April 6, 2014.

U.S. Department of Health and Human Services. (1999b.). *Older adults and mental health. Mental health: A report of the Surgeon General.* http://www.surgeongeneral.gov/library/mentalhealth/chapter5/sec1.html, Accessed 12.11.09.

Unützer, J., et al. (2009). Health care costs associated with depression in medically ill fee-for-service Medicare participants. *Journal of the American Geriatrics Society, 57*, 506.

Wetterling, T., et al. (2001). The severity of alcohol withdrawal is not age dependent. *Alcohol and Alcoholism (Oxford, Oxfordshire), 36*, 75.

Whooley, M., & Simon, G. (2000). Managing depression in medical outpatients. *New England Journal of Medicine, 343*, 1942.

You, S. K., et al. (2009). Spirituality, depression, living alone, and perceived health among Korean older adults in the community. *Archives of Psychiatric Nursing, 23*, 309.

36

Soldiers and Veterans*

Randy L. Moore, Nanci A. Swan

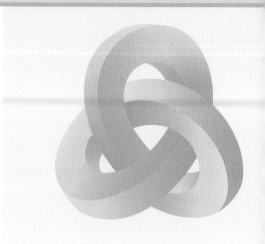

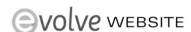 WEBSITE

http://evolve.elsevier.com/Keltner

LEARNING OBJECTIVES

- Recognize the criteria and terminology used in *DSM-5* for posttraumatic stress disorder (PTSD).
- Describe the primary symptoms of PTSD.
- Describe the neurologic alterations associated with PTSD.

- Explain the mechanism of damage causing traumatic brain injury (TBI).
- Identify criteria for TBI.
- Describe neurologic alterations associated with TBI.
- Identify treatment options for patients with PTSD and TBI.

And there went out another horse that was red: and power was given to him that sat thereon to take peace from the earth, and that they should kill one another …

Revelation 6:4

Many Americans have seen the movie *Saving Private Ryan*. In this movie, viewers were plunged into the horrors of war almost before they could start munching on their popcorn. Up until the 1960s, Hollywood glossed over such brutal realities. Men were shot, staggered a step or two, and then fell—to die quickly, quietly, and often without a trace of blood. Beginning in the late 1960s, movie directors became intent on *realism*. Whether or not cinematic realism is healthy is deserving of careful debate. That discussion aside, *Saving Private Ryan*, winner of five Academy Awards, eliminated all illusions of a clean kill. In the early scenes of the movie, the realistic carnage at the D-Day landing created visceral reactions in most moviegoers. Young men were seen blown asunder with legs no longer attached to bodies and heads rendered unrecognizable. Screams of the dying mixed with cries for "momma" caused all but the most steeled to turn a head or close an eye. Many in the audience wondered if such inhuman destruction of other humans was possible. And, if so, could anyone survive such brutality and ever be the same?

American soldiers today are subject to such mayhem. Almost daily our newspapers report of a suicide bomber self-exploding and taking 10, 20, or more people with him. In these all-too-frequent scenarios, often only pieces of human flesh can be retrieved with identification of the dead not always possible. However, more likely for our servicemen is the potential to be injured or killed by an improvised explosive device (IED) carefully hidden along some isolated desert highway. The moviegoers' question remains relevant for mental health providers and for Americans in general: "Can anyone witness such carnage and just pick up their lives where they left off?" The answer for many soldiers is a resounding "no."

Readers of this chapter may find themselves in harm's way, although more likely you may find yourself caring for the survivors. This care can occur close to the point of impact or more remotely after these symptoms have fully developed. Bombings are no longer an attack that occurs in faraway lands and are viewed only in the news—on April 15, 2013, a bombing occurred at the end of the Boston Marathon that killed 3 people and injured another 264 people. Additionally, mass shootings are gaining favor among people intent to do harm. The last five mass shootings as of this writing are recorded here: Newtown, Connecticut, December 14, 2012, 27 people killed; University of Texas, August 5, 2012, 6 killed and 3 injured; Aurora, Colorado, July 20, 2012, 12 killed; Norway, July

---

* The previous edition of this chapter was written by Norman L. Keltner and John P. McGuinness.

22, 2011, 77 killed; Tucson, Arizona, January 8, 2011, 6 killed and 13 injured (including then U.S. Representative Gabrielle Giffords). Added to these shootings was a mass stabbing at a school in Murraysville, Pennsylvania on April 9, 2014 that injured at least 20 people. These examples are provided to express the reality that we may come to face.

Soldiers who are exposed to combat are changed persons. The challenge is to ensure that the changes are in a positive direction. Unfortunately, this is not always the case. Two overarching war-caused conditions have emerged as soldiers filter back from duty in Iraq and Afghanistan: posttraumatic stress disorder (PTSD) and the so-called signature wound of this war, traumatic brain injury (TBI). This chapter addresses these two related diagnostic injuries because nurses, particularly psychiatric nurses, will be providing care for more and more of these veterans. The accompanying case of a soldier on his second tour of duty in Iraq is typical of the experiences and symptoms found in PTSD.

NORM'S NOTES

Most of our nation honors our military and veteran population and remembers their families around Memorial Day and Veteran's Day. One could argue that keeping these patriots in the forefront of our minds should be occurring daily. After all these years, brothers, sisters, friends, and neighbors still remember. Subsequently, in 2009, an Army psychiatrist killed 13 people at Fort Hood, Texas. During his trial someone suggested he suffered from PTSD. Not true!... That kind of sloppy thinking is exactly what the editors of the *DSM* have clarified. Hearing about a battle is not the same as being in a battle. Go figure! This is a serious chapter about men and women who have risked their lives for their country and who have been injured doing so. Keep this in mind as you read.

CASE STUDY: POSTTRAUMATIC STRESS DISORDER

Specialist Gomez, a 22-year-old infantryman, was brought to Combat Stress Control after an incident in which he was found by hospital staff "choking" a middle-aged civilian Iraqi man who was also convalescing on the same hospital ward at an Air Force Theater Hospital in northern Iraq. At that time, Specialist Gomez was serving his second combat tour of duty and had just been injured in the fifth IED explosion he had personally experienced as a member of a five-man team out on patrol in their Bradley Fighting Vehicle. One team member was killed outright. Another team member subsequently died of the injuries he sustained. Two other team members sustained major injuries, including severed limbs. Specialist Gomez was not sure why he survived and sustained only minor contusions and ruptured eardrums.

In his initial interview at Combat Stress Control, he described "flashbacks" that he was having of the recent explosion, even though he was also having difficulty remembering certain events. He had been in the Air Force Theater Hospital for 2 days. He had asked hospital staff to move him to a different ward because he was afraid that he might injure someone

because of the anger, rage, and guilt (at being alive) he was experiencing. He related how he was having great difficulty in distinguishing who was or was not "the enemy." Bed space was limited at the hospital, and he could not be moved to another area.

On his return home 4 months later, Specialist Gomez sought a referral to the Mental Health Clinic at his army base because he was constantly irritable and having difficulties in his relationship with his fiancé, with whom he was living. She was upset with his tendencies to become easily startled "by the smallest thing" and his inability to relax and not be on guard all the time. She felt he was not the same man with whom she had fallen in love and was displeased with his being constantly moody and distant. He was no longer excited about the plans to marry and start a family they had made before his most recent deployment.

Specialist Gomez also described difficulties he was having in going to and staying asleep. He stated that he seldom slept for more than 2 or 3 hours, even after drinking a fifth of liquor. Also, he realized that there was nothing he could do to stop combat-related nightmares he experienced on a nightly basis. He was having intrusive thoughts of his combat experiences many times per day, but he also was having some difficulty remembering certain events and places he had been while in Iraq. He was avoiding most social events, including a unit cookout because the smell of grilling hamburgers reminded him of the burning flesh he had smelled while in Iraq.

OVERVIEW

Since October 2001, more than 2.5 million U.S. troops have been deployed to Operations Iraqi Freedom (OIF) and Enduring Freedom (OEF) in Iraq and Afghanistan (Crawford, 2013). More than 6600 deaths of U.S. soldiers have occurred, and another 48,000 have been injured (Institute of Medicine, 2013). One third of these returning service members have mental health issues (Stiglitz & Bilmes, 2008), and the Institute of Medicine data reveal that 4% to 20% of these men and women have PTSD.

Many soldiers have served their time in "hell" only to be redeployed, as happened to Specialist Gomez in the previous case study. Others have had their tours extended, a particularly demoralizing order when plans to return home were dashed by decision makers thousands of miles away. In a RAND Corporation (2008) of roughly 2000 servicemen randomly selected from across the United States, it was found that most had exposure to trauma, 50% reported having a friend killed or seriously wounded in battle, almost 50% had seen dead and seriously injured civilians, and 10% reported being injured to the point of needing hospitalization (Lew et al., 2008; Tanielian & Jaycox, 2008). Hoge et al. (2004) painted an even grimmer picture in their report—more than 90% of soldiers had seen dead bodies or body parts or both, and more than 50% reported responsibility for killing an enemy combatant. The above-cited RAND report concluded that 18.5% of all returning servicemen from the war zone met criteria for PTSD or depression, 19.5% met criteria for TBI, and more than one third of those surveyed with mild TBI had an overlap of PTSD (Lew et al., 2008). Converting these percentages into numbers showed that about 300,000 soldiers were experiencing PTSD and 320,000 may have experienced TBI. In a large study of OIF and OEF veterans (289,328 soldiers) using the Veterans Healthcare Administration services, Seal and colleagues (2009) found that 37% had a mental health diagnosis, with 22% having PTSD. There is a concern of underreporting because of stigma associated with certain "labels." It is possible that the psychological burden of combat has been significantly underestimated (Sammons & Batten, 2008).

The military mission in Iraq ended in December 2011. The end of the war in Afghanistan is just over the horizon. Hundreds of thousands of service members have redeployed to home. Although some continue their service to the United States, many have completed their obligated service and returned to their civilian lives. Although statistics can be mind-numbing, nurses should always be aware that these are real people with real hopes and real dreams with real families praying for their safe return. These statistics should also forewarn us that a large wave of soldiers with PTSD and TBI is crossing the threshold of the health care system.

AMERICAN DEATHS IN WAR	
U.S troop deaths: Iraq and Afghanistan	>6600
U.S. service member injuries	>48,000
Previous U.S. war deaths (by war)	
Civil War	>620,000
World War II	>406,900
Korean War	>36,000
Vietnam War	>58,000

From American Deaths through History (n.d.). From the War of Independence to Operation Enduring Freedom—blood spilled from sea to shining sea. *Military Factory*. <http://www.militaryfactory.com/american_war_deaths.asp> Accessed June 7, 2013.

POSTTRAUMATIC STRESS DISORDER

The constellation of symptoms that comprise PTSD has existed for as long as men have fought and under many names. During the American Civil War, it was known as *soldier's heart*. In World War I, it was called *shell shock*, and during World War II, it was known as *battle fatigue*. *Posttraumatic stress disorder* is a relatively recent term. It was coined about 30 years ago in recognition of the symptom complex manifested by Vietnam War veterans. PTSD first appeared in the third edition of *DSM* published in 1980. From there, the term trickled into professional publications with perhaps the first medical and nursing articles printed in 1980 (Horowitz et al.) and 1983 (Keltner et al.), respectively. Although coined only around 1980, the term *PTSD* is widely understood and employed in dialogue in the United States as the impact of war

has stressed families, pressured health care agencies, and affected the national equilibrium.

The term *posttraumatic stress disorder* is worth examining. First, *DSM* considers it a "disorder," a mental diagnosis that is distinct from other mental disorders. Second, it is expressed as "stress"—stress caused by experiencing "trauma." Finally, "post" suggests that the reaction occurs after the exposure to trauma and can be delayed for years before surfacing. Solomon and Mikulincer (2006) reported a lag time of 20 years for PTSD to manifest in some Israeli soldiers exposed to combat. *DSM-5* has also restricted the use of the diagnosis. Criterion A1 focuses on the event—it must pose actual or threatened death or serious injury or threaten the physical integrity of the person or others. Criterion A2 focuses on the person's response—horror, helplessness, or fear. Table 36-1 provides specific criteria as established by the American Psychiatric Association; italicized examples come from the case of Specialist Gomez presented earlier in the chapter.

TABLE 36-1	MAJOR SYMPTOMS OF POSTTRAUMATIC STRESS DISORDER

1. Reexperiencing
- Recurrence and intrusive thoughts—*"intrusive thoughts of his combat experiences many times"*
- Recurring dreams
- Flashbacks
- Psychological distress related to symbols/remembrance of event—*"anger, rage, and guilt"*
- Physiologic distress related to symbols/remembrance of event

2. Avoidance
- Avoidance of trauma-related thoughts
- Avoidance of trauma-related activities—*"avoiding most social events ... burning flesh"*
- Amnesia for trauma—*"difficulty remembering certain events and places"*
- Feeling detached or estranged—*"constantly moody and distant"*
- Restricted affect—*"not the same man"*
- Sense of foreshortened future—*"no longer excited about plans they had made"*

3. Hyperarousal
- Insomnia—*"difficulties in going to and staying asleep"*
- Irritability—*"beginning to choke a middle-aged civilian Iraqi"*
- Difficulty concentrating
- Hypervigilance—*"inability to relax and not be on guard all the time"*
- Exaggerated startle reflex—*"she was upset about his tendencies to become easily startled"*

Note: Italicized text relates to the case of Specialist Gomez (Keltner & Dowben, 2007).
Adapted from National Institute of Mental Health (n.d.). *Post-traumatic stress disorder.* <http://www.nimh.nih.gov/health/topics/post-traumatic-stress-disorder-ptsd/index.shtml> Accessed June 10, 2013.

Primary Symptoms of Posttraumatic Stress Disorder

The primary symptoms of PTSD are psychological: reexperiencing of trauma, avoidance of trauma-reminding phenomena, and hyperarousal.

Reexperiencing of the traumatic event comes in several forms. The event might be replayed over and over (*recurrence*), or it might inject itself into an otherwise non–trauma-related stream of thought. The latter is referred to as *thought intrusion*. Other manifestations of reexperiencing include troubled sleep. *Repetitive dreams* that replay the event or some distortion of the event render the soldier unable to find escape even in sleep. *Flashbacks* (dissociative reactions) take reexperiencing to yet another level. During flashbacks, the veteran relives the event while awake. Soldiers suggest that for a short period of time, they think they are back in the battle environment. Some may demonstrate reflex behaviors during this period that approximate behavior expected on the battlefield.

Avoidance is another cardinal symptom of PTSD. Soldiers who experience this symptom *avoid trauma-related thoughts* and *avoid activities* that are trauma-related or reminiscent of the traumatic event. Just as flashbacks might be considered a psychological extension of repetitive dreams, soldiers with PTSD may go beyond thought avoidance to actual *amnesia* for the event in question. Although avoiding trauma-related activities reflects a conscious problem-solving effort to prevent discomfort, some individuals extend that avoidance psychologically with feelings of *detachment* or *estrangement*. This feeling of unreality can be meaningfully constructed as an attempt to avoid pain. These negative alterations in mood and cognition can also include persistent and exaggerated negative beliefs, a negative emotional state, and the inability to experience positive emotions.

Hyperarousal is the third cardinal symptom diagnostic of PTSD. As might be assumed, the soldier is on edge or *hypervigilant*. He scans the environment for threats and often overreacts to stimuli or exhibits an *exaggerated startle reflex*. For example, many veterans have described diving for safety after hearing a car backfire. Being continuously on guard is exhausting, yet because he is on guard, sleep escapes him, and *insomnia* develops. Self-destructive or reckless behavior can occur. Finally, hypervigilance, overreactions, and lack of sleep take their toll, leaving the soldier tired and *irritable*. Tired, irritable, hypervigilant, and easily startled people are difficult to live with. Marriages and relationships that survive deployment often break up under the strain of this emotional rollercoaster. The stress family members feel related to the combat veteran experiencing PTSD has been called "secondary traumatization" (Galovski & Lyons, 2004). Numbing, arousal, and anger are predictive of family distress. The family members must also be targeted for improving their psychological well-being. Finally, few employers are willing to maintain the employment of a person with acute PTSD.

Symptom Delay

As Solomon and Mikulincer (2006) pointed out, the delay in symptoms or at least in diagnosis can stretch out over decades. Seal and colleagues (2009) suggested a variety of reasons why this might be true. Their suggestions include the following psychosocial parameters peculiar to PTSD:

1. The term *posttraumatic* may literally be true in that it may take time for the traumas of war to surface.
2. The stigma of a mental illness may cause some to "fight" the symptoms or self-medicate (e.g., with alcohol) until doing so no longer works.
3. Physical or other mental health problems may obscure PTSD.

Comorbidities

PTSD is often accompanied by another mental health disorder, such as depression, anxiety, or substance abuse. Older veterans with PTSD tend to have a comorbid depression, whereas younger soldiers tend to have a drug and alcohol abuse comorbidity. Based on the report by Weinberger (1987), one would suspect various windows of vulnerability to psychiatric syndromes. Weinberger found that psychiatric manifestations resulting from head injuries during war could be reliably predicted based on the age of the soldier. Stated another way, age at the time of neural insult had a high reliability in predicting the kind of psychiatric problem that emerged after injury. Weinberger stated that when looking at age of onset of various psychiatric disorders, one would usually see a consistent pattern of emergence.

AGE OF ONSET OF PSYCHIATRIC DISORDERS

DISORDER	AGE OF ONSET (YEARS)
Conduct disorders	~10-20
Schizophrenia type	Teens to mid-20s
Affective disorders	Late 20s to 40s
Dementia	50s to late 70s

From Weinberger, D.R. (1987). Implications of normal brain development for the pathogenesis of schizophrenia. *Archives of General Psychiatry*, *44*, 660.

Applying these observed epidemiologic trends, Weinberger suggested that brain injury at any given time along this continuum would most likely result in a psychiatric disorder consistent with what is found in the general population. It is not surprising that young soldiers (defined as 16 to 24 years old in Seal's study) would have more conduct problems (i.e., drinking and drug use) and that older soldiers (approximately 40 years old) would have more depression.

Neurologic Alterations Associated with Posttraumatic Stress Disorder

PTSD is not just a psychological problem. Distinguishable neuroanatomic and neurochemical changes seem to be linked to this disorder. Following is a brief review of these neural alterations.

Neuroanatomic Changes in Posttraumatic Stress Disorder

Soldiers with PTSD are thought to have experienced changes in their prefrontal cortex and various limbic structures (i.e., amygdala and hippocampus). Although much research has focused on discovering neuroanatomic alterations through the use of various brain scanning technologies such as computed tomography (CT), magnetic resonance imaging (MRI) including functional MRI, and positron emission tomography (PET), for the purposes of this brief discussion, such changes can be reduced to simply this: individuals with PTSD tend to have reduced volume in key brain areas (Bremner et al., 1999; Driessen et al., 2004). A recurring theme in these studies is alterations in function of the amygdala. Rauch et al. (2000) demonstrated exaggerated amygdala responses to general negative stimuli in brains affected with PTSD, essentially dissociated hyperresponsivity. The amygdalae are nuclei located deep in the temporal lobe (continuous with basal ganglia; see Chapter 4) and have a major role in memory and emotions. The prefrontal cortex is the site of our center of inhibition, sometimes referred to as the "chief executive officer (CEO)" of the brain, and is responsible for cognitive analysis and abstract thought—it is the part of the brain that says "keep that thought to yourself" or "I probably shouldn't have sex with this person I don't know." Brain research suggests this area does not reach maturation until 25 years of age. The effective prefrontal cortex inhibits the amygdala as well, so that most of us do not overreact to every loud noise or punch someone just because they startle us. It is suggested that this ability to mute stimuli is diminished in brains with PTSD because of a compromised prefrontal cortex (Vasterling et al., 2009). The hippocampus is also affected. Rauch et al. (2000) noted a reduction in right hippocampus volume by 8% (MRI measurement) in Vietnam veterans with a diagnosis of PTSD. These investigators further noted that this reduction in hippocampal volume has been replicated four times in published literature with volume reductions reaching 26%. As student nurses know, the hippocampi are the primary neural structures responsible for memory and learning. Hippocampal function also includes *contextualization*—the ability to put an event in context (Vasterling et al., 2009). If one is more "on guard" because of diminished inhibition of the emotion center (i.e., the amygdalae) and has diminished ability to contextualize life occurrences ("this is a safe area," "this place is not safe"), a recipe for disaster lurks. Stated another way, impaired amygdala function opens the opportunity for overreaction, whereas impaired hippocampal function compounds that tendency with an inability to "read" the environment correctly.

Neurochemical Changes in Posttraumatic Stress Disorder

Two biochemical systems are affected by large doses of stress: the sympathetic nervous system (SNS) and the corticotropin-releasing hormone (CRH) system. These two systems work synergistically, with the SNS providing the body with the energy demanded by the stressor and the CRH system providing the body with the tools required to contain the stress reaction (Harvey et al., 2006). CRH neurons are predominantly located in the paraventricular nucleus of the hypothalamus. Tracts extend to the anterior pituitary gland, and when CRH is released there, it results in the liberation of adrenocorticotropic hormone (ACTH). On reaching the adrenal cortex, ACTH causes the discharge of the glucocorticoid cortisol into the systemic circulation. This stimulation by ACTH also activates the release of epinephrine and norepinephrine from the adrenal medulla. When abundant epinephrine and norepinephrine is released, as occurs during stress, this activates the SNS with subsequent stimulation of the adrenal medulla releasing even more norepinephrine and epinephrine.

Adaptive physiologic responses to stress include increases in glucose, heart rate, blood pressure, and respiratory rate (Selye, 1946). Elevated cortisol and norepinephrine and epinephrine increase alertness and vigilance and diminish interest in sex (Chrousos & Gold, 1992). Although all of these elevations are adaptive at times, prolonged elevations that can occur during combat may result in a system continually "turned on," morphing alertness into hyperalertness with insomnia and vigilance into hypervigilance. In one postmortem research study, researchers noted the activation of CRH neurons by measuring the amount of CRH–messenger RNA (mRNA). The results showed that patients with a diagnosis of Alzheimer's disease (n = 10) had higher than normal CRH-mRNA levels, and patients with a diagnosis of depression (n = 7) had even higher levels (Raadsheer et al., 1995). Finally, prolonged elevations of cortisol are associated with accelerated apoptosis (programmed cell death) of hippocampal neurons—the very structure needed for previously mentioned contextualization (Vaidya & Duman, 2001).

Treatment for Posttraumatic Stress Disorder

Treatment is frequently symptom specific and may include a short course of antipsychotics, antidepressants, antianxiety medications, or prazosin. Selective serotonin reuptake inhibitors (SSRIs) including sertraline and paroxetine are approved by the U.S. Food and Drug Administration for treatment of PTSD. Prazosin has been used typically for the treatment of hypertension; however, it works by blocking the brain's response to norepinephrine. This drug has not been approved by the FDA for treatment of PTSD and its use is considered off-label (Mayo Clinic Staff, 2011b). Psychotherapy is also used either in combination with drugs or alone. Different types of psychotherapy include cognitive therapy; behavioral therapy, specifically exposure therapy, and eye movement desensitization and reprocessing.

Posttraumatic Stress Disorder Resilience Factors

While countries will continue to find ways to send its young into harm's way, considerable work is being done to see what might be protective factors. Some of these include social support, coping self-efficacy ("belief that you can do it"), and hope, including optimism and expecting the positive (National Center for PTSD, 2010).

The U.S. Army has recognized the importance of trying to prepare soldiers for the atrocities they will see and has developed Resiliency Training, including institutional, operational, and family modules as well as military resilience trainer and facilitator modules. Although this training will not prove to be a magic bullet, it will insert one more tool into the toolkit of the warriors who are sent into harm's way. The Navy and Marine Corps version is called the Stress Resilience Training System, and the Air Force has Trauma and Resiliency Training Seminars.

DSM-5 DIFFERENTIAL DIAGNOSIS LIST

PTSD
Adjustment disorder
Acute stress disorder
Anxiety disorder
Obsessive-compulsive disorder
Major depressive disorder
Personality disorder
Dissociative disorder
Conversion disorder
Psychotic disorder
Traumatic brain injury
PTSD, Posttraumatic stress disorder.

From American Psychiatric Association (2013). *Diagnostic and statistical manual of mental disorders* (5th ed.). Arlington, Virginia: APA.

TRAUMATIC BRAIN INJURY

Between October 2001 and April 2014, more than 4400 American soldiers were killed fighting in Iraq (OIF), and more than 2300 died while serving in OEF (www.icausualities.org; accessed April 23, 2014). In contrast to previous wars, a predominance of deaths and injuries were directly linked to explosions, particularly blast injuries (Okie, 2006). Improvements in battle armor, emergency care on the battlefield, and better helmets have saved soldiers who would have most surely died in those previous conflicts; however, this improved protection has had an unforeseen consequence—a tremendous increase in the number of soldiers with TBI (Warden, 2006). TBI has been designated as the "signature wound or injury" of the most recent wars (Uomoto, 2012; Wallace, 2009). Although

an overall improvement in body protection has been achieved, the head is still vulnerable to explosive blasts of air. A soldier with TBI often has not been touched by anything other than the force of the blast. Because mild TBI often is not associated with an obvious wound or because the soldier may have other wounds that take priority (e.g., a hemorrhaging leg wound), TBI may be completely overlooked. Many of these soldiers have been sent back to the battlefield because no obvious injury was detectable. TBI has emerged as the most pressing emergency needs of OEF ad OIF veterans (Sammons & Batten, 2008). Box 36-1 outlines the characteristics of the "typical" victim of TBI (Hoge et al., 2008).

Defining Traumatic Brain Injury

When a soldier is said to have experienced a TBI, typically a mild TBI or concussion is meant. Mild TBI is defined as loss of consciousness for less than 30 minutes with posttraumatic amnesia lasting less than 24 hours. Moderate TBI is defined as a loss of consciousness more than 1 hour and posttraumatic amnesia lasting more than 24 hours (Martin et al., 2008). TBIs can be defined as head injuries caused by blunt trauma or acceleration/deceleration (blast) forces that manifest in one or more of the ways outlined in Box 36-2. As noted earlier in the chapter, the blasts that affect troops often come from IEDs. In such cases, a blast of air hits a person in a wave of pressure, and a lowering of the pressure occurs as the blast wave passes (Zeitzer & Brooks, 2008). Additionally, just as a tidal wave also rushes back to sea, a reversal of air pressure back toward the victim occurs. This increase, decrease, and then increase of pressure has an injurious impact on the brain and is directly

---

BOX 36-1 CHARACTERISTICS OF SOLDIERS WITH TRAUMATIC BRAIN INJURY

Engaged in high combat intensity
Injured by a blast
Experienced more than one explosion
Younger
Lower rank
Male

From Hoge, C.W., et al. (2008). Mild traumatic brain injury in U.S. soldiers returning from Iraq. *The New England Journal of Medicine, 358,* 453.

BOX 36-2 CRITERIA FOR MILD TRAUMATIC BRAIN INJURY

1. Any period of confusion, disorientation, or impaired consciousness
2. Any dysfunction of memory around the time of injury
3. Loss of consciousness, if any, lasts less than 30 minutes
4. Onset of observed neurologic or neuropsychological signs and symptoms

Adapted from U.S. Centers for Disease Control and Prevention (2003). Report to Congress on mild TBI after injury in the United States: steps to prevent a serious public health problem. Atlanta: CDC.

related to the force of the initial explosion. All of these pressures and intensities are magnified when soldiers are in vehicles or buildings in which the blast wave can "bounce" around. Nonetheless, most soldiers make a good recovery (Warden, 2006). Many soldiers with a mild TBI experience resolution of overt symptoms in days or, at most, weeks (Bigler, 2008). Symptoms subside within a year in 85% or more of affected soldiers (Zeitzer & Brooks, 2008). A small but significant number report lingering problems (Wood, 2004).

CASE STUDY: TRAUMATIC BRAIN INJURY

Joe Johnson is a 43-year-old African-American veteran who achieved the rank of E-6. He joined the Alabama National Guard as a young man to supplement his income. As a "weekend warrior," he was able to obtain a good civilian job. Because it was a civil service position, he enjoyed support for his part-time military career that some Guard members and reservists do not have.

Similar to many once-per-month soldiers, Mr. Johnson never really anticipated being activated and sent to war. Although it is made clear from day one that activation is a risk, many generations of these soldiers have never been seriously threatened by this life-changing order.

Mr. Johnson was activated and eventually sent to Iraq. In his 9 months there, his unit experienced more than 35 IED attacks. He escaped serious injury in all but one of these attacks, although fellow unit members were seriously wounded and killed. He recounts standing by helplessly as a young soldier from home bled to death because the medics were unable to stem hemorrhaging of blood. This and other traumatic stressors gave rise to PTSD. His final IED experience tossed his Humvee into the air, rendering him unconscious and amnesic for the event. He was discharged from the military with diagnoses of PTSD and TBI.

Mr. Johnson presents to the advanced practice registered nurse with the following complaints: memory loss, memory problems, irritability, cognitive difficulties (e.g., "I ain't as sharp as I used to be"), fatigue, anxiety, attention impairment, and deficient word finding. He also admits he would like to "rip off the head" of a man who he perceives is picking on him. When asked if he had worked with this person before activation, he responds, "Yeah, but we didn't have no problem then." When Mr. Johnson was asked if he had taken into account that he might have changed, too, he appeared dumbfounded by the consideration. In addition to these symptoms and concerns, Mr. Johnson admits to all of the classic PTSD symptoms: reexperiencing, avoidance, and hyperarousal.

Primary Symptoms of Traumatic Brain Injury

Many key symptoms have been associated with TBI. Cognitive problems include memory disturbances, decreased attention span, language problems, apathy, inability to "tune out" extraneous stimuli, and reduced efficiency of information processing. Physical problems such as headaches, dizziness, and blurred vision create added difficulties. Behavioral problems also affect the person and his family. For example, irritability, anxiety, depression, fatigue, and sleep difficulties are very prominent. Perhaps the most exasperating experience for

family and friends is the victim's inability to recognize these deficiencies in himself (Zeitzer & Brooks, 2008). Table 36-2 lists symptoms and syndromes associated with TBI. Table 36-3 lists prevalence and incidence rates for selected psychiatric disorders associated with more severe TBIs.

Neurologic Alterations Associated with Traumatic Brain Injury

As with PTSD, TBI is not just a psychological problem. Changes, although subtle at times and apparently not as long lasting, can be determined in brains with TBI as well. Following is a brief review of what is known or suspected about the neurologic consequences of exposure to explosions and other blunt trauma to the head.

Neuroanatomic Changes in Traumatic Brain Injury

Because TBI is thought to be less enduring than PTSD, it has also been thought that persistent pathology is less likely to occur. More recent evidence has shown this assumption to be erroneous. As more sophisticated technologies such as MRI and PET scans are used, long-term patterns of brain alterations have been noted. These changes tend to be subtle, requiring a different level of imaging than typically provided by CT and MRI. A technique called *diffusion tensor imaging* (DTI), a form of MRI, provides this level of visualization. DTI is able to produce neural tract images. Magnetoencephalography, a noninvasive functional imaging technique, measures brain waves to identify injured gray matter. This device has been used in conjunction with DTI, which measures damage in white matter, to determine potential TBI (Huang et al., 2009). In TBIs, the acceleration and deceleration forces cause a shearing of axons resulting in injury (Zeitzer & Brooks, 2008). These injuries can be so microscopic that only the most sophisticated imaging technologies can reveal and measure these pathologies. Symptomatic white matter changes can be noted on DTI in patients with mild TBI that are very similar to white matter abnormalities seen in patients with early Alzheimer's dementia (Fakhran et al., 2013). Axonal injuries include tearing of axons, disconnection of axons, microhemorrhages in frontal and temporal lobes, and hippocampal axonal and hemorrhagic damage (Vasterling et al., 2009).

Neurochemical Changes in Traumatic Brain Injury

Kokiko and Hamm (2007) described a biphasic model of neurochemical changes in TBI: an acute phase followed by a chronic phase. During the acute phase, the neural insult causes the activation of large amounts of glutamate. Glutamate, the most abundant excitatory neurotransmitter in the brain, increases neuron firing. This overfiring of neurons, known as *excitotoxicity*, causes the nonprogrammed death of neurons. Neuronal death enhances the axonal injury noted in the previous section. The hippocampus is particularly sensitive to these developments. The acute phase with its increased levels of excitatory transmitters and neuron destruction is followed by the chronic phase. In this phase, related to loss of neurons, catecholamine and acetylcholine synthesis declines. In keeping with current models of psychopathology, a decrease

TABLE 36-2	SYMPTOMS AND SYNDROMES ASSOCIATED WITH MILD TRAUMATIC BRAIN INJURY	
COGNITIVE	**PHYSICAL**	**EMOTIONAL AND BEHAVIORAL**
Attention problems	Appetite changes	Aggression
Executive dysfunction	Fatigue	Alcohol abuse
Planning	Headaches	Avolition
Abstract reasoning	Loss of urinary control	Attention-deficit/hyperactivity disorder
Problem solving	Pain	Decreased affective oscillation
Insight, judgment	Decreased libido	Disinhibition
Impaired judgment and decision making	Seizures	Irritability
Impaired self-awareness	Sensitivity to light	Major depression
Memory problems	Sleep disturbances	PTSD
Working memory problems	Weight changes	Psychosis
Word-finding difficulties	Vertigo	
	Visual impairment	

PTSD, Posttraumatic stress disorder.
Adapted from Jorge, R.E. (2005). Neuropsychiatric consequences of traumatic brain injury: a review of recent findings. *Current Opinion in Psychiatry, 18*, 289; Keltner, N.L., & Cooke, B.B. (2007). Traumatic brain injury: war related. *Perspectives in Psychiatric Care, 43*, 223; Kim, E., et al. (2007). Neuropsychiatric complications of traumatic brain injury: a critical review of the literature (a report of the ANPA Committee on research). *The Journal of Neuropsychiatry and Clinical Neurosciences, 19*, 106; Mathias, J.L., & Wheaton, P. (2006). Changes in attention and information-processing speed following severe traumatic brain injury (TBI). *Brain Injury, 20*, 569; Zeitzer, M.B., & Brooks, J.M. (2008). In the line of fire: traumatic brain injury among Iraq war veterans. *AAOHN Journal, 56*, 347.

TABLE 36-3	POSTTRAUMATIC BRAIN INJURY PSYCHIATRIC DISORDERS ASSOCIATED WITH BRAIN INJURY	
PSYCHIATRIC DISORDER	**INCIDENCE (%)**	**PREVALENCE (%)**
Post-TBI psychosis	20	Unknown
Post-TBI depression	15-33	18-61
Post-TBI mania	9	1-22
Post-TBI PTSD	13-27	3-59

Note: Kim and colleagues reviewed approximately 32 studies to support these findings.
PTSD, Posttraumatic stress disorder; *TBI*, traumatic brain injury.
Adapted from Keltner, N.L., & Cooke, B.B. (2007). Traumatic brain injury: war related. *Perspectives in Psychiatric Care, 43*, 223; Kim, E., et al. (2007). Neuropsychiatric complications of traumatic brain injury: a critical review of the literature (a report of the ANPA Committee on research). *The Journal of Neuropsychiatry and Clinical Neurosciences, 19*, 106.

in catecholamines would contribute to disturbances in affect, whereas a reduction in acetylcholine would foster cognitive deficits.

TREATING POSTTRAUMATIC STRESS DISORDER AND TRAUMATIC BRAIN INJURY

One question surrounding PTSD and TBI is whether a person can have both related to the same trauma. A major consideration for answering this question with a "no" is the fact that core symptoms for PTSD such as reexperiencing, thought intrusion, flashbacks, and avoidance all are based on "remembering" the trauma. A core symptom of TBI is amnesia for the event. Straightforward reasoning would

suggest that one cannot reexperience, flashback, and avoid something that one cannot remember. That logic aside, the consensus of opinion is that PTSD and TBI can and do coexist. Kim and colleagues (2007) found that 25% of veterans with TBI also met diagnostic criteria for PTSD. According to Warden (2006), soldiers who had been involved in a blast injury were more likely to experience TBI and PTSD. This combination diagnosis is now referred to as "postdeployment multisymptom disorder"(Uomoto, 2012). Anecdotal reports suggest an even higher comorbidity. This chapter addresses treatment considerations for both diagnoses.

Treating Posttraumatic Stress Disorder

The goals for treating PTSD include the following (Davidson, 2006; Dowben et al., 2007):

- Reducing primary symptoms (see Table 36-1)
- Improving functioning
- Strengthening resilience
- Relieving comorbid symptoms
- Preventing relapse

Antidepressants, particularly SSRIs, are very effective for treating the symptoms of PTSD. SSRIs not only have proven effectiveness for core symptoms but also are beneficial for comorbid expressions of depression and anxiety (Vieweg et al., 2006). Paroxetine and sertraline are often prescribed, but other SSRIs have proven effective as well (Friedman, 2006). Venlafaxine and mirtazapine are agents that can be used when SSRIs fail—with the added property of causing a reduced incidence of sexual side effects.

Antipsychotics and mood stabilizers are frequently prescribed. Antipsychotics can be used to supplement SSRIs (Davis et al., 2006) or for overt psychotic symptoms. Individuals with PTSD may present with both psychosis and subsyndromal symptoms. Because many of these individuals experience mood fluctuations and irritability, medications muting the intensity of these behaviors are important. Drugs such as divalproex and carbamazepine are prescribed in these situations.

Treating Traumatic Brain Injury

Individualized and integrative care is required to care for today's returning veterans (Batten & Pollack, 2008). Early and competent assessment at the time of injury is vital. In November 2006, the U.S. Defense and Veterans Brain Injury Center organized a panel that developed clinical practice guidelines for treatment of TBI. They developed guidelines for field evaluation and treatment including education, rest and release of duty requirements, and evacuation parameters (Wallace, 2009).

Pharmacotherapy of TBI presents another variable. The very nature of TBIs indicates an alteration in brain function. This pathology adds a dimension to drug response that may not occur in the general population. One soldier might respond in an expected manner, whereas another might respond in a very unique way. Patients with TBI, again related to the brain injury, can be overly sensitive to psychotropic medications (Tenuvuo, 2006). Because of variance in sensitivity, it is important to "start low and go slow" (Ashman et al., 2006). However, some patients do not respond to normal dosage, again presumably related to TBI. The conundrum of being on guard for hypersensitive patients while possibly treating a drug-resistant patient can make finding the right drug at the right dosage a long and tedious process for patient, clinician, and family members.

Typically, treatment is symptom-based: nonopioid (if at all possible) pain medication for headaches, antidepressants for depression, antipsychotics for psychosis, mood stabilizers for mood swings and irritability, cognitive enhancers for cognitive problems, and anxiolytics for anxiety.

As noted, cognitive symptoms are common disabilities associated with TBIs. Methylphenidate (dopamine reuptake inhibitor) is recommended for attention problems, decreased alertness, and slowed mental processing (Tenuvuo, 2006; Neurobehavioral Guidelines Working Group et al., 2006). Donepezil (cholinesterase inhibitor) is occasionally prescribed for attention deficits.

Depression is a common problem as well and is treated with sertraline and other SSRIs. A tricyclic antidepressant such as amitriptyline may be ordered for some patients. A guiding principle for pharmacotherapy is the minimization of anticholinergic and sedative effects (Cooke & Keltner, 2008). Anxiety may be even more common among these patients than depression. Most often, anxiety is treated with a short-term benzodiazepine such as lorazepam and with an SSRI. It is hoped that the patient will reach a point where the benzodiazepine can be eliminated from the regimen.

Manic symptoms are rare. If they do develop, traditional dosages of lithium or divalproex are recommended (Cooke & Keltner, 2008). Psychosis is also unlikely as a sequela of TBI. Should hallucinatory or delusional thinking develop, atypical antipsychotics are most likely to be prescribed. Finally, and perhaps most concerning, are the aggressive symptoms that are common in patients with TBI. Because aggressive behaviors increase safety risks and because these behaviors frighten

others, it is important for the patient, the family, and the nurse to deal with this symptom quickly. Pharmacotherapy includes beta blockers for potentially out-of-control behaviors. Methylphenidate has also proven to be an effective tool for agitation (Ashman et al., 2006; Neurobehavioral Guidelines Working Group et al., 2006). Other medications proven to be effective for aggression include divalproex and lithium (Cooke & Keltner, 2008). There are some questionable uses of neuroprotective treatment with neurotropic factors, antioxidants, and glutamate agonists, which may prevent axonal loss. There have been similar investigations in patients experiencing diffuse axonal injury (Inglese et al., 2005).

Family Considerations

Soldiers come from families and go back to families. As with most serious medical and psychiatric conditions, it is the family that is typically left standing. After the military command makes its visit and medals are pinned on soldiers, the family must pick up the pieces of a life changed by war. Because of the impact of the war on families and the impact of families on recovery, Box 36-3 has been carefully referenced for the best evidence-based approach for family education. A careful reading and rereading will be beneficial.

NORM'S NOTES

War is as old as mankind. I finished nursing school in the mid-1960s. Back in the day, it took about 6 weeks to learn if you had passed the state nursing examination. I found out in a matter of days. **Why?** The Army had my tests graded by hand and within a week of taking my state boards I had a license and a letter from the United States Army. I was to be a soldier. **Why?** Vietnam! Although I was never shot at, I took care of many soldiers whose lives would never be the same. War leaves lasting memories. Fast forward 40 years—Randy Moore served a tour in Iraq. He also has firsthand knowledge of the traumas of war. Men and women remained ravaged by war. Family emotions endure a crucible. This chapter closes the book and rightly so. Maybe it is the last thing you should think about as you finish the course. Men and women continue to die or are traumatized daily as they carry out their duty to protect and defend the United States. As a nation and as healthcare professionals, we must learn to do a better job of providing mental health care to these individuals. **Why?** If we learned anything from previous wars, it is this: Unless we learn to deal with these issues now, we will have to deal with them later.

? CRITICAL THINKING QUESTIONS

1. Many nurses in the United States are against the wars in Iraq and Afghanistan. Do you think they should voice their reservations to veterans with PTSD and TBI?
2. It was discussed that some people believe PTSD and TBIs are mutually exclusive phenomena. Can you make an argument to support this view?

BOX 36-3 FAMILY CAREGIVING AND TRAUMATIC BRAIN INJURY

CAREGIVER PROBLEMS AND NEEDS	POTENTIAL INTERVENTIONS OR STRATEGIES FOR CAREGIVER PROBLEMS
Cognitive and behavioral impairments of people with TBI (Anderson et al., 2009; Kreutzer et al., 2009b; Sander et al., 2009)	Encourage or develop programs to increase family and social support of caregivers or family members (Hanks et al., 2007; Kendall & Terry, 2009).
Judgment and safety-related concerns regarding travel and finances for people with TBI (Kreutzer et al., 2009a)	Offer problem-solving skill training programs for caregivers or family members (Rivera et al., 2007)
Need more information about physical, cognitive, medical, and behavioral status and prognosis of people with TBI (Smith & Smith, 2000)	Offer programs to improve coping skills of caregivers or family members (Knight et al., 1998)
Lack of information regarding how to access outpatient and community-based services (Turner et al., 2007) and how to navigate the health care system effectively to meet the needs of a loved one with TBI (Smith & Smith, 2000)	Provide information regarding physical, cognitive, medical, and behavioral status and prognosis of people with TBI (Kreutzer et al., 1994; Rodgers et al., 2007)
Lack of free time to meet caregivers' needs (Marsh et al., 1998a)	Develop programs that improve socialization of caregivers or family members (Rodgers et al., 2007)
Decreased initiative, emotional withdrawal, and fatigue in people with TBI (Koskinen, 1998)	Identify marital counseling sources (Tyerman & Booth, 2001)
Physical impairment and dependency in people with TBI (Marsh et al., 1998b)	Community-based programs conducted by interdisciplinary professionals to assist in setting shared goals and formulating priorities for rehabilitation (Smith et al., 2006)
Social isolation of people with TBI, leading to caregivers' isolation (Marsh et al., 1998b)	Develop web-based family treatment programs to enhance family problem solving and reduce behavioral and social problems of people with TBI (Wade et al., 2008)
Negative impact on caregivers' physical health (Marsh et al., 1998b)	Assist with physical, emotional, financial, domestic, transportation, and respite support networks (Turner et al., 2007)
Marital discord (Tyerman & Booth, 2001)	Telephone interventions to offer psychosocial support (Brown et al., 1999)
	Encourage caregivers to allocate time for themselves (e.g., shopping, exercise)
	Develop materials for caregivers regarding how to access outpatient and community-based services

TBI, Traumatic brain injury.

▮ STUDY NOTES

1. American soldiers are exposed to great carnage, and that exposure cannot help but leave a lasting impression.
2. Two major disabilities associated with the wars in Iraq and Afghanistan are PTSD and TBI.
3. The primary symptoms of PTSD are reexperiencing, avoidance, and hyperarousal.
4. Many soldiers with PTSD also have a comorbid disorder. Substance abuse, anxiety, and depression are common comorbidities.
5. Significant neurochemical changes (e.g., chronic overactivity of the sympathetic nervous system and the corticotropin-releasing system) are a direct result of the traumatic stress soldiers experience in war.
6. TBIs are called the signature wounds of recent wars and are directly linked to exposure to explosions.
7. Often, a soldier with TBI was "only hit" by a blast of air.
8. The diagnosis of TBI typically refers to what has historically been identified as a mild concussion.
9. The overarching categories of TBI symptoms are cognitive, physical, and emotional/behavioral. Amnesia is a key symptom.
10. Neurochemically, TBI causes elevations of glutamate, resulting in overfiring of neurons.
11. Both PTSD and TBI are treated with psychotropic medications based on symptoms (e.g., antidepressants for symptoms of depression).
12. "After the military command makes its visit and medals are pinned on soldiers, it is the family that will pick up the pieces of a life changed by war."

REFERENCES

American Deaths through History. (n.d.). From the War of Independence to Operation Enduring Freedom—blood spilled from sea to shining sea. *Military Factory.* http://www. militaryfactory.com/american_war_deaths.asp, Accessed 07.06.13.

American Psychiatric Association. (2013). *Diagnostic and statistical manual of mental disorders* (5th ed.). Arlington, Virginia: APA.

Anderson, M. I., et al. (2009). Differential pathways of psychological distress in spouses vs. parents of people with severe traumatic brain injury (TBI): Multi-group analysis. *Brain Injury, 23,* 931.

Ashman, T., et al. (2006). Neurobehavioral consequences of traumatic brain injury. *The Mount Sinai Journal of Medicine, New York, 73,* 999.

Batten, S. V., & Pollack, S. J. (2008). Integrative outpatient treatment for returning service members. *Journal of Clinical Psychology, 64,* 928.

Bigler, E. D. (2008). Neuropsychology and clinical neuroscience of persistent post-concussive syndrome. *Journal of the International Neuropsychological Society, 14,* 1.

Bremner, J. D., et al. (1999). Neural correlates of memories of childhood sexual abuse in women with and without posttraumatic stress disorder. *The American Journal of Psychiatry, 156,* 1787.

Brown, R., et al. (1999). Distance education and caregiver support groups: Comparison of traditional and telephone groups. *The Journal of Head Trauma Rehabilitation, 14,* 257.

Chrousos, G. P., & Gold, P. W. (1992). The concepts of stress and stress system disorders: Overview of physical and behavioral homeostasis. *JAMA, 4,* 1244.

Cooke, B. B., & Keltner, N. L. (2008). Traumatic brain injury: War related: Part II. *Perspectives in Psychiatric Care, 44,* 54.

Crawford, N. C. (2013, March 20). The Iraq war: Ten years in ten numbers. *Foreign Policy: The Middle East Channel.* http:// mideast.foreignpolicy.com/posts/2013/03/20/the_iraq_war_ ten_years_in_ten_numbers, Accessed 07.06.13.

Davidson, J. R. (2006). Pharmacologic treatment of acute and chronic stress following trauma: 2006. *The Journal of Clinical Psychiatry, 67*(Suppl. 2), 34.

Davis, L. L., et al. (2006). Long-term pharmacotherapy for post-traumatic stress disorder. *CNS Drugs, 20,* 465.

Dowben, J. S., Grant, J. S., & Keltner, N. L. (2007). Psychobiological substrates of posttraumatic stress disorder: Part II. *Perspectives in Psychiatric Care, 43,* 146.

Driessen, M., et al. (2004). Posttraumatic stress disorder and fMRI activation patterns of traumatic memory in patients with borderline personality disorder. *Biological Psychiatry, 55,* 603.

Fakhran, S., Yaeger, K., & Alhilali, L. (2013). Symptomatic white matter changes in mild traumatic brain injury resemble pathologic feature of early Alzheimer dementia. *Radiology, 269,* 249.

Friedman, M. (2006). *Post traumatic and acute stress disorder.* Kansas City, MO: Compact Clinicals.

Galovski, T., & Lyons, J. (2004). Psychological sequelae of combat violence: A review of the impact of PTSD on the veteran's family and possible interventions. *Aggression and Violent Behavior, 9,* 447.

Hanks, R. A., Rapport, L. J., & Vangel, S. (2007). Caregiving appraisal after traumatic brain injury: The effects of functional status, coping style, social support and family functioning. *NeuroRehabilitation, 22,* 43.

Harvey, B. H., et al. (2006). Cortical/hippocampal monoamines, HPA-axis changes and aversive behavior following stress and restress in an animal model of post-traumatic stress disorder. *Physiology & Behavior, 87,* 881.

Hoge, C. W., et al. (2004). Combat duty in Iraq and Afghanistan, mental health problems, and barriers to care. *The New England Journal of Medicine, 351,* 13.

Hoge, C. W., et al. (2008). Mild traumatic brain injury in U.S. soldiers returning from Iraq. *The New England Journal of Medicine, 358,* 453.

Horowitz, M. J., et al. (1980). Signs and symptoms of posttraumatic stress disorder. *Archives of General Psychiatry, 37,* 85.

Huang, M. X., et al. (2009). Integrated imaging approach with MEG and DTI to detect mild traumatic brain injury in military and civilian patients. *Journal of Neurotrauma, 26,* 1213.

Inglese, M., et al. (2005). Diffuse axonal injury in mild traumatic brain injury: A diffusion tensor imaging study. *Journal of Neurosurgery, 103,* 298.

Institute of Medicine. (2013). *Returning home from Iraq and Afghanistan: Assessment of readjustment needs of veterans, service members, and their families.* http://www.iom.edu/Reports/2013/ Returning-Home-from-Iraq-and-Afghanistan.aspx.

Jorge, R. E. (2005). Neuropsychiatric consequences of traumatic brain injury: A review of recent findings. *Current Opinion in Psychiatry, 18,* 289.

Keltner, N. L., & Cooke, B. B. (2007). Traumatic brain injury: War related. *Perspectives in Psychiatric Care, 43,* 223.

Keltner, N. L., Doggett, R., & Johnson, R. (1983). For the Viet Nam veteran the war goes on. *Perspectives in Psychiatric Care, 21,* 108.

Keltner, N. L., & Dowben, J. S. (2007). Psychobiological substrates of posttraumatic stress disorder: Part I. *Perspectives in Psychiatric Care, 43,* 97.

Kendall, E., & Terry, D. (2009). Predicting emotional well-being following traumatic brain injury: A test of mediated and moderated models. *Social Science & Medicine, 69,* 947.

Kim, E., et al. (2007). Neuropsychiatric complications of traumatic brain injury: A critical review of the literature (a report of the ANPA Committee on research). *The Journal of Neuropsychiatry and Clinical Neurosciences, 19,* 106.

Knight, R. G., Devereux, R., & Godfrey, H. P. (1998). Caring for a family member with a traumatic brain injury. *Brain Injury, 12,* 467.

Kokiko, O. N., & Hamm, R. J. (2007). A review of pharmacological treatments used in experimental models of traumatic brain injury. *Brain Injury, 21,* 269.

Koskinen, S. (1998). Quality of life 10 years after a very severe traumatic brain injury (TBI): The perspective of the injured and the closest relative. *Brain Injury, 12,* 631.

Kreutzer, J. S., Serio, C. D., & Bergquist, S. (1994). Family needs after brain injury: A quantitative analysis. *The Journal of Head Trauma Rehabilitation, 9,* 104.

Kreutzer, J. S., et al. 2009a. Caregivers' concerns about judgment and safety of patients with brain injury: A preliminary investigation. *PM & R, 1,* 723.

Kreutzer, J. S., et al. 2009b. Caregivers' wellbeing after traumatic brain injury: A multicenter prospective investigation. *Archives of Physical Medicine and Rehabilitation, 90,* 939.

Lew, H. L., et al. (2008). Overlap of mild TBI and mental health conditions in returning OIF/OEF service members and veterans. *Journal of Rehabilitation Research and Development, 45,* xi.

Marsh, N. V., et al. 1998a. Caregiver burden at 1 year following severe traumatic brain injury. *Brain Injury, 12,* 1045.

Marsh, N. V., et al. 1998b. Caregiver burden at 6 months following severe traumatic brain injury. *Brain Injury, 12,* 225.

Martin, E. M., et al. (2008). Traumatic brain injuries sustained in Afghanistan and Iraqi wars. *The American Journal of Nursing, 108,* 40.

Mathias, J. L., & Wheaton, P. (2006). Changes in attention and information-processing speed following severe traumatic brain injury (TBI). *Brain Injury, 20,* 569.

Mayo Clinic Staff. (2011, April 8a.). *Post-traumatic stress disorder (PTSD).* http://www.mayoclinic.com/health/post-traumatic-stress disorder/DS00246/DSECTION=risk-factors.

Mayo Clinic Staff. (2011, April 8b.). *Post-traumatic stress disorder (PTSD): Treatments and drugs.* http://www.mayoclinic.com/health/post-traumatic-stress%20disorder/DS00246/DSECTION=treatments-and-drugs, Accessed 07.06.13.

National Center for PTSD. (2010, June 28). *Effects of disasters: Risk and resilience factors.* http://www.ptsd.va.gov/public/pages/effects_of_disasters_risk_and_resilience:factors.asp, Accessed 07.06.13, http://www.ptsd.va.gov/public/types/disasters/effects_of_disasters_risk_and_resilience:factors.asp, Accessed 21.03.14.

National Institute of Mental Health. (n.d.). *Post-traumatic stress disorder.* http://www.nimh.nih.gov/health/topics/post-traumatic-stress-disorder-ptsd/index.shtml, Accessed 10.06.13.

Neurobehavioral Guidelines Working Group, et al. (2006). Guidelines for the pharmacologic treatment of neurobehavioral sequelae of traumatic brain injury. *Journal of Neurotrauma, 23,* 1468.

Okie, S. (2006). Reconstructing lives—A tale of two soldiers. *The New England Journal of Medicine, 355,* 2609.

Raadsheer, F. C., et al. (1995). Corticotropin-releasing hormone mRNA levels in the paraventricular nucleus of patients with Alzheimer's disease and depression. *The American Journal of Psychiatry, 152,* 1372.

Rand Corporation. (2008). *Invisible wounds of war: Psychological and cognitive injuries, their consequences, and services to assist recovery* (T. Tanielian & L. H. Jaycox, Eds.). Santa Monica, CA: The Center for Military Health Policy Research and the Rand Corporation, http://www.rand.org/content/dam/rand/pubs/monographs/2008/RAND_MG720.pdf (accessed 23.04.14).

Rauch, S., et al. (2000). Exaggerated amygdala response to masked facial stimuli in posttraumatic stress disorder: A functional MRI study. *Biological Psychiatry, 47,* 769.

Rivera, P., et al. (2007). Predictors of caregiver depression among community-residing families living with traumatic brain injury. *NeuroRehabilitation, 22,* 3.

Rodgers, M. L., et al. (2007). Adapting multiple-family group treatment for brain and spinal cord injury intervention development and preliminary outcomes. *American Journal of Physical Medicine & Rehabilitation, 86,* 482.

Sammons, M. T., & Batten, S. V. (2008). Psychological services for returning veterans and their families: Evolving conceptualizations of the sequelae of war-zone experiences. *Journal of Clinical Psychology, 64,* 921.

Sander, A. M., et al. (2009). A web-based videoconferencing approach to training caregivers in rural areas to compensate for problems related to traumatic brain injury. *The Journal of Head Trauma Rehabilitation, 24,* 248.

Seal, K. H., et al. (2009). Trends and risk factors for mental health diagnoses among Iraq and Afghanistan veterans using Department of Veterans Affairs health care, 2002–2008. *American Journal of Public Health, 99,* 1651.

Selye, H. (1946). The general adaptation syndrome and the diseases of adaptation. *Journal of Clinical Endocrinology, 6,* 117.

Smith, J. E., & Smith, D. L. (2000). No map, no guide. Family caregivers' perspectives on their journeys through the system. *Care Management Journals, 2,* 27.

Smith, M. J., et al. (2006). The impact of community rehabilitation for acquired brain injury on carer burden: An exploratory study. *The Journal of Head Trauma Rehabilitation, 21,* 76.

Solomon, Z., & Mikulincer, M. (2006). Trajectories of PTSD: A 20-year longitudinal study. *The American Journal of Psychiatry, 163,* 659.

Stiglitz, J. E., & Bilmes, L. J. (2008). *The three trillion dollar war: The true cost of the Iraq Conflict.* New York: WW Norton & Company.

Tanielian, T., & Jaycox, L. H. (2008). *Invisible wounds of war: Psychological and cognitive injuries, their consequences, and services to assist recovery.* Santa Monica, CA: RAND.

Tenuvuo, O. (2006). Pharmacological enhancement of cognitive and behavioral deficits after traumatic brain injury. *Current Opinion in Neurology, 19,* 528.

Turner, B., et al. (2007). A qualitative study of the transition from hospital to home for individuals with acquired brain injury and their family caregivers. *Brain Injury, 21,* 1119.

Tyerman, A., & Booth, J. (2001). Family interventions after traumatic brain injury: A service example. *NeuroRehabilitation, 16,* 59.

U.S. Centers for Disease Control and Prevention. (2003). *Report to Congress on mild TBI after injury in the United States: Steps to prevent a serious public health problem.* Atlanta: CDC.

Uomoto, J. M. (2012). Best practices in veteran traumatic brain injury care. *The Journal of Head Trauma Rehabilitation, 27,* 241.

Vaidya, V. A., & Duman, R. S. (2001). Depression-emerging insights from neurobiology. *British Medical Bulletin, 57,* 61.

Vasterling, J. J., Verfaellie, M., & Sullivan, K. D. (2009). Mild traumatic brain injury and posttraumatic stress disorder in returning veterans: Perspectives from cognitive neuroscience. *Clinical Psychology Review, 29,* 674.

Vieweg, W. V., et al. (2006). Posttraumatic stress disorder: Clinical features, pathophysiology, and treatment. *The American Journal of Medicine, 119,* 383.

Wade, S. L., et al. (2008). Preliminary efficacy of a Web-based family problem-solving treatment program for adolescents with traumatic brain injury. *The Journal of Head Trauma Rehabilitation, 23,* 369.

Wallace, D. (2009). Improvised explosive devices and traumatic brain injury: The military experience in Iraq and Afghanistan. *Australasian Psychiatry, 17,* 218.

Warden, D. (2006). Military TBI during the Iraq and Afghanistan wars. *The Journal of Head Trauma Rehabilitation, 21,* 398.

Weinberger, D. R. (1987). Implications of normal brain development for the pathogenesis of schizophrenia. *Archives of General Psychiatry, 44,* 660.

Wood, R. L. (2004). Understanding the "miserable minority": A diathesis-stress paradigm for post-concussional syndrome. *Brain Injury, 18,* 1135.

Zeitzer, M. B., & Brooks, J. M. (2008). In the line of fire: Traumatic brain injury among Iraq war veterans. *AAOHN Journal, 56,* 347.

DSM-5 Classification*

Before each disorder name, ICD-9-CM codes are provided, followed by ICD-10-CM codes in parentheses. Blank lines indicate that either the ICD-9-CM or the ICD-10-CM code is not applicable. For some disorders, the code can be indicated only according to the subtype or specifier.

ICD-9-CM codes are to be used for coding purposes in the United States through September 30, 2014. ICD-10-CM codes are to be used starting October 1, 2014.

Following chapter titles and disorder names, page numbers for the corresponding text or criteria are included in parentheses.

Note for all mental disorders due to another medical condition: Indicate the name of the other medical condition in the name of the mental disorder due to [the medical condition]. The code and name for the other medical condition should be listed first immediately before the mental disorder due to the medical condition.

NEURODEVELOPMENTAL DISORDERS (31)

Intellectual Disabilities (33)

319	(——.——)	Intellectual Disability (Intellectual Developmental Disorder) (33)
		Specify current severity:
	(F70)	Mild
	(F71)	Moderate
	(F72)	Severe
	(F73)	Profound
315.8	(F88)	Global Developmental Delay (41)
319	(F79)	Unspecified Intellectual Disability (Intellectual Developmental Disorder) (41)

Communication Disorders (41)

315.39	(F80.9)	Language Disorder (42)
315.39	(F80.0)	Speech Sound Disorder (44)
315.35	(F80.81)	Childhood-Onset Fluency Disorder (Stuttering) (45)
		Note: Later-onset cases are diagnosed as 307.0 (F98.5) adult-onset fluency disorder.
315.39	(F80.98)	Social (Pragmatic) Communication Disorder (47)
307.9	(F80.9)	Unspecified Communication Disorder (49)

Autism Spectrum Disorder (50)

299.00	(F84.0)	Autism Spectrum Disorder (50)
		Specify if: Associated with a known medical or genetic condition or environmental factor; Associated with another neurodevelopmental, mental or behavioral disorder
		Specify current severity for Criterion A and Criterion B: Requiring very substantial support, Requiring substantial support, Requiring support
		Specify if: With or without accompanying intellectual impairment, With or without accompanying language impairment, With catatonia (use additional code 293.89 [F06.1])

Attention-Deficit/Hyperactivity Disorder (59)

——.——	——.——	Attention-Deficit/Hyperactivity Disorder (59)
		Specify whether:
314.01	(F90.2)	Combined presentation
314.00	(F90.0)	Predominantly inattentive presentation
314.01	(F90.1)	Predominantly hyperactive/impulsive presentation
		Specify if: In partial remission
		Specify current severity: Mild, Moderate, Severe
314.01	(F90.8)	Other Specified Attention-Deficit/Hyperactivity Disorder (65)
314.01	(F90.9)	Unspecified Attention-Deficit/Hyperactivity Disorder (66)

Specific Learning Disorder (66)

——.——	——.——	Specific Learning Disorder (66)
		Specify if:
315.00	(F81.0)	With impairment in reading (*specify* if with word reading accuracy, reading rate or fluency, reading comprehension)
315.2	(F81.81)	With impairment in written expression (*specify* if with spelling accuracy, grammar and punctuation accuracy, clarity or organization of written expression)

*From American Psychiatric Association. (2013). *Diagnostic and statistical manual of mental disorders* (5th ed.). Arlington, VA: APA.

315.1	**(F81.2)**	With impairment in mathematics (*specify* if with number sense, memorization or arithmetic facts, accurate or fluent calculation, accurate math reasoning)

Specify current severity: Mild, Moderate, Severe

Motor Disorders (74)

315.4	**(F82)**	Developmental Coordination Disorder (74)
307.3	**(F98.4)**	Stereotypic Movement Disorder (77)

Specify if: With self-injurious behavior, Without self-injurious behavior

Specify if: Associated with a known medical or genetic condition, neurodevelopmental disorder, or environmental factor

Specify current severity: Mild, Moderate, Severe

Tic Disorders

307.23	**(F95.2)**	Tourette's Disorder (81)
307.22	**(F95.1)**	Persistent (Chronic) Motor or Vocal Tic Disorder (81)

Specify if: With motor tics only, With vocal tics only

307.21	**(F95.0)**	Provisional Tic Disorder (81)
307.20	**(F95.8)**	Other Specified Tic Disorder (85)
307.20	**(F95.9)**	Unspecified Tic Disorder (85)

Other Neurodevelopmental Disorders (86)

315.8	**(F88)**	Other Specified Neurodevelopmental Disorder (86)
315.9	**(F89)**	Unspecified Neurodevelopmental Disorder (86)

SCHIZOPHRENIA SPECTRUM AND OTHER PSYCHOTIC DISORDERS (87)

The following specifiers apply to Schizophrenia Spectrum and Other Psychotic Disorders where indicated:

[a]*Specify* if: The following course specifiers are only to be used after a 1-year duration of the disorder: First episode, currently in acute episode; First episode, currently in partial remission; First episode, currently in full remission; Multiple episodes, currently in acute episode; Multiple episodes, currently in partial remission; Multiple episodes, currently in full remission; Continuous; Unspecified

[b]*Specify* if: With catatonia (use additional code 293.89 [F06.1])
[c]*Specify* current severity of delusions, hallucinations, disorganized speech, abnormal psychomotor behavior, negative symptoms, impaired cognition, depression, and mania symptoms

301.22	**(F21)**	Schizotypal (Personality) Disorder (90)
297.1	**(F22)**	Delusional Disorder[a,c] (90)

Specify whether: Erotomanic type, Grandiose type, Jealous type, Persecutory type, Somatic type, Mixed type, Unspecified type

Specify if: With bizarre content

298.8	**(F23)**	Brief Psychotic Disorder[b,c] (94)

Specify if: With marked stressor(s), Without marked stressor(s), With postpartum onset

295.40	**(F20.81)**	Schizophreniform Disorder[b,c] (96)

Specify if: With good prognostic features, Without good prognostic features

295.90	**(F20.9)**	Schizophrenia[a,b,c] (99)
—.—	(—.—)	Schizoaffective Disorder[a,b,c] (105)

Specify whether:

295.70	**(F25.0)**	Bipolar type
295.70	**(F25.1)**	Depressive type
—.—	(—.—)	Substance/Medication-Induced Psychotic Disorder[c] (110)

Note: See the criteria set and corresponding recording procedures for substance-specific codes and ICD-9-CM and ICD-10-CM coding.

Specify if: With onset during intoxication, With onset during withdrawal

—.—	(—.—)	Psychotic Disorder Due to Another Medical Condition[c] (115)

Specify whether:

293.81	**(F06.2)**	With delusions
293.82	**(F06.0)**	With hallucinations
293.89	**(F06.1)**	Catatonia Associated With Another Mental Disorder (Catatonia Specifier) (119)
293.89	**(F06.1)**	Catatonic Disorder Due to Another Medical Condition (120)
293.89	**(F06.1)**	Unspecified Catatonia (121)

Note: Code first 781.99 (R29.818) other symptoms involving nervous and musculoskeletal systems.

298.8	**(F28)**	Other Specified Schizophrenia Spectrum and Other Psychotic Disorder (122)
298.9	**(F29)**	Unspecified Schizophrenia Spectrum and Other Psychotic Disorder (122)

BIPOLAR AND RELATED DISORDERS (123)

The following specifiers apply to Bipolar and Related Disorders where indicated:

[a]*Specify*: With anxious distress (*specify* current severity: mild, moderate, moderate-severe, severe); With mixed features; With rapid cycling; With melancholic features; With atypical features; With mood-congruent psychotic features; With mood-incongruent psychotic features; With catatonia (use additional code 293.89 [F06.1]); With peripartum onset; With seasonal pattern

—.—	(—.—)	Bipolar I Disorder[a] (123)
—.—	(—.—)	Current or most recent episode manic

296.41	**(F31.11)**	Mild
296.42	**(F31.12)**	Moderate
296.43	**(F31.13)**	Severe
296.44	**(F31.2)**	With psychotic features
296.45	**(F31.73)**	In partial remission
296.46	**(F31.74)**	In full remission
296.40	**(F31.9)**	Unspecified
296.40	**(F31.0)**	Current or most recent episode hypomanic
296.45	**(F31.73)**	In partial remission
296.46	**(F31.74)**	In full remission
296.40	**(F31.9)**	Unspecified
—.—	(—.—)	Current or most recent episode depressed
296.51	**(F31.31)**	Mild
296.52	**(F31.32)**	Moderate
296.53	**(F31.4)**	Severe
296.54	**(F31.5)**	With psychotic features
296.55	**(F31.75)**	In partial remission
296.56	**(F31.76)**	In full remission
296.50	**(F31.9)**	Unspecified
296.7	**(F31.9)**	Current or most recent episode unspecified
296.89	**(F31.81)**	Bipolar II Disorder[a] (132)

Specify current or most recent episode: Hypomanic, Depressed

Specify course if full criteria for a mood episode are not currently met: In partial remission, In full remission

Specify severity if full criteria for a mood episode are not currently met: Mild, Moderate, Severe

301.13	**(F34.0)**	Cyclothymic Disorder (139)

Specify if: With anxious distress

—.—	(—.—)	Substance/Medication-Induced Bipolar and Related Disorder (142)

Note: See the criteria set and corresponding recording procedures for substance-specific coded and ICD-9-CM and ICD-10-CM coding.

Specify if: With onset during intoxication, With onset during withdrawal

293.83	(—.—)	Bipolar and Related Disorder Due to Another Medical Condition (145)

Specify if:

	(F06.33)	With manic features
	(F06.33)	With manic- or hypomanic-like episode
	(F06.33)	With mixed features
296.89	**(F31.89)**	Other specified Bipolar and Related Disorder (148)
296.80	**(F31.9)**	Unspecified Bipolar and Related Disorder (149)

DEPRESSIVE DISORDERS (155)

The following specifiers apply to Depressive Disorders where indicated:

[a]*Specify*: With anxious distress (*specify* current severity: mild, moderate, moderate-severe, severe); With mixed features; With melancholic features; With atypical features; With mood-congruent psychotic features; With mood-incongruent psychotic features; With catatonia

(use additional code 293.89 [F06.1]); With peripartum onset; With seasonal pattern

296.99	**(F34.8)**	Disruptive Mood Dysregulation Disorder (156)
—.—	(—.—)	Major Depressive Disorder[a] (160)
—.—	(—.—)	Single episode
296.21	**(F32.0)**	Mild
296.22	**(F32.1)**	Moderate
296.23	**(F32.2)**	Severe
296.24	**(F32.3)**	With psychotic features
296.25	**(F32.4)**	In partial remission
296.26	**(F32.5)**	In full remission
296.20	**(F32.9)**	Unspecified
—.—	(—.—)	Recurrent episode
296.31	**(F33.0)**	Mild
296.32	**(F33.1)**	Moderate
296.33	**(F33.2)**	Severe
296.34	**(F33.3)**	With psychotic features
296.35	**(F33.41)**	In partial remission
296.36	**(F33.42)**	In full remission
296.30	**(F33.9)**	Unspecified
300.4	**(F34.1)**	Persistent Depressive Disorder (Dysthymia)[a] (168)

Specify if: In partial remission, In full remission

Specify if: Early onset, Late onset

Specify if: With pure dysthymic syndrome; With persistent major depressive episode; With intermittent major depressive episodes, with current episode; With intermittent major depressive episodes, without current episode

Specify current severity: Mild, Moderate, Severe

625.4	**(N94.3)**	Premenstrual Dysphoric Disorder (171)
—.—	(—.—)	Substance/Medication-Induced Depressive Disorder (175)

Note: See the criteria set and corresponding recording procedures for substance-specific codes and ICD-9-CM and ICD-10-CM coding.

Specify if: With onset during intoxication, With onset during withdrawal

293.83	(—.—)	Depressive Disorder Due to Another Medical Condition (180)

Specify if:

	(F06.31)	With depressive features
	(F06.32)	With major depressive-like episode
	(F06.34)	With mixed features
311	**(F32.8)**	Other Specified Depressive Disorder (183)
311	**(F32.9)**	Unspecified Depressive Disorder (184)

ANXIETY DISORDERS (189)

309.21	**(F93.0)**	Separation Anxiety Disorder (190)
312.23	**(F94.0)**	Selective Mutism (195)
300.29	(—.—)	Specific Phobia (197)
		Specify if:
	(F40.218)	Animal

(F40.228)		Natural environmental
(——.——)		Blood-injection-injury
(F40.230)		Fear of blood
(F40.231)		Fear of injections and transfusions
(F40.232)		Fear of other medical care
(F40.233)		Fear of injury
(F40.248)		Situational
(F40.298)		Other
300.23	**(F40.10)**	Social Anxiety Disorder (Social Phobia) (202)

Specify if: Performance only

300.01	**(F41.0)**	Panic Disorder (208)
——.——	**(——.——)**	Panic Attack Specifier (214)
300.22	**(F40.00)**	Agoraphobia (217)
300.02	**(F41.1)**	Generalized Anxiety Disorder (222)
——.——	**(——.——)**	Substance/Medication-Induced Anxiety Disorder (226)

Note: See the criteria set and corresponding recording procedures for substance-specific codes and ICD-9-CM and ICD-10-CM coding.

Specify if: With onset during intoxication, With onset during withdrawal, With onset after medication use

293.84	**(F06.4)**	Anxiety Disorder Due to Another Medical Condition (230)
300.09	**(F41.8)**	Other Specified Anxiety Disorder (233)
300.00	**(F41.9)**	Unspecified Anxiety Disorder (233)

OBSESSIVE-COMPULSIVE AND RELATED DISORDERS (235)

The following specifiers apply to Obsessive-Compulsive and Related Disorders where indicated:

ªSpecify if: With good or fair insight, With poor insight, With absent insight/delusional beliefs

300.3	**(F42)**	Obsessive-Compulsive Disorderª (237)

Specify if: Tic-related

300.7	**(F45.22)**	Body Dysmorphic Disorderª (242)

Specify if: With muscle dysmorphia

300.3	**(F42)**	Hoarding Disorderª (247)

Specify if: With excessive acquisition

312.39	**(F63.2)**	Trichotillomania (Hair-Pulling Disorder) (251)
698.4	**(L98.1)**	Excoriation (Skin-Picking) Disorder (254)
——.——	**(——.——)**	Substance/Medication-Induced Obsessive-Compulsive and Related Disorder (257)

Note: See the criteria set and corresponding recording procedures for substance-specific codes and ICD-9-CM and ICD-10-CM coding.

Specify if: With onset during intoxication, With onset during withdrawal, With onset after medication use

294.8	**(F06.8)**	Obsessive-Compulsive and Related Disorder Due to Another Medical Condition (260)

Specify if: With obsessive-compulsive disorder-like symptoms, With appearance preoccupations, With hoarding symptoms, With hair-pulling symptoms, With skin-picking symptoms

300.3	**(F42)**	Other Specified Obsessive-Compulsive and Related Disorder (263)
300.3	**(F42)**	Unspecified Obsessive-Compulsive and Related Disorder (264)

TRAUMA- AND STRESSOR-RELATED DISORDERS (265)

313.89	**(F94.1)**	Reactive Attachment Disorder (265)

Specify if: Persistent
Specify current severity: Severe

313.89	**(F94.2)**	Disinhibited Social Engagement Disorder (268)

Specify if: Persistent
Specify current severity: Severe

309.81	**(F43.10)**	Posttraumatic Stress Disorder (includes Posttraumatic Stress Disorder for Children 6 Years and Younger) (271)

Specify whether: With dissociative symptoms
Specify if: With delayed expression

308.3	**(F43.0)**	Acute Stress Disorder (280)
——.——	**(——.——)**	Adjustment Disorder (286)

Specify whether:

309.0	**(F43.21)**	With depressed mood
309.24	**(F43.22)**	With anxiety
309.28	**(F43.23)**	With mixed anxiety and depressed mood
309.3	**(F43.24)**	With disturbance of conduct
309.4	**(F43.25)**	With mixed disturbance of emotions and conduct
309.9	**(F43.20)**	Unspecified
309.89	**(F43.8)**	Other Specified Trauma- and Stressor-Related Disorder (289)
309.9	**(F43.9)**	Unspecified Trauma- and Stressor-Related Disorder (290)

DISSOCIATIVE DISORDERS (291)

300.14	**(F44.81)**	Dissociative Identity Disorder (292)
300.12	**(F44.0)**	Dissociative Amnesia (298)

Specify if:

300.13	**(F44.1)**	With dissociative fugue
300.6	**(F48.1)**	Depersonalization/Derealization Disorder (302)
300.15	**(F44.89)**	Other Specified Dissociative Disorder (306)
300.15	**(F44.9)**	Unspecified Dissociative Disorder (307)

SOMATIC SYMPTOM AND RELATED DISORDERS (309)

300.82	**(F45.1)**	Somatic Symptom Disorder (311)
		Specify if: With predominant pain
		Specify if: Persistent
		Specify current severity: Mild, Moderate, Severe
300.7	**(F45.21)**	Illness Anxiety Disorder (315)
		Specify whether: Care seeking type, Care avoidant type
300.11	**(——.——)**	Conversion Disorder (Functional Neurological Symptom Disorder) (318)
		Specify symptom type:
	(F44.4)	With weakness or paralysis
	(F44.4)	With abnormal movement
	(F44.4)	With swallowing symptoms
	(F44.4)	With speech symptom
	(F44.5)	With attacks or seizures
	(F44.6)	With anesthesia or sensory loss
	(F44.6)	With special sensory symptom
	(F44.7)	With mixed symptoms
		Specify if: Acute episode, Persistent
		Specify if: With psychological stressor (specify stressor), Without psychological stressor
316	**(F54)**	Psychological Factors Affecting Other Medical Conditions (322)
		Specify current severity: Mild, Moderate, Severe, Extreme
300.19	**(F68.10)**	Factitious Disorder (includes Factitious Disorder Imposed on Self, Factitious Disorder Imposed on Another) (324)
		Specify Single episode, Recurrent episodes
300.89	**(F45.8)**	Other Specified Somatic Symptom and Related Disorder (327)
300.82	**(F45.9)**	Unspecified Somatic Symptom and Related Disorder (327)

FEEDING AND EATING DISORDERS (329)

The following specifiers apply to Feeding and Eating Disorders where indicated:
[a]*Specify* if: In remission
[b]*Specify* if: In partial remission, In full remission
[c]*Specify* current severity: Mild, Moderate, Severe, Extreme

307.52	**(——.——)**	Pica[a] (329)
	(F98.3)	In children
	(F50.8)	In adults
307.53	**(F98.21)**	Rumination Disorder[a] (332)
307.59	**(F50.8)**	Avoidant/Restrictive Food Intake Disorder[a] (334)
307.1	**(——.——)**	Anorexia Nervosa[b,c] (338)
		Specify whether:
	(F50.01)	Restricting type
	(F50.02)	Binge-eating/purging type
307.51	**(F50.2)**	Bulimia Nervosa[b,c] (345)
307.51	**(F50.8)**	Binge-Eating Disorder[b,c] (350)
307.59	**(F50.8)**	Other Specified Feeding or Eating Disorder (353)
307.50	**(F50.9)**	Unspecified Feeding or Eating Disorder (354)

ELIMINATION DISORDERS (355)

307.6	**(F98.0)**	Enuresis (355)
		Specify whether: Nocturnal only, Diurnal only, Nocturnal and diurnal
307.7	**(F98.1)**	Encopresis (357)
		Specify whether: With constipation and overflow incontinence, Without constipation and overflow incontinence
——.——	**(——.——)**	Other Specified Elimination Disorder (359)
788.39	**(N39.498)**	With urinary symptoms
787.6	**(R15.9)**	With fecal symptoms
——.——	**(——.——)**	Unspecified Elimination Disorder (360)
788.3	**(R32)**	With urinary symptoms
787.6	**(R15.9)**	With fecal symptoms

SLEEP-WAKE DISORDERS (361)

The following specifiers apply to Sleep-Wake Disorders where indicated:
[a]*Specify* if: Episodic, Persistent, Recurrent
[b]*Specify* if: Acute, Subacute, Persistent
[c]*Specify* current severity: Mild, Moderate, Severe

780.52	**(G47.00)**	Insomnia Disorder[a] (362)
		Specify if: With non-sleep disorder mental comorbidity, With other medical comorbidity, With other sleep disorder
780.54	**(G47.10)**	Hypersomnolence Disorder[b,c] (368)
		Specify if: With mental disorder, With medical condition, With another sleep disorder
——.——	**(——.——)**	Narcolepsy[c] (372)
		Specify whether:
347.00	**(G47.419)**	Narcolepsy without cataplexy but with hypocretin deficiency
347.01	**(G47.411)**	Narcolepsy with cataplexy but without hypocretin deficiency
347.00	**(G47.419)**	Autosomal dominant cerebellar ataxia, deafness, and narcolepsy
347.00	**(G47.419)**	Autosomal dominant narcolepsy, obesity, and type 2 diabetes
347.10	**(G47.429)**	Narcolepsy secondary to another medical condition

Breathing-Related Sleep Disorders (378)

327.23	**(G47.33)**	Obstructive Sleep Apnea Hypopnea[c] (378)
——.——	**(——.——)**	Central Sleep Apnea (383)
		Specify whether:
327.21	**(G47.31)**	Idiopathic central sleep apnea
786.04	**(R06.3)**	Cheyne-Stokes breathing
780.57	**(G47.37)**	Central sleep apnea comorbid with opioid use
		Note: First code opioid use disorder, if present.
		Specify current severity
——.——	**(——.——)**	Sleep-Related Hypoventilation (387)
		Specify whether:

327.24	**(G473.34)**	Idiopathic hypoventilation
327.25	**(G47.35)**	Congenital central alveolar hypoventilation
327.26	**(G47.36)**	Comorbid sleep-related hypoventilation
		Specify current severity
——.——	(——.——)	Circadian Rhythm Sleep-Wake Disorders[a] (390)
		Specify whether:
307.45	**(G47.21)**	Delayed sleep phase type (391)
		Specify if: Familial, Overlapping with non-24-hour sleep-wake type
307.45	**(G47.22)**	Advanced sleep phase type (393)
		Specify if: Familial
307.45	**(G47.23)**	Irregular sleep-wake type (394)
307.45	**(G47.24)**	Non-24-hour sleep-wake type (396)
307.45	**(G47.26)**	Shift work type (397)
307.45	**(G47.20)**	Unspecified type

Parasomnias (399)

——.——	(——.——)	Non-Rapid Eye Movement Sleep Arousal Disorders (399)
		Specify whether:
307.46	**(F51.3)**	Sleepwalking type
		Specify if: With sleep-related eating, With sleep-related sexual behavior (sexsomnia)
307.46	**(F51.4)**	Sleep terror type
307.47	**(F51.5)**	Nightmare Disorder[b,c] (404)
		Specify if: During sleep onset
		Specify if: With associated non-sleep disorder, With associated other medical condition, With associated other sleep disorder
327.42	**(G473.52)**	Rapid Eye Movement Sleep Behavior Disorder (407)
333.94	**(G25.81)**	Restless Legs Syndrome (410)
——.——	(——.——)	Substance/Medication-Induced Sleep Disorder (413)
		Note: See the criteria set and corresponding recording procedures for substance-specific codes and ICD-9-CM and ICD-10-CM coding.
		Specify whether: Insomnia type, Daytime sleepiness type, Parasomnia type, Mixed type
		Specify if: With onset during intoxication, With onset during discontinuation/withdrawal
780.52	**(G47.09)**	Other Specified Insomnia Disorder (420)
780.52	**(G47.00)**	Unspecified Insomnia Disorder (420)
780.54	**(G47.19)**	Other Specified Hypersomnolence Disorder (421)
780.54	**(G47.10)**	Unspecified Hypersomnolence Disorder (421)
780.59	**(G47.8)**	Other Specified Sleep-Wake Disorder (421)
780.59	**(G47.9)**	Unspecified Sleep-Wake Disorder (422)

SEXUAL DYSFUNCTIONS (423)

The following specifiers apply to Sexual Dysfunctions where indicated:
[a]*Specify* whether: Lifelong, Acquired
[b]*Specify* whether: Generalized, Situational
[c]*Specify* current severity: Mild, Moderate, Severe

302.74	**(F52.32)**	Delayed Ejaculation[a,b,c] (424)
302.72	**(F52.21)**	Erectile Disorder[a,b,c] (426)
302.73	**(F52.31)**	Female Orgasmic Disorder[a,b,c] (429)
		Specify if: Never experienced an orgasm under any situation
302.72	**(F52.22)**	Female Sexual Interest/Arousal Disorder[a,b,c] (433)
302.76	**(F52.6)**	Genito-Pelvic Pain/Penetration Disorder[a,c] (437)
302.71	**(F52.0)**	Male Hypoactive Sexual Desire Disorder[a,b,c] (440)
302.75	**(F52.4)**	Premature (Early) Ejaculation[a,b,c] (443)
——.——	(——.——)	Substance/Medication-Induced Sexual Dysfunction[c] (446)
		Note: See the criteria and corresponding recording procedures for substance-specific codes and ICD-9-CM and ICD-10-CM coding.
		Specify if: With onset during intoxication, With onset during withdrawal, With onset after medication use
302.79	**(F52.8)**	Other Specified Sexual Dysfunction (450)
302.70	**(F52.9)**	Unspecified Sexual Dysfunction (450)

GENDER DYSPHORIA (451)

——.——	(——.——)	Gender Dysphoria (452)
302.6	**(F64.2)**	Gender Dysphoria in Children
		Specify if: With a disorder of sex development
302.85	**(F64.1)**	Gender Dysphoria in Adolescents and Adults
		Specify if: With a disorder of sex development
		Specify if: Posttransition
		Note: Code the disorder of sex development if present, in addition to gender dysphoria.
302.6	**(F64.8)**	Other Specified Gender Dysphoria (459)
302.6	**(F64.)**	Unspecified Gender Dysphoria (459)

DISRUPTIVE, IMPULSE-CONTROL, AND CONDUCT DISORDERS (461)

313.81	**(F91.3)**	Oppositional Defiant Disorder (462)
		Specify current severity: Mild, Moderate, Severe
312.34	**(F63.81)**	Intermittent Explosive Disorder (466)
——.——	(——.——)	Conduct Disorder (469)
		Specify whether:
312.81	**(F91.1)**	Childhood-onset type

312.32	**(F91.2)**	Adolescent-onset type
312.89	**(F91.9)**	Unspecified onset
		Specify if: With limited prosocial emotions
		Specify current severity: Mild, Moderate, Severe
301.7	**(F60.2)**	Antisocial Personality Disorder (476)
312.33	**(F63.1)**	Pyromania (476)
312.32	**(F63.3)**	Kleptomania (478)
312.89	**(F91.8)**	Other Specified Disruptive, Impulse-Control, and Conduct Disorder (479)
312.9	**(F91.9)**	Unspecified Disruptive, Impulse-Control, and Conduct Disorder (480)

SUBSTANCE-RELATED AND ADDICTIVE DISORDERS (481)

The following specifiers and note apply to Substance-Related and Addictive Disorders where indicated:

[a]*Specify* if: In early remission, In sustained remission

[b]*Specify* if: In a controlled environment

[c]*Specify* if: With perceptual disturbances

[d]The ICD-10-CM code indicated the comorbid presence of a moderate or severe substance use disorder, which must be present in order to apply the code for substance withdrawal.

Substance-Related Disorders (483)

Alcohol-Related Disorders (490)

——.——	(——.——)	Alcohol Use Disorder[a,b] (490)
		Specify current severity:
305.00	**(F10.10)**	Mild
303.90	**(F10.20)**	Moderate
303.90	**(F10.20)**	Severe
303.00	(——.——)	Alcohol Intoxication (497)
	(F10.129)	With use disorder, mild
	(F10.229)	With use disorder, moderate or severe
	(F10.929)	Without use disorder
291.81	(——.——)	Alcohol Withdrawal[c,d] (499)
	(F10.239)	Without perceptual disturbances
	(F10.232)	With perceptual disturbances
——.——	(——.——)	Other Alcohol-Induced Disorder (502)
291.9	**(F10.99)**	Unspecified Alcohol-Related Disorder (503)

Caffeine-Related Disorders (503)

305.90	**(F15.929)**	Caffeine Intoxication (503)
292.0	**(F15.93)**	Caffeine Withdrawal (506)
——.——	(——.——)	Other Caffeine-Induced Disorder (508)
292.9	**(F15.99)**	Unspecified Caffeine-Related Disorder (509)

Cannabis-Related Disorders (509)

——.——	(——.——)	Cannabis Use Disorder[a,b] (509)
		Specify current severity:
305.20	**(F12.10)**	Mild

304.30	**(F12.20)**	Moderate
304.30	**(F12.20)**	Severe
292.89	(——.——)	Cannabis Intoxication[c] (516)
		Without perceptual disturbances
	(F12.129)	With use disorder, mild
	(F12.229)	With use disorder, moderate or severe
	(F12.929)	Without use disorder
		With perceptual disturbances
	(F12.122)	With use disorder, mild
	(F12.222)	With use disorder, moderate or severe
	(F12.922)	Without use disorder
292.0	**(F12.288)**	Cannabis Withdrawal[d] (517)
——.——	(——.——)	Other Cannabis-Induced disorders (519)
292.9	**(F12.99)**	Unspecified Cannabis-Related Disorder (519)

Hallucinogen-Related Disorders (520)

——.——	(——.——)	Phencyclidine Use Disorder[a,b] (520)
		Specify current severity:
305.90	**(F16.10)**	Mild
304.60	**(F16.20)**	Moderate
304.60	**(F16.20)**	Severe
——.——	(——.——)	Other Hallucinogen Use Disorder[a,b] (523)
		Specify the particular hallucinogen
		Specify current severity:
305.30	**(F16.10)**	Mild
304.50	**(F16.20)**	Moderate
304.50	**(F16.20)**	Severe
292.89	(——.——)	Phencyclidine Intoxication (527)
	(F16.129)	With use disorder, mild
	(F16.229)	With use disorder, moderate or severe
	(F16.292)	Without use disorder
292.89	(——.——)	Other Hallucinogen Intoxication (529)
	(F16.129)	With use disorder, mild
	(F16.229)	With use disorder, moderate or severe
	(F16.929)	Without use disorder
292.89	**(F16.983)**	Hallucinogen Persisting Perception Disorder (531)
——.——	(——.——)	Other Phencyclidine-Induced Disorder (532)
——.——	(——.——)	Other Hallucinogen-Induced Disorder (532)
292.9	**(F16.99)**	Unspecified Phencyclidine-Related Disorder (533)
292.9	**(F16.99)**	Unspecified Hallucinogen-Related Disorder (533)

Inhalant-Related Disorder (533)

——.——	(——.——)	Inhalant Use Disorder[a,b] (533)
		Specify the particular inhalant
		Specify current severity:
305.90	**(F18.10)**	Mild
304.60	**(F18.20)**	Moderate
304.60	**(F18.20)**	Severe
292.89	(——.——)	Inhalant Intoxication (538)
	(F18.129)	With use disorder, mild
	(F18.229)	With use disorder, moderate or severe
	(F18.929)	Without use disorder

——.——	(——.——)	Other Inhalant-Induced Disorder (540)
292.9	(F18.99)	Unspecified Inhalant-Related Disorder (540)

Opioid-Related Disorders (540)

——.——	(——.——)	Opioid Use Disorder[a] (541)
		Specify if: On maintenance therapy, In a controlled environment
		Specify current severity:
305.50	(F11.10)	Mild
304.00	(F11.20)	Moderate
304.00	(F11.20)	Severe
292.89	(——.——)	Opioid Intoxication[c] (546)
		Without perceptual disturbances
	(F11.129)	With use disorder, mild
	(F11.229)	With use disorder, moderate or severe
	(F11.929)	Without use disorder
		With perceptual disturbances
	(F11.122)	With use disorder, mild
	(F11.222)	With use disorder, moderate or severe
	(F11.922)	Without use disorder
292.0	(F11.23)	Opioid Withdrawal[d] (547)
——.——	(——.——)	Other Opioid-Induced Disorder (549)
292.9	(F11.99)	Unspecified Opioid-Related Disorder (550)

Sedative-, Hypnotic-, or Anxiolytic-Related Disorders (550)

——.——	(——.——)	Sedative, Hypnotic, or Anxiolytic Use Disorder[a,b] (550)
		Specify current severity:
305.40	(F13.10)	Mild
304.10	(F13.20)	Moderate
304.10	(F13.20)	Severe
292.89	(——.——)	Sedative, Hypnotic, or Anxiolytic Intoxication (556)
	(F13.129)	With use disorder, mild
	(F13.229)	With use disorder, moderate or severe
	(F13.929)	Without use disorder
292.0	(——.——)	Sedative, Hypnotic, or Anxiolytic Withdrawal[c,d] (557)
	(F13.229)	Without perceptual disturbances
	(F13.232)	With perceptual disturbances
——.——	(——.——)	Other Sedative-, Hypnotic-, or Anxiolytic-Induced Disorder (560)
292.9	(F13.99)	Unspecified Sedative-, Hypnotic-, or Anxiolytic-Related Disorder (560)

Stimulant-Related Disorders (561)

——.——	(——.——)	Stimulant Use Disorder[a,b] (561)
		Specify current severity:
——.——	(——.——)	Mild
305.70	(F15.10)	Amphetamine-type substance
305.60	(F14.10)	Cocaine
305.70	(F15.10)	Other or unspecified stimulant
——.——	(——.——)	Moderate
304.40	(F15.20)	Amphetamine-type substance
304.20	(F14.20)	Cocaine
304.40	(F15.20)	Other or unspecified stimulant
——.——	(——.——)	Severe
304.40	(F15.20)	Amphetamine-type substance
304.20	(F14.20)	Cocaine
304.40	(F15.20)	Other or unspecified stimulant
292.89	(——.——)	Stimulant Intoxication[c] (567)
		Specify the specific intoxicant
292.89	(——.——)	Amphetamine or other stimulant, Without perceptual disturbances
	(F15.129)	With use disorder, mild
	(F15.229)	With use disorder, moderate or severe
	(F15.929)	Without use disorder
292.89	(——.——)	Cocaine, Without perceptual disturbances
	(F14.129)	With use disorder, mild
	(F14.229)	With use disorder, moderate or severe
	(F14.929)	Without use disorder
292.89	(——.——)	Amphetamine or other stimulant, With perceptual disturbances
	(F15.122)	With use disorder, mild
	(F15.222)	With use disorder, moderate or severe
	(F15.922)	Without use disorder
292.89	(——.——)	Cocaine, With perceptual disturbances
	(F14.122)	With use disorder, mild
	(F14.222)	Without use disorder, moderate or severe
	(F14.922)	Without use disorder
292.0	(——.——)	Stimulant Withdrawal[d] (569)
		Specify the specific substance causing the withdrawal syndrome
	(F15.23)	Amphetamine or other stimulant
	(F14.23)	Cocaine
——.——	(——.——)	Other Stimulant-Induced Disorder (570)
292.9	(——.——)	Unspecified Stimulant-Related Disorder (570)
	(F15.99)	Amphetamine or other stimulant
	(F14.99)	Cocaine

Tobacco-Related Disorders (571)

——.——	(——.——)	Tobacco Use Disorder[a] (571)
		Specify if: On maintenance therapy, In a controlled environment
		Specify current severity:
305.1	(Z72.0)	Mild
305.1	(F17.200)	Moderate
305.1	(F17.200)	Severe
292.0	(F17.203)	Tobacco Withdrawal[d] (575)
——.——	(——.——)	Other Tobacco-Induced Disorder (576)
292.9	(F17.209)	Unspecified Tobacco-Related Disorder (577)

Other (or Unknown) Substance-Related Disorders (577)

—.—	(—.—)	Other (or Unknown) Substance Use Disorder[a,b] (577)
		Specify current severity:
305.90	(F19.10)	Mild
304.90	(F19.20)	Moderate
304.90	(F19.20)	Severe
292.89	(—.—)	Other (or Unknown) Substance Intoxication (581)
	(F19.129)	With use disorder, mild
	(F19.229)	With use disorder, moderate or severe
	(F19.229)	Without use disorder
292.0	(F19.23)	Other (or Unknown) Substance Withdrawal[d] (583)
—.—	(—.—)	Other (or Unknown) Substance-Induced Disorders (584)
292.2	(F19.99)	Unspecified Other (or Unknown) Substance-Related Disorder (585)

Non-Substance-Related Disorders (585)

312.31	(F63.0)	Gambling Disorder[a] (585)
		Specify if: Episodic, Persistent
		Specify current severity: Mild, Moderate, Severe

NEUROCOGNITIVE DISORDERS (591)

—.—	(—.—)	Delirium (596)
		[a]**Note:** See the criteria set and corresponding recording procedures for substance-specific codes and ICD-9-CM and ICD-10-CM coding.
		Specify whether:
—.—	(—.—)	Substance intoxication delirium[a]
—.—	(—.—)	Substance withdrawal delirium[a]
292.81	(—.—)	Medication-induced delirium[a]
293.0	(F05)	Delirium due to another medical condition
293.0	(F05)	Delirium due to multiple etiologies
		Specify if: Acute, Persistent
		Specify if: Hyperactive, Hypoactive, Mixed level of activity
780.09	(R41.0)	Other Specified Delirium (602)
780.09	(R41.0)	Unspecified Delirium (602)

Major and Mild Neurocognitive Disorders (602)

Specify whether due to: Alzheimer's disease, Frontotemporal lobar degeneration, Lewy body disease, Vascular disease, Traumatic brain injury, Substance/medication use, HIV infection, Prion disease, Parkinson's disease, Huntington's disease, Another medical condition, Multiple etiologies, Unspecified
[a]*Specify* Without behavioral disturbance, With behavioral disturbance. *For possible major neurocognitive disorder and for mild neurocognitive disorder, behavioral disturbance cannot be coded but should still be indicated in writing.*
[b]*Specify* current severity: Mild, Moderate, Severe. *This specifier applies only to major neurocognitive disorder (including probable and possible).*

Note: As indicated for each subtype, an additional medical code is needed for probable major neurocognitive disorder or major neurocognitive disorder. An additional medical code should *not* be used for possible major neurocognitive disorder or mild neurocognitive disorder.

Major or Mild Neurocognitive Disorder Due to Alzheimer's Disease (611)

—.—	(—.—)	Probable Major Neurocognitive Disorder Due to Alzheimer's Disease[b]
		Note: Code first **331.0 (G30.9)** Alzheimer's disease
294.11	(F02.81)	With behavioral disturbance
294.10	(F02.80)	Without behavioral disturbance
331.9	(G31.9)	Possible Major Neurocognitive Disorder Due to Alzheimer's Disease[a,b]
331.83	(G31.84)	Mild Neurocognitive Disorder Due to Alzheimer's Disease[a]

Major or Mild Frontotemporal Neurocognitive Disorder (614)

—.—	(—.—)	Probable Major Neurocognitive Disorder Due to Frontotemporal Lobar Degeneration[b]
		Note: Code first **331.19 (G31.09)** frontotemporal disease.
294.11	(F02.81)	With behavioral disturbance
294.10	(F02.80)	Without behavioral disturbance
331.9	(G31.9)	Possible Major Neurocognitive Disorder Due to Frontotemporal Lobar Degeneration[a,b]
331.83	(G31.84)	Mild Neurocognitive Disorder Due to Frontotemporal Lobar Degeneration[a]

Major or Mild Neurocognitive Disorder with Lewy Bodies (618)

—.—	(—.—)	Probable Major Neurocognitive Disorder With Lewy Bodies[b]
		Note: Code first **331.82 (G31.83)** Lewy body disease.
294.11	(F02.81)	With behavioral disturbance
294.10	(F02.80)	Without behavioral disturbance
331.9	(G31.9)	Possible Major Neurocognitive Disorder With Lewy Bodies[a,b]
331.83	(G31.84)	Mild Neurocognitive Disorder With Lewy Bodies[a]

Major or Mild Vascular Neurocognitive Disorder (621)

—.—	(—.—)	Probable Major Vascular Neurocognitive Disorder[b]
		Note: No additional medical code for vascular disease.
290.40	(F01.51)	With behavioral disturbance
290.40	(F01.50)	Without behavioral disturbance
331.9	(G31.9)	Possible Major Vascular Neurocognitive Disorder[a,b]
331.83	(G31.84)	Mild Vascular Neurocognitive Disorder[a]

Major or Mild Neurocognitive Disorder Due to Traumatic Brain Injury (624)

——.——	(——.——)	Major Neurocognitive Disorder Due to Traumatic Brain Injury[b]
		Note: For ICD-9-CM, code first **907.0** late effect of intracranial injury without skull fracture. For ICD-10-CM, code first **S06.2X9S** diffuse traumatic brain injury with loss of consciousness of unspecified duration, sequela.
294.11	(F02.81)	With behavioral disturbance
294.10	(F02.80)	Without behavioral disturbance
331.83	(G31.84)	Mild Neurocognitive Disorder Due to Traumatic Brain Injury[a]

Substance/Medication-Induced Major or Mild Neurocognitive Disorder[a] (627)

Note: No additional medical code. See the criteria set and corresponding recording procedures for substance-specific codes and ICD-9-CM and ICD-10-CM coding.
Specify if: Persistent

Major or Mild Neurocognitive Disorder Due to HIV Infection (632)

——.——	(——.——)	Major Neurocognitive Disorder Due to HIV Infection[b]
		Note: Code first **042 (B20)** HIV infection.
294.11	(F02.81)	With behavioral disturbance
294.10	(F02.80)	Without behavioral disturbance
331.83	(G31.84)	Mild Neurocognitive Disorder Due to HIV Infection[a]

Major or Mild Neurocognitive Disorder Due to Prion Disease (634)

——.——	(——.——)	Major Neurocognitive Disorder Due to Prion Disease[b]
		Note: Code first **046.79 (A81.9)** prion disease.
294.11	(F02.81)	With behavioral disturbance
294.10	(F02.80)	Without behavioral disturbance
331.83	(G31.84)	Mild Neurocognitive Disorder Due to Prion Disease[a]

Major or Mild Neurocognitive Disorder Due to Parkinson's Disease (636)

——.——	(——.——)	Major Neurocognitive Disorder Probably Due to Parkinson's Disease[b]
		Note: Code first **332.0 (G20)** Parkinson's disease.
294.11	(F02.81)	With behavioral disturbance
294.10	(F02.80)	Without behavioral disturbance
331.9	(G31.9)	Major Neurocognitive Disorder Possibly Due to Parkinson's Disease[a,b]
331.83	(G31.84)	Mild Neurocognitive Disorder Due to Parkinson's Disease[a]

Major or Mild Neurocognitive Disorder Due to Huntington's Disease (638)

——.——	(——.——)	Major Neurocognitive Disorder Due to Huntington's Disease[b]
		Note: Code first **333.4 (G10)** Huntington's disease.
294.11	(F02.81)	With behavioral disturbance
294.10	(F02.80)	Without behavioral disturbance
331.83	(G31.84)	Mild Neurocognitive Disorder Due to Huntington's Disease[a]

Major or Mild Neurocognitive Disorder Due to Another Medical Condition[a] (641)

——.——	(——.——)	Major Neurocognitive Disorder Due to Another Medical Condition[b]
		Note: Code first the other medical condition.
294.11	(F02.81)	With behavioral disturbance
294.10	(F02.80)	Without behavioral disturbance
331.83	(G31.84)	Mild Neurocognitive Disorder Due to Another Medical Condition[a]

Major or Mild Neurocognitive Disorder Due to Multiple Etiologies (642)

——.——	(——.——)	Major Neurocognitive Disorder Due to Multiple Etiologies[b]
		Note: Code first all the etiological medical conditions (with the exception of vascular disease).
294.11	(F02.81)	With behavioral disturbance
294.10	(F02.80)	Without behavioral disturbance
331.83	(G31.84)	Mild Neurocognitive Disorder Due to Multiple Etiologies[a]

Unspecified Neurocognitive Disorder (643)

799.59	(R41.9)	Unspecified Neurocognitive Disorder[a]

PERSONALITY DISORDERS (645)

Cluster A Personality Disorders

301.0	(F60.0)	Paranoid Personality Disorder (649)
301.20	(F60.1)	Schizoid Personality Disorder (652)
301.22	(F21)	Schizotypal Personality Disorder (655)

Cluster B Personality Disorders

301.7	(F60.2)	Antisocial Personality Disorder (659)
301.83	(F60.3)	Borderline Personality Disorder (663)
301.50	(F60.4)	Histrionic Personality Disorder (667)
301.81	(F60.81)	Narcissistic Personality Disorder (669)

Cluster C Personality Disorders

301.82	(F60.6)	Avoidant Personality Disorder (672)
301.6	(F60.7)	Dependent Personality Disorder (675)
301.4	(F60.5)	Obsessive-Compulsive Personality Disorder (678)

Other Personality Disorders

310.1	(F07.0)	Personality Change Due to Another Medical Condition (682) *Specify* whether: Labile type, Disinhibited type, Aggressive type, Apathetic type, Paranoid type, Other type, Combined type, Unspecified type
301.89	(F60.89)	Other Specified Personality Disorder (684)
301.9	(F60.9)	Unspecified Personality Disorder (684)

PARAPHILIC DISORDERS (685)

The following specifier applies to Paraphilic Disorders where indicated:
[a]*Specify* if: In a controlled environment, In full remission

302.82	(F65.3)	Voyeuristic Disorder[a] (686)
302.4	(F65.2)	Exhibitionistic Disorder[a] (689) *Specify* whether: Sexually aroused by exposing genitals to prepubertal children, Sexually aroused by exposing genitals to physically mature individuals, Sexually aroused by exposing genitals to prepubertal children and to physically mature individuals
302.89	(F65.81)	Frotteuristic Disorder[a] (691)
302.83	(F65.51)	Sexual Masochism Disorder[a] (694) *Specify* if: With asphyxiophilia
302.84	(F65.52)	Sexual Sadism Disorder[a] (695)
302.2	(F65.4)	Pedophilic Disorder (697) *Specify* whether: Exclusive type, Nonexclusive type *Specify* if: Sexually attracted to males, Sexually attracted to females, Sexually attracted to both *Specify* if: Limited to incest
302.81	(F65.0)	Fetishistic Disorder[a] (700) *Specify:* Body part(s), Nonliving object(s), Other
302.3	(F65.1)	Transvestic Disorder[a] (702) *Specify* if: With fetishism, With autogynephilia
302.89	(F65.89)	Other Specified Paraphilic Disorder (705)
302.9	(F65.9)	Unspecified Paraphilic Disorder (705)

OTHER MENTAL DISORDERS (707)

294.8	(F06.8)	Other Specified Mental Disorder Due to Another Medical Condition (707)
294.9	(F09)	Unspecified Mental Disorder Due to Another Medical Condition (708)
300.9	(F99)	Other Specified Mental Disorder (708)
300.9	(F99)	Unspecified Mental Disorder (708)

MEDICATION-INDUCED MOVEMENT DISORDERS AND OTHER ADVERSE EFFECTS OF MEDICATION (709)

332.1	(G21.11)	Neuroleptic-Induced Parkinsonism (709)
332.1	(G21.19)	Other Medication-Induced Parkinsonism (709)
333.92	(G21.0)	Neuroleptic Malignant Syndrome (709)
333.72	(G24.02)	Medication-Induced Acute Dystonia (711)
333.99	(G25.71)	Medication-Induced Acute Akathisia (711)
333.85	(G24.01)	Tardive Dyskinesia (712)
333.72	(G24.09)	Tardive Dystonia (712)
333.99	(G25.71)	Tardive Akathisia (712)
333.1	(G25.1)	Medication-Induced Postural Tremor (712)
333.99	(G25.79)	Other Medication-Induced Movement Disorder (712)
——.——	(——.——)	Antidepressant Discontinuation Syndrome (712)
995.29	(T43.205A)	Initial encounter
995.29	(T43.205D)	Subsequent encounter
995.29	(T43.205S)	Sequelae
——.——	(——.——)	Other Adverse Effect of Medication (714)
995.20	(T50.905A)	Initial encounter
995.20	(T50.905D)	Subsequent encounter
995.20	(T50.905S)	Sequelae

OTHER CONDITIONS THAT MAY BE A FOCUS OF CLINICAL ATTENTION (715)

Relational Problems (715)

Problems Related to Family Upbringing (715)

V61.20	(Z62.820)	Parent-Child Relational Problem (715)
V61.8	(Z62.891)	Sibling Relational Problem (716)
V61.8	(Z62.29)	Upbringing Away From Parents (716)
V61.29	(Z62.898)	Child Affected by Parental Relationship Distress (716)

Other Problems Related to Primary Support Group (716)

V61.10	(Z63.0)	Relationship Distress With Spouse or Intimate Partner (716)
V61.03	(Z63.5)	Disruption of Family by Separation or Divorce (716)
V61.8	(Z63.8)	High Expressed Emotion Level Within Family (716)
V62.82	(Z63.4)	Uncomplicated Bereavement (716)

Abuse and Neglect (717)

Child Maltreatment and Neglect Problems (717)

Child Physical Abuse (717)

Child Physical Abuse, Confirmed (717)

995.54	(T743.12XA)	Initial encounter
995.54	(T74.12XD)	Subsequent encounter

Child Physical Abuse, Suspected (717)
995.54 **(T76.12XA)** Initial encounter
995.54 **(T76.12XD)** Subsequent encounter
Other Circumstances Related to Child Physical Abuse (718)
V61.21 **(Z69.010)** Encounter for mental health services for victim of child abuse by parent
V61.21 **(Z69.020)** Encounter for mental health services for victim of nonparental child abuse
V15.41 **(Z62.810)** Personal history (past history) of physical abuse in childhood
V61.22 **(Z69.011)** Encounter for mental health services for perpetrator of parental child abuse
V62.83 **(Z69.021)** Encounter for mental health services for perpetrator of nonparental child abuse

Child Sexual Abuse (718)
Child Sexual Abuse, Confirmed (718)
995.53 **(T74.22XA)** Initial encounter
995.53 **(T74.22XD)** Subsequent encounter
Child Sexual Abuse, Suspected (718)
995.53 **(T76.22XA)** Initial encounter
995.53 **(T76.22XD)** Subsequent encounter
Other Circumstances Related to Child Sexual Abuse (718)
V61.21 **(Z69.010)** Encounter for mental health services for victim of child sexual abuse by parent
V61.21 **(Z69.020)** Encounter for mental health services for victim of nonparental child sexual abuse
V15.21 **(Z62.810)** Personal history (past history) of sexual abuse in childhood
V61.22 **(Z69.011)** Encounter for mental health services for perpetrator of parental child sexual abuse
V62.83 **(Z69.021)** Encounter for mental health services for perpetrator of nonparental child sexual abuse

Child Neglect (718)
Child Neglect, Confirmed (718)
995.52 **(T74.02ZA)** Initial encounter
995.52 **(T74.02XD)** Subsequent encounter
Child Neglect, Suspected (719)
995.52 **(T76.02XA)** Initial encounter
995.52 **(T76.02XD)** Subsequent encounter
Other Circumstances Related to Child Neglect (719)
V61.21 **(Z69.010)** Encounter for mental health services for victim of child neglect by parent
V61.21 **(Z69.020)** Encounter for mental health services for victim of nonparental child neglect
V15.42 **(Z62.812)** Personal history (past history) of neglect in childhood
V61.22 **(Z69.011)** Encounter for mental health services for perpetrator of parental child neglect
V62.83 **(Z69.021)** Encounter for mental health services for perpetrator of nonparental child neglect

Child Psychological Abuse (719)
Child Psychological Abuse, Confirmed (719)
995.51 **(T74.32XA)** Initial encounter
995.51 **(T74.32XD)** Subsequent encounter
Child Psychological Abuse, Suspected (719)
995.51 **(T76.32XA)** Initial encounter
995.51 **(T76.32XD)** Subsequent encounter
Other Circumstances Related to Child Psychological Abuse (719)
V61.21 **(Z69.010)** Encounter for mental health services for victim of child psychological abuse by parent
V61.21 **(Z69.020)** Encounter for mental health services for victim of nonparental child psychological abuse
V15.42 **(Z62.811)** Personal history (past history) of psychological abuse in childhood
V61.22 **(Z69.011)** Encounter for mental health services for perpetrator of parental child psychological abuse
V62.83 **(Z69.021)** Encounter for mental health services for perpetrator of nonparental child psychological abuse

Adult Maltreatment and Neglect Problems (720)

Spouse or Partner Violence, Physical (720)
Spouse or Partner Violence, Physical, Confirmed (720)
995.81 **(T74.11XA)** Initial encounter
995.81 **(T74.11XD)** Subsequent encounter
Spouse or Partner Violence, Physical, Suspected (720)
995.81 **(T76.11XA)** Initial encounter
995.81 **(T76.11XD)** Subsequent encounter
Other Circumstances Related to Spouse or Partner Violence, Physical (720)
V61.11 **(Z96.11)** Encounter for mental health services for victim of spouse or partner violence, physical
V15.41 **(Z91.410)** Personal history (past history) of spouse or partner violence, physical
V61.12 **(Z69.12)** Encounter for mental health services for perpetrator of spouse or partner violence, physical

Spouse or Partner Violence, Sexual (720)
Spouse or Partner Violence, Sexual, Confirmed (720)
995.83 **(T74.21XA)** Initial encounter
995.83 **(T74.21XD)** Subsequent encounter
Spouse or Partner Violence, Sexual, Suspected (720)
995.83 **(T76.21XA)** Initial encounter
995.83 **(T76.21XD)** Subsequent encounter
Other Circumstances Related to Spouse or Partner Violence, Sexual (720)
V61.11 **(Z69.81)** Encounter for mental health services for victim of spouse or partner violence, sexual
V15.41 **(Z91.410)** Personal history (past history) of spouse or partner violence, sexual

V61.12	(Z69.12)	Encounter for mental health services for perpetrator of spouse or partner violence, sexual

Spouse or Partner Neglect (721)
Spouse or Partner Neglect, Confirmed (721)

995.85	(T47.01XA)	Initial encounter
995.85	(T74.01XD)	Subsequent encounter

Spouse or Partner Neglect, Suspected (721)

995.85	(T76.01XA)	Initial encounter
995.85	(T76.01XD)	Subsequent encounter

Other Circumstances Related to Spouse or Partner Neglect (721)

V61.11	(Z69.11)	Encounter for mental health services for victim of spouse or partner neglect
V15.42	(Z91.412)	Personal history (past history) of spouse or partner neglect
V61.12	(Z69.12)	Encounter for mental health services for perpetrator of spouse or partner neglect

Spouse or Partner Abuse, Psychological (721)
Spouse or Partner Abuse, Psychological, Confirmed (721)

995.82	(T74.31XA)	Initial encounter
995.82	(T74.31XD)	Subsequent encounter

Spouse or Partner Abuse, Psychological, Suspected (721)

995.82	(T76.31XA)	Initial encounter
995.82	(T76.31XD)	Subsequent encounter

Other Circumstances Related to Spouse or Partner Abuse, Psychological (721)

V61.11	(Z69.11)	Encounter for mental health services for victim of spouse or partner psychological abuse
V15.42	(Z91.411)	Personal history (past history) of spouse or partner psychological abuse
V61.12	(Z69.12)	Encounter for mental health services for perpetrator of spouse or partner psychological abuse

Adult Abuse by Nonspouse or Nonpartner (722)
Adult Physical Abuse by Nonspouse or Nonpartner, Confirmed (722)

995.81	(T74.11XA)	Initial encounter
995.81	(T74.11XD)	Subsequent encounter

Adult Physical Abuse by Nonspouse or Nonpartner, Suspected (722)

995.81	(T76.11XA)	Initial encounter
995.81	(T76.11XD)	Subsequent encounter

Adult Sexual Abuse by Nonspouse or Nonpartner, Confirmed (722)

995.83	(T74.21XA)	Initial encounter
995.83	(T74.21XD)	Subsequent encounter

Adult Sexual Abuse by Nonspouse or Nonpartner, Suspected (722)

995.83	(T76.21XA)	Initial encounter
995.83	(T76.21XD)	Subsequent encounter

Adult Psychological Abuse by Nonspouse or Nonpartner, Confirmed (722)

995.82	(T74.31XA)	Initial encounter
995.82	(T74.31XD)	Subsequent encounter

Adult Psychological Abuse by Nonspouse or Nonpartner, Suspected (722)

995.82	(T76.31XA)	Initial encounter
995.82	(T76.31XD)	Subsequent encounter

Other Circumstances Related to Adult Abuse by Nonspouse or Nonpartner (722)

V65.49	(Z69.81)	Encounter for mental health services for victim of nonspousal adult abuse
V62.83	(Z69.82)	Encounter for mental health services for perpetrator of nonspousal adult abuse

Educational and Occupational Problems (723)
Educational Problems (723)

V62.3	(Z55.9)	Academic or Educational Problem (723)

Occupational Problems (723)

V62.21	(Z56.82)	Problem Related to Current Military Deployment Status (723)
V62.29	(Z56.9)	Other Problem Related to Employment (723)

Housing and Economic Problems (723)
Housing Problems (723)

V60.0	(Z59.0)	Homelessness (723)
V60.1	(Z59.1)	Inadequate Housing (723)
V60.89	(Z59.2)	Discord With Neighbor, Lodger, or Landlord (723)
V60.6	(Z59.3)	Problem Related to Living in a Residential Institution (724)

Economic Problems (724)

V60.2	(Z59.4)	Lack of Adequate Food or Safe Drinking Water (724)
V60.2	(Z59.5)	Extreme Poverty (724)
V60.2	(Z59.6)	Low Income (724)
V60.2	(Z59.7)	Insufficient Social Insurance or Welfare Support (724)
V60.9	(Z59.9)	Unspecified Housing or Economic Problem (724)

Other Problems Related to the Social Environment (724)

V62.89	(Z60.0)	Phase of Life Problem (724)
V60.3	(Z60.2)	Problem Related to Living Alone (724)
V62.4	(Z60.3)	Acculturation Difficulty (724)
V62.4	(Z60.4)	Social Exclusion or Rejection (724)
V62.4	(Z60.5)	Target of (Perceived) Adverse Discrimination or Persecution (724)
V62.9	(Z60.9)	Unspecified Problem Related to Social Environment (725)

Problems Related to Crime or Interaction with the Legal System (725)

V62.879	(Z65.4)	Victim of Crime (725)
V62.5	(Z65.0)	Conviction in Civil or Criminal Proceedings Without Imprisonment (725)

V62.5	**(Z65.1)**	Imprisonment or Other Incarceration (725)
V62.5	**(Z65.2)**	Problems Related to Release From Prison (725)
V62.5	**(Z65.3)**	Problems Related to Other Legal Circumstances (725)

Other Health Service Encounters for Counseling and Medical Advice (725)

V65.4	**(Z70.9)**	Sex Counseling (725)
V65.40	**(Z71.9)**	Other Counseling or Consultation (725)

Problems Related to Other Psychosocial, Personal, and Environmental Circumstances (725)

V62.89	**(Z65.8)**	Religious or Spiritual Problem (725)
V61.7	**(Z64.0)**	Problems Related to Unwanted Pregnancy (725)
V61.5	**(Z64.1)**	Problems Related to Multiparity (725)
V62.89	**(Z64.4)**	Discord With Social Service Provider, Including Probation Officer, Case Manager, or Social Service Worker (725)
V62.89	**(Z65.4)**	Victim of Terrorism or Torture (725)
V62.22	**(Z65.5)**	Exposure to Disaster, War, or Other Hostilities (725)
V62.89	**(Z65.8)**	Other Problem Related to Psychosocial Circumstances (725)
V62.9	**(Z65.9)**	Unspecified Problem Related to Unspecified Psychosocial Circumstances (725)

Other Circumstances of Personal History (726)

V15.49	**(Z91.49)**	Other Personal History of Psychological Trauma (726)
V15.59	**(Z91.5)**	Personal History of Self-Harm (726)
V62.22	**(Z91.82)**	Personal History of Military Deployment (726)
V15.89	**(Z91.89)**	Other Personal Risk Factors (726)
V69.9	**(Z72.9)**	Problem Related to Lifestyle (726)
V71.01	**(Z72.811)**	Adult Antisocial Behavior (726)
V71.02	**(Z72.810)**	Child or Adolescent Antisocial Behavior (726)

Problems Related to Access to Medical and Other Health Care (726)

V63.9	**(Z75.3)**	Unavailability or Inaccessibility of Health Care Facilities (726)
V63.8	**(Z75.4)**	Unavailability or Inaccessibility of Other Helping Agencies (726)

Nonadherence to Medical Treatment (726)

V15.81	**(Z91.19)**	Nonadherence to Medical Treatment (726)
278.00	**(E66.9)**	Overweight or Obesity (726)
V65.2	**(Z76.5)**	Malingering (726)
V40.31	**(Z91.83)**	Wandering Associated With a Mental Disorder (727)
V62.89	**(R41.83)**	Borderline Intellectual Functioning (727)

GLOSSARY

absence seizure A type of generalized seizure in which there is an abrupt loss of consciousness (usually lasting <10 seconds); these seizures are nonconvulsive in nature and might not be noticed by others.

abstinence syndrome Physical signs and symptoms that occur when the addictive substance is reduced or withheld; also referred to as *withdrawal.*

abstract thinking The ability to find meaning in proverbs; the ability to conceptualize.

abuse Excessive use of a substance that differs from societal norms and causes clinically significant impairment.

acceptance The allowance of respect of individuality.

acetylcholine (ACh) A neurotransmitter synthesized by choline acetyltransferase from acetyl coenzyme A and choline. It is found in the peripheral nervous system at the myoneural junction; in the autonomic ganglia for parasympathetic or sympathetic systems; and in the parasympathetic postganglionic synapses, including cranial nerves III, VII, IX, and X. Acetylcholine is found in the spinal cord, basal ganglia, and numerous sites within the cerebral cortex. Cortical ACh is synthesized primarily in the nucleus basalis of Meynert and in the septal area near the hypothalamus.

acrophobia Fear of high places.

active listening Verbal and nonverbal skills used by the examiner to demonstrate interest and concern to the patient.

acupressure Use of pressure to restore balance by stimulating meridians.

acupuncture Ancient Chinese health practice that involves puncturing the skin with hair-thin needles at particular locations on the patient's body called *acupuncture points.* Acupuncture is believed to help reduce pain or change a body function. Sometimes the needles are twirled, giving a slight electric charge.

acute stress disorder The development of characteristic anxiety, dissociative, and other symptoms that occur within 1 month after exposure to an extreme traumatic stressor.

addiction Psychological and physiologic symptoms indicating that an individual cannot control his or her use of psychoactive substances.

advocacy Negotiating with others to develop, improve, and provide services for a patient.

affect Emotional range attached to ideas; outwardly demonstrated; feeling, mood, or emotional tone.

   appropriate a. Emotional tone in harmony with the accompanying idea, thought, or verbalization.

   blunted a. Disturbance manifested by a severe reduction in the intensity of affect.

   flat a. Absence or near-absence of any signs of affective expression.

   inappropriate a. Incongruence between the emotional feeling tone and the idea, thought, or speech accompanying it.

   labile a. Rapid changes in emotional feeling tone, unrelated to external stimuli.

affective disorders Group of psychiatric diagnoses characterized by mood disturbances on a continuum of depression to mania.

aggression Forceful verbal or physical action—that is, the motor counterpart of the affect of anger, rage, or hostility.

agitation Anxiety associated with severe motor restlessness.

agnosia Difficulty in recognizing familiar objects; a symptom of organic brain disease.

agnostic One who is uncertain about whether there is a god (Greek *a,* no; *gnosis,* knowledge).

agonist In pharmacology, a substance that acts with, enhances, or potentiates a specific receptor type.

agoraphobia Fear of being in a place or situation in which escape might be difficult or embarrassing or in which help might be unavailable in case of a panic attack.

agranulocytosis A significant decrease in white blood cell count, which can have serious or lethal consequences. Clozapine can cause agranulocytosis.

agraphia Loss of the ability to write.

AIDS dementia complex A dementia attributed to HIV infection.

akathisia Motor restlessness, generally expressed as the inability to sit still, caused by the dopamine blockade by certain types of neuroleptic medications; an extrapyramidal side effect (EPSE).

alcoholic Individual whose compulsive use of alcohol causes problems at home, at work, or socially and who continues to use alcohol despite these adverse consequences.

Alcoholics Anonymous (AA) Self-help organization that uses a 12-step program to assist alcoholics to achieve and maintain sobriety; Al-Anon assists the spouses of alcoholics; Alateen assists the teenage children of alcoholics.

alertness Awareness and attentiveness to surroundings.

alternative therapy Broad range of healing philosophies and approaches that mainstream Western medicine does not commonly use, accept, study, understand, or make available.

Alzheimer's disease More correctly referred to as *dementia of the Alzheimer type* (DAT). DAT is the most common type of dementia. The characteristic symptoms are amnesia, aphasia, apraxia, and agnosia. It is a cognitive mental disorder resulting in dementia that is related to a progressive deterioration of brain tissue, described as plaques and neurofibrillary tangles.

ambivalence Opposing impulses or feelings directed toward the same person or object at the same time.

amenorrhea Absence of menstruation.

amnesia Partial or total inability to recall past information.

   anterograde a. Recent memory loss, as in the early stages of Alzheimer's disease.

   global a. Total memory loss, as in advanced stages of Alzheimer's disease.

   retrograde a. Remote memory loss, as in later stages of Alzheimer's disease.

   short-term a. Memory loss observed in alcoholic blackouts.

amygdala Cluster of nuclei in the medial temporal lobe involved with endocrine and behavioral functions and that plays a role in food and water intake, drive behavior, and emotions connected with those behaviors. In animal studies, electrical stimulation of the amygdala causes defensiveness, rage, or aggression.

analytic worldview Perception of the world that values detail to time, individuality, and possessions.

anergia Absence of energy caused by changes in brain chemistry, anatomy, or both.

anger Normal emotional response to the perception of a frustration of desires or threat to one's needs.

anhedonia Loss of pleasure in activities or interests previously enjoyed; a symptom noted in depression and schizophrenia.

anorexia nervosa Disorder characterized by a refusal to eat over a long period, resulting in emaciation, amenorrhea, disturbance in body image, and intense fear of becoming obese.

Antabuse (disulfiram) Drug given to alcoholics that blocks the breakdown of acetaldehyde, producing nausea, vomiting, dizziness, flushing, and tachycardia if alcohol is consumed.

antagonist In pharmacology, a substance that blocks a receptor.

anterior commissure White matter tract that connects the olfactory structures bilaterally as well as the temporal lobes and the amygdala.

anticholinergic effect Effect caused by drugs that block ACh receptors. Common anticholinergic effects include dry mouth, blurred vision, constipation, and urinary hesitancy.

antisocial personality Personality disorder with the essential feature of a pervasive pattern of blatant disregard for social norms.

anxiety Nonspecific, unpleasant feeling of discomfort, with physiologic and psychological symptoms that generally result from a perception of a threat to safety and security.

anxiety disorders Patterns of symptoms and behaviors in which anxiety is either the primary disturbance or a secondary problem that is recognized when the primary symptoms are removed.

anxiolytic Antianxiety drug.

apathy Lack of feeling, interest, or emotion; indifference that is occasionally a mechanism for avoiding intense emotion.

aphasia Difficulty in searching for words.

  motor a. Impaired speech as a result of an organic brain disorder in which understanding remains.

  nominal a. Difficulty in finding the correct words in their appropriate sequence.

  sensory a. Loss of ability to comprehend the meaning of words.

appropriate Suitable or fitting for a particular person, purpose, occasion, or situation, such as appropriate affect, response, or attire.

apraxia Inability to perform previously known, purposeful, skilled activities in the absence of loss of motor function.

assault Legally, any behavior that physically or verbally presents an immediate threat of physical injury to another individual.

assertiveness Direct expression of feelings and needs in a way that respects the rights of others and self.

asylum (1) Place of safety or sanctuary; a refuge; (2) institution for the care of the mentally ill; often associated with mistreatment and callousness.

atheist One who believes that there is no deity (Greek *a*, no; *theos*, God).

attention-deficit/hyperactivity disorder (ADHD) Relatively common disorder of childhood onset characterized by inattention, impulsiveness, and overactivity.

attitude Pattern of mental views and feelings accumulated through past experiences and affected by present stimuli; a manner, disposition, tendency, or orientation with regard to a person or situation.

atypical depression Subtype of depression occurring more often in younger individuals; expressed by atypical symptoms—for example, increased appetite, weight gain, hypersomnia.

autism (1) Preoccupation with self without concern for external reality; a self-made private world of the individual with schizophrenia; (2) a disorder of markedly abnormal or impaired development in social interactions and communication occurring in early childhood.

autistic thinking Thoughts, ideas, or desires derived from internal, private stimuli or drives that are often incongruent with reality.

autonomic nervous system Division of the peripheral nervous system that is involuntary and innervates the viscera, heart, blood vessels, smooth muscle, and glands. It is divided into the parasympathetic (craniosacral) and sympathetic (thoracolumbar) systems.

avolition Lack of motivation.

axon Long process from the neuronal cell body that transmits impulses away from the cell.

B

balance Process by which patients are helped to achieve independence while conforming to norms.

basal ganglia Large nuclei, including the caudate nucleus, putamen, and globus pallidus, which are responsible for modulating voluntary movement.

battery Touching of the person of another, of his or her clothes, or anything else attached to his or her person without consent.

behavior Any observable, recordable, and measurable movement, response, or act of an individual (verbal and nonverbal).

behavior therapy Therapeutic approach that helps the patient modify behavior by changing old patterns of behavior.

binge Eating an unusually large amount of food in a relatively short period.

binge eating Disorder in which an individual regularly eats large amounts of food in a discrete period of time. Bingeing occurs without purging.

biofeedback The use of a machine to communicate physical changes; used to train a person to reduce anxiety and modify behavioral responses.

biologic variations Physical differences between individuals or differences in body structure, skin color, other visible characteristics, enzymatic and genetic variations, electrocardiographic patterns, susceptibility to disease, nutritional preferences and deficiencies, and psychological characteristics.

bipolar disorder Affective or mood disorder characterized by at least one episode of mania, with or without a history of depression.

biracial Individual who crosses two racial and cultural groups.

bizarre Markedly unusual in appearance, thought, style, character, or behavior; absurd.

blackout Period in which a drinker functions socially but for which the drinker has no memory.

blocking Unconscious interruption in train of thought.

blood-brain barrier Guards the brain from fluctuations in body chemistry; regulates the amount and speed with which substances in the blood enter the brain.

borderline personality disorder Personality disorder with the essential feature of a pervasive pattern of unstable self-image, interpersonal relations, and mood.

bradykinesia Slow or retarded movement.

brainstem Vital structure that carries all information to and from the cerebral cortex and spinal cord. Because the brainstem is also responsible for respiration, its function is essential for life. It consists of the midbrain, pons, and medulla.

bulimia Compulsive binge eating accompanied by purging and an overconcern with body shape and weight. It is characterized by an insatiable craving for food, resulting in episodes of continuous eating and often followed by purging, depression, and self-deprivation.

bulimia nervosa Disorder characterized by binge eating, compensatory behavior, and overconcern with body shape and weight.

bureaucracy Excessive rules and structure that get in the way of efficient, responsive, and creative nursing care solutions.

burnout Spiraling process of decreased effectiveness.

C

case management Collaborative process for meeting health needs through the use of a variety of services in a cost-effective manner.

catalepsy State of unconsciousness in which immobility is constantly maintained.

catatonia Immobility as a result of psychological causes.

catatonic behavior Motor anomalies in nonorganic disorders, such as schizophrenia.

catecholamines Derived from the amino acid tyrosine, these substances include dopamine, norepinephrine, and epinephrine. Catecholamines are a subcategory of the monoamines, which also include serotonin and histamine. Catecholamines and their synthesis products are widely distributed in the central and peripheral nervous systems.

caudate Basal ganglia nucleus that protrudes into the anterior horn of the lateral ventricle.

cerebral cortex Narrow ribbon of gray matter that lies on the surface of the cerebrum. The gray matter lies on top of the white matter. The reverse is true in the spinal cord.

child abuse Harmful physical, emotional, sexual, or verbal behavior inflicted on a child.

cholinergics Substances that stimulate the cholinergic system. In the peripheral nervous system, cholinergic drugs constrict the pupil, increase the production of saliva and respiratory secretions, slow the heart, and increase gastrointestinal peristalsis and urinary output.

chorea Greek term for dance. The choreas are demonstrated as hyperkinetic disorders characterized by involuntary, unpredictable, and random movements of the trunk, head, face, and limbs.

chromosome The self-replicating genetic structure of cells containing the cellular DNA that bears in its nucleotide sequence the linear array of genes. Eukaryotic genomes (such as humans have) consist of many chromosomes whose DNA is associated with different types of proteins.

circumstantiality Digression of inappropriate thoughts into ideas, eventually reaching the desired goal.

cirrhosis Disease of the liver; characterized by the development of scar tissue in the liver. The person most likely to develop cirrhosis is a middle-aged man with chronic alcoholism.

civil law The part of the legal system concerned with the legal rights and duties of private persons. Civil lawsuits can recapture monetary loss from professionals who have been guilty of false imprisonment, defamation of character, assault and battery, or negligence.

clang associations Speech pattern characterized by words similar in sound but not in meaning that conjure up new thoughts; noted in types of schizophrenia.

clarification Communication skill that helps define a patient's responses through the use of direct questions.

claustrophobia Fear of closed places.

clinical depression Another term for major depressive disorder that defines the disturbance of a person's mood.

clinical supervision Formal meeting among psychiatric nursing peers to examine attitudes, reactions, and conflicts with patients on the unit and to find new ways of approaching patient problems.

clonic State in which rigidity and relaxation succeed each other.

closed-ended questions Questions that generally elicit a "yes" or "no" response. Useful in gathering factual data.

clouding of consciousness Incomplete clarity of mind, with disturbance in perception and attitude (e.g., stupor).

codependency Stress-related preoccupation with an addicted person's life, leading to extreme dependence on that person.

cognition Act or process of knowing and perceiving.

cognitive disorders Disorders that affect consciousness, memory, and other thought processes.

cognitive dissonance A state that arises when two opposing beliefs exist at the same time.

cognitive processes Processes that pertain to perception, judgment, memory, and reasoning.

coma State of depressed consciousness wherein even extreme stimulation of the reticular activating system does not elicit a response.

command hallucinations Hallucinations that tell the patient to take some specific action, such as to kill himself or herself or someone else.

common law/case law The term *common law* is applied to the body of principles that has evolved and continues to evolve and expand from judicial decisions that arise during the trial of actual court cases; law based on the outcome of cases.

communication Process that is the matrix for thought and relationships among all people, regardless of cultural heritage.

community meeting Meeting that is held in the therapeutic milieu and in which joint problem solving by community members is encouraged.

community mental health Application of the principles of psychiatric care to communities and groups of people. The goal of this effort is to maintain health, prevent mental illness when possible, and, if treatment is indicated, treat the individual closer to his or her support systems.

Community Mental Health Centers Act Legislation initiated in 1963 authorizing federal funds for the construction of comprehensive mental health centers.

community worldview Community needs and concerns are more important than individual ones. Quiet, respectful communication is valued as well as meditation and reading as a learning style.

comorbidity Simultaneous existence of medical and psychiatric problems, each complicating the other.

complementary therapy Same as *alternative therapy*, but denotes therapy used as an adjunct to, rather than as a replacement for, conventional treatment.

complex partial seizure Formerly referred to as *temporal lobe* or *psychomotor seizure*; seizure typically begins with a clouding of consciousness followed by some meaningless movement such as lip smacking or hand clapping; brief periods of forgetfulness are common.

comprehension Capacity to perceive and understand.

compulsion Uncontrollable impulse to perform an act or ritual repeatedly; might be in response to an obsession (unwilled, persistent thought), as in obsessive-compulsive disorder. The act or ritual serves to decrease anxiety. Examples of rituals include hand washing, cleaning, and checking (e.g., checking to see whether door is locked).

concrete communication Inability to think and communicate abstractly.

concrete thinking Use of literal meaning without ability to consider abstract meaning (e.g., "don't cry over spilled milk" might be interpreted as meaning, "Okay, I'll cry over the sink.")

confabulation Unconscious filling of gaps in memory with imagined or untrue experiences that the person believes but have no basis in reality.

confidentiality Treating the information about and from patients in a private manner; information about patients is confidential and requires patient approval before disclosure.

conflict Differing perspectives among staff or patients regarding various aspects of treatment.

confused state Bewildered, perplexed, or unclear. The type and degree of confusion should be specified.

congruence Accordant states. An example is mood congruence, in which the person's visible emotional state correlates with his or her mood or feeling state.

consciousness State of awareness.

conservator Guardian; a legally appointed person who controls the affairs of a gravely disabled person, including the right to consent to or refuse psychiatric treatment.

consultant-liaison nurse Psychiatric mental health nurse who provides expert consultation for patients and staff in other parts of the hospital agency.

consumer Person in treatment for psychiatric services.

continuum of care Levels of care through which an individual can move depending on his or her needs at a given point in time.

contralateral Opposite side of the body.

conversion Process by which a psychological event, an idea, a memory, or an impulse is represented by a bodily change or symptom, such as blindness or paralysis.

coping mechanism Any effort directed at stress management.

corporate compliance Health care provider's responsibility to comply with governmental laws and regulations.

corpus callosum Major connecting and communicating pathway between the brain hemispheres.

cortisol Glucocorticoid hormone found in the adrenal cortex that is involved in carbohydrate and protein metabolism. Cortisol hypersecretion occurs in many depressed individuals. Excretion of this hormone is not suppressed in many persons with major depression after an injection of dexamethasone.

creed Set formula that states the religious and spiritual beliefs of a community of faith (Latin, *credo*, I trust, believe).

criminal law Part of the legal system concerned with crime that is defined in state and federal statutes.

crisis A 4- to 6-week period of severe emotional disorganization following a major stressful event (e.g., divorce, job loss) as a result of the failure of coping mechanisms, lack of support, or both.

cultural awareness Process whereby the nurse acknowledges his or her cultural biases and recognizes that other individuals, groups, or communities have their unique cultural similarities and differences.

cultural competence Process whereby the nurse has developed cultural awareness, knowledge, and skills to promote effective and quality health care for patients.

cultural diversity Variety of cultural groupings; might include age, gender, socioeconomic status, religion, race, and ethnicity.

cultural negotiation Nurse's ability to work with a patient's cultural belief system to develop culturally appropriate interventions.

cultural preservation Nurse's ability to acknowledge, value, and accept a patient's cultural beliefs.

cultural repatterning Nurse's ability to incorporate cultural preservation and negotiation to identify patient needs, develop expected outcomes, and evaluate outcome plans.

cultural values Unique, individual expressions of beliefs related to culture that have been accepted as appropriate over time for persons in that culture.

culturally diverse nursing care Modification of nursing approaches to provide culturally competent care.

culture The internal and external manifestation of beliefs, values, and norms of an individual, group, or community that are used as premises for daily life and functioning.

cupping Alternative cultural or medical treatment that uses a small glass or cup to conduct the moxibustion treatment.

custodial care Process of caring for hygienic and nutritional needs in an institution but not providing treatment for a mental disorder.

cyclothymia Chronic mood disturbance of at least 2 years' duration involving numerous hypomanic episodes and numerous periods of depression. It does not meet the criteria for a manic episode or major depression.

D

deinstitutionalization Shift in treatment location from large public hospitals to community settings.

delirium Disorder with alterations in consciousness and changes in cognition, usually caused by a general medical condition or substances. Typically, delirium develops over a short period and is treatable. It is (usually) a reversible bewildered state of clouded consciousness, generally accompanied by restlessness, disorientation, and fear. It might include periods of hallucinations.

delusion Fixed, false belief, inconsistent with the person's intelligence and culture; unamenable to reason.

bizarre d. Absurd belief.

nihilistic d. False belief that the self, part of the self, or another object has ceased to exist.

paranoid d. Oversuspiciousness leading to persecutory delusions.

persecution d. False belief that one is being persecuted.

reference d. False belief that the behavior of others in the environment refers to oneself; derived from ideas of reference in which one wrongly believes that he or she is being talked about.

somatic d. False belief involving functioning of one's body.

dementia Disorder that causes pronounced memory and cognitive disturbances. Typically, dementias are gradual in onset and progressive in course.

dendrites Many projections from the neuron that transmit impulses to the cell body.

denial Avoidance of disagreeable realities or threats by ignoring or refusing to recognize them; an unconscious defense mechanism that might or might not be adaptive.

deoxyribonucleic acid (DNA) Molecule, primarily located in the nucleus of the cell, that encodes genetic information.

dependence State in which a person must take a usual or an increasing dose of a drug to prevent the onset of abstinence symptoms, withdrawal, or both.

depersonalization Feeling of unreality or strangeness related to one's self, body parts, bodily functions, or external environment (out of body experience).

depression Lowered or saddened mood state.

derailment Gradual or sudden deviation in train of thought, without thought-blocking.

derealization Distortion of spatial relationships so that the environment becomes distorted or unfamiliar.

devaluation Criticism of others that defends against one's own feelings of inadequacy.

dexamethasone suppression test (DST) Diagnostic test for clinical depression that measures the function of the hypothalamic-pituitary-adrenal (HPA) axis.

diencephalon Posterior part of the forebrain; includes the thalamus, hypothalamus, epithalamus, and metathalamus.

disinhibition State in which a person is unable to suppress urges or statements that might be socially unacceptable (e.g., telling a dirty joke in an inappropriate situation).

disoriented Disturbance in orientation of time, place, or person.

displacement Shift of emotion from an object or a person who incites the emotion to a less threatening source; an unconscious defense mechanism that might or might not be adaptive.

dissociation (1) Removal from conscious awareness of painful feelings, memories, thoughts, or aspects of identity; (2) splitting or separation of any group of mental or behavioral processes from the rest of the person's consciousness or identity.

dissociative reaction Process by which an individual blocks off part of his or her life from conscious recognition because of severe anxiety.

distractibility Inability to concentrate attention.

dopamine Brain neurotransmitter that influences muscle movement and emotions. The dopamine theory states that individuals with schizophrenia might have too much dopamine, which might account for their sensoriperceptual alterations. Research has refined this theory.

double bind Conflicting demands by significant individuals in a person's life. The person cannot meet both demands, so he or she is doomed to failure.

dysarthria Difficulty in articulation.

dyskinesia Disturbed coordination and motor activity, usually producing a jerky motion; an EPSE of neuroleptic medications related to their effect on dopamine receptors. (See also *tardive dyskinesia.*)

dyslexia Difficulty in reading.

dysphagia Difficulty in swallowing.

dysphoria Disorder of affect similar to, but less severe than, that demonstrated in major depression.

dysthymia Clinical syndrome similar to, but less severe than, that demonstrated in major depressive disorder. Chronic mood disturbance involving a depressed mood for at least 2 years, more days than not.

dystonia Rigidity in muscles that control posture, gait, or ocular movement; an EPSE of neuroleptic medications that block dopamine.

E

echolalia Speech pattern characterized by repeating the words of one person by another; noted in types of schizophrenia.

echopraxia Imitation of the body position of another.

ecologic worldview Perception of the world based on the belief that there is interconnectedness between a person and the earth and that people have a responsibility to take care of the earth.

electroconvulsive therapy (ECT) Form of somatic therapy that uses electrically induced seizures to relieve a person's intractable depressive symptoms.

emaciated Made excessively thin by lack of nutrition.

emotion Complex feeling state with psychological, somatic, and behavioral components related to affect and mood.

empathy Objective understanding of how patients feel or how they see their situations.

enkephalins Widely distributed opioid-like neuropeptides that are part of the endorphin family. These substances mediate pain perception, taste, olfaction, arousal, emotional behavior, vision, hearing, neurohormone secretion, motor coordination, and water balance.

environmental control Ability of an individual to control nature by planning activities and tasks to assist in maintaining optimal balance in life.

epidemiology Study of the frequency and distribution of disease conditions in the population.

epilepsy Disorder of the central nervous system (CNS) in which the major symptom is a seizure. The seizure is caused by a temporary disturbance of brain impulses.

ethnicity Characteristic of a group whose members share a common social and cultural heritage passed on to each successive generation.

ethnocentrism Acknowledging and valuing one's own culture only.

ethnopharmacology Study of pharmacogenetic, pharmacodynamic, and pharmacokinetic influences based on different ethnic, racial, and cultural groups.

etiology Study of the causes of diseases, including both direct and predisposing causes.

euphoria Sense of elation or well-being; elevation of mood; complete lack of tension. It is most notable in the manic phase of bipolar disorder.

euthymia Normal, homeostatic mood state.

excitement Excited motor activity.

existentialism Philosophy that emphasizes the individual's ability and responsibility to make one's existence meaningful by making choices in the face of life's deep pain and uncertainty.

expansive mood Elevated, unrestrained expression of feelings.

extrapyramidal side effects (EPSEs) Involuntary muscle movements resulting from the effects of neuroleptic drugs on the extrapyramidal system. These drugs cause a dopamine blockade that creates a dopamine-ACh imbalance. EPSEs include akathisia, akinesia, dystonia, drug-induced parkinsonism, and neuroleptic malignant syndrome.

extrapyramidal system Outside the pyramidal (voluntary) tract; coordinates involuntary movements.

eye contact Occasional glancing into a person's eyes to demonstrate interest during an interaction.

F

faith Traditionally, the creed that one follows within one's religious community, but the term can be used more broadly to describe one's total life view, religiously based or not.

family system Field of influence exerted on one another by family members because of their complex interaction.

fantasy Imaginary sequence of events, common in childhood; appropriate as long as the person is aware of reality.

fear Anxiety as a result of consciously recognized and realistic danger.

feedback Articulation of one's perception of what another person has said or meant. This process requires at least two people.

flashbacks Cognitive, emotional, and physical reexperiencing of traumatic events.

flight of ideas Speech pattern demonstrated by a rapid transition from topic to topic, frequently without completing any of the preceding ideas; prominent in manic states.

free association In a therapeutic context, saying anything that comes to mind.

fugue Period of personality dissociation with memory loss.

G

gait Manner of progression in walking. For example, in an ataxic gait, the foot is raised high and the sole strikes down suddenly.

gamma-aminobutyric acid (GABA) Inhibitory amino acid neurotransmitter formed during the citric acid cycle from its precursor, glutamic acid. GABA receptors are widely distributed in the CNS and produce neuronal hyperpolarization through an influx of chloride ions. Drugs that increase the GABA level reduce anxiety and seizures.

gender identity disorder A profound discomfort with one's own gender and a strong and persistent identification with the opposite gender.

general leads Interactive skills that facilitate the communication process by encouraging the patient to continue.

generalized seizure Seizure that involves both hemispheres of the brain at the onset of the seizure. Consciousness is usually impaired.

genes The fundamental physical and functional units of heredity. A gene is located in a sequence of nucleotides located in a particular position on a particular chromosome. There are about 30,000 different human genes.

genetic vulnerability (1) Tendency to inherit traits, behaviors, and biologic characteristics of one's ancestors; (2) predisposition that increases the risk of exhibiting a psychiatric disorder.

global memory loss Total memory loss, as in advanced stages of Alzheimer's disease.

globus pallidus Gray matter structure located medial to the putamen. This portion of the basal ganglia is smaller and triangular in shape. It is subdivided into the globus pallidus externa and globus pallidus interna.

glutamate Major excitatory transmitter in the CNS with receptors throughout the brain. Glutamate stimulation of N-methyl-D-aspartate (NMDA)–activated channels permits excessive inflow of calcium ions and production of free radicals, which might cause neuronal death.

grand mal seizure Type of generalized seizure in which there is loss of consciousness and convulsions. This type of seizure is most frequently known as epilepsy by laypersons.

gravely disabled Describes a person who is unable to provide food, clothing, or shelter for himself or herself because of a mental illness.

gray matter Composed of the cell bodies and dendrites of neurons.

grimacing Contortion of facial muscles; might be an EPSE.

gyri Convolutions of gray matter on the cerebrum.

H

half-life The amount of time it takes the body to metabolize and excrete a drug. Half-lives can range from minutes to weeks.

hallucination False sensory perceptions not associated with real external stimuli; might involve any of the five senses: auditory, visual, olfactory, gustatory, or tactile.

auditory h. "Hearing voices" or noises that others do not hear. Most prevalent in schizophrenia. The sounds might be perceived as thoughts or voices coming from any type of transmitter or from the patient's mind. The messages might be condemning and accusatory or complimentary and encouraging. It is critical that the examiner be aware that the messages might be directing the patient toward harming self or others, so the message content cannot be ignored.

tactile h. False sensory perception on the skin or scalp. Common in alcohol withdrawal. Hallucinations might also be an effect of certain types of drugs, such as amphetamines, hallucinogens, and cannabis.

visual h. "Seeing things" that others do not see. May be associated with organic conditions.

herbaceutical Plant or plant part that produces and contains chemical substances that act on the body.

here and now focus Assisting patients to understand how their current behaviors influence daily living.

holistic Pertaining to totality or the whole (holistic care).

homeless Without a home. Homeless individuals, including whole families, might live on the street exclusively or might make use of community shelters, halfway houses, cheap hotels, or board-and-care homes.

homeopathy Unconventional Western medicine system based on the principle that "like cures like" (i.e., that the same substance in large doses produces the symptoms of an illness and in very minute doses cures it). Homeopathic physicians believe that the more dilute the remedy, the greater its potency. Homeopathic practitioners use small doses of specially prepared plant extracts and minerals to stimulate the body's defense mechanisms and healing processes to treat illness.

hostile Feeling intense anger and resentment, exhibited by destructive behavior.

hot or cold treatments Cultural-medical approaches to maintaining or returning a person to a state of wellness. These approaches do not refer to the temperature of a treatment but to the fact that a specific, defined approach is appropriate for each state of wellness or illness.

human immunodeficiency infection Spectrum of illness caused by HIV that ranges from acutely or chronically HIV-infected adults to infants in the neonatal period.

human immunodeficiency virus (HIV) Virus that has been isolated and recognized as the causative agent of acquired immunodeficiency syndrome (AIDS). HIV is classified as a lentivirus in a subgroup of the retroviruses.

human immunodeficiency virus, type 1 (HIV-1) Retrovirus identified as the cause of AIDS.

humanist Individual who emphasizes people, rather than other parts of the observable world or religion.

Huntington's disease Genetically transmitted disease that includes motor and cognitive changes.

hydrotherapy Use of water (wet sheet packs, 2- to 10-hour baths) for psychotherapeutic purposes.

hyperactivity (hyperkinesis) Restless, aggressive, often destructive activity; prominent in manic states.

hypersomnia Increased and prolonged sleeping.

hypoactivity (hypokinesis) Decreased activity or retardation (psychomotor retardation); slowing of psychological and physical functions.

hypomania Clinical syndrome similar to, but less severe than, that demonstrated in a full-blown manic episode.

hypothalamus Group of nuclei in the diencephalon that influences eating behavior, temperature regulation, emotional expression, and autonomic system. Dopaminergic neurons in the hypothalamus control lactation.

I

idealization Defense mechanism characterized by viewing others as perfect; exalting others.

ideas of reference Belief that some events have a special meaning (e.g., people laughing are perceived as laughing at the patient).

idiopathic Without known cause.

illogical (thinking) Contains erroneous conclusions or internal contradictions (irrational thoughts).

illusion Misinterpretation of a sensory input; observed in alcoholic withdrawal and delirious states.

impaired parent Parent whose nurturing capabilities are compromised or absent, related to psychiatric or substance abuse disorders.

incidence The rate at which a certain condition occurs, such as the number of new cases of a specific mental disorder occurring during a certain period.

independence Taking actions for one's behalf, rather than asking others to do so.

individual responsibility Owning one's tasks, needs, feelings, and thoughts and taking action to address these responsibilities and needs.

indoklon therapy Convulsive therapy similar to ECT; however, convulsions are induced by ether rather than by electrical stimulus.

informed consent Providing the patient with information about a specific treatment, including its benefits, side effects, and possible risks, that will enable the patient to make a competent and voluntary decision.

insight   Recognition of motivational sources behind one's thoughts, actions, or behavior.

insomnia   Inability to sleep or disrupted sleep patterns.

intellectual functioning   Individual's general fund of knowledge, orientation, memory, mastery of simple mathematical equations, and capacity for abstract thinking.

intellectualization   An (unconscious) defense mechanism; a process of thinking excessively about the philosophical or theoretical basis of a subject to the extent that anxiety-provoking issues are avoided.

internal capsule   Broad band of myelinated fibers that separate the lentiform nuclei from the caudate nucleus and thalamus. Corticospinal (motor or pyramidal) tracts travel through the internal capsule, cerebral peduncles, and cerebral pyramids into the spinal cord, where they constitute the lateral corticospinal pathway. Damage to any of these structures can result in hemiparesis or hemiplegia.

involuntary commitment   Commitment status in which a person who has the legal capacity to consent to mental health treatment refuses to do so and is involuntarily detained for treatment by the state.

ipsilateral   Same side of body.

irrational beliefs   Beliefs that are not logical but that influence feelings and behaviors.

J

judgment and comprehension   Ability to understand, recall, mobilize, and integrate constructively previous learning in meeting new situations.

K

kinesics   Study of body movements.

Korsakoff's psychosis   Organic mental disorder with memory loss related to chronic and excessive alcohol abuse.

Kraepelin   German psychiatrist who initiated a classification system for psychiatry in 1896. He used the term *dementia praecox.*

L

labile   Mood, affect, or behavior that is subject to frequent, extreme, or unpredictable changes.

least restrictive alternative   Environment that provides the necessary treatment requirements in the least restrictive setting possible. For example, a hospital setting is more restrictive than a board-and-care setting. If the board-and-care setting provides the necessary treatment requirements for a person, that environment represents the least restrictive alternative.

lentiform nuclei   Putamen and globus pallidus of the basal ganglia.

lesion   Injury to tissue.

Lewy bodies   Eosinophilic cytoplasmic inclusions seen in neuromelanin-containing neurons in Parkinson's disease or dementia.

ligand   An ion, a molecule, or a molecular group that binds to another chemical entity to form a larger complex.

limit setting   Holding individuals to established norms with the intent of assisting them to function more constructively.

limited or special power of attorney   Written document in which one person, the principal, authorizes another person, the attorney-in-fact, to act on the principal's behalf. In a limited power of attorney, the attorney-in-fact is granted only powers specifically defined in the document.

lipid solubility   Ability of a substance to dissolve in fat.

lithium   Element or salt used in the treatment and prevention of manic episodes.

locus ceruleus   Small nucleus ("blue spot") in the pontine tegmentum whose neurons are the major source of norepinephrine in the brain; present bilaterally.

loose association   Pattern of speech in which a person's ideas slip off track onto another that is completely unrelated or only slightly related.

M

magical thinking   Belief that thoughts, words, or actions can cause or prevent an occurrence by some magical means.

malingering   Deliberate feigning of an illness.

malpractice   Negligence by a professional. Malpractice is a civil action that can be brought against a nurse if he or she has breached a standard of care that a reasonably prudent nurse would meet.

managed care   Health care system that arranges the relationship among payers, providers, and consumers; monitors and influences the behavior of the mental health providers and the outcomes of care and reimburses for services.

mania   Disordered mental state of extreme excitement, hyperactivity, euphoria, and hyperverbal behavior.

master-servant rule   As applied to the employer-employee relationship, this rule holds the employer responsible for the acts of employees as long as the employees are acting within the scope of their employment or authority.

medially   Toward the midline.

medulla   Approximately 3 cm long; the most caudal portion of the brainstem. It controls respiration and supplies innervation to the tongue and palate.

melancholic depression   Subgroup generally seen in older individuals, often misdiagnosed as dementia; more often associated with dexamethasone nonsuppression. Depression usually worse in the morning, early morning awakening, psychomotor retardation or agitation, excessive or inappropriate guilt, and significant anorexia or weight loss are symptoms of melancholia.

memory   Function by which information stored in the brain is later recalled to the conscious mind.

meninges   Outer lining of the CNS composed of the dura mater, arachnoid, and pia mater.

mental disorder   A clinically significant behavioral or psychological syndrome or pattern … associated with present distress or disability.

mental retardation   Lack of intelligence so great that it interferes with social and occupational performance.

mental status examination (MSE)   Record of current findings that includes a description of a patient's appearance, behavior, motor activity, speech, alertness, mood, cognition, intelligence, reactions, views, and attitudes.

meridian   Lines in a body that are representative of psychological or physical body functions. Cultural healers stimulate meridians and release harmful toxins or illness-producing spirits through the use of alternative treatment approaches such as moxibustion, cupping, coining, or skin scraping.

mesocortical tract   Dopaminergic tract that projects from the ventral tegmental area near the substantia nigra to the neocortex, particularly the prefrontal cortex; involved in motivation, planning, behavior, attention, and social behavior.

mesolimbic tract   Catecholaminergic neuronal tract (mostly dopaminergic) with cell bodies located in the ventral tegmental area of the midbrain and axons that project to the hippocampus, entorhinal cortex, amygdala, anterior cingulate gyrus, nucleus accumbens, and other limbic regions.

metabolic tolerance   Process that occurs when the body is more efficient at metabolizing a substance.

midbrain   Most rostral division of the brainstem. It contains important structures such as the cerebral aqueduct, superior and inferior colliculi, red nuclei, substantia nigra, cerebral peduncles, and oculomotor and trochlear cranial nerve nuclei.

milieu   Environment or setting.

milieu management   Purposeful manipulation of the environment to promote a therapeutic atmosphere.

milieu therapy   Use of the environment to promote optimal functioning in a group or individual.

minority   Social, religious, ethnic, occupational, or other group that constitutes less than a numeric majority of the population.

model of care   Philosophy of causative and curative factors of mental illness that drives the nature of the care activities offered.

monoamine   Category of neurotransmitters that contain one amino group and are derived from amino acids. Subcategories of monoamines include the catecholamines (dopamine, norepinephrine, epinephrine), which are derived from tyrosine, and the indolamine serotonin, which is derived from tryptophan. Histamine is categorized as a monoamine but is biochemically different. Monoamine-synthesizing neurons are primarily found in the brainstem but have a wide net of influence because of the ubiquitous distribution of their axonal projections.

monoamine oxidase   Enzyme that metabolizes monoamines such as dopamine, norepinephrine, and serotonin.

monoamine oxidase inhibitors (MAOIs) Antidepressant drugs that increase the bioavailability of certain neurotransmitters by interfering with their metabolism.

mood Individual's internal state of mind that is exhibited through feelings and emotions.

mood disorder Diagnostic category in *DSM-5* that includes depressive disorders and bipolar disorders.

moxibustion Alternative cultural medical treatment approach that uses moxa and heat to release illness-producing spirits from the body, mind, or spirit.

mutism Refusal to speak.

N

NANDA North American Nursing Diagnosis Association.

narcissism Extreme self-centeredness and self-absorption (narcissistic personality disorder).

narcotherapy Induction of a state of sedation by intravenous administration of sedatives (e.g., amobarbital) or stimulants (e.g., methylphenidate).

National Alliance on Mental Illness A grassroots mental health organization that is dedicated to building hope in people with mental illness, advocating for access to services, treatment, supports, and research.

National Institute of Mental Health Government organization in the National Institutes of Health concerned with mental health issues in the United States.

natural cause of illness Belief that everyone and everything in the world is interrelated and that a disruption of this connectedness causes illness or disease.

nature argument Argument that proposes a specific mental disorder is caused by biologic factors (e.g., neurotransmitter irregularities, pathoanatomy) rather than by psychodynamic factors (e.g., related to upbringing, life events, or other stressors).

naturopathic physician Alternative care practitioner who holds a doctor of naturopathy (ND) degree.

naturopathy Discipline that views disease as a manifestation of alterations in the processes by which the body naturally heals itself and emphasizes health restoration rather than disease treatment. Naturopathic physicians use an array of healing practices that include diet and clinical nutrition; homeopathy; acupuncture; herbal medicine; hydrotherapy (use of water in a range of temperatures and methods of applications); spinal and soft tissue manipulation; physical therapies involving electric currents; ultrasound and light therapies; therapeutic counseling; and pharmacology.

negativism Motiveless resistance to all instruction.

negligence Failure to do that which a reasonably prudent and careful person would do under the circumstances or doing what a reasonable and prudent person would not do.

neologism Speech pattern characterized by the production of unknown words; noted in some types of schizophrenia.

neurocognitive disorders Class of disorders of mental functioning caused either by permanent brain damage or temporary brain dysfunction. Cognition, emotions, and motivation are affected.

neurofibrillary tangle Mass of abnormal filamentous material located within the cell body of neurons. These tangles occur in several brain disorders, including Alzheimer's disease, and are composed of cytoskeletal components.

neuroleptic Antipsychotic medication.

neuron Nerve cell.

neurotransmitter Chemical found in the nervous system (e.g., norepinephrine, serotonin, dopamine) that facilitates the transmission of nerve impulses across synapses between neurons.

nihilistic ideas Thoughts of nonexistence and hopelessness.

N-methyl-D-aspartate (NMDA) receptor Glutamate receptor that is the primary mechanism for controlling synaptic plasticity and memory function. NMDA receptors are thought to be present in all or almost all neurons in the CNS.

noncompliance Failure to take medication as prescribed.

nonviolence Solving conflictual situations by methods other than verbal or physical aggression.

norepinephrine Catecholamine neurotransmitter that is primarily synthesized in neurons of the locus ceruleus in the pons. Deficiencies of norepinephrine are linked to depression.

norepinephrine and dopamine reuptake inhibitors (NDRIs) Class of antidepressants; the only antidepressants that primarily block the reuptake of dopamine.

norm Expected behavior for a given therapeutic setting.

nucleus accumbens This nucleus is adjacent to the medial and ventral portions of the caudate and putamen. The neurons in this nucleus project to both the globus pallidus and the substantia nigra; a major component of the "reward pathway."

nucleus basalis of Meynert Located bilaterally, directly beneath the anterior commissure, the major brain site for the production of ACh. Fibers from this nucleus project diffusely to the cerebral cortex.

nurse-patient interaction Purposeful use of the relationship between the patient and nurse for achieving patient treatment goals.

nursing diagnosis Statement that describes a patient's potential or actual problem or response to illness treatable by nurses.

nurture argument This argument proposes that a specific mental disorder is caused by psychodynamic factors (e.g., related to upbringing, interactions, life events, or other stressors) rather than by biologic factors (e.g., neurotransmitter irregularities, pathoanatomy).

O

obesity Abnormal increase in the proportion of fat cells, mainly in the viscera and subcutaneous tissues of the body.

objectivity Process of remaining open, unbiased, and emotionally separate from a patient.

obsession Pathologic persistence of an unwilled thought, feeling, or impulse to the extent that it cannot be eliminated from consciousness by logical effort.

obsessive-compulsive disorder Disorder in which recurrent obsessions (thoughts) alternate with compulsions (behaviors) in an effort to decrease anxiety.

occupational therapy Uses the activities of daily living to help people with mental disabilities achieve maximum functioning and independence at home and in the workplace.

oculogyric crisis Involuntary tonic muscle spasms of the eye. The eyes usually roll upward in a fixed stare. This frightening dystonic reaction is caused by antipsychotic drugs.

olfactory Pertaining to the sense of smell.

open posture Relaxed yet attentive position with arms uncrossed; enhances patient's trust in the examiner.

open-ended statement Statement that elicits further exploration of the patient's problem by encouraging communication; can also be in the form of a question.

openness Atmosphere in which people are free to express their thoughts and feelings without fear of ridicule or censure.

opportunistic illnesses Illnesses that develop when the immune system is inactive or suppressed.

orientation Conscious awareness of person, place, and time.

P

panic State of extreme, acute, intense anxiety, accompanied by disorganization of personality and function.

paranoia Extreme suspiciousness of others and their actions.

paranoid thinking Oversuspicious thinking that might lead to persecutory delusions or projectile behavior patterns.

parkinsonism Cause (e.g., brain injury, antipsychotic drugs, carbon monoxide) of parkinsonism symptoms is known or suspected.

parkinsonism symptoms Masked facies, muscle rigidity, and shuffling gait. Symptoms are common in patients taking neuroleptic drugs; EPSEs are related to dopamine blockade.

Parkinson's disease Also known as *idiopathic parkinsonism*, where the cause is unknown. It pathologically manifests as a loss of dopaminergic neurons in the substantia nigra and clinically exhibits a variety of motor and nonmotor signs and symptoms.

partial seizure Usually involves one hemisphere of the brain at the onset of the seizure.

passive aggression Anger expressed indirectly through subtle and evasive ways.

pedophilia Intense sexual arousal or desire and acts, fantasies, or other stimuli involving children.

perception Awareness of objects and relationships that follows stimulation of peripheral sense organs.

perseveration   Pattern of speech characterized by repetition of the same word or idea in response to different questions.

personal control   Exerting limits on one's own impulses to act in a manner that is contrary to one's best interests, treatment goals, or personal needs.

personality disorder   Exaggerated, inflexible, and pervasive behavior patterns destructive to the individual and others.

pervasive developmental disorder (PDD)   Any one of several conditions characterized by multiple social and cognitive delays.

petit mal seizure   Variant of absence seizures characterized by three spikes per second and a wave pattern on electroencephalogram.

pharmacodynamic tolerance   Tolerance seen when higher blood levels are required to produce a given effect.

phobia   Exaggerated, pathologic fear of some specific type of stimulus or situation.

phobic disorder   Severe phobic behavior patterns that render the individual dysfunctional. Avoidance of the feared object or situation serves to assuage anxiety.

physical or emotional security   Feeling safe from emotional, verbal, and physical assault.

postpartum depression   Subtype of depression in the postpartum period occurring 30 days or less after childbirth.

posttraumatic stress disorder (PTSD)   Development of characteristic symptoms (e.g., intense fear, helplessness, reexperiencing of events) after exposure to an extreme traumatic stressor.

preconscious   Memories that can be recalled to consciousness with some effort.

precursor   Something that precedes. For example, tyrosine is a precursor to dopamine in the synthesis of dopamine in the body.

premorbid   State before onset of a disorder.

prevalence   Estimate of the frequency of a disease condition in the population (e.g., ADHD affects 5% of children).

primary appraisal   Judgment an individual makes about an event.

primary gain   Relief or expression of anxiety through symptoms of a disorder.

privacy   Allowance of physical and emotional space for self and others.

probable cause   Sufficient credible facts that would induce a reasonably intelligent and prudent person to believe that a cause of action exists.

process recording   Written record of an encounter with a patient that is as nearly verbatim as possible, including both verbal and nonverbal behaviors of the nurse and the patient.

professional chaplain   Also known as a spiritual care professional; one who has extensive postgraduate clinical training to offer spiritual care within a health care organization.

projective identification   Defense mechanism characterized by placement of feelings on another to justify one's own expression of feelings.

proxemics   Study of how people perceive and use environmental, social, and personal space in interactions with others.

pseudodementia   A depressive condition of older adults characterized by impaired cognitive function.

psychiatric rehabilitation   Promotion of the patient's highest level of functioning in the least restrictive environment.

psychoeducation   Strategy of teaching patients and families about disorders, treatments, coping techniques, and resources, based on the observation that people can be more effective participants in their own care if they have knowledge.

psychomotor retardation   Markedly slowed speech and body movements.

psychoneuroimmunology   Field of research focusing on the interactions of mind, environment, and bodily function, particularly immune system function.

psychopathology   Study of underlying processes, both biologic and psychosocial, that lead to mental disorders.

psychosis   Inability to recognize reality, complicated by severe thought disorders and the inability to relate to others.

psychosocial adversity   Environmental conditions such as poverty, unemployment, or overcrowded living conditions that do not support optimal development of a child.

psychotherapeutic management   Model for nursing care that balances the three primary intervention models used by psychiatric nurses: therapeutic nurse-patient relationship, psychopharmacology, and milieu management.

psychotic depression   Subtype of depression in which a person experiences delusions and hallucinations; often misdiagnosed as schizophrenia or schizoaffective disorder.

psychotropic drugs   Medications used in the treatment of mental illness.

purge   Compensation for calories consumed by self-induced vomiting, laxative abuse, diuretics, or enemas.

pyramidal system   Motor system for voluntary movement.

R

race   Breeding population that primarily mates within itself.

raphe nuclei   Nuclei located along the midline of the brainstem (*raphe*, seam). Serotonin is synthesized from these cells.

reactive depression   Depressed mood related to a life event (e.g., divorce, losing one's job).

reappraisal   Appraisal made after new or additional information has been received.

receptor   A specialized area on a nerve membrane, blood vessel, or muscle that receives the chemical stimulation to activate or inhibit normal actions of nerves, blood vessels, or muscles.

recovery   Defined by the Substance Abuse and Mental Health Services Administration as "a process of change through which individuals improve their health and wellness, live a self-directed life, and strive to reach their full potential."

recreational therapist   Assists patients in finding leisure interests so that they can learn to balance work and play.

relational worldview   Perception of the world grounded in the belief in spirituality and the significance of relationships and interactions among individuals.

religion   Defined structures, rituals, beliefs, and values through which communities frequently address spiritual concerns.

religiosity   Preoccupation with religious ideas or content.

resiliency   Capability to withstand stressors without permanent dysfunction or developmental delay.

respect for the individual   Acknowledgment and allowance of the rights of others to be unique.

restraint   Physical control of a patient to prevent injury to the patient, staff, and other patients.

reuptake   Physiologic process that occurs when a neurotransmitter is taken up into the presynaptic neuron after having been released into the synapse. Some psychotropic drugs are designed to prevent the reuptake of a specific neurotransmitter to increase the synaptic presence of that neurotransmitter.

rigidity   Assumption of a stiff, rigid posture.

S

satisfaction   Relaxation of the tension of physiologic needs.

schizophrenia   Syndrome, illness, or mental health disorder characterized by hallucinations or delusions or both. Symptoms generally reflect a progressive deterioration and disorganization of the individual's personality structure, affect, and cognition.

scientific cause of illness   Belief that there are specific concrete explanations for every illness and disease. This explanation involves the entrance of pathogens such as viruses, bacteria, and germs into the body.

seasonal affective disorder (SAD)   Subtype of depression occurring in late autumn or winter and lasting until spring.

seclusion   Process of placing a patient alone in a specially designed room for protection and close observation.

secondary appraisal   Evaluation an individual makes about potential actions to be taken.

secondary gain   Attention and support received from others while ill.

selective serotonin-norepinephrine reuptake inhibitors (SNRIs)   Class of antidepressants; block the reuptake of serotonin and norepinephrine. At higher doses, the reuptake of dopamine is also inhibited.

selective serotonin reuptake inhibitors (SSRIs)   Class of antidepressants; potent blockers of serotonin reuptake, increasing the level of serotonin in the synapse.

self-mutilation   The intentional act of tissue destruction to one's own body with the purpose of shifting overwhelming emotional pain to a more acceptable physical pain.

serotonin (5-HT)   Monoamine neurotransmitter from the indolamine family. It is derived from the amino acid tryptophan.

shuffling gait (parkinsonian gait) Style of walking typically demonstrated by individuals whose dopamine stores have been blocked or depleted as a result of Parkinson's disease or antipsychotic medications.

smudging Common sacred rite of purification and cleansing practiced by many Native American nations. It includes the burning of cedar and sage for the purpose of fanning smoke with an eagle feather over or near the patient. It is seen as purifying the spirit and preparing the patient for a difficult spiritual journey such as illness or death and is also used for other spiritual rituals.

social organization Culture around particular units, such as family, racial, or ethnic groups; religious groups; and community or social groups.

social skills group Group that helps psychiatric patients learn, practice, and develop skills for dealing with people in social situations.

socialization skills Skills necessary for negotiating daily interpersonal issues (e.g., acknowledging responsibility for one's behavior, using eye contact appropriately, interacting with others for purposes of sharing and support).

somatic therapy Therapeutic approach that uses physiologic or physical interventions to effect behavioral changes. For example, ECT is a somatic treatment.

somatization Conversion of mental states or experiences into bodily symptoms; associated with anxiety.

soul Nonphysical, transcendent part of human beings involving their mind and will.

space Refers to distance and intimacy needs of culturally unique individuals in human interaction.

spirituality Awareness of relationships with all creation, an appreciation of presence and purpose that goes beyond the five senses and the physical world; includes a sense of meaning and belonging. It is often inclusive of religion.

splitting Inability to integrate good and bad aspects of self and others; person views self and others as all good or all bad.

status epilepticus Repetitive seizures; usually refers to repetitive grand mal seizures.

statutory law Statutory law is written law emanating from a legislative body. These laws are written by state and federal legislative authorities and passed in accordance with state and federal law.

steady state Desired state in anticonvulsant and other therapies, when the serum concentration of the drug is consistent and is maintained at a therapeutic level.

step system Process by which inpatients gain privileges and responsibilities based on their progress.

stereotyping Assumption that all people in similar cultural, racial, ethnic, or other groups think and act alike.

stereotypy Continuous repetition of speech or physical activities.

stressor Stimulus perceived by the individual or the organism as challenging, threatening, or damaging.

striatum Basal ganglia that include the caudate and putamen.

substance-induced mood disorder Disorder that results from the disturbance or alteration of a person's mood caused by the ingestion of a prescribed or nonprescribed drug or medication or by exposure to a toxic substance.

substantia nigra Literally, black substance; a pigmented area of the midbrain where dopamine is synthesized.

substrate The material or substance on which an enzyme acts.

suicidal ideation Individual's thinking about and inclination toward self-injury or self-destruction.

suicidal plan Specific method designed to inflict self-injury or self-destruction as verbalized by an individual.

suicide Self-inflicted death.

sulcus Groove separating gyri. Deep sulci are referred to as fissures.

synapse Microscopic space between two neurons.

T

tangentiality Inability to have goal-directed associations of thought; never gets to desired goal from desired point.

tardive dyskinesia Extrapyramidal syndrome that usually emerges late in the course of long-term antipsychotic drug therapy; includes grimacing, buccolingual movements, and dystonia (impaired muscle tonus); might be irreversible.

teamwork Staff working together to achieve agreed-on goals for the unit and for patient care.

terror State of extreme tension.

theist One who believes in God, without necessarily conforming to a particular set of religious beliefs; from the Greek word for God, *theos*.

therapeutic In the psychotherapeutic management model, the communication of respect, a desire to help, and understanding to another person. Understanding includes knowledge of mental mechanisms, coping strategies, and stressors. Active listening is a crucial component of being therapeutic.

therapeutic communication Interactive verbal and nonverbal strategies that focus on the needs of the patient and facilitate a goal-directed, patient-oriented communication process.

therapeutic listening Listening that is focused on the patient and obtains therapeutically useful information about the patient.

therapeutic milieu Treatment environment managed in such a way that the environment itself is therapeutic.

therapy Means, usually with words, to cure or manage the course of another person's mental disorder. Nurses who practice psychotherapy are trained in a specific therapy model (e.g., psychoanalysis, cognitive therapy).

thinking Process of following a goal-directed flow of ideas, symbols, and associations to a logical conclusion in accordance with the person's developmental stage.

thought disorder Thinking characterized by loose associations, neologisms, and illogical constructs and conclusions.

time Either a physical quantity measured by a clock or patterns and orientations that relate to social processes.

time-out Disengaging a child from a specific situation (e.g., directing the child to sit in a chair facing away from others so that the child might regain self-control).

tolerance Need for increasing amounts of a substance to achieve the same effects.

tonic State of continuous tension.

transference Unconscious emotional reaction to a current situation that is based on previous experiences.

transinstitutionalization A product of deinstitutionalization. A shifting of the care of mental patients to jails, prisons, nursing homes, and board-and-care facilities.

tricyclic antidepressants (TCAs) Antidepressants that block the reuptake of norepinephrine and serotonin into the presynaptic neuron.

tuberoinfundibular tract Dopaminergic system with neurons in the arcuate nucleus of the hypothalamus that project to the pituitary stalk. This tract controls the secretion of prolactin.

tyramine Substance derived from the amino acid tyrosine and found in many common foods, such as aged cheeses, yogurt, and avocados. Tyramine-rich foods can cause a hypertensive crisis in a person being treated with MAOIs.

tyrosine Amino acid that is the precursor to dopamine.

U

unconscious Memories, conflicts, experiences, and materials that have been repressed and cannot be recalled at will.

undoing Defense mechanism by which a person symbolically acts out to reverse a previously committed act or thought; a common ritual in obsessive-compulsive disorder.

unit norm Expected behavior for a given therapeutic setting.

unnatural cause of illness Belief that outside forces such as a spell or a hex being cast on the sick person are the cause or the source of illness or disease.

V

validation Process of confirming an individual's intent by questioning the content of his or her message.

vascular dementia Results from the interruption of blood flow to the brain, which causes anoxia, ischemia, and subsequent infarction.

ventral tegmental area (VTA) Located in the midbrain, this region is dorsomedial to the substantia nigra and ventral to the red nuclei. The nuclei in this area produce dopamine. The efferent pathways from the VTA include the mesocortical and mesolimbic tracts.

ventricle System of connected brain cavities that are filled with cerebrospinal fluid, including the lateral ventricles (in the central portion of the telencephalon), the third ventricle (which runs between the thalami), the fourth ventricle (in the pons and medulla), and the connecting cerebral aqueduct (in the midbrain).

vesicle Storage sac at the synaptic terminal.

voluntary commitment Situation whereby the patient or his or her conservator or guardian requests psychiatric treatment and signs an application for that treatment. This person is also free to sign himself or herself out of the hospital.

W

Wernicke's area Sophisticated auditory association cortex located within the planum temporale that interprets spoken language.

Wernicke's encephalopathy Confusion and ophthalmoplegia caused by thiamine deficiency; most common in alcoholics. It results in necrosis and hemorrhage in the mammillary bodies and periventricular structures of the brainstem.

Western medicine Conventional clinicians use this term to describe the medicine practiced by the holders of Doctor of Medicine (MD) or Doctor of Osteopathy (DO) degrees, some of whom might also practice complementary and alternative medicine. Other terms for conventional medicine are allopathic medicine, regular medicine, mainstream medicine, and biomedicine.

white matter Substance in the brain composed of myelinated neuronal axons.

withdrawal (1) Act or process of turning inward to avoid a perceived environmental threat; (2) physiologic response to cessation of an addictive substance.

word salad Speech pattern characterized by an incoherent mixture of words or phrases.

Note: Page numbers followed by *f* indicate figures, *b* indicate boxes and *t* indicate tables.